W0193106

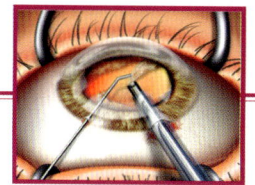

Phacoemulsification Surgery

Defined to Refined Approach

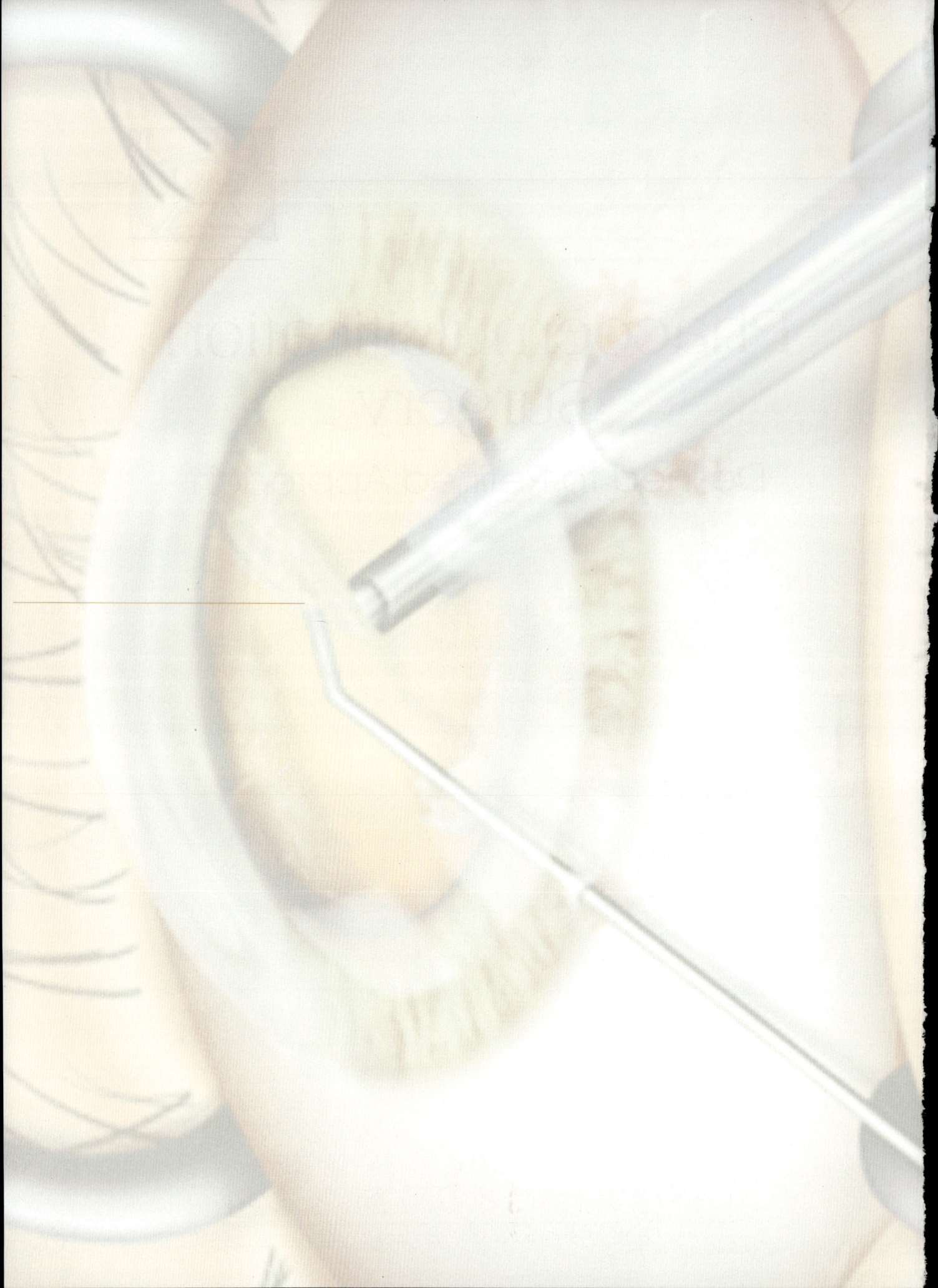

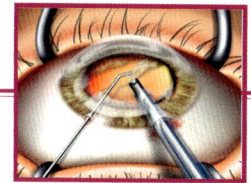

Phacoemulsification Surgery

Defined to Refined Approach

Col JKS Parihar SM, VSM
Senior Adviser Ophthalmology
Professor and Head
Department of Ophthalmology
Army Hospital (Research and Referral)
Delhi Cantt

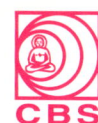

CBS Publishers & Distributors Pvt Ltd

New Delhi • Bengaluru • Pune • Kochi • Chennai

Phacoemulsification Surgery
Defined to Refined Approach

ISBN: 978-81-239-1971-3

Copyright © Author and Publisher

First Edition: 2011

Published by Satish Kumar Jain and produced by Vinod K. Jain for

CBS Publishers & Distributors Pvt Ltd

CBS Plaza, 4819/XI, Prahlad Street, 24 Ansari Road, Daryaganj, New Delhi 110 002, India
Ph: 23289259, 23266861/67   Fax: +91-11-23243014   Website: www.cbspd.com
e-mail: delhi@cbspd.com;
cbspubs@vsnl.com;
cbspubs@airtelmail.in.

Branches

- Bengaluru: Seema House 2975, 17th Cross, K.R. Road,
  Banasankari 2nd Stage, Bengaluru 560 070, Karnataka
  Ph: +91-80-26771678/79   Fax: +91-80-26771680   e-mail: bangalore@cbspd.com

- Pune: Bhuruk Prestige, Sr. No. 52/12/2+1+3/2 Narhe, Haveli
  (Near Katraj-Dehu Road Bypass), Pune 411 051, Maharashtra
  Ph: +91-20-64704058/64704059/32342277   Fax: +91-20-24300160   e-mail: pune@cbspd.com

- Kochi: 36/14 Kalluvilakam, Lissie Hospital Road,
  Kochi 682 018, Kerala
  Ph: +91-484-4059061-65   Fax: +91-484-4059065   e-mail: cochin@cbspd.com

- Chennai: 20, West Park Road, Shenoy Nagar,
  Chennai 600 030, Tamil Nadu
  Ph: +91-44-26260666, 26208620   Fax: +91-44-45530020   e-mail: chennai@cbspd.com

Printed at: Manipal Press Limited, Manipal, Karnataka

List of Contributors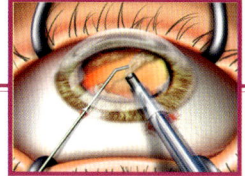

Col JKS Parihar SM, VSM, MBBS, MS (Ophthal), DOMS, DNB, MAMAS
Senior Adviser, Ophthalmology and Anterior Segment Microsurgery
Professor and Head
Department of Ophthalmology
Army Hospital (Research and Referral), Delhi Cantt, (Post Graduate Institute of Medical Sciences, Affiliated to Delhi University)
jksparihar@gmail.com

Late Colonel Rangin Banerji MS, DO, FRCS
Formerly, Senior Adviser and Professor of Ophthalmology
Command Hospital (EC)
Kolkata, West Bengal

Prof SK Angra MS, FAMS
Formerly, Professor of Ophthalmology and Head, Cornea Services,
RP Centre for Ophthalmic Sciences
All India Institute of Medical Sciences, New Delhi
A 58, Swastha Vihar, New Delhi

Dr SB Kelkar MS, DOMS
Director, Professor
National Institute of Ophthalmology
Ghole Road, Shivaji Nagar, Pune
Maharashtra

Dr VK Saini MS
Director, Medical Education
Ministry of Health, Govt of MP
Bhopal, Madhya Pradesh

Dr (Mrs) S Biseria Gupta MS
Director, Professor and Head
Regional Institute of Ophthalmology
Gandhi Medical College
Bhopal, Madhya Pradesh

Col RP Gupta MS, FRF
Professor and Head
Dept of Ophthalmology
DY Medical College
Pune, Maharashtra

Dr Pushpa Varma MS
Professor and Head
Dept of Ophthalmology
MGM Medical College
Indore, Madhya Pradesh

Dr (Mrs) Purshottma Sadhotra MS
Professor and Head
Dept of Ophthalmology
Acharya Shri Chander College of Medical Sciences and Hospital (ASCOMS)
Sidhra, Jammu Tawi
Jammu and Kashmir

Col Neelam Puthran MS
Professor and Head
Department of Ophthalmology
Yenepoya Medical College, Deralakatte
Mangalore, Karnataka

Dr MPS Sachdeva MD
Chairman and Senior Consultant
Centre for Sight
Safdarjung Enclave, New Delhi

Dr US Tiwari MS
Professor and Head
Dept of Ophthalmology, GR Medical College
Gwalior, Madhya Pradesh

Dr M Shrivastava MS
Professor and Head
Dept of Ophthalmology, NSCB Medical College
Jabalpur, Madhya Pradesh

Dr Ulka Shrivastava MS
Professor of Ophthalmology
Dept of Ophthalmology
MGM Medical College
Indore, Madhya Pradesh

Jeewan S Titiyal MD
Professor of Ophthalmology and Head Cornea Services
RP Centre for Ophthalmic Sciences
All India Institute of Medical Sciences, New Delhi

Brig AP Kamath
Professor, Ophthalmology
Commandant MH
Chennai, Tamil Nadu

Col FEA Rodrigues MS
Prof and Head, Department of Ophthalmology
Father Muller Medical College, Mangalore
Karnataka
drfear4393@hotmail.com

Brig A Banerji MS
Professor and Head
Department of Ophthalmology
AFMC, Pune, Maharashtra

Dr Sanjivani Ambekar MS
Professor and Head
Dept of Ophthalmology, BJ Medical College
Pune, Maharashtra

Col VS Gurunadh MS, DOMS
Professor Ophthalmology, AFMC, Pune, Maharashtra

Dr S Natarajan DO
Director, Senior Consultant Ophthalmology
Aditya Jyot Eye Hospital Pvt. Ltd.
Plot No. 153, Road No. 9, Major Parmeshwaran Road
Opp S.I.W.S. College Gate No. 3, 400031, Wadala West,
Wadala, Mumbai, Maharashtra

R K Shrivastava MS
Consultant Ophthalmology, ESI Hospital
Indore, Madhya Pradesh

Surgeon Cdr TR Bera MS
Formerly, Associate Professor and Classified Specialist
Ophthalmology
Command Hospital (EC) and Post Graduate Institute of
Medical Sciences, affiliated to West Bengal University of
Heath Sciences, Kolkata, West Bengal

Col V Mathur MS
Senior Adviser and Professor of Ophthalmology
Command Hospital (EC) and Post Graduate Institute of
Medical Sciences, affiliated to West Bengal University of
Heath Sciences, Kolkata, West Bengal

Surgeon Cdr T Choudhary MS
Classified Specialist and Associate Professor
Ophthalmology
INHS Asvani, Mumbai (Post Graduate Institute of Medical
Sciences, affiliated to MUHS, Nashik) Maharashtra

Tanuj Dada MD
Associate Professor of Ophthalmology and Glaucoma
Services, RP Centre for Ophthalmic Sciences
All India Institute of Medical Sciences, New Delhi

Rajesh Sinha MD, DNB, FRCS
Associate Professor of Ophthalmology and Kerato
Refractive Services
RP Centre for Ophthalmic Sciences
All India Institute of Medical Sciences, New Delhi

Lt Col Shantanu Mukerjee MS
Classified Specialist and Assistant Professor
Ophthalmology
Army Hospital (Research & Referral),
Delhi Cantt
(Post Graduate Institute of Medical Sciences, affiliated
to Delhi University)

Lt Col Sandipan Bandopadhyay MS
Classified Specialist and Assistant Professor
Ophthalmology, Army College of Medical Sciences
Base Hospital, Delhi Cantt

Lt Col Santosh Kumar MS
Associate Professor Ophthalmology
AFMC Pune, Maharashtra

Rashmi Akshikar MS, DNB, MRCOPHTH
Member of Royal College of Ophthalmology
London, UK
Speciality Registrar in Ophthalmology
Queen Elizabeth 2 Hospital Welwyn Garden City-Herts
London (UK)

Affilations: Royal Society of Medicine London (UK)
South Wales Ophthalmological Society(SWOS)
South Wales Paediatric Ophthalmological Society
(SWOPOS)

Lt Col SK Mishra VSM,MS
Classified Specialist and Assistant Professor
Ophthalmology
Army Hospital (Research & Referral) Delhi Cantt (Post
Graduate Institute of Medical Sciences, affiliated to Delhi
University)

Lt Col Anirudh Singh MS
Associate Professor and Classified Specialist
Ophthalmology
Command Hospital (WC) (Post Graduate Institute of
Medical Sciences, affiliated to West Bengal University of
Heath Sciences) Chandimandir, Haryana

Lt Col Sandeep Gupta MS
Graded Specialist Ophthalmology
Military Hospital Mhow, Madhya Pradesh

Lt Col Nitin Vichare MS
Classified Specialist and Assistant Professor
Ophthalmology, Army College of Medical Sciences
Base Hospital, Delhi Cantt

Major Jaya Kaushik MS
Graded Specialist and Assistant Professor
Ophthalmology
Army Hospital (Research & Referral), Delhi Cantt (Post
Graduate Institute of Medical Sciences, affiliated to Delhi
University) arnavjaya@gmail.com

Surgeon Lt Commander AS Parihar MS
Graded Specialist, Ophthalmology
INHS Kalyani, Vishakhapatnam, Andhra Pradesh

Major SK Dhar MS
Graded Specialist Ophthalmology
Military Hospital, Jammu, Jammu and Kashmir

Major S Meneria VSM, MS
Graded Specialist Ophthalmology
Military Hospital, Jhansi, Uttar Pradesh

Foreword

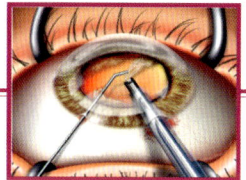

Dr MC Nahata MBBS, DOMS, MS
Formerly:
Member, Public Service Commission
Dean, GR Medical College, Gwalior (MP)
Prof and Head, Department of Ophthalmology
MGM Medical College, Indore (MP)

125, Kanchan Bagh
Indore 452001, MP

Swami Vivekananda has said that "Every one (including the physician) has a social obligation to consider. At the expense of the patient and the society he is able to complete his education. It is his duty to repay that loan as selfless service to the humanity. Serve with knowledge that in serving other person we serve no other person but God himself", he maintained.

Col JKS Parihar has followed the path of selfless service with knowledge as suggested by Swamiji. The monograph reveals how Col Parihar has become ophthalmic surgeon instead a cardiothoracic one for the benefit of the society and also recapitulates his association with many ophthalmic surgeons of the country in various capacities. In the monograph *Phacoemulsification Surgery* he very aptly described the intricacies and details of the procedure including anaesthesia and machines used therein. The language used is simple and lucid making it possible for even the young and budding Ophthalmologists to understand and even develop confidence to undertake surgery without hesitation and reservation. It is an established fact that all surgeries have the risk of complications and phacoemulsification is no exception to this dictum. The author has very specifically enumerated the causes of such unwanted eventualities and given appropriate advice to prevent such happening by preparing oneself.

In the career of an ophthalmic surgeon, occasion are not few when he has to undertake surgery on his kith and kin, VIPs and Elite of the society. In a situation like the one, the surgeon cannot remain normal evident by the palpitation he gets which he alone knows and feels, Col Parihar's guideline if followed will be for the benefit both of the patient and surgeon. The author of the monograph, one of the senior-most eminent ophthalmologists is a teacher of quality, a skillful artistic surgeon and a research scholar of repute besides being a social worker and above all a human being, he has been decorated with innumerable awards, honours, recognitions and assistance for the research projects needed for the betterment of ophthalmic science, which he carried out successfully. The monograph which he has presented to the society is an asset for the benefit of ophthalmologists both senior and young as well as to the social worker. It is a great effort by the author and his associates which kindles the light for the betterment of the society and great cause of prevention of blindness.

MC Nahata

Foreword

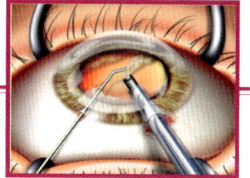

Air Marshal (Rtd) MS Boparai, AVSM

Professor Emeritus

National Academy of Medical Sciences (India)

Member Board of Management

Baba Farid University of Health Sciences, Punjab

Former Prof of Ophthalmology and

Director/Commandant

Armed Forces Medical College, Pune

boparaiorbit@gmail.com

915 Defence Colony
Sector 17B, Gurgaon
Haryana 122001, India

It is always a pleasure for a teacher to see his student evolve into a professional of eminence and so it is a matter of pride for me to be associated with this book authored by Col JKS Parihar SM, VSM.

Col Parihar has accumulated a large body of work in his career in the Armed Forces and we are proud of his achievements even prior to the publication of this book. This work, however, is evidence of his coming of age as a teacher and elder statesman in the field. A work such as this is a labour of love and hard work and reflects the attention to documentation and critical analysis over a 30-year long career. Indeed it is fascinating that a complete spectrum of total transformation spreading from historical and conventional technique of cataract surgery by ICCE to the latest technique of advanced phaco and its concurrent applications has been witnessed and performed by him in true sense. Having seen the progress of the author over the years, I am sure he has motivated many students to grow and spread the culture of excellence and dedication over the Armed forces fraternity. This publication is sure to extend a similar philosophy all over the country and students and practitioners alike will find it a comforting companion in all situations.

I wish the author and the book all the best.

MS Boparai

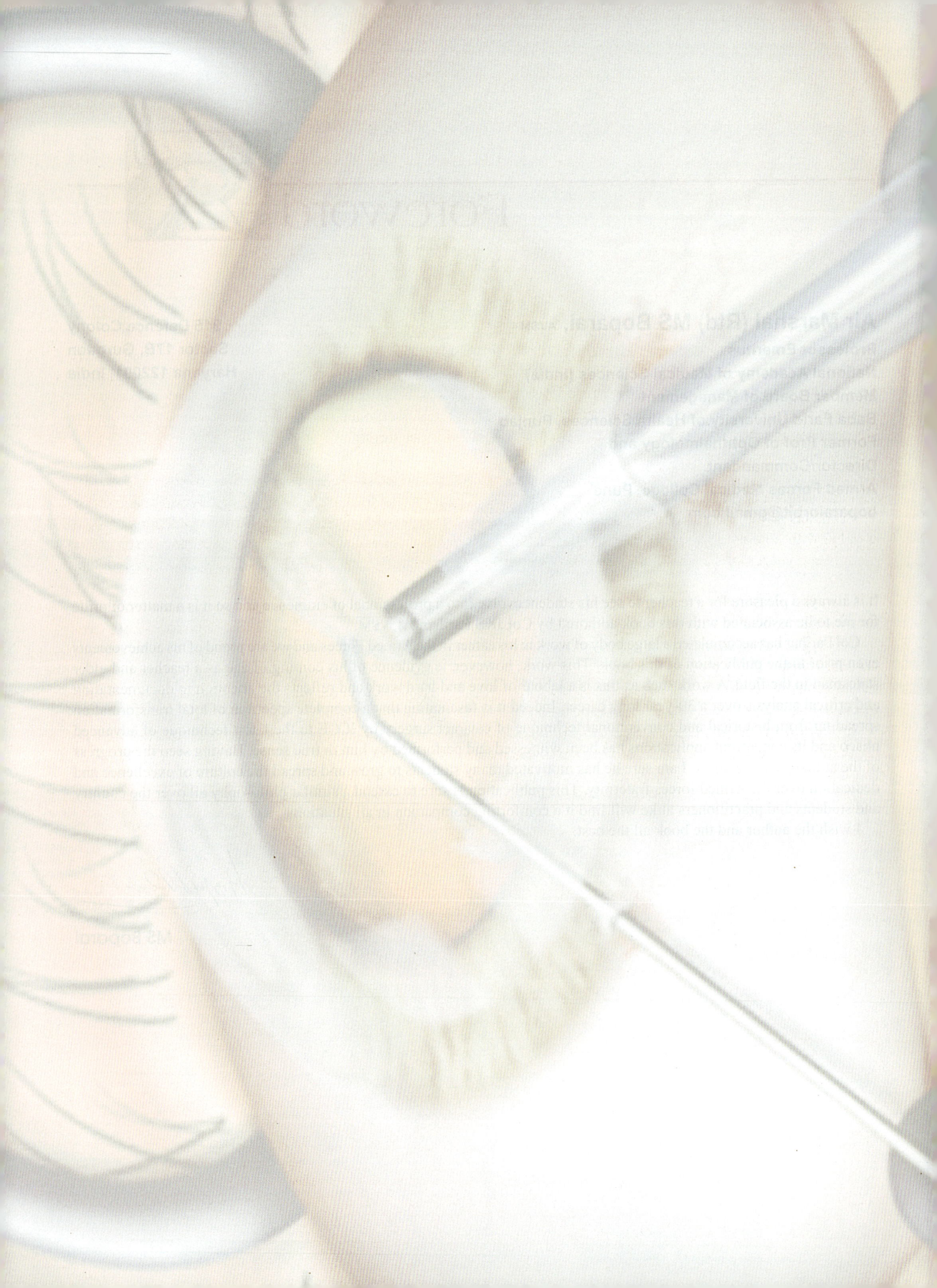

Preface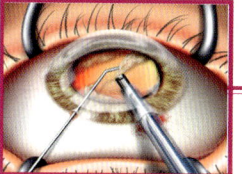

The mystery and chemistry of *Phacoemulsification Surgery* remains the most fascinating part of my life. I have lived up each and every moment of life with this technique since 1995, the beginning of my days with this coveted surgical technique. As I passed through my personal Phaco journey of 17 long years, I developed a desire to pen down my experiences of handling every aspect of phacoemulsification technique. I wanted the younger generation of ophthalmologists to understand the nuances and finer practical methodologies so that they are able to cover the steep learning curve associated with this technique and do not pass through the constraints experienced by me.

This book is aimed to provide comprehensive input about finer details of various aspects of phacoemulsification surgery to young ophthalmologists, postgraduate students and post-doctoral fellows in advanced ophthalmic anterior segment surgeries. The language of this book has been kept lucid so that the facts are clearly understood and grasped. The contents of this book have been designed with the intention to provide useful practical tips of surgical technique coupled with inherent flavour of theoretical aspects of such fascinating and most sought after ophthalmic surgery of modern era, yet comprehensive enough to be a center piece in phacoemulsification surgery training programs around the world.

Chapters on latest designs of multifocal and accommodative IOL implants as well as on advanced phacoemulsifier machines have been incorporated to maintain the pace with rapid advancement in the subject. The book also provides knowledge about concurrent surgical procedures where phacoemulsification surgery is clubbed with glaucoma and corneal transplant procedures. An exhaustive and analytical approach to cataract associated with other complex ocular problems is worth considering. A sincere effort has been made to cover the other side of the coin by compiling the views as well as on the table experience of patients undergoing this surgery.

All our efforts are made to take care of all the details published in this text but omissions and commissions do happen. I sincerely take the responsibility for all such lapses and would be obliged if I am made aware of these.

I hope this text and manual will fill in the need of lucid text on modern techniques of cataract surgery.

Col JKS Parihar

Acknowledgments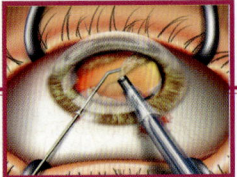

I acknowledge contribution of the entire paramedical staff of the department for providing untiring, selfless and wholehearted congenial environment in the department and operation theatre so as to enable me to perform all kind of complex surgical procedures as well as the documenting surgical videos and digital imaging used in this publication.

I extend my sincere gratitude to Col Arindam Chatterjee, Lt Col Sameer Kumar and Dr Bipin Rai, for providing excellent editorial expertise.

The editorial staff of CBS Publishers particularly Mr YN Arjuna deserves special thanks. My most sincere gratitude is due to Mr Chand S Nagar and Ms Nishi Verma of limited colours for providing excellent graphics, editing of colour plates and designing the format of the book. Undoubtedly, I would like to recall immense contribution of Late Mr BR Sharma who was the guiding force to produce and publish this textbook through CBS Publishers.

Words cannot express my feelings towards my beautiful wife Yogeshwari, daughter Aparna and son Ashwini who sacrificed their genuine wish to enjoy life during the period of drafting this monograph and through their dedication and inspiration in making sure I finally finished this work.

I dedicate this book to my parents, Dr Keshav Singh Parihar and Mrs Urmila Devi Parihar for their sincere efforts to make me competent enough to attain present position.

Col JKS Parihar

Contents

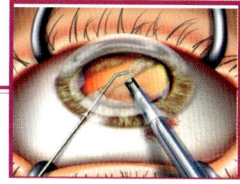

UNIT 1

BASICS OF PHACOEMULSIFICATION SURGERY

UNIT 2

PHACO INCEPTION AND INSTRUMENTATION

UNIT 3

BASIC SURGICAL TECHNIQUES IN PHACOEMULSIFICATION

UNIT 4

VARIOUS TECHNIQUES OF NUCLEOTOMY IN PHACOEMULSIFICATION

UNIT 5

VARIOUS TECHNIQUES OF IRRIGATION AND ASPIRATION IN PHACOEMULSIFICATION

UNIT 6

INTRAOCULAR LENS IMPLANTS

UNIT 7

PHACOEMULSIFICATION IN CHALLENGING SITUATIONS

UNIT 8

PHACOEMULSIFICATION AND CONCURRENT PROCEDURES

UNIT 9

ADVANCEMENT IN PHACOAPPLICATIONS

UNIT 10

CONTEMPORARY ISSUE IN PHACOEMULSIFICATION SURGERY

Basics of
Phacoemulsification Surgery

1

Kaleidoscopic View of Cataract and Phacoemulsification Surgery: Sutureless to Sutureless Surgery

Dr Rashmi Akshikar and Col JKS Parihar SM, VSM

History is not a dead record, and evolution is its living story. Tracing the pages of yesteryears of cataract surgery enlightens us not only about the evolution of facts, observations, mechanics and technologies, but of a more maturing thought process which stands the test of time and is a trailblazer in this whole process of evolution.

Cataract is a suffusion of coagulated humours (like a waterfall). It was this belief that formed the basis of couching as a procedure to cure cataract and as long as this belief prevailed, the procedure of couching prevailed, untill the mid seventeenth century.

Couching meaning as a 'pillow would couch on the sofa'; likewise the lens lie in the inferior vitreous. Couching definitely was the earliest cataract surgery (5th Century BC) It was the first documented by the Hindu surgeon 'Sushruta' in his 'Sushruta Samhita'.It was highlighted by the use of a needle, which pierced the posterior limbus and depressed the lens from the visual axis. A variation of the same was reclination, wherein the inferior zonules lay intact and the lens lay hinged on them, popping now and then in the visual axis.

It was documented that Alexander the Great brought couching to Europe. However, excavations from Babylonia, Greece and Egypt reveal bronze instruments used in couching, indicating its presence in Europe as well. Celsius in 29 AD documented practising breaking of cataract by using needles–'needling and in his De re Medicina'. Interestingly enough, the earliest evidence of the consumer protection act can be traced to the code of Hammurabi (1750 AD) which punished the surgeon by cutting off his arm if an eye was lost in couching. Though now practised only in some bush lands of Africa, the procedure did present modern ophthalmology with the concept of 'pars plana vitrectomy'.

'Cataract is the opacification of crystalline lens' – Rolfinck – 1650. After an erratic evolution of 3000 years,

the ocular anatomy and physiology was finally enlightened, when in the year 1 AD, Celsius, Ruffles and Galen all described the structure of lens with its anterior capsule and zonular structures. However, Celsius thought the lens to be the seat of vision. His teachings prevailed for nearly 1500 years until in 1515, Francisco Manrolycus clearly established the optical function of the lens. And Rolfinck correctly stated its opacification to be cataract. Both these concepts gave rise to a great furore in the scientific world, which took a hundred years to subside. However what evolved out of this furore was the acceptance of the fact that, cataract could be cured by removing the lens out of the eye and vision could still be retained. Aphakia was acceptable, as vision without the lens was possible. In 1707, Mario Antoinette showed vision was possible with Aphakia in animals. In 1722, Charles St. Yves performed the first intracapsular cataract extraction, though inadvertently, on a dislocated cataractous lens. In 1753, Samuel Sharp of London milked out the entire lens through an intact incision by using thumb pressure. The technique of ICCE was officially born and is here to stay. Later this milking out of lens was done by the use of a suction cup – the erisiphakes or grasping forceps. ICCE was greatly popularised by the vast experiences of McNamara, Molrony and Smith. Col Smith, the giant of ICCE, as he was referred to, performed a record 50 to 100 ICCE surgeries per day while serving in Punjab. He popularised his highly acclaimed Smith-Indian technique.

The paper 'A new way of curing Cataract' presented by 1752 by Dr Jacques Daniel in 1752 brought about a major revolution in cataract surgery and thus began the age of extra capsular surgery. Surprisingly, ECCE developed more as a technique than a concept, for it came at a time when the posterior capsule was still thought as a vitreous face. The ECCE technique, refined and came to the forefront, but not the extracapsular concept. This was the underlying reason why it was largely replaced by ICCE in the early

20th century. The other obvious reason was that mature cataract was an absolute essentiality retaining cortical matter causing severe inflammatory reaction in the eye. The technique demanded certain surgical skills. However, ECCE resurged and this was thanked to three men:

    (i) **Harold Scheie:** Who in 1960 standardised and popularised aspiration for congenital and traumatic soft cataracts.

   (ii) **Charles Kelman:** Who in 1966 thought of aspirating hard cataracts and Phacoemulsification was born.

  (iii) **Cornelius Binkhort:** Who was methodically innovating and developing Harold Ridley's artificial intraocular lens.

Furthermore, the reasons for ECCE were made obvious by retinal surgeons. De John Craig's drawings illustrated a definite decrease in the incidence of cystoid macular oedema, retinal detachment and retinal holes with the extra-capsular technique.

The beginning of the later half of the 20th century was the period of the most happenings in ophthalmology. The 1970 and 1980 decades saw ophthalmology conferences and meetings with the great debate 'ICCE versus ECCE'. In those days, ECCE was less popular (approximately 15% as compared to 85% in the favour of ICCE). Even well-established surgeons like Dr Maumenee, Dr Jerry Emery and Dr Norman Jaffe were more inclined towards ICCE as compared to ECCE. However, there were definite trends towards shifting to ECCE particularly in high risk and young cases having high myopia and in cases having a history of retinal detachment in the contralateral eye. The winds of change were evident.

ARTIFICIAL INTRAOCULAR LENS: A REVOLUTION IN THE EVOLUTION

The evolution of IOL has been a fascinating exercise in the field of ophthalmology. As usual with any invention, initial experiences are bound to be disappointing but sustained efforts and zeal ultimately leads to final success. The earliest reference in history is of an attempt made by Tadini in the 18th century. He had attempted to implant a well-polished sphere. This attempt was later described by Casanova.

The next significant attempt to perform implantation was unsuccessfully made in 1795 by Cassamator, a Dresden ophthalmologist.

Sir Harold Ridley was inspired by the comment of his student, who, while he was doing ICCE, suggested that he should replace the crystalline lens with an artificial lens.

Sir Harold Ridley, an ophthalmologist working with RAF, during II world war, discovered that canopy pieces from a crashed windshield of an aircraft, lay inert in the eyes of the injured pilot. The material was *polymethyl-methacrylate*. Inspired by this he performed the first successful implant of artificial IOL made of PMMA, on 29th Nov, 1949. This was a milestone in the revolution of cataract surgery and the evolution of cataract surgery. However, Ridley's initial lens was fraught with problems because of its weight (112 mg) and an improper design.

The PMMA caused no inflammatory reaction in the eye, though implanting the IOL in the AC was not without complications. This brought ECCE again to the centre stage. The obvious benefits of ECCE and IOL were, that a cataract extraction, at an early stage, was possible and unilateral operability very much acceptable. But more so the operated eye was closest to a normal eye both anatomically and functionally, as never before.

After Ridley's attempt at IOL implantation, during the next fifty years a large number of different lens styles and designs were developed.

GLIMPSES OF EVOLUTION OF PHACOEMULSIFICATION SURGERY

A surgeon's experiences that are encountered during the initial period of phacoemulsification surgery are as following:

A Big Question and a Bigger Quest: Evolution of Small Incision Cataract Surgery

Dr. Charles Kelman raised the relevant question, if cataract could be removed through the same sised incision as that for a prophylactic iridectomy?

The question definitely acted as a trailblazer in the evolution of cataract surgery. The quest, however, began with a simple observation by Charles Kelman that an eye with a prophylactic iridectomy was much less irritated postoperatively and required a much less hospital stay than the conventionally operated eye.

Kelman concluded the answer to be, a small incision procedure would be ideal to remove a cataract through that small an incision.

Cryofreeze removal of the cataract came to Kelman's mind and inspired by the neurosurgical cryoprobe, he devised the cryostylet. The cryostylet worked on the peltier effect and used no coolants, but used electricity to achieve freezing. The procedure was unable to decrease the incision size considerably and more so the incidence of posterior capsular rupture was high. Kelman abandoned it.

Aspiration of Cataract

After the failure of the cryostylet procedure, attention was diverted towards the aspiration method as a probable method of future for small incision cataract surgery as congenital and traumatic cataracts were being extracted through a very small incision by contemporary surgeons. As such, aspiration had stood the test of time and continues to do so in the evolution of cataract surgery. The Persians were the first to suck out cataract through needles. The eleventh century Arabian ophthalmologist Ammar Ibn Ali invented the aspiration needle and also advocated scleral approach to aspirate the cataractous lens. From Ammar's needle to the modern day phaco probe, aspiration has evolved through many devices.

This drew Kelman's attention to modify the procedure of aspiration for small incision surgery.

The stepping-stone was Kelman's encapsulation sac devised in 1962. Till then, devices as Fuchs suction syringe were in vogue for the congenital and traumatic cataracts. The encapsulation sac required an incision of the size of 2 mm, macerated with the help of micro-dissectors wherein the lens was enclosed. The procedure was extremely traumatic and unrefined and was soon abandoned. However, the concept stayed on.

The dental drill inspired Kelman to try rotational devices to fragment the lens. The devices had a rotating shaft, rotating needle surrounded by irrigation aspiration tubes. However, dental drilling was different from cataract extraction, for the tooth was fixed to the root, the lens was not. Thus, the lens rotated on drilling, instead, fragmenting and denuding the corneal endothelium. Not only the edges of the lens abraded the endothelium, but also its fragments caused a sun blast effect to further destroy it. The rotating device caused ensnarement and disinsertion of the iris and often a complete inadvertent iridectomy.

Learning from these failures, an attempt was made to devise an instrument that would keep the lens stationary. The micro-blender was the first of this style, with two needles turning in opposite directions, thus nullifying, the spin. Then came the slow rotorshaped as a cock screw, and the bident that would grasp the lens while a rotary device fragmented it. All of them failed.

Failure of rotary devices shifted the focus to oscillating devices. Imagination again came handy and an oscillating Handpiece was made from an electric toothbrush. It moved along a 45°–90° arch, rocked the lens vigorously and was soon abandoned. With rotation and oscillation long gone, the next to be tried were vibrators, both high and low frequency, but with no use.

From a series of these sad failures surfaced the principles of intra-cameral surgery. Clearly motion was not the thing for intra-cameral surgery, more so a device in slow motion caused more damage than a rapid one. Further, these devices needed to be stabilised by using both the hands, when manoeuvring in the anterior chamber thus incapacitating the surgeon.

Linear Acceleration: A Journey from Plunger to the Probe

Where other motions failed, linear acceleration paved the path to success. What it did was, it made penetrating the lens possible without overcoming its standing inertia. Thus,

during the procedure, the lens remained stationary. As a result here we had a high frequency solid plunger tip accelerating at 240000g's, with irrigation flow around it and encased in a sleeve. This was the design of the ultrasonic probe, which proved to be the forerunner of the first phacoemulsifier.

What the probe lacked and was later added to the phacoemulsifier was an aspiration system. Also the tip of the probe was fairly blunt and accumulated a lot of heat. This was due to many reasons such as occlusion of the irrigation by lens particles, a faulty design of the irrigation system itself and a high emission of ultrasonic radiation due to a large tip mass. All these were rectified in the phacoemulsifier.

First Phacoemulsifier

The first phacoemulsifier which was used on animals had several undermentioned interesting features:

It was an assembly of various individual components like a separate table. A dental tartar removal device was modified and attached to provide suction and irrigation.

An aspiration system was added subsequently to hold the lens firmly against a vibrating tip. The design of the aspiration needle was of a lumen, narrowest at the tip and wider at a distance away from it. Thus, the lens fragment was sucked away causing no occlusion or interruption to the irrigation flow. This also eliminated the heat build up at the needle tip. Also the irrigation tube opening was close to the needle tip which further reduced the heat accumulation.

Ultrasonic Handpiece

The first generation Handpieces were very heavy weighing about 500 grams and it was too difficult to manoeuver with them due to their obvious large size and shape like that of a flashlight. A three-dimensional parallelogram was exclusively designed to overcome the problems of stabilising and rotational movements of Handpiece during surgery.

This was the modification of the plunger. Firstly, the plunger tip was replaced by a sharp longitudinal needle. This kept the lens stationary as well as reduced the emission of ultrasonic radiations into the anterior chamber well below safety limits. The needle vibrated 20,000 times per second with a stroke amplitude of 0.003 in air. However, the initial grades of phacoemulsifier were unsuitable for hard cataract since the ultrasonic stroke was very small and was not capable enough to negotiate with hard cataract effectively. Subsequently, the heavy and bulky magnetostrictive Handpiece was replaced with smaller, lighter and high frequency piezoelectric crystals producing 40000 cycles which was found to be more effective and widely accepted by other ophthalmic surgeons.

Most interesting component of the first phacoemulsifier was a three-dimensional parallelogram which supported the heavy phaco handpiece during surgery. In addition a separate, irrigation aspiration handpiece without any vibration was developed for removing the peripheral soft cortical matter. Also its lumen could be placed away from posterior capsule.

Problems of Thermal Injury Effects

The original handpiece was magnetostrictive, heavy and used to produce significant heat energy. Hence, the problem of heat build up and thermal injury was very significant. To overcome this situation, the original magnetostrictive handpiece was equipped with a water cooling system. The water used for cooling around and out of magnetostrictive plates used to be nonsterile. Hence, a specific device was designed to keep nonsterile water away from the sterile irrigation fluid. Any failure in this isolation mechanism would have created unpleasant situation of infection. However, the invention of air-cooled piezoelectric crystals eliminated the need for separate water cooling devices. The insulating device like sleeves protects incision and cornea from thermal injury. Over and above, such sleeves provide space for movement of irrigating fluid as well as additional cooling effects. Silicone and teflon are preferred materials for sleeves. Among these two, silicone is more acceptable.

Phaco tips

The original tips were made up of steel. These tips were heavy, fragile with short longevity. Another significant problem was to have flaking from chipped tip. However, steel tips were replaced subsequently by titanium which still holds good both in terms of proven inert material and practically no reactions inside the eye due to this metal.

Irrigation/Aspiration Handpiece

Initially, the complete process of phacoemulsification including cortical aspiration and final wash used to be completed by using a single phaco handpiece. However, the need for modified tips was realised at initial stage only due to persistent problems of engagement of posterior capsule during I/A procedure. Sir Kelman had modified the tip by having a blind terminal end and lumen on the side of tip. A separate irrigation and aspiration handpiece without any vibrating tip had become the reality later on.

The Cavitron/Kelman Phacoemulsifier Aspirator System

Three generations of instruments were developed from 1970 to 1976. The basic aim was to have an ideal phacoemulsification machine which should not only be capable of handling different types of cataracts effectively without jeopardising the safety, but would also be able to maintain essential integrity of intraocular structures.

The MODEL 8000 V is the best representation of these early machines. It was highlighted by an irrigation system which was a gravity flow system, with a pinch valve controlled by a footswitch. The irrigation solution bottle was suspended at a height of 65 cm. Suction was provided by a peristaltic pump. The aspiration had an inbuilt mechanism to limit the vacuum, thereby avoiding excessive collapse or shallowing of the anterior chamber. An additional aspect of the system was the vent control, in order to break the vacuum. The acoustic vibrator in the ultrasonic handpiece, fragments the lens at a frequency of 40 kHz. The ultrasonic handpiece was provided with a cooling system working on negative pressure to combat heat generated during energy conversion. Assembling the ultrasonic handpiece was important, as both sterile and nonsterile fluids were present in the same handpiece.

The front panel of the instrument in its upper half displayed a footswitch position indicator, a four position rotatory vacuum select switch, vent and cooling fault indicator, an ultrasonic power control switch and an elapsed time indicator. The lower half of the front panel had vacuum control port, peristaltic pump and an irrigation pinch valve.

Glimpses of Evolution of Surgeons Experiences Encountered during Initial Period of Phacoemulsification Surgery

First Kelman Technique

It was performed in 1967, on a selected group of 12, mostly elderly with mature hard cataracts and diseased retinas. The first surgery was on a 60-year-old woman with dense mature cataract and severe diabetic retinopathy. The time taken was 4 hours with more than an hour of ultrasonic vibration, and almost 3 litres of irrigation fluid was used. But the cornea collapsed into the probe almost 30 times. This had resulted in severe striate which lasted for more than one month, However, the cornea responded and cleared eventually in due course of time and there was a ray of hope.

The foundation was definitely laid now with development of a modality of fragmentation—the phacoprobe. But still to be worked on was a sophisticated and balanced irrigation-aspiration system as well as a technique to bring the nucleus into the anterior chamber. One can only imagine, the great courage and determination of Sir Charles Kelman under significant constraints of experience, lack of good machine, operating microscope, non-availability of viscoelastics and good drugs for intra and postoperative need in those days. However, the process of the evolution of small incision cataract surgery and a revolution in the speciality of ophthalmology had begun.

Journey from Operating Loupe to Operating Microscope (Magnification and Visualisation)

In the early seventies, operating loupes was the standard method of magnification which was not adequate for such complex surgical technology of phacoemulsification. From our own experience we can imagine the difficulties of making rhexis or even capsulotomy and other basic steps of phaco like washing of cortical material under loupe without coaxial magnification and red reflex even today. It is absolutely impossible to detect small rent or zonulysis under loupe without red reflex, indeed a very horrifying thought for us, but it was a reality for a Phaco surgeon in those days.

Few microscopes that were available for surgery, were basically of industrial grade and without quality of depth perception, having inadequate magnification and no coaxial illumination and hence no red reflex.

The first microscope which was used by Sir Charles Kelman was a table top dissecting microscope having very poor quality of illumination. However, his first reasonably good microscope was an ENT microscope in which he managed to get depth perception and red reflex through additional coaxial light. This kind of modification continued for quite some time until proper ophthalmic operating microscope was made available.

Intraoperative Constraints and the Way Those Were Conquered

Miosis

Intraoperative miosis is still a big problem. A good and sustained mydriasis is an essential prerequisite of successful phaco surgery. Any tissue handling or even vibrating tip may cause miosis. Imagine those initial days of phacosurgery, when heavy handpieces, no viscoelastics, no mydriatic and over and above surgery without operating microscope was the reality. Needless to stress, a modern Phaco surgeon would not have dared to perform phaco even in a dream in those situations. Sir Kelman invented to perform large sector iridectomy to handle miosis (modern surgeons perhaps got the idea to stretch pupil or perform sphincterotomy in case of a miotic pupil from this only). However, this iridectomy was not totally foolproof since iris capture and chaffing was a frequent and annoying problem. The next answer to this problem was anterior chamber phaco which is still performed by beginners inspite of the possibility of increased loss of endothelial cell count. However, this problem was finally overcome by the invention and practice of mydriatics in the infusion fluids.

Phaco in Precapsulorrhexis Era

Most of us are aware of the fact that conventional anterior capsulotomy is not an ideal choice for good and smooth phacoemulsification. The inventors of phaco had faced serious complications like rent and zonulysis due to traction of flaps of the anterior capsule and very soon realised the need for some different ways to make capsular opening. While working on animal eyes, it was an accidental observation by Sir Kelman that a relatively blunt cystitome did not cut the capsule but tore it in the form of a triangle. Indeed it was a fascinating and brilliant observation which turned to be the beginning of the era of modern capsulotomy by the name of Christmas Tree Opening. The same accidentally formed triangular capsulotomy, particularly in case of mature or in paediatric cataract, still holds manageable even for the performing of foldable IOL implantation.

Constraints of Instability of Anterior Chamber

Initial phacoemulsifiers did not have proper mechanics to adjust suction as per the need of the phacoprocedure. This had resulted in the inherent problem of sudden and unpredictable surge leading to the collapsing of anterior chamber, repeated corneal touch, and severe loss of endothelial cells. This problem was overcome by the invention of the fluid control valve system which was based on the clinical experience of monitoring the mechanism of flow in arteries by the creation of an electric current from the ions in the event of blood flow through the arteries.

Posterior Capsule Tear

The success and failure of phaco surgeons swing over integrity of 6 to 7 micron thickness of the posterior capsule which is still a matter of biggest concern.

The first generation ultrasonic handpieces and phacoemulsifier systems had an inherent constraint of effective system of fluidics, vacuum as well as of US energy delivery system. Over and above, other factors like nonavailability of good operating microscopes, instrumentation, viscoelastics and inadequate surgical expertise were compounding factors to have higher incidence of posterior capsule tear. Surgeons preferred to perform phaco in anterior chamber to avoid injury to the posterior capsule until newer generation phacoemulsifiers were made available.

Cold phaco: The Hot New Thing

In the last few decades, phaco technology has further evolved in strides to achieve superior fluidics, titrable power, easily useable Handpieces, but most of all an effort to minimise the heat build up at the phaco tip and thus achieve a cold phaco.

The state-of-the-art ALCON legacy phaco machine has had three major upgrades since its release. The latest being the NEOSONIX Handpiece which blends traditional linear acceleration with oscillation to tackle denser cataracts (two degree oscillation at 100 Hz). Also the new steerable silicon encapsulated I/A tip provides more flexibility and continuous fluid outflow, to maintain a more stable anterior chamber. Not to mention the new software options allowing surgeons to preprogram power and aspiration settings for each step. To mention a few others is the STAAR Surgical's sonic wave which uses a frequency of just 40–400 Hz, thus decreasing the thermal energy output and the Dodick photolysis system which introduces Q-switched Nd:YAG laser energy instead of standard ultrasound waves to break cataract. Also, we have the Allergan Sovereign which delivers phaco power in short bursts or pulses, instead of linear fashion.

Evolution in mechanics can be exemplified in the form of the Bausch and Lomb Millennium, where phaco and vacuum power is controlled by dual linear 'foot pedal'. The concentrix pump also delinks functions of vacuum and ultrasound, thus giving the surgeon independent control over each. And the quest continues for perfection.

IMPORTANT LANDMARKS IN THE EVOLUTION OF CATARACT SURGERY

Illumination evolved from projection lamps with blue filters, to magnifying telescopic loupes and then the microscope.

Development of metallurgy saw good steel instruments in early 19th century. The forerunner was von Graefe's knife. von Graefe also introduced superior incision and iridectomy. With ab-externo incisions, the knife lost to scissors, scalpels and razor blades. Further came the diamond and ruby microblades. Modern corneal scissors are similar to Daviel's keratomes.

In 1867, Henry Willard Williams of Boston used sutures for the first time in cataract surgery. Suturing was uncommon till the early 19th century, the Kat silk 6–0 used was 150 microns and crude. Later, it was replaced by a single strand virgin silk, 50 microns, shedding in 3 weeks. These were swaged on a traumatic hollow needle to minimise reactivity. Deadly nightshade or belladonna atropa was used since 1796 to dilate pupils, atropine was extracted later in 1831.

In 1884, cocaine drops were used as topical anaesthesia in cataract surgery.

Antibiotics and corticosteroids came into use in 1950 and revived ECCE, along with iridectomy.

Choice, an assistant to Ridley, along with Binkhorst capitalised on lighter, anterior chamber lenses, the Choices mark 4 lenses and Binkhorst iris clip lens. At the same time, suturing improved with 10–0 nylon sutures, as thin as 12 microns.

John Pearce, in 1970 developed small incision microsurgery, and IOL implantation in posterior chamber.

Galand in Liege, refined it to endocapsular implantation.

Fankhause in 1983 developed, the YAG laser capsulotomy.

At the same time, foot pedal control in microscopes and a USG A - SCAN were also developed.

Viscoelastics were introduced as late as 1990 by Craig and Artola.

Continuous curvilinear capsulorrhexis was introduced in 1990 by Gimble and Neuhman.

The next milestone in the journey of this evolution is, vision at 91 as good as at 19.

BIBLIOGRAPHY

1. Kelman CD, Cooper IS: Cryosurgery of retinal detachment and other ocular conditions. The Eye, Ear, Nose and Throat Monthly 42: 42–46, 1963.
2. Cryogenic surgery: N Engl/Med 268: 1963.
3. Kelman CD: Symposium; phacoemulsification. History of emulsification and aspiration of senile cataracts. Transactions American Academy of Ophthalmology and Otolaryngology 78: OP7–OP9, 1974.
4. Apple AJ, Sims J. Harold Ridley and the Invention of the Intraocular Lens. Survey of Ophthalmology. 1996; 2001–2002.
5. Ridley NHL. Intraocular acrylic lenses. Trans Ophthalmol Soc UK and Oxford Ophthalmol Congress. 1951; LXXI: 617–21.
6. Ridley NHL. Further observations on intraocular acrylic lenses in cataract surgery. Trans Am Acad Ophthalmol Otolaryngol. 1953; 57:98–106.
7. Ridley NHL. Intraocular acrylic lenses after cataract extraction. Lancet. 1952; 1:118–19.
8. Apple DJ. Sir Harold Ridley receives England's highest honor. Surv Ophthalmol. 2000; 44:542.
9. Apple DJ, Peng Q. Harold Ridley knighted. Ophthalmology 2000; 107:412–13.
10. Apple DJ. Sir Nicholas Harold Ridley: All's well that ends well. Am J Ophthalmol. 2002; 133:131–33.
11. Williams HP. Sir Harold Ridley's vision. Br J Ophthalmol 2001; 85:1022–1023.
12. Vail D. Discussion of Ridley H: Further observations on intraocular acrylic lenses. Trans Am Acad Ophthalmol Otolaryngol 1953; 57:104.
13. Apple DJ, Mamalis N, Loftfield K, Googe JM, Novak LC, Kavka-Van Norman D, et al. Complications of intraocular lenses: A historical and histopathological review. Surv Ophthalmol 1984; 29:1–54.
14. Apple DJ, Kincaid MC, Mamalis N, Olson RJ. Intraocular lenses; evolution, designs, complications, and pathology. Baltimore, MD: Williams and Wilkins. 1989. 370–377.
15. Choyce DP. Intraocular Lenses and Implants. London, UK: HK Lewis & Co. 1964. 1–211.
16. Ridley NHL. Television in ophthalmology. Proc XVI Intern Congress Ophthalmol. 1950; pp 1397–1404.

2

Preoperative Clinical Evaluation for Phacoemulsification Cataract Surgery

Dr. Aradhana Singh and Col JKS Parihar SM, VSM

INTRODUCTION

The history of cataract surgery dates back to almost 20 centuries. The initial method of cataract extraction was by couching, the first written description of which has been given by the ancient Indian surgeon Sushruta (circa 600 BC). It was followed through the middle ages up to early 1900s. The father of modern cataract surgery Jacques Daviel introduced the incisional extraction of the cataract in 1753 but surgeons still continued to practise the virtues of couching for another 150 years. Between the years 1753 to 1862 three major milestones altered the direction of cataract surgery. The introduction of the initial surgical incision to the upper part of the eye, the introduction of pharmacologic mydriasis and the addition of preliminary iridectomy improved the prognosis of postoperative cataract surgery results. Daviel described the method for the Extracapsular Cataract Extraction (ECCE) technique. Daviel and Samuel Sharp are credited with cataract surgery involving taking out of the entire lens with the capsule intact. The ICCE was being practised as the surgeons recognised that Daviel's operation had dangers of vitreous loss and bound down pupils, due to inflammation. The ICCE was further modified by Colonel Henry Smith famed for the Smith Indian linear sliding manouvre of lens expression. This was followed by the technique of Verhoeff using the Verhoeff's capsular forceps which minimised the vitreous loss. P Stoewer used a suction device. This was followed by the use of chemical zonulysis as demonstrated by Jose Barraquer. Mechanical zonulysis was brought in vogue by Christiaen and Luca. Cryoextraction was introduced by Krawawicz. ICCE was in its heyday in the early 1970s. But, it was short-lived as it lived for only a century owing to the introduction of the intraocular lens which replaced it and at the same time revolutionised the whole concept of cataract surgery. The ICCE concept of cataract removal occupied the innovative surgeons belonging to the first 65 years of the 20th century. Contact lens development from 1940s to 1970s enhanced aphakic rehabilitation of the patients. The first intraocular lens implantation was done by Harold Ridley on 29th November, 1949. This was further enhanced by the technique of ECCE which provided a stable posterior capsule for the support of the intraocular lens. The work of Cornelius Binkhorst and Jan Worst aimed at proving the need of ECCE for better placement of the intraocular lens. This was further improved by Charles Kelman with the advent of the phacoemulsification system.

THEORY OF PSEUDOPHAKOS: METHODS OF CORRECTION OF APHAKIA

Since a spectacle lens and a contact lens are safe appliances because they can be replaced, if defective, what accounts then for the current popularity of IOL? This is explained by examining the three available methods of optical correction of aphakia:

(a) Spectacle lens in front of the eyes
(b) Contact lens
(c) IOL

Constraints and Demerits of Aphakic Corrections by Spectacle Lens

- Magnification of image sizes by about 25%
- Spherical aberration – Pin cushion distortion
- Poor coordination of manual movements due to the above reasons
- Restriction of visual fields – small sizes of aphakic fields of vision
- Ring scotoma
- Unrefracted field of vision outside spectacle lens
- Aesthetically unfavorable and cumbersome

Contact Lens

Advantages:
- Only 7% magnification
- No appreciable spherical aberration
- No ring scotoma or restriction of field of vision

Disadvantage:
- Difficult to use in children and elderly
- Unsuitable for certain professions—farmers, miners, etc.

IOL

Disadvantage

Error of power calculation cannot be changed once implanted.

Advantages

- 0.20% minification of image
- Normal field of vision
- No spherical aberration
- No problem of insertion and removal.

SIGNIFICANCE OF PREOPERATIVE CLINICAL EVALUATION FOR CATARACT SURGERY

Cataract extraction is the most commonly performed surgery in the geriatric age group, i.e. above 60 years of age.

A detailed and precise preoperative history is more important than the actual surgery itself. A thorough history gives a clue about the cause of cataract. There is a wide variation in the decision of ophthalmologists, as far as cataract removal goes, i.e. the decision from non-removal to removal, no matter what the status of cataract is. The important question is whether the operation will benefit the patient. Here the question of evaluation for cataract surgery comes. Before deciding to operate on a person for cataract, various issues have to be dealt with. Preoperatively the patient has to be evaluated physically as well as mentally to be prepared for the surgery. The article by Reeves and associates raises important questions, namely, can a self-administered questionnaire help determine which patients need a preoperative history and physical examination before cataract surgery? And how thorough should that history and physical examination be? Even though most cataract patients are at higher risks of perioperative complications due to advanced age, most eye procedures are minimally invasive and are considered low risk. The ideal questionnaire would be brief, yet thorough. Future researchers may want to use psychometric techniques to evaluate usefulness of each individual question to achieve this. Questions about specific symptoms such as those associated with systemic conditions like heart failure and uremia might supplement questions about already diagnosed medical problems.

HISTORY TAKING

History is generally elicited systematically in the following order:

Symptoms

A detailed history of the presenting complaint should be taken.

(a) Patients commonly present with painless progressive diminution of vision, aging from few months to few years. Traumatic cataracts may present with shorter duration, which may vary from few hours to few weeks after the injury depending on the severity of injury. Pain may be associated with complicated cataracts (e.g. cataracts secondary to uveitis) or in complications of cataracts (as seen in phacomorphic or phacolytic glaucoma).

Painless progressive diminution of vision is also a common symptom of open angle glaucoma. Hence, the above condition must be ruled out.

(b) The refraction of the eye may change depending on the quantity and type of cataract. Nuclear sclerosis induces myopia and, hence explains the reason behind the so-called "second sight" in presbyopes. Distant vision usually improves with concave lenses in such cases, but the near vision does not. Patients with posterior subcapsular cataract have their near vision affected more as compared to the distant vision. Diurnal variation of vision may also occur. Patients with central posterior subcapsular cataract have better vision at night as a result of pupillary dilatation.

(c) Halos may also form an important part of the symptoms of cataract. Lenticular halos must be differentiated from glaucomatous halos (by Fincham's test).

(d) Glare is a common symptom of posterior sub-capsular cataracts. It is due to scattering of light by the cataract.

Associated History

Depending on the age group, specific history associated with cataract may be elicited.

(a) **Senile age group:** History of exposure to sun (U-V rays) is important, as this is the commonest cause of senile cataract. History of various systemic illnesses has to be taken. History of diabetes is important both as a cause of cataract and for postoperative management after cataract surgery. A history of hypertension and other systemic illnesses like ischaemic heart disease and pulmonary disorders is taken as a preoperative work up. The severity of other co-morbidities will determine the type of anaesthetic management and extent of intra and postoperative monitoring.

(b) **Presenile age group:** These patients are in the 3rd and 4th decades of life. The common predisposing factors leading to cataract in these patients are diabetes, myotonic dystrophy, atopic dermatitis, and neurofibromatosis type II traumatic cataracts due to direct trauma, electric shock, ionising radiation or lightning strike can also occur in this group as a result of occupational hazard.

Toxic cataracts are a result of intake of various drugs. Drugs commonly causing cataract are steroids, chlorpromazine, busulfan, amiodarone, miotics and gold.

Secondary cataract can result due to uveitis, angle closure glaucoma, high myopia and hereditary fundus dystrophies like retinitis pigmentosa and Leber's amaurosis.

(c) **Congenital:** Congenital cataract in the pediatric age group is a major cause of childhood blindness. In the pediatric cataract population examined, approximately half of the patients were diagnosed in the first year of life. Over 18% had a positive family history of cataract. Identification of the genes that cause pediatric and congenital cataract should help clarify the etiology of some sporadic and unilateral cataracts. Hence, family history of congenital cataract and consanguinity of marriage is important in this age group.

Other causes of congenital cataract are intrauterine infections like rubella in the first trimester. Congenital rubella is associated with cataracts in 15% of cases. After the gestational age of 6 weeks, the virus is incapable of crossing the lens capsule, so the lens is unaffected if maternal infection occurs after this period. Other intrauterine causes leading to cataract are the TORCH organisms.

Various metabolic disorders associated with congenital cataract are galactosemia, mannosidosis, neonatal hypocalcemia, and hypoglycemia and galactokinase deficiency. Various systemic syndromes associated with neonatal cataracts are Lowe's syndrome, chromosomal disorders like Down syndrome (trisomy 21), Patau syndrome (trisomy 13), Edwards' syndrome (trisomy 18) and Turner's syndrome.

SYSTEMIC EXAMINATION

Before proceeding onto ocular examination, a quick systemic examination must be carried out. An adequate systemic evaluation helps in the assessment of the physical status of an individual who has to undergo surgery. Since majority of the patients are above 60 years of age systemic evaluation is important in order to avoid unrelated complications following cataract surgery.

General examination includes evaluation of pulse, blood pressure, lymph node, assessment of pallor, oedema, clubbing, etc. The patient should also be assessed for features of specific disorders like Marfan's syndrome and storage disorders like Hurler's and Hunter's syndrome.

Systemic review of the cardiovascular, respiratory, Nervous systems as well as the abdomen must not be neglected.

OCULAR EXAMINATION

A systematic and thorough approach to the ocular examination is important to assess the preoperative status of the eye. This helps in decision-making of whether or not to operate on the eye. It also gives an indication about the postoperative visual prognosis.

The ocular examination is carried out in the following order:

Visual Acuity

Visual acuity is one of the most important aspects of ocular examination. It is determined for both near and distant visions. The degree of visual impairment caused by cataract should be estimated. In a clinical practice, the measurement of visual acuity is considered synonymous with the measurement of "minimum resolvable". The threshold of the minimum resolvable is between 30 seconds and 1 minute of arc. Therefore, all the clinical tests employed to measure the visual acuity take the above principle into consideration. Based on this basic principle many visual acuity charts have been developed. In mature cataracts the visual acuity varies from perception of light to hand movements close to the face. In immature cataracts, the acuity may vary from counting fingers to 6/9.

The various visual tests for distant vision can be grouped as:

Detection Acuity Tests

These assess without correctly recognising the ability to detect the smallest stimulus. Common detection acuity tests are:

(i) Dot visual acuity test
(ii) Catford drum test
(iii) Boek Candy beads test
(iv) STYCAR graded ball's test
(v) Schwarting metronome test.

Recognition Acuity Tests

These are designed to assess the ability to recognise the stimulus or to distinguish it from other competing stimuli. These include:

Direction Identification Tests

(i) Snellen's E-chart test

(ii) Landolt's C-chart test

(iii) Sjögren's hand test

(iv) Arrows test

Letter Identification Tests

(i) Snellen's letter chart test

(ii) Sheridan's letter test

(iii) Flook's symbol test

(iv) Lipman's HOTV test

Picture Identification Charts (Miniature Toy Test)

(i) Alien's picture cards test

(ii) Beale Collins picture charts test

(iii) Domino cards test

(iv) Light house test

(v) Miniature toy test of Sheridan

Tests based on Picture Identification on Behavioural Pattern

(i) Cardiff acuity cards test

(ii) Bailey Hall cereal test

The resolution acuity tests are mainly carried out in infants.

Resolution Acuity Tests

(i) Optokinetic nystagmus (OKN) test

(ii) Preferential looking test (PLT)

(iii) Two alternative forced choice (2-AFC) test

(iv) Operent variation looking (OPL) test

(v) Teller acuity cards (TAC) test

(vi) Visually evoked response (VER)

Measurement of Visual Acuity for Near

Near vision is tested by asking the patient to read a near vision chart, which consists of a series of different sizes of printer type arranged in increasing order and marked accordingly. Commonly used near vision charts are as follows:

(i) **Jaeger's chart:** Jaeger in 1867 devised the near vision chart, which consisted of the ordinary printers' fonts of varying sizes used at that time. Printers' fonts have changed considerably since then, however, it is now the general custom to use various sizes of modern fonts, which approximate Jaeger's original choice. In this chart prints are marked from 1 to 7 and accordingly patient's acuity is labelled as Jl to J7 depending upon the print that he can read.

(ii) **Roman test-types:** The Jaeger's charts made from the modern fonts deviate considerably from the original standard, but they are probably sufficiently accurate for all practical purposes. However, to overcome this theoretical problem the 'Faculty of Ophthalmologists of Great Britain' in 1952 devised another near vision chart. It consists of 'Times Roman' type fonts with standard spacing. According to this chart, the near vision is recorded as N5, N6, N8, N10, N12, N18, N36 and N48.

(iii) **Snellen's near vision test-types:** Snellen introduced the so-called 'Snellen's equivalent for near vision' on the same principles as his distant types. The graded thickness of the letters of different lines is about 1/17th of the distant vision chart letters. In this event, the letters equivalent to 6/6 lines subtend an angle of 5 minutes at an average reading distance (35 cm/14 in.). The unusual configuration of letters of this chart, however, cannot be constructed from the available printer's fonts. It can only be reproduced by a photographic reduction of the standard Snellen's distant vision test types to approximately I/17th of their normal size. Further, such a test has never become popular. The graded sizes of pleasing types of passages from literature, the reading of which helps in the interpretation are habitually employed.

(iv) Two important methods useful in subjective test of the resolving power of the eye in moderate cataracts are: (a) Laser interferometer and (b) Potential visual acuity meter.

(a) **Laser interferometer:** Laser interferometer is mounted on a slit lamp. Laser generated interference fringes are used. A small He-Ne laser provides a collimated beam that is optically divided. The two beams of light are projected into the eye through a dilated pupil. The intersections of beams produce interference fringes that can be imaged on the macula. Changing the angular separation of the two beams can vary the size of the laser fringes. Coarse fringe patterns are used at first and are gradually reduced in size until the patient can no longer discern them. The laser interferometer resolving power of an eye can be converted to standard visual acuity with a simple table that theoretically indicates the maximal visual acuity possible. It has some limitations, as it is a subjective test requiring patient's co-operation, thus eliminating very old and very young patients. It also overpredicts the vision in the amblyopic eye. It is useful in moderate cataracts and in some degree of maculopathy.

(b) **Potential visual acuity meter:** Potential visual acuity meter consists of a slit lamp attachment that can project an entire visual acuity chart onto the retina. It emits 0.1 mm beam of light through relatively clearer areas of the cataract. This test is easier to perform than laser interferometry. However, it can overpredict vision in cystoid macular oedema and epiretinal membranes because sensory elements of retina are relatively undisturbed.

Visual Fields

Visual fields examination is carried out for mild or moderate cataracts. It is an important test to distinguish visual loss due to glaucoma or from that due to cataract. Both peripheral and central field analyses are done. In the present day field analysis is carried out by automated perimetry.

Torch Light Examination

Torch light examination of the eyes involves the evaluation of extraocular movements that gives a general idea of the function of the 3rd, 4th and 6th cranial nerves. The squint evaluation is carried out by cover, cover-uncover and alternate cover tests. The status of the orbit is examined to rule out any exophthalmos or enophthalmos. The lacrimal system patency and status is determined by regurgitation test or sac syringing test. It is also important to rule out any local infection at this stage.

Slit Lamp Biomicroscopy (Figs 2.1 to 2.7)

The next step in the examination is **Slit Lamp Biomicroscopy**. The status of lids and adenexa are noted to rule out any local infections like meibomitis, blepharitis and dacrocystitis, which should be managed preoperatively. The conjunctiva is examined for any congestion, papillae, follicles and degenerative conditions like pterygium. Any abnormality indicating active inflammation or infection is treated. The health of the cornea is assessed. The common endothelial abnormality like guttata is an indication of poor endothelium and hence can lead to corneal damage intraoperatively. An endothelial dystrophy of the Fuchs's type influences the prognosis and the choice of surgery. There is no sure way to distinguish cases of cornea guttata that remain unchanged indefinitely from those that are merely a prelude to full-blown Fuchs's dystrophy.

The other features assessed are sensation, surface, shine, clarity and surrounding structures of the cornea. The anterior chamber depth and contents are examined to rule out angle closure glaucoma and any uveitis. The iris colour and pattern are examined. Any rubeosis iridis which is an indication of concealed (by cataract) diabetic retinopathy and central retinal vein occlusion should be ruled out.

The pupillary reaction and the size of pupil are noted. Any relative afferent pupillary defect is to be looked for to determine the status of optic nerve/retina and hence, the visual prognosis postoperatively.

The type and degree of cataract is determined only after pupillary dilatation on a slit lamp. This is important in deciding upon the type of cataract surgery.

Intraocular Pressure

Intraocular pressure determination is done both by indentation and by more accurate applanation methods. Schiotz tonometer (indentation principle) is commonly used in a diagnostic camp scenario. In a clinical setup the Goldman's tonometer or non-contact tonometer are preferred. In children the TONO-PEN or the PERKIN'S hand-held applanation tonometer is used. Glaucoma resulting from a phacolytic process, a subluxated lens, uveitis, hemolytic process, etc. will alter the technique of surgery. For instance, a trabeculectomy may be planned in addition to cataract extraction in cases of glaucoma.

Gonioscopy

Gonioscopy is done to rule out narrow angles, angle recession (in cases of trauma), peripheral anterior synechiae, or neovascularisation (Fig. 2.8).

Presence of any of the above will alter the technique of surgery.

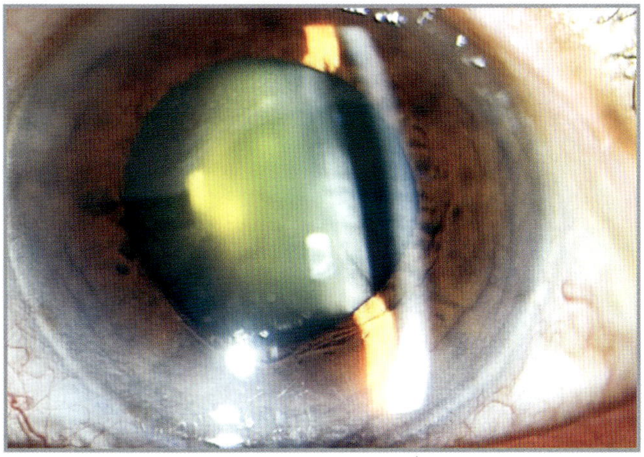

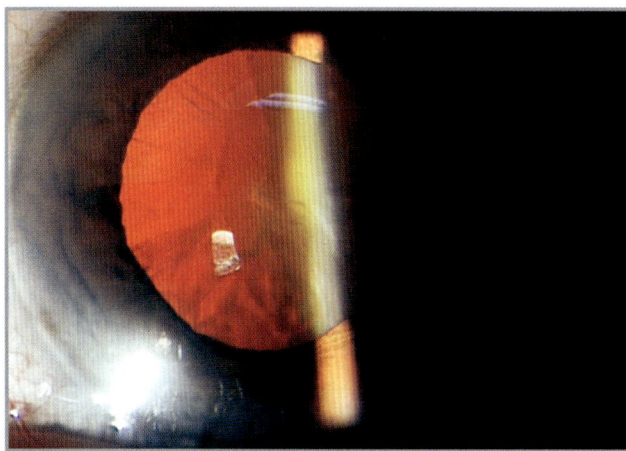

Fig. 2.1: Slit lamp biomicroscopy: Preoperative evaluation grade III cataract

Fig. 2.2: Slit lamp biomicroscopy: Preoperative evaluation of cataract under indirect illumination

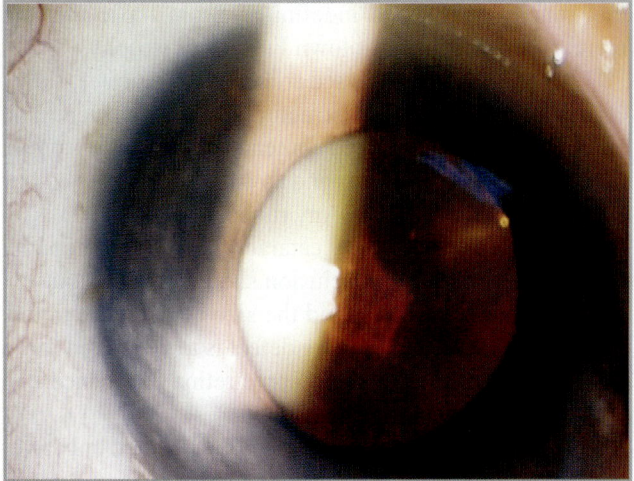

Fig. 2.3: Slit lamp biomicroscopy: Preoperative evaluation of posterior subcapsular cataract under indirect illumination

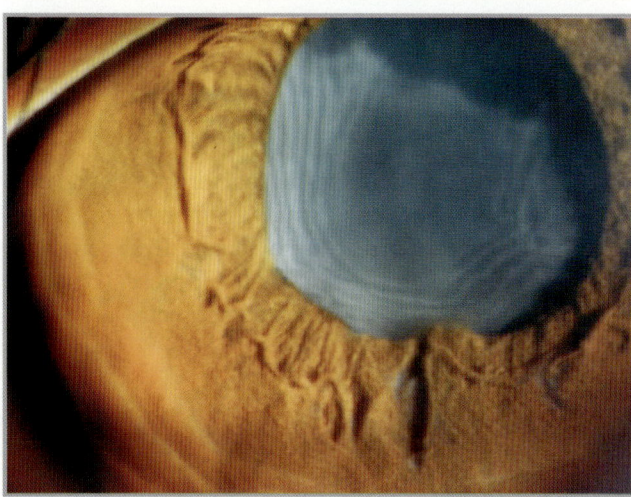

Fig. 2.4: Slit lamp biomicroscopy: Preoperative evaluation of traumatic cataract

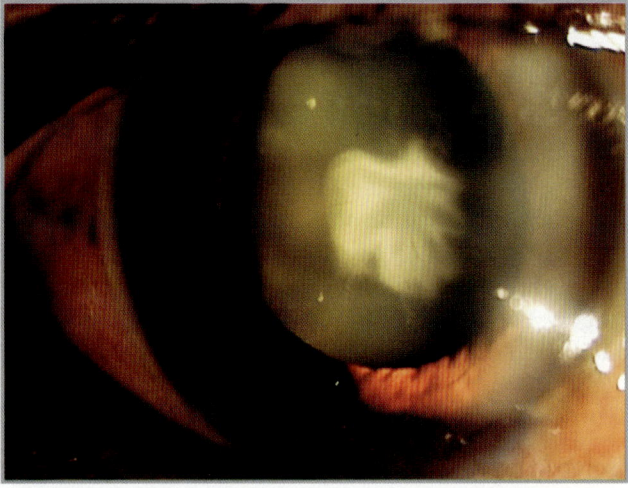

Fig. 2.5: Slit lamp biomicroscopy: Preoperative evaluation of traumatic cataract

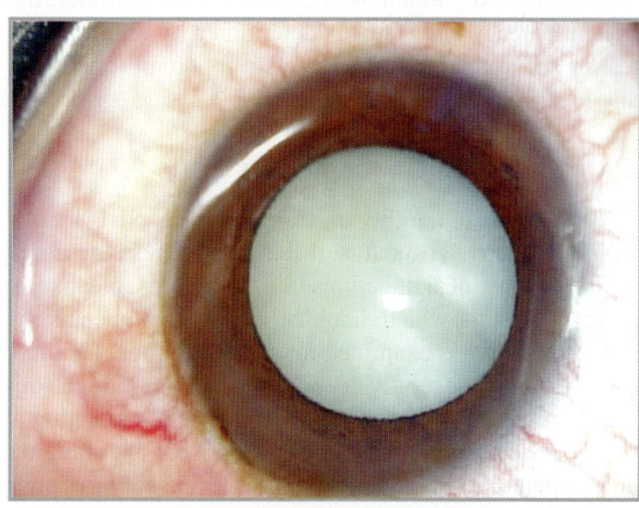

Fig. 2.6: Hypermature cataract

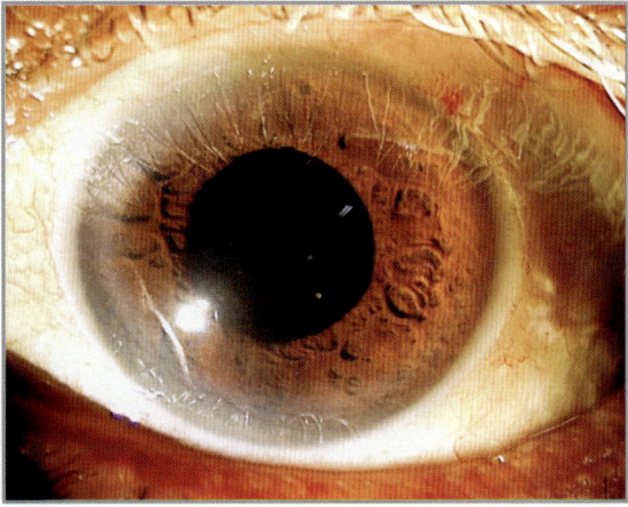

Fig. 2.7: Slit lamp biomicroscopy: Postoperative evaluation

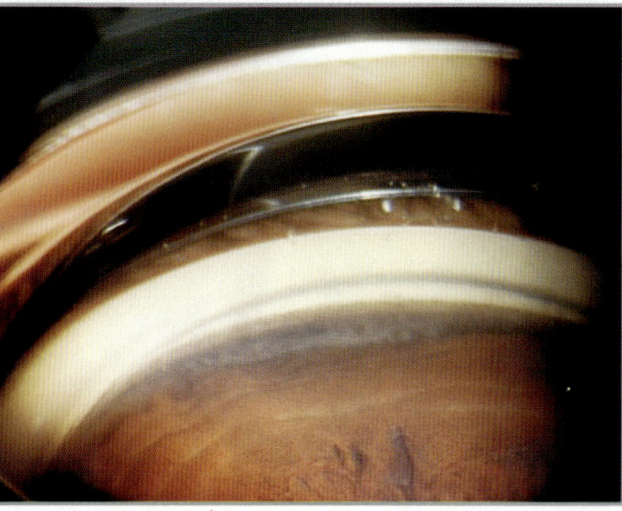

Fig. 2.8: Gonioscopic evaluation posttraumatic angle recession

Fundus Examination

Fundus examination is carried out after the pupillary dilatation. Unless the cataract is almost mature a reasonably adequate fundus examination is possible. Any retinal abnormalities like degeneration of retina/macula (ARMD), inflammations of retina, anatomical anomalies (coloboma) will alter the postoperative visual prognosis. The fundus examination is carried out by both direct and indirect ophthalmoscopy. Indirect ophthalmoscopy gives a better view of the fundus in hazy media as compared to the direct ophthalmoscopy.

Other important ocular examinations include:

Macular Function Tests

The special macular function tests mentioned below are not routinely performed, nevertheless, it is worthwhile noting them down in case of a doubtful macular pathology.

(a) Two light discrimination test

(b) Colour perception test

(c) Blue field entoptoscopy: This test involves observation of leucocytes flowing in macular capillaries, which appear as "flying corpuscles" when seen under bright blue light.

(d) Amsler grid test evaluates the 10 degree of visual field surrounding fixation. A patient with early macular lesion will report distorted lines in the Amsler charts.

(e) Photo stress test: In this test, the patient fixates the light of a pen torch held about 3 cm away for 10 seconds. The photo stress recovery time is measured by the time taken to read any 3 letters of the pretest acuity line. In a patient with macular pathology, the photo stress time will be longer than 50 seconds.

Other important tests are B-scan, glare disability and contrast sensitivity tests.

B-scan

B-scan is done in cases of dense cataracts in which the fundus is not visualised and in which a retinal pathology is suspected.

Glare Disability

Glare disability test is carried by the Muller-Nadler vision tester and the brightness acuity tester. This test may be optional depending upon the requirement of the specific case.

Contrast Sensitivity

Contrast ensitivity function is measured using a Pelli-Robson contrast sensitivity chart, Arden grating, Cambridge low contrast gratings and the Vistech chart. This test may be optional depending upon the requirements of the specific case.

Electrophysiological Tests

Electrophysiological tests such as Electroretinogram (ERG) and Electrooculogram (EOG) are done in special situations. Trauma might lead the clinician to order an ERG because of the possibility of detecting a retinal detachment or siderosis bulbi. EOG is useful in evaluation of hereditary degenerative diseases like retinitis pigmentosa. Visually evoked potential (VEP) provides a way to predict relative visual acuity in eyes with opaque media.

INTRAOCULAR LENS IMPLANT POWER CALCULATION

Today cataract surgery with IOL implantation is a successful procedure. It is minimally invasive, rehabilitation is quick and the complication rate is low. In addition, the refractive outcome is excellent and vision can be improved to a level better than what it was before the formation of cataract. The main factor in a good refractive outcome is precise IOL power calculation. The calculation is normally based on corneal keratometry and ultrasound axial length measurement which is a well-established field of ocular biometry. Recently an instrument was commercially introduced for IOL power calculation. The axial length measurement is based on Partial Coherence interferometry (PCI), the same principle is used to examine the posterior part of the ocular wall in optical coherence tomography.

Accurate IOL power calculation is an important step in modern day cataract surgery. Once the IOL is implanted, the patient must live with any mistake that may have been committed or be subjected to removal and reimplantation of the IOL which in itself has many intra- and postoperative complications. Devices like A-scan have made it convenient to accurately determine the axial length of the eye. In the past, in the absence of ultrasonography IOL power was determined using intelligent guesswork and taking into consideration various factors like preoperative refraction and the age of patient, etc. however, now various formulae have been developed for IOL power calculation based on biometry. Biometry consists of keratometric reading (K), axial length of the eye (AL), perhaps with a measurement of anterior chamber depth. Various computer programmes have been developed for easy calculations. The formulae used in IOL power calculation are broadly divided into 2 groups, viz; theoretical and regression formulae.

A commonly used formula in today's practice is the SRK-II formula which is a regression formula. In addition to the modified SRK-II formula, a number of other formulae have been developed which are:

• Second generation modified theoretical and empirical formulae.

• Combination of theoretical and empirical formulae.

Evaluation of IOL power calculation and its applied aspects will be discussed in detail subsequently as separate chapters.

PREOPERATIVE INVESTIGATIONS

Routine investigations like haemoglobin and blood sugar levels are checked in older patients Additional investigations like ECG, chest X-ray and serum creatinine may be done if the patient has any significant medical history or if the patient is undergoing surgery under general anesthesia.

In cases of congenital cataract, additional special investigations like serological tests for intrauterine TORCH infection, urine analysis for reducing substances like milk feed, urine chromatography for amino acids, calcium levels and chromosomal analysis are to be done to rule out any syndromes associated with congenital cataract.

PREPARATION OF THE PATIENT FOR THE SURGERY

Preparation of the patient preoperatively is as important as the surgery itself. It is the surgeon's approach to the patient which makes a difference. The patient should be made aware of the various risks and complications associated with the surgery. After a thorough assessment of the patient, the visual prognosis should be explained to the patient in case of any posterior segment pathology or amblyopias. A calm and sympathetic attitude to the patient helps the surgeon to gain the patient's confidence. This will also help to reduce the patient's anxiety to a large extent. The surgeon must impart that it is a team effort with the surgeon as the head. Informed consent (IC) is taken routinely before any surgery. IC was developed as an ethical guideline 150 years ago and has evolved over the past 85 years to its current standardised form. It is the first and foremost legal document designed to protect the physician from the patient. The IC form is signed by the patient, spouse or next of kin. In cases of individuals below 16 years of age the IC is signed by the parents or guardian.

Although cataract surgery is accompanied by a low rate of adverse medical events, most patients undergoing surgery are elderly and commonly have medical conditions that put them at an increased risk of intra- and postoperative complications.

Medical malpractice litigation in cataract surgery has increased severalfold in the past 25 years. In response risk of litigation, physicians have made changes in their practices that include increasing time spent with their patients, more detailed record keeping and prescribing of additional tests and treatment procedures. In assessing the effectiveness of cataract surgery, the importance of the patient's perspective has been recognised. Besides, the clinical outcomes like visual acuity, assessments, etc. are directed at subjective measures of vision related functioning and patient's satisfaction and the structure and process of care are also very important.

REFERENCES

1. Norman. S. Jaffe, Mark. S. Jaffe and Gary. F. Jaffe. Cataract Surgery and its complications. 6th Edition. 2–17.
2. Erin. N. Marcus, Steven Gayer and Douglas R. Anderson. EDITORIAL. Medical Evaluation of Patients Before Ocular Surgery. Am J. Ophthalmology. May 2003. 136(2). 338–339.
3. Jack.J.Kanski. Clinical Ophthalmology. A Systematic Approach. Fourth Edition. 157–182.
4. M.G. Wirth, I.M. Russell-Eggitt, J.E. Craig, J.E. Elder and D.A. Mackey. Aetiology of Congenital and Paediatric Cataract in an Australian Population. Br.J. Ophthalmology. 2002. 86. 782–786.
5. A.K.Khurana.Theory and Practice of Optics and Refraction. First Edition. 31–51 and 246–253.
6. Leclaire et al. A new glare test for clinical testing: results comparing normal subjects and variously corrected aphakics. Arch. Ophthal. 1982. 100. 153–158.
7. Ja'nos Ne'meth, Orsolya Fekete and Norbert Pesztenlehrer. Optical and Ultrasound Measurement of Axial Length and Anterior Chamber Depth for Intraocular Lens Power Calculation. J Cataract Refract Surg 2003. 29:85–88.
8. Haigis W, Lege B, Miller N, Schneider B. Comparison of immersion ultrasound biometry and partial coherence interferometry for intraocular lens power calculation according to Haigis. Graefes Arch Clin Exp Ophthalmol 2000; 238:765–773.
9. Drexler W, Findl O, Menapace R, et al. Partial coherence interferometry: a novel approach to biometry in cataract surgery (letter). Am J Ophthalmol 1998; 126:524–534.
10. Fercher AF, Hitzenberger CK, Drexler W, et al. In vivo optical coherence tomography. Am J Ophthalmol 1993; 116: 113–114.
11. Carlos Argento, Mari'a Jose Costino, Daniel Badoza. Intraocular lens power calculation after refractive surgery. J Cataract Refract Surg 2003; 29:1346–1351.
12. Irwin Y. Cua, Mujtaba A. Qazi, Steven F.Lee, Jay S. Pepose. Intraocular lens calculations in patients with corneal scarring and irregular astigmatism. J Cataract Refract Surg 2003; 29:1352–1357.
13. Daniel Scanlan, Farhan Siddiqui, Gail Perry, Cindy M.L. Hutnik. Informed consent for cataract surgery: What patients do and do not understand. J Catarct Refract Surg 2003; 29: 1904–1912.
14. Marvin F Kraushar, Margaret F. Turner, Westfield, NJ. Medical Malpractice Litigation in Cataract Surgery. Arch Ophthalmol 1987; 105:1339–1343.
15. M D Nijkamp, H J M Sixma, H Afman, F Hiddema, S A Koopmans, B van den Borne, F Hendrikse, R M M A Nuijts. Quality of care from the perspective of the cataract patient: the reliability and validity of the QUOTE-Cataract. Br J Ophthalmol 2002; 86: 840–842.
16. Sherman W. Reeves, James M. Tielsch, Joanne Katz, Eric B. Bass, and Oliver D. Schein. A Self-administered Health Questionnaire for the Preoperative Risk Stratification of Patients Undergoing Cataract Surgery. Am J Ophthalmol May 2003; 135(5):599–606.

3

Surgical and Applied Anatomy of Lens

Dr M Shrivastava, Col JKS Parihar SM,VSM and Dr Doma Wanchugh

INTRODUCTION

Key to success of phacoemulsification surgery and an ultimate outcome depends upon an understanding of basic instrumentation, surgical technique and its application in a judicious manner during phaco surgery. Undoubtedly, the next most important factor remains the precise knowledge of the surgical anatomy of the lens and its correlation with various steps of phaco procedures. For anterior segment surgeons, the basic understanding of the cornea, lens and the anterior chamber is a very crucial and significant factor. Better understanding of the lens anatomy facilitates smooth and successful completion of the procedure. This involves all the steps of phaco including rhexis, hydroprocedures, nucleus management and irrigation/aspiration.

APPLIED SURGICAL ANATOMY

The lens is a transparent, biconvex crystalline structure placed between the iris and the vitreous with the help of suspensory ligaments (zonular fibres) in the patellar fossa, which is a saucer-shaped depression. The posterior surface of the lens capsule is attached to the vitreous in a circular area by ligamentum hyloideocapsulare (Wiegart's ligament). Inside this circle, between the hyaloid face and the lens capsule is a small potential space called the retrolental or Berger's space.

The Human Crystalline Lens can be Broadly divided into Four Parts

(i) Lens capsule: Anterior/Equatorial and Posterior having variations in anatomical structures.
(ii) Central hard nucleus,
(iii) Epinucleus plate, which may have a variable thickness
(iv) Lens cortex.

Biomicroscopic Slit Lamp Evaluation of the Lens

The concentric layers from front to back are:
(i) **Capsule:** Anterior/equatorial and posterior having variations in anatomical structures.
(ii) **Superficial cortex:** It can be further subclassified into 3 layers in the beam of a slit lamp:
- Superficial cortical clear zone or subscapular clear zone
- first zone of disjunction
- Second cortical clear zone or the subclear zone of cortex
(iii) **Deep cortex:** It is stratified into 2 perinuclear zones which autofluorescence a brilliant green under an exciting blue light.
- Bright light scattering zone
- Relatively clear zone
(iv) **Nucleus:** It shows the following stratifications:
- Central part represents embryonic nucleus and lacks scattering of light
- Anterior and posterior peripheral light scattering areas.
(v) **Grading of nuclear hardness:** Grading of nuclear hardness is a very important structural evaluation prior to the phacoemulsification cataract surgery. The machine parameters are to be adjusted as per the grading of the lens nucleus. Nucleus can be graded as follows (Figs 3.1 to 3.5):

Grade I – Whitish/green yellow
Grade II – Yellow
Grade III – Amber
Grade IV – Brown
Grade V – Black

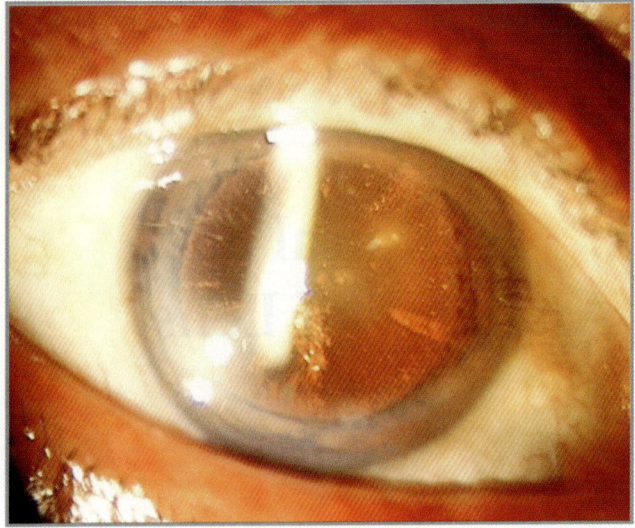

Fig. 3.1: Nucleus grading: Grade I (whitish/green yellow) cataract

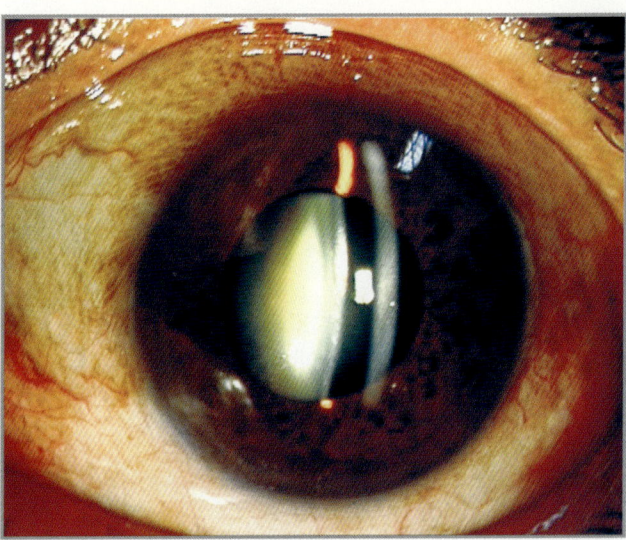

Fig. 3.2: Nucleus grading: Grade II (yellowish-white) cataract

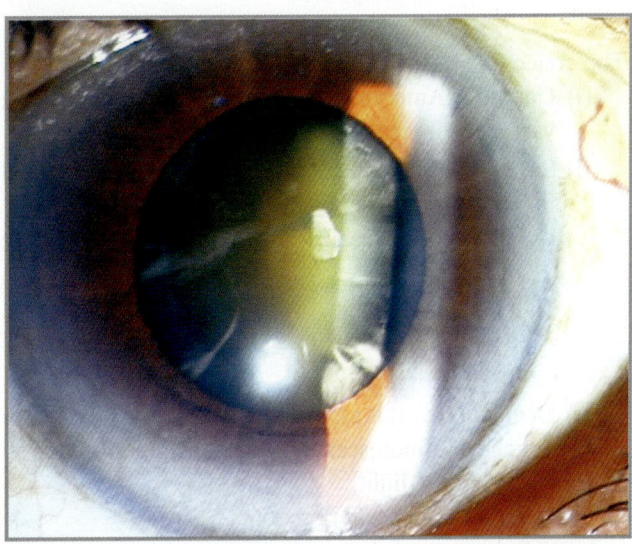

Fig. 3.3: Nucleus grading: Grade III (amber colour) cataract

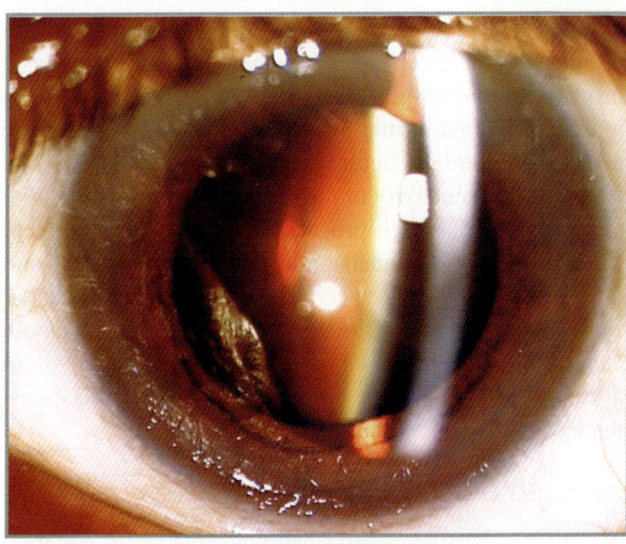

Fig. 3.4: Nucleus grading: Grade IV (brown) cataract

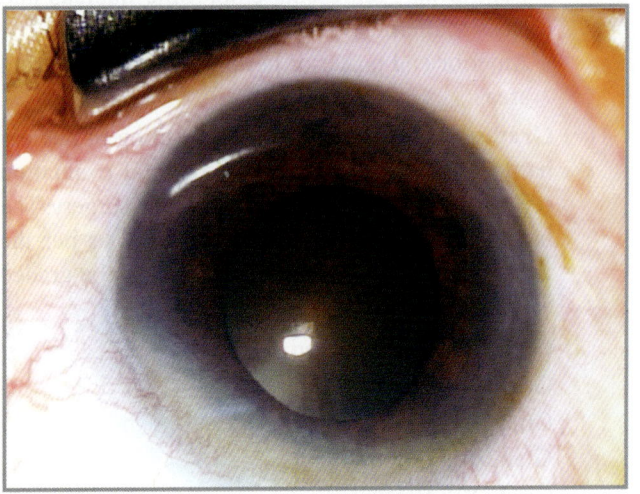

Fig. 3.5: Nucleus grading: Grade V (black) cataract

APPLIED EMBRYOLOGY OF THE LENS

Formation of Optic Vesicle and Optic Stalk

In the 3rd week of gestation, the region of the neural plate which forms the prosencephalon shows a linear thickened area on either side which becomes depressed to form the optic sulcus. As the sulcus deepens, the walls of the procencephalon overlying the sulcus bulge out to form the optic vesicle. The proximal part of the optic vesicle becomes elongated and constricted to form the optic stalk.

Formation of the Lens Placode (27 days of Gestation)

The part of the surface ectoderm overlying the optic vesicle becomes thickened to form the lens placode at about 27 days of gestation.

Formation of the Lens Vesicle

The lens placode is converted into a lens vesicle which consists of a single layer of cells covered by a basal lamina.

Primary Lens Fibres

The apices of the cells of the posterior wall of the lens vesicle grow towards the anterior lens capsule, obliterating the lumen of the lens vesicle. These elongated cells are known as the primary lens fibres and they attach to the apical surface of the anterior lens epithelium and their nuclei disappear. They form the embryonic nucleus.

Secondary Lens Fibres

Derived from the equatorial cells of the anterior epithelium, these fibres follow concentric patterns, thus, giving the lens a laminated appearance.

Secondary lens fibres can be further classified as per the period of development as undermentioned:
  (i) Foetal nucleus: Lens at birth
  (ii) Infantile nucleus: Lens at puberty
  (iii) Adolescent nucleus: Lens nucleus and fibres between puberty and early adulthood
  (iv) Adult nucleus: Status of lens in early adult life
  (v) Cortex: Continuously growing and regenerating. These fibres belong to the youngest lens fibres.

Tunica Vasculosa Lentis

Though the lens remains an avascular structure since it is developed, blood vessels are an essential component of its developmental stage. The lens receives nourishment during embryonic and foetal life through tunica vasculosa lentis which is an essential vascular capsule. Mesenchymal tissue surrounding the primitive lens is responsible to form tunica vasculosa lentis. This receives an abundant blood supply from the hyaloid artery at a very early stage. However, tunica vasculosa lentis regresses later and the vascular capsule disappears before birth. The lens now gets its nutrition by diffusion from the aqueous and the vitreous humour. In very rare circumstances, rudimentary blood vessels may be seen in the lens. However, it does not produce any unwanted or unpleasant situation during phaco surgery.

Lens Capsule

Lens capsule resembles a bag which is membranous and non-cellular which encapsulates the lens. Lens capsule is formed as a result of the accumulation of basal laminae tissue originated from the lens on its external aspect.

Changes in the Configuration and Shape of a Lens during Development

  (i) Embryonic primitive lens: Anteroposteriorly elongated.

  (ii) At the 7th–8th week: Spherical
  (iii) Embryonic (Delayed stage): Ellipsoid.
  (iv) Foetal: Spheroidal. The anteroposterior diameter is nearly at par with that of an adult nucleus. However, equatorial diameter is almost two-thirds of an adult nucleus.

ANATOMY OF LENS

Macroscopic Anatomic Features

  (a) **Colour of the lens**
      At birth (Up to 25–30 years): Transparent and colourless.
      After 30 years: It acquires a definite yellow tinge and becomes amber-coloured.
  (b) **Consistency** of the lens cortex is softer than the nucleus.
  (c) **Weight**
      At 0–9 yrs: 135 mg
      At 40–50 yrs. 255 mg
  (d) **The thickness** (Axial or anteroposterior diameter):
      At birth: 3.5 mm
      Adult: 5 mm
  (e) **Radius**
      The anterior surface: 10 mm.
      The posterior surface: 6 mm.
      The anterior surface is less convex than the posterior one. These two surfaces meet at the equator. The centres of the anterior and posterior surface are called the anterior and the posterior poles respectively. The anterior pole is about 3 mm from the back of the cornea.
  (f) **The equatorial diameter of the lens**
      At birth: 6.5 mm
      Second decade onwards: 9 to 10 mm.
  (g) **The refractive index of the lens**
      1.39 (Nucleus—1.42, Cortex— 1.38)
  (h) **The refractive power** 16–17 dioptres.
  (j) **The accommodative power**
      (i) At birth: 14–16 dioptres
      (ii) At 25 years: 7–8 dioptres
      (iii) At 50 years: 1–2 dioptres

Macroscopic Anatomy

  (a) **The lens capsule:** It is a thin, transparent, hyaline collagenous material which surrounds the lens completely. The capsule is produced continuously throughout life by the basal area of the lens epithelium and is the thickest basement membrane in the body. The thickness of lens capsule varies from 07 micron to 11 micron at different parts, which varies according to age and site. It is thicker anteriorly than posteriorly and at the equator than at the poles, and is thinnest at the posterior pole.

On light microscopy it appears as a homogeneous material and stains with PAS. Ultramicroscopy shows a lamellar appearance with fine filaments.

(b) **Anterior lens epithelium:** It consists of a single layer of cuboidal nucleated epithelial cells which lie deep to the anterior capsule. The epithelium is responsible for all the metabolic, synthetic and transport processes of the lens. These cells become columnar in the equatorial region and elongate to form new lens fibres throughout life. There is no posterior epithelium as these cells fill the cavity of the lens vesicle during development.

Zones of the lens epithelium

- **Central zone:** It consists of cuboidal cells. Their nuclei are round and located slightly apically. They are stable cells and do not normally mitose. However, they do so in response to a wide variety of injurious insults including uveitis. Metaplasia of these cells can lead to anterior subcapsular cataract like shield cataract in atopic dermatitis and glaucomflecken seen after an attack of acute congestive close angle glaucoma.
- **Intermediate zone:** It consists of smaller and more cylindrical cells located peripherally to the central zone. These cells mitose occasionally.
- **Germinative zone:** It consists of columnar cells and are located just preequatorialy. These cells divide actively to form new cells which migrate posteriorly to form lens fibres. These cells are extremely susceptible to irradiation. Dysplasia of these cells can lead to posterior subcapsular cataract as seen in radiation cataract, myotonic dystrophy and neurofibromatosis.

Lens Fibres

(a) **Formation:** Initially, they are formed from the posterior epithelium which runs from posterior to anterior to fill the lens vesicle. Later. the cells of the equatorial region of the anterior lens epithelium form the lens fibres. The superficial fibres are elongated with the nuclei being relatively anteriorly placed. These nuclei form a line which is convex at the equator called the lens or nuclear bow.

(b) **Structure of lens fibres:** On cross section, the lens fibres are almost hexagonal in shape and are bound together by ground substance. The nuclei of these lens fibres disappear later on. There are interlocking processes between cells with zonulae occludens present.

(c) **Structural arrangement of lens fibres:** The initial fibres of the foetal nucleus are arranged in such a way that they terminate in two Y-shaped sutures in the anterior and posterior surfaces of the lens. Later,

growth of the lens fibres becomes more irregular and it forms dendritic patterns.

(d) **Zonal arrangement of lens fibres:** Nucleus contains the oldest fibres and forms the central part of the lens. It has the following zones from inside outwards:
   (i) Embryonic nucleus
   (ii) Foetal nucleus: corresponds to lens from 3 months of gestation till birth.
   (iii) Infantile nucleus: corresponds to lens from birth till puberty.
   (iv) Adolescent nucleus: corresponds to nucleus from puberty till adult life.
   (v) Adult nucleus: corresponds to lens in adult life.
       The size of the embryonic and foetal nucleus always remains same while that of the adult nucleus increases.
   (vi) Cortex: It is the part of the lens which lies just outside the adult nucleus and comprises the youngest lens fibres.

The Lens Zonules

(a) **Development:** They develop from the neuroectoderm in the ciliary region. Initially they are a continuation of the internal limiting membrane over the non pigmented epithelium of the developing ciliary processes. Later they are synthesised by the ciliary epithelial cells. The zonules reach the lens and merge with the anterior and posterior capsules by the 5th month of gestation.

(b) **Function:** They hold the lens in position and allow the ciliary muscle to act upon it.

(c) **Structure:** The zonular fibres are transparent and each fibre has a diameter of 0.35 to 1.0 micron. They are composed of glycoprotein and mucopolysaccharides.

Structurally, they are of 3 types:
   (i) First type fibres—Thick, wavy and lie near the vitreous.
   (ii) Second type fibres—Thin and flat.
   (iii) Third type fibres—Very fine and run a circular course.

(d) **Gross appearance:** The ciliary zonules extend from the ciliary body to the equator of the lens. On cut section, they are arranged in a triangular form, with the base of the triangle towards the equator of the lens and the apex towards the ciliary body. The canal of Hannover is a space between the anterior and the posterior zonular fibres which is devoid of lens fibres.

(e) **Arrangement of the zonular fibres:** The main fibres are:

(i) **Orbiculoposterior capsular fibres:** They are the most posterior and the innermost zonular fibres. They arise from the Ora serrata and are inserted in the posterior capsule of the lens with hyaloideocapsular ligament. They are second type fibres.

(ii) **Orbiculoanterior capsular fibres:** They are the thickest and the strongest zonular fibres and are the first type of fibres. They arise from the pars plana of the ciliary body and are inserted anterior to the equator.

(iii) **Cilioposterior capsular fibres:** They are the most numerous. They arise from the valleys and a few from the sides of the ciliary processes and are inserted into the posterior capsule anterior to the attachment of the orbiculoposterior fibres.

(iv) **Cilio-equatorial fibres:** They arise from the valleys of the ciliary processes and are inserted at the equator. They are the third type of fibres. They are more in young age and decrease with increasing age.

(v) **Auxiliary fibres:** They anchor the individual portions of the zonules and provide strength to the main fibres. They also hold the various portions of the ciliary body together.

(f) **Recent concepts of the zonular fibres:** Main zonular fibres: The suspensory zonular complex has been divided into following zones:

(i) **Pars orbicularis:** The fibres arise from the posterior end of the pars plana and pass forward over the pars plana as a feltwork.

(ii) **Zonular plexus:** On reaching the posterior end of the pars plicata, the zonular fibres form zonular plexuses, which pass through the valleys of the ciliary processes. These plexuses are firmly attached to the bases of the ciliary valleys by fibres known as tension fibres.

(iii) **Zonular fork:** After reaching the anterior margin of the pars plicata, the zonular plexuses consolidate into zonular bundles which proceed towards the lens.
The point of angulation of the zonules at the midzone of the ciliary valleys is called zonular fork.

(iv) **Zonular limbs:** At the zonular fork, the zonular fibres are divided into 3 limbs—the anterior, equatorial and posterior ones—running to the anterior, equatorial and the posterior lens capsule respectively.

• *Anterior zonular limb:* Analogous to the orbiculoanterior capsular fibres. They are inserted at 1.5 mm from the equator as an irregular double row of bundles. These fibres decrease with age and are inserted more centrally.

• *Equatorial zonular fibres:* Analogous to cilioequatorial fibres. They are inserted into the capsule of the equatorial region.

• *Posterior zonular limb:* Analogous to orbiculoposterior capsular fibres and the cilioposterior capsular fibres. They are inserted into the posterior capsule from the posterior edge of the equator to about 1.25 mm.

(v) **Hyaloid zonule:** This is a single layer of zonules connecting the anterior hyaloid at the border of the patellar fossa with the pars plana and the pars plicata. The space between the hyaloid zonule and the posterior zonule is the canal of Petit.

(vi) **Hyalocapsular zonule:** It is a circular band of zonular fibres present at the site of attachment of the anterior hyaloid membrane to the posterior lens capsule at the rim of the patellar fossa. It probably corresponds to the ligament of Wiegrt.

(vii) **Circumferential zonular spindles:**
• *Anterior ciliary girdle:* These fibres bind the ciliary processes with the anterior hyaloid membrane of the vitreous.
• *Posterior ciliary girdle:* It is present on the middle of the pars plana. It binds the pars plana with the anterior hyaloid membrane.

CONGENITAL/DEVELOPMENTAL ANOMALIES OF THE LENS

Lens may have several anomalies in the structure, configuration as well as its position in the eye. Such derangements may influence phaco surgery performance adversely. Most of the time, lens may be associated with multiple and other congenital anomalies including nystagmus, microphthalmos or other colobomas including uveal and optic nerve involvements. The application of phaco energy, machine settings and surgical technique needs very minute, meticulous and cautious attention at each and every step of the procedure. The risk of intraoperative complications and postoperative behaviour may also have several constraints. Additional surgical procedures like use of CTR rings may be an essential requirement. Hence, it is worth considering the correlating adverse impact of abnormal lens development with performance of phacosurgery. Each and every problem will be dealt with in detail in subsequent chapters.

Developmental Cataract

These may be present at birth or develop later. It has a tendency to affect the particular zone which was being formed when this process was interrupted. Following are the clinical types:

(i) **Punctate cataract**
   - Cataracta caerulea or blue dot cataract
   - Sutural cataract/anterior axial embryonic cataract
   - Cataracta centralis pulverulenta

(ii) **Zonular cataract or lamellar cataract:** It accounts for 50% of all clinically significant congenital cataracts. A zone around the embryonic nucleus becomes opaque as development is interfered with at a later stage. Linear opacities like spokes of a wheel may run outwards towards the equator and are called riders. These cataracts are usually bilateral. They may be of genetic or environmental origin. The lack of vitamin D is an important factor.

(iii) **Fusiform cataract:** It is an anteroposterior spindle-shaped opacity. It is genetically determined.

(iv) **Nuclear cataract:**
   - *Embryonal nuclear cataract:* The central nucleus is opaque as development is interfered with at a very early stage.
   - *Progressive congenital cataract:* Due to German measles in the mother in the 2nd or 3rd months of gestation. The whole lens becomes opaque and is associated with other congenital anomalies like congenital heart disease, microphthalmos, microencephaly, mental retardation, deafness and dental anomalies.

(v) **Coronary cataract:** It is a developmental cataract occurring at puberty. It appears as club-shaped opacities near the periphery of the lens and hence vision is not affected.

(vi) **Anterior capsular (polar) cataract:** This may be developmental or acquired.

(vii) **Posterior capsular (polar) cataract:** It is due to the persistence of the posterior part of the vascular sheath of the lens.

Abnormal Shape or Size

(i) **Coloboma of lens:** There is a notch-shaped defect usually in the inferior margin. It is due to defective development of part of the suspensory ligament.

(ii) **Cataract associated with anterior persistent hyperplastic primary vitreous:** The eye is usually microphthalmic and a total cataract is associated with a developmental anomaly due to persistence of the primary vitreous and the hyaloid arterial system.

(iii) **Spherophakia, microphakia and microspherophakia:** They are variants in the shape of the lens.

(iv) **Lenticonus:** The surface of the lens is more conical than spherical. It is more commonly posterior than anterior and is seen in Alport's syndrome.

(v) **Ectopia lentis:** It is a congenital dislocation or subluxation of the lens, usually upwards and bilateral. Partial lens displacement is called subluxation and complete displacement is called dislocation. It is sometimes associated with Marfan's syndrome or homocystinuria. The basic defect is a breakage or weakening of the zonules.

Apart from poor vision, patients complain of uniocular diplopia and glare. There may be myopia, astigmatism and reduced amplitude of accommodation. Signs include an obvious lens displacement though this may only be seen through a dilated pupil. There may be iridodonesis and phacodonesis along with a deep anterior chamber. Vitreous may henmate into the anterior chamber and glaucoma due to pupillary blockage, is common.

Phaco Inception and Instrumentation

4

Road to Phacoemulsification Surgery: How to Carve a Smooth Learning Curve

Col JKS Parihar SM, VSM **and Lt Col Anirudh Singh**

For most of the modern day ophthalmic surgeons, there lies no elaboration of the basic point that phacoemulsification cataract surgery is the bread and butter and those who do not convert from conventional to phacoemulsification cataract surgery, may be left behind. The pearls of conversion lie in patience, perseverance and an eye for detail. Many books had been written in the last 6–7 years about how to convert to phacoemulsification but even these have undergone radical changes in the light of modern equipment and techniques.

It is said that the words of wisdom lie side by side with the words of caution. Thus, although phacoemulsification surgery gives better and accurate results than a conventional surgery yet the surgeon who foregoes the intricacies of the surgery can land up in greater trouble vis. a vis a conventional cataract surgery.

We have compiled the factors to be considered in conversion from conventional to phacoemulsification cataract surgery based on our experiences as well as the experiences of our teachers and colleagues.

   I. Be thorough with the theory of phacoemulsification procedures, phacoemulsification machine and its dynamics as well as associated complications and their management.

  II. Beginning with phaco be ideal: Be an ideal learner, not an idol surgeon.

    (a) Ideal patient

    (b) Ideal cataract

    (c) Ideal phacomachine

    (d) Ideal operating microscope

    (e) Ideal OT environment with proper OT table and operating stool

    (f) Ideal surgeon with ideal assistance

    (g) Ideal anaesthesia

    (h) Learn from an ideal teacher (not the least).

  III. Surgery: Gradual transition and knowing when to stop, convert and proceed.

  IV. Keep two devils around (a competent anaesthesiologist and a surgeon to handle severe complication maybe a VR surgeon or any experienced and proficient surgeon to handle such eventualities) he may not be in the OT at that time but should be accessible at the time of eventualities at a short notice.

THEORY OF PHACOEMULSIFICATION PROCEDURES

Like in any surgical procedure, a precise knowledge of various steps is essential and the consequences of ignoring such minute details can be disastrous. It is imperative that the surgeon is aware of every step and can use his presence of mind to judge the consequences thereof. We think it will be of solace to many that the learning curve of phacoemulsification is pretty long, so don't despair and be perseverant.

Observe the surgery keenly with an eye on minute details by watching the videos of the experienced surgeons as well as surgeons who are in transition. We will not elaborate this aspect any further as it will be dealt with in greater detail in the following chapters.

BEGINNING TO PHACO

Ideal Patient

Initially if an ideal patient is selected the learning surgeon can concentrate better on his surgery leading to better results thus maintaining confidence. It will also clear him from any anxiety or guilt in the event of any eventuality during the surgery. Moreover, with the threat of CPA (Consumer Protection Act) looming large, selecting an ideal patient will ensure that the surgeon is protected in the learning phase. We have compiled a list of factors to be considered in selecting an ideal patient. They are:

(i) Age 50–60 yrs (more the age, harder the nucleus)
(ii) Not over anxious or oversensitive. You know it when you give your peribulbar or when IV line is started and the patient literally jumps from the OT table.
(iii) No systemic/ocular illness.
(iv) No deep set eyes (to give optimal accessibility to the intraocular structures and provide a sufficiently large area for manipulation)
(v) Not one-eyed
(vi) Should not have a strong orbicularis action which may create problem during prolonged surgery by a beginner or while managing unpleasant complications.
(vii) Begin with right eye to face right direction and dimension.
(viii) Not a bread earner in the family.
(ix) Not too educated (we have known of patients questioning the surgeon about the steps of surgery), so be sure that you select a patient with low education background. Mind you, our patients are under L.A. so they are aware if you ask for surgical advice from your seniors or speaking aloud about the difficulty or complications encountered.

Ideal Cataract

Selecting an ideal cataract will help the budding surgeon in mastering the steps without getting stuck in the first few cases. The golden rule is 'not too hard and not too soft'. So, let's see what are the points for an ideal cataract:

(i) Good pupillary dilatation (>6.5 mm required)
(ii) Corneal clarity
(iii) Red glow should be present even though faint (helps in capsulorrhexis and also to evaluate the extension of the hard portion of the nucleus, the size of which is proportional to the hardness of the cataract)
(iv) Grade of nucleus (should be Grade II or III).
Grade II or III is a moderately hard senile cataract with a nucleus that permits simple manipulations, without requiring more time or energy of ultrasound. This type of cataract is often characterised by an epinucleus and by cortex thick enough to absorb the effects of the maneuvers on the nucleus and avoid excessive stimulation of the surrounding structures.
Grade I will be a pain initially as nuclear cracking is difficult and Grade IV–V will require more power and more time for cracking thus may lead to a sequel of complications and even disaster.

(v) Do not consider eyes with uveitis, glaucoma or with a history of trauma.

Ideal Phacomachine (Peristaltic versus Ventury)

This is one point which has undergone a radical change due to the advent of better and more sophisticated machines. The earlier surgeons used to stress on only the peristaltic machines for phaco but now this holds no ground as the surgeon is supposed to be proficient in both peristaltic and ventury machines. The present day ventury machines have far advanced and better safety controls. Many of the surgeons have started on ventury and have become masters in this field. But there are still many who will opt for peristaltic for initial few cases before switching on to the ventury system. It is ultimately the surgeon's confidence and availability of the machine which decides this factor.

Peristaltic machines although more forgiving to the learning surgeon is less effective for aspirating the cracked nuclear fragments and so in effect takes longer time. Ventury with its preset vacuum is very effective for aspirating the cracked nuclear pieces but at the same time the learning surgeon has to be careful to keep the probe at mid iris level and avoid tearing the posterior capsule.

For peristaltic machine, power should be around 30% for grade II nuclear sclerosis and vacuum set at around 45–60 mmHg in the sculpting phase. In the aspirating stage, power can be 20–30%, vacuum has to be around 100–150 mmHg. Finally in irrigation and aspiration stage vacuum has to be 400–450 mmHg. The flow rate varies from 15 to 30 ml/mt at different stages.

For ventury machines, power should be 20–30% for grade II nuclear sclerosis and vacuum set at around 20–30 mmHg in the sculpting phase. In the aspirating stage power can be the same or less but vacuum has to be around 120–130 mmHg. Finally in irrigation and aspiration stages, vacuum has to be 300–350 cc/min.

Basic, Intermediate or High End Machine?

Another major point of contention is what type of peristaltic or ventury machine is available, and also a major consideration is the surgeon's capability and confidence. However, every surgeon should be proficient in basic and intermediate machines before moving on to high end machines.

Ideal Microscope

The significance of having a good microscope cannot be downplayed, especially in phaco, where the quality of optics and illumination along with depth perception and zoom capacity of microscope are of primal importance in appreciating the fine nuances of phacoemulsification cataract surgery at every surgical step. Learning to work under a magnification of 8–10 × and then moving to 12–16 × for capsulorrhexis and then, again moving back to around 12 × for phacoemulsification surgery is the ideal situation. The common mistake is working under a constant high magnification even during sculpting and aspiration, as the surgeon is bound to loose depth perception leading to its sequel of complications. The focus of the microscope has to be constantly changed while operating. The focus has to be over the conjunctival vessels while giving the initial incision, then shifted to the anterior capsule while doing capsulorrhexis, then over the pupillary plane while sculpting and then again over the base of the trench created while cracking, moving back to iris plane while aspirating the fragments and then moving the focus to posterior capsule while irrigation-aspiration is on.

An observer microscope has additional benefits where the teacher can guide you through the steps and at the same time reconfirm the correctness of your steps.

Another associated point is whether you can manage common complications using your own microscope or you need to shift to a higher end ophthalmic microscope. Therein lies the significance of working under an ideal microscope with optimum qualities as elaborated above.

Ideal Operation Theatre Environment with Proper OT Table and Operating Stool

An ideal OT environment is required for an uninterrupted and yet, efficient handling of an anxious patient and an even more anxious learning surgeon. A quiet and peaceful atmosphere in the OT can work wonders on the frayed nerves of both the surgeon and the patient.

The patient has to be comfortable and the surgeon should have a proper OT table with adjustable height so that the patient can be better placed under the microscope. The phaco warrior has to have his comfortable throne, i.e. operating stool as sciatica is known to be very common due to prolonged compression by the edge of a hard stool. An ideal OT stool should have an adjustable height so that the surgeon can be more comfortable and adjust his feet position on the controls for the microscope as well as on the foot pedal of the phacomachine.

Ideal Surgeon with Ideal Assistance

The surgeon will undoubtedly have anxiety before starting to phaco but he has to be convinced about the benefits to the patient and embark on this crusade with full enthusiasm. As in any crusade the armamentarium has to be of superior quality and the warrior has to have a definite plan with alternative plans for any eventualities, similarly the phaco warrior has to know his machine and has definite ideas of the steps he will undertake and proceed. It is also of immense importance that the surgeon knows what to do in the event of any complication.

The phaco warrior (sounds better, does not it?) has to learn to be ambidextrous and practise using his left hand more often in day-to-day activities like shaving with the left hand, opening the door with the left hand or opening the lock with key in the left hand. Gradually, the surgeon will learn to simultaneously use both his hands which is an absolute necessity in the present day bimanual phaco surgery.

The surgeon has to be proficient in extracapsular cataract surgery and should learn the basic steps like capsulorrhexis, hydrodissection, hydrodelineation, rotation of the nucleus and irrigation aspiration with the I/A probe.

An ideal assistance during the surgery is a must and a learning Phaco surgeon with a learning assistant can be a deadly combination. An ideal assistant is one who has already assisted experienced Phaco surgeons and can judge by the surgeon's gestures about the requirement of instruments at each stage of the surgery. Well-trained and meticulous OT staff will be able to better assist and efficiently tackle any unforeseen complication or sequel of surgery.

Ideal Anaesthesia

Though we give peribulbar in all our initial cases and now switch over to topical anaesthesia for last four years, yet the importance of a good and adequate peribulbar cannot be ignored at least by the learning Phaco surgeon. 5–6 ml of anaesthetic mixture (bupivacaine 0.5% + lignocaine 2% in equal amounts mixed with hylase) is usually enough. Wait for 5–10 minutes for adequate plane of anaesthesia and start your case. You will not like an uncooperative patient when you are learning the finer steps of surgery or are concentrating on capsulorrhexis where a slight movement of the patient can spell trouble. Only when you have done a sizeable number of cases (at least 100–150 cases) should you attempt a topical anaesthesia.

Ideal Teacher

An ideal teacher during the learning phase can be a boon to the surgeon when guidance is required at each and every step of phacoemulsification surgery. It works wonders on the learning surgeon's confidence when he knows that he will be bailed out of any tricky situation whatsoever during the surgery. Proper guidance as well as correcting one's mistakes at the initial inception stage is crucial to the development of a good phaco surgeon.

PHACOEMULSIFICATION SURGERY: GRADUAL TRANSITION AND KNOWING WHEN TO STOP / CONVERT AND PROCEED

With the above factors of ideal patient, ideal cataract, ideal machine and the ideal surgeon in mind, the learning surgeon should start his surgery. The transition should be gradual and the surgeon has to have immense patience. Do not despair if you have to convert back to extracapsular cataract surgery or small incision cataract surgery midway, it happens to all of us initially. Remember learning is okay but the ultimate benefit to the patient should always be kept in mind. Be absolutely thorough in all the steps as even minimum error during anyone of the various phases of the operation can change the results of the successive manoeuvres and increase the difficulties to such a degree that the final outcome of surgery may be compromised. Even the smallest details, which are apparently insignificant, play an important role in the success of the planned operation and, therefore, every step requires maximum care and attention. Few pearls to be remembered during the planning for surgery are:

(a) Scleral entry is better initially as converting to small incision cataract extraction in the event of any complication is easier.

(b) Do not proceed further with your phaco if your capsulorrhexis has been incomplete or has gone out. For beginners, this is the first black hole where the edge of capsulorrhexis will invariably go to the equator during the nucleus manipulation and can lead to posterior capsular rent or more seriously nucleus drop. It is better to go back to the conventional technique in such a case. Once you are proficient in phaco you will be able to manage even with an incomplete capsulorrhexis.

(c) Do a good hydro-dissection and hydro-delineation and ensure nuclear rotation. You can use the side port to inject fluid under the 12 o'clock capsule. If hydrodissection is incomplete and rotation is difficult, it will create more stress on the zonular fibres leading to capsular dehiscence.

(d) Nuclear sculpting should be done adequately to make a tunnel of about 1½ phaco probe width and 2½ phaco probe deep. Only then, the nucleus will crack for easy aspiration. Remember dawn like appearance (faint red glow visible through mid of trench) at the floor of trench is indeed a goodluck sign for both the surgeon and the patient.

(e) Phaco the nucleus pieces in the mid iris plane and do not go after the pieces deeper than this plane. Also avoid doing phaco in the anterior chamber as it is quite traumatic to the corneal endothelium. Mid zone of anterior chamber is most safe for phaco surgery as it has the maximum depth in the centre due to maximum concavity of corneal dome (2.5 to 3 mm). Lens has maximum thickness in the centre (4–4.5 mm) as well as the posterior capsule has maximum concavity at this point, hence you can achieve a very good safety zone if phaco is being restricted up to the central zone at iris plane or just below it.

THE TWO DEVILS: ANAESTHESIOLOGIST AND AN EXPERIENCED SURGEON

Both of them are indispensable while learning this art and they can bail you out in case unforeseen and severe complications should arise. Our patients are elderly and can have any serious cardiac mishap in case of prolonged surgery or otherwise. The anaesthesiologist proves helpful in such circumstances and besides his presence is a legal requirement. The role of a good and experienced surgeon to guide you or to fish you out of troubled waters is well understood by the learning surgeon by now.

CONCLUSION

Learn and perfect one step at a time till you are fully confident before moving on to your first case of phaco. To summarise, the sequence of steps to begin with are in the order of ease of learning curve and to ease out from probabilities of complications.

(a) Construction of side port entry.
(b) Insertion of IOL through tunnel.
(c) Scleral tunnel
(d) Secondary nucleus rotation (after making initial trench)
(e) Trypan Blue enhanced capsulorrhexis
(f) Capsulorrhexis
(g) Hydrodissection and hydrodelineation.
(h) Construction of initial trenching in lower half.
(i) Rotation of nucleus and make superficial trenches in subsequent quadrants.
(j) Emulsification and aspiration of second and third fragment.
(k) Corneal tunnel.
(l) Primary rotation of nucleus (prior to sculpting)
(m) Co-axial cortical irrigation/aspiration
(n) Chopping
(o) Bimanual cortical irrigation/aspiration
(p) Posterior capsulorrhexis
(q) IOL insertion in the bag following rent
(r) Concurrent procedures like phacotrab
(s) Phaco in hard cataract /difficult situations

Remember go step by step and you can do it.

And once again last, but not the least, is the realisation that the learning curve for phacoemulsification surgery is steep and there is no shortcut to the same. The path to learning phacoemulsification has its own ups and downs but challenges should make you more determined in your quest. Be perseverant, patient and keep on learning from each situation and each case and you can really become a phaco warrior.

5

Basics of Various Phacoemulsifier Machines

Col JKS Parihar SM, VSM and Brig. AP Kamath

INTRODUCTION

Phacoemulsification was a big leap towards complete transformation of the manner in which cataract surgery was performed. It opened possibilities towards unbelievable achievement of 'no suture cataract surgery' resulting in near emmetropia. At the time when the concept of removing cataractous lens through a tiny incision with the help of ultrasonic power was put forward by Dr Charles Kelman, intracapsular cataract surgery (ICCE) was a well established procedure, requiring 180 degrees limbal incision and resultant postoperative astigmatism and aphakia. In addition, the patient required long hospital stay and had to be bedridden for several days. Phacoemulsification started a new era of truly revolutionised day-care cataract surgery. The Basic concept of using ultrasound energy nearly remaining unchanged over the last four decades shows how advanced the concept was. The last few years have shown tremendous advancement in the phacodynamics and machine technology as well as in surgical techniques, quality and designs of IOL implants.

This chapter will discuss in length the various terms and concepts used in phacoemulsification, the mechanism of the phaco machine and how it works. It is essential to have the basic concepts clear in one's mind to get the maximum out of the machine. It is well said that once you consume liquor, you enjoy for a few moments, however, later, the drink overpowers you. In the same manner, you should govern the machine instead of the machine governing you. Hence, it is essential to understand the basics of the phaco machine, troubleshooter tips and advantages of specific types of machine being preferred by you.

Phacoemulsification consists of two elements:

  (i) Ultrasound energy to emulsify the nucleus

  (ii) Fluidic circuit for removal of emulsified lens matter through a small incision while maintaining the anterior chamber.

This fluidic circuit is supplied by an elevated irrigating bottle, which helps in maintaining the anterior chamber. Irrigating lines bring fluid from the bottle into the anterior chamber passing through infusion lines into the sleeve of phaco tip, cooling it in the process. Fluid leaves the anterior chamber via aspiration line. The circuit is regulated by a pump, which not only removes fluid from the anterior chamber but also the emulsified lens materials by driving nuclear fragments towards the phaco tip. Maintaining constant intraocular pressure and stable anterior chamber depth require equilibrium between the fluid infused into the eye and the amount of fluid aspirated. In order to exploit the potential of a phaco machine, a surgeon must understand the logic behind types of pump systems and settings of various parameters of a phaco machine.

PHACO: OVERVIEW OF FLUIDICS

It is important to understand the anterior chamber dynamics and the correct meaning of various terms used in the phaco-emulsification before starting the actual surgical procedure.

Various terms used are:
- Inflow
- Aspiration flow rate
- Incisional outflow
- Vacuum
- Rise time
- Post occlusion surge
- Venting
- Reflux

Inflow

Fluid entering the anterior chamber from irrigating bottle is termed inflow. Inflow rate is determined by the bottle height, bore of the tubing, bore of the irrigation line of phaco handpiece and resistance encountered at the phaco sleeve. It is measured in cc/min. Higher the bottle height, higher will be the inflow rate. Similarly, large bore tubing and decreased resistance will increase the inflow. Inflow determines the pressure head in the anterior chamber. Inflow greater than or equal to outflow maintains stable anterior chamber and intraocular pressure during phacoemulsification.

Aspiration Flow Rate

Aspiration flow rate that is frequently termed as flow rate means rate at which fluid flows out of the eye. It is the quantity of fluid aspirated during given time. It is measured in cc per min (cc/min). Fluid entering anterior chamber is aspirated by a pump mechanism. Aspiration flow causing the fluid to leave the eye tends to decrease the pressure in the anterior chamber. To maintain stable intraocular pressure during the surgery, the inflow rate should at least equal to or if possible exceed the aspiration flow rate. Maintaining the bottle height proportionate to the aspiration flow rate is necessary, as higher aspiration rate demands higher bottle height otherwise the anterior chamber will collapse.

Aspiration flow rate is the only measurable component of the outflow. Fluid leaking from the main or side port incision cannot be measured. Aspiration flow rate coupled with the pump mechanism is constantly monitored by the machine in real time giving the surgeon factual data at any given moment.

Incisional Outflow

Fluid also moves out of the eye either through main phaco incision or from the side port incisions at variable rates. It is the non-measurable part of the outflow. The main incision is calibrated for the size of the phaco tip (3.2 mm, 2.8 mm or smaller). Incision is constructed to be watertight as the lips of the wound envelope the tip of phaco probe, fluid leaks from around the tip. A smaller incision can compress the sleeve around the phaco tip causing obstruction to the inflow as well as increasing the chances of the wound burn. The incisional outflow can significantly be reduced by using special design sleeves such as micro seal by Bausch and Lomb.

Vacuum

Vacuum is the negative pressure that provides the holding force. Vacuum is generated by the aspiration pump as the pump acts to draw the fluid out of the aspiration line tubing. In peristaltic type of pumps, occlusion of the phaco tip by nuclear fragments or other materials leads to the creation of a negative pressure in the aspiration line as continuing pump action draws more fluid out, while in venturi pumps, vacuum is generated in the rigid chamber (cassette) then propagated down the aspiration line as far as to the phaco tip. Higher vacuum gives better holding power. Maximum vacuum can be preset by the surgeon on the panel and the machine after achieving this preset value interrupts the pump action.

Rise Time

Rise time means how fast the vacuum builds up to its maximum preset value. It is inversely proportional to the aspiration flow rate. If the flow rate is increased then the rise time is reduced and preset vacuum levels are reached faster. Rise time also denotes the reaction time available to the surgeon in case the inadvertent materials are aspirated in the phaco tip. Rapid increase of rise time associated with high flow rate gives proportionately less reaction time to the surgeon. Peristaltic pumps have better regulation of the rise time compared to other pumps.

Rise time is also linked to the compliance of the tubing of the machine. Tubing in the aspiration line has to be compressible when they pass over the roller beads of the peristaltic pumps. This compressible nature of the tubing decreases the rate of vacuum rise and thus increases the rise time. Vacuum pumps can utilise the comparatively rigid tubing and hence have shorter rise time. Thus, peristaltic pumps give greater reaction time to the surgeon.

Post occlusion Surge

In the occluded state, with any pump design, vacuum is generated in the tubing. In an unmodulated system, when occlusion breaks, fluid rushes into the tubing to equilibrate the pressure difference between the anterior chamber and the lumen of the tube, which is called post occlusion surge. During the period of occlusion, the walls of tubing tend to collapse in proportion to the increase in vacuum which is transmitted down the aspiration line. With release of occlusion, the tubing re-expands and often rebounds, which results in a large post occlusion surge with resultant collapse of the anterior chamber. Compliance of the tubing plays an important part with less compliant tubing having less of the surge. An experienced surgeon while aspirating nuclear fragments reduces vacuum just before occlusion breaks.

Modern phaco machines adopt various measures to reduce the surge. Some machines have a power sensing transducer in the vacuum line. At the first sign of power fluctuation, the fluid from a bottle higher than the irrigating bottle is allowed into the vacuum line. Other machines adopt similar sensing devices that stop the pump for brief seconds, when occlusion break is detected.

Venting

It is the mechanism in which air or fluid is injected in to the aspiration line to eliminate the vacuum in the tubing. It is activated to return the pressure to the atmospheric level when pedal is moved from position 2 to position 1. Thus, venting brings back the system to atmospheric pressure.

Venting is also initiated when vacuum level exceeds the preset levels.

Reflux

It is the mechanism which helps the surgeon to release the inadvertently caught material at the tip. Reflux mode activated through the pedal causes positive pressure in the aspiration line and reversal of the flow thus releasing the materials. Reflux action is a component of peristaltic system.

ESSENTIAL COMPONENTS OF PHACOEMULSIFIER

A surgeon should be familiar with the various components of the machine he is handling to extract maximum from it. He should be aware of the type of the machine he is using as well as its attachments to utilise them to the fullest.

1. The main console consists of the following components:
   (a) Fluidic pump systems
   (b) Irrigation system
   (c) Panel display board to control and monitor functions of the machine
   (d) Additional attachment system: For bipolar cautery, vitrectomy
2. Phaco handpieces and tips
3. Compressor for ventury system

Fluidic Pump System

Traditionally, two basic types of pumps are used in phaco machines, i.e. peristaltic or constant flow pump and vacuum or constant pressure pump.

(i) **Peristaltic system** (Fig. 5.1): In this pump, roller beads that rotate against compressible tubing generate the flow. This milks the fluid along the lumen and the creates a pressure gradient between pump and anterior chamber. These are also known as positive displacement pumps. An advantage of these pumps is that flow rate and vacuum can be regulated independently of each other. Flow rate is directly proportional to the rotational speed of pump and is independent of the pressure in line

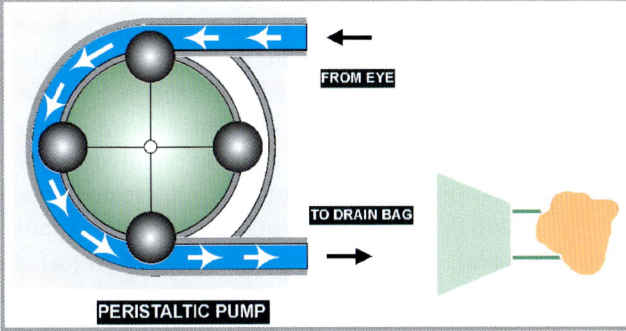

Fig. 5.1: Fluidic pump system: Peristaltic system

via elevated irrigating bottle. The rotational speed of the pump head is determined by the flow rate. Hence, when the tip is occluded, the surgeon can control the speed of vacuum build up via pump speed control. The rate of vacuum build up is inversely proportional to the rotation speed of the pump head. If the flow rate is halved, the rise time is doubled. A longer rise time gives a surgeon more time to react in cases of inadvertent incarceration of iris/lens capsule. To prevent the vacuum build up rising above preset value, various measures are used. In some machines, the pump stops once preset vacuum is reached. In some machines it is overcome by venting air/ fluid into the aspiration line. Hence, in peristaltic pump one can directly control flow rate and indirectly the vacuum.

(ii) **Vacuum pumps:** This group includes venturi pump, diaphragm pump and rotary vane system. In these, vacuum is generated in a rigid chamber (cassette) in the machine using a pump, e.g. venturi, the diaphragm pump or rotary vane pump. The pressure generated travels down along the aspiration tubing as far as the phaco tip. The pressure difference between the tip and the chamber generates flow when tip is unoccluded. When tip is occluded the flow ceases and the vacuum is transmitted down the aspiration line to the tip. Because rollers are not used to collapse the tubing as with peristaltic pump, vacuum pumps can apply more rigid tubing with less compliance. Thus, lower compliance coupled with short time required for the vacuum transfer from cassette to tip results in low rise time. Linear control of vacuum in vacuum pumps indirectly controls the flow rate. In vacuum pumps, flow rate is affected by the height of the irrigating bottle as higher pressure head from higher bottle pushes fluid through the open circuit more rapidly.

In venturi pump, compressed gas is blown across the opening of variable diameter connected to the cassette. By changing the volume of the gas pressure gradient is created which is transmitted via the cassette down the aspiration line. Diaphragm pumps utilise a membrane moved by a motor to create the pressure difference. Eccentrically rotating lamellae fitted in the rotary vane system create the outward force and generate vacuum to draw the fluid out of the aspiration line.

Low rise time in vacuum pumps is a potential liability as it gives less time to the surgeon to react if unwanted material is inadvertently incarcerated in the aspiration port causing potentially permanent damage. Most vacuum pumps do not allow attenuation of rise time, but recent machines such as Storz-Millennium allow a surgeon to set time delay for full vacuum build up when the foot pedal moves in position 2. In addition, the particular machine has dual linear control of vacuum and ultrasound in two planes of pedal movement (pitch and yaw) so that the surgeon can activate the phaco power at safer vacuum levels before reaching the set maximum vacuum.

(iii) **Scroll pump:** This new system developed by Bausch and Lomb surgicals contains two circular elements, fitted into each other in such a way that inner and outer components are moved opposite to each other. When the two elements rotate opposite to each other the force generated causes the fluid inside the system to be pushed out and the new fluid is aspirated inside. Thus, a negative force is created which acts as a vacuum. Advantage of this system is that since no tubing is needed inside the system, compliance is minimal. Thus, tighter control of vacuum can be achieved.

Irrigation System

Irrigation line originates from the bottle placed at a height. Gravity helps the fluid to flow into the eye. This height from the eye level of the patient as well as the bore of the tube determines rate of flow in the irrigation line. Approximately, 10 mm Hg hydrostatic pressure is produced intraocularly for every 15 cm bottle height above the eye. This irrigation line is passed through the clamp, which is released when the foot pedal is taken to position 1 starting the flow in the handpiece. Bottle height should be adjusted by the surgeon for the aspiration flow set.

Panel Display Board to Control and Monitor Functions of the Machine

The settings of the machine are displayed on the monitor. This LCD display screen shows the maximum preset values as well as the real time actual phaco power and vacuum being utilised. The machines give characteristic sounds when irrigation is activated, vacuum is activated, when maximum preset vacuum is reached and when phaco energy is being applied. Surgeon should be familiar with these sounds to control the functions effectively intraoperatively by foot pedal. It is well said that phaco is a surgery that is done with two feet, two hands, two eyes and two ears.

Additional Attachment System

(i) **Bipolar cautery:** Leads for bipolar cautery in surgeries where homeostasis is required following lifting of conjunctival flap as in scleral tunnel for phaco surgery.

(ii) **Vitrectomy probe:** Vitrector probe to do anterior vitrectomy as in cases with posterior capsular rent.

Phaco Handpiece and Tips and Sleeves

The phaco handpiece houses an ultrasonic transducer, a device that converts electrical energy to mechanical vibratory energy (Fig. 5.2).

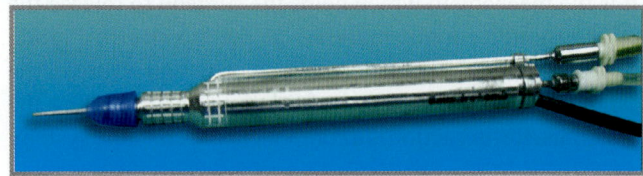

Fig. 5.2: Phaco handpiece with a tip and a sleeve

The transducers are of two types:
(i) Magnetostrictive
(ii) Piezoelectric

The first ophthalmic phaco handpieces were of magnetostrictive type. They were inefficient and generated a lot of heat which required water cooling. This water cooling had to be separated from the irrigation line. Inadvertent breakdown of the barrier between the two carried the risk of infection. Present phaco handpieces use piezoelectric transducers. These crystals are embedded in the handpieces and are generally two to three in number.

The frequency at which a phaco handpiece is set to work, depends on the design and material used. Hence, frequency is fixed for a given machine and depends on the manufacturer. Most machines utilise piezoelectric crystals oscillating between approximately 20,000 to 60,000 times per second. This ultrasound energy is transmitted to the phaco needle, which then vibrates at the same frequency. Adjustment of power settings on the machine affects the stroke length, i.e. the distance travelled by the tip during one cycle. Maximum stroke length on most machines is about five microns. Once the maximum ultrasound power is preset on the machines front panel, a surgeon can then titrate with linear pedal control the percentage of the preset maximum power.

The Physical Mechanisms

The physical mechanisms that break nuclear material when phaco tip is used are:

(i) **The jack hammer like effect:** With the actual to and fro movement, the phaco tip breaks the nucleus mechanically. This is called as the jack hammer effect which is more evident on the hard nucleus.

(ii) **Cavitation effect:** The effect of rapidly retreating phaco tip on return part of cycle creates a void within fluid just in front of retreating tip (cavitation bubble). As the tip retreats more, the size of the cavitation bubble increases until it implodes. The mechanical and thermal forces that occur during such an implosion are large and destructive and tend to break down molecular bonding in the nucleus in the immediate vicinity.

(iii) **Acoustic breakdown:** of lenticular material as a result of forward propagating acoustic waves generated by the tip.

Linear Control of Power

Phaco energy is generally controlled in linear mode with foot pedal in position 3. As the pedal is pressed down, more energy is applied which increases in the linear mode until the maximum preset power is reached. When the foot pedal is pressed down fully maximum power set on the panel is reached. Thus, when maximum preset power is 70%, pressing down the foot pedal halfway will give the 35% of the phaco power.

Pulse/Burst Mode

Most machines have the option to apply the power in pulses—usually the pulses occur at variable rates between 1–10 pulses per second. While the active tip pushes the material away, when power is interrupted flow draws the material back in contact with the tip ready for another short pulse of power. As a result, less power is consumed for a given volume of material. Modern machines have a software that allows burst mode, which in its basic setting gives 20 milliseconds burst followed by 1–2 second pause. These have the option of linear control of burst frequency in foot pedal position 3. With frequency increasing until continuous phaco is reached, white star phaco by allergan uses ultrasound bursts with relatively longer intervals. It is claimed that this allows the phaco tip to cool between bursts removing the need for constant irrigation around the tip.

Phaco Tips

Depending upon the design of distal bevel angle, the phaco tips are classified into 0°, 15°, 30° and 45°. The design of a phaco tip plays an important role in its effectiveness. A 45° tip is more efficient in sculpting a hard nucleus due to jack hammer mechanism whereas, efficiency of a 0° tip is due to micro cavitations effect. A fine balance has to be struck by manufacturers between these two factors in order to ensure that a given tip is efficient. Some tips have bell-shaped end (Cobra tip) or bent at tip (Kelman tip). These are more efficient due to more mechanical effect as well as microcavitations effect.

Standard Tip

It is a straight shaft 19 G bore needle with outer diameter of 1.1 mm and inner diameter of 0.9 mm. It is the most common tip used in cataract surgery. It is available in bevel angles of 0°, 15°, 30° and 45°. The 0° tip has no bevel

outside but there is internal 60° bevel which provides the cutting angle (Fig. 5.3).

The 0° tip gives the best hold on the nuclear fragments. The 30° tip is most commonly used as it gives best balance between the holding capability and the cutting edge as it presents more cross-sectional area to the cataract than the 0° tip. The 45° tip gives best cutting efficiency in hard cataracts but it has less efficient occlusion.

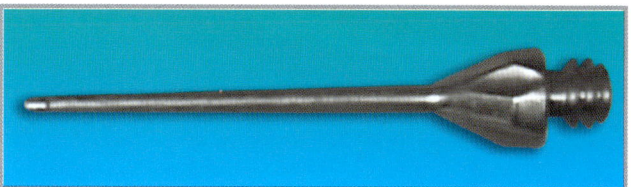

Fig. 5.3: Standard tip (19 G bore needle with an outer diameter of 1.1 mm and an inner diameter of 0.9 mm)

Kelman (Bent) Tip

It has 19 G needle similar to the standard tip but the distal end is bent to give it increased cutting ability. There is also a transverse motion in addition to the normal longitudinal motion of the phaco tip. The bent edge is more in contact with the nucleus, thus enabling the phaco power to be transmitted in a better way, especially to the posterior part of the nucleus. This tip is better for the divide and conquer technique of phacoemulsification. Kelman tip is more effective in cutting hard grade 4 nucleus as it is able to deliver energy in a better way towards the periphery. Because of the downward curve, the design is more ergonomic providing lesser stress on the wound by keeping the handpiece more aligned to the incision. Though, it is more efficient yet, if the surgeon is inexperienced it can cause more complications [(Figs. 5.4(a) and b)].

Micro Tip

As the name suggests, these needles are of smaller diameters requiring smaller entry wound for them. These needles have outer diameters of 0.9 mm with internal diameters of 0.5 to 0.7 mm (average 0.6 mm). These needles have an increased mass compared to the standard tip facilitating better transmission of the phaco power (Fig. 5.5).

Compared to the standard tip, the overall diameter is 35% less, whereas the inner diameter is 48% smaller. Alongwith smaller incisions, they have increased visibility and manoeuvrability. These tips provide precise cutting for the lower average ultrasonic power used. Because of smaller internal lumen, these tips provide enhanced surge protection.

Mackool Tip

Mackool tip contain thin polymer tubing inside the infusion sleeve separating it from the vibrating needle. This polymer, about 50–75 micron thick has a very less friction

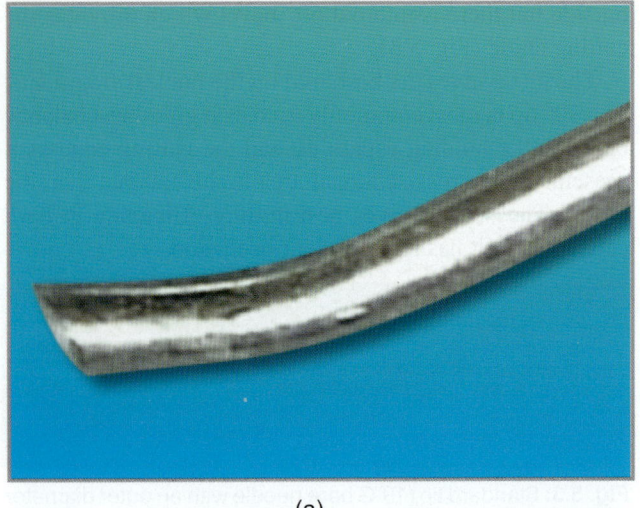

(a)

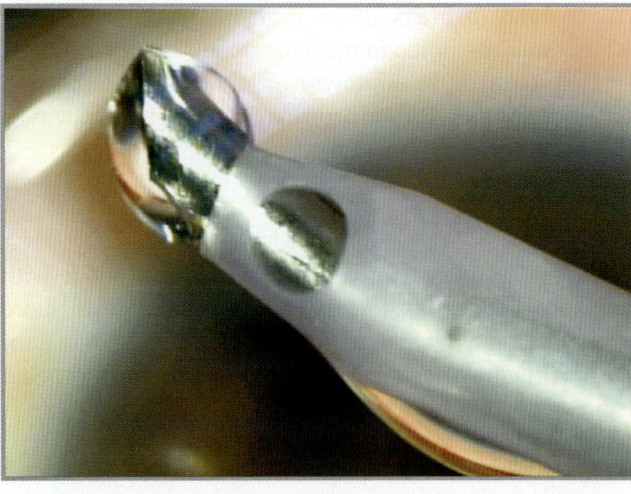

(b)

Fig. 5.4: Kelman (bent) tip

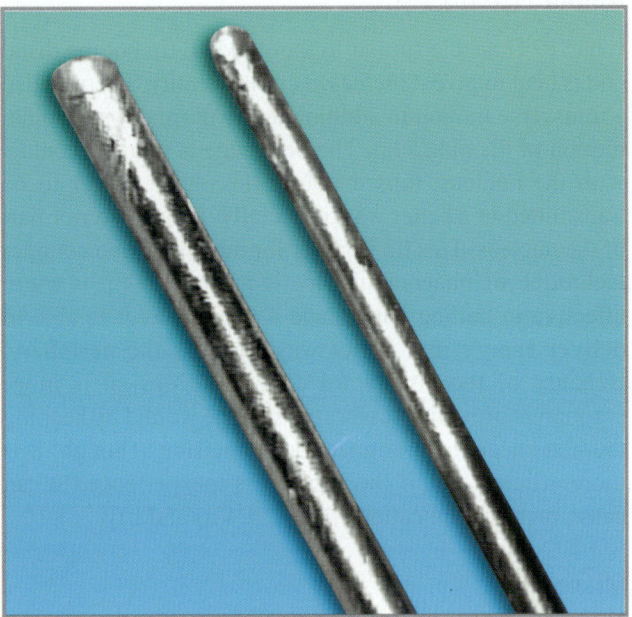

Fig. 5.5: Phaco tips: Standard tip (19 G bore needle with outer diameter 1.1 mm and inner diameter of 0.9 mm) and Micro tips (0.9 /0.65 mm)

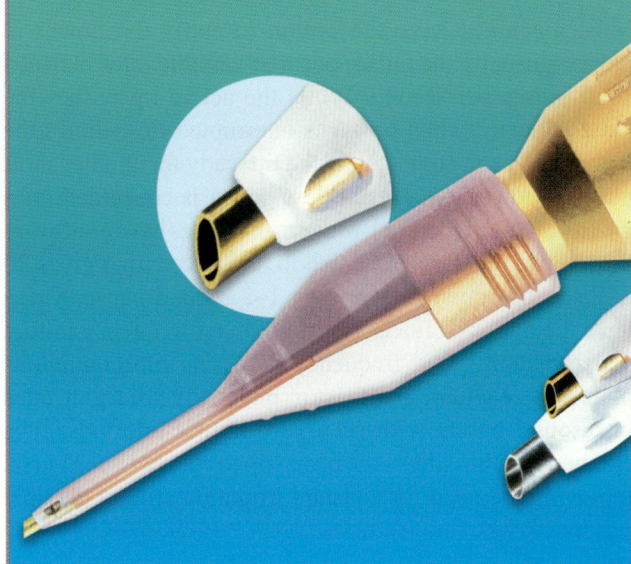

Fig. 5.6: Mackool handpiece with Mackool tip

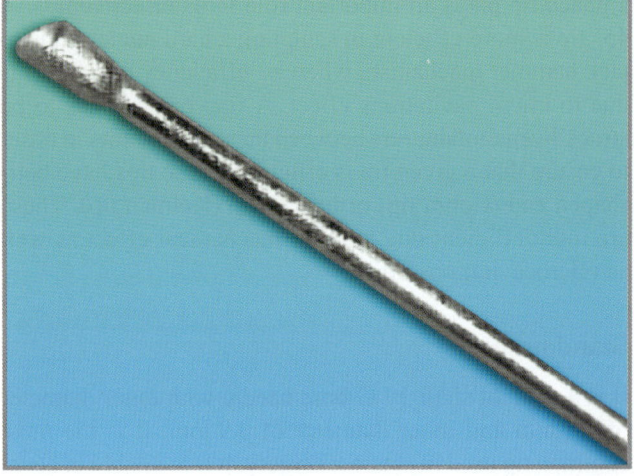

Fig. 5.7: Flared tip

coefficient. The vibrating needle generates less heat when surrounded by this polymer, thus heat transmission is reduced. This has greater advantage in comparison with slightly increased infusion sleeve thickness.

Mackool tip are available in both standard as well as micro tip version. Kelman (bent) tip are also provided by the Mackool features (Fig. 5.6).

Flared Tip (Fig. 5.7)

These tip have their distant edges enlarged to form a bell-shaped feature and they have their internal lumen's reduced. The distal end is enlarged to 1.14 mm in standard tip. This design is also available in the micro-tip version. This design gives larger distant area for better transfer of the phaco energy to the nuclear fragments due to increased mass of the tip end increasing both jack hammer and cavitation effect.

Flared tips are available in Mackool system also.

Aspiration Bypass (ABS) Tip

Among one of the Alcon's new innovations, **Turbosonic® ABS™** bypass phaco tip with 0.18 mm bypass port on the side of the phaco tip is one (Fig. 5.8).

This phaco tip is unique with a small hole of 0.18 mm diameter at the distal end of the phaco needle. This extra opening provides continuous outflow throughout nucleus emulsification, even during full occlusion. When main port is not occluded, the outflow from the side opening is negligible due to very high resistance by the smaller diameter of the hole. The ABS port is activated once the primary aspiration port is occluded. This flow from ABS port cools down the phaco needle, the incision site and also the entire anterior chamber by replacing the fluid continuously. This continuous flow lessens the chances of surge after occlusion breaks improving the chamber stability. This system changes the occlusion break response from static – dynamic to dynamic – dynamic (Figs 5.8 to 5.10).

The ABS port system design is also available in Mackool tip .

Microflow Tips

These needles, designed by Bausch and Lomb, are similar to a standard phaco needle having grooves on the outer shaft (Fig. 5.11).

Grooves help cool down the tip, thus reducing the chances of causing wound burns.

Cobra Tips

These tips have increased width at their distal extremity. These tips have an increased tendency to heat up.

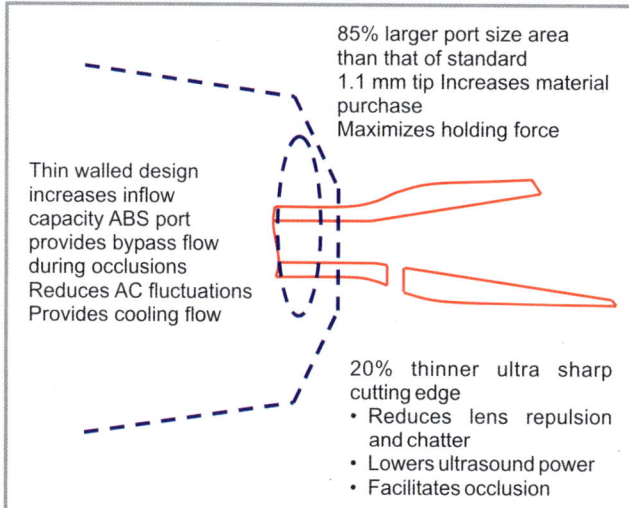

Fig. 5.8: Physics of ABS tip

Diaphragm Tips

It has a constriction of the internal lumen at the distal end which acts like a diaphragm giving less surge on release of the occlusion. They can be used with high vacuum settings.

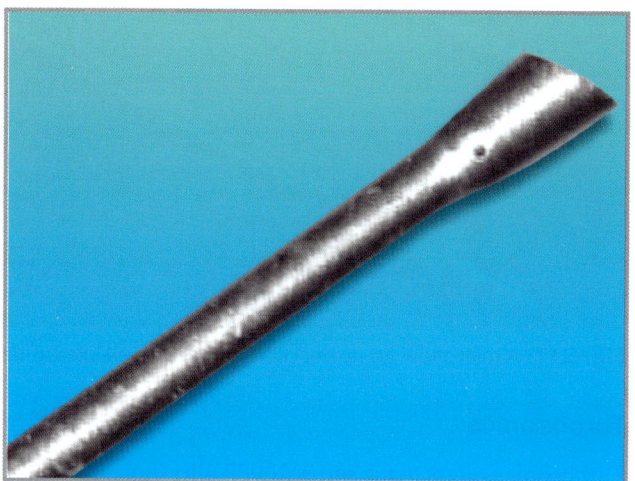

Fig. 5.9: ABS Tip

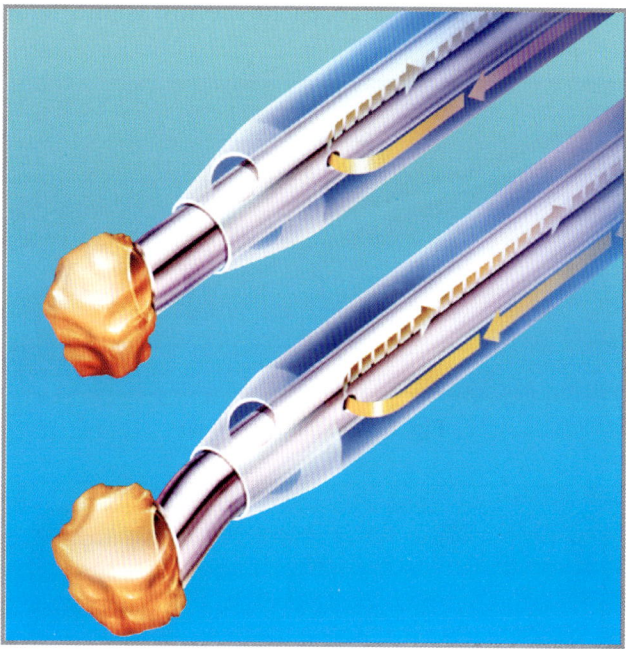

(a)

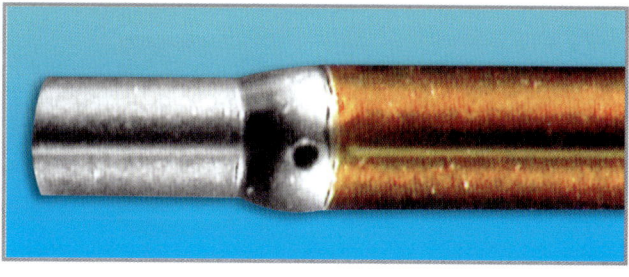

(b)

Fig. 5.10: (a) ABS Tip, (b) Mackool ABS

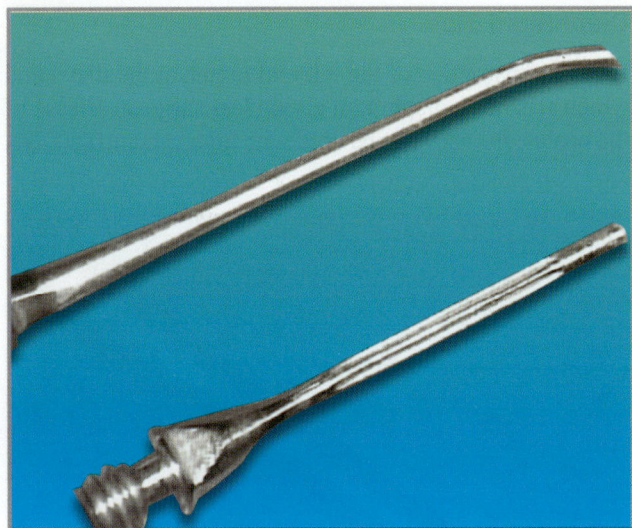

Fig. 5.11: A microflow tip (lower) compared with a Kelman tip

Tip type	Cassette type	Port area (mm²)	Vacuum (mm Hg)	Holding force factor
1.1 mm	Standard	0.656	150	98
1.1 mm	MaxVac	0.656	250	164
Micro tip	Standard	0.342	250	86
Micro tip	MaxVac	0.342	350	120
Mackool-0.9 mm	MaxVac	0.342	350	120
0.9 mm ABS	MaxVac	0.342	400	137
1.1 mm ABS	MaxVac	0.656	400	262
Flared/ ABS-0.9mm	MaxVac	0.985	500	493

Turbosonics

Turbosonics refers to the series 20000 ultrasonic tip design and has the following (Fig. 5.12):
- Special hydrodynamically tapered hub design
- Harmonically balanced to the ultrasonic hand piece

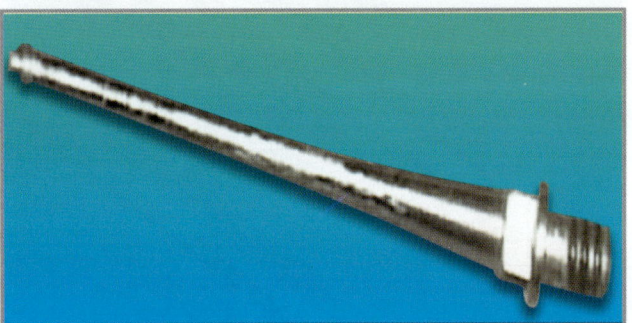

Fig. 5.12: Turbosonics tip

Wrench

Specially designed wrenchs are essentially required to tighten or adjust the phaco tip in the phaco handpiece [Fig. 5.13(a) and (b)].

Phaco Sleeves

Phaco sleeves are made up of silicon polymer. Sleeves are of immense value and functions (Fig. 5.14).

  (i) Act as thermal insulators or vibrating phaco tip and hence, minimise the risk of direct thermal corneal/ incision burn.
 (ii) It provides space for irrigating fluid all around phaco tip, thereby providing additional cooling effect as well as a third port for irrigation fluid during coaxial phacoemulsification surgery.
(iii) Silicone sleeves around aspiration/irrigation handpiece provide irrigation fluid for aspiration of cortical matter.

Irrigation and Aspiration Handpiece

Irrigation and aspiration handpiece is used for removal of cortical matter after removal of nucleus and epinucleus. It

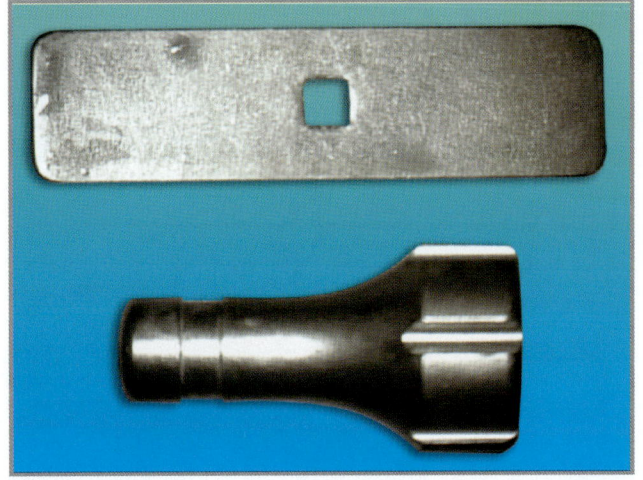

(a)

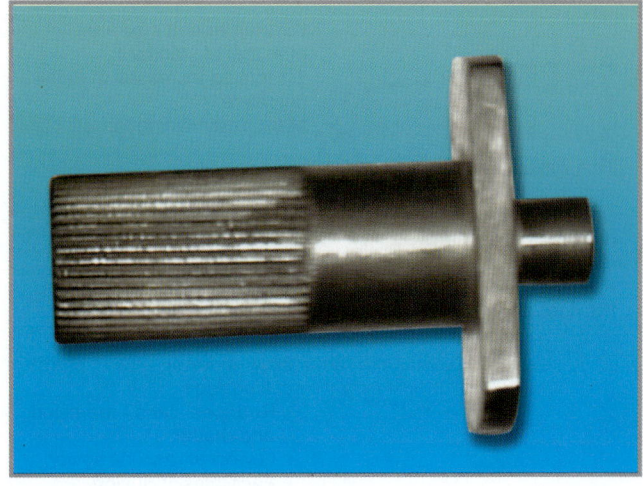

(b)

Fig. 5.13: (a) and (b) Wrench

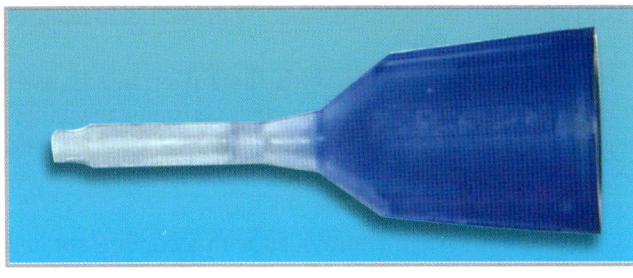

(a)

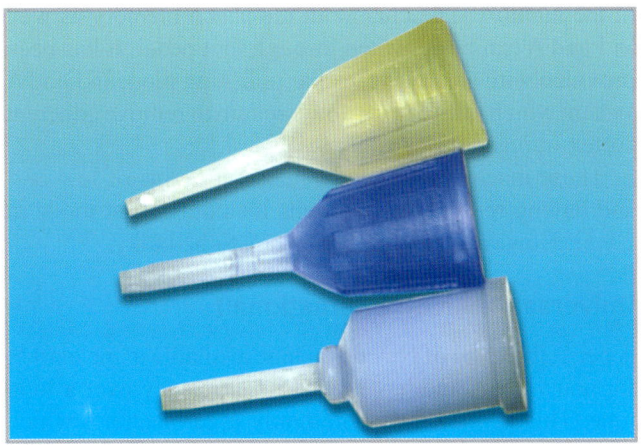

(b)

Fig. 5.14: (a) and (b) Phaco sleeves

has a metal tip covered with either silicon or metal sleeve. The aspiration port is of diameter 0.3 mm. This small diameter can catch cortical matter while providing with necessary resistance to fluid outflow while working with high vacuum (400 mm Hg). This hole size struck a balance between the vacuum necessary to remove the cortical matter while preventing sudden collapse of the anterior chamber by providing enough resistance for fluid outflow. This also gives enough time to the surgeon to act in case there is inadvertent catching of the posterior capsule or the iris into the hole.

Two-handed irrigation aspiration system (Bimanual I and A) separates the irrigation line from the aspiration line. Separate handpieces are provided for them. Irrigation and aspiration lines can be connected to them separately. The tip size is smaller so that they can be inserted from the side port incision removing the need to enlarge the incision in case of microincisional cataract surgery (Fig. 5.15).

The tip are slightly bent so that they are easier to handle. These tip are of great help to remove the sub-incisional cortex by providing greater manoeuvrability. Because of the smaller size of irrigating holes sudden collapse of anterior chamber can occur.

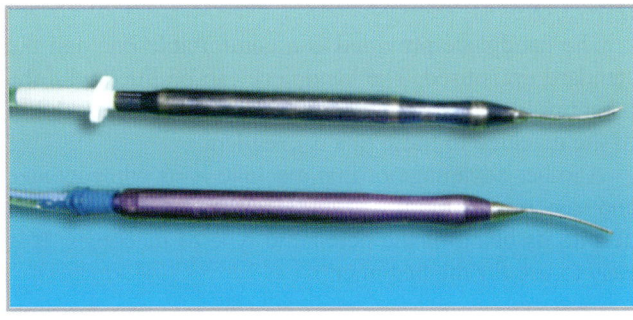

(a)

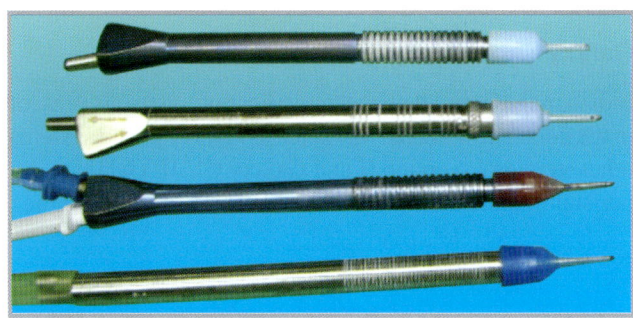

(b)

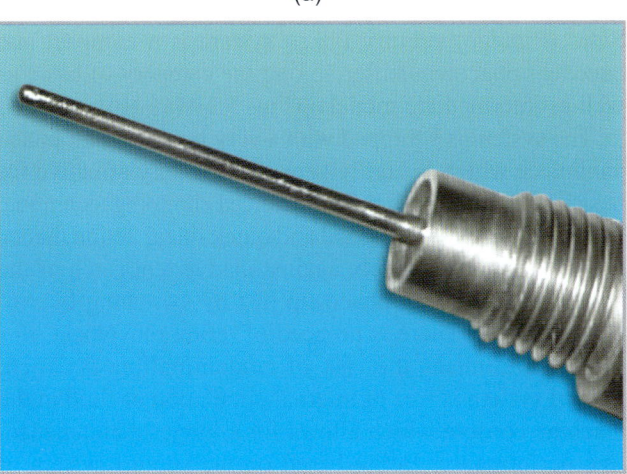

(c)

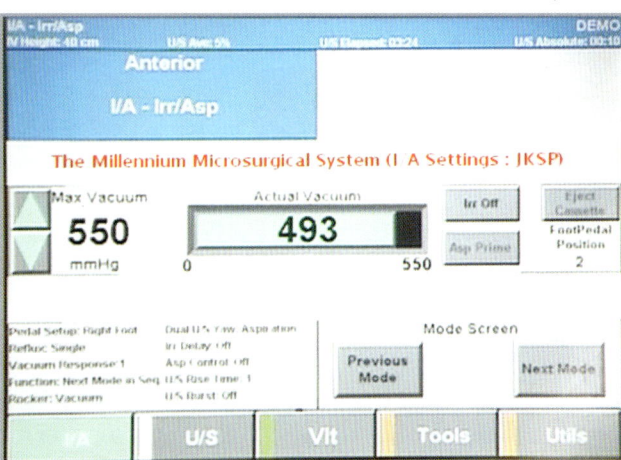

(d)

Fig. 5.15: (a) Bimanual irrigation and aspiration handpiece, (b) and (c) Coaxial irrigation aspiration system, (d) I/A settings for coaxial irrigation aspiration system

Foot Pedal

The control pedal, generally speaking, has four positions. called position 0, 1, 2 and 3 (Fig. 5.16).

At position 0 the system is at rest. When the operator moves the pedal to position 1, the irrigation starts. It is accompanied by a voice alarm or a specific noise which starts from the machine the volume of which can be controlled by the operator. With foot pedal in position 2, the pump mechanism starts and vacuum builds up. This draws the nuclear and other materials towards the phaco tip. With foot position 3, surgeon starts the ultrasound energy which is coupled with the excursion of the foot pedal linearly.

Understanding Phaco Machines

A phaco surgeon should be well aware of the advantages and limitations of his machine as well as specific functions his machine is providing to get the best out of it. He should be comfortable with the machine. Here, we are describing the commonly available machines in the commercially market (We do not have any proprietary interest with any of the systems). All available systems carry several good points. including basic functions and service system or advanced technology. It is further stressed that our view should only be considered on technical merit not as a recommendation or adverse comments.

Galaxy (Appasamy/India)

Indian manufactured phacoemulsification system is present in the domestic markets. Marketed as Galaxy phaco systems it has version I, version II and Galaxy CV II. Galaxy I is a peristaltic machine while Galaxy II is a venturi machine.

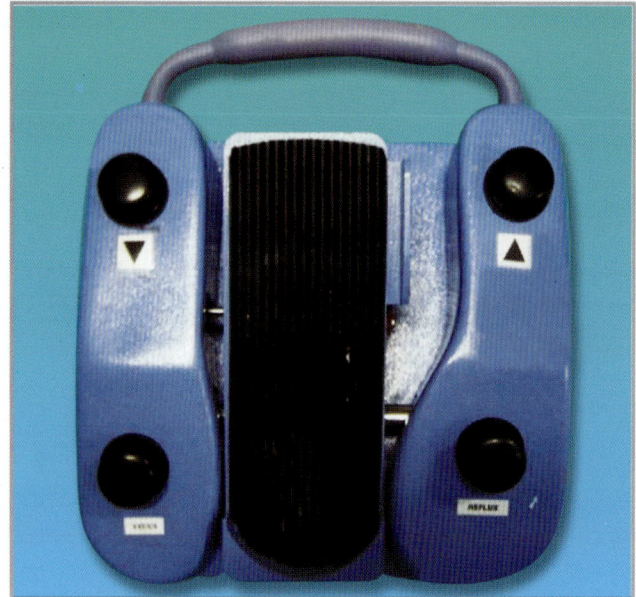

Fig. 5.16: Foot pedal

Galaxy CV II is an advanced model with additional features [(Figs 5.17(a) to (f)].

Galaxy I is provided with the roller beads over which the tubing passes. As with other peristaltic machines, it gives independent control of the aspiration flow rate and vacuum. It has a delayed rise time and is useful to new phaco surgeons.

The venturi system is provided with a compressor and has the linear as well as the pulse mode. Machine parameters for upto four different surgeons can be entered in the memory. The change in the phaco memory as well as I and A can be activated through foot pedal. It has been provided with a unique capsular polishing mode in I and A system which utilises very low vacuum to remove adherent cortex in posterior capsule.

These machines have advantages in terms of low cost and having reasonable functions including burst mode in CV II. However, handpiece appears to be bulky.

Universal II (Alcon International)

A peristaltic type of phaco machine available in the market for many years and has proven its efficiency over a long time. This is one of the commonly used machines which has very good fluidics control for the peristaltic pump.

Provided with the pump and with the roller beads this machine can achieve good vacuum with the occlusion (Fig. 5.18).

The handpiece provided is a comfortable one and the standard tip is used. The handpiece can be fitted with the other tips like micro tips or micro flow needles. Adaptability of the machine to these tips is excellent.

Another advantage of this machine is its compact size and easy transportability. Fluidics of the machine is good despite its being of the peristaltic type of machines. It is easy to use for the beginner.

Storz (Protégé) Venturi Phaco System

Storz (Protégé) ventury Phaco system is a compact and excellent phacoemulsifier among the category of basic as well as intermediate models [(Figs 5.19 (a), (b)].

The system is equipped with a very light, elegant phaco handpiece which is highly versatile and very effective for basic sculpting as well as for advanced chopping technique.

Foot pedal provides good and quick linear action, hence provides enhanced safety against inadvertent catch of the posterior capsule by phaco tip just by switching over to the position 1. There is no need of reflux movement, this further minimises the risk of contamination. As such, venturi system is free of internal circulation of fluid in the machine console which allows for a longer maintenance-free performance. Being based on the venturi system, it facilitates excellent irrigation and aspiration potential. A strong aspiration potential with good safety allows precise handling of any kind of cortex.

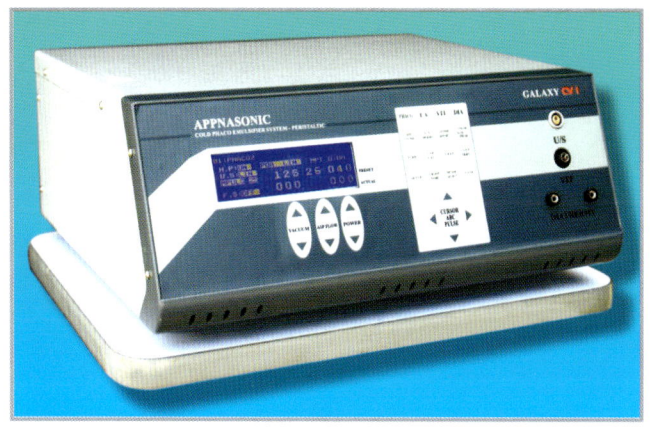

(a)

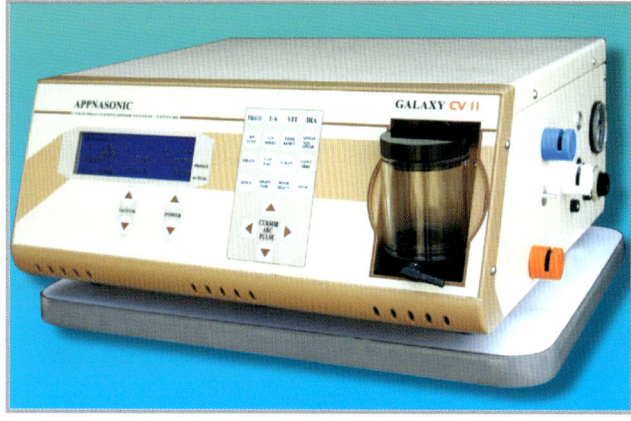

(b)

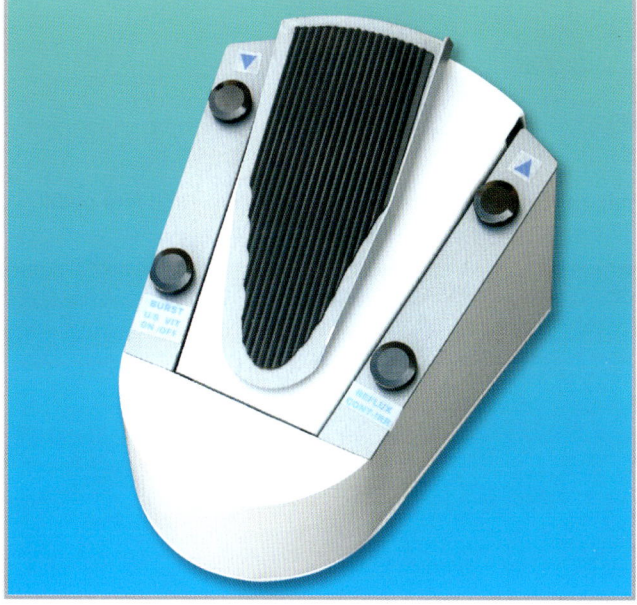

(c)

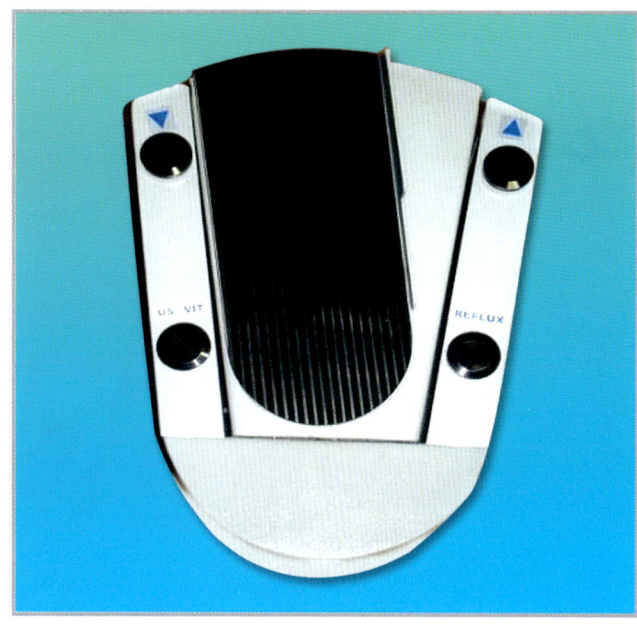

(d)

(e)

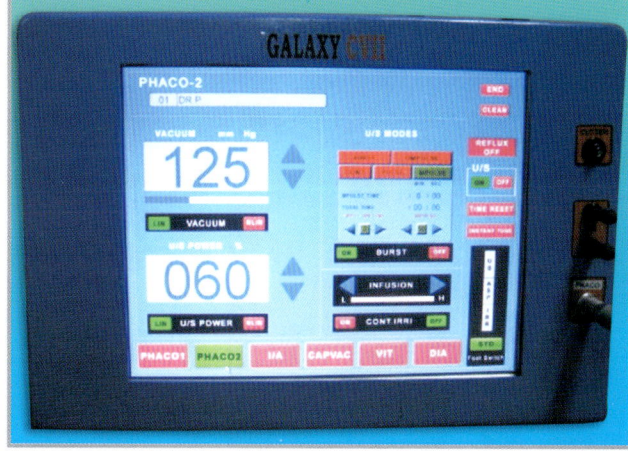

(f)

Fig. 5.17: (a) Galaxy I peristaltic machine (Appasamy/India), (b) Galaxy II venturi machine (Appasamy/India), (c) Galaxy hand-piece and coaxial IA system, (d) Foot pedal Galaxy (Appasamy/India), (e) Foot pedal Galaxy (Appasamy/India), (f) Galaxy CV II (Appasamy/India)

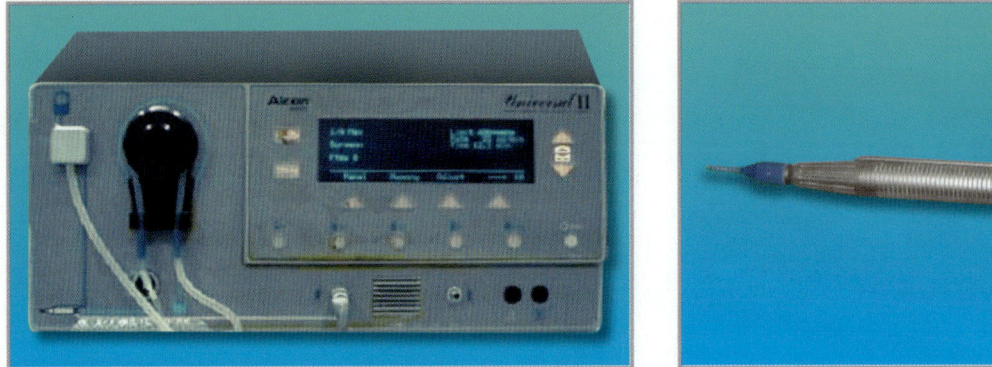

(a)

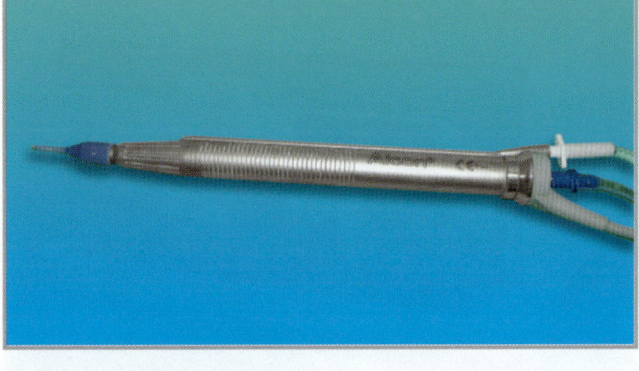

(b)

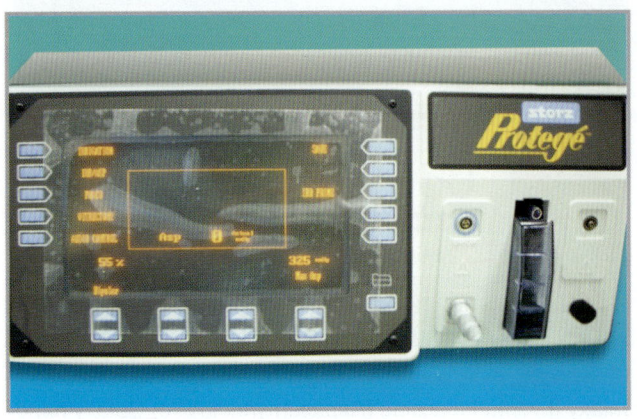

(c)

Fig. 5.18 (a) Universal II peristaltic machine (Alcon international), (b) Universal II handpiece, (c) Universal II foot pedal

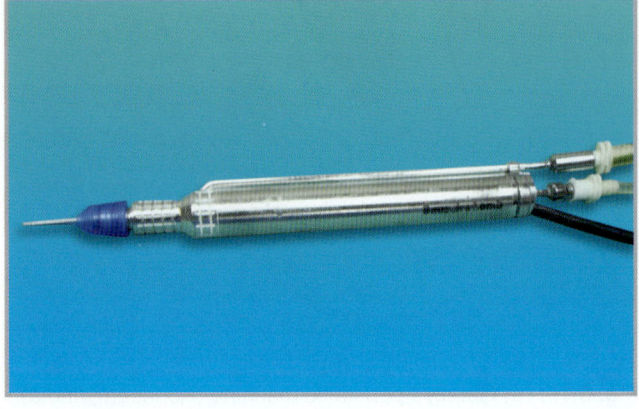

(a)

(b)

Fig. 5.19: (a) Storz (Protégé) Venturi phaco system, (b) Protégé handpiece

I myself have admired its performance in over 6000 phacosurgeries of all kinds and belonging to all grades of surgery. Undoubtedly, this system is one of the best bid on overall functions and cost combinations.

The Alcon Series 20000 Legacy Advantec

Introduced as successor of series 10000 by Alcon it has many added advantages and new features. It has been upgraded over the period to have better versatility with newer developments. The latest version of the 20000 series is called as Advantec. It has better and faster computing microprocessors for real time adjustments intraoperatively. Provided with four piezoelectric crystals, it provides variable frequencies between 20–80 KHz. Special feature of the system is the inbuilt constant admittance tuning which ensures that power of the ultrasound remains at the optimal level at any given time and density of cataract.

The machine is fitted with the peristaltic type of pump. Its unique feature is the part 'aspiration cartridge' in which a part of flexible tubes are replaced by rigid channels providing more accurate control of the fluid dynamics.

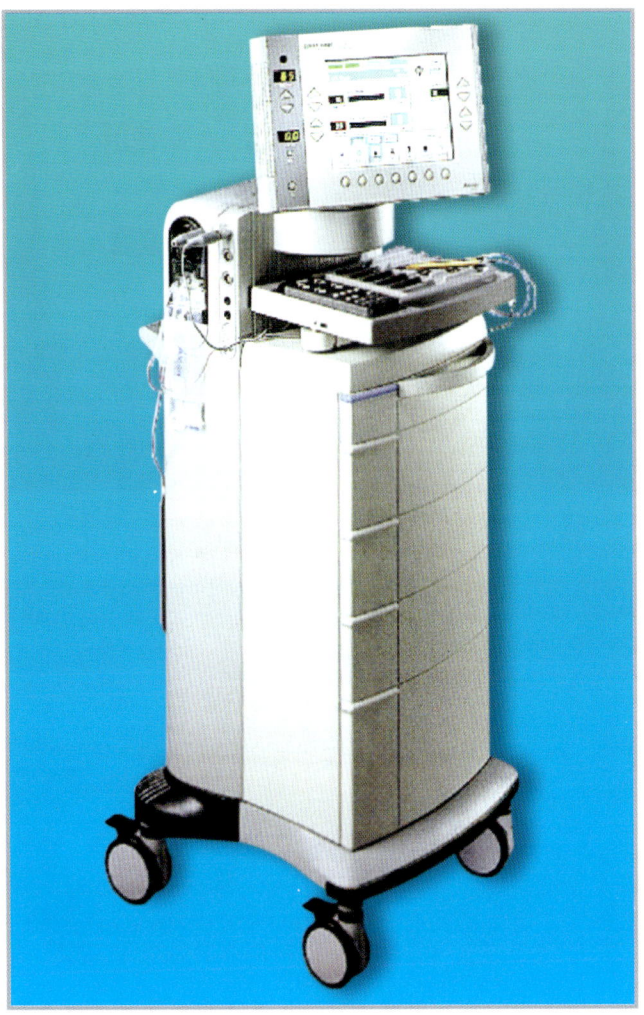

Fig. 5.20: The Alcon series 20000 Legacy Advantec

The Maxvac system is also developed to provide maximum protection of the surge and maintain the chamber. The tubes of Maxvac system are rigid with greater wall thickness and smaller internal diameter thus having lower compliance of system. This combination of features of aspiration cartridge with Maxvac system provides better fluidics management.

Sets of different phaco tips termed turbosonic tips have been developed for Advantec. Legacy inherits a wide variety of sophisticated turbosonics tip configurations, which provide the surgeon unsurpassed flexibility by allowing the user to make tip selection based on technique and the cataract type rather than using a "one size fits all" approach. These tips are available in different sizes and designs giving a wide variety of choices to the surgeon. These turbosonic tips are designed with tapering proximal ends, which reduce fluid resistance and turbulence in aspiration.

These tips are available as:
- Standard tips (turbosonics tip) either straight or Kelman (bent) variety
- Turbosonics microtips with external diameters of 0.9 mm with internal diameters of 0.6 mm
- Turbosonic aspiration bypass system (ABS)
- Flared tips with Flared ABS

Advantec is provided with Neosonix handpiece. It is a newer advance in the phaco technology where the tip is provided with the rotationary movement along with traditional longitudinal movement. This provides greater holding force to the tip by decreasing the repulsion thus requiring less energy for cataract removal.

Advantec is also available with Mackool system in which rigid polymer sleeve covers the tip inside the irrigation sleeve. This sleeve reduces friction and heat generation at the cost of slightly increasing the sleeve diameter, but this brings down heat transfer and wound burn.

Advantec hardware and software reduces the amount of energy entering the eye by allowing the legacy to deliver bursts of energy—in short or long pulses—with variable periods of rest. This reduction in energy allows harder cataracts to be tackled with greater ease (Fig. 5.20).

Alcon Infinity

One of the newest additions from Alcon laboratories is the introduction of a high end phacoemulsifier named Infinity.

It is a triple function system which utilises:
- Traditional ultrasound
- OZil handpiece for tortional phaco
- AquaLase: Pulsed water jet system for soft cataract

This system has been provided with different high end functions for a different variety of cataracts. The special handpiece called OZil torsional handpiece and its software are available on Infinity vision system of Alcon. It utilises a unique side to side shearing effect which almost eliminates repulsion, increases cutting efficiency and followability to very high levels compared to the traditional phaco.

Aqualase uses pulses of balanced salt solution at 50 Hz to 100 Hz to dissolve the cataract. This modality may potentially demonstrate advantages in terms of safety and prevention of secondary posterior capsular opacification.

AMO (Allergan Medical Optics) Sovereign with White Staar

White Staar technology, brought out by AMO is a new rapid-pulsed phaco system that permits cataract surgery with reduced heat, where high aspiration is used with modification of phaco power and is ideally suited to small-incision surgery.

It is a peristaltic pump system provided with an advanced system called shield system. It has a special sensor which modifies aspiration flow and vacuum in real time on the basis of the inputs from the aspiration line. This can help to use high vacuum in the phaco setting minimizing the use of ultrasound (Fig. 5.21).

Sovereign is provided with the ability to pulse much more rapidly. A short burst of phaco followed by a long interval allows the tip to cool down reducing the need for constant irrigation of the tip. This technology gives true cold phaco. The phaco interval between the successive burst of energy causes breakdown of the cataract. This is called 'transient cavitation' technology.

Opticon 2000 Pulsar Minimal Stress

Pulsar is fitted with a peristaltic pump which has a very effective surge suppression system to maintain the anterior chamber. Excellent anterior chamber stability is achieved with this system.

The traditional ultrasound handpiece with four piezoelectric crystals is with a frequency of 40 KHz. The system is fitted with a system called Stroke Ruler where the actual stroke length is measured in real time and is adjusted to the set level if the tip faces more resistance as in cases of hard cataract, by maintaining the constant stroke length. Therefore, there is an overall decrease in the power used.

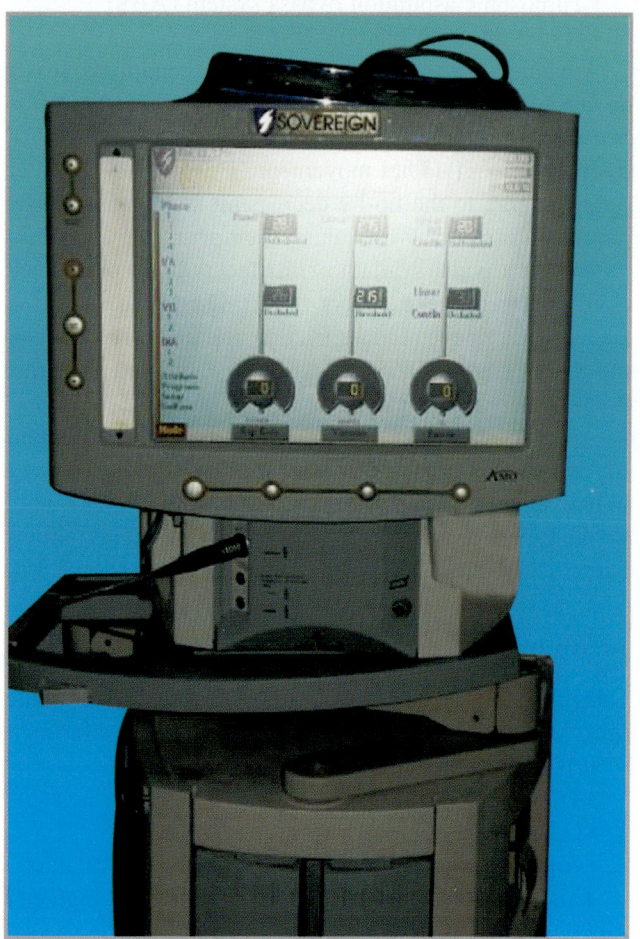

(a)

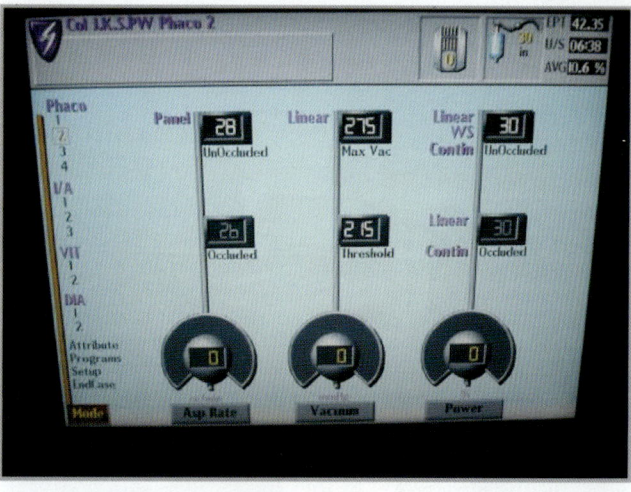

(b)

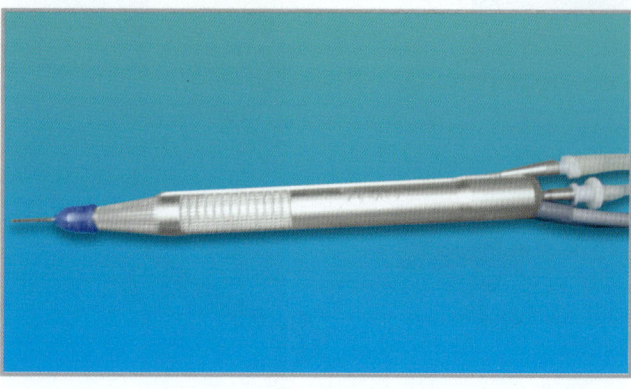

(c)

Fig. 5.21: (a) AMO (Allergan Medical Optics) Sovereign with White Staar, (b) AMO (Allergan Medical Optics) Sovereign with White Staar, (c) Sovereign Handpiece

The handpiece is called slim 4 handpiece which is smaller and lighter for better adaptability by the surgeon.

The Millennium Microsurgical System

The Millennium Microsurgical System from Bausch and Lomb has three notable features (Fig. 5.22):

(i) Dual linear control

(ii) Concentrix fluidics control technology and

(iii) Micro-phaco burst capabilities.

The new Millennium system provides the vacuum creation and ultrasound energy at dual control mode. A surgeon is provided with special foot pedal where greater vertical pressure corresponds to the greater creation of vacuum while horizontal excursion provides the ultrasound power. Thus, the surgeon can give ultrasound energy at the desired vacuum level when occlusion is achieved. This in turn can reduce surge.

Fluid system uses Concentrix system which has a scroll pump. It contains two circular elements, fitted into each other in a way that the inner and outer components are moved opposite to each other. When the two elements rotate opposite to each other, force is generated causing the fluid within the system to be pushed out and the new fluid is aspirated inside. Thus, negative force is created which acts as a vacuum. Since no tubing is needed inside the system, compliance is minimal. Thus, tighter control of vacuum can be achieved.

Combined Phacoemulsification and Posterior Segment Surgery System

Different machines which have combined phacoemulsification along with the vitrectomy mode are available in the market.

(i) DORC (Fig. 5.23)

(ii) Alcon Accurus

(iii) The Millennium Microsurgical System from Bausch and Lomb.

These systems are venturi systems provided with a compressor. They are basically vitrectomy machines used for posterior segment surgeries. The vitrector and the functions for retinal surgeries like that for air injection or viscous fluid injection are provided in the machine.

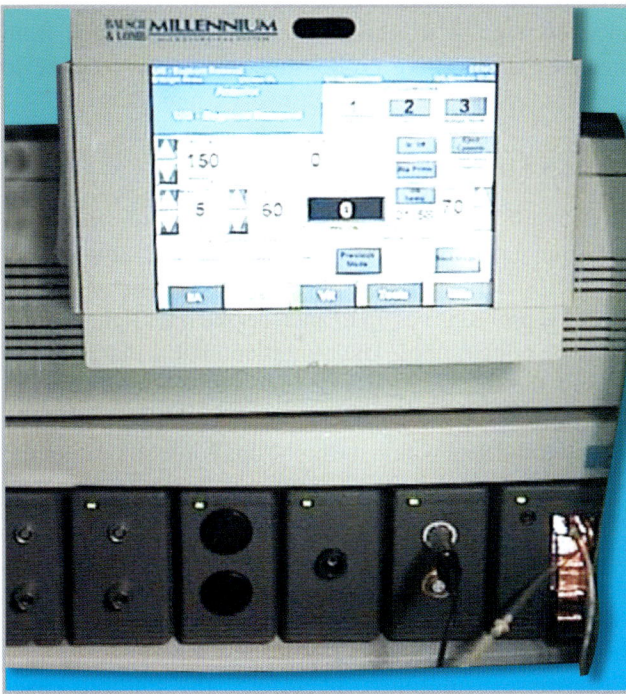

(a)

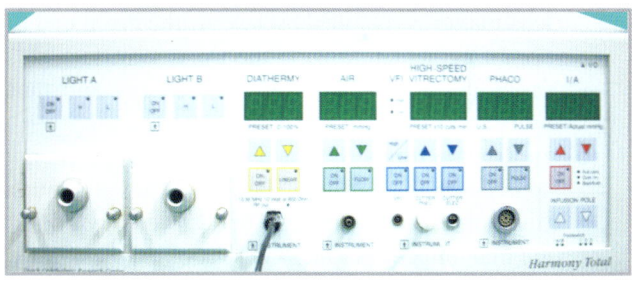

(a)

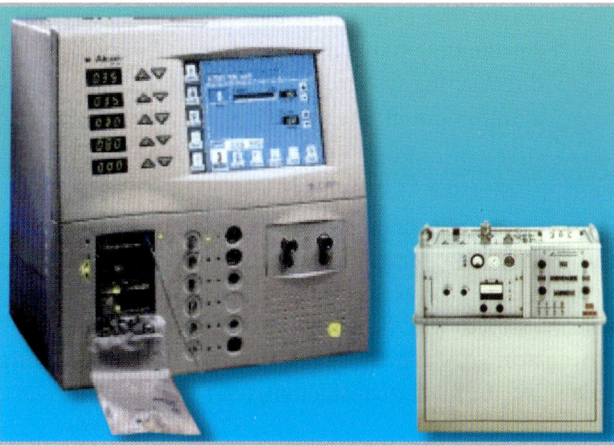

(b)

Fig. 5.23: (a) Combined phacoemulsification and posterior segment surgery system: DORC, (b) Combined phacoemulsification and posterior segment surgery system: Alcon Accurus

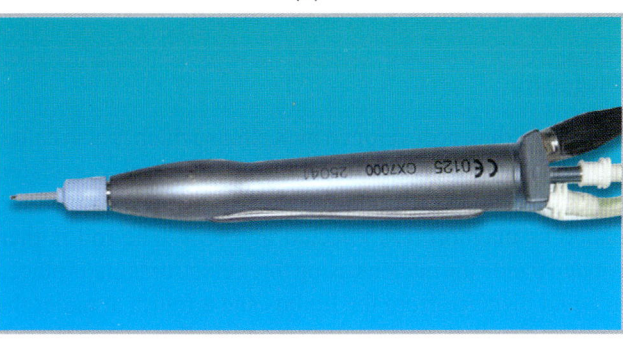

(b)

Fig. 5.22: (a) The millennium microsurgical system, (b) The millennium handpiece

The phaco mode is a standard linear or pulse mode phaco useful for phacofragmentation. In our view, the phaco is a subsidiary function in these machines and these machines are referred to as posterior segment surgery system and additional phacomachines rather than as primary phaco machines (Fig. 5.23).

NEWER DEVELOPMENTS IN PHACO SURGERY

Laser Phaco

One of the latest developments in cataract surgery has been the invention of devices that utilise laser energy for the removal of cataract. Laser cataract surgery has opened new avenues for cataract removal with fewer chances of complications related to excessive heat injury. Laser phacoemulsification as such will be dealt with in detail in separate chapters.

Currently Nd: YAG and Erbium YAG laser are the two types of laser used in laser phaco system.

There are two types of laser phaco systems using Nd: YAG laser:

(a) **Direct acting system:** This system uses Nd: YAG laser through a 1.8 mm diameter tip. Laser energy tracks along a fibre and across an open area called photofragmentation zone, which is a 2.5 mm zone into which nuclear material is aspirated. Resulting lens matter is removed by I/A. At the distal end of photofragmentation zone the tip is bent forwards providing a back stop for laser energy and thus prevents damage to non-target organ.

(b) **Indirect acting system:** In this system the energy source is pulsed Nd: YAG laser transmitted through fibreoptic into the probe. The laser energy strikes the titanium target which causes optical breakdown and plasma formation. Thus titanium target acts as a transducer converting laser energy into shock waves that ablate the nucleus and also shield the surrounding tissue of patient's eye. As compared to direct acting system, the requirement of laser energy is minimum in this system.

Systems using Erbium Laser

Erbium laser phacoemulsification is effective for lenses with mild to moderate nuclear sclerosis. Advantages of Erbium laser phacoemulsification are less energy transmission to eye, no heating of anterior chamber, high protection of corneal endothelium, smooth cutting capability, useful for capsulotomy.

Limitations of Erbium Laser Phaco System

- Fibre material in Erbium laser phaco systems is made up of zincorium fluoride and sapphire. Zincorium fluoride is sensitive to hydroscopic change, so cannot be autoclaved. Fibre is very expensive. Sapphire fibre can be autoclaved but it is brittle and has relatively low transmission power.
- Inability to remove dense nuclei.
- High cost.

Future development in laser phaco system may help to make small incision cataract surgery more accessible to more number of surgeons.

Dodick ARC Photolysis

This phacoemulsification system (ARC Laser Corporation) uses an Nd:YAG laser instead of ultrasound to break up a cataractous lens. Nd: YAG laser (1064 nm laser) is made to fall on the titanium mirror. The shock waves which are produced cause breakdown of the lens matter. Ocular tissues are not directly exposed to the laser light and heat produced is minimal. "It is impossible to produce a corneal-scleral burn with this laser apparatus," Dr Dodick said in an interview. "Also, the infusion can be separated from the laser emulsifying probe, thus making it possible to perform the operation through two 1.2 mm incisions."

Photon Laser Phacolysis

The Photon Laser Phacolysis system uses an Nd: YAG 1064 nm laser to produce photo-acoustic ablation of cataract material under aspiration. The ski-shaped distal tip of the probe curves up to intersect the laser light emitted from the optical fibre. The aspiration inlet is placed in the face of the tip, creating a photon trap. Thus, all rays of laser photons that enter the aspiration port are internally reflected and kept within the probe tip. While some minimal heating of tissue occurs, the heat is very rapidly removed by aspiration and the temperature of the probe tip rises, approximately by 1°C.

The peak intensity of the Photon Laser Phacolysis system is more than 10,000 times below that required for the onset of plasma generation, the operative action during posterior capsulotomy. Therefore, the Photon Laser Phacolysis system represents an exceptionally safe modality in terms of capsular integrity.

Phacofly

This procedure is developed by Kelman which is also called as KELMAST (Kelman electromagnetically assisted surgical technique). In this procedure, a tiny magnetic rod called as magnorbit is injected into lens. The rod is then rotated inside the nucleus using three electromagnets placed at equal distance from the limbus and a fourth at under the patient's head. As the nucleus is emulsified it is aspirated. After complete aspiration of lens matter a rounded bead is introduced for polishing the bag. The intact capsular bag allows the injection of clear collagen till visualisation of retinal vessels occurs through a lens placed over ocular part of the microscope. At this stage, the patient is emmetropic.

Phaconit

This is new technique in which cataract is removed through 0.9 mm incision using a phaco tip without infusion sleeve. The irrigating chopper is used through the side port with the left hand providing irrigation. The assistant pours water continuously at the site of incision to cool the phaco tip. Thus, cataract is removed through 0.9 mm incision.

Cold Phaco

White Staar Phaco by Allergan uses ultrasound bursts with relatively longer intervals. Instead of a continuous phaco mode, energy is delivered in short bursts followed by long intervals. Thus, it utilises less phaco energy. It is claimed that this allows the phaco tip to cool between bursts removing the need for constant irrigation around the tip.

STAAR Surgical's Sonic Wave

One of the recent new machines for cataract extraction is the Wave (STAAR Surgicals). The Wave is designed as an instrument that combines phaco technology with new features and a new user interface. Innovations in energy delivery, high vacuum tubing, and digitally recordable procedures with video overlays make this, one of the most technologically advanced and theoretically safest machines available. The Sonic Wave uses sonic energy in the range of 40 Hz to 400 Hz in addition to the 40,000 Hz range that ultrasonic phaco machines generally employ. The lower energy generally produces less heat, reducing the risk of corneal burns. The ultrasound handpiece is a lightweight (2.25 ounces) 2-crystal, 40 kHz piezo-electric auto-tuning handpiece that utilises a load compensating ultrasonic driver. One of the unique features of the Wave is its ability to adjust vacuum as a function of ultrasound power. This feature is termed auto-correlation (A/C) mode. It enables lens fragments to be engaged at low vacuum levels in the foot position.

1. Vacuum levels are proportionally increased with increases in ultrasound power in foot position
2. Proportional increases in vacuum allow for faster aspiration of lens fragments by overcoming the repulsive forces generated by ultrasound energy at the tip.

The Sonic Wave also employs, the Ultra Vac coiled tubing which is designed to stabilise the anterior chamber and to prevent post-occlusion surge, which can cause anterior chambers to dimple and collapse.

SuperVac tubing increases vacuum capability to up to 650 mm Hg while significantly increasing AC stability. The AC is maintained by achieving a positive fluid balance between infusion flow and aspiration flow.

NeoSonix

NeoSonix technology is a hybrid modality involving low frequency oscillatory movement that may be used alone or in a combination with standard high frequency ultrasonic phaco. Softer grades of nuclear sclerosis may be completely addressed with the low frequency modality, while denser grades will likely require the addition of ultrasound. In the NeoSonix mode, the phaco tip has a variable rotational oscillation up to 2°, at 120 Hz. Thus in addition to the longitudinal movement of the tip it also has the rotatory movement. This helps in less chattering of the nuclear fragments and repulsion of the fragments by the tip is less, providing better hold and less utilisation of phaco energy.

The Catarex Technology

A fundamentally new and different technology which utilises a high speed motor with a 1.5 mm diameter partially shielded impeller probe. This technology utilises a rotation based vortex flow in the capsular bag.

Technique involves a 1.5 mm hole punched into the capsule via an electrosurgical probe. The lens is hydro-dissected, and the impeller probe placed at the opening of the capsule. The bag remains distended via the inflow and without moving the tip at all, the hard lens material is emulsified and removed with no ultrasound at all. It is the final step leading to the refillable liquid polymer injectable lens substitute. This surgery is far faster than phaco—it can be done within 2 minutes—and far safer too. Presently, this technology is useful in the softer nucleus.

Torsional Phaco

Alcon laboratories has come out with a new modality called torsional phaco. The special handpiece called OZil torsional handpiece and its software are available on Infinity vision system of Alcon. It utilises a unique side to side shearing effect which almost eliminates repulsion, increases cutting efficiency and followability to very high levels compared to the traditional phaco. In torsional mode, the handpiece oscillates from side to side at about 32,000 times per second. This side to side motion shears off nucleus pieces without repelling them, thus eliminating chatter.

The unique design with the angled tip design makes the velocity at the tip three times to that of its shaft. Therefore, the amount of energy being released at the tip is much greater than the amount of the heat generated at the incision. The torsional phaco can be combined with the traditional linear ultrasound so that combination of power can be delivered for faster and safer removal of nucleus. This technique is far more useful in hard cataracts.

Aqualase

Research has led to the development of a fluid-based cataract extraction system. Another non-thermal modality,

Aqualase uses pulses of balanced salt solution at 50 Hz to 100 Hz to dissolve the cataract (Fig. 5.24).

This modality may potentially demonstrate advantages in terms of safety and prevention of secondary posterior capsular opacification. Aqualase represents an innovative and potentially advantageous modality for cataract extraction. It is commercially available already and has been found to be useful for soft cataracts.

I myself have experienced the aqualase technology just recently. We have used aqualase successfully in Indian cataracts up to grade 3. Aqualase is very effective while performing sculpting whereas chopping needs special attention since a fluid wave is preceded by nucleus emulsification at least 1 mm ahead of the tip. Hence, a good pupillary dilatation is prerequisite to this technology.

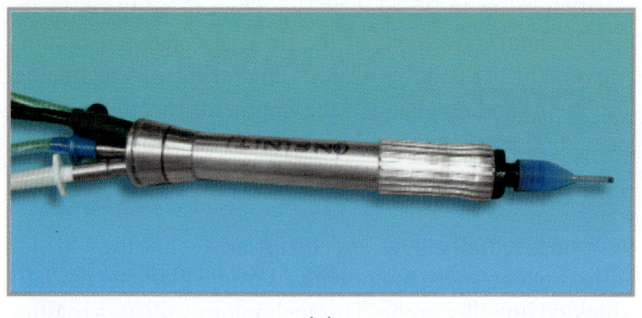
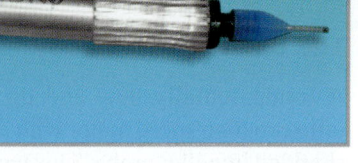

(a)

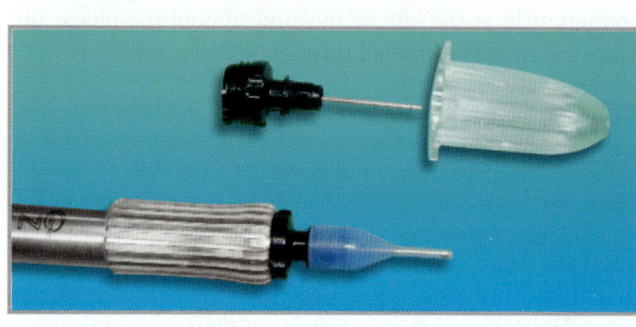

(b)

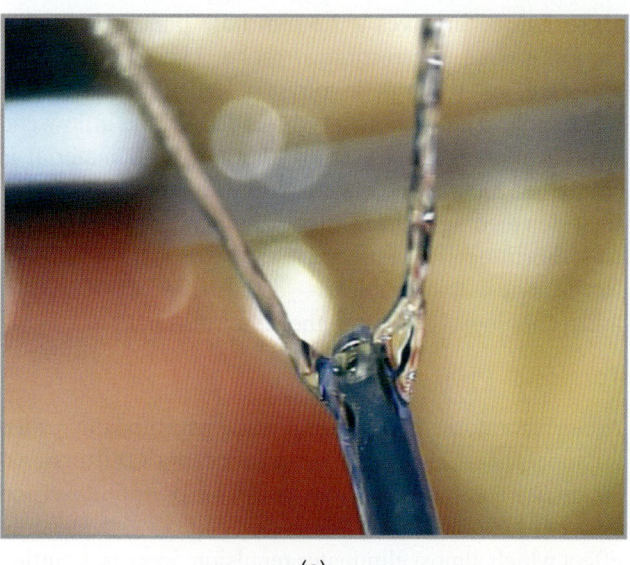
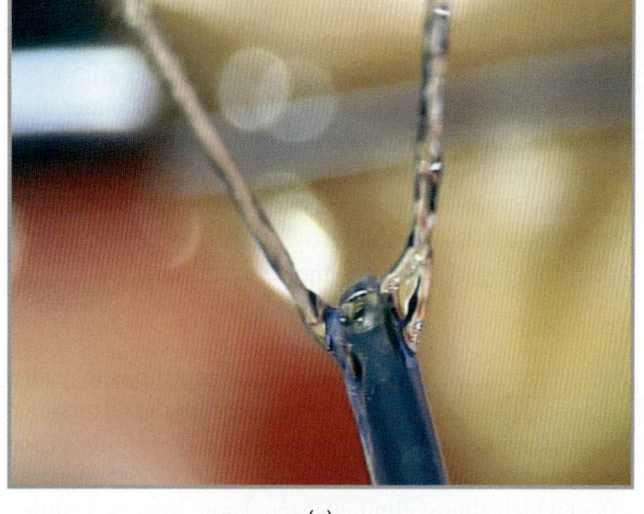

(c)

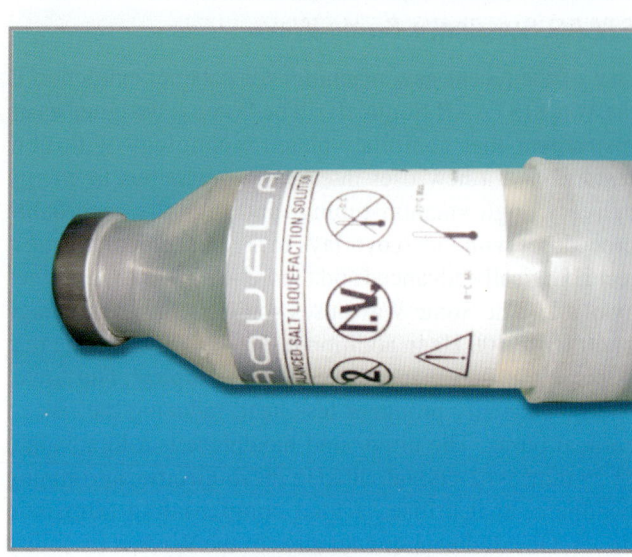

(d)

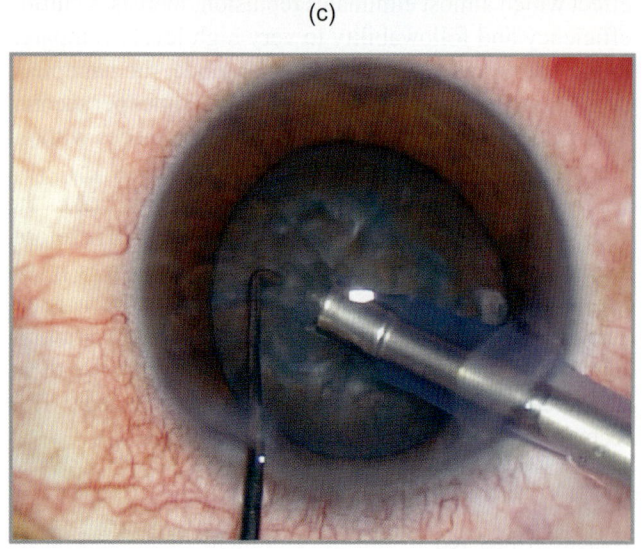

(e)

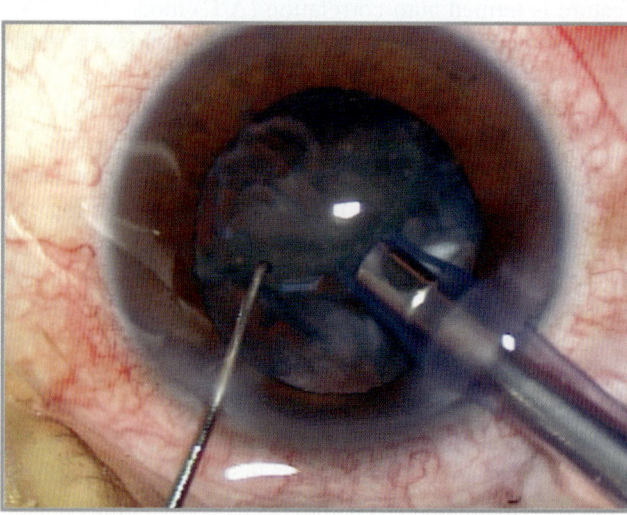

(f)

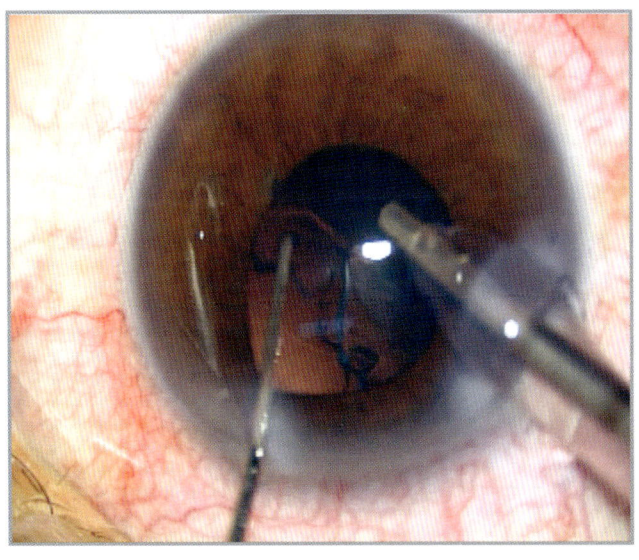

(g)

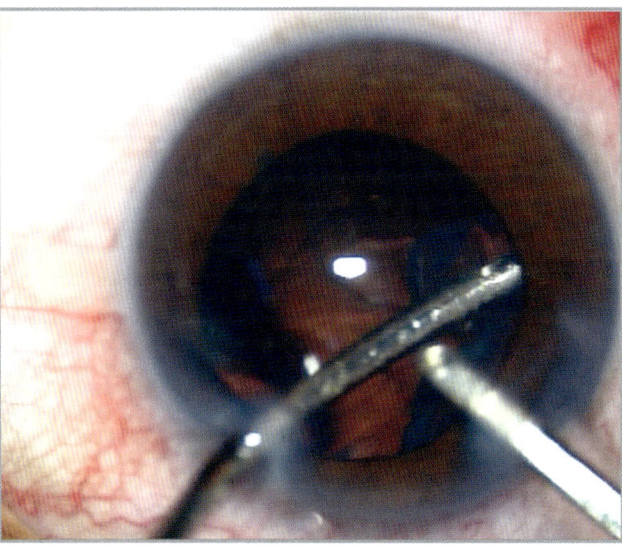

(h)

Fig. 5.24: (a) Aqualase: Phacoemulsification Surgery system, (b) Aqualase: Phacoemulsification handpiece and tip, (c) Aqualase: Handpiece and tip, (d) Aqualase: Balanced salt liquefaction solution, (e) Aqualase: Stop and chop, (f) Aqualase: Fragment removal, (g) Aqualase: Cortical plate removal (h) Aqualase: Cortical plate removal by bimanual I/A

Postoperative recovery has been found very satisfactory. Corneal clarity on very next day has been remarkable. Corneal endothelial cell loss is very minimal (less than 3%) following application of aqualase technology.

WHAT IS STILL IN THE FUTURE

- Developments are continuing and soon the coupled phaco will be available. However, simply using in infrasound works only on Grade 2–3 cataracts. It still does not function on the *Indian hard* cataract.
- However, a modification on the standard systems using a new, indigenously developed at BARC, is the high resistance clear Teflon sleeve for the phaco that permits easy transference to Microphaco for all.

CONCLUSION

All the goods are in a basket. Choose your phaco machine as per experience, quantum and quality of work and, of course, financial status. A Bullock cart can't match a Mercedes and a Mercedes can't match a Bullet train and none of them can match a supersonic jet. Obviously, a jet pilot can't ride a Bullock Cart and vice versa.

6

Instrumentation in Phacoemulsification Surgery

Dr Sanjivani Ambekar, Col JKS Parihar SM, VSM and Dr KS Basra

INTRODUCTION

Undoubtedly the significance of modifying and innovating new ophthalmic surgical instruments to meet the challenges of rapidly advancing technology in the field of modern cataract surgery cannot be undermined. One cannot expect an excellent outcome without having a good operating microscope, phacomachine, and surgical instruments apart from surgical expertise. Quality of instruments is of utmost importance for a smooth, quick, and precise surgical outcome. Substandard instrumentation is likely to damage ocular tissues during surgical procedures.

It is worth considering for each and every phaco surgeon to familiarise himself with a quality and the types of instruments suited to his own requirements. An attempt is being made to acquaint oneself with this specific need. However, it is always better to choose surgical instruments which should appropriately be tailor-made for specific and personalised surgical technique and preference.

Characteristic Features of Good Surgical Instruments

(i) A good surgical instrument is a useful adjuvant to perform the surgical procedure in an efficient, undisrupted and precise manner with enhanced ease of manipulation and surgical comfort.

(ii) Instrument should be made up of alloy metals having properties of being non-corrosive, and nontoxic to ocular tissue and should allow quick and safe manoeuvres under the operating microscope. The tip of the instrument should have dimensions proportionate to the tissue being handled.

(iii) It should be light in weight, handy and made up of non-corrosive and non-reflective metals under the illumination of operating microscope light.

(iv) It should have adequate tensile strength to overcome resistance within the tissues.

(v) All instruments being used in a given surgical procedure should ideally have uniform working distance from the tip of each instrument so as to provide quick and smooth completion of the surgical procedure.

(vi) The instrument should have an appropriate handle which should be able to maintain the equilibrium between surgical performance and intraoperative ease to handle such an instrument by having the balanced distribution of instrument's weight.

WHAT TYPES OF SURGICAL INSTRUMENTS SHOULD BE PREFERRED

Steel and Its Alloy

For several decades, surgical instruments made up of steel and subsequently, of steel alloy, enjoyed supremacy in the field of any surgical discipline despite the risk of rust formation and metal infiltration into the ocular tissue. However, with the advent of operating microscope and microsurgical procedures there was added need for much more sophisticated, smaller, light weight and precise microsurgical instruments to perform the given task of microsurgery in an accomplished and fine manner. The steel alloy instruments were found unsuitable to achieve such standards. The need to refine forceps, to provide sharper cutting tools, and to have more accurate needle holders was paramount. The titanium metal is an ideal substitute for all queries related to constraints of steel alloy encountered during microsurgical procedures.

Titanium Instruments

Titanium and its alloy came into practice in the early seventies. Modern titanium instruments have gone into complete transformation in terms of alloy contents, design, and innovations in ergodynamics of instrumentation. A close interaction between instruments manufacturers and ophthalmic surgeons has definitely contributed in a very significant manner to improve and produce designs as per the need of the latest surgical techniques.

Advantages Over Steel Alloy

(i) Titanium and its alloys are without any doubt far superior in terms of high precision and are more refined than those of stainless steel.

(ii) It is lighter than stainless steel, resists corrosion, is capable of maintaining its efficacy over repeated sterilisations, and can have a non-reflective surface.

(iii) Titanium alloys such as 6 AL-4V is found to have several physical properties like non-magnetic, higher grades of metallic hardness and durability, as well as a low thermal conductivity.

Disadvantage

The titanium instruments does not provide a sustained sharp edge as compared to any other alloy metals. However, the sharpness of titanium instruments can be enhanced by resurfacing the tips and sharp edges by diamond polishing.

Selective Preferences of Instruments: Titanium *vs* Metal

Sharp and fine instruments may be of titanium, whereas coarse instruments like cannulae, speculum, dialler may be of steel. However, it is preferred to have all instruments made of titanium.

Diamond and Sapphire Blades

Steel instruments and blades are synonymous with the standard instrumentation in the field of surgery [Fig. 6.1 (a) and (b)].

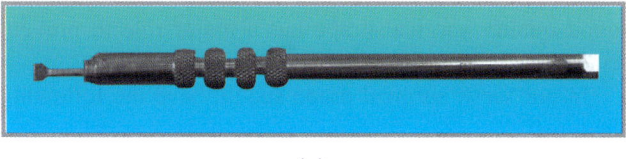

(a)

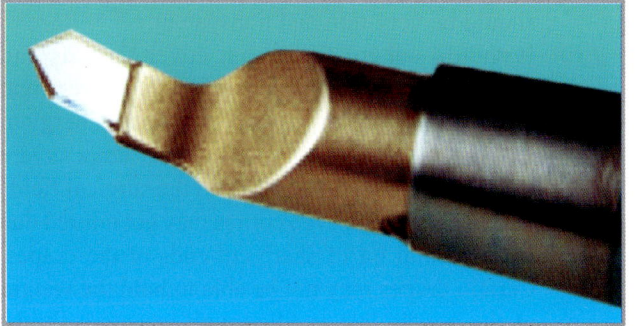

(b)

Fig. 6.1: Diamond blade

Steel blades were routinely used for different types of incisions in ophthalmic practice including the field of cataract surgery. The same trend continues with the phacoemulsification surgery. Though, titanium has taken over steel in case of microsurgical instrumentation, steel blades continue to its remain the first preference for most of the surgeons due to its easy availability, good results and cost efficacy factors of such blades. Despite such wide acceptance of steel blades, a need was always felt to have a superior type of material for incision due to the fact of the emerging problem of intraoperative stripping of endothelium and considerable resistance of the Bowman membrane during construction of incision.

New Horizon of Precision and Perfection of Sharpness: Diamond as Material for Ophthalmic Instruments and Knives and Blades

To overcome the problems and constraints of steel and its alloys, particularly in case of blades and knives, diamond was found to be a very effective and useful alternative. The superior quality of diamond being a sharp and the most precise cutting structure available had taken over wide acceptance rapidly by becoming the surgeon's first preference in phacoemulsification and other ophthalmic microsurgical procedures.

Notwithstanding the emergence of disposable high grade steel blades has been found to be very effective as single use blades, diamond blades continue to enjoy preference. Despite its superiority and precision of high order, diamond blades required several modifications in its design and quality of material as well as based on the surgeons' experiences and modifications in surgical techniques. Diamond ophthalmology blades are much sharper than the best steel blades. These blades have undergone significant modifications and innovations in terms of design, bevel, angulations, and edges of tips and quality of sharpness, precision and durability.

Newer designs are facilitating protection to the sharp tip by retraction of blade via a bayonet mechanism, into the knife handle when it is not in use or during the process of cleaning and sterilisation. Hence safety and longevity of sharp surfaces and edges can be maintained for longer durations. Further, the introduction of 'Luer Lock' adaptor is an excellent safety measure during stocking and transportation of diamond knives. This system is equally beneficial during cleaning, flushing of fluid jet stream that is possible through the handle without exposing the sharp tip of blade.

Despite initial higher cost, the diamond blade turns to be a good deal in the long term if maintained and used properly.

Evolution of Diamond Blades

The first generation diamond blades were bevelled from the superior surface, however, their sides were not bevelled.

This kind of surface was restricting side to side manoeuverability in case of subsequent extension of wound. Incision was prone to have lacerations on the flap.

Second generations blade were redesigned to have bevelled sides to resolve constraints of wound stripping.

Third generation diamond blades are further modified to sharp surfaces in all dimensions of crescent blades. These modifications have improved precision and efficacy of the surgeon.

Salient Features (Diamond Blades)

(i) Diamond is one of the most hard and sharp materials available for surgical blades.

(ii) Diamond incision has identical configuration of cutting surfaces in all the dimensions, hence, wound healing is rapid and produces least incision related induced astigmatism.

(iii) Least friction on the tissue being cut.

(iv) Minimal cutting pressure is required. Cutting edge and quality of incision remains identical and precise even after several incisions.

(v) Diamond knives can provide precise thickness and length of the incision by virtue of its having the ability to preset the blade depth at any given desired setting.

Salient Features (Sapphire Blades)

Quality of incision is superior than that of steel, however, inferior than that of diamond blades. Less durable as compared to diamond blades.

Relatively more fragile to autoclaving.

Economically less costly.

Types of Diamond/Sapphire Blades

Different types of diamond blades are available to meet the requirements of the particular kind of incision.

- Keratome 2.8, 3.0 and 3.2 mm.
- Trapezoid pattern 3.2 mm crescent blade for scleral tunnel configuration,
- 1 mm keratome, angulated, single edged, or trapezoid pattern micro blades for MICS incision.
- Sharp tip 15 degree, single edged blade for side port incision.
- Blades are available with titanium or polycarbonate handles with adjustable micro keratome to adjust depth of the incision.

Stainless Steel Microsurgical Blades

Present generation stainless steel microsurgical blades are very much in demand due to marked improvements in quality and design as well as inherent advantages of their cost-effectiveness and capability of constructing consistent, good and precise surgical incision which is very much

superior to the conventional stainless steel blades and close to that of diamond blades.

Disposable Surgical Instruments

Disposable surgical instruments are gaining popularity over conventional microsurgical instruments and cannulae due to better performance as well as cost-effectiveness as there is no need of repairs with disposables, which turns out to be costly and time-consuming. Use of disposables greatly reduces the risk of contamination and hence, is a very useful tool to reduce the incidence of endophthalmitis.

Resposable Instruments

Resposable instrument is a term given to surgical instruments having replaceable tip or cannulae with metal handles. Such types of instruments enjoy merits of being conventional as well as disposable surgical instruments. Such kind of instruments are much cheaper than standard surgical instruments and can be reusable for a small number of procedures. Various types of instruments like speculums, microsurgical blades, needle holders, scissors, forceps, diallers and choppers can be made available in this category.

PHACOINSTRUMENTATION CAN BE GROUPED AS PER SURGICAL STEPS

Surgical Drape

Modern phacoemulsification surgery is based on high vacuum, high flow of fluids and less energy. Undoubtedly, exposure to fluids is a major issue with cataract surgery in the present era, particularly in relation to the incidence of endophthalmitis.

Contamination of surgical fields from soiled lids and adjacent fields are essentially crucial factors in regard to higher probability of subsequent intraocular infections. A good quality surgical drape has a major role to prevent endophthalmitis.

In our view, surgical drape should have the following features:

(i) Drape should be thin, nontoxic and biodegradable.

(ii) Drape covering the central area of surgical field should be very thin and transparent.

(iii) It should adhere firmly but cover the lids and adjacent areas smoothly. However, its removal should not create any discomfort or skin allergy to the patient. We have noticed certain drapes were too thick and would not stick to the surgical fields during procedure; even cornea may get injured due to accidental hit of sharp cut ends of the drapes. Certain drapes may not be able to hold the weight of the pouch, that is filled with irrigating fluids, hence may shift from its normal position and may create inconvenience during surgery.

Speculum

Quality of the speculum leads to an excellent outcome. Good speculum should be able to provide adequate exposure of palpebral fissures so as to facilitate appropriate and precise instrumentation without compromising comfort of the patient and it should not produce undue pressure on the eyeball. Speculum should be light and able to hold the eyelids under gentle pressure. Too heavy speculum will evert eyelids or will shift during procedures due to its own weight.Too tight speculum leads to severe pressure on the eyeball as well as restrict manoeuvrability of instrumentation. Too loose speculum will not allow control of lid movement, particularly in case of surgery under topical anaesthesia which is a standard practice in reputed institutions. I myself prefer to use solid blade titanium speculum in all types of anterior segment procedures. We found this type of speculum very handy during topical phaco, besides, it holds drape in a proper position. However, every surgeon should have his own preference on the type and quality of instrumentation (Fig. 6.2).

Incision

The preparation of various types of incisions is considered to be a very specific and crucial manoeuvre in phacoemulsification surgery. The success of phaco procedures is exclusively based on precise and excellent incision, rhexis, and hydroprocedures. Besides, an excellent incision is the most significant factor in relation to the final visual outcome and pattern and quantum of astigmatism. In standard phacoemulsification, one needs to construct side port or incision for second instrumentation along with main incision in the form of scleral or clear corneal tunnel incision. In

certain situations, such tunnels may require extension or may get converted into conventional incisions. Following types of blades are in routine practise in phacoemulsification surgery [Fig. 6.3(a)].

(i) MVR, 15 degree angulated or 1 mm keratomes blades for side port /Second Incision.
(ii) 2.8/3.00/3.2 mm crescent keratomes for clear corneal valve incision.
(iii) Trapezoid Scleral tunnel blades.
(iv) 5.00/5.25/5.50 or 6.0 mm blades for extension of tunnel.

Side Port Incision

The preparation of a side port incision is considered to be an essential manoeuvre in phacoemulsification for bimanual instrumentation. This type of incision offers several advantages including [Fig. 6.3(b) and (c)]:

- Stabilising the globe; injecting viscoelastics without compromising integrity of the anterior chamber;
- Most crucial to handle bimanual manoeuvring of lens nucleus throughout the procedure.

Construction of side port incision can be done either as paracentesis or as small valve incision. Paracentesis can be done with the help of MVR (microvitreoretinal) knife or by 15 degree angulated side port blade. The author (JKSP) prefers to construct two small corneal valve incisions of 1 mm each with the help of either 15 degree angulated blades or specially designed 1 mm blade which is generally used in bimanual micro phaco. 1 mm diamond blades can also be used for this purpose.

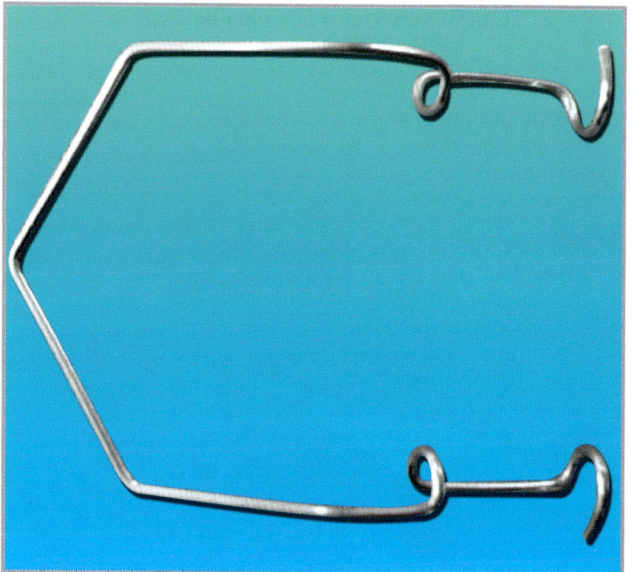

(a)

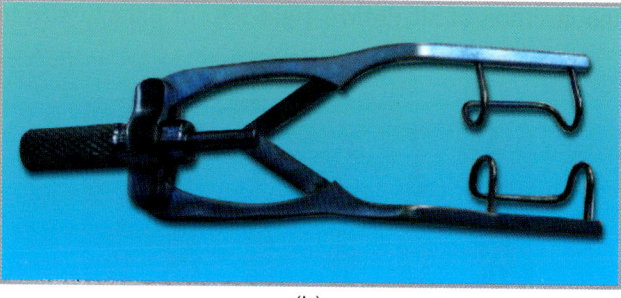

(b)

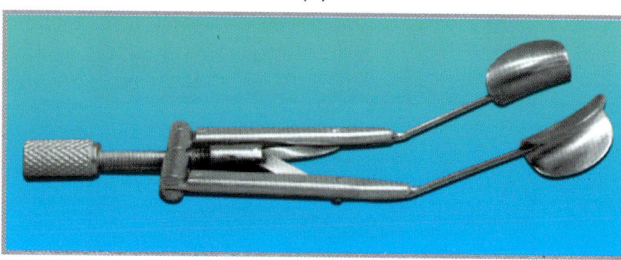

(c)

Fig. 6.2: (a) Barraquer Eye Speculum Fenestrated open blades, (b) Eye Speculum Solid blades (More suitable for temporal placement), (c) Liebermann–Tennant Eye Speculum Fenestrated open blades for temporal placement

However, the author prefers to convert one of the small incisions, subsequently into 2.8 mm valve incision as the main incision. It is essential to have the incision plane parallel to the iris plane in both the incisions.

The simultaneous construction of a two-valve incision allows coherent bimanual manoeuvre during rhexis and hydroprocedures as it acts well as a release valve if required to decompress the AC at any time.

Construction of Corneal Valve Incision

Corneal valve incision has become very popular and almost the standard incision for modern phacoemulsification technique due to obvious reasons of its simplified technique no need of conjunctival dissection and very comfortable surgical manipulations during topical as well as in case of no anaesthesia cataract surgery. Details of the surgical technique and other details have been discussed separately under incision techniques [Fig. 6.3(d) to (g)].

Corneal valve incision can be constructed with the help of calibrated diamond knife (preset to 250 microns) or metal blades. Most surgeons prefer to construct 2.8 mm initially for the purpose of nucleus management which is subsequently extended upto 3 or 3.2 mm by respective size keratomes for IOL implantation.

However, as described earlier, the author prefers to construct two incisions of 1 mm each as initial valve incisions and one of which is subsequently being converted into the main corneal valve incision of 2.8 mm.

A 5.5 mm extender blade will be required for the extension of incision for insertion of 5.5 mm phaco profile all PMMA IOL.

Whereas, 6.0 mm blade is essentially required for the enlargement of incision so as to make it appropriate for the insertion of all PMMA rigid IOL of 6.0 mm size in case of special situations or at the eventuality of any complication where foldable IOL implantation may not be feasible.

Instruments used for Scleral Tunnel Incision

Scleral tunnel incision finds itself at lower preference in the modern phacosurgery due to increasing popularity of topical anaesthesia and quick, smooth surgery through clear corneal incision. Over and above, an absolute quiet eye is less common following scleral tunnel incision due to handling of conjunctiva and sclera. Despite these limitations scleral tunnel is more astigmatic free and ideal for the case with corneal endothelial and stromal involvements. This is also preferred with concurrent glaucoma and cataract surgeries. Despite my definite preference towards corneal incision, it is recommended that every surgeon should choose incision of his own choice.

Recommended Instruments for Scleral Tunnel

3.2/3.0 mm, trapezoid, Crescent blades made up of steel or diamond are essential for this kind of incision. Diamond knife should be calibrated to 300 microns so as to provide 40–50% of the scleral thickness of sclera, a requisite for external scleral incision.

In case of metal blades, initial groove may be made with the help of 11 no. blade on bard parker handle or with the help of razor blade fragment. Straight crescent micro-knife of 3.0/3.2 mm width angled at 60° allows ease of handling; unlike a straight blade. The final entry to the chamber is being made with the help of 2.8/3.0/3.2 mm keratome blade which is usually angled at 45° for ease of handling by the surgeon. Straight keratomes can also be used.

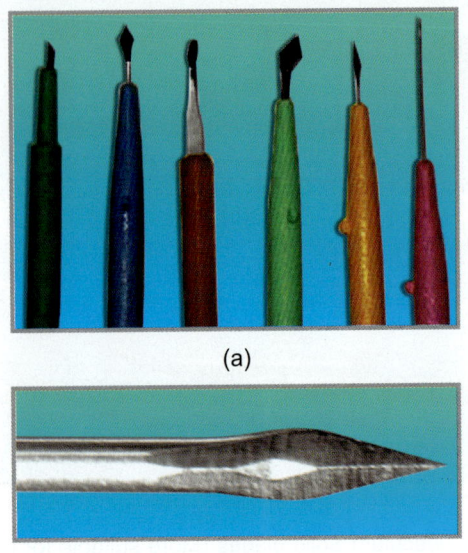

(a)

(b)

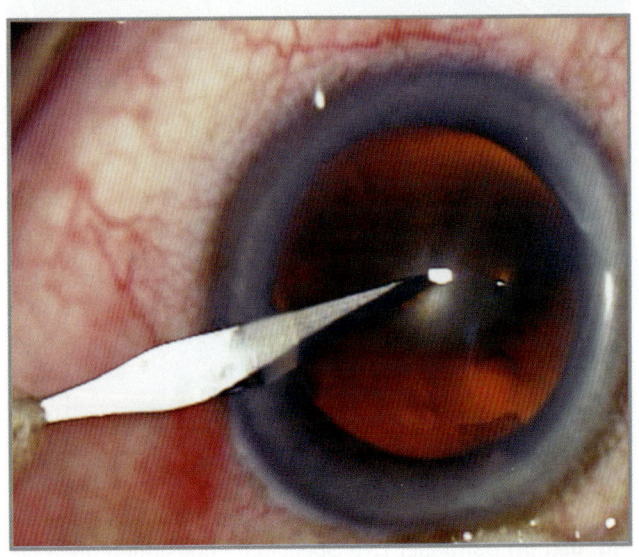

(c)

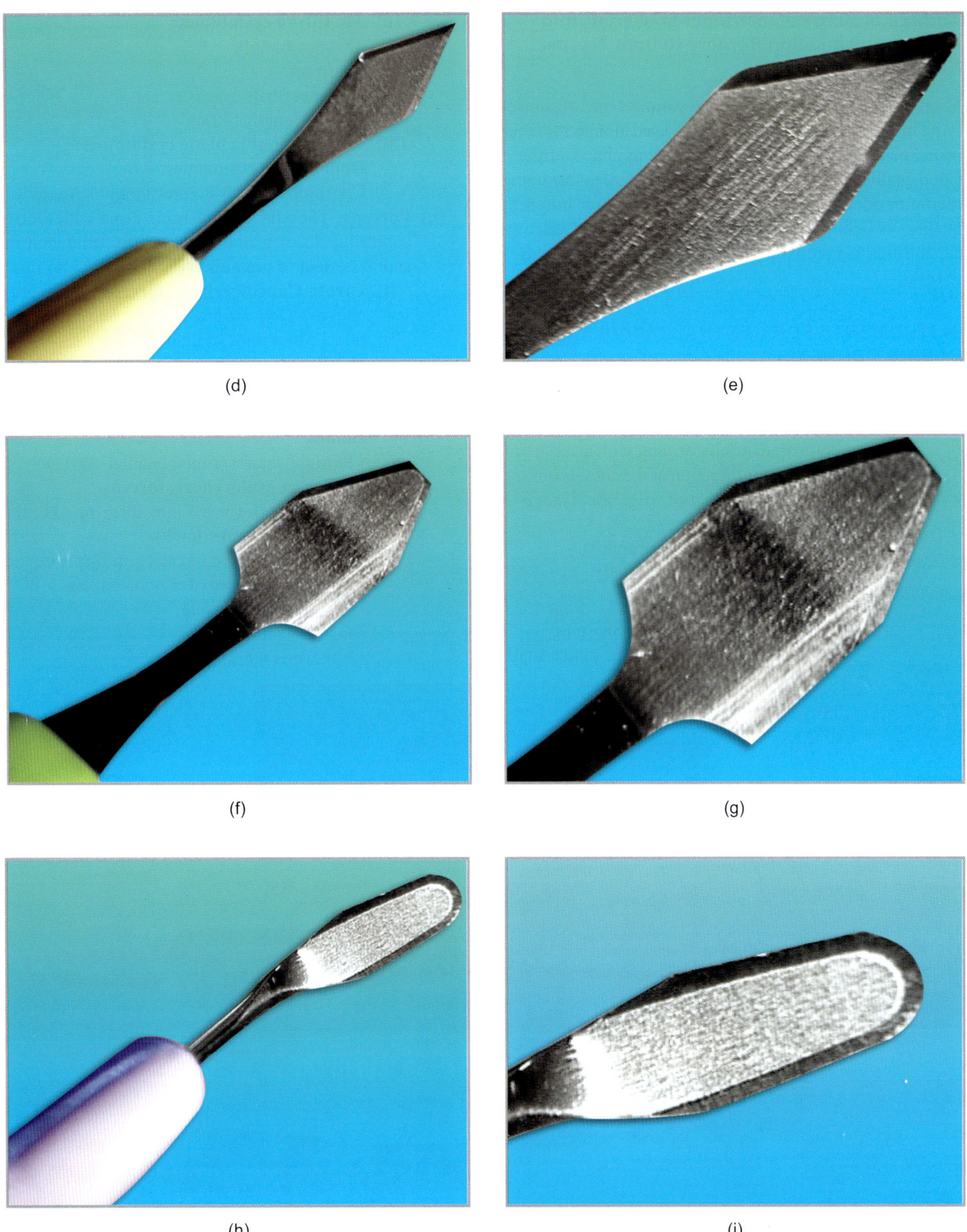

Fig. 6.3: (a) Various types of blades used in phacoemulsification surgery, (b) MVR blade for side port incision, (c) 15 degree angled blade for initial /side port incision, (d) and (e) 2.8 mm keratome for the construction of corneal valve incision, (f) and (g) 5.5 mm extender blade for the extension of incision for insertion of 5.5 mm phaco profile all PMMA IOL, (h) and (i) 3.2/3.0 mm, trapezoid, crescent blade for scleral tunnel incision

Additional Surgical Instruments used during Phacoemulsification Surgery to hold Tissue/IOL/Suture

Micro forceps (Colibri/Limbs) and various types of suture-tying or plane forceps are essentially used alongwith other instruments as and when required during phaco surgery. Good quality nonreflective titanium micro forceps are being recommended for these purposes due to their inherent qualities of light weight, non toxic and smooth manoeuvring capabilities as compared to the steel forceps [Fig. 6.4(a) to (e)].

INSTRUMENTS FOR CENTRAL CURVILINEAR CAPSULORRHEXIS

(a) Cystotomes, (b) Forceps and (c) Coaxial forceps

(a) **Cystotomes: irrigating or nonirrigating:** Can be either preprepared or self-forming with a variety of angulations, with the direction of the cutting surface equal to or opposite to that of irrigation. Gauge—varies from 22–30 G.
Irrigating cystotomes (formed, straight)
Irrigating cystotomes (formed, angled)

(i) **Kratz angled cystotomes:**
   - 60 degree angle
   - Angled 12 mm from tip
   - Sharp tip
   - 22 gauze shaft

(ii) **Mc Intyre cystotomes:**
   45 degree angle
   Sharp tip
   22 gauze shaft
   Overall length 14 mm

(iii) **Kelman double blade cystotomes:**
   Double edge cystotomes:
   Capsulorrhexis cystotome straight/Angled

(b) **Forceps:** They have converging arms with a disc capturing tip or a blunt lock-in tip, produced in stainless steel or titanium with sharp or blunt tips.

(i) **Utrata Capsulorrhexis forceps** [Fig. 6.5(a) and (e)]: Delicate grasping tips and extremely thin 11 mm long straight shanks
   - Tip length—11 mm, 45° angled
   - Iris stop platform, 8.5 mm from tip.

(ii) **Utrata capsulorrhexis forceps straight shanks**
   - Straight shanks, round handle.

(iii) **Masket capsulorrhexis forceps**
   Iris step platform 8.5 mm form tip, 11 mm long curved shanks Jaffe's
   Nevyas Adv: There forceps grip firmly on the flap even in abnormal conditions, e.g.
   - Non-uniform capsule
   - Insufficient mydriasis
   - Abnormal working angle.

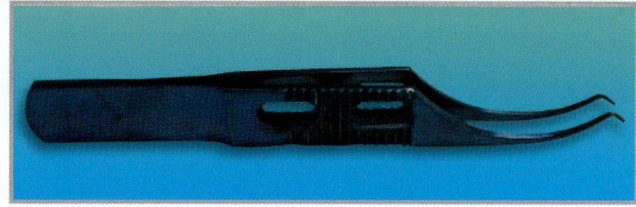

(a)

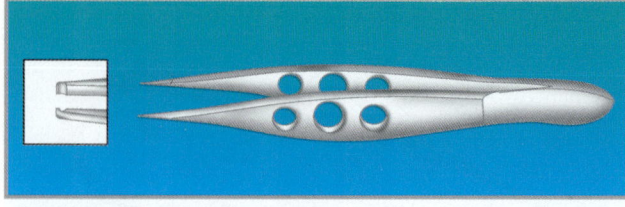

(b)

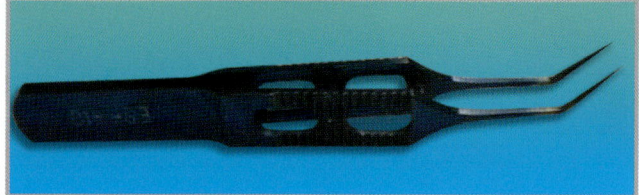

(c)

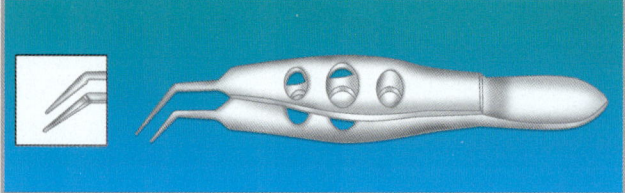

(d)

(e)

Fig. 6.4: (a) Micro Colibri corneo scleral forceps 1 x 2 teeth, 0.12 mm with tying platform, (b) and (c) Pierse type micro forceps with platform overall length 85 straight, (d) and (e) McPherson fragment forceps smooth jaws 5 mm long, 7.5 mm angled ideal for IOL and 8-0 to 11-0 sutures

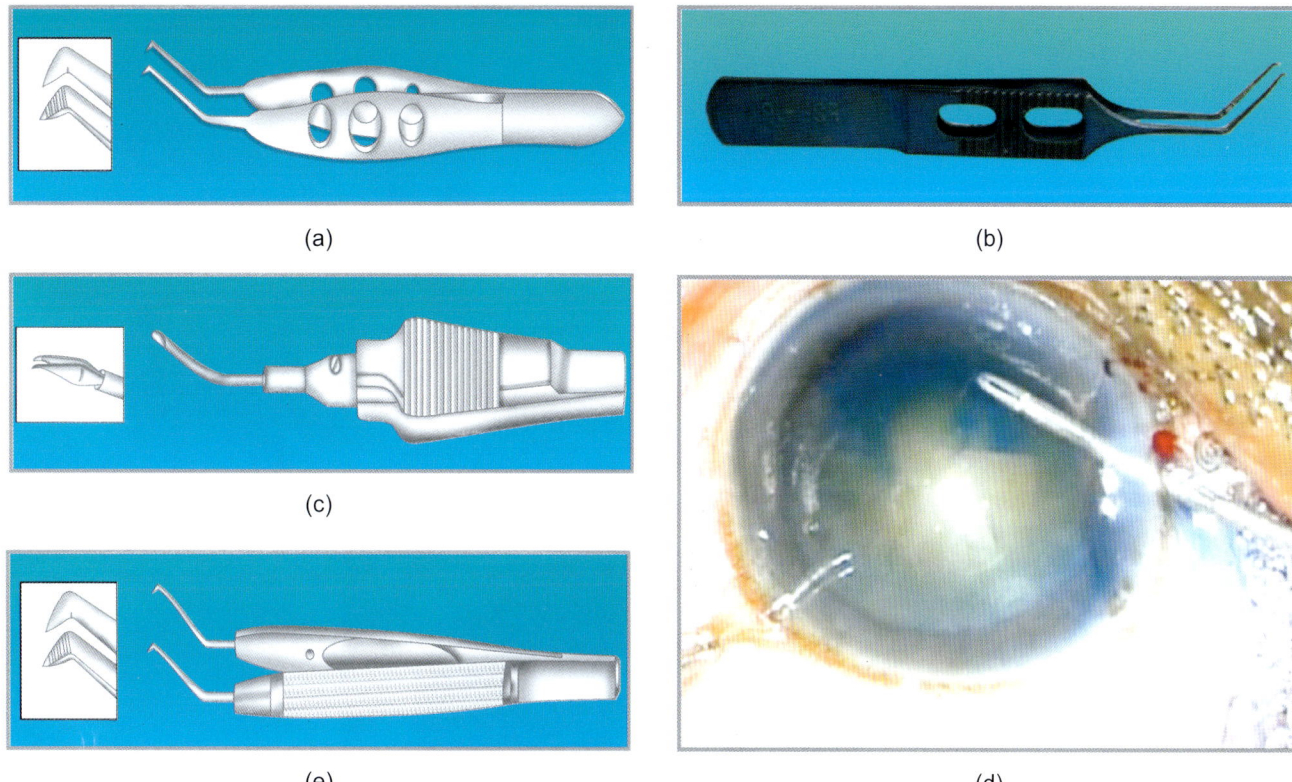

Fig. 6.5: (a) and (b) Utrata capsulorrhexis forceps, (c) Utrata capsulorrhexis forceps straight shanks, (d) Microsurgical capsulorrhexis forceps (Appasamy /India), (e) One tip sharp and one tip blunt

(c) **Coaxial forceps:** Principles of forceps used in endovitreal surgery.

Caporossi co-axial forceps: Blunt tip and is built around a man drill with very small diameter (27 G)

Dossi forceps: Larger (21 G) with sharper edges.

Advantages

• Can be used through an opening of 1.0 to 1.4 mm thereby leading to chamber maintenance better control of rhexis.
• All the advantages of capsulorrhexis forceps.
• Capsulorrhexis forceps with one sharp tip and one blunt tip

Cross Action Capsulorrhexis Forceps

A more specific example of the application of such principles is in the inamura cross action capsulorrhexis forceps. The use of a cross action mechanism positions the fulcrum within the incision, minimising the amount of gap and thereby reducing the amount of viscoelastic loss from the anterior chamber. Furthermore, a fulcrum closer to the instrument tip provides more exquisite control of the action, while allowing continual tip alignment. The use of serrations at the tip enhances the grip of the anterior capsule tissue, thereby facilitating the procedure of complete curvilinear capsulorrhexis.

IRRIGATING CANNULA FOR HYDROPROCEDURES

Different types of irrigating cannulae are essentially required to achieve excellent hydroprocedures which is of utmost significance for smooth conclusion of phacoemulsification surgery. Three types of irrigating cannulae are basically used during hydroprocedures:

(i) Hydrodissection cannula
(ii) Hydrodelineation cannula
(iii) Stromal hydration cannula

(i) Hydrodissection Cannula

Hydrodissection refers to the injection of balanced salt solution/Ringer's lactate under the anterior capsular flap until the fluid courses around the equator at the cortico-epinuclear plane, flows under the epinucleus and separates the epinucleus from its cortical attachments. The endpoint of this procedure is the convex "fluid-wave" seen crossing the field away from the point of injection. On completion of the procedure, the nucleus should rotate freely in the capsular bag [Fig. 6.6(a) to (c)].

Hydrodissection is best performed using a 25 gauge cannula with a blunt round tip, though opinions vary with different surgeons preferring cannula ranging from 25 to 30 G. This cannula is placed on a 2 cc syringe filled with balanced salt solution/Ringer's lactate.

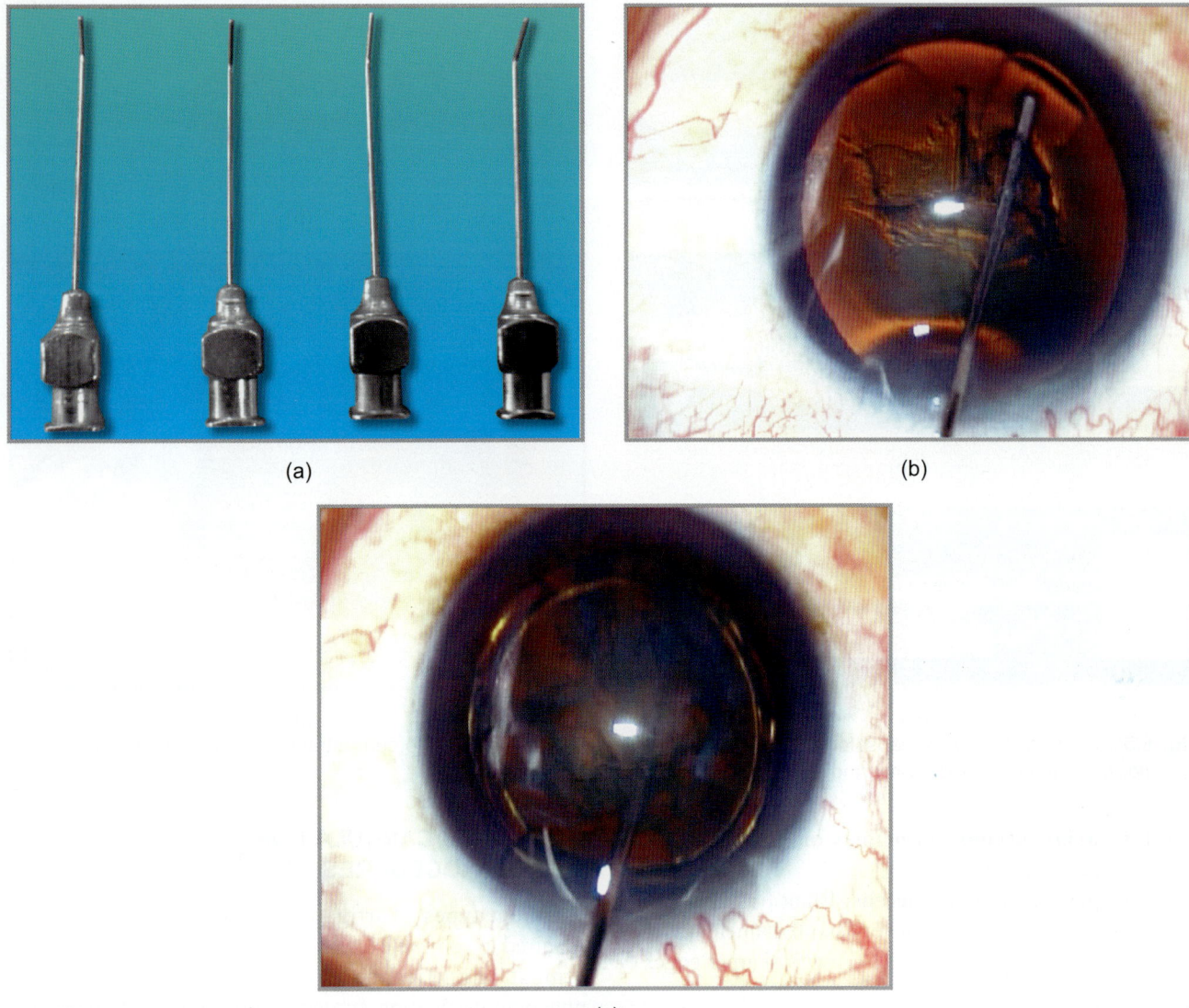

Fig. 6.6: (a) Hydroprocedure cannula, (b) Placement of hydrodissection cannula, (c) Hydrodissection (golden ring)

The tip of the cannula is passed under the edge of the anterior capsule obtained after CCC and advanced for 1 mm. Care is taken to keep the cannula perpendicular to the capsulotomy edge. Now, a minimal amount of fluid is injected in a spurt. A distinct fluid wave can be seen progressing centrally from the point of injection. This wave is due to the fluid interface coursing all around the cortex at the corticoepinuclear plane, in the process breaking the corticoepinuclear adhesions. Ultimately, the fluid emerges into the anterior chamber from the end opposite to the point of injection.

(ii) Hydrodelineation Cannula

Hydrodelineation should follow hydrodissection. The preferred cannula for hydrodelamination is a 26 G or 25 Gauze cannula with a blunt tip to embed the cannula into the nucleus without significant posterior stress. However, for the ease of use, most of the surgeons perform hydrodelamination with the same cannula that they have used for hydrodissection. In this procedure, the cannula is pushed into the mass of the nucleus just central to the edge of the CCC in a tangential position till it meets with resistance. At a particular point, the nucleus will stop giving way and care is to be taken here, to resist the temptation of digging deeper with an aim to reduce the phacoable nucleus. The posterior push, if applied, causes zonular stress and irreparable zonular damage.

(iii) Stromal Hydration Cannula

Stromal hydration is an important step to achieve hydrosealing to the incision lips. The cannula should be able to push a gentle pressure wave of fluid jet into stromal layer at the incision site (Fig. 6.7).

The cannula should be hard enough to sustain fluid manoeuvre and able to allow fluid to get into stromal layers. The preferred cannula for stromal hydration is a 24 G or

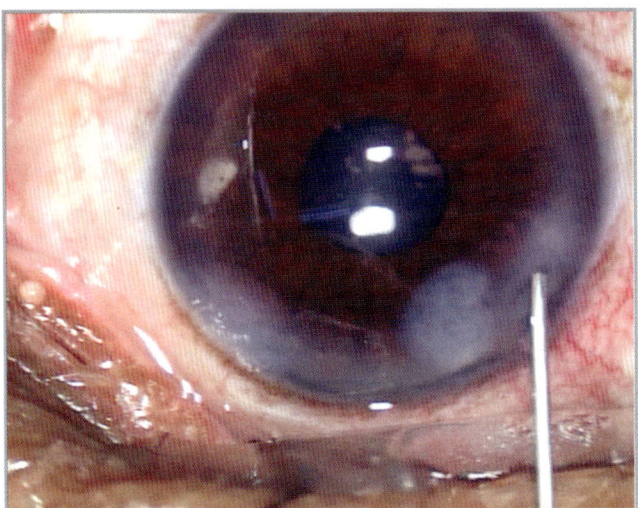

Fig. 6.7: Stromal hydration cannula

25 Gauze cannula with a round and blunt pointed tip to embed the cannula into the stroma under slight and gentle stress.

INSTRUMENTS USED ALONG WITH PHACOEMULSIFICATION TIP

Sculpting/Divide and Conquer Technique of Nucleotomy

Rotation of Nucleus

Rotation of nucleus can be done with the help of a second instrument. A good quality dialler or Y pusher is an ideal choice for this purpose. Choppers can also be used.

Splitting/Cracking of Nucleus

Two instruments (either a phaco probe and a chopper or 2 choppers or diallers) are required for this manoeuvre dialler should have a blunt tip on a 1 mm long shaft with a 75 or 90 degree angulation. Choppers should have blunt tips but sharp posterior surfaces and angulations of 75 to 90 degree. The instrument should be able to have access right up to the roof of the trench.

The instruments should be able to apply force in opposite directions on the wall of the trench in such a manner that the centre tends to depress slightly and the periphery of the nucleus should lift upwards.

Instruments for Chopping Technique of Nucleotomy

Chopper

One of the main uses of a chopper is in the Nagahara chop technique and in the stop and chop technique, in which the chopper is brought from the 6 o'clock position towards the phaco tip (which is in the nucleus as close to the incision as possible). Optimum tip length is 1.5 to 1.75 mm.

Nagahara Karate Chopper

- Tip length — 1.5 mm
- Its end is spear-shaped for ease of insertion into the nucleus (Fig. 6.8).

Agarwal's phaco chopper has a 1 mm fully cutting edge.

Appasamy Phaco chopper

A 0.75 mm blunt polished tip which does not damage the posterior capsule.

Gillum phaco splitter and side port splitter
Steinert nucleus chopper: Mackorl
Uses of a chopper:
- Nucleus rotation
- Nucleus cracking (divide and conquer)
- For feeding nucleus fragments to phaco probe
- Keep fragments away from corneal endothelium.

Other instruments that can be used are:

Sinskey lens manipulating hook: A 0.2 mm diamond blunt tip cyclodialysis spatula (castroviejo's)

Parihar's Lateral Chopper

Specially designed for lateral incision phaco surgery without changing or shifting the surgeon's position. Very useful with internuclear or peripheral chopping in cases of hard cataract.

IOL DELIVERY SYSTEMS (HOLDER AND FOLDER)

(a) Forceps: (holder and folder)
(b) Injectors: (Silicon-plate haptic lenses have to be delivered by this system.)

Forceps

(i) **Folder:** Used to fold the lens along the diameter Direct action or cross action [Fig. 6.9(a) to (e)].
(ii) **Holder:** To insert the folded lens into the capsular bag.
Direct action or cross action.

Two basic techniques are currently used for insertion of foldable IOL with forceps.

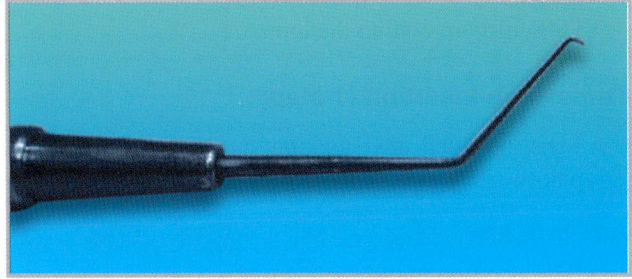

Fig. 6.8: Nagahara Karate Chopper

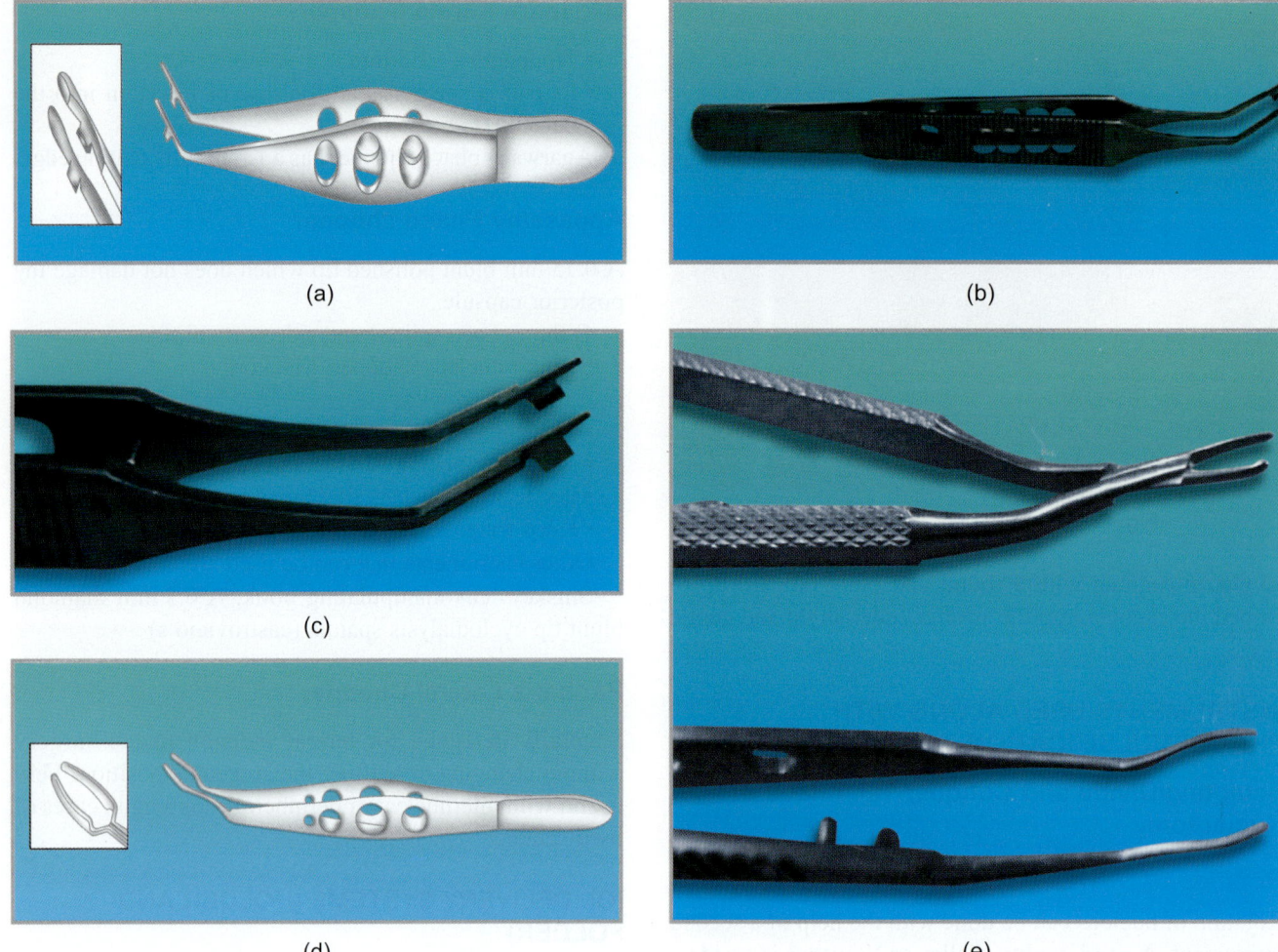

Fig. 6.9: (a), (b) and (c) Lens folding forceps for acrylic foldable lens with notches, (d) and (e) Neuhann lens holding forceps for foldable IOL implant

Longitudinal Insertion (2 step technique)

Lens is folded such that loops are along the greatest axis of the instrument.

Advantages

- Easy insertion.
- Good control

Disadvantages

- Difficulty in folding and gripping with insertion forceps.
- Difficulty in rotating the loop.

Transverse Insertion (1 step)

- Lens is folded after making sure that the loops are placed transversely.

Advantages

- IOL insertion in one manoeuvre .
- Good control of folding and unfolding.

Disadvantages

- Difficult to insert through the incision, leading to tissue trauma.
- Greater chances of loop damage.
- Difficult to insert both loops inside rhexis.
- Higher risk of posterior capsule or rhexis rupture.
- Greater endothelial damage.

Insertion of Foldable Lenses with Injector

IOL implant injector systems have become an integral component of IOL surgery. These devices provide excellent opportunity to implant IOL through a very small incision by the nontouch technique. Hence, possibility of preoperative contamination of IOL becomes quite less as compared to manual insertion with the help of IOL holding/folding forceps delivery system. Despite several advantages, there are certain under-mentioned inherent constraints with the injector systems.

(i) Lens can be damaged while loading and unloading.

(ii) Each lens make requires a different injector.

(iii) If injector is used with open loops, the loops and/ or lens can be damaged.

(iv) Stretching of incision edges with injector.

(v) Unpredictable delivery of IOL may take place in the anterior chamber or in the bag which may lead to an injury to the posterior capsule.

Various types of injector systems are available for different types of IOL implants. Most reputed companies have designed specific types of injector for their own IOL implants. Both metallic and disposable injectors are available for IOL implantation. IOL implant delivery systems are described subsequently in detail in a separate chapter.

Special instruments used in phaconit (Needle incision technique) are discussed along with MICS surgery in a separate chapter.

CONCLUSION

Instrumentation is one of the most significant and integral components of modern surgical field which has a perfect blend of skill and technology to produce unbelievable results. A close and perfect coordination among ophthalmic surgeons, engineers and surgical equipment and instrument manufacturers is an essential demand of the day. A conscientious surgeon should not settle down with existing resources only. A close look and composite effort to combine virtual three-dimensional digital graphic imaging, ergo dynamic factors of instrumentations and newer modifications in the field of surgical technology is the need of the day, which will ultimately lead to greater heights and towards the final aim and result of all times—the eagles vision in all conditions.

BIBLIOGRAPHY

1. Kelman CD. Phacoemulsification and aspiration. Am J Ophthalmol 1967;64:23–33.
2. Pierse JD. Summary of instrument development. Adv Ophthalmol 1970;22:273.
3. Pierse JD, Steele AD, Walter DO. The introduction of titanium alloys in ophthalmic microsurgical instruments. Br J Ophthalmol 1976;60:597–598.
4. Christ FR, Buchen SY, Deacon J, et al. Biomaterials used for intraocular lenses. In: Wise DL, Trantolo DJ, Altobelli DE, et al, eds. Encyclopaedic handbook of biomaterials and bioengineering. Part B: Applications. Vol 2. New York, Basle, Hong Kong: Marcel Dekker, 1995;1261–1313.
5. Pierse JD. Diamonds: Their design for and influence on modern microsurgery. Dev Ophthalmol 1981;1:15–2.
6. Duckworth and Kent. Ophthalmic titanium surgical instruments catalogue: new dimensions. 1998–1999 edition.
7. Steinert RF, Brint SF, White SM, et al. Astigmatism after small incision cataract surgery: a prospective, randomised, multicentre comparison of 4 and 6.5 mm incisions. Ophthalmology 1991;98:417–423.

7

Optical Aspects of Intraocular Lens Power Calculation in Different Situations (Including Applied)

Col JKS Parihar SM,VSM, Lt. Col S Bandopadhyay and Dr Pradeep Misra

INTRODUCTION

Today cataract surgery with IOL implantation is a successful procedure. It is minimally invasive, rehabilitation is quick, and complication rate is low. In addition, the refractive outcome is excellent and vision can be improved to a better level than what it was before cataract formation. The main factor for attaining a good outcome and optimal postoperative refraction is precise and accurate IOL power calculation. Once the IOL is implanted, the patient must live with any mistake that may have been committed or be subject to removal and reimplantation of the IOL which in itself has many intra- and postoperative complications. The intraocular lens power is calculated using the standard formula and is dependent on accurate measurements of the axial eye length, the corneal radius, and the anterior chamber depth. The importance of ocular biometry is well documented. Devices like A-scan have made it convenient to accurately determine the axial length of the eye. In the absence of ultrasonography in the earlier days, IOL power was determined using intelligent guesswork on the basis of concept of Standard and IDEM lenses and taking into consideration various factors like preoperative refraction and the age of patient, etc.

The corneal radius is typically measured using keratometry, while the anterior chamber length is measured by slit lamp illumination. Ultrasound, using either immersion techniques or applanation where the ultrasound transducer is placed on the surface of the cornea, is used to assess the axial eye length. The applanation technique is most commonly used. Recently, partial coherence interferometry has been introduced as an alternative technique to measure the axial length of the eye. This technique relies on a laser Doppler technique to measure the echo delay and the intensity of infrared light reflected back from tissue interfaces. The measurement of the corneal radius is performed by using traditional keratometry principles and measurement of the anterior chamber depth by slit lamp illumination. The IOL Master (Carl Zeiss) is a device approved by the US Food and Drug Administration (FDA). It includes a software that uses the above measurements to calculate the intraocular lens power according to standard formula. This technique, which is thought to be more accurate and precise than ultrasound biometry, may ultimately contribute to improved post-surgical refraction. Partial coherence interferometry may also be referred to as optical (or ocular) coherence biometry or laser Doppler interferometry.

CALCULATING THE APPROXIMATE IOL POWER WITHOUT BIOMETRY (PRE-BIOMETRY ERA)

This only has an historical importance for these methods were used when A-scan and keratometer were not available.

This is, essentially a guesswork approach to determine the IOL power. The different approaches to this guesswork lens calculation are:
1. IDEM lenses
2. Standard lens
3. Emmetropia lens.

IDEM Lens

The concept was developed by Gernet and Zorkendorfer and it had shown that the power of natural lens is 23.70 D. The crystalline lens is located 6 mm behind the corneal apex while the PC IOL is further forward, hence the power of PC IOL should be weaker than that of the crystalline lens. Therefore, a + 20 D PC IOL will restore the preoperative refraction. The power of IOL for other site of implantation can be calculated on the basis of its distance from the corneal apex, e.g. – Angle supported AC IOL – +17 D

Iris clip IOL +18 D

PC IOL +20 D

This method has an important limitation that is, an IDEM lens will restore the preoperative refractive state of the eye only if the preoperative crystalline lens power is indeed +23.70 D. This, however, is not always the case. As the total refractive power of the eye depends on multiple factors like the axial length, corneal curvature, lens power, anterior chamber depth, hence, even if the eye is emmetropic the crystalline lens power may not be 23.7 D. Due to this an error of +/– 2 is common.

Standard Lens

The concept here is that the lens is 2 D stronger than IDEM lenses, thus rendering the eye to be about 1.5 D myopic as compared to its primary state of refraction. Since this concept was most commonly used before biometric calculation became popular, these lenses were called standard lens.

Emmetropia Lens

The emmetropia lens concept was a further refinement on the IDEM lens concept. Here the primary refraction, that is, the refraction of the eye before cataract developed, is taken into consideration. For this, a careful refractive history that shows the refraction and spectacle correction should be available with old records.

Power of PC IOL in hypermetropia = Power of IDEM lens + (Preoperative refractive error × 1.25)

Power of PC IOL in myope = Power of IDEM lens – (Preoperative refractive error × 1.25)

However, this method is also fraught with errors due to the following reasons:

(a) The refractive history may not always be available or inaccurate.

(b) This is assessed on the IDEM concept, which does not take into account the other parameters (axial length, corneal curvature, etc.) on which the total refractive power of the eye depends.

THEORETICAL AND REGRESSION FORMULAE FOR POWER CALCULATIONS OF IOL IMPLANTS

This concept of IOL power calculation here depends on formulae, in which the parameters required are essentially keratometric reading (K), with a USG measurement of axial length (AL) and in some cases, the anterior chamber depth (ACD).

Various computer programmes and normograms have been developed for accurate IOL power calculation.

The formula for power calculations is essentially of two types:
1. Theoretical formula
2. Regression formula

Theoretical Formula

These formula's are essentially based on geometric optics as applied to schematic eye with the aim to calculate the IOL power, which will lead to postoperative emmetropia.

These formula's are based on following variables:
(i) The axial length of eyeball
(ii) Average keratometric reading
(iii) The estimated postoperative anterior chamber depth (ACD)

It was in 1967 that Fyodorov and coworkers, first presented a theoretical formula based on geometric optics. Subsequently, a number of formulae followed of which, the best known are of Binkhorst, Colenbrander, Thijssen. These theoretical formula's, while appearing different in the first glance, are essentially the same, except for other then the correction factor. Also, an assumed value for ACD was used in these formula's.

These formula's are as follows:

1. Fyodorov $P = \dfrac{N - LK}{\dfrac{(L - C)\,(1 - CK)}{N}}$

2. Colenbrander $P = \dfrac{N}{LC} - \dfrac{N}{\dfrac{N - C}{K}}$

3. Binkhorst $P = \dfrac{1000\dfrac{(NR)}{0.333} - L}{(L - C)\dfrac{(NR)}{0.333} - C}$

P = Lens implant power for emmetropia
N = Aqueous and vitreous refractive index
L = Axial length
K = Corneal curvature
C = Postoperative anterior chamber depth (mm)
R = Radius of curvature (mm)

These theoretical formulae can essentially be represented by the following formula which is essentially the algebraic transformation of theoretical formula:

$$P = \frac{N}{LC} - \frac{NK}{N - KC}$$

The theoretical formulae were originally used for iris-supported lens for which it gave accurate value. However, when PC IOL implantation became popular these formulae showed the following shortfalls:

(i) They tend to predict too large an emmetropic value in short eyes (less than 22 mm) and too small a value in long eyes (>24.5 mm)

(ii) These formulae require ACD calculation, which itself is derived from guesswork.

Hence, accuracy of the IOL power depends on the accuracy of this guesswork. For iris supported IOL this guesswork of ACD was reliable, while for PC IOL the ACD was more unpredictable.

Regression Formula

The shortfalls of the theoretical formula were mitigated by the use of a linear regression technique to determine a linear formula for predicting the emmetropic implant power. This technique makes use of the experience of a surgeon already familiar with implant surgery to find the relationship between preoperative axial length, corneal power, implant power and postoperative refractive error.

When a large number of implant cases are studied and are fed into a regression analysis, an accurate linear formula can be determined to calculate the IOL power from AL (axial length) and K (keratometric) value. The ACD (anterior chamber depth) value is incorporated as a constant and the value of which is itself derived from the regression analysis.

A number of regression formulae are available out of which SRK (Sanders, Retzlaff and Kraft)—formula is the most popular.

SRK I Formula

P = A–2.5 L – 0.9 K
P = IOL power
A = Constant specific for each type and design of lens
K = Average keratometry in dioptres
L = Axial length in mm

For 1 mm change in axial length, the lens power changes by 2.5 D and for change in 1 D in K reading, the lens implant power changes by 0.9 D. The constant A is greater when the lens is closer to the retina. Therefore, it is highest with PC IOL and least with AC IOL.

This performs well for eyes between axial lengths of 22–24.5 mm. For eyes less than 22 mm, the regression formula tends to predict a lesser value and for longer eyes, a higher value.

Hence, this formula was further modified to solve this error of regression formula.

SRK II Formula

The basic equation is the same as SRK I formula but depending on the axial length of the eye, the following adjustments are made:

If AL is <20 mm –P +3 D
If AL 20–20.99 mm –P +2 D
If AL 21–21.99 mm –P +1 D
If AL 22–24.5 mm –P
If AL >24.5 mm –P –0.5 D

Where P is the IOL power derived by SRK I formula.

Modified SRK II Formula

In this formula, the power P derived by SRK I formula is adjusted as follows, which gives a more predictable value as compared to SRK II formula.

If AL is <20 mm –P + 1.5 D

If AL 20–20.99 mm –P + 1 D
If AL 21–21.99 mm – P +0.5 D
If AL 22–24.5 mm – P
If AL 24.5–26 mm – P –1 D
If AL is >26 mm – P–1.5 D

Subsequently, other modern formula's were developed which can be grouped as follows:

 (i) Second generation theoretical formula
 (ii) Second generation modified empirical formula
 (iii) Combination of theoretical and empirical formula

Holladay Formula

It represents a further refinement of second generation theoretical formula's. It uses both axial length and corneal power to predict the position of the implant. The Holladay formula would not suffer from the problems of a linear formula describing a nonlinear system because it is a nonlinear formula. This formula also incorporates the surgeon factor, which the surgeon can modify by studying his own cases, it is a feedback loop by which a surgeon can improve upon his IOL power calculation accuracy.

Holladay Formula and Constants

Recommended constants and measured values
 n_c = Refractive index of cornea = 4/3
 K = Average K reading (dioptres)
 n_a = Refractive index of aqueous = 1.336
 R = Average corneal radius (mm) = 337.5/K
 RT = Retinal thickness factor = 0.200 mm
 AL = Measured ultrasonic axial length (mm)

Chosen values

 V = Vertex distance of pseudophakic spectacles (mm), default = 12 mm
 Ref = Desired postoperative spheroequivalent refraction (dioptres)
 SF = "surgeon factor" = distance from aphakic anterior iris plane to optical plane of IOL (mm)

Definitions of Other Variables

AG = Anterior chamber diameter from angle to angle (mm)
ACD = Anatomic anterior chamber depth (mm), distance from corneal vertex to anterior iris plane
Aim = Modified axial length (mm) = ultrasonic axial length (AL) + retinal thickness factor (RT)
I = Power of IOL (dioptres)
ARef = Actual postoperative spheroquivalent refraction (dioptres)

Equations

Eq 1. Rag = R, if R < 7 mm, then Rag = 7 mm
Eq 2. AG = 12.5 AL/23.45, if AG > 13.5 mm, then AG = 13.5 mm

Eq 3. $ACD = 0.56 + Rag - \{SQRT [Rag\ Rag - (AG\ AG/4)]\}$

IOL power (I) from desired postoperative refraction (Ref)

Eq 4. $I = 1000\ n_a\{n_aR - (n_c - 1)\ Aim - 0.001\ Ref\ [V(n_aR - (n_c1)\ Aim) + Aim\ R]\}\ (Aim - ACD - SF)(n_aR - (n_c - 1)\ (ACD + SF) - 0.001\ Ref\ \{V\ [n_aR - (n_c - 1)(ACD + SF)] + (ACD + SF)\ R\}$

Resultant refraction (Ref) from IOL power (I)

Eq 5. $Ref = 1000\ o,\ [n_aR - (n_c - 1)\ Aim] - I\ (Aim - ACD - SF)(n_aR - (n_c - 1)(ACD + SF)]\ n_a(V(n_aR - (n_c - 1)\ Aim) + Aim\ R) - 0.001\ I\ (Aim - ACD - SF)\ [V(n_aR - (n_c - 1)(ACD + SF) + (ACD + SF)\ R]$

Reverse solution: "Surgeon Factor" (SF) from IOL power (I) and actual stabilised postoperative refraction (A Ref)

Eq 6. $AQ = (n_c - 1) - \{(0.001\ A\ Ref\ [V(n_c - 1) - R])\}$

Eq 7. $BQ = ARef\ 0.001\ [(Aim\ V(n_c - 1)] - \{R[Aim - (VnJ)]\} - \{[(n_c - 1)\ Aim] + (n_aR)\}$

Eq 8. $CO.! = 0.001\ ARef\ \{[V(n_aR) - (n_c - 1)\ Aim] + (Aim\ R)\}$

Eq 9. $COj = \{1000\ n_a[(n_aR) - (n_c - 1)\ Aim] - CW^{\wedge}/I$

Eq 10. $CQ_3 = (Aim\ N_aR) - (0.001\ ARef\ Aim\ V\ R\ N_a)$

Eq 11. $CW = CW_3 - CW_2$

Eq 12. $SF = \{[(-BQ) - SQRT\ (BQ\ BQ) - (4\ AQ\ CQ)]\}/(2\ AQ) - ACD$

$K = 46\ D$

$AL = 22\ mm$ $Aim = 22.2\ mm$

Numeric Example

$V = 12\ mm$ $Ref = -0.50000\ D$

$I = 21.45970\ D$ $ARef = -0.5000$

$SF = +0.50000\ mm$

$AQ = 0.331665\ BQ$

Forward solution for T and Ref

$Rag = R = 7.33696\ mm$

$AG = 11.72708\ mm$

$ACD = 3.48676\ mm$

$I = 21.45970\ D$

$Ref = -0.50000\ D$

Reverse Solution for "SF"

$CQ_3 = 218.91391\ CQ = 63.39617\ SF = +0.50000\ mm$

SRK/T Formula

This formula was developed in 1990, another second-generation theoretical formula was optimised with regression technique; hence it does not suffer the drawback of SRK I formula, which describes a nonlinear system in a linear equation.

While, the Holladay formula estimates the position of the implant; which even the SRK/T does, but in addition, also provides for a retinal thickness correction factor.

Sanders and coworkers, found that they could get a better fit in all their data by varying the retinal thickness factor according to the axial length, which is as follows:

Retinal thickness correction factor=(0.65696–0.02029) axial length.

Error in the given measurement, constitutes a larger problem than inaccuracies in formula's; any of the modern formula's (SRK II, Holladay, SRK/T) can be used with accuracy.

CALCULATING THE APPROPRIATE IMPLANT POWER BY VARIOUS METHODS

Taking the Measurement needed to Predict the IOL Power

The measurement/variables which are taken for IOL power calculation are:

(a) Corneal curvature – refractive power of the cornea

(b) Axial length of the eye

(c) Anterior chamber depth (not required for the modern regression formula).

(a) Corneal Curvature

The refractive power of cornea is measured by a keratometer or an ophthalmometer.

(i) Keratometry is a measurement of the curvature of the anterior surface of cornea across 2 mm–3 mm long fixed chord that lies in the optical zone of cornea.

(ii) Anterior surface of cornea acts as a convex mirror and the size of image formed varies with the curvature.

(iii) The two principle meridians are averaged to obtain a spherical equivalent.

(iv) Average of three readings should be taken for accuracy.

(v) It is necessary to obtain central fixation.

The keratometers commonly used are:

(i) Bausch and Lomb keratometer and

(ii) Javal-Schiotz keratometer

(i) Bausch and Lomb Keratometer

Based on the principle of constant object size and variable image (Figs 7.1 to 7.3), an examiners view of mires A after alignment, B when measuring the horizontal meridian, C mires in oblique astigmatism, D alignment of mires in oblique astigmatism

Practical points during measurement of corneal curvature:

• The instrument should be calibrated by calibration spheres provided by manufacturers

• Chin should be on the chinrest and head against the headrest. The eye which is not being examined should be covered by an occluder.

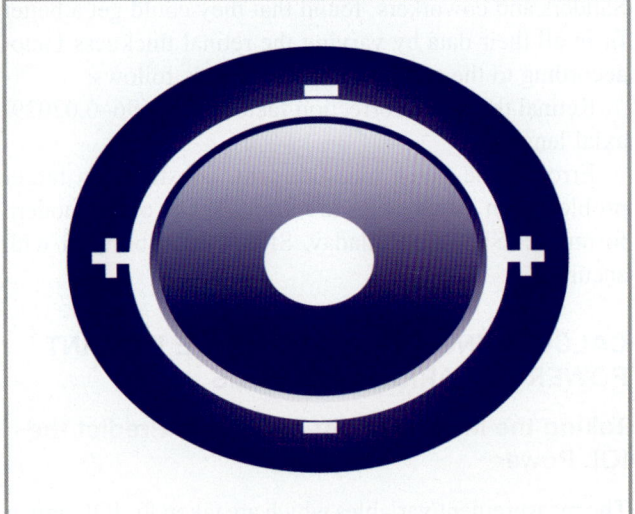

Fig. 7.1

Fig. 7.3

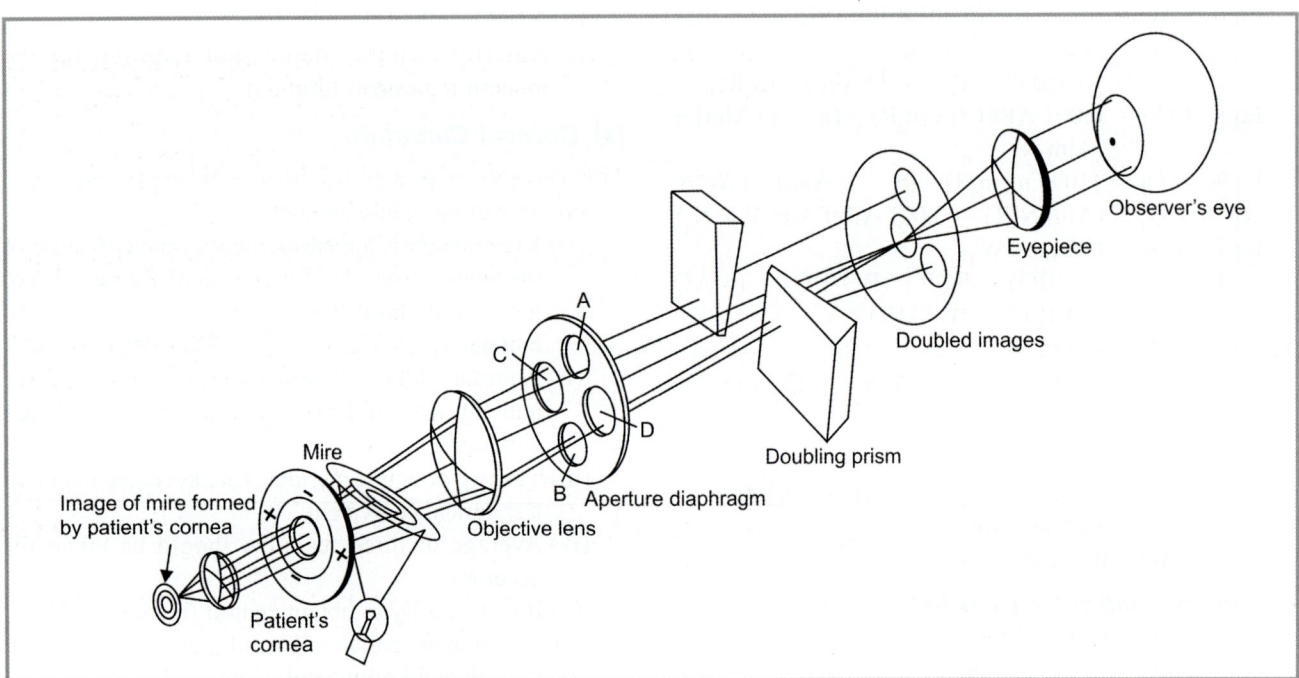

Fig. 7.2: Optical system of Bausch and Lomb keratometer

- Patient pupil and the projective knob are at the same level.
- Mire is focused on the centre of cornea and a clear image of mire is obtained
- For horizontal measurement, the + signs are made to coincide and for the vertical meridian, the – signs are made to coincide.
- In case of oblique astigmatism, the entire instrument is rotated till the + signs are aligned.

(ii) Javal-Schiotz Keratometer

Based on the principle of variable object size (Mires) and constant image (corneal) size (Figs 7.4 to 7.6).

Practical points during measurement:

(i) Calibration of the instrument.

(ii) Patient positioning, so that the eye is at the level of the telescope (T) of the instrument.

(iii) Mires are focused on the centre of cornea and adjusted so that edges meet.

(iv) Reading is first taken in the horizontal meridian then the instrument is rotated by 90° and the measurement is taken again.

(v) For oblique astigmatism, the instrument is rotated till central line coincides.

(vi) An error of 0.1 mm in radius of curvature results in a refractive error of approx. 0.5 D.

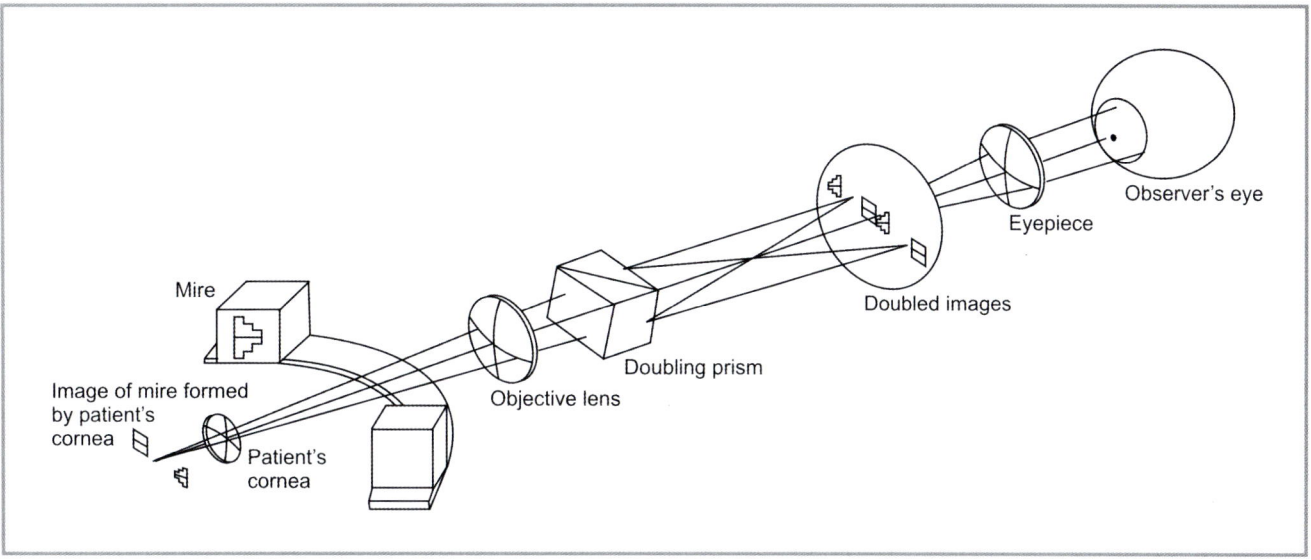

Fig. 7.4: Line diagram of Javal-Schiotz keratometer

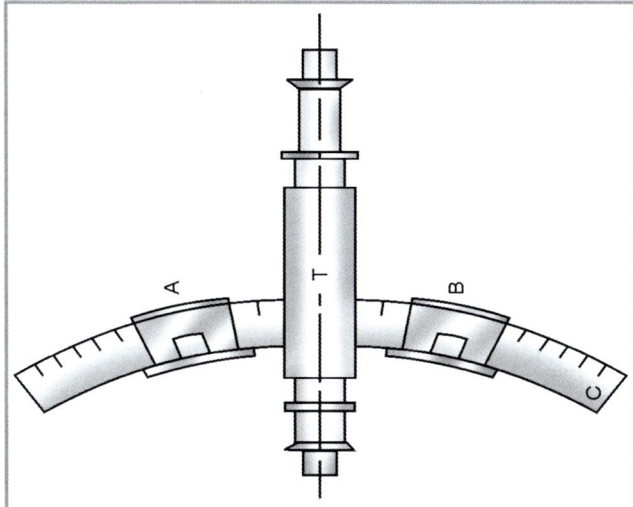

Fig. 7.5: Structure of Javal – Schiotz keratometer – mires A and B on the arc

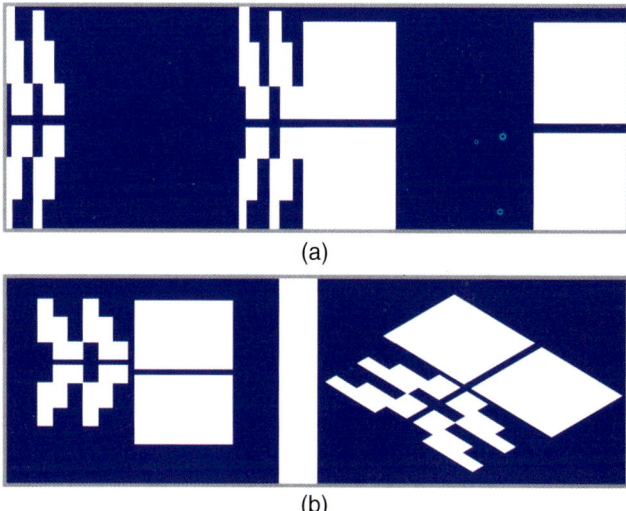

Fig. 7.6: (a) Mires–examiner's view (b) Mire in oblique astigmatism

(b) Axial Length of the Eye

Done by A-scan USG, different modes of coupling between the transducer and eye are used, e.g. steridrape waterbath, contact lens, fluid filled crystal transducer with membrane at one end. But the most commonly used transducer is solid probe that resembles the prism of an applanation tonometer.

- A high degree of accuracy is required in the measurement as an error of 1 mm leads to a miscalculation of 3.00 D.
- The probe can be hand-held or mounted on a slit lamp like an applanation tonometer and this gives more reliable results.
- Avoid corneal compression during measurements
- The probe should be perpendicular to the retina, only then, it will give the accurate axial length.

Characteristics of a Good A-Scan (Fig. 7.7)

- A tall echo from the cornea
- Tall echoes from anterior and posterior lens surfaces
- Tall sharply rising echo from the retina
- Medium to low echo from the sclera and orbital fat, respectively

Machine should be set accurately, depending on the status of the eye, e.g. right/left, phakic/pseudophakic/aphakic. Repeated readings should be consistent.

Anterior Chamber Depth

This is required for theoretical formula. As these are not used the AC depth is not measured. Also measuring the ACD is fraught with problems as the preoperative ACD does not correlate with the postoperative ACD.

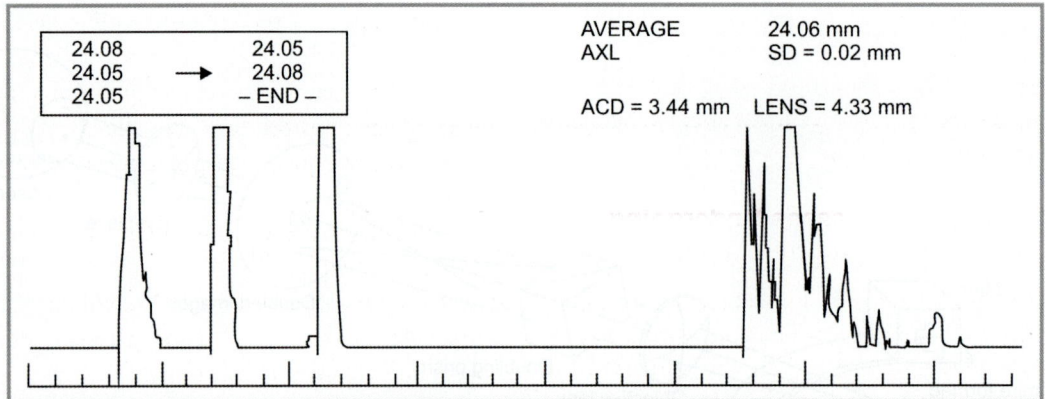

Fig. 7.7: Characteristics of a good A-Scan

- Postoperative ACD changes with the type, design and positioning of IOL.
- ACD also changes with age as the crystalline lens grows in size.

After carrying out the above measurement one can proceed to IOL power calculation. Following criteria can be checked to assess the accuracy of your measurement:

Repeat the measurement if:

(i) Axial length <22.0 mm or >25.0 mm

(ii) Average corneal power <40 D or >47 D

(iii) Between the eyes, difference in
- Average corneal power >1.0 D
- Axial length >0.3 mm
- Emmetropic implant power >1 D

Sources of error in axial length measurement

(a) Improper calibration

(b) Decentration of probe

(c) Corneal indentation

(d) Pattern of echo selection not proper

Sources of error in keratometry

(a) Improper calibration of equipment

(b) Improper positioning of patient

(c) Decentration of mires on the eye

Individual Variations

The variation in the position of implant can cause a change in the postoperative refraction to differ from what was predicted.

If the implant sits more posteriorly, there will be a hyperopic shift in postoperative refraction. This can occur in the following conditions.

(a) Lax posterior capsule

(b) A small zonular dialysis

If the implant sits more anteriorly, there will be a myopic shift, like when A in the bag PC IOL is placed in the sulcus.

Many surgeons have noticed that the SRK formula consistently leads to errors on the myopic or hypermetropic side and, therefore, prefer to calculate their own A-constant.

Sources of error in the formula's

A linear equation like SRK I formula describing a non-linear system (optical system) is accurate for average size eyes, but becomes inaccurate as the axial length deviates from normal.

Also the first generation formula does not take into consideration the retinal thickness factor and the lenticular thickness. These factors are taken care in the SRK/T formula.

BIOMETRY IN SPECIAL SITUATIONS

Aphakic Eyes

Biometry is required for secondary IOL implantation. Immersion technique of biometry is the method of choice for aphakes rather than the noncontact technique.

Pseudophakic Eyes

Biometry is required in cases needing an IOL exchange. In most modern biometers, options are available for phakics, pseudophakics or aphakics.

Paediatric Biometry and IOL Power Calculation

In the first year of life, the eyeball grows rapidly. Hence there will be a myopic shift if an IOL is implanted in this age group as the globe increases in size. Hence, the aim is to implant an IOL with 60–75% under correction, depending upon the child's age. Younger the child, more the under correction. The calculation for IOL to be implanted is made, taking into consideration the standard adult axial length as 23 mm and the standard IOL power as 22 D.

Guidelines for the Choice of IOL Power

(i) Children less than two years of age
- Do biometry and under correct by 20%, or
- Use only the axial length measurement
- Axial length and suggested IOL diopteric power

   17 mm : + 28 D

   18 mm : + 27 D

19 mm : + 26 D
20 mm : + 24 D
21 mm : + 22 D

(ii) **Children between 2 and 8 years of age:** Do biometry and under correct by 10%.

IOL Power calculation in cases Undergoing Cataract Extraction with Keratoplasty

It is difficult to get an accurate keratometric reading on pathological the cornea. The transplanted cornea are often flatter than host cornea. Over and above, graft suturing also produces induced astigmatism which is quite high and irregular in nature. Hence, it is better to choose a lens power relatively greater than what the formula predicts. It is better to err in myopic direction.

We have designed our own standardisation of presumed IOL power in these cases by taking into consideration the axial length of the affected eye and keratometric readings of the fellow eye. The result of this formula is further modified by deducting +3.5 to +4 dioptre from the outcome depending upon the graft size. This much myopic shift, reasonably corrects surgically induced hypermetropic astigmatism to a great extent.

However, each surgeon must develop his or her own approach regarding lens power calculation in such cases. Also, the IOL value of the other eye can act as a guide if it is normal.

Biometry and IOL Power Calculation after Keratorefractive Surgery

IOL power calculation, based on routine biometry is inaccurate in cases of keratorefractive surgery. This incorrect result is due to an assumption which is used in keratometer or corneal topography system that is like comparing the cornea to a sphere, centrally and taking the posterior radius of curvature of cornea 1.2 mm steeper than the anterior radius and a refractive index of 1.3375. These assumptions are no longer true after the cornea undergoes keratorefractive surgery. After PRK, LASIK the anterior surface of cornea is flattened with little or no effect on the posterior curvature. The methods to calculate the IOL power under these circumstances are:

(a) Calculation method
(b) Trial hard contact lens method
(c) Corneal topography/keratometric method

(a) Calculation Method

It is the most accurate method. In this method, the change in refraction at the corneal plane is subtracted from the original K reading prior to the procedure, to obtain a calculated postoperative K reading. Hence, it is mandatory to have the keratometry readings and refraction prior to

the keratorefractive procedure as well as the postprocedure stabilised refraction should also be available.

Mean preoperative K – Change in refraction at corneal plane = Mean postoperative K value

Convert the pre- and postoperative refraction into spherical equivalents.

Convert this spheroequivalent refraction at spectacle plane to corneal pane.

Change in refraction at corneal plane = Preoperative spheroequivalent at corneal plane – Postoperative spheroequivalent at corneal plane

Subtract this change in refraction at corneal plane from mean preoperative K value to get the mean postoperative K value. Based on this K value the IOL power is accurately calculated.

(b) Trial Hard Contact Lens Method

The method is also reliable but may not be useful in all cases. In this method the spheroequivalent refraction is determined by normal refraction and the refraction is repeated with a hard contact lens.

If the SER (spheroequivalent refraction) with contact lens is equal to that with normal refraction, K reading of cornea is equal to that of base curve of plano contact lens.

If a patient has a myopic shift with the contact lens, the base curve of contact lens is greater than that of the cornea by a magnitude equal to the amount of the shift, and the opposite is true if the contact lens refraction shows a hyperopic shift.

This is an accurate method but cataract itself may prevent refraction.

(c) Corneal Topography/Keratometric Method

These systems are based on the assumption that the posterior radius of curvature of the cornea averages 1.2 mm less than the anterior surface. This is no longer true in corneas subjected to refractive surgeries. During corneal topography there is always an overestimation of 1 D for a change of 7 D (approximately by 14%). Therefore, whatever be the change in postoperative K reading, it is under corrected by 14% to get an accurate postoperative K.

In difficult cases, standard calculation schemes are overemployed and new mathematical algorithms are necessary to adequately address these problems. Ray-tracing algorithms and other complex mathematical computation schemes are of increasing interest and will gradually replace conventional calculation formula's for the determination of intraocular lens power. The present system of IOL constants works by simply moving the position of an IOL power prediction curve for the utilised formula up or down. For each formula, the shape of this power prediction curve is mostly fixed. The larger the IOL constant, the more IOL power each formula will recommend for the same set of measurements. And the smaller the IOL constant, the less the IOL power and the same formula will be recommended for the same set of measurements. It is essential to note that the shape of this curve remains the same. Other than the lens constant, these formula's treat all IOLs as if they were exactly the same and make similar assumptions for all eyes regardless of individual differences. In reality, two eyes with exactly same axial lengths and same keratometry may require completely different IOL powers. This is due to two additional variables: the actual (not assumed) distance of the lens from the cornea (known as the effective lens position) and the individual geometry of each lens model. Commonly used lens constants simply do not take this into account. These include:

    (i) SRK/T formula – uses "A-constant"

    (ii) Holladay 1 formula – uses "Surgeon Factor"

    (iii) Holladay 2 formula – uses "Anterior Chamber Depth" (ACD)

    (iv) Hoffer Q formula – uses "Anterior Chamber Depth" (ACD)

These standard IOL constants are mostly interchangeable. Knowing one, it is possible to calculate the other. In this way, surgeons can move from one formula to another for the same intraocular lens implant. The shape of the power prediction curve generated by each formula remains the same no matter which IOL is being used. However, variations in keratometer, ultrasound machine settings, and surgical techniques (such as the creation of the capsulorrhexis) can all have an impact on the refractive outcome as independent variables. "Personalising" the lens constant for a given IOL and formula can be used to make global adjustments for a variety of practice-specific variables.

Also, consider that 3rd generation 2-variable formulae (SRK/T, Hoffer Q and Holladay 1) assume that the distance from the principal plane of the cornea to the thin lens equivalent of the IOL is in part related to the axial length. That is to say, short eyes will have shallower anterior chambers and long eyes will always have deeper anterior chambers. We now know that this is not necessarily so. In reality, short eyes most commonly have perfectly normal anterior chamber anatomy in the psuedophakic state. What these eyes have is large lenses. Take out the lens and the anterior chamber dimensions, 80% of the time, are not all that different from an eye of normal axial length. Think about it when you do phaco for a patient with a short axial length and prior angle closure—what does the resultant anatomy look like? It looks just like a normal eye; and that is why all 3rd generation 2-variable formula's have a limited axial length range of accuracy. The Holladay 1, for example, works well for eyes of normal to moderately long axial lengths, while the Hoffer Q has been reported to work better for shorter axial lengths.

Haigis formula

A recent exception to all of this is the Haigis formula, which comes as part of the IOL Master Software package. Rather than moving a fixed formula-specific IOL power prediction curve up (more IOL power recommended) or down (less IOL power recommended), the Haigis formula uses three constants (a0, a1 and a2) to set both the position and the shape of a power prediction curve.

    d = the effective lens position

    where,

    d = a0 + (a1 * ACD) + (a2 * AL)

ACD is the measured anterior chamber depth of the eye (corneal vertex to the anterior lens capsule) and AL is the axial length of the eye; the distance from the cornea vertex, to the vitreoretinal interface.

The a0 constant, basically moves the power prediction curve up, or down, in much the same way as the A-constant, Surgeon Factor, or ACD does for the Holladay 1, Holladay 2, Hoffer Q and SRK/T formula's.

The a1 constant is tied to the measured anterior chamber depth.

The a2 constant is tied to the measured axial length.

In this way, the value for d is determined by a function, rather than a single number. The a0, a1 and a2 constants are derived by multivariable regression analysis from a large sample of surgeons and IOL-specific outcomes for a wide range of axial lengths and anterior chamber depths. The resulting a0, a1 and a2 constants are such that they closely match actual observed results of a specific surgeon and the individual geometry of an intraocular lens implant. This means that a portion of the mathematics of the Haigis formula is individually adjusted for each surgeon/IOL combination.

IOL Calculation using the Hoffer Q Formula

The Hoffer Q formula was published in 1993 [HOFFER, 1993], based on the earlier work of Kenneth J. Hoffer, M.D.

    The Hoffer Q IOL power P

    P = f (A, K, Rx, pACD)

    is a function of

    A : axial length, K : average corneal refractive power (K-reading)

    Rx : refraction

    pACD : personalised ACD (ACD-constant)

    Likewise, the Hoffer Q refractive error

    Rx = f (A, K, P, pACD)

    depends on A, K, P and pACD.

For the calculations, the corneal radii R1C and R2C in [mm] are converted into K in [D] according to:

    K = 0.5 (K1 + K2) with K1 = 337.5/R1C and

    K2 = 337.5/R2C

The personalised ACD (pACD) is set equal to the manufacturer's ACD-constant, if the calculation was selected to be based on the ACD-constant. In case, the

A-constant was chosen, pACD is derived from the A-constant [Hoffer, 1998], according to [Holladay et al, 1988].

pACD = ACD const = 0.58357 * A const – 63.896.

FINAL SELECTION OF IMPLANT POWER

After the measurements have been obtained and the implant power formula chosen has been applied, the surgeon armed with the calculated emmetropising and ametropising values for the patient must make the final decision as to what strength implant to place in the patient's eye. The following factors should be considered:

Fellow Eye Refraction and Cataract, if any

If the refractive error of the opposite eye lies between – 2.0 D and +2.0 D, emmetropia should be aimed for. These patients can usually tolerate an anisometropia of 2 D. If the refractive error is more than ±2.0 D and both eyes have got cataract, stepwise reduction can be done by choosing suitable implant powers, e.g. –4.0 D pre-operative refraction can be reduced by aiming for 2 D under correction in one eye and then emmetropia in the other.

Lifestyle of Patient

Active patients are best served by near emmetropia, sedentary patients may prefer myopia.

Hedging

It has been found that the actual postoperative refraction varies by more than 1 D from the calculated refraction in over 10% of the cases and so it is preferable to hedge towards myopia.

PREOPERATIVE SELECTION OF LENS POWER

Choosing the correct implant power is very important for patient satisfaction after implant surgery. The important steps in calculating the appropriate lens power for cataract surgery are as follows:

1. Determine the target postoperative status of the eye.
2. Take the necessary measurements to predict the appropriate lens power.
3. Finally calculate the IOL power from the appropriate measurements.

Step 1: Determine the target postoperative refractive state.

Ideally, emmetropia should be the goal, however, following factors come into consideration:
  (a) The refractive error of the other eye
  (b) The visual acuity of the other eye
  (c) The refractive error with which the patient has been living for most of his life
  (d) The occupation and lifestyle of the patient

These factors should be taken into consideration for optimal patient comfort, and this decision comes with experience, however, certain guidelines are given below:

A high myope or a high hyperope will more readily accept Plano than a low (–2.5) myope as he/she would not be used to reading with spectacle.

Elderly people with indoor habits/ lifestyle will like to be slightly myope 1–2 D.

People with outdoor occupation/lifestyle will prefer to be Plano. When the vision in the other eye is good (will not require cataract surgery in near future), the following guidelines can be followed:

1. Refractive error of the fellow eye to be between – 2.00 and +2.00 D. These are good candidates for emmetropia as the eye can easily tolerate an anisometropia of 2 D.
2. Refractive error of the other eye to be more than – 2.00 D. The operated eye should be made 1.5–2.00 D closer to Plano than the other eye, as a higher degree of anisometropia may not be tolerated.
3. Refractive error of other eyes more than +2.00 D. 2–3 D towards Plano can be done in such cases.

If both eyes are cataractous, emmetropia or slight myopia should be the aim depending on the lifestyle of the patient.

Hypermetropia, usually is not tolerated by most of the patients.

Also, there is another concept of monovision in which one eye is made emmetropic and the other eye is made slightly (1.00–1.50 D) myopic so that the patient is corrected for both near and distance vision. However, with the use of multifocal IOL and the probability of further improvement in multifocal lens design, tackling the above problem will become easy.

RECOMMENDATIONS FOR SELECTION OF IOL IN THE OPERATING ROOM

1. OT staff should be made aware of the importance of proper IOL power.
2. The surgeon should make himself conversant with the availability of the primary and back-up implants in the stock. Corresponding AC IOL power should also be calculated, preoperatively for use in case of need.
3. All relevant documents like OT list and case sheets should have endorsement of specifications of IOL implant including type (rigid/foldable/hydrophobic/hydrophilic/manufacturer), IOL power since each and every IOL may have different A constant, and ACD which may alter respective IOL power.
4. Avoid using varieties of IOL styles.
5. Ensure correctness of IOL implant and its power from relevant documents prior to the IOL implantation.

REFERENCES AND BIBLIOGRAPHY

1. Norman.S.Jaffe, Mark.S.Jaffe and Gary.F.Jaffe. Cataract Surgery and its complications. 6th edition. 2–17.
2. Ridley H: Intraocular acrylic lense. Transophthalmol soc UK 71:617–621,1951.
3. Holladay JJ et al: J cataract refract surgery 13.4, 1988.
4. Jack.J.Kanski. Clinical Ophthalmology. A systematic approach. Fourth Ed. 157–182.
5. Alpar JJ, FechnerPU: Fechners intraocular lens, New York,1986, Stratton.
6. Erin.N.Marcus, Steven Gayer and Douglas R Anderson. Editorial Medical evaluation of patients before Ocular surgery. Am J Ophthalmology. May 2003. 136(2). 338–339.
7. Ellingson FT. The uveitis, glaucoma hyphaema syndrome associated with the mark VIII anterior chamber lens implant J AM Intraocular implant soc, 1978.4:50–3.
8. Binkhorst RD: The optical design of intraocular lens implant. Ophthalmic surgery 6(3):17–31, 1975.
9. M.G.Wirth, I.M. Russell-Eggitt, J.E.Craig, J.E.Elder and D.A.Mackey. Aetiology of Congenital and Paediatric cataract in an Australian population. Br. J. Ophthalmology. 2002. 86: 782–786.
10. Ja'nos Ne'meth, Orsolya Fekete and Norbert Pesztenlehrer. Optical ans Ultrasound measurement of Axial length and Anterior Chamber Depth for Intraocular Lens Power calculation. J Cataract Refract Surg 2003.29:85–88.
11. Colenbrander MD, Calculation of the power of an iris clip lens for distant vision, Br J Ophthalmol 57:735–740,1973.
12. Sanders DR, Retzlaff J, Kraft MC, Comparison of the SRK II formula and other second generation formula, J cataract refractive surgery 14:136–141,1988.
13. Leclaire et al. A new glare test for clinical testing: results comparing normal subjects and variously corrected aphakics. Arch.Ophthal. 1982. 100 153–158.
14. Fyodorov SN, Galin MA, Linksz A, Calculation of the optical power of intraocular lense, Invest Ophthalmol14:625–28, 1975.
15. Sanders DR, Kraff MC: Improvement of intraocular lens calculation using empirical data, J Am Intraocular implant soc 8:263–267, 1980.
16. Drexler W, Findl O, Menapace R, et al. Partial coherence interferometry: a novel approach to biometry in cataract surgery (letter). Am J Ophthalmology 1998;126:524–534.
17. Linksz A: Optical complication of aphakia.In Theodore FH, editor, complication after cataract surgery, Boston, 1964, Little, Brown & Co.
18. Fercher A F, Hitzenberger CK, Drexler W et al. In vivo optical coherence tomography. Am J Ophthalmol 1993; 116:113–114.
19. Haigis W, Lege B, Miller N, Schneider B. Comparison of immersion ultrasound biometry and partial coherence interferometry for intraocular lens power calculation according to Haigis. Graefes Arch Clin Exp Ophthalmol 2000; 238:765–773.
20. Girad Lj and others. Intraocular implants and contact lense: A comparison of the visual function of monocular aphakia patients treated by intraocular implants and contact lens, Arch Ophthalmol, 68:763–775,1962.
21. Daniel Scanlan, Farhan Siddiqui, Gail Perry, Cindy M L Hutnik. Informed consent for cataract surgery: what patients do and do not understand. J Cataract Refract Surg 2003; 29:1904–1912.
22. Sherman W Reeves, James M Tielsch, Joanne Katz, Eric B Bass, Oliver D Schein. A self-administered health questionnaire for the preoperative risk stratification of patients undergoing cataract surgery. Am J Ophthalmol May 2003; 135(5) 599–606.
23. Thijssen JM. The emmetropic and the iseikonic implant lens. Computer calculation of the refractive power and its accuracy, Ophthalmogica 171: 467–468,1975.
24. Sanders DR et al, Development of the SRK/T IOL power calculation formula; J cataract refractive surg 16:333–340, 1990.
25. Retzlat J : A new intraocular lens calculation formula, J Am intraocular implant Soc 6: 148–152,1980.
26. Retzlaff J : Posterior chamber implant power calculation regressive formula, J Am Intraocular implant soc 6; 268–270, 1980.
27. M D Nijkamp, H J M Sixma, H Afman, F Hiddema, S A Koopmans, B van den Borne, F Hendrikse, R M M A Nujits. Quality of care from the perspective of the cataract patient: the reliability and validity of the QUOTE-Cataract. Br J Ophthalmol 2002; 86:840–842.
28. Marvin F Kraushar, Margaret F Turner, Westfield N J. Medical malpractice litigation in cataract surgery. Arch Ophthalmol 1987; 105:1339–1343.
29. Irwin Y Cua, Mujtaba A Qazi, Steven F Lee, Jay S Pepose. Intraocular lens calculations in patients with corneal scarring and irregular astigmatism. J Cataract Refract Surg 2003; 29:1352–1357.
30. Carlos Argento, Maria Jose Costino, Daniel Badoza. Intraocular lens power calculation after refractive surgery. J Cataract Refract Surg 2003; 29:1346–1351.
31. Lowe Rf, Clark BA. Posterior corneal curvature, Br J Ophthalmol 1973; 57; 46470.

8

Application of Viscoelastic Substances in Phacoemulsification Surgery

Dr RK Shrivastava and Ulka Shrivastava

INTRODUCTION

Viscoelastic substances play an important role in the successful performance of many intraocular anterior segment surgeries, especially in extracapsular cataract extraction and phacoemulsification.

Microsurgery as such requires a lot of manipulation involving a risk of intraocular tissue damage. Therefore, it should not only be offensive, i.e. the desired action on the tissue, but also defensive, i.e. the prevention of undesired side effects on surrounding tissues.

Viscosurgery (as called by Balazs) aims at preventing mechanical damage to tissue, providing a wider space for surgical manipulation and avoiding adhesions, postoperatively.

Viscoelastic substances serve the dual purpose of protection of the tissue surface and maintenance of sufficient space for manipulation within the eye and, therefore have been indispensable in certain surgical procedures.

HISTORY

Viscoelastics have been developed as an extremely useful adjuvant in various types of ophthalmic procedures including cataract extraction, intraocular lens (IOL) implantation and exchange, keratoplasty, glaucoma surgeries and vitreoretinal procedures.

In 1958, Balazs developed hyaluronic acid (HA) as a vitreous substitute, but sodium hyaluronate was first used in ophthalmic surgery in 1976 as a replacement for vitreous and aqueous humour.

Since then, ophthalmic surgical procedures have undergone considerable advancements and these agents facilitate important intraocular manipulation during various ophthalmic surgical procedures.

USE OF VISCOELASTIC SUBSTANCES IN CATARACT SURGERY

Viscoelastics have been classified as devices (not drugs) by the the US Food and Drug Administration, popularly known as Ophthalmologic Viscoelastic Devices (OVDs).

Use of viscoelastics is very important in certain procedures in which the maintenance of anatomic spaces and atraumatic tissue manipulation are required. They also have lubricating, wetting and protective qualities.

The most common surgical application of viscoelastics in ophthalmology is cataract extraction.

OVDs are helpful in each step of modern cataract surgery, which can be explained under the following heads:

(a) **Protection of corneal epithelium:** Viscoelastic substance is placed on the cornea and offers prolonged protection of the epithelium without altering visibility.

(b) **Control of capillary oozing:** When viscoelastic substance is placed over the area of capillary oozing, it controls the oozing by mechanical action.

(c) **Anterior chamber maintenance during wound making:** Viscoelastic substance is injected into the anterior chamber which prevents the collapse of the chamber and damage to the iris by instruments during wound-making.

(d) **Helpful in performing an intact and successful capsulorrhexis:** In performing a good capsulorrhexis, viscoelastics play a very important role by maintaining the anterior chamber and providing excellent visibility.

(e) **Cleavage of lens structures:** During phacoemulsification viscoelastics are injected into the cleavage plane between the lens nucleus and the cortex. This greatly facilitates phacoemulsification of the nucleus.

Such "viscodissection" is specially useful in the case of cataracts with a soft nucleus.

(f) **Viscoexpression:** The technique of nuclear viscoexpression is useful after capsulorrhexis during ECCE.

(g) **Nuclear emulsification:** During phacoemulsification, the viscoelastic does not leak out and thus maintains the anterior chamber. Also because of their low cohesiveness, they remain in the anterior chamber.

(h) **Capsular bag filling during IOL implantation:** During IOL implantation, viscoelastic is injected into the capsular bag. It allows to keep the bag well opened and formed, thus allowing the easy IOL implantation. OVD is also helpful in correct positioning, centring and allowing for possible IOL rotation manoeuvres.

(j) **Protection of corneal endothelium:** Viscoelastics are very helpful in protecting the corneal endothelium from mechanical trauma, particularly in IOL insertion and contact with neighbouring tissues and surgical instruments.

Moreover, OVDs adhere to the corneal endothelium, thus protecting the corneal endothelial cells. Healon and Healon GV provide excellent endothelial protection because of their scavenger effect by which they capture free radicals released during phacoemulsification and their chemical receptors on the corneal endothelium. They maintain space for manipulation, coat the endothelium and implant to avoid direct contact, protect the endothelium from compressive and shear forces.

This adherent layer affords greater protection for the endothelial cells during surgery.

(k) **High elasticity:** This also protects from the possible impacts of the lens material against the endothelium.

The phaco-tip being in a closed system, its vibrations are transmitted to the internal structures of the eye but viscoelastics provide a smothering shield against them.

Physical trauma to endothelium due to IOL can also be reduced by coating the IOL with a viscoelastic substance before implantation.

VISCOELASTIC SUBSTANCES

Viscoelastic substances have dual properties; they act as viscous liquids as well as elastic solids or gels.

Each commercial preparation varies in physical, chemical and rheologic properties, which affect the clinical behaviour of the material.

Physical Properties

(i) **Optical:** As transparency is the main requisite, viscoelastics should be optically clear and should not impair the visibility inside anterior chamber. Similarly, refractive index should not deviate much from that of aqueous, and for easier distinction it should slightly be different in colour from aqueous.

(ii) **Coatability:** The coating ability of the substance is characterised by measuring the surface tension and the contact angle. Lower surface tension and lower contact angle indicate a better ability to coat.

(iii) **Viscosity:** Viscous or viscoplastic substances, by virtue of their slow flow velocity, are deposited onto tissue or implant surfaces and remain adhered as ideal surface tactical tools and provide tissue lubrication.

As space tactical tools, they are useful in maintaining space against vitreous pressure.

(iv) **Elasticity and Pseudoplasticity:**
- **Pseudoplasticity:** Is the ability of the substance to be passed through a small channel, e.g. a fine cannula, a 30 gauge needle, or the pores of the trabecular meshwork.
- **Elasticity:** Enables the substance to regain its original shape after mechanical compression.

Elastic material does not spread into covering layers, and it is easily wiped off. It is useful as space expander even in open cavities and sub compartments.

(v) **Viscoelasticity:** Viscoelastic response to a mechanical force depends on the velocity of the impact. Viscous flow results when slow velocity rearrangement of molecular configuration occurs. Similarly, when high velocity deformation of molecular chains occur, the energy is stored as elasticity.

(vi) **Cohesiveness:** It is the degree to which a material adheres to itself due to the function of molecular weight and elasticity.

We should choose a viscoelastic material considering the type of surgical procedure and the cohesive characteristics of the viscoelastic.

(vii) **Non-cohesive (or dispersive) viscoelastics:** Adhere to ocular surfaces, thereby providing a protective coating to the tissues and remain in position without excessive leakage during irrigation.

Thus, viscoelastics with low cohesive properties are advantageous during iris plane and anterior chamber phacoemulsifications, particularly where endothelial protection is critical, for example, cases of Fuch's endothelial dystrophy.

The disadvantage is that more time and effort is required for removal of the viscoelastics.

In contrast, **cohesive viscoelastics** adhere more to themselves than to the ocular surfaces; and thus aspiration from the eye becomes easy.

The more cohesive viscoelastics are desirable when our principal goals are anterior chamber maintenance tissue manipulation and easy removal as they have the ability to maintain a deep anterior chamber against high positive vitreous pressure.

Cohesive viscoelastics are effective during capsulorrhexis, IOL implantation and particularly while unfolding a very fine foldable lens.

Some market preparations like Duovisc contain separate syringes, allowing the surgeon to use different viscoelastic materials according to the particular steps in a surgical procedure.

(viii) **Protectability and maintenance of shape:** It protects the endothelium and separates the tissues to maintain the shape.

Chemical Properties

A viscoelastic substance should be:
  (i) Inert
 (ii) Iso-osmotic
(iii) Free of particulate matter
(iv) Non-pyogenic, non-antigenic, non-toxic
 (v) Hydrophilic
(vi) Non-allergenic
(vii) Reabsorbed without inflammation
(viii) Dilutable
(ix) Sterile
 (x) Having no interference with wound healing

VISCOELASTIC AGENTS

Sodium Hyaluronate

Balazs introduced sodium hyaluronate in 1965. It is a naturally occurring glycosaminoglycan (mucopolysaccharide) consisting of a long, unbranched chain of alternating N-acetyl-glycosamine and sodium gluconate. In the eye, it is normally present in high concentrations in:

(a) The vitreous humour.
(b) The connective tissue of the trabecular meshwork, where it may influence the aqueous outflow.
(c) Corneal endothelium is naturally covered with a layer of sodium hyaluronate and endothelial cells bind high molecular weight hyaluronate.

It is extracted from a number of sources including:
  (i) The dermis of rooster combs
 (ii) Umbilical cords and
(iii) Culture of streptococci

(d) Physiological Properties: In buffered physiological sodium chloride solution without any preservatives:
  (i) Viscosity is 10,00,000 to 30,00,000 centipoises.
 (ii) pH is 7.2 + 0.1 mm
(iii) Density is 1.004
(iv) Chain length is approximately 10,000 nm
 (v) Molecular weight is 1.1 to 1.8×10^6.

 (vi) Its transition from viscous to elastic behaviour occurs at low concentrations and low velocities.
(vii) It can easily be injected through a 30-gauge cannula and retain its original shape in aqueous.
(viii) It is at least 400,000 times more viscous than aqueous.
 (ix) It is synthesised within the plasma membrane without involvement of any protein template and is released directly into the extracellular matrix.
 (x) In the musculoskeletal system and eye, it acts as a natural biologic lubricant and thus as a shock absorber.
 (xi) It plays an important role during embryonic development and growth, by stabilising cells and tissues.

It has two fractions:
  (i) IF-NaHA – one which causes inflammation
 (ii) NIF-NaHA – non-inflammatory fraction

(e) **Advantages**
  (i) Non-inflammatory.
 (ii) Non-allergic, as it is a biologic product.
(iii) No carcinogenic effects.
(iv) Does not support bacterial growth.
 (v) Can be stored at room temperature for 1 month.
 (vi) In pure form, postoperative raise in IOP is less than others.
(vii) Creates and maintains space in anterior chamber. Because of pseudoplasticity, it is easy to insert and remove through a narrow 30 gauge cannula.

(f) **Disadvantages**
  (i) Autoclaving is not possible
 (ii) All sodium hyaluronate products require refrigeration and so it remains unaltered even after 3–5 years at 2–8°C. Prior to its use, it should be acclimatised to room temperature
(iii) Postoperative rise in IOP: Mechanisms of rise in IOP.
   • Mechanical obstruction to outflow.
   • Decreased outflow facility with sodium hyaluronate that is relieved with hyaluronidase.
(iv) Poor coatability.

(g) **Commercial Preparations**
  (i) Healon (Pharmacia and UpJohn)
 (ii) Healon-GV (Pharmacia and UpJohn)
(iii) AMVISC (Chiron Vision)
(iv) AMVISC PLUS (Chiron Vision)
 (v) AMO VITRA X (Allergan)
 (vi) Provisc (Alcon)
(vii) Viscoat (Alcon)
(viii) IAL (Low molecular weight NaHA)

(ix) Opegan (Low molecular weight NaHA)

(x) Duovisc (6+7) (Alcon)

Chondroitin Sulphate

It is a naturally occurring glycosaminoglycan that consists of repeating disaccharide subunits of N-acetyl-galactosamine and sodium gluconate.

Unlike NaHA, sulphate group of chondroitin sulphate results in a double negative charge per repeating disaccharide subunit compared with the single negative charge per subunit in HA, which allows it to better coat positively charged implant surfaces and reduce electrostatic interactions between an intraocular lens and the endothelium.

(a) **Sources are:**
   (i) Shark fin cartilage
   (ii) Genetic engineering
   (iii) It is also a part of the extracellular matrix in humans and is the main polysaccharide component of harder connective tissue such as cartilage.
   Within ocular tissues – the greatest concentration is in cornea.

(b) **Properties of Chondroitin Sulphate**
   (i) Molecular weight – 25,000
   (ii) pH –7.3
   (iii) Osmolality – 700 mOsm/kg for 20%
                    1050 mOsm/kg for 50%
   (iv) Buffer solvent – Physiologic buffer
   (v) Colour – Yellow
   (vi) No pseudoplasticity – Chondroitin sulphate is not a pseudoplastic fluid. Instead, it maintains a constant viscosity at various shear rates.

(c) **Advantages:** Better viscosity

(d) **Disadvantages:** Requires a large bore cannula for injecting.

(e) **Commercial Preparations**
   (i) CDS-1   (20%)
   (ii) CDS-2   (50%)
   (iii) Viscoat (1:3 mixture of 4% CDS and 3% NaHA)
   (iv) Ocugel (HPMC and Chondroitin sulphate)

Hydroxypropylmethyl Cellulose (HPMC)

(a) It was introduced by Fechner in 1976.

(b) The active ingredient is highly purified hydroxyl-propyl-methyl-cellulose (HPMC).

(c) It consists of long chains of glucose molecules with replacement of the hydrogen of hydroxyl groups by medroxypropyl (up to 29%) and hydroxypropyl (up to 8.5%) side chain which results in increased hydrophilicity.

(d) **Sources are**
   (i) Wood pulp
   (ii) Cotton
   Widely found in nature forming skeleton of most plant structures and plant cells.

(e) **Advantages**
   (i) Low cost
   (ii) Easy to prepare
   (iii) Can be autoclaved
   (iv) Highly hydrophilic and easily diluted, so it can be easily irrigated from the eye. Therefore, it is mainly used as a surface protective tool.

(f) **Disadvantages:** It requires a large bore cannula for injecting.

(g) **Commercial Preparations**
   (i) Medrocel (1% cellulose).
   (ii) Moisol (2% HPMC).
   (iii) Viscomet (1 ml = 20 mg).
   (iv) Occucoat (2% HPMC) – Storz ophthalmicus
   (v) Hymecel.
   (vi) Visilon
   (vii) Cellugel (2% HPMC) – Alcon.
   (viii) Ocugel (Combination of HPMC and Chondroitin sulphate).

Polyacrylamide

(a) Polymer of acrylamide.

(b) Composed of long chains of carbon atoms similar to fatty acids, carotenoids and natural rubber.

(c) It has been used in electrophoresis and chromatography for years.

(d) **Advantages:** A low contact angle produces more coatability.

(e) **Disadvantage:** It requires long time for elimination from body.

(f) **Commercial Preparation:** Orcolon: Manufactured by Optical Radiation Corporation, Azusa (CA). It is a synthetic viscoelastic solution that consists of 0.5% polyacrylamide.

Collagen

(a) Human placental collagen (Type IV) has been found to be a useful viscoelastic substance.

(b) Collagen is a protein, whereas the other viscoelastic substances are polysaccharides.

(c) **Source:** A 2% solution is obtained as supernatant after centrifugation for removal of fibrillar material.

(d) **Disadvantage:** May cause allergic reactions as it is a protein.

(e) **Commercial Preparations**
   (i) Collagel (Human collagen) (Domilens, Quebec, Canada).
   (ii) Visco-collagen (synthetic).

NEWER VISCOELASTICS

(a) Poly TEGMA-40

(i) It contains 40% triethylenglycol monome-thacrylate.

(ii) It is a hydrophilic polymer.

(iii) It is characterised by high biological tolerance after its implantation into the anterior chamber

(iv) It might be considered as a potential visco-elastic substance in humans.

(b) Poly GLYMA

(i) Glycerol monomethacrylate.

(ii) Polyglyma proved unsuitable for intracameral use.

CONCLUSION

Ophthalmic viscosurgical devices (OVDs) or viscoelastic substances are excellent pharmaceutical devices in anterior segment surgery. The viscoelastics have revolutionised the intraoperative protection of corneal endothelium and other structures against ultrasonic, mechanical, or irrigation trauma as well as augmented greater postsurgical structural integrity and visual outcome following anterior segment surgery.

The combination of viscodispersive and cohesive viscoelastics has been found to provide superior protection, space maintenance and intraoperative ease as compared to the singular application of visco dispersive or cohesive viscoelastics. Despite several advantages, viscoelastics tend to develop a transient rise in intraocular pressure following intraocular surgery due to their cohesive property which may exert increased resistance at aqueous outflow channels. Hence, a meticulous removal of viscoelastics is essential to minimise the possibility of the transient rise in intraocular pressure.

BIBLIOGRAPHY

1. M. Holzer. Effect of healon5 and 4 other viscoelastic substances on intraocular pressure and endothelium after cataract surgery. Journal of Cataract & Refractive Surgery; 27, (2) 213–218.

2. Mester U, Hauck C, Anterist N, Löw M Comparison of Four Viscoelastic Substances for Cataract Surgery in Eyes with Cornea guttata Kohnen, T (ed): Modern Cataract Surgery. Dev Ophthalmol. Basel, Karger, 2002, vol 34, 25–31.

3. Olson, Randall J., "A Brief Review of Viscoelastics," Clinical Research Forum, Mar. 15, 1990, p. 19.

4. Glasser et al., "A Comparison of the Efficacy and Toxicity of and Intraocular Pressure Response to Viscous Solutions in the Anterior Chamber," Arch. Ophthalmol. (104), Dec. 1986, pp. 1819–1824.

5. Glasser et al., "Endothelial Protection and Viscoelastic Retention During Phacoemulsification and Intraocular Lens Implantation," Arch. Ophthalmol. (109), Oct. 1991, pp. 1438–1440.

6. Arshinoff SA, Jafari M. A new classification of ophthalmic viscosurgical devices (OVDs). J Cataract Refract Surg. 2005; 31:2167–2171.

7. Arshinoff SA. Dispersive and cohesive viscoelastic materials in phacoemulsification. Ophthalmic Pract. 1995; 13:98–104.

8. Arshinoff SA. Dispersive-cohesive viscoelastic soft shell technique. J Cataract Refract Surg. 1999; 25:167–173.

9. Arshinoff SA. Using BSS with viscoadaptives in the ultimate soft-shell technique. J Cataract Refract Surg. 2002; 28:1509–1514.

10. Arshinoff S. Using viscoelastics to solve problems in cataract surgery. Video presented at: The ASCRS/ASOA Symposium on Cataract, IOL and Refractive Surgery; April 16–22, 1998; San Diego, CA.

11. Arshinoff SA. Using viscoelastics to manage problems in cataract surgery. In: Fishkind WJ, ed. Complications in Phaco-emulsification: Avoidance, Recognition and Management. Thieme: New York; 2002:182–193.

12. Arshinoff SA. The ultimate soft shell technique (USST) and Acrys of Monarch injector cartridges. Letter. J Cataract Refract Surg. 2004; 30:1809–1810.

13. Arshinoff SA. USST and no cycloplegic drops before cataract surgery. Letter. J Cataract Refract Surg. 2004; 30:941–942.

14. Arshinoff SA. Capsular dyes and the USST. Letter. J Cataract Refract Surg. 2005; 31:259–260.

15. Chang DF, Campbell JR. Intraoperative floppy iris syndrome associated with tamsulosin. J Cataract Refract Surg. 2005; 31:664–673.

16. Arshinoff SA. Modified SSTÐUSST for tamsulosin-associated intraocular floppy-iris syndrome [published correction to title appears in J Cataract Refract Surg. 2006; 32:1076]. J Cataract Refract Surg. 2006; 32:559–561.

17. Arshinoff SA. Phaco slice and separate. J Cataract Refract Surg. 1999; 25:474–478.

18. Arshinoff SA, Wong E. Understanding, retaining, and removing dispersive and pseudo-dispersive OVDs. J Cataract Refract Surg. 2003; 29:2318–2323.

19. Hütz WW, Eckhardt HB, Kohnen T. Comparison of viscoelastic substances used in phacoemulsification. J Cataract Refract Surg. 1996; 22(11):955–959.

20. Georg Rainer, Rupert Menapace, Oliver Findl, Barbara Kiss, Vanessa Petternel, Michael Georgopoulos, Barbara Schneider. Intraocular pressure rise after small incision cataract surgery: a randomised intraindividual comparison of two dispersive vis-coelastic agents Br J Ophthalmol 2001; 85:139–142 (February).

21. Rainer G, Menapace R, Findl O, Georgopoulos M, Kiss B, Petternel V 1: Intraocular pressure after small incision cataract surgery with Healon5 and Viscoat. J Cataract Refract Surg. 2000 Feb; 26(2):271–6.

22. Rainer G, Menapace R, Findl O, Sacu S, Schmid K, Petternel V, Kiss B, Georgopoulos M.Effect of a fixed dorzolamide-timolol combination on intraocular pressure after small-incision cataract surgery with Viscoat. J Cataract Refract Surg. 2003 Sep; 29(9):1748–52.

23. Holzer MP, Tetz MR, Auffarth GU, Welt R, Völcker HE. Effect of Healon5 and 4 other viscoelastic substances on intraocular pressure and endothelium after cataract surgery. J Cataract Refract Surg. 2001 Nov; 27(11):1711–2.

24. Oshika T, Eguchi S, Oki K, Yaguchi S, Bissen-Miyajima H, Ota I, Sugita G, Miyata K. Clinical comparison of Healon5 and Healon in phacoemulsification and intraocular lens implantation; Randomised multicentre study. J Cataract Refract Surg. 2004 Feb; 30(2):357–62.

25. Miller KM, Colvard DM. Randomised clinical comparison of Healon GV and Viscoat.: J Cataract Refract Surg. 1999 Dec; 25(12):1630–6.

26. Ravalico G, Tognetto D, Baccara F, Lovisato A.Corneal endothelial protection by different viscoelastics during phacoemulsification. J Cataract Refract Surg. 1997 Apr; 23(3):433–9.

27. Maár N, Graebe A, Schild G, Stur M, Amon M. Influence of viscoelastic substances used in cataract surgery on corneal metabolism and endothelial morphology: comparison of Healon and Viscoat. J Cataract Refract Surg. 2001 Nov; 27(11):1756–61.

28. Koch DD, Liu JF, Glasser DB, Merin LM, Haft E.A comparison of corneal endothelial changes after use of Healon or Viscoat during phacoemulsification. Am J Ophthalmol. 1993 Feb 15; 115(2):188–201.

29. Schwenn O, Dick HB, Krummenauer F, Christmann S, Vogel A, Pfeiffer N Healon5versus Viscoat during cataract surgery: intraocular pressure, laser flare and corneal changes.Graefes Arch Clin Exp Ophthalmol.2000 Oct; 238(10):861–7.

30. Kiss B, Findl O, Menapace R, Petternel V, Wirtitsch M, Lorang T, Gengler M, Drexler W. Corneal endothelial cell protection with a dispersive viscoelastic material and an irrigating solution during phacoemulsification: low-cost versus expensive combination. J Cataract Refract Surg. 2003 Apr; 29(4):733–40.

31. Behndig A, Lundberg B. Transient corneal edema after phacoemulsification: comparison of 3 viscoelastic regimens. J Cataract Refract Surg. 2002 Sep; 28(9):1551–6.

Basic Surgical Techniques in Phacoemulsification

9

Anaesthesia Techniques in Phacosurgery

Col JKS Parihar SM, VSM, Maj Jaya Kaushik and Maj Swadheen Menaria VSM

INTRODUCTION

As in any surgical procedure, anaesthesia and analgesia are important and crucial factors attained in cataract surgery. The need of intra and immediate postoperative anaesthesia and analgesia have significantly contributed towards achieving desirable results after cataract surgery. It is also important to attain immobility of the ball during the intraoperative period. Despite the fact that the growing acceptance and demand of topical anaesthesia in phacoemulsification cataract surgery, the conventional anaesthesia technique like peribulbar is loosing ground and facial with retrobulbar has practically attained obsolete status. All beginners and less experienced surgeons have to rely upon conventional anaesthesia techniques. Undoubtedly combined procedures for concurrent glaucoma and cataract will also need conventional anaesthesia.

Over and above, despite all favourable factors for topical anaesthesia, some patients will definitely need conventional premedications or anaesthesia even in the hands of most experienced phaco surgeons. Hence, a detailed overview on various anaesthesia techniques is still relevant and worth considering.

OBJECTIVES OF ANAESTHETIC PROCEDURES IN PHACOEMULSIFICATION SURGERY

1. Ideal Anaesthesia /Analgesics

The surgeon strives to achieve the following parameters during the procedure:
- (a) Immobility of the globe and the eyelids
- (b) Control of IOT
- (c) Anaesthesia of the globe, eyelids and adnexa
- (d) Control of blood pressure
- (e) Relaxation of patient
- (f) Avoiding untoward incidents, i.e. occulocardiac reflex
- (g) Smooth reversal of anaesthesia.

ROLE OF PREOPERATIVE (PREANAESTHESIA) MEDICATIONS IN PHACOEMULSIFICATION SURGERY

Irrespective of the type of anaesthesia, the patient is administered preoperative medication which plays an important role in the procedure by mainly reducing anxiety and unwanted psychological stress on the patient. This can be achieved by administering anxiolytics such as alprazolam or diazepam a night prior to surgery.

On the day of the procedure, the patient can be premedicated with short acting intravenous drugs such as midzolam and alfentanil. Also oral medication with benzodiazepines may too be effective.

The use of premedication is also not without its share of side effects such as confusion, disorientation, and reduced patient cooperation.

Premedication had a significant role during the era of ICCE, since a large incision and exposed vitreous phase in ICCE demanded a very high degree of immobility of the eyeball during surgery and the immediate postoperative period, good analgesia and a comfort level for both the patient and the surgeon. The premedication continues in practice with ECCE and with PC IOL implant, probably due to continuation of the previous thought process of the same generation during the transition phase. The advent of peribulbar anaesthesia has shown significant decline in premedication. The beginning of the phacoemulsification era in our country in the early nineties continued to enjoy the privilege of being dependency on medication. Seemingly, old habits, good or bad, do not pass away soon. Another reason appears to be a steep and prolonged learning curve associated with phacosurgery. Lack of experience and a high incidence of dreaded intraoperative complications prompted surgeons to persistently rely on premedication schedule.

The growing preference for topical anaesthesia, MICS and the invention of newer phacomachines have witnessed phacosurgery as a customised outdoor and a no patch no prick procedure. A patient demands complete consciousness, both during and soon after the surgery. He expects to walk in for surgery and move out himself without any assistance after surgery. Most patients prefer to resume their activities at the earliest. In modern times, even surgeons are happy to complete a surgical procedure within 15 minutes and as a result, premedication is gradually losing in popularity. However, a good number of cases still need premedication for phacoemulsification surgery due to obvious reasons of personality or associated systemic diseases.

Premedication Protocol as practised by the Author (JKSP)

The author does not recommend any kind of premedication as a most surgeries are routinely performed under topical anaesthesia alone. However, hypertensives, overanxious and very apprehensive personalities, definitely deserve a mild tranquillizer just an hour before the commencement of surgery. In rare situations, intravenous analgesics and sedatives may be of benefit. All younger patients, particularly females are significantly benefited by intraoperative analgesics.

Local Anaesthesia in Phacoemulsification Surgery

Local anaesthetics are a class of similar compounds that reversibly block conduction in peripheral and central nervous tissues when applied in appropriate concentrations. Local anaesthetics cause both sensory and motor paralyses in the innervated area.

A multitude of local anaesthesia techniques and drugs are available to the surgeon in the present day scenario. As mentioned earlier, these include a combination of facial and retrobulbar, peribulbar and topical anaesthesia. It is worth considering to evaluate the various aspects of such agents and techniques for a better understanding of the role of anaesthesia in modern surgery.

For a local anaesthetic to be used successfully in ophthalmic anaesthesia, it must have—potency, rapid onset, desirably long duration of both sensory and motor block, minimal systemic toxicity.

History

The era of local anaesthesia commenced in 1964 when Koller described the local anaesthetic effect of cocaine and introduced it for use in ophthalmology. Since, cocaine, an alkaloid isolated in 1860 from the leaves of an Andean mountain shrub-Erythroxylon coca, has serious CNS toxicity and causes sloughing of the corneal epithelium, its use in ophthalmology is limited. This prompted the German chemical industry to seek less toxic synthetic substitutes and resulted in the discovery of procaine in 1905, which became the prototype for current local anaesthetics. The most widely used agents in ophthalmology today are lidocaine, tetracaine and bupivacaine.

General Mechanism of Action

Local anaesthetic agents block the generation and conduction of nerve impulses. All excitable cells have ionic disequilibria across semipermeable membranes providing the potential energy for impulse conduction. The Na-K ATPase, a membranes bound enzyme, maintains the ionic disequilibrium in nerve cells, pumping out three sodium (Na^+) ions for every two of potassium (K^+) that are absorbed. During an action potential, Na^+ channels open briefly, allowing a small quantity of Na^+ to flow into the cell, causing depolarisation. Local anaesthetics block impulses by inhibiting individual Na^+ channels, thereby preventing the action potential to be generated. The pharmacological effects also depend on the temperature and pH of the medium. Recent work by Franks and Lieb, suggests a more precise theory of both local and general anaesthetic actions. Challenging the well-entrenched, "lipid hypothesis", these authors suggest that anaesthetics operate not indiscriminately on membrane lipids but precisely on certain sensitive membrane proteins regulating ionic channels that govern the responses of nerve cells. If the nerve cell anaesthetic sensitive proteins are isolated, "designer anaesthetics" could be synthesised to lock onto the sites specifically in order to enhance an anaesthetic sensitivity and minimise its toxicity.

Successful ophthalmic anaesthesia depends upon the knowledge of pharmacological properties of commonly used local agents.

The commonly used local anaesthetic agents are as follows:

Amide Linked Agents

Lidocaine Hydrochloride

Lidocaine hydrochloride (Xylocaine) is the first of the amide-linked local anaesthetics.

It is the most widely used agent, both in topical and retro/peribulbar block anaesthesia. It is commonly used in 2% or 4% concentrations for regional anaesthesia. It has a rapid onset of action, but it is of a relatively short duration.

Topical: 2–4% (preferably 2%)
Retro/peribulbar: 1–2%

Mechanism of action

Lidocaine causes reversible inhibition of nerve impulse generation and conduction, at free nerve endings of cornea (topical application) and nerves within the cone (retro/peribulbar block), respectively. This is due to the blockade of sodium channels which results in the inhibition of sodium influx and depolarisation.

On topical application, its good lipid solubility allows fast passage across the cornea and acts on the anterior chamber structures.

Lidocaine consists of a lipophilic (hydrophobic) aromatic ring group joined to a more hydrophilic base, a tertiary amine, by an intermedius, producing compounds that are more hydrophobic, thus increasing the duration and potency of the agents.

Site of action

Topical: Naked nerve endings in cornea and conjunctiva, penetrate through cornea into the anterior chamber and act on the iris and ciliary body neurons.

Regional: Branches of ophthalmic division of the trigeminal nerve as they pass through the supraorbital fissure/infraorbital fissure/annulus of zinn.

Onset/Duration of action

Lidocaine is an amide compound and is not degraded in the eye by the plasmatic or tissue esterases but mainly in the liver, therefore it has a longer duration.

Topical: Action begins within 2–5 minutes and lasts for 15–20 minutes.

Retro/peribulbar: Action begins within 10 minutes and lasts for 60–120 minutes.

Side effects

Local: Burning is mainly due to the acidic nature of the solution (pH-6–6.5), alteration of tear film temporarily. It rapidly crosses corneal epithelium and stroma and therefore temporary epithelial and stromal oedema can be seen even after the use of unpreserved solution.

Systemic: Drowsiness and mental clouding is occasionally seen after systemic absorption following retro/peribulbar block.

Mepivacaine Hydrochloride

Occasionally used in some countries, it is also an amide-linked anaesthetic. Because of poor corneal penetration it is not preferred for topical anaesthesia but it can be used in peri/retrobulbar block in 0.25–0.75% concentration. Also, in intracameral injection, in a dose of 0.4 ml as 2% concentration of unpreserved solution after topical anaesthesia with Lidocaine or Bupivacaine, it has been found to be safe to the endothelium.

The duration of action of the 2% mepivacaine hydrochloride (carbocaine) solution is about 50% longer than lidocaine because of its lesser vasodilator property.

Onset/Duration of action

Topical: Action starts within 1–3 minutes and lasts 10–15 minutes.

Regional block: Action starts within 10 minutes and lasts 80–160 minutes.

Side effects

Causes more burning on topical application than lidocaine (pH–5–5.6). Drowsiness and mental clouding is seen occasionally after regional block.

Applied aspects

Not used commonly, however, presently it is being evaluated world over for intracameral use along with topical agents for longer postsurgical analgesia.

Bupivacaine Hydrochloride

It is also an amide compound like lidocaine but it is the most lipid soluble agent of this class, which has excellent corneal penetration and passage into the anterior chamber. Bupivacaine hydrochloride (Marcaine, Winthrop) has higher lipid solubility and protein-binding properties than mepivacaine and therefore is more potent and has a longer duration of action. It can be used in topical and in peri-retrobulbar block.

The 0.75% solution is usually used for topical whereas 0.25–0.75% can be used for retro/peribulbar block anaesthesia. Epinephrine does not extend its duration of action. It allows excellent postoperative analgesia compared with shorter-acting agents.

Mechanism of action

Blocks Na^+ ion channels in nerve endings of cornea when used topically, thus inhibiting the generation of impulses. When used in retro/peribulbar blocks, it acts upon the motor nerves supplying the extraocular muscles, orbicularis oculi and the sensory neurons from the cornea and conjunctiva by temporarily inhibiting the conduction of impulses.

Site of action

Topical: Naked nerve endings in cornea and conjunctiva.

Peri/retrobulbar block: Branches of the ophthalmic division of trigeminal nerve (sensory) as they pass through the supraorbital fissure/infraorbital fissure/annulus of zinn and the branches of the occulomotor, abducent and trochlear nerves supplying the extraocular muscles.

Onset and Duration of action

Topical: Action starts within 5–10 minutes and lasts for 20–30 minutes.

Regional block: Onset occurs within 10 minutes and lasts for 180–360 minutes.

Side effects

Local (on topical use): Similar to lidocaine

Systemic: Drowsiness and mental clouding are seen occasionally after regional blocks.

Applied aspects: Because of its longer duration, if mixed with lidocaine, the duration of anaesthesia is increased.

Etidocaine Hydrochloride

It is also an amide linked anaesthetic.

Mechanism of action: Similar to lidocaine

Site of action: Similar to lidocaine

Onset/Duration of action

It has a slightly rapid onset and longer duration of action than lidocaine.

Side effects: Similar to lidocaine

Applied aspects

Etidocaine hydrochloride (Duranest) is a modification of lidocaine with prolonged duration and rapid onset, and is presently being used only in some countries.

Ropivacaine: It is also an amide linked anaesthetic with properties similar to lidocaine, except that it has less cardiac and CNS side effects.

Ester Linked Compounds

Tetracaine

This is the first of the ester-linked anaesthetic but fell into disrepute due to is corneal toxicity. Also it leads to toxicity in people with esterase deficiency. It is used as 0.5% solution, (pH 5–6, pKa 3.7)

Mechanism of action

Basic mechanism of action remains same as it is also a sodium channel blocker, but it is rapidly hydrolysed by the plasmatic and tissue esterases within the eye, and therefore has a shorter duration of action.

Site of action: Similar to other topical agents.

Onset/Duration of action

Action starts within 0.5 minutes and lasts for 10–15 minutes.

Side effects

It is more toxic to cornea than other topically used anaesthetics. In esterase deficient individuals, it can lead to serious adverse effects as it is not degraded within the eye.

Applied aspects: It is seldom used nowadays.

Proparacaine

It is another ester-linked anaesthetic used in ophthalmic surgery. It is used in 0.5% concentration, as a topical agent.

Mechanism of action: similar to tetracaine

Site of action: Similar to tetracaine

Onset/Duration of action

Action starts within 0.25 minutes and lasts for 5–10 minutes.

Side effects

It is not degraded to PABA, and is therefore considered safer than other ester-linked agents. It is also less irritating and painful than benoxinate, another ester-linked anaesthetic.

Applied aspects

It is increasingly being used nowadays for office examination techniques due to its quick onset and short duration of action.

Benoxinate

It is similar to other ester-linked agents. It is also being used widely for office procedures but remains to be more toxic to cornea and should be used cautiously.

Onset/duration of action

Onset occurs within 15 seconds and lasts for 5–10 minutes. It is used as a 0.4 solution (pH 5–6, pKa 2.2)

Anaesthetic Cocktails

Combining local anaesthetic solutions is common clinical practice. A fast-onset shorter-acting agent such as lidocaine is often combined with a long-acting but slow-onset agent such as bupivacaine. For a local anaesthetic to be successfully and safely used in ophthalmic anaesthesia, it must have potency, rapid onset of action, long duration of sensory and motor block and minimal systemic toxicity. The individual profile of an agent is determined mainly by its physicochemical characteristics.

In addition to the physicochemical properties, latency also depends on the concentration. Lidocaine has a more rapid onset of action than bupivacaine, and 0.75%. bupivacaine causes a more rapid anaesthetic effect than 0.25% bupivacaine. Procaine has a short duration of action, lidocaine, an intermediate duration and bupivacaine, the longest duration. The duration of sensory and motor blockade can be considerably enhanced by judicious combination of lidocaine and bupivacaine along with diluted vasoconstrictors such as epinephrine. This permits the ophthalmologist to perform complicated intraocular procedures and minimise postoperative pain and discomfort.

The enzyme hyaluronidase promotes the spread of the local anaesthetic solution through the tissues. It causes a reversible hydrolysis of extracellular hyaluronic acid.

Demerits of Cocktails

Despite several advantages, anaesthetic cocktails carry certain disadvantages and demerits.

(i) **Cardiovascular arrhythmia/hypertension:** Cardiovascular arrhythmia may occur when local anaesthetic agents with epinephrine are used during general anaesthesia with halothane. Patient receiving monoamine oxidase inhibitors or tricyclic antidepressants may experience severe and prolonged hypertension with local anaesthetics containing epinephrine thus vasoconstrictions are best avoided.

(ii) **Toxicity to the corneal endothelium damage:** Many commercially available solutions of epinephrine contain sodium bisulfite, a preservative that may be highly toxic to the corneal endothelium. Endothelial damage, which may result in bullous keratopathy, can be prevented if a non-preserved solution is used. The solution should be diluted to a concentration not exceeding 1:5000, because epinephrine is both an a and b receptor agonist.

VARIOUS TECHNIQUES OF INFILTRATIVE ANAESTHESIA IN CATARACT SURGERY

1. Facial
2. Retrobulbar anaesthesia
3. Peribulbar anaesthesia
4. Subconjunctival/sub-Tenon's anaesthesia.

Facial Anaesthesia (Fig. 9.1)

Different approaches and techniques

During the process of eye surgery it is important to restrain the eyelid to prevent its squeesing action. This is achieved with the help of the same anaesthetic mixture described above. Various procedures to achieve this have been described namely:

(i) **O'Brien akinesia:** The condyloid process of the mandible is palpated just in front of the tragus of the ear by asking the patient to open and close his or her mouth. By use of a 1 inch, 27 gauge disposable needle infiltration is carried out just in front of the tragus of the ear over the condyloid process of the mandible thus blocking special nerves at the proximal trunk of the nerve.

(ii) **Van Lint akinesia:** Anaesthetic drug is infiltrated around the terminal branches of the facial nerve. Van lint akinesia is obtained by infiltration anaesthesia in the region of the terminal branches of the facial nerve. Several millilitres of anaesthetic mixture are injected 1 cm temporally to the lateral canthus down to bone using a 1.5 inch, 22 or 25 gauge, disposable needle.

(iii) **Atkinson's akinesia:** Atkinson akinesia involves an injection made along the inferior edge of the zygomatic bone and then upward across the zygomatic arch towards the top of the ear. The injection is begun at the inferior edge of the zygomatic bone at a point slightly posterior to a vertical line drawn from the lateral margin of the orbit. A 1.5 inch, 23 gauge needle with a rounded point is used to inject the anaesthetic mixture as it advances close to the bone and then across the zygomatic arch to just in front of the top of the ear. About 3 ml of drug is injected along the inferior edge of zygomatic arch.

(iv) **Nadbath-Ellis technique:** The facial nerve is blocked as it emerges from the stylomastoid foramen and enters the parotid gland. The anterosuperior border of the mastoid process and the posterior border of the ramus of the mandible are identified by palpation. The tympanomastoid fissure can be palpated at the superior end of the anterior border of the mastoid bone. A 5/8 inch, 25 or 26 gauge disposable needle attached to syringe containing 4 ml of the anaesthetic mixture is

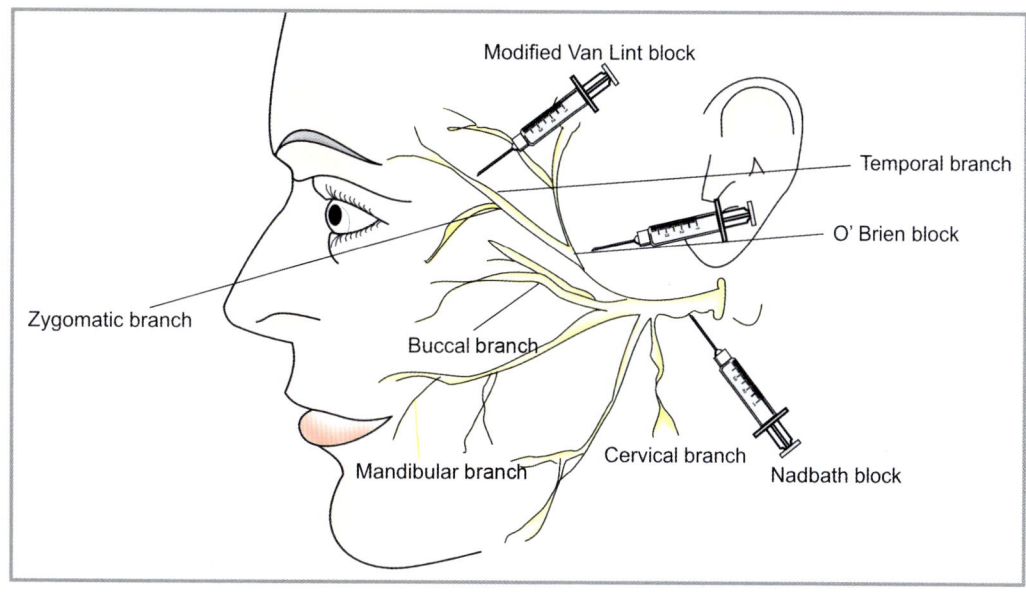

Fig. 9.1: Surface anatomy of various techniques of infiltrative anaesthesia

inserted perpendicularly into the area 1 or 2 mm below the auricle.

Disadvantages of various methods of facial block

(i) The disadvantages of the Van Lint akinesia block are: Discomfort, proximity to the eye, and common postoperative ecchymoses.

(ii) The major disadvantage of the Nadbath-Ellis block is: Proximity of the injection to important structures such as the carotid artery and the glossopharyngeal nerve.

Retrobulbar Anaesthesia

Historical Background

Retrobulbar block was first used in 1884 by Knapp in New York, for enucleation of the eyeball, which was also the very same year in which cocaine was discovered by Koller who was an Austrian ophthalmology resident at that time. In the early 19th century, the use of retrobulbar anaesthesia was pioneered by Atkinson by a blunt 35 mm needle.

This remained the standard approach for anaesthesia for more than 80 years.

Technique

This procedure involves at the onset, conjunctival anaesthesia with 1% amethocaine instillation repeated every minute thrice. Anaesthesia and akinesia of eye are obtained by injecting the local anaesthetic solution (2% xylocaine plus 0.5% bupivacaine with hyalase) in the retrobulbar space within the muscle cone. A 23 gauze, 2.5 cm, sharp edged round tipped needle is inserted halfway between the lateral canthus and the lateral limbus in the lower conjunctiva. Between the inferior and lateral rectus it is directed posteriorly till the orbital septum, then the needle is directed towards the apex of the orbit and advanced till it meets the resistance in the intermuscular septum. After puncturing this structure, the needle is in the retrobulbar space where 1.5 to 2 ml of the anaesthetic mixture is injected. The globe is subsequently compressed to ensure even distribution of the drug and maintenance of hemostasis.

Site and Mechanism of Action

The aim is to block the oculomotor nerve before they enter the four rectus muscles in the posterior intraconal space. Proper technique of this procedure ensures block of all extraocular muscles except the superior oblique, paralyses the ciliary ganglion, and anaesthesises the entire globe.

Actions of Retrobulbar Anaesthesia

Paralyses the ciliary ganglion block, produces following beneficial actions:

(i) Anaesthetises the entire globe

(ii) Extrinsic and intrinsic akinesia of eyeball

(iii) Analgesia of eyeball

(iv) Mydriasis due to intrinsic akinesia/paralysis of sphincteric pupillae

(v) Ciliary body paralysis leading to lowering of IOP

(vi) Reduction in the vitreous volume

(vii) Mild proptosis due to reduction in the muscle tone

(viii) Inhibiton of oculocardiac reflex causing bradycardia post traction on the eye.

Merits of Retrobulbar Anaesthesia

(i) Excellent akinesia and anaesthesia

(ii) Quick onset of block

(iii) Low volume of anaesthetic agent ensures low IOP during surgery

(iv) Loss of visual acuity helps prevent patient from seeing through the procedure.

Demerits of Retrobulbar Anaesthesia

Retrobulbar block has largely been replaced by peribulbar block technique due to high incidence of complications which include:

(i) Accidental intravascular injection of the drug leading to anaphylaxis

(ii) Retrobulbar haemorrhage

(iii) Chemosis or subconjunctival oedema

(iv) Penetration or perforation of the globe

(v) Central spread of drug causing central depression neurological deficit and at times, death may ensure.

(vi) Optic nerve atrophy due to direct damage to the optic nerve or central retinal artery, injection into the optic sheath or haemorrhage within the nerve sheaths

(vii) Retinal vessel occlusion

(viii) Grand Mal seizures

(ix) Contralateral amaurosis

(x) Pulmonary oedema

(xi) Respiratory depression or arrest. Serious complications can result from a retrobulbar injection including globe perforation, central spread of local anaesthetic, retrobulbar haemorrhage, retinal vascular occlusion, optic nerve trauma, and optic atrophy.

(xii) Perforation of the globe occurs more frequently in elongated myopic eyes and in deep set eyes.

(xiii) The direct spread of anaesthetic to the central nervous system is explained by the demonstration of anatomic pathways from the subdural space of the optic nerve to the chiasm states this central spread should be suspected if there is an onset of any of the following: mental confusion or loss of contact with the patient, signs of extraocular paresis or amaurosis of the contralateral eye, shivering bordering to convulsive behaviour, nausea or vomiting, dysphagia, sudden swings in the cardiovascular vital signs, dyspnea, or respiratory depression.

(xiv) Retrobulbar haemorrhages are not uncommon but vary in severity. Venous haemorrhages usually spread slowly and are often limited. An arterial haemorrhage causes a rapid and taut orbital swelling, marked proptosis with immobility of the globe, elevated IOP, inability to separate the eyelids, and massive ecchymosis of the lids and conjunctiva. The increased orbital pressure may tamponade the small nutrient vessels in the optic nerve, resulting in severe visual loss and late optic atrophy in the absence of retinal vascular occlusion. Management includes lateral canthotomy, digital pressure, osmotic diuresis, and anterior para-centesis (although this is controversial). Cataract surgery should not be attempted when a serious retrobulbar haemorrhage occurs.

(xv) Strabismus after cataract surgery is not uncommon. Typically, the patient reports diplopia immediately upon removal of the patch.

(xvi) Recently, postoperative diplopia has been reported to be caused by the effect of the local anaesthesia on the extraocular muscles. Experimental injection of 0.75% bupivacaine hydrochloride into human extraocular muscles at the time of cataract surgery can produce postoperative strabismus, postopera-tive diplopia, and ptosis.

(xvii) Postoperative ptosis is frequent. The cause is multi-factorial. It is probably more common in patients in whom the levator aponeurosis is already unhealthy, including degenerative conditions of the aponeurosis with disinsertion in the tarsal plate, dehiscence, and rarefaction.

Peribulbar Anaesthesia

Peribulbar anaesthesia is the most commonly used procedure for attaining anaesthesia and akinesia of the eye, It has largely replaced retrobulbar blocks and GA in many eye surgeries. Peribulbar anaesthesia can be achieved by the administration of one or two injections, one in the temporal side and one in the nasal side of eyeball. Prior to this, the conjunctival sac is anaesthetised with 1% amethocaine. The author has preference to single injection inferotemporal approach that results in excellent results with least complications for several of years.

Historical Background

It was in 1994 when Davis and Mandel described the efficacy of this technique. The risks of damage to orbital structures was decreased but larger amount of anaesthetic agent was needed. Nowadays, it is the most widely used technique in ophthalmic surgery. Prior to this, parabulbar technique was described by Bergman in 1993. It was also known as Sub Tenon's Block or pinpoint anaesthesia or medial episcleral block and was later modified by Greenbaum and Aleman by using a flexible cannula.

Mechanism of Action

The peribulbar and retrobulbar spaces are not anatomically distinct compartments, when the anaesthetic agent is instilled in the peribulbar space it also reaches the retrobulbar space. Therefore, after 10 minutes of ocular compression, minimal orbicularis function and good overall anaesthetic action are observed.

Different Approaches

(i) **Infratemporal injection:** Here the lid is retracted manually with the needle being inserted between the lateral canthus and the lateral limbus. The needle is advanced horizontally past the equator of the globe. It is then pointed medially to avoid the bony orbital margin where the anaesthetic drug is injected.

(ii) **Nasal injection:** Using the same needle, the conjunctiva is pierced over the nasal side medial to the caruncle. It is then directed deep horizontally parallel to the medial orbital wall, where the drug is injected.

Role of External Pressure Application Following Peribulbar Infiltration

Most cataract surgeons today apply external pressure to the globe for several minutes or more after administering a local anaesthetic. This can be accomplished in several ways. One method is to apply digital pressure either continuously or intermittently (to prevent vascular occlusion) for 5 or more minutes. The mechanism for the hypotension induced by digital pressure is not clear but Hildreth reported a loss of fluid from the vitreous and the expression of aqueous to be the main cause.

A device commonly used in lowering IOP is the Honanballoon (Lebanon Corp Lebanon, IN) a pneumatic balloon that is placed over the closed eyelid and secured in place with an adjustable headband. A pressure of 30 mm Hg for 15 to 20 minutes usually results in a soft eye for extracapsular surgery. The application of pressure to the eye may cause slowing of the heart rate owing to the oculoavagal reflex therefore all patients should be monitored for signs of bradycardia while pressure is being applied to the globe.

Duration

The block usually takes approximately 10–15 minutes to be effective. The indicators of which are:

(i) Ptosis

(ii) Akinesia of eyeball

(iii) Inability to fully close the eye, once opened

If however anaesthesia does not take effect even after 10–15 min an additional amount of 2–3 ml of the drug needs to be instilled

Advantages and Disadvantages of the Peribulbar Block

Merits
(i) Risk of complications low
(ii) All advantages of retrobulbar anaesthesia are present

Demerits
(i) All disadvantages of retrobulbar block are present, but they occur less frequently
(ii) Quality of akinesia and anaesthesia may not be as good
(iii) Block takes longer to act
(iv) Chemosis occurs in 80% cases
(v) More than one injection is not a infrequent occurrence

Parabulbar/Subconjunctival/Sub-Tenon's Anaesthesia

This block was reintroduced into the clinical practice as a simple, safe and effective technique because of continuing concerns over serious complications of sharp needle blocks. The conjunctiva is anaesthesised with an LA following which a bridle suture is placed 7–8 mm from the corneal limbus between 1 and 2 o'clock position.

A mixture of 2.5–3.5 ml 2% lidocaine, 0.5% bupivacaine plus 1500U hyaluronidase is forced posteriorly with the help of a Greenbaum cannula.

Advantages
(i) Less painful than retrobulbar block
(ii) No serious complications associated with this technique
(iii) No increase in IOL with administration of LA
(iv) Surgery can begin almost immediately
(v) Lasts for 60 min and supplemental anaesthesia can be given
(vi) Globe can be voluntarily moved at surgeons instructions
(vii) Low dose and less volume of anaesthesia is used.

Disadvantages
(i) The LA must be injected into the capsule. Double perforation of the conjunctiva resulting in the anaesthetic leaking out, which decreases the effectiveness of the block.
(ii) Since the eye can be moved during the procedure, it is important that stabilising sutures or forceps are used.
(iii) Dissection of capsule must be carried out under sterile conditions.

TOPICAL ANAESTHESIA

Topical anaesthesia for cataract surgery was first employed at the end of the 19th century shortly after discovering the pharmacological properties of cocaine. Modern surface anaesthesia in cataract surgery began in the year 1991 with Dr Fichman performing a series of phacoemulsifications under surface anaesthesia using 5% tetracaine eyedrops. Presently, the use of 0.5 ml of 1% lignocaine is the most popular method for attaining anaesthesia.

Mechanism/Site of Action/Duration of Action

Application of the anaesthetic agent in the lower fornix alone produces a detectable level of anaesthetic agent in the anterior chamber along with providing sufficient analgesia thus suppressing iris and ciliary body pain. During intraoperative period, the drops should be applied every 15–20 minutes or whenever required till the surgery gets over. Motor fibres are blocked only if high drug concentrations are used. Mydriasis is achieved due to paralysis of intraocular muscles but there is no way of paralysing the extraocular muscles or achieving akinesia of eyeballs. The absence of ocular akinesia makes small incision surgeries mandatory such as phacoemulsification. Features of various topical anaesthetic agents are summarised as follows:

Agent	Concentration	Onset of action (Mts)	Duration (Mts)
Amides			
Lidocaine	4 %	2–5	15–20
Bupivacaine	0.5–2%	5–10	20–30
Esters			
Tetracaine	0.5%	0.25	5–10
Proparacaine	0.5%	0.25	5–10

Advantages and Disadvantages of Topical Anaesthesia

Advantages
(i) Risk of needle insertion is absent
(ii) No risk of haemorrhage or hyphema
(iii) Maintenance of functional vision
(iv) Patients remains conscious
(v) No postoperative diplopia or ptosis.

Disadvantages
(i) No akinesia of eyes
(ii) Patient may distract during surgery by talking
(iii) Anaesthesia may not be adequate if complications occur.

Adverse Effects of Topical Anaesthesia

(i) Alteration of lacrimation or tear film stability

(ii) Epithelial toxicity—with delayed wound healing in some cases

(iii) Endothelial toxicity—occurs due to preservative benzalkonium

(iv) Allergic reactions—contact dermatitis, most commonly to proparcaine.

SURFACE KERATOPATHY

Prerequisites for Phacoemulsification Surgery under Topical Anaesthesia

(i) Smaller incisions to permit good anterior chamber maintenance

(ii) Quick, precise and perfect atraumatic surgery

(iii) No too sharp instruments while handling the conjunctiva and cornea.

(iv) Avoid touching the iris

(v) Clear corneal chopping.

CONCLUSION

The quest for better anaesthetic agent and technique has kept on changing its goals with the advent of faster and less traumatic approaches in cataract surgery.

With phacoemulsification, the requirement of ocular immotility during surgery has lost the importance which was attached to it earlier. This becomes more relevant now, with the development of SICS and MICS. Only two small incisions are made and the instruments are used as levers to stabilise and guide the eyeball.

The longer postsurgical analgesia is also not required. In fact, any pain soon after the surgery when the analgesic effect has decreased, may suggest some complication. Surgeries have now become sutureless, thus allowing no pad and bandage and almost immediate return to daily work. The paralysis of ocular motility is, therefore, no longer desired.

Topical anaesthesia has emerged as a well respected technique, overcoming most of the side effects of painful injections and complications of regional blocks.

BIBLIOGRAPHY

1. O'Brien CS. Local anaesthesia in Ophthalmic Surgery. Trans Sect Ophthalmol AMA 1927; 78:237–53.
2. Knapp H. On cocaine and its use in ophthalmic and general surgery. Arch Ophthalmol 1884; 13:402–48.
3. Norman S Jaffe, Cataract Surgery and its complications Pg. 33–41. Eugene Wolfe, Anatomy of Eye and Orbit, Pg. 254,325.
4. Atkinson WS. Use of hyaluronidase with local anaesthetic in ophthalmology: Preliminary report. Arch Ophthalmol 1949; 42:628–31.
5. Mindel JS. Value of hyaluronidase in ocular surgical akinesia. Am J Ophthalmol 1978; 85:643–46.
6. Wood M. Local anaesthetic agents. In: Wood M, Wood AJJ, eds. Drugs and anaesthesia. Baltimore: Williams and Wilkins, 1990:319–46.
7. Wong D, Hunter JM, Mostafa SM. Local anaesthesia for ophthalmic surgery. In: Mostafa SM, ed. Anaesthesia for ophthalmic surgery. New York:Oxford University, 1991: 249–75.
8. Hamilton RC. Complications of ophthalmic regional anaesthesia. Ophthalmol Clin North Am 1998; 11:99–114.
9. Hamilton RC, Gimbel HV, Javitt JC. The prevention of complications of regional anaesthesia for ophthalmology. Ophthalmol Clin North Am 1990; 3:111–25.
10. Robert L Stamper, Zahal, Meltra. Regional Anesthesia for intraocular surgeries, Ophthalmology Clinics of North America,. 1990; 3: 1.
11. Ali-Melkkila T, Virkkila M, Leino K, Palve H:Regional anaesthesia for cataract surgery: comparison of three techniques. British Journal of Ophthalmology, 1993, Vol 77, 771–773.
12. Wagle AA, Wagle AM, Bacsal K, Tan CS, Chee SP, Au Eong KG. Practice preferences of ophthalmic anaesthesia for cataract surgery in Singapore.Singapore Med J. 2007 Apr; 48(4):287–90.
13. Bloom LU, Scheie. The warming of LA to decrease discomfort, ophthal, surgery. 1984; 15,603.
14. Gioia L, Cabrini L, Gemma M, Fiori R, Fasce F, Bolognesi G, Spinelli A, Beretta L. Sedative effect of acupuncture during cataract surgery: prospective randomised double-blind study. J Cataract Refract Surg. 2006 Nov; 32(11):1951–4.
15. Kim MS, Cho KS, Woo H-M, Kim JH. Effect of hand massage on anxiety in cataract surgery using local anaesthesia. J Cataract Refract Surg 2001; 27:884–90.
16. Kaplan LL, PBA, Ahn JC, Stanley, Subarachnoid injection as a complication of Retrobulbar anaesthesia. Ophthal Surgeries, 1988; 19:374.
17. Chang JL. Jopzates, Brainstem anaesthesia following RBB, Anesthesiology. 1984; 61:789.
18. Puustjarvi T, Purhonen S. Permanent blindness following retrobulbar hemorrhage after peribulbar anaesthesia for cataract surgery. Ophthalmic Surg 1992; 23:450–2.
19. Ahn JC, Stanley JA. Subarachnoid injections as a complication of retrobulbar anaesthesia. Am J Ophthalmol 1987; 103:225–30.
20. Davis DB, Mandel HR. Post Peribulbar anaesthesia, an alternative to Retrobulbar Anesthesia. J Cataract, Refractive Surgeries 1982; 13:761.
21. Schneider M, Faulborn J, Von Hochstetter AHC. Posterior peribulbar Anesthesia for eye surgery. Eur J Anaesth 1989; 6:425–30.
22. Davis DB, Mandel MR. Efficacy and complication rate of 16224 consecutive peribulbar blocks: a prospective multi-centre study. J Cataract Refract Surg 1994; 20:327–37.
23. Mount AM, Seward HC. Scleral perforations during peribulbar anaesthesia. Eye 1993; 7:766–7.
24. Rathi V, Basti S, Gupta S. Globe rupture during digital massage after peribulbar anaesthesia. J Cataract Refract Surg 1997; 23:297–9.

25. Murdoch IE. Peribulbar versus retrobulbar anaesthesia. Eye 1990; 4:445–9.

26. Ugur B, Dundar SO, Ogurlu M, Gezer E, Ozcura F, Gursoy F. Ropivacaine versus lidocaine for deep-topical, nerve-block anaesthesia in cataract surgery: a double-blind randomised clinicaltrial.Clin Experiment Ophthalmol. 2007 Mar; 35(2):148–51.

27. Kim MS, Cho KS, Woo H-M, Kim JH. Effect of hand massage on anxiety in cataract surgery using local anaesthesia. J Cataract Refract Surg 2001; 27:884–90.

28. Reinhardt S, Burkhardt U, Nestler A, Wiedemann R. Use of piritramide for analgesia and sedation during peribulbar nerve block for cataract surgery. Ophthalmologica 2002; 216:256–60.

29. Puri P, Verma D, McKibbin M. Management of ocular perforations resulting from peribulbar anaesthesia. Indian J Ophthalmol 1999; 47:181–83.

30. Ripart J, Lefrant JY, Lalourcey L, et al. Medial canthus (caruncle) single injection periocular anaesthesia. Anesth Analg 1996; 83:1234–8.

31. Ripart J, Prat-Pradal D, Charavel P, Eledjam JJ. Medial canthus single injection episcleral (sub-Tenon) anaesthesia anatomic imaging. Clin Anat 1998; 11:390–5.

32. Ripart J, Metge L, Prat-Pradal D, et al. Medial canthus single injection episcleral (sub-Tenon) anaesthesia computed tomography imaging. Anesth Analg 1998; 87:43–5.

33. Ripart J, L'Hermite J, Nouvellon E, et al. Regional anaesthesia for ophthalmic surgery performed by single episcleral (sub-Tenon) injection: a 802 cases experience. Reg Anesth 1999; 24:A59

34. Ripart J, Lefrant JY, Vivien B, et al. Ophthalmic regional anaesthesia: medial canthus episcleral (Sub-Tenon) anaesthesia is more efficient than peribulbar anaesthesia: a double blind randomised study. Anesthesiology 2000; 92:1278–85.

35. de la Marnieere E, Maye R, Albertim, Batissc JL, Baltenneck. Comparison between Greenbachs Parabulbar Anaesthesia and Ripart's subtenon anaesthesia in the anterior. segment surgery. J Fr Ophthalmol 2002; 25:161–5.

36. Stevens JD. A new local anesthetics techniques for cataract extraction by one quadrant sub-Tenon's infiltration. Br J Ophthalmol 1992; 76:670–4.

37. Freiman BJ. Friedberg MA. Globe Perforation associated with sub Tenon's anaesthesia. Am J Ophthalmol 2001; 131:520–1

38. Fichman RA. Use of topical anaesthesia alone in cataract surgery. J Cataract Refract Surg 1996; 22:612–4.

39. Gombos K, Jakubovits E, Kolos A, Salacz G, Nemeth J. Cataract surgery anaesthesia: is topical anaesthesia really better than retrobulbar ? Acta Ophthalmol Scand. 2007 May; 85(3):309–16.

40. Johnston RL, Whitefield LA, Giralt J, Harrun S, Akerele T, Bryan SJ, Kayali N, Claoue CM. Topical versus peribulbar anaesthesia, without sedation, for clear corneal phacoemulsification. J Cataract Refract Surg 1998; 24:407–10.

41. Dinsmore SC. Drop, then decide approach to topical anaesthesia. J Cataract Refract Surg 1995; 21:666–71.

42. Chuang LH, Yeung L, Ku WC, Yang KJ, Lai CC. Safety and efficacy of topical anaesthesia combined with a lower concentration of intracameral lidocaine in phacoemulsification: paired human eye study. J Cataract Refract Surg. 2007 Feb; 33(2):293–6.

43. Ugur B, Dundar SO, Ogurlu M, Gezer E, Ozcura F, Gursoy F. Ropivacaine versus lidocaine for deep-topical, nerve-block anaesthesia in cataract surgery: a double-blind randomized clinicaltrial.Clin Experiment Ophthalmol. 2007 Mar; 35(2):148–51.

44. Amiel H, Koch PS. Tetracaine hydrochloride 0.5% versus lidocaine 2% jelly as a topical anaesthetic agent in cataract surgery: comparative clinical trial. J Cataract Refract Surg. 2007 Jan; 33(1):98–100.

45. Kwok AK, Lai TY, Lee VY, Yeung YS, Chu KO, Pang CC. Effect of application duration of 2% lidocaine jelly on aqueous lidocaine concentration for topical anaesthesia in cataract surgery. Graefes Arch Clin Exp Ophthalmol. 2006 Sep; 244(9):1096–100.

46. Chuang LH, Yeung L, Ku WC, Yang KJ, Lai CC. Safety and efficacy of topical anaesthesia combined with a lower concentration of intracameral lidocaine in phacoemulsification: paired human eye study. J Cataract Refract Surg. 2007 Feb; 33(2):293–6.

47. Kongsap P, Wiriyaluppa C. A comparison of patient pain during cataract surgery with topical anaesthesia in Prechop Manual Phacofragmentation versus phacoemulsification. J Med Assoc Thai. 2006 Jul; 89(7):959–66.

48. Habib NE, Mandour NM, Balmer HG. Effect of midazolam on anxiety level and pain perception in cataract surgery with topical anaesthesia J Cataract Refract Surg. 2004 Feb; 30(2):437–43.

49. Liu DT, Lee VY, Chan WM, Lam DS.Pain induced by phacoemulsification without sedation using topical or peribulbar anaesthesia. J Cataract Refract Surg. 2006 Jan; 32(1):2.

50. Rosenthal KJ. Deep, topical, nerve-block anaesthesia. J Cataract Refract Surg 1995; 21:499–503.

51. Bloomberg LB, Pellican KJ. Topical anaesthesia using the Bloomberg Supernumb Anesthetic Ring. J Cataract Refract Surg 1995; 21:16–20.

52. Unal M, Yucel I, Sarici A, Artunay O, Devranoglu K, Akar Y, Altin M.Phacoemulsification with topical anaesthesia: Resident experience.J Cataract Refract Surg. 2006 Aug; 32(8):1361–5.

53. Harman DM. Combined sedation and topical anaesthesia for cataract surgery. J Cataract Refract Surg 2000; 26:109 13.

54. Maclean H, Burton T, Murray A. Patient comfort during cataract surgery with modified topical and peribulbar anaesthesia. J Cataract Refract Surg 1997; 23:277–83.

55. Nielsen PJ. Immediate visual capability after cataract surgery: topical versus retrobulbar anaesthesia. J Cataract Refract Surg 1995; 21:302–4.

56. Boezaart A, Berry R, Nell M: Topical anaesthesia versus retrobulbar block for cataract surgery: the patients' perspective J Clin Anesth. 2000; 12:58–6.

57. Ang CL, Au Eong KG, Lee SS, Chan SP, Tan CS. Patients' expectation and experience of visual sensations during phacoemulsification under topicalanaesthesia. Eye. 2006 May 19.

58. Venkatesh R, Muralikrishnan R, Au Eong KG. Visual sensation during phacoemulsification using topical versus regional anaesthesia. J Cataract Refract Surg. 2005 Oct; 31(10):1855–6.

59. Leo SW, Lee LK, Au Eong KG. Visual experience during phacoemulsification under topical anaesthesia: a nationwide

survey of Singapore ophthalmologists. Clin Experiment Ophthalmol. 2005 Dec; 33(6):578–81.

60. Douglas K Newman:Visual experience during phacoemulsification cataract surgery under topical anaesthesia Br J Ophthalmol 2000; 84:13–15.

61. Voon LW, Au Eong KG, Saw SM, Verma D, Laude A. Effect of preoperative counselling on patient fear from the visual experience during phacoemulsification under topical anaesthesia: Multicentre randomised clinical trial. J Cataract Refract Surg. 2005 Oct; 31(10):1966–9.

62. Jonas JB, Pakdaman B, Sauder G. Frequency and predicting factors of surgical complications in cataract surgery performed under topical anaesthesia.Acta Ophthalmol Scand. 2006 Feb; 84(1):151–2.

63. Hadden PW, Scott RC.Cardiac arrest during phacoemulsification using topical anaesthesia in an unsedated patient. J Cataract Refract Surg. 2006 Feb; 32(2):369. No abstract available.

64. O'brien PD, Ho SL, Fitzpatrick P, Power W. Risk factors for a postoperative intraocular pressure spike after phacoemulsification.Can J Ophthalmol. 2007 Feb; 42(1):51–5.

65. Eke T, Thompson JR. Serious complications of local anaesthesia for cataract surgery: a 1 year national survey in the United Kingdom. Br J Ophthalmol. 2007 Apr; 91(4): 470–5.

66. Gordon RA, Kerr JH, Taylor R. A laboratory and clinical evaluation of mepivacaine (carbocaine). Can Anaesth Soc J 1960; 7:290–6.

67. Iamsukhon M, Kulpapangkorn P, Hirunwiwatkul P, Tulvatana W. Effectiveness of oxygenation under the drape in phacoemulsification with intraocular lens implantation: a randomised clinical trial. J Med Assoc Thai. 2006 Mar; 89(3):343–9.

68. Jonas JB, Pakdaman B, Sauder G. Cataract surgery under systemic anticoagulant therapy with coumarin. Eur J Ophthalmol. 2006 Jan-Feb; 16(1):30–2.

69. Cagini C, De Carolis A, Fiore T, Iaccheri B, Giordanelli A, Romanelli D. Limbal anaesthesia versus topical anaesthesia for clear corneal phacoemulsification. Acta Ophthalmol Scand. 2006 Feb; 84(1):105–9.

70. Jonas JB, Hugger P, Sauder G. Topical anaesthesia for transpupillary silicone oil removal combined with cataract surgery. J Cataract Refract Surg. 2005 Sep; 31(9):1781–2.

71. O'Brien PD, Fitzpatrick P, Power W. Patient pain during stretching of small pupils in phacoemulsification performed using topical anaesthesia. J Cataract Refract Surg. 2005 Sep; 31(9):1760–3.

10

Phaco Incisions: Good Beginning, Full Success: Wound Construction for Sutureless Cataract Surgery

Dr US Tewari MS and Col JKS Parihar SM, VSM

INTRODUCTION

The observations made by Thrasher and Boerner (1984) are remarkable. They observed that a 9.00 mm posterior limbal incision would induce less astigmatism as compared to a 6.00 mm conventional limbal incision. On the basis of these observations, Richard Kratz developed the scleral pocket incision that consisted of scleral tunnel and a corneal wedge. The incision had to be closed with 10–0 nylon sutures such as a running shoelace, X-stitch, horizontal mattress suture of Shepherd, horizontal anchor suture of Masket or the infinity suture of Howard Fine.

However, Michael McFarland was the first surgeon to perform sutureless cataract surgery. He initiated this procedure in January 1990 after observing that the scleral tunnel wounds appeared to be watertight. McFarland became convinced that suture was superfluous to a properly configured wound. Subsequently, Paul Ernest recognised that internal corneal lip was far more important than the long scleral tunnel. This lip was also intended to prevent hyphaemas that occurred in 5 to10% of patients undergoing scleral tunnel incision, and to prevent delayed filtering blebs.

RELEVANT SURGICAL ANATOMY

The limbus is more than the border zone between the cornea and sclera; it has multiple functions including nourishment of the peripheral cornea, corneal wound healing, immunosurveillance of the ocular surface, hypersensitivity responses, and it contains the pathways of aqueous humor outflow and thus is involved in control of intraocular pressure. It is also the site of surgical incisions into the anterior chamber for cataract and glaucoma surgery.

Anatomical Limbus

It refers to a circumcorneal transition zone of conjunctivocorneal and corneoscleral junction.

Surgical Limbus

These landmarks characterise it:
(a) Anterior limbal border: It overlies termination of the Bowman's membrane.
(b) Midlimbal border: It is a junction of blue zone with white area. It overlies termination of Descemet's membrane. It is the preferred site of incision for entry into the eye.
(c) Post limbal border: It is one mm posterior to midlimbal line. It overlies the scleral spur.

Basic Concepts Related to Postcataract Surgery Astigmatism

It is well established that:
(a) Surgery leads to flattening of the meridian along the incision, i.e. a conventional incision from 10 to 2 o'clock position will induce against the rule astigmatism (ATR).
(b) Suture induced astigmatism is temporary. Sutures cannot prevent astigmatic decay (Fig. 10.1).
(c) Surgically Induced Astigmatism (SIA) depends on several factors.
    (i) Following factors are under surgeon's control:
        • Incision length

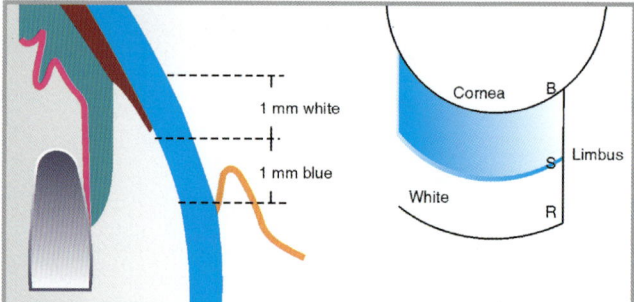

Fig. 10.1: Surgical anatomy of limbus

- Site of incision
- Wound configuration
- Sutures—only temporary astigmatism

(ii) Factors beyond the surgeon's control
- Wound healing
- Tissue elasticity
- Concurrent diseases, etc.

(d) Preoperative Astigmatism is an important factor.

One must remember that incision size is the major determinant whereas site and wound configuration are contributory.

Surgically Induced Astigmatism (SIA) can be calculated by several methods such as vector analysis method, subtraction method, etc. A simple method that can be used for calculating SIA is 'Algebraic Subtraction' method. For example, if Preoperative astigmatism is 1 dioptre with the rule, and postoperative astigmatism is 0.5 dioptre against the rule then surgically induced astigmatism is 1.5 dioptre. This represents a total shift towards against the rule by 1.5 D.

Surgeon can calculate SIA in his own cases and make necessary modifications in his technique.

(e) Concept of self-sealing wound

The features of an incision that make it self-sealing are:

(i) Creation of corneal valve and

(ii) Making of a squares tunnel incision that means moving posterior from limbus to sclera increases appositional surfaces to enhance wound healing [Figs 10.2(a) to (d)].

It is basically the inner lip of the wound, which functions as a valve with the normal IOP. This lip gets pushed up against the dome of the cornea, thus sealing the wound. Usually 1.75 mm is adequate for the formation of a good corneal valve. It should be uniform throughout its whole length. A ragged or irregular lip will not function as a good valve.

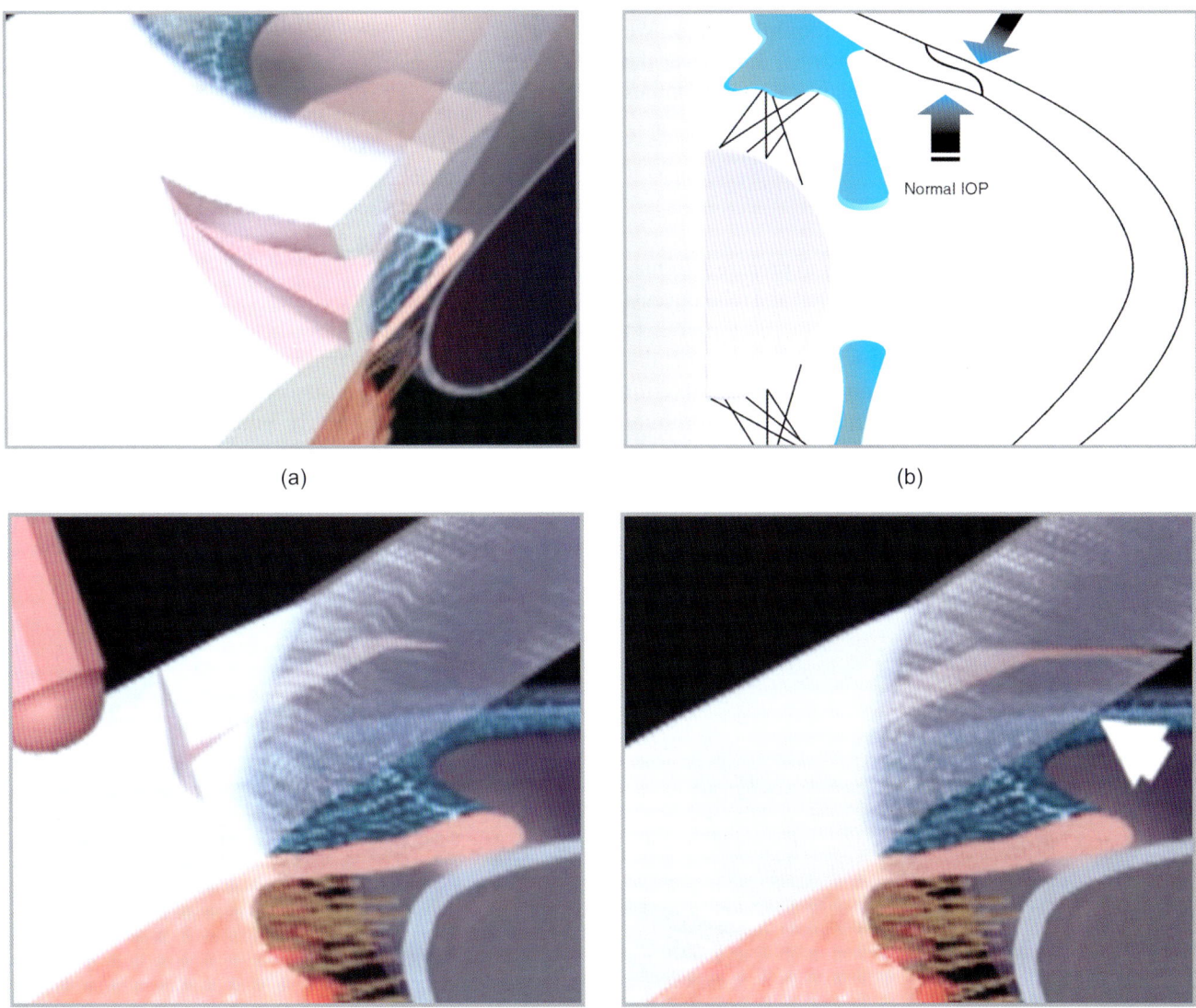

(a)

(b)

(c)

(d)

Figs 10.2(a) to (d): Concept of self sealing valve

Instruments (for scleral pocket incision/clear corneal incision):

   (i) 15 degree MVR blade for making side port
   (ii) Keratome (2.8–5.2 mm) steel or diamond blade
   (iii) Crescent knife 2.2 mm Steel or diamond knife

Bevelled up Keratomes and crescents are commonly used as they ride down the tissues; hence making the dissection easier.

Prerequisites

Sharp instruments and a tense eyeball are the prerequisites for a good incision, so viscoelastic should be injected from the side port to obtain adequate IOP.

Preparation of the Surgical Field

There is no doubt that using 0.5% providone-iodine (Betadine) has a positive effect, not only on decreasing flora on the lids and eyes of the patient but also in decreasing the incidence of postoperative endophthalmitis. We routinely evert the lashes with steristrips, drape over the meibomian orifices and place a wick in the lateral canthus to disallow pooling of fluids.

Technique

Conjunctival Flap

Conjunctiva is detached from limbus to prepare a fornix-based flap. Tenon's attachment is severed and relaxing cuts are made on either side of the flap. Cauterise posterior to the proposed site of incision that will keep the tunnel dry as the blood vessels traverse from posterior to anterior direction. Keep the use of cautery to the minimum (Fig. 10.3).

Excessive cautery can lead to tissue shrinkage and ischaemia, and thereby induce more astigmatism and delayed wound healing, respectively.

Side port entry/Incision: A side port should be made by a 15 degree or similar blade. Now, inflate the anterior chamber by a viscoelastic substance (Fig. 10.4).

Scleral Pocket Incision

Place incision at least 2 mm behind conjunctival attachment, i.e. at the posterior limbal border. After gaining sufficient experience and confidence, one can place incision even posterior. In shallow anterior chamber, the entry should be relatively anterior so as to facilitate manoeuvrability. The shape of the external incision can be straight or frown depending on the confidence level of the surgeon. The frown incision is more stable and astigmatism-friendly (Fig. 10.5).

One can use Bard parker knife with 11 number blade to make a 0.3 mm groove. The edge of crescent knife can be used as a practical guide. Initially, make an oblique incision to avoid complications such as scleral disinsertion, premature entry or button holing of the scleral flap. The ideal way is to use a guarded diamond knife (provided one can afford this luxury).

To dissect the scleral tunnel, use a crescent knife. Engage the tissue with the tip of the crescent knife, maintain the same plane while dissecting the tunnel and follow the contour of the globe while dissecting sides. Also remember that an instrument such as a crescent knife with bevel up tends to ride down the tissue, thereby premature entry is more likely than the button holing (Fig. 10.6).

As one approaches the cornea, the tip of the blade should be tilted anteriorly to follow the anterior curve of limbus. Please note that the internal incision should be larger than the external one. Go on dissecting to clear the cornea so as to make a tunnel of nearly 3 mm.

The anterior chamber entry is made with the help of a 3.2 mm keratome after identifying the anterior limit of the tunnel by the dimple down technique (Fig. 10.7). Take care not to hit the iris or lens while entry is being made.

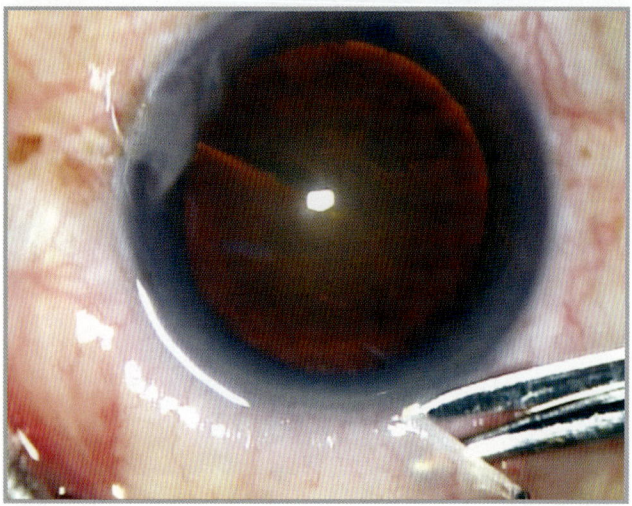

Fig. 10.3: Conjunctival flap

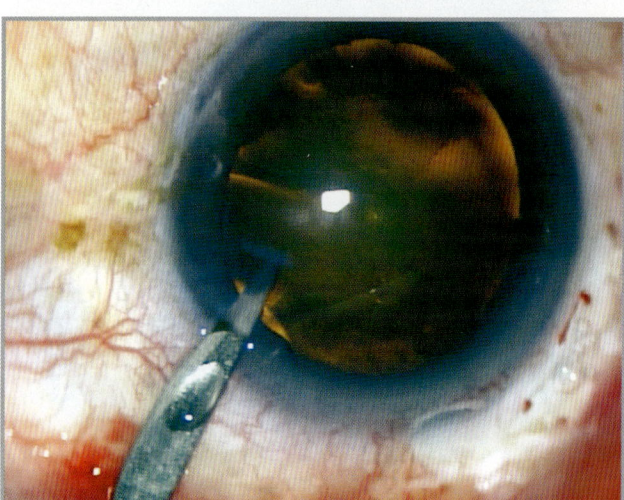

Fig. 10.4: Side port entry

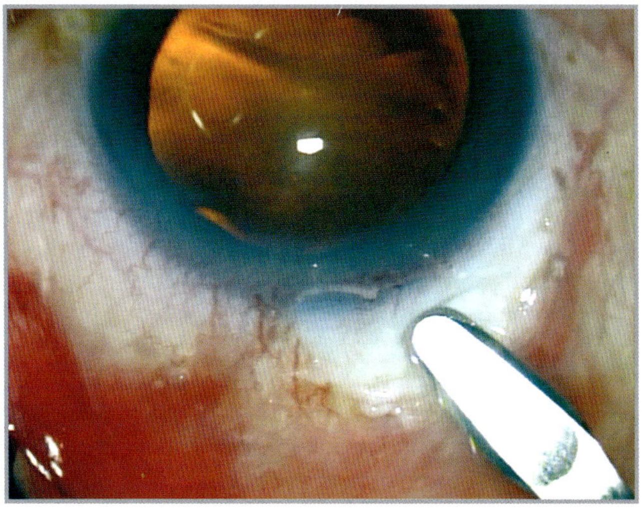

(a)

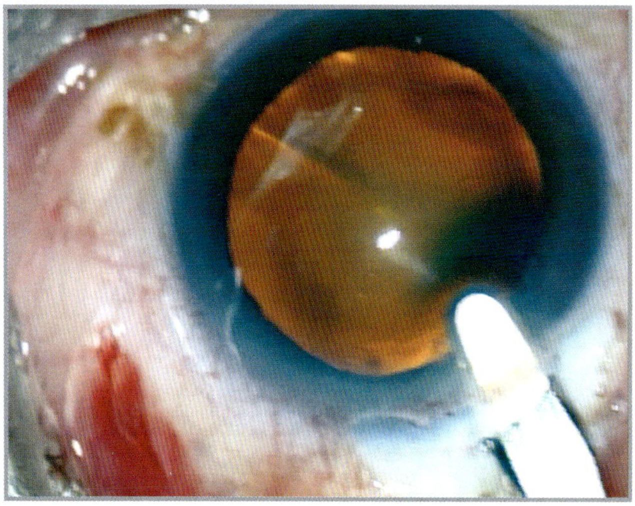

(b)

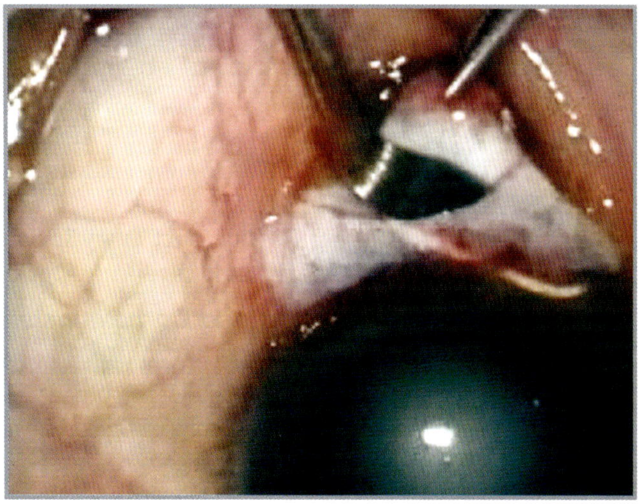

(c)

Figs 10.5: (a), (b) Initiating scleral pocket incision, (c) Dissecting sides of tunnel

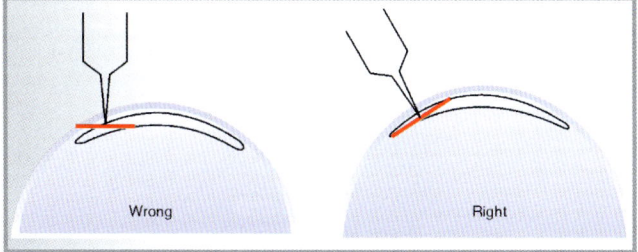

Fig. 10.6: Dissecting tunnel from sides

Enlarging the Section

This is performed with the help of a 3.2 mm keratome. The section is enlarged by cutting the tissue while moving the keratome inwards so as to have a better control to maintain the plane of tunnel. Avoid touching the iris, as it will cause constriction of pupil. It should be performed after capsulotomy and before hydroprocedures.

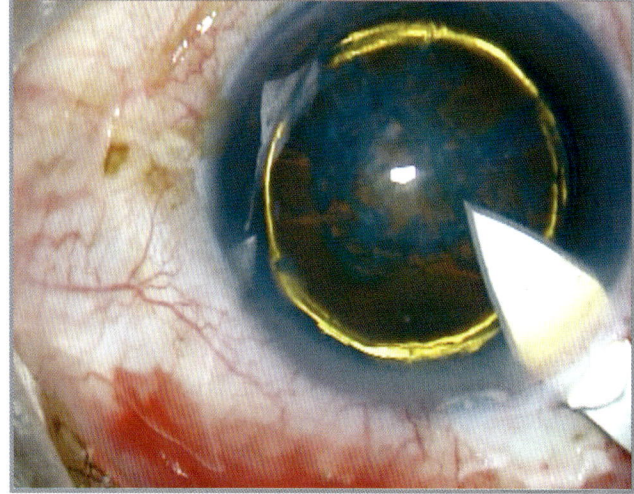

Fig. 10.7: Dimple down technique for entry into anterior chamber

Complications

(i) **Scleral disinsertion:** If initial cut is more than 80–90% deep it results in wound gap leading to astigmatism. If it occurs it should be sutured at the end of phacoemulsification. It is managed by putting radial suture to appose the edge of scleral groove.

(ii) **Torn edges:** It occurs when a surgeon moves his knife parallel to the floor rather than being along the curvature of eyeball. The knife has to tilt a little towards the side of motion of blade. It can be avoided by pressing the keratome against the globe and pointing the tip upwards.

(iii) **Thin and shredded flap (torn or fragment):** If a thin flap is detected early before the tunnel has reached the cornea then stop, deepen the initial groove and dissect again in deeper plane or alternatively, another groove is made 1 mm in front of the initial groove.

(iv) **Too long corneal valve:** It happens when a sharp crescent knife is used in a pressurised eye. If the tunnel is too long it perforates the globe ½ mm behind.

(v) **Premature entry**
- **Early perforation of cornea** can be due to too deep initial groove or too sharp knife or failure to move knife in accordance with the curvature of cornea, which may result in premature entry into AC resulting in unstable AC, repeated iris prolapse, miosis and difficult surgery. If it is recognised in time, make another groove 1 mm in front of the initial incision.
- If premature entry has already been made, further course depends on the type of cataract and the degree of mydriasis. In case of soft cataract, with fully dilated pupil and no iris prolapse, proceed with the surgery as planned. If pupil is semi-dilated or there is repeated iris prolapse or the cataract is hard, you can either convert to EECE or suture the initial incision and complete the nucleotomy from corneal temporal incision if initial tunnel is made at 12 O'clock.

When and How to Convert?

For a novice, the following situations call for conversion to conventional ECCE/IOL surgery:
1. Posterior capsule rent/ zonular dehiscence
2. Small pupil
3. Failure to tip the nucleus out of the bag
4. Hazy cornea jeopardising visibility
5. Very hard nucleus

The technique of conversion is simple: Just make a radial cut from one end of the tunnel right up to the anterior chamber that can be enlarged along the limbus. If necessary, cut from another end of the tunnel and enlarge it. The wound should be closed by a single horizontal suture or infinity or anchor suture.

Clear Corneal Incision

If temporal corneal incision is placed, it has advantage of:
1. Being compatible with topical anaesthesia since painful cautery is not required
2. Reduced surgical time and cost effectiveness due to elimination of conjunctiva and scleral steps and additional instruments
3. Avoiding scleral dissection errors such as thin flap, premature entry, etc.
4. Increased visibility due to enhanced red reflex
5. Superior astigmatic result because it is located in periphery of cornea away from the optical axis
6. Ease of surgery as:
   (a) Deep set globe and prominent glabellar ridge do not interfere
   (b) Less pooling of water in fornix
   (c) Less chance of oar locking of instruments
   (d) No bridle sutures are required
   (e) It neutralises drag on incision by gravity and lid blink.

Side port entry/Incision: Similar to conjuctival flap. (Fig. 10.8).

Hinged Corneal Incision

Initial perpendicular groove is made at 0.60 mm or more depth and 3.2 mm wide and tunnel is made parallel to iris at half corneal thickness, i.e. 0.30 mm in anterior one-third of corneal stroma. It is more resistance to external pressure than uniplanar and biplanar incisions (Figs 10.9 and 10.10).

Wound Closure

Self sealing incision does not require sutures, because when eye is pressurised with a balanced salt solution through the

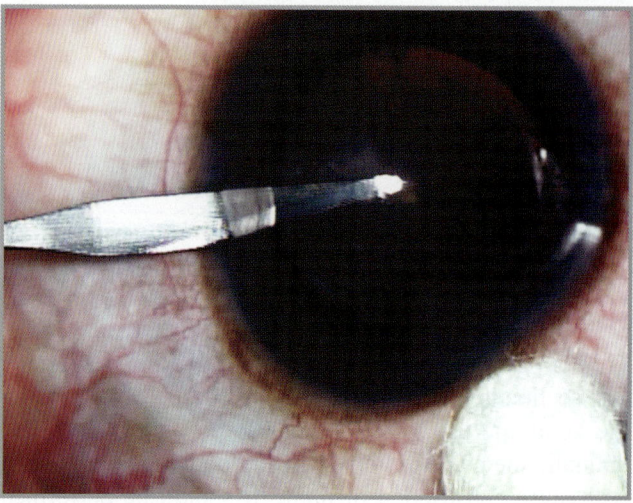

Fig.10.8: Side port entry/Incision

side port incision to a normal IOP, higher pressure inside AC forces two lips of internal opening against each other and closes them making it watertight. Internal corneal lip should be of adequate length all along, i.e. 2 mm approximately.

Types and Technique of Wound Closure

Wound integrity should be checked in all cases by depressing the posterior lip of incision. If there is a leakage through incision, stromal hydration at ends should be done which creates oedema, pulling tissues tight against each other and helps in a leakproof closure of the wound. If the wound is still leaky, 1 or 2 sutures depending upon size of incision should be placed with 10–0 monofilament nylon (Fig. 10.11).

Suturing techniques can be a radial or horizontal technique. Both may be either interrupted or continuous.

Continuous sutures equalise tension across the wound, whereas interrupted sutures may give better control by individual suture cutting.

Radial Sutures

Radial sutures are placed to approximate the edges of the incision which pulls scleral flap and cornea to new unphysiological position and disturb internal entry site leading to astigmatism.

Horizontal Sutures

It does not attempt to approximate edges of incision but it simply flattens scleral tunnel and makes incisions watertight. Horizontal sutures cause fewer disturbances of internal entry incision which is why, are less likely to cause astigmatism than radial sutures.

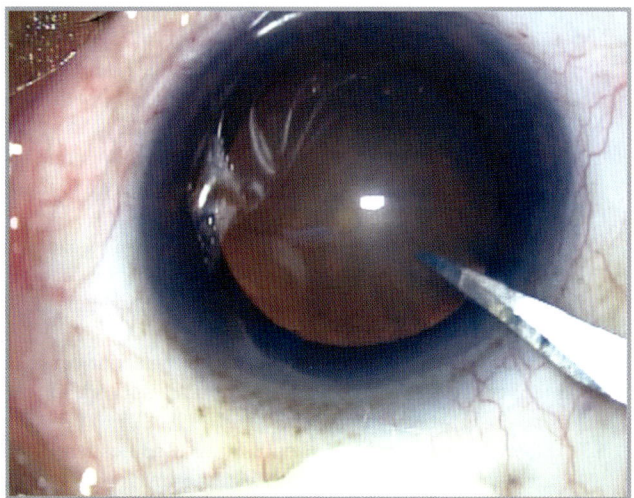

Fig. 10.9: Side port entry/incision prior to the construction of hinged corneal incision

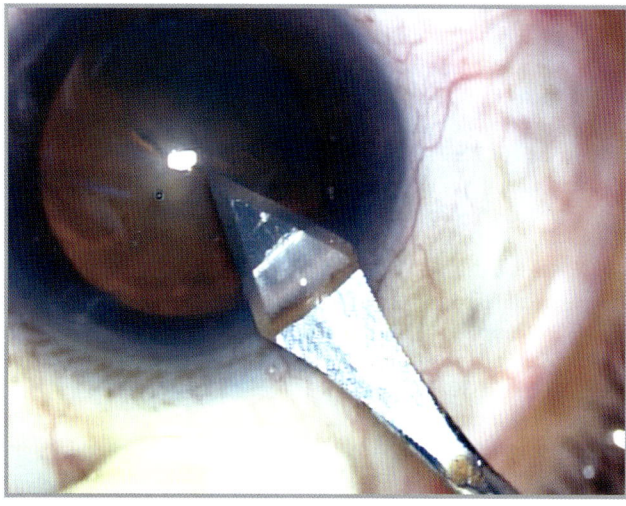

Fig. 10.10: Clear corneal incision (2.80 mm keratome entry)

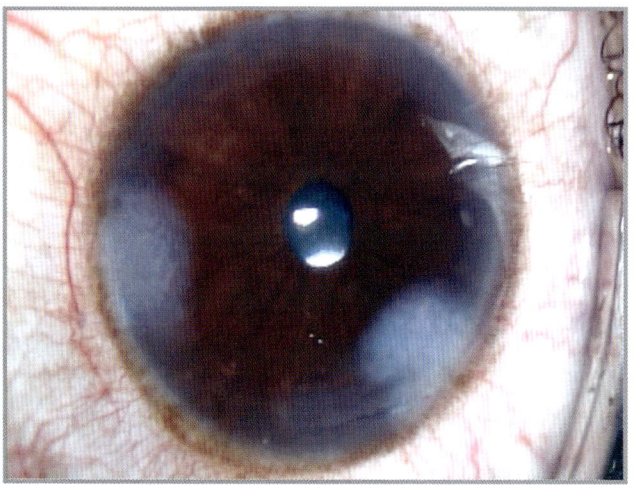

(a)

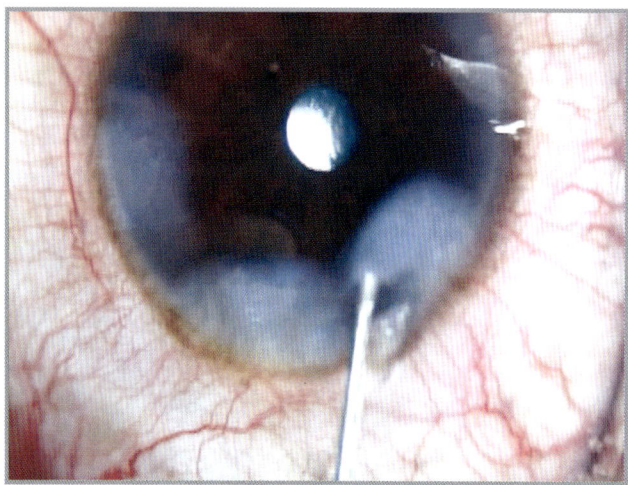

(b)

Fig. 10.11: (a), (b) Stromal hydration

Infinity Sutures

It sutures the roof of scleral tunnel that in cross section resembles the symbol for infinity. The first loop covers 40% of the tunnel width, with the needle entering at the right end of incision and exiting at the centre. The suture is then brought further left with the needle entering at the left end of incision and exiting at the centre. The two ends of sutures are pulled up tightly, tied and the suture ends are cut.

BIBLIOGRAPHY

1. Girard L J, Hoffman RF. Scleral tunnel to prevent induced astigmatism. Am J Ophthalmol 1984; 97: 450–456.
2. Kratz RP, Colveard DM, Mazzoceo TR,Davidson B. Clinical evaluation of terry surgical keratometer. Am Intraocular Implant Soc J 1990; 6: 249–251.
3. Jack A Singer. Frown incision for minimising induced astigmatism after small incision cataract surgery with rigid optic intraocular lens implantation. J Cataract Refract Surg 1991; 17: 677–688.
4. Mishra P. Small incision cataract surgery- Non Phaco SICS. Indian Intaocul Implant Refract J 2003; 1:9–15.
5. Kapoor Sashi. Incisions . Emmetropia, J Intraocular Implant and Refract Society 1999; 2: 17–25.
6. Mishra P. Cataract surgery in children. Cyber lectures, www.indmedica.com/ophthal 2000; 1–5.
7. Mody Kirit , Singh Gagan J. Small incision non-phaco cataract surgery. Emmetropia, J Intraocular Implant and Refract Society 1999; 2:9–11.
8. Kumar Ravindra. Small incision cataract surgery without phaco- my experience. Emmetropia, J Intraocular and Refract Society 1999; 2: 53–55.
9. Mishra P. Microvectis Technique. In: Singh Kamaljeet,ed, Small Incision Cataract Surgery.Jaypee Brothers, NewDelhi, 2002, pp 113–116.
10. Mishra P.Incision in Non phaco SICS, Orissa journal ophthal 2000; I I:30–32.
11. Manual small incision cataract surgery, Aravind eye hospital, Madurai, 2000.
12. Luther F. The phacosandwich Technique. In Rozakis cataract surgery: Alternative small incision technique.Thorofare,N.J. Slack Inc.71–110.
13. Kansas P. Phaco fracture In Rozakis cataract surgery: Alternative small incision technique. Thorofare, N.J. Slack Inc.45–70.
14. Hennig A, Kumar J,Yorston D et al. Sutureless cataract surgery with nucleus extraction. Br J Ophthalmol 2003; 87:266–270.
15. Thomas R, Kuriakose T, George R. Towards achieving small incision cataract surgery 99.8% of time. Indian J Ophthalmol 2000; 48:145–51.
16. Natchiar G. Manual small incision cataract surgery. Madurai, India: Aravind Publication,2000.
17. Goel R, Malik KPS. Techniques of Nuclear delivery in Nonphaco small incision cataract surgery. Ophthalmol Today 2003; IV:92–94.
18. Dandona L, Dandona R, Naduvilath TJ. Population based assessment of the outcome of cataract surgery in an urban population in southern India. Am J Ophthalmol 1999; 127:650–658.
19. Prajna NV, Chandrakanth KS, Kim R. et al. The Madurai intraocular lens study II: clinical outcomes. Am J Ophthalmol 1998; 125:14-25.
20. Holladat JT, Cravy TV, Koch DD, Calculating the surgically induced refracting change following ocular surgery. J Cataract Refract Surg 1992; 18:429–443.
21. Wright M, Chawla H, Adams A. Results of small incision extracapsular cataract surgery using the anterior chamber maintainer without viscoelastics. Br J Ophthalmol 1999; 83:71–75.
22. Peng Q, Hennig A, Vasavada AR et al. Posterior capsular plaque: a common feature of cataract surgery in the developing world. Am J Ophthalmol 1998; 125:621–626.
23. Haberle H, Anders N, Drosch S et al. Modification of no stitch technique in extracapsular cataract extraction by a single radial suture. Effect on postoperative astigmatism.
24. Morlet N, Minassian D, Dart J. Asigmatism and the analysis of its surgical correction. Br J Ophthalmol 2001; 85: 1127–38.

11

Capsulorrhexis

Dr S Biseria Gupta and Col JKS Parihar SM, VSM

INTRODUCTION

In the latter half of the last century various types of capsulotomy were popular. There were some inherent problems in these techniques, especially with reference to phacoemulsification like peripheral extension and decentration of the intraocular lens implanted in the bag. To overcome this problem in the mid 1980's, Howard Gimble (North America) presented his continuous tear capsulotomy. Almost at the same time, Thomas Neuhann (West Germany) independently developed the technique he called circular capsulorrhexis. Both the surgeons agreed to call their invention "continuous curvilinear capsulorrhexis".

Introduction of capsulorrhexis marked the new era of compartmentalisation in cataract surgery. It is now accepted, as the standard technique of making anterior capsular opening as against the once popular method of capsulotomy. The term capsulorrhexis is derived from the Greek word "rhexis", which means, "tearing". Achieving a proper size capsulorrhexis is mandatory for a problem-free phacoemulsification. Capsulorrhexis dictates the rest of the phacoemulsification procedure and hence its importance cannot be overstressed. It is one of the most difficult steps to master and every beginner should understand the basics of the technique.

Since capsulorrhexis involves tearing instead of cutting, a smooth circular opening is created which retains the lens capsular mechanical properties. Unlike capsulotomy, which is easily extended towards the periphery, it is almost impossible to tear the smooth continuous margin of capsulorrhexis.

ADVANTAGES OF AN INTACT CAPSULORRHEXIS

Intraoperative

(i) The smooth margin and absence of edges and tags make the steps like aspiration irrigation trouble-free.

(ii) The margins can be stretched considerably without causing distortion.

(iii) Intraoperative stress on the zonules is minimal and is distributed evenly.

(iv) During phacoemulsification (closed chamber surgery) the capsular bag is ballooned up pushing the posterior capsule posteriorly and the rhexis margins are stretched horizontally, thus providing enough space to manoeuvre away from the cornea and reduce a risk of engaging the posterior capsule.

(v) Hydrorocedures and nuclear management inside the capsular bag are no longer plagued by the risk of posterior extension of the capsular tears.

(vi) The bag fixation of the IOL prevents decentration and irregular astigmatism.

(vii) In event of posterior capsular rents it is still possible to safely implant IOL in the sulcus or do **rhexis fixation** (optic capture in side rhexis margin with haptics in the ciliary sulcus).

Postoperative

(i) Uniform distribution of forces within the capsular bag prevents decentration and dislocation of the IOL.

(ii) Possibility of iris contact, pigment dispersion and postoperative inflammation is reduced.

MECHANICS OF CAPSULORRHEXIS

After creation of the capsular flap, depending on the direction of application of the force, anterior capsulorrhexis can be completed by tearing, either by stretching or by shearing.

Stretching

Force sufficient to overcome the strength of the capsule is applied on the anterior capsular flap. The direction of the force applied is perpendicular to the direction of the tear, i.e. centripetal (towards the centre of the pupil), as shown in the figure, to prevent it from going towards the periphery. It is very difficult to control the process of tearing as the rhexis has the tendency to run towards the periphery with a force less than what is needed to tear the flap in the right direction (Fig. 11.1a).

Shearing

The force is applied in the direction of least resistance, i.e. perpendicular to its plane. This means that only a minimal force is required to tear the capsule and hence lesser chances of peripheral extension exist (Fig. 11.1b).

TECHNIQUES OF CAPSULORRHEXIS

The two popular techniques of capsulorrhexis currently in use are:
- (a) Bent needle or cystotome (Fig. 11.2)
- (b) Utrata forceps (Fig. 11.3)

Bent needle or Cystotomes Technique of Capsulorrhexis

Before starting the capsulorrhexis, it is desirable to make the anterior capsule flat by making the anterior chamber deep by injecting a viscoelastic substance. In this technique a bent 26 G needle or cystotome with a very sharp cutting tip is brought to rest at the centre of the capsule, inserted just below the capsule and raised, thus creating an initial puncture in the anterior capsule.

This puncture is made either in the centre or somewhere within the desired diameter of the capsulorrhexis. In the same motion, a curved slit is created. From this point the circular tear is started by lifting and pushing or pulling the central point of the anterior capsule depending on the direction in which the surgeon wishes to start.

This manoeuvre creates a flap which is turned upon itself. The base of this flap is engaged with the needle tip and torn in a circular manner by applying the tear force accordingly. Care should be taken not to perforate the

capsule and engage the cortex as this could reduce the visibility of the capsule and make the procedure difficult.

As the tear is brought around full circle the needle tip is repositioned in a similar manner at least 5 to 6 times over the flap to provide better control. The capsulorrhexis is completed by bringing the two ends together from outside inwards. Throughout the procedure, the anterior chamber should be deep.

Utrata Forceps Technique

Alternatively, forceps (Utrata) can be used for creating the flap and grasping the capsule. It was introduced by Utrata.

In this technique, the corneal incision required is larger (3 mm) to allow movement of the forceps. The anterior chamber is filled with a viscoelastic and the anterior capsular flap is created with a cystotome or Utrata forceps itself. The flap is then grasped with the forceps and traction is applied to tear it circularly. The direction of traction should be inwards to avoid peripheral extension.

CAPSULAR STAINING TECHNIQUES

(a) Attempts to enhance the visualisation of the anterior capsule to facilitate capsulorrhexis in white cataracts or cataracts with no red glow, started in 1993 when Hoffen and McFarland used sub capsular injection of fluorescein. Since then, many dyes have been tried. Some of these dyes are as follows:
  - (i) Autologus blood
  - (ii) Fluorescein sodium
  - (iii) Gentian violet
  - (iv) Methylene blue
  - (v) Trypan blue
  - (vi) Indocyanine green
(b) Two techniques were used to stain the anterior capsule—one under the air bubble over the capsule and the subcapsular injection. Over the years, it was demonstrated that trypan blue and ICG are not only safe for staining of the anterior capsule for capsulorrhexis, but they also do not leak into the vitreous like fluorescein (Fig. 11.4).

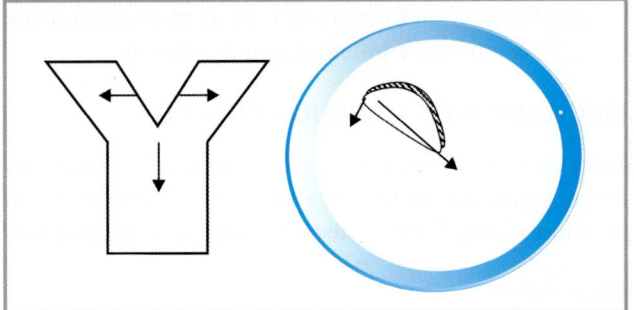
(a)

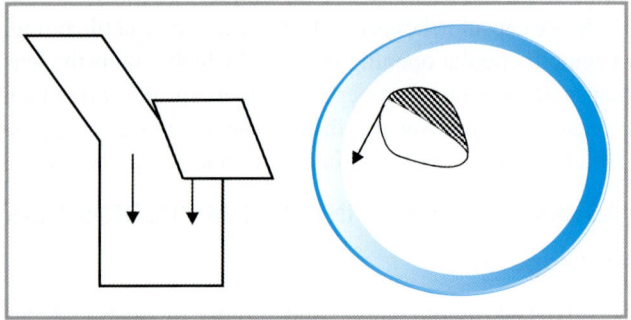
(b)

Fig. 11.1: (a) Tearing by stretching (b) Tearing by shearing

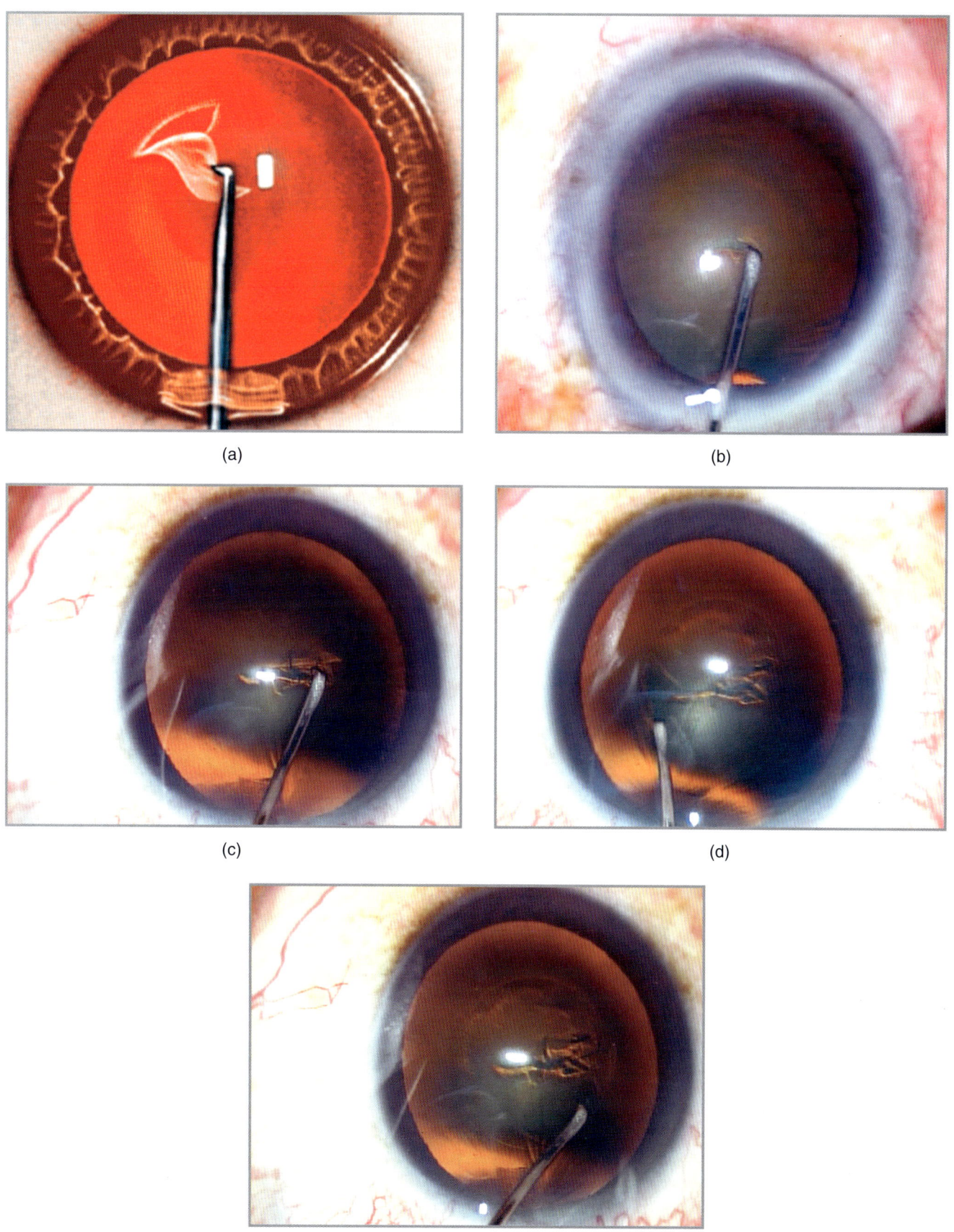

(a)

(b)

(c)

(d)

(e)

Fig. 11.2: (a) Creation of anterior capsular flap by cystotome, (b) to (e) Techniques of capsulorrhexis: bent needle or cystotomes technique

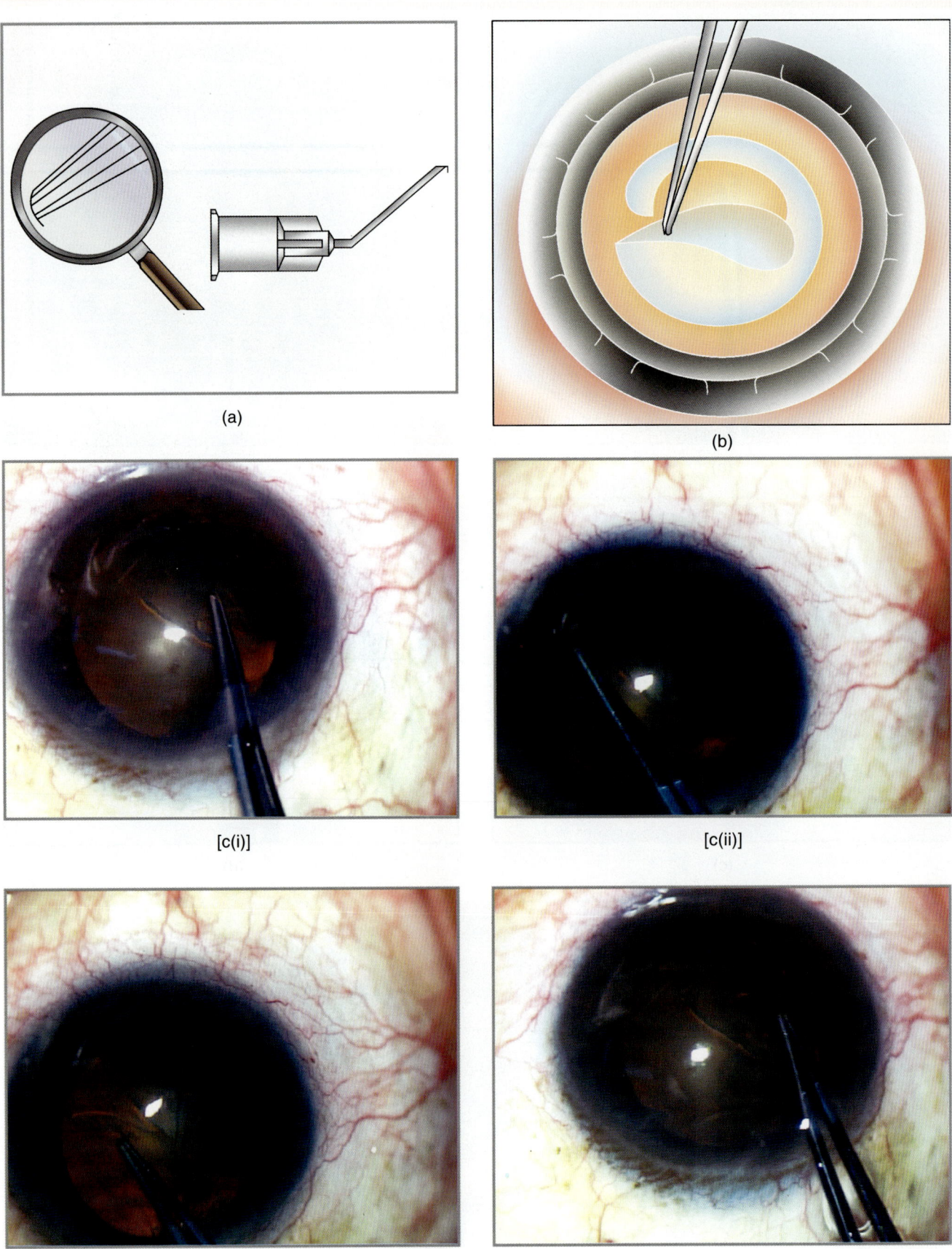

(a)

(b)

[c(i)]

[c(ii)]

[c(iii)]

[c(iv)]

Fig. 11.3: (a) Utrata forceps and cystotome, (b) Capsulorrhexis using utrata forceps, (c) (i) Commencing capsulorrhexis using utrata forceps (ii), (iii) and (iv) Capsulorrhexis using utrata forceps (anticlock movement)

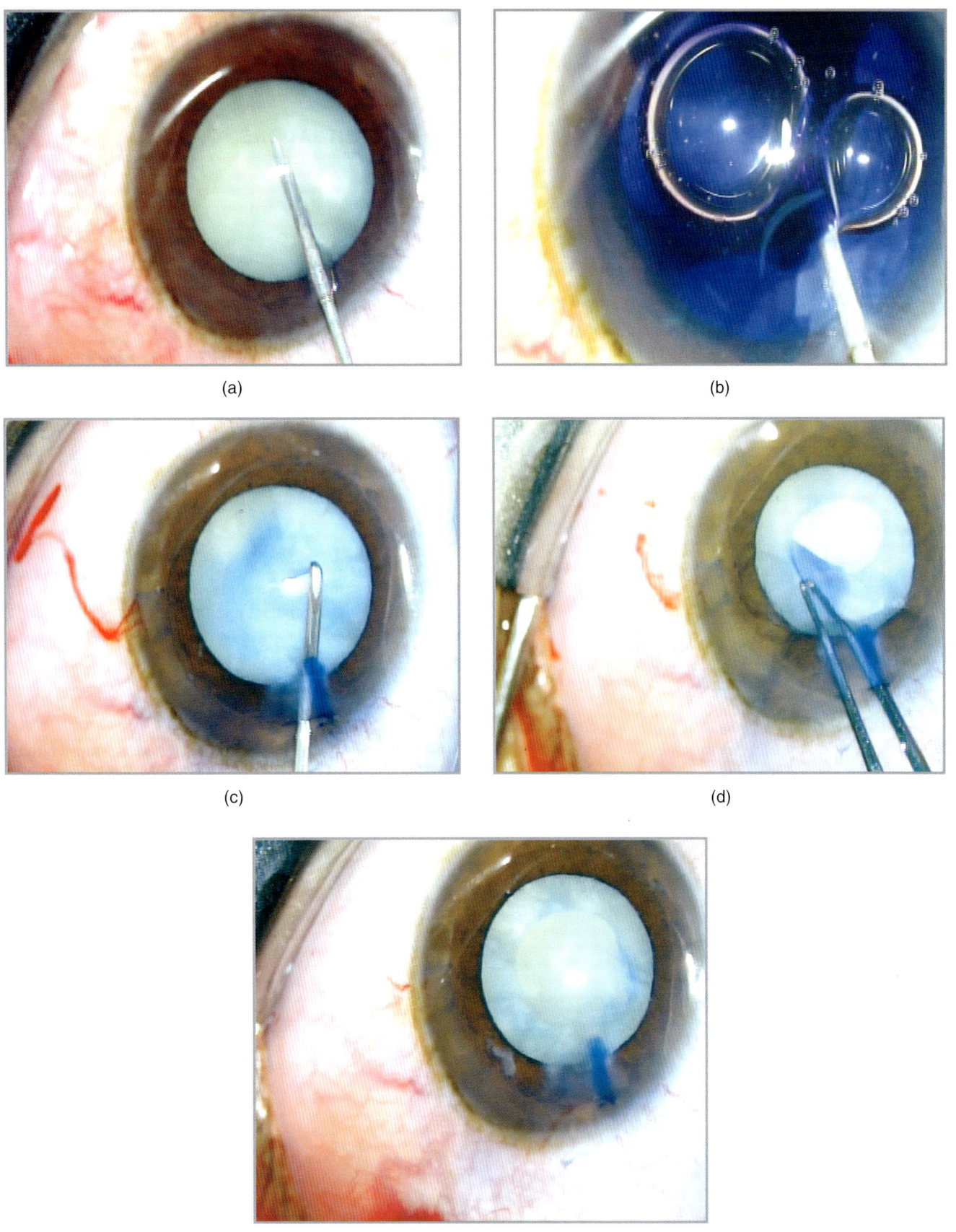

(a)

(b)

(c)

(d)

(e)

Fig. 11.4: (a) Capsular staining techniques of capsulorrhexis: Insertion of 26 gauze needle into the anterior chamber, (b) Capsular staining under air bubble with trypan blue, (c) to (e) Capsular staining assisted capsulorrhexis

Trypan blue is used in the concentration of 0.1% and ICG 0.5%. Trypan blue is the dye preferred by most surgeons as compared to ICG because of the following factors:

(i) Better contrast
(ii) Cheaper
(iii) No need for reconstitution
(iv) No endothelial staining

It should, however, be noted that these dyes stain the foldable hydrophilic acrylic lenses requiring explantation and lens exchange, hence should not be used in cases where such lens is being implanted.

Staining of anterior capsule under air bubble is the favoured method as it is safer and recommended for cases with high intralenticular pressure. The safety and usage of trypan blue for capsular staining is well established now. Staining of the capsule also offers the advantage of visibility of the rhexis margin during rest of the phacoemulsification procedure thus increasing the safety by reducing the risk of inadvertent damage to the rhexis margin, and better cortical cleaning.

A capsulorrhexis opening of 5 to 6 mm is considered adequate. An ideal capsulorrhexis is one, which is well centreed and just overlaps the optics of the IOL (Fig. 11.5).

TIPS FOR MAKING AN IDEAL SIZE CAPSULORRHEXIS

(i) Loosen the speculum and drapes should not pull on ocular adnexa.
(ii) Liberal use of viscoelastics whenever needed to keep the anterior chamber deep.
(iii) Frequent regrasping of the capsular flap near the origin.
(iv) Use of soft shell technique.
(v) Stabilisation of the globe by a second instrument when using topical anaesthesia.
(vi) Use of forceps gives better control.
(vii) Correctly assess or measure the size of pupillary dilatation.

(viii) Use of an optical zone marker to judge the rhexis size.
(ix) Capsular staining technique for cataract with poor glow and pediatric cataract.

DIFFICULT SITUATIONS

Rhexis Escape

One of the major problems encountered during capsulorrhexis is rhexis escape, i.e. tendency of peripheral extension. Such a problem can arise at any step.
Tips for managing rhexis escape:

(i) Deepen the anterior chamber with viscoelastic.
(ii) Attempt to direct the flap towards the centre of the pupil with cystotome or forceps.
(iii) The above manoeuvre is not always successful, under such circumstances it is advisable to redirect the flap back to the initial route by making a cut at the escape point with microsurgical scissors or
(iv) Start a new rhexis at other position and then merge with the original rhexis at the escape point.

Stellate Burst

A Stellate opening may occur when the needle tip or the cystotome is blunt. Such an opening is managed by tearing in both directions from the most peripheral edges to achieve a continuous capsulorrhexis as shown in the Fig. 11.6.

Small Rhexis

Sometimes, the size of rhexis achieved is smaller than desired or during the process of capsulorrhexis it is noted that the diameter of the rhexis is smaller than desired. If such a condition is encountered capsulorrhexis may be spiralled out till the intended diameter is achieved and then the tear is brought inwards to complete the rhexis. Alternately, a small cut may be given with micro scissors and the capsular flap is spiralled out to achieve the desired diameter.

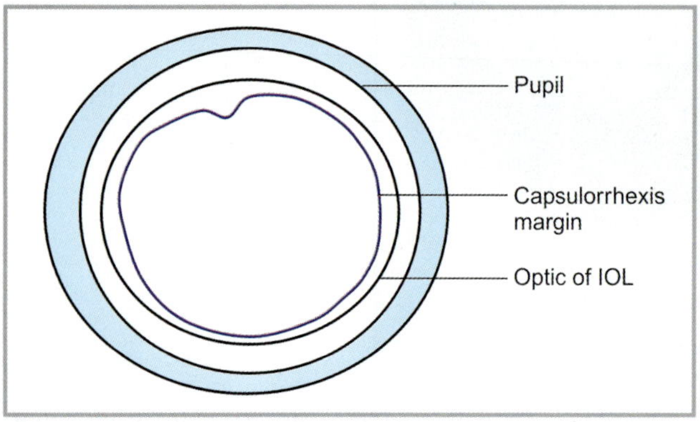

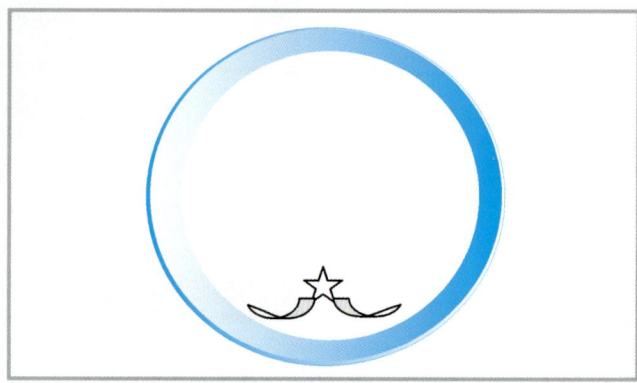

Fig. 11.5: Ideal capsulorrhexis

Pupil

Capsulorrhexis margin

Optic of IOL

Fig. 11.6: Management of Stellate opening

No Red Glow

Absence of red reflex is a challenging situation for any surgeon performing capsulorrhexis. In our country it is a rather commonly encountered situation. Under such circumstances visualisation of the leading edge of the capsular flap is very difficult and errant capsular tearing frequently occurs and is difficult to control. When confronted with such a situation one of the following modifications or a combination of these modifications may be of great help:

   (i) Increasing magnification
   (ii) Dimming of operating room lights
   (iii) Use of air
   (iv) Use of high density viscoelastics
   (v) Endoilluminator
   (vi) Tangential light (endoilluminator) placed at limbus
   (vii) Two stage CCC approach (debulking and removal of lens through small rhexis followed by enlargement of rhexis)
   (viii) Capsular staining with dye.

Small Pupil

There are many patients with conditions like diabetes, uveitis, etc. where the pupil fails to dilate. Performing capsulorrhexis when the pupillary size is smaller than the desired rhexis size may end up in disaster. For performing safe rhexis one may follow different techniques or a combination. Tips for performing safe capsulorrhexis with small pupil area are as follows:

   (i) Start Capsulorrhexis from the centre
   (ii) Visualising the tear by retracting the pupil with the second instrument
   (iii) Two stage CCC approach
   (iv) Iris retractors
   (v) Sphincterotomies

Pediatric Cataract

The capsule in pediatric cataract is extremely elastic and very difficult to handle. Capsulorrhexis in such cases have very high propensity for peripheral extension. Tips for capsulorrhexis in pediatric cases are:

   (i) High density viscoelastic
   (ii) Pronounced centripetal direction of tearing
   (iii) Capsular staining for better visualisation.

Complications and Pit Falls of Capsulorrhexis and their Remedies

   (i) Difficulty in removal of 12 O' clock cortical matter can be managed with bent J-shaped cannula or a bimanual I/A or even dialling of IOL, releases the cortical matter.
   (ii) **In case with decentred capsular opening**, the IOL may get decentreed following fibrosis of the capsule. It can be prevented by centring the rhexis by removal of excess capsule.
   (iii) **Discontinuity of anterior capsular rim with peripheral extension** may be seen in Stellate opening and intumescent swollen lens. Debulking of cortical matter helps in such cases and the base of the capsular tear can be pulled centripetally. Such manoeuvres may help in some cases only and hence, such a condition is better anticipated and prevented.
   (iv) **Capsular contraction syndrome** (Fig. 11.7) is seen commonly in capsulorrhexis, especially in cases with small rhexis. It is characterised by fibrous dysplasia of residual lens epithelium resulting in extreme reduction in size of the anterior capsular opening and the equatorial bag diameter. It may result in malposition of the capsular opening and displacement of IOL. It is common in pseudo-exfoliation, advanced age, uveitis and myotonic dystrophy. This condition can be treated by early radial YAG laser capsulotomies. Large capsulorrhexis by reducing the epithelial cells, decreases the chance of capsular contraction.
   (v) **Capsular bag distension** or **capsular block** means fluid hyper distension of the capsular bag. It occurs because of blockage of anterior capsular opening by IOL optic. The source of this fluid is unclear. A self-limiting condition can be permanently cured by making a small opening with YAG laser in the anterior or posterior capsule.

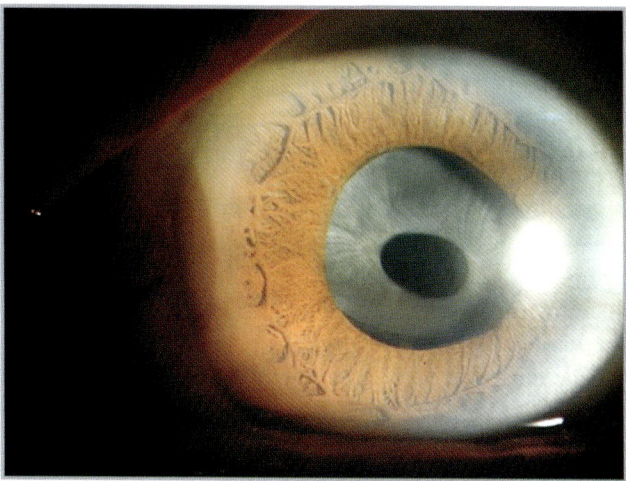

Fig. 11.7: Capsular contraction syndrome

12

Hydroprocedures in Phacoemulsification

Surg Cdr Tarun Choudhary and Col JKS Parihar SM, VSM

INTRODUCTION

Lead Kindly light …

Keep thou my feet: I do not ask to see

The distant scene: one-step enough for me.

These five words from a church hymn are as relevant for phacoemulsification as they are in any other walk of life. If we approach the art of phacoemulsification one step at a time, the road to conversion to phacoemulsification will be littered with less pitfalls and setbacks.

An important steps in the procedure of phacoemulsification are the hydroprocedures, which have stood the test of time and have become a critical and integral step in modern, safe phacoemulsification.

Hydroprocedures, essentially encompass two procedures: hydrodissection and hydrodelineation. The succeeding paragraphs will aim at giving the reader a thorough scientific understanding of the above-named procedures and their variations as practised in phacoemulsification today.

CONCENTRIC ANATOMY OF THE LENS

A detailed description of the anatomy and embryology of the lens is beyond the scope of this chapter. However, it is prudent to reinforce our knowledge about the basic anatomy of the lens so as to get a better understanding of the various hydroprocedures.

The lens is derived from the outer embryonic surface ectoderm. A chemical induction process causes the cluster of surface ectoderm cells to evolve into the lens vesicle. The cytoplasmic processes of the growing cells eventually obliterate the lumen of the vesicle, forming the lens nucleus. An anterior displacement of the lens epithelial cells that formerly lined the posterior capsule occurs. This is the reason why there are no cells lining the posterior capsule of the normal crystalline lens after the embryonic stage.

The formation of all subsequent fibres around the embryonic nucleus occurs at the equatorial lens bow. It is called so because of the bow-like arrangement of the nuclei of the cells (Fig. 12.1). The anterior lens epithelial cells slowly migrate towards the equator. As they reach the equator they undergo a more rapid mitotic division.

The cytoplasmic processes of the cells forming the lens bow elongate resulting in laying down of new cortical fibres. As new fibres are formed, the cell nuclei gradually disappear. Thus, the centre or the nucleus of the lens does not have cell nuclei.

The lens present at birth is 6 to 8 mm in diameter and 4 mm in thickness. It consists of the embryonic and foetal nucleus. The adult lens has a diameter of 9.6 mm ($\pm$ 0.4 mm) and a thickness of 4.2 mm ($\pm$ 0.5 mm). The weight of an adult is about 225–235 mg and it has a yellowish tinge which intensifies with age.

The lens nucleus basically consists of three components: the capsule, the epithelium and the lens substance. The lens substance is in turn composed of two separate entities,

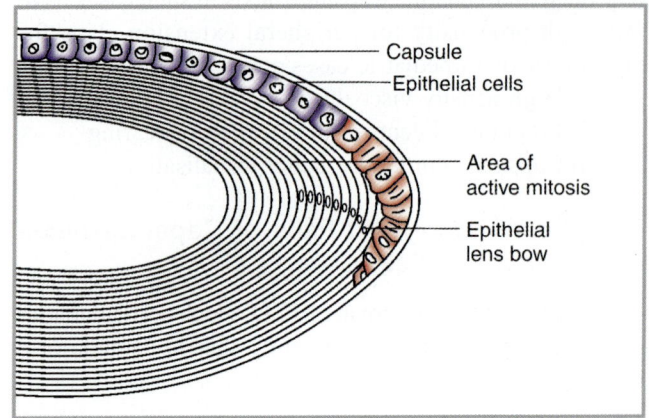

Fig. 12.1: Mitosis of anterior epithelial cells and formation of cortical fibres in lens

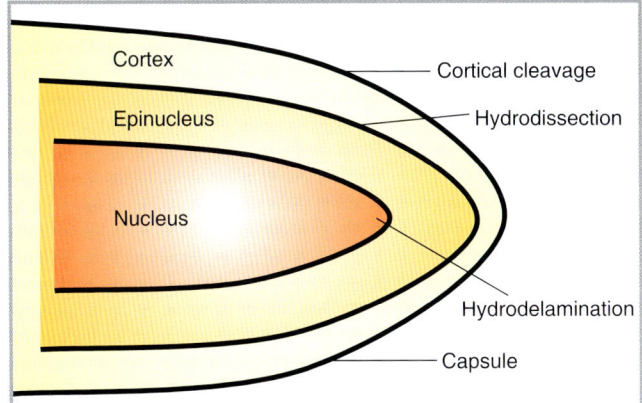

Fig. 12.2: Layers of crystalline lens and planes of hydroprocedures

viz: the Cortex and the Nucleus, which are formed due to the continuous growth of the lens epithelium. The water content of the lens is the highest in the outer layers of the cortex, whereas the protein content increases as one moves towards the nucleus. With growth, new lens fibres are added to the cortex and cortical compaction occurs. This central compaction is a gradual transition with the intermediate region between the cortical fibres and the hard nucleus made up of compact waterless cortical fibres with no cellular nuclei. This intermediate zone which engulfs the hard core is called the epinucleus (Fig 12.2).

HYDRODISSECTION

Introduction

KJ Faust introduced the term "hydrodissection" and also described the technique for ECCE, he recognised its applicability to phacoemulsification. Since then, the procedure has been referred to by different names by various surgeons. Subtle modifications of this procedure led to the advent of "cortical cleaving hydrodissection" by Howard Fine and "hydro free hydrodissection" by HV Gimbel, the details of which will be discussed subsequently.

In the times gone by, when the technique of phacoemulsification was in its infancy, most of the surgeons desisted from carrying out hydrodissection. In fact the cortico-epinuclear adhesions which the hydrodissection aims at breaking were referred to as the "third hand" in phacoemulsification. This was in the pre-CCC era when phacoemulsification was accomplished with can-opener capsulotomy and at the iris plane. Here the "third hand" was required to hold on to the nucleus while sculpting was in progress so that it did not prolapse into the anterior chamber.

In modern day phacoemulsification, lots of reasons have been propagated for the need to carry out hydrodissection. With the present day machines all other reasons are superfluous except for the fact that hydrodissection is essential to rotate the nucleus. Hydrodissection breaks the cortico-epinuclear adhesions to make the nucleus free-floating in the capsular bag. This allows placing the part of the nucleus to be worked upon at 6'O'Clock.

Definition

Hydrodissection refers to the injection of balanced salt solution/Ringer's lactate under the anterior capsular flap until the fluid courses around the equator at the cortico-epinuclear plane, flows under the epinucleus and separates the epinucleus from its cortical attachments.

The end point of this procedure is the convex "fluid-wave" seen crossing the field away from the point of injection. On completion of the procedure, the nucleus should rotate freely in the capsular bag. Any other outcome indicates an incomplete or improper hydrodissection and warrants a repeat hydrodissection. Other signs of a good hydrodissection are a shallowing of the anterior chamber, dullness of the red glow and, as mentioned earlier, a free rotation of the nucleus.

Technique

As the anterior chamber would have been filled with viscoelastic for CCC, a part of this viscoelastic must be removed from the anterior chamber before hydrodissection. If hydrodissection is attempted with an anterior chamber full of viscoelastic, the posterior capsule can "blow out", sinking the nucleus into the vitreous.

Hydrodissection is best performed using a 25 gauge cannula with a blunt rounded tip, though opinions vary with different surgeons preferring cannulas ranging from 25 to 30 G. This cannula is placed on a 2 cc syringe filled with balanced salt solution/Ringer's lactate.

The tip of the cannula is passed under the edge of the anterior capsule obtained after CCC and advanced for 1 mm. Care is taken to keep the cannula perpendicular to the capsulotomy edge (Fig. 12.3). Now, a minimal amount of fluid is injected in a spurt. A distinct fluid wave can be seen progressing centrally from the point of injection. This wave is due to the fluid interface coursing all around the cortex at the cortico-epinuclear plane, in the process breaking the cortico-epinuclear adhesions. Ultimately, the fluid emerges into the anterior chamber from the end opposite to the point of injection. Two to three such injections are made in separate quadrants of the lens, injecting a spurt of little fluid every time. There is no hard and fast rule as to the exact meridian in which the injections are to be made.

While injecting, very light pressure is applied on the central nucleus to prevent what I call "hydro-phimosis". This phenomenon is generally seen in cases with a relatively small CCC, where an excess amount of fluid has been injected or the fluid has been injected slowly and

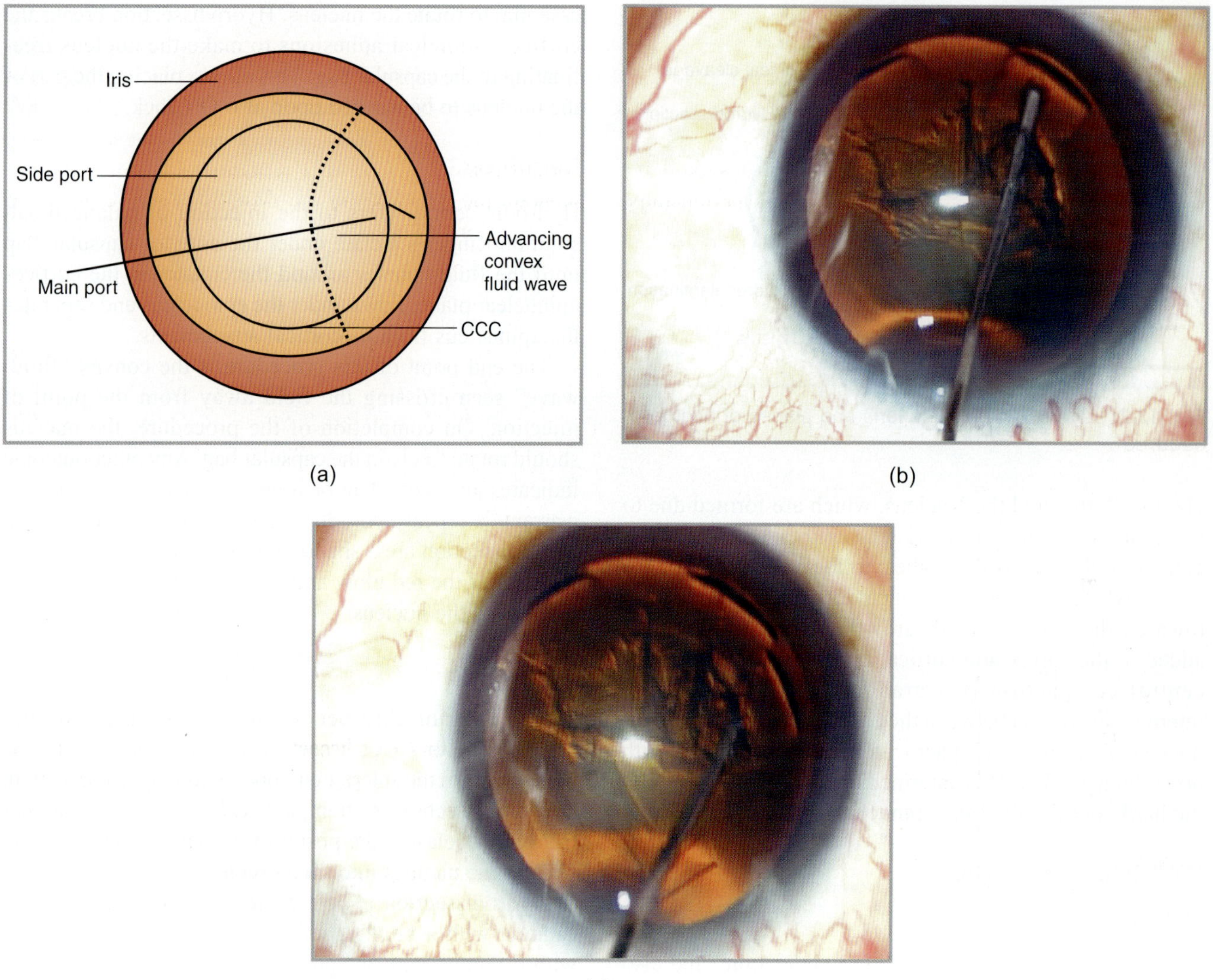

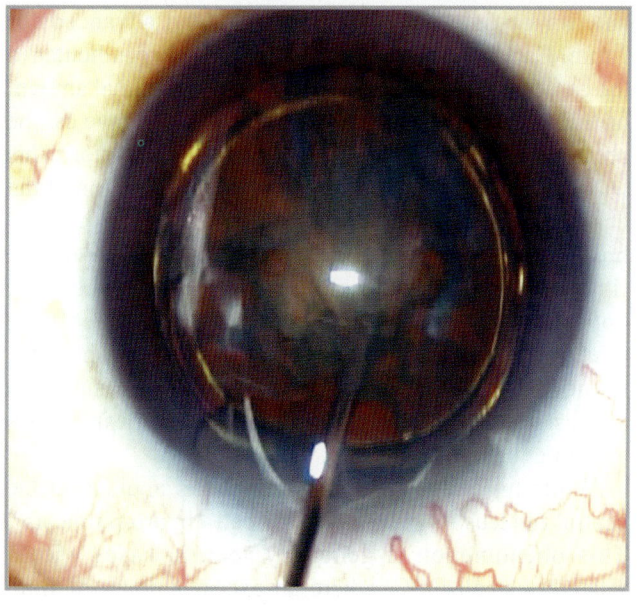

(a)

(b)

(c)

Fig. 12.3: (a), (b) and (c) Placement of hydrodissection cannula

Fig. 12.4: Hydrodissection (fluid wave)

not in a spurt. Here, the fluid accumulates behind the nucleus between the epinucleus and the cortex and does not emerge into the anterior chamber from the site opposite to that of the injection. This causes a stretch of the posterior capsule, which might "blow out" posteriorly. Conversely, the collected fluid pushes up the lens pouting it out of the CCC and leading to an extremely shallow anterior chamber or even lenticulo-corneal touch. Many a surgeon has been a mute witness to the nucleus sinking into the vitreous after hydrodissection, without them having as much as touched the phacoemulsification machine.

Also, after every injection of the fluid, the nucleus is slightly tapped before the next injection is made in a separate quadrant so that any trapped retronuclear fluid is squeezed out into the anterior chamber. After two to three such hydrodissections, an attempt is made to rotate the nucleus by embedding a dialler tip into the nucleus just inside the edge of the capsulotomy and twirling the dialler slowly. While rotating the nucleus, the principle of torque has to be kept in mind. If you recall your physics text, torque is defined as the product of force and lever arm (Torque = Force × Lever arm). Thus, to ensure that minimal force is required to rotate the nucleus, the lever arm (distance between the centre of the nucleus and the point where the dialler has been embedded) should be maximum. Thus, the dialler should be embedded peripherally as close to the edge of the CCC as possible. It is to be remembered that at the time of rotation, no posterior pressure or centrifugal force should be applied. A nicely hydrodissected nucleus will rotate freely like a top with the minimum of effort. A failure to rotate the nucleus calls for repeat hydrodissection and not use of excess force.

Hydrodissection in Posterior Polar Cataracts

Posterior polar cataracts offer a challenge for phacoemulsi-fication. They are one of the most common types of congenital and presenile symptomatic cataracts. They morphologically consist of a circular plaque with concentric whorls on the central posterior capsule. They are generally bilateral though may be asymmetrical. The posterior central opacity extends anteriorly from the posterior capsule into the posterior cortex. Posterior polar cataracts may be stationary or progressive. They are usually autosomal dominant (haptoglobin focus of chromosome 18) with sporadic cases arising due to new mutations. The exact pathogenesis is not known with the cataract being attributed to persistence of the hyaloid artery or an invasion of the lens by mesoblastic tissue.

Posterior polar cataracts are to be differentiated from posterior subcapsular cataracts and posterior lenticonus. Posterior subcapsular cataracts would have a minimal clear zone between the cataract and the posterior capsule. Posterior lenticonus is a unilateral, sporadically occurring porous opacity which has a posterior protuberance of the posterior curvature of the lens.

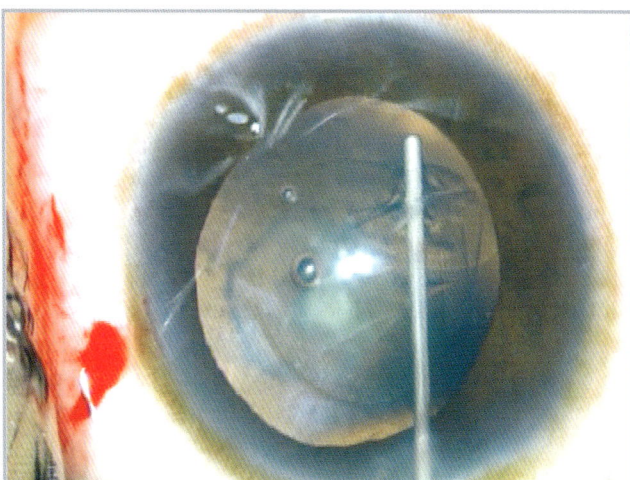

Fig. 12.5: Hydrodissection (fluid wave) in posterior polar cataracts

Posterior polar cataracts are more prone to have a posterior "blow out" during hydrodissection with the posterior capsular rent typically being circular and corresponding to the rim of the opacity. This is thought to be due to excessive tight adherence of plaque to otherwise normal posterior capsule. The hydrodissection does not separate the plaque from the posterior capsule but pulls the posterior capsule along. The other school of thought is that the posterior capsule lying under the opacity is exceedingly thin, thus rupturing it even with a small spurt of fluid wave. The only deliverance in such situations is conservancy. It is better in such situations to err on the side of safety and underdo the hydrodissection rather than overdo it. Some surgeons who trench the nucleus before cracking it do minimal hydrodissection. They believe that the fluid flow from the phaco tip during sculpting forms the desired cleavage between the cortex and the epinucleus. Still, doing hydrodissection in a posterior polar cataract is a situation which gives even the most skilled phaco surgeons a skipped heartbeat.

Modifications of Hydrodissection

(i) **Viscodissection:** Use of viscoelastics has been tried for viscodissection of the capsule from the nucleus but is not favoured as the procedure tends to displace the nucleus into the anterior chamber.

(ii) **Cortical cleaving hydrodissection:** It was assumed that cortex by its natural tendency was adherent to the capsule. Fine challenged this concept and argued that he could not find any cortex adherent to the undersurface of the circular piece of anterior capsule that he removed after doing a CCC. It implied that cortex was not necessarily attached to a capsule and it may be possible to separate the two of them. In cortical cleaving hydrodissection, the cannula is lifted to tent up the anterior capsule before injecting the fluid. The fluid which comes out of the cannula hits the tented up anterior capsule, courses along its posterior surface, thus dissecting the capsule from the posterior cortex. Most of the surgeons doing phacoemulsification today do cortical cleaving hydrodissection, though they loosely refer to it as only hydrodissection.

The advantage cited for cortical cleaving hydrodissection is that with this technique, the entire cortex is adherent to the nucleus and once the nucleus is removed by phaco, there is no cortical clean-up and aspiration required. This reduces the extent of irrigation-aspiration to be done. Also the thorough removal of the cortex by cortical cleaving hydrodissection not only decreases the number of lens epithelial cells that have a potential to proliferate but also may decrease the potential for a lens induced (phacogenic) inflammation.

(iii) Hydro-free dissection: Gimbel proposed the routine application of a lifting and tenting of the anterior capsular edge along with a sideways sweeping motion of the cannula under the capsular flap prior to injecting the fluid. He named this technique hydro-free dissection. It has been seen that hydro-free dissection followed by injection of the fluid under the anterior capsule gives the cleanest possible cleavage in the quadrant where the hydrodissection has been carried out. Some cortical fibres may remain attached to the capsule in other quadrants as the fluid wave follows the path of least resistance and dissects into cortical lamellae at the pole when it meets the radial fibres coming from the opposite side. Since the quadrant of hydrodissection is the cleanest, it is advised by some surgeons to start the hydro-dissection in the subincisional area with a J-shaped cannula to minimise the difficult cortical clean-up of the subincisional area.

HYDRODELAMINATION

Introduction and Definition

Hydrodelamination is also known by other names like hydrodelineation, hydrodemarcation, hydrofragmentation, etc. Anis introduced the term hydrodelineation and described it as an incremental injection of fluid directly into the lens matter within the confines of the capsular bag. It is in fact a concentric dismantling of the cataract.

The aim of hydrodelamination is to divide the nucleus into two concentric parts—the outer epinucleus and the inner hard nucleus. It is the inner hard nucleus that requires the attention of the phaco power whereas the outer

epinucleus is soft and can be easily taken care of by aspiration without phaco power, thus saving on phaco-time, energy and effort.

An added advantage of performing hydrodelamination is the safety it imparts to the phaco procedure. The central hard nucleus is not only hard in terms of its physical state but also hard to phacoemulsify. The central hard nucleus, once broken into pieces with phaco, has sharp edges capable of cutting the anterior or posterior capsule during manipulation in the process of phacoemulsification. Hydrodelamination divides the nucleus into an outer cushion and an inner hard nucleus. The cushion of epinucleus acts as a sponge and shock absorber, thereby forming a zone of comfort between the capsule and the hard nuclear edges, preventing capsular rents and tears.

Technique

The sequence of hydroprocedures used to be a topic of debate in earlier days but now there is a consensus that hydrodelineation should follow hydrodissection. The preferred cannula for hydrodelamination is a 26 G cannula with a blunt pointed tip to embed the cannula into the nucleus without significant posterior stress. However, for ease of use, most of the surgeons perform hydrodelamination with the same cannula that they have used for hydrodissection. In this procedure, the cannula is pushed into the mass of the nucleus just central to the edge of the CCC in a tangential position till it meets with resistance. At a particular point, the nucleus will stop giving way and care is to be taken here to resist the temptation of digging deeper with an aim to reduce the phacoable nucleus. The posterior push, if applied, causes zonular stress and irreparable zonular damage.

At the place where the cannula has come to a stop, the cannula is withdrawn a fraction of a millimetre and a spurt of minimal amount of fluid is injected into the tract formed by the cannula. The end point is signalled by what has been classically described as a golden ring/halo. Sometimes, only a dark separation plane may be seen and in other cases only a partial ring may be seen. A partial ring necessitates a re-hydrodelamination. A number of surgeons, including the author, avoid hydrodelamination in grade II or III cataracts. This is for the simple reason that with the present machines available, it is possible to phaco less dense cataracts with minimal power and high suction. The whole nucleus follows into the phaco tip at these high parameters. In case of soft cataracts, when hydrodelamination is done, the cannula progresses to a greater depth before coming to a stop. Thus, we have a thicker epinuclear shell and a thin central core nucleus. This thick epinucleus causes a lot of struggle coming out through the aspiration port and sometimes, requires even controlled light phaco power application.

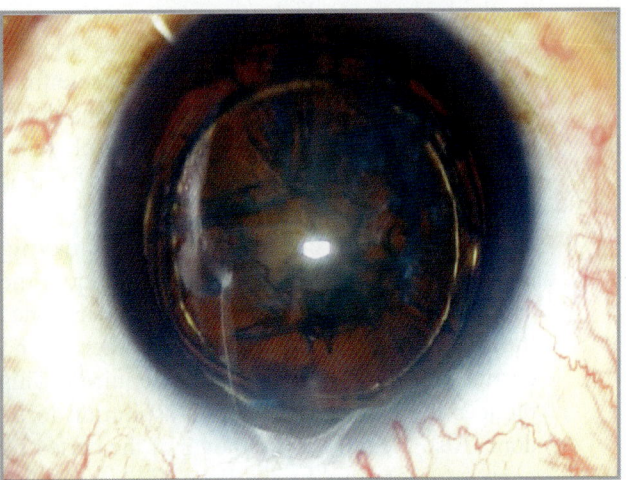

Fig. 12.6: Hydrodelamination (multiple golden rings) (fluid is pushed into epinucleus /cortex after golden ring formation)

Hydrosonic

Hydrosonic is an ultrasonically driven needle placed into the body of the nucleus. With successive injections of balanced salt solution or Ringer's lactate, hydrosonic is used to fragment the nucleus into sections or lamellae which can be emulsified with greater ease and with less ultrasonic energy being delivered to the eye. This technique has not gained in popularity due to the inordinately large time it takes to accomplish the task vis-à-vis the minimal benefits offered.

BIBLIOGRAPHY

1. Allarakhia L, Pearce JL: A new cannula for hydrodissection. Ophthalmic Surg 1989, 20:295–7.
2. Auffarth GU, Newland TJ, Wesendahl TA, Apple DJ. Nd:YAG laser damage to silicone intraocular lenses confused with pigment deposits on clinical examination. Am J Ophthalmol. 1994 15; 118(4):526–528.
3. Apple DJ, Solomon KD, Tetz MR, Assia EI, Holland EY, Legler UF, Tsai JC, Castaneda VE, Hoggatt JP, Kostick AM. Posterior capsule opacification. Surv Ophthalmol. 1992 37(2):73–116.
4. Assia E, Apple DJ: Side view analysis of the lens, I: the crystalline lens and the evacuated bag, Arch Ophthalmol 1992, 110:89–93 .
5. Blaydes JE, Fritz KJ, Fogle JA: New techniques of viscosurgery with phacoemulsification. J Am Intraocul Implant Soc 1985, 11:395–7.
6. Blumenthal M, Ashkenazi I, Assia E, Cahane M. Small-incision manual extracapsular cataract extraction using selective hydrodissection.Ophthalmic Surg. 1992; 23:699–701.
7. Blumenthal M, Assia E, Schochot Y. Lens anatomical principles and their technical implications in cataract surgery. Part I: The lens capsule. J Cataract Refract Surg. 1991 Mar; 17(2):205–210.
8. Drews RC, et al: Hydrodissection in extracapsular cataract extraction.Eur J Implant Refract Surg 1098,1:99–100.
9. Drews RC, et al: Hydrodissection of the lens at surgery. Dev Ophthalmol 1987, 14:152–4.
10. Durham DG, Gills JP. Three thousand YAG lasers in posterior capsulotomies: an analysis of complications and comparison to polishing and surgical discissions. Trans Am Ophthalmol Soc. 1985; 83:218–235.
11. Emery JM, McIntyre DJ: Extracapsular Cataract Surgery. St Louis, Mosby,1983,38–40
12. Emery JM, Wilhelmus KA, Rosenberg S: Complications of phacoemulsification.Ophthalmology 1978,85:141–50.
13. Faust KJ: Hydrodissection of soft nuclei. J Am Intraocul Implant Soc 1984,10:75–7.
14. Fine IH: Cortical Cleaving Hydrodissection. J Cataract Refract Surgery 1992, 18:508–12.
15. Frezzotti R, Caporossi A. Pathogenesis of posterior capsular opacification. Part I. Epidemiological and clinico-statistical data. J Cataract Refract Surg. 1990; 16(3):347–352.
16. Fourman S, Apisson J. Late-onset elevation in intraocular pressure after neodymium-YAG laser posterior capsulotomy. Arch Ophthalmol. 1991; 109(4):511–513.
17. Gimbel HV: Evolving techniques of cataract surgery: Semin Ophthalmol, 1992, 7:193–207.
18. Gimbel HV. Hydrodissection and hydrodelineation Int Ophthalmol Clin.1994; 34:73-90.
19. Green WR, McDonnell PJ. Opacification of the posterior capsule. Trans Ophthalmol Soc U K. 1985; 104 :727–739.
20. Hurvitz LM. Posterior capsular rupture at hydrodissection (letter). J Cataract Refract Surg. 1991; 17:866.
21. Holweger RR, Marefat B. Intraocular pressure change after neodymium:YAG capsulotomy. J Cataract Refract Surg. 1997 23(1):115–121.
22. Hara T, Hara T: Endocapsular Phacoemulsification and aspiration (ECPEA): recent surgical techniques and clinical results. Ophthalmic Surg 1987, 20:469–75.
23. Javitt JC, Tielsch JM, Canner JK, Kolb MM, Sommer A, Steinberg EP. National outcomes of cataract extraction. Increased risk of retinal complications associated with Nd:YAG laser capsulotomy. The Cataract Patient Outcomes Research Team. Ophthalmology. 1992 Oct; 99(10):1487–1498.
24. Kelman CD: The history and development of phacoemulsification. Int Ophthalmol Clin 1994, 34:1–12.
25. KelmanCD: Symposium: phacoemulsification.Summary of personal experience. Trans Am Acad Ophthalmol Otolaryngol 1984, 78:35–38.
26. Koch DD, Liu JF. Multilamellar hydrodissection in phacoemulsification and planned extracapsular surgery. J Cataract Refract Surg.1990; 16:559–562.
27. Koch DD, Liu JF, Gill EP, Parke DW 2nd. Axial myopia increases the risk of retinal complications after neodymium-YAG laser posterior capsulotomy. Arch Ophthalmol. 1989 Jul; 107(7):986–990. [PubMed]
28. Kershner RM. Capsular rupture at hydrodissection (letter). J Cataract Refract Surg. 1992; 18:423.
29. Ladas ID, Baltatzis S, Panagiotidis D, Zafirakis P, Kokolakis SN, Theodossiadis GP. Topical 2.0% dorzolamide vs oral acetazolamide for prevention of intraocular pressure rise after neodymium:YAG laser posterior capsulotomy. Arch Ophthalmol. 1997; 115(10):1241–1244.
30. Lewis H, Singer TR, Hanscom TA, Straatsma BR. A prospective study of cystoid macular edema after neodymium: YAG laser posterior capsulotomy. Ophthalmology. 1987; 94(5):478–482.
31. Magno BV, Datiles MB, Lasa MS, Fajardo MR, Caruso RC, Kaiser-Kupfer MI. Evaluation of visual function following neodymium:YAG laser posterior capsulotomy. Ophthalmology. 1997; 104(8):1287–1293. [PubMed]
32. Miyake, K. et al. New classification of capsular block syndrome. J Cataract Refract Surg. 1998;24: 1230–1234.
33. Milauskas AT. Posterior capsule opacification after silicone lens implantation and its management. J Cataract Refract Surg. 1987 Nov; 13(6):644–648.
34. McDonnell PJ, Zarbin MA, Green WR. Posterior capsule opacification in pseudophakic eyes. Ophthalmology. 1983 Dec; 90(12):1548–1553.
35. Moisseiev J, Bartov E, Schochat A, Blumenthal M. Long-term study of the prevalence of capsular opacification

following extracapsular cataract extraction. J Cataract Refract Surg. 1989 Sep; 15(5):531–533.

36. Newland TJ, Auffarth GU, Wesendahl TA, Apple DJ. Neodymium:YAG laser damage on silicone intraocular lenses. A comparison of lesions on explanted lenses and experimentally produced lesions. J Cataract Refract Surg. 1994 Sep; 20(5):527–533.

37. Nishi O. Incidence of posterior capsule opacification in eyes with and without posterior chamber intraocular lenses. J Cataract Refract Surg. 1986 Sep; 12(5):519–522.

38. Nishi O, Nishi K. Intercapsular cataract surgery with lens epithelial cell removal. Part III: Long-term follow-up of posterior capsular opacification. J Cataract Refract Surg. 1991 Mar; 17(2):218–220.

39. Ng DT, Rowe NA, Francis IC, et al: Intraoperative Complications of 1000 phacoemulsification procedures: a prospective study. J Cataract refract Surg 1989, 15:7–84.

40. Ota I, Miyake S, Miyake K. Dislocation of the lens nucleus into the vitreous cavity after standard hydrodissection.Am J Ophthalmol. 1996; 121:706–708.

41. Peng Q, Apple DJ, Visessook N, et al. Surgical prevention of posterior capsule opacification. Part 2: enhancement of cortical clean up by focusing on hydrodissection. J Cataract Refract Surg. 2000; 26:188–197.

42. Powell SK, Olson RJ. Incidence of retinal detachment after cataract surgery and neodymium: YAG laser capsulotomy. J Cataract Refract Surg. 1995 (2):132–135.

43. Ranta P, Kivelä T. Retinal detachment in pseudophakic eyes with and without Nd:YAG laser posterior capsulotomy. Ophthalmology. 1998; 105(11):2127–2133.

44. Steinert RF, Puliafito CA, Kumar SR, Dudak SD, Patel S. Cystoid macular edema, retinal detachment, and glaucoma after Nd:YAG laser posterior capsulotomy. Am J Ophthalmol. 1991; 112(4):373–380.

45. Smith RT, Moscoso WE, Trokel S, Auran J. The barrier function in neodymium-YAG laser capsulotomy. Arch Ophthalmol. 1995; 113(5):645–652.

46. Seibel B: Phacodynamics: Mastering the tools and techniques of phacoemulsification surgery.Thorofare, NJ Slack Inc, 1996, ed 2

47. Simcoe CW: Irrigating spatula for nuclear separation. J Am Intraocul Implant Soc 1981, 7: 172.

48. Sellman TR, Lindstrom RL. Effect of a plano-convex posterior chamber lens on capsular opacification from Elschnig pearl formation. J Cataract Refract Surg. 1988; 14(1):68–72.

49. Thurmond JA; A simple method of nucleus removal during extracapsular surgery. J Am Intraocul Implant Soc 1981, 7: 376–7.

50. Tetz MR, Apple DJ, Price FW Jr, Piest KL, Kincaid MC, Bath PE. A newly described complication of neodymium-YAG laser capsulotomy: exacerbation of an intraocular infection. Case report. Arch Ophthalmol. 1987; 105(10): 1324–1325.

51. Vasavada AR, Singh R, Apple DJ, et al. Effect of hydrodissection on intraoperative performance: randomised study. J Cataract Refract Surg. 2002; 28:1623–1628.

52. Vasavada AR, Goyal D, Shastri L, Singh R. Corticocapsular adhesions and their effect during cataract surgery. J Cataract Refract Surg. 1991; 17:866.

53. Yeoh R. The "pupil snap" sign of posterior capsule rupture with hydrodissection in phacoemulsification (letter).Br J Ophthalmol. 1996:80:486.

Various Techniques of Nucleotomy in Phacoemulsification

13

Divide and Conquer

Col JKS Parihar SM, VSM

INTRODUCTION

Charles Kelman introduced the technique of phaco-emulsification in 1967, and ever since, it has undergone a number of modifications. All these modifications were made with the sole aim of achieving the highest degree of safety, while minimising energy requirement as well as reducing real surgical time period.

In the last three decades, phacoemulsification has undergone significant transformation of technique right from anterior chamber phacoemulsification to iris plane, mono manual technique to present bimanual handling of cataractous lens. There are several variants in bimanual phacoemulsification techniques. Among all these, the basic technique remains that of multiple fragmentation of lens nucleus by ultrasonic or mechanical mode followed by emulsification and aspiration of small fragments. Hence, the ultimate theme remains: divide the lens into multiple small pieces, separate them and gradually keep emulsifying and aspirating them out. There is no hard and fast rule to do so. Most of the variants of different techniques are based on grading of nuclear hardness density and colour of cataractous lens and probable requirement of ultrasonic energy during emulsification as discussed earlier. Hence a single case may have a combination of different methods as per requirement at that particular time. A good phaco surgeon should have the ability to handle the machine effectively rather than the phacomachine dictating its own terms. This is akin to driving a sports car or a fighter aircraft where you have a moving target with several obstacles. Frequent application of different modes of the machine is like trying to achieve the maximum fuel efficiency while operating in top gear, which should remain the sole aim of an efficient phaco surgeon. An excellent phaco surgeon should have

1. Sound and crystal clear understanding of the applied anatomy of the lens, anterior segment and lens, particularly in relation to the density, configuration of lens structures in various types and gradings of nuclear thicknesses.
2. Maximum movements of left hand with chopper or any other instrument for lens manipulation.
3. Use of a phaco tip for cutting, cracking posterior plate and suction in different modes.
4. Nuclear segmentation and rotation.
5. Rely more upon I/A rather on ultrasound energy.
6. Nuclear fragment removal.
7. Strong grip of instruments restricts mobility of manoeuvre. A free pen grip was advocated for smooth functioning. However I experienced that a rolling grip (like rolling glass pellets) of instruments including of Dialler, Chopper/I/A or phaco handpiece while performing the procedure enhances surgical efficacy in any given situation.
8. Tremendous flexibility of movements of shoulder, elbow, and wrist as well as of foot pedal control is of immense value to attain an excellent outcome.
9. Last but not the least, the flexibility of mind and overall attitude, willingness to adapt and react according to the situation is very crucial and an essential need to attain superiority in phaco techniques.

APPLIED ANATOMY OF THE LENS AND ITS APPLICATION WITH NUCLEOTOMY TECHNIQUES

Applied anatomy of the lens has already been described earlier in detail in a separate chapter. However, a crisp review of the salient and important features of applied anatomy in relation to nucleotomy is worth considering.

"Z" Security (Most secured zone) zone of phacoemulsification surgery: Mid pupillary plane.

The anterior chamber has maximum depth at its centre. The lens also possesses maximum thickness of about 5 mm in the central zone which is gradually becoming less at the periphery. Over and above, pupillary margins are also well away during the entire procedure. Hence, any manoeuvre performed at this particular zone provides maximum security against probable insult to the corneal endothelium as well as to posterior capsule during the entire procedure of phacoemulsification. It is something like playing carpet to carpet with the middle of the cricket bat while maintaining guard on the middle stump and leaving any ball which is outside the off stump. No sixer, only doubles or boundaries.

Grading of the Hardness of the Nucleus

The curvature and density of lens nucleus varies as per the age of the patient. Initially, the lens nucleus is soft in density and smaller in size and is surrounded with the epinucleus and soft cortical plate. However, as age advances or in cases of progressive nuclear sclerosis and cataract, the volume and hardness of nucleus increases resulting in thinning of epinucleus and cortical plate. Hence the safety zone between nucleus and posterior capsule is further narrowed down. Since, the classical sculpting movements should confine upto the margins of the nucleus as well as upto 75 to 80% of its thickness, thus the amount of desired ultrasonic energy as well as the length and thickness of the trench will depend upon density grading of the nucleus. In the same manner the chopping technique will also vary as per grading of the nucleus. The increasing density of nucleus will follow the higher convexity of the posterior pole and thus the phaco tip movement will also vary and have to be angled more during trenching, which is directly proportionate to the hardness of the lens nucleus.

Harder the Nucleus, Higher the Risk of Complications

The structural changes linked with hardness of the nucleus is not only confined to the nucleus but also involves the posterior capsule as it is thinning and there are fragile zonules and fluid vitreous as well, thus dense nucleus carries much higher risk of intraoperative complications.

TECHNIQUE OF PHACOEMULSIFICATION SURGERY

The basic principle of nucleotomy remains ultrasonic/ mechanical fragmentation of lens nucleus while maintaining the cortical plate intact and final aspiration/removal of smaller lens fragments and cortical matter at the end.

One needs to quickly change and apply modified technique depending upon the given situation and type of nucleus. The initial era of phaco had experienced more stress on ultimate removal of lens nucleus based on energy applications. Hence first and second generation phacoemulsifier and phacotechniques were based on more energy delivery and cutting ability of tip and handpiece in toto. The stress on fluidics and aspiration and irrigation, hydroprocedures was relatively less. The advent of chopping was the beginning of era of fluidics and less reliant on ultrasonic energy application. The present generation of phacoemulsifier and phaco techniques rely exclusively on fluidics, aspiration and irrigation while aiming minimal or no energy application even for hard cataracts. The torsional and aqualase techniques are examples of this concept.

Widely accepted techniques of phacoemulsification are as follows:

(Co-Axial/Bimanual Phacoemulsification).

1. Nuclear sculpting and trenching (Divide and Conquer/Howard Gimbel)/Two (Maloney) or four trench (John Shepard) methods.
2. Chopping
3. Stop and Chop
4. Flipping of nucleus
5. Endocapsular phacoemulsification
6. Supranuclear phacoemulsification
7. Phacoaspiration for ultrasoft, traumatic and paediatric cataracts.

Each and every technique will be discussed as a separate chapter subsequently.

DIVIDE AND CONQUER (SCULPTING/TRENCHING)

Dr Howard V. Gimbel, MD, MPH, FRCSC: True Portraits of Modern Ophthalmology

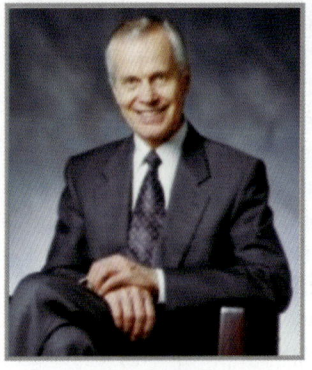

Sculpting or trenching which is popularly known as the divide and conquer technique of nucleotomy (DCN) was introduced by Dr Howard V. Gimbel, MD, MPH, FRCSC in 1986, as a modification in existing nucleotomy technique at that time. In addition to the development of DCN, Dr Gimbel has also invented the technique of Continuous-Tear Capsulotomy which is popularly known as capsulorrhexis. The combination of capsulorrhexis and DCN technique is the most basic and safest way of handling any kind of nucleus and it has totally transformed phacoemulsification surgery as the most secure, safe and widely accepted technique of handling cataract the world over.

He has also promoted the concept of cataract surgery as a day care out door procedure which has resulted in saving of human and hospital resources to a great extent.

Born into a pioneering farm family in Calgary in 1934, Dr. Gimbel was destined to be the torchbearer of phaco-emulsification technique in the 21st century. After obtaining a B.A. degree in Physics from Walla College, College Place, Washington, Dr Gimbel obtained a degree in medicine in 1960 and a Masters in Public Health in 1978, from Loma Linda University, Loma Linda, California. He joined residency in ophthalmology at White Memorial Medical Centre in Los Angeles. Dr. Gimbel began his practice in ophthalmology in 1964 at Calgary. He had commenced outpatient cataract surgery in 1980.

The concept of day care cataract surgery as an out door procedure was conceived and promoted by him all over the world which has resulted in saving of human and medical care resources to a great extent.

He had opened the Gimbel Eye Surgical Centre in 1984 which had witnessed a glorious era for several decades. Dr Gimbel carries a unique distinction of holding various teaching appointments at the University of Calgary and the University of California, San Francisco and as of Professor and Chairman of the Department of Ophthalmology at Loma Linda University, California in 2000. In addition to his significant involvement with clinical medicine, he has been actively participating as a guest speaker world wide in his field of interest.

Apart from his contribution in cataract surgery, Dr Gimbel had also introduced keratorefractive radial keratotomy procedure in 1984 and Excimer laser refractive surgery in Canada in 1990.

Dr Gimbel had received several awards during his illustrious career. Of these, the most prominent is the Alberta Order of Excellence in 1992 for his phenomenal contribution towards research, innovations, academics and promotion of cataract surgery health care system par excellence. He is also the recipient of Binkhorst Medal conferred by the American Society of Cataract and Refractive Surgery in 1994. He enjoys the privilege of being included in the scroll of distinction as one of the "25 Most Influential Ophthalmologists of the 20th Century" by the American Society of Cataract and Refractive Surgery.

His immense popularity and dedication towards research and care of human kind led to huge financial donations which were effectively utilised by the Gimbel Eye Foundation for the promotion of research, academics and health care service activities.

One must admit, Dr Gimbel's contribution is one of the most significant one in the present era towards the promotion of phacoemulsification surgery.

EVOLUTION OF DIVIDE AND CONQUER (SCULPTING/TRENCHING) TECHNIQUE OF NUCLEOTOMY/NUCLEOFRACTIS (DCN)

Dr Howard Gimbel derived this technique in 1986. Most of the techniques of nuclear fragmentation are only modifications of his technique. The basic theme of this method remains multiple segmentation of lens nucleus followed by gradual removal through capsulorrhexis. This procedure is one of the safest procedure, remains a time tested method for safe and successful completion of phaco-emulsification. Maloney had further modified Gimbel's technique as fractional 2:4 phaco having two equal halves of the nucleus initially, followed by division into quadrants and emulsification. Present popularity of phacoemul-sification as a widely acknowledged surgical technique for cataract surgery lies upon the foundation of good results based on Gimbel's technique and devotion. This procedure has resulted in significant reduction in surgical time and amount of ultrasonic energy utilised for emulsification.

Dr Gimbel's Technique of DCN

Dr Gimbel had used the technique of Trench Divide and Conquer (TDC/DCN) Nucleofractis in soft to moderate grade of cataract. The modified variation of Trench Divide and conquer technique popularly known as crater DCN was specially designed for the management of hard cataracts.

After constructing scleral tunnel incision, remaining initial steps of the continuous curvilinear capsulorrhexis (CCC) and hydrodissection and hydrodelineation were performed in a usual manner. Needless to stress the advantages of free rotation of the nucleus and epinucleus, which enhances the efficacy of DCN as well as reduces stress on the zonules while rotational manoeuvres are being employed.

Dr Gimbel preferred to use 30 or 45 degree tip to cons-truct a deep trench. He had used a cyclodialysis spatula or nucleus rotator as the second instrument through a paracentesis or side port incision.

The peculiarity of sculpting in this technique was a construction of a deep trench by sculpting, which was away from the centre of the nucleus and towards the right side of it as compared to the present trend of making trench in to the centre of the nucleus. A cyclodialysis spatula or nucleus rotator was simultaneously placed over the mid of anterior surface of the lens as a second instrument. The trench was completed by gradual and sequential movements of phaco tip until the adequate depth of trench was achieved. A visible red reflex through the trench and an adequate width.

The next step happened to be the fracturing of the nucleus into two halves. While maintaining the phacoemulsifier settings on irrigation mode only (foot position 1), the phaco tip and the second instrument were placed deeply in the groove right upto the floor of the trench and against the both walls of such a manner so as to produce mechanical splitting of the nucleus into two hemi sections of different sizes (the right fragment is larger than the left obviously due to right sided position of the phaco tip at the time of commencement of trenching). The splitting was achieved by the virtue of divergent force applied on the opposite walls of the trench.

Once complete splitting of the nucleus is achieved in two pieces, the next step remains to hold the smaller left piece of the nucleus with the help of that phaco tip which was embedded into the nucleus at the 5 o'clock position. This smaller piece was further converted into multiple arrangements by gentle manipulations created by movements of the phaco tip and second instruments in proximity.

The entire contents of the nucleus would then be subsequently emulsified ensuring nuclear fragments position at the iridocapsular plane. Removal of the residual cortex was fashioned in a standard manner with the help of I/A mode.

The DCN technique adopted by Dr Gimbel had certain variations in terms of position of the second instrument and phaco tip while nudging it into the nucleus. Down slope sculpting was one such kind of modification in which the second instrument was nudged inferiorly at 6 O'clock position thus to ensure sculpting of the nucleus in the superior portion; hence maintaining good visibility and access to posterior structures while performing nucleotomy particularly parallel and close to the posterior capsule. Despite such close proximity to the posterior surface, posterior capsule remains away from the phaco tip in this technique since nucleus material is always preceding to the vibrating phaco tip. This kind of nucleotomy maintains close and natural relations with the anatomy and internal configuration of the nucleus, particularly with posterior concave curvature of the lens. Hence surgical manoeuvre of sculpting remains compatible with the nucleus configuration and thereby enhances intraoperative safety.

MULTIDIRECTIONAL DIVIDE AND CONQUER (MDC) TECHNIQUE

Down-slope Sculpting

As described earlier, adequate thicknesses of posterior plate is essential throughout the period of sculpting and subsequent nucleofractis in a conventional divide and conquer nucleofractis (DCN) technique. Thick, sticky and cheesy cortex and small pupil may not be suitable for conventional DCN. The drawback of DCN is that the nucleofractis is being done in a parallel plane against the natural down slope configuration of the lens fibres in the nucleus. In contrast to it, the down slope technique of DCN follows the natural course of lens fibres during nucleotomy and fractis, hence provides several additional advantages over conventional DCN. To achieve nucleotomy following

course of lens fibres, lens nucleus is being nudged inferiorly at 6 o'clock position with the help of dialler through the side port. Once nucleus is nudged at the inferior pole, the sculpting is commenced by placing a phaco tip at the superior pole and proximal to the centre of it. While ensuring sculpting from just inside the continuous curvilinear capsulorrhexis at superior pole to the centre of lens, the action follows the course of action in a concave slope which is parallel to the configuration of posterior aspect of lens nucleus and posterior capsule as well. The particular position of the second instrument at inferior pole of the nucleus facilitates sculpting throughout the down slope of the nucleus right upto the deepest layers of lens fibres. Hence sculpting action is very much unlikely to produce any undue stress on the posterior capsule during sculpting.

Merits

(i) Very useful in cases of small pupil, hard nucleus as well as in cases of sticky and very cheesy cortex.

(ii) Safe, effective and quick since the process of sculpting continues to follow the course of lens fibres and the posterior capsule as well.

(iii) Least possibilities of entrapment and inadvertent posterior capsule tear.

(iv) Down slope sculpting in the upper pole of the lens and little proximal to the centre of it, significantly minimises the risk of inadvertent rupture of the posterior capsule.

Demerits

(i) Great care and meticulous attention is required while performing nucleotomy through small rhexis so as to avoid any break or extension of rhexis due to inadvertent trauma to the rhexis margins.

(ii) Undue pressure to be avoided on zonules while attempting intracapsular inferior displacement of the nucleus for superior pole sculpting. This may lead to zonulysis of superior quadrant zonules. Adequate Hydrodissection is of immense value to facilitate in the bag manipulation of nucleus while ensuring least stress on the upper zonular apparatus.

(iii) While attempting sculpting towards posterior pole, a surgeon should ensure to maintain a moderate force and speed along with gentle posterior push on the phaco tip so as to avoid sculpting of soft cortical material and probable injury to the inferior zonules.

Phacosweep Technique

Phacosweep technique is a variation of the conventional unidirectional sculpting technique.

A conventional phaco tip creates a trench in a vertical direction only ahead of the vibrating end of the phaco tip. Hence, cracking and splitting of the nucleus can only be achieved in a vertical plane. Thus, multiple nucleotomy may not be possible without repeated rotations of the nucleus. However, by virtue of curved angulation, the kelman tip offers additional advantage of ultrasonic emulsification in both vertical and horizontal directions, that too, without attempting multiple rotations of the nucleus. While keeping angulated portion of the tip in the vertical direction, vertical groove can be constructed whereas, horizontal groove can be constructed by just shifting the angulated portion of the tip perpendicular to the vertical groove. The angulated kelman tip follows the natural contour and curvatures of the lens nucleus; hence it offers better safety against any inadvertent rupture of the posterior capsule. This simultaneous horizontal and vertical groove construction without rotating the lens nucleus and subsequently the nucleotomy technique together is popularly known as the Phacosweep technique.

Down slope MDC, initiates nucleotomy from debulking the superior part of the lens while nudging inferior pole of it, whereas in the phaco sweep technique, it initiates nucleotomy after constructing vertical groove.

After achieving desired depth upto the deeper layers, the angulated portion of the kelman tip is directed horizontally to achieve lateral sweeping motion, thereby to construct a small lateral groove just at the inferior portion of the initially constructed vertical trench. The tip is subsequently turned to the opposite direction to also create a lateral groove on the other side. Hence, a good and adequate depth of horizontal as well as vertical trenches can be achieved, that to without rotating the nucleus. These simultaneous vertical and horizontal trenches provide excellent debulking of the central core nucleus. The next step is to fashion a horizontal crack in the nucleus by exerting gentle pressure on the wall of the grooves in an inferior portion and providing support and stabilising the nucleus at the superior pole. Horizontal splitting is achieved by manipulating two instruments in the deeper portion of the central groove. Hence phacosweep achieves multidirectional nucleotomy in the inferior portions. These fragments are subsequently emulsified by getting them into the most secured midpupillary and central zone of corneal dome. The next step is to get superior portion of the nucleus into the central zone and the completes the process of nuclear emulsification. Hence, phacosweep enjoys the privilege of minimal stress on the zonules during nucleotomy which is of immense significance and merit while handling, cheesy and sticky cortex, nonrotating nucleus, small pupil or subluxated lens, where repeated nuclear rotation may lead to zonular stress and threat of impending intraoperative complications.

DIVIDE AND CONQUER AS PRACTICED BY THE AUTHOR

The modern technique of DCN has gone through several transformations since its inception by Dr Gimbel. These modifications are mainly based on evolution of different kinds of nucleotomy techniques as well as tremendous improvements in the machine technology, particularly the invention of fluid dynamics and micropulse techniques. Such modifications were exclusively aiming application of less energy, more vacuum yet retaining higher degree of safety and efficacy. The author too has experienced significant changes in-his technique of handling lens nucleus. To begin with conventional DCN, the author has shifted to direct chop under topical via through a transition phase of various hybrid techniques. In a lighter way, phaco surgeons have become less powerful (using very less ultrasonic energy), bonsai (using a narrow bore and a curved phaco tip) and swimming in a pool with life jacket on (applying more fluidics and using micro pulses).

The Author's Technique

Bottle Height

The moderate bottle height of around 50–65 cm above the patient head is an ideal situation for nucleotomy by the divide and conquer technique. A very high bottle height will positively infuse more fluid in the anterior chamber which will produce undue push on the lens diaphragm, making it deeper. Such inherent deepening and the potential risk of making the phaco probe stand more vertical results in higher chances of posterior capsule rupture as well as of corneal burn.

Incisions, Rhexis and Hydroprocedures

After constructing clear corneal incision at 10–11 O'clock position, (temporal for right eye and nasal for left eye respectively) a side port incision is made around 100 to 110 degree away from the main incision. A moderately large continuous curvilinear capsulorrhexis (CCC) of around 6–6.5 mm size with inferior descent is being constructed.

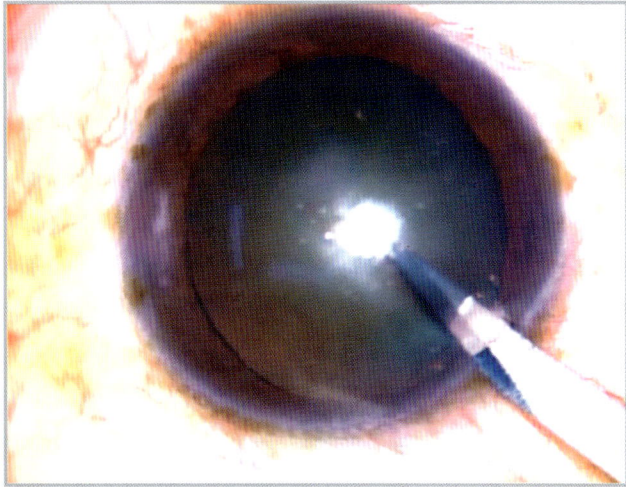

Fig. 13.1: DCN: Primary incision at 10–11 o'clock position for subsequent clear corneal incision, (temporal for right eye and nasal for left eye, respectively)

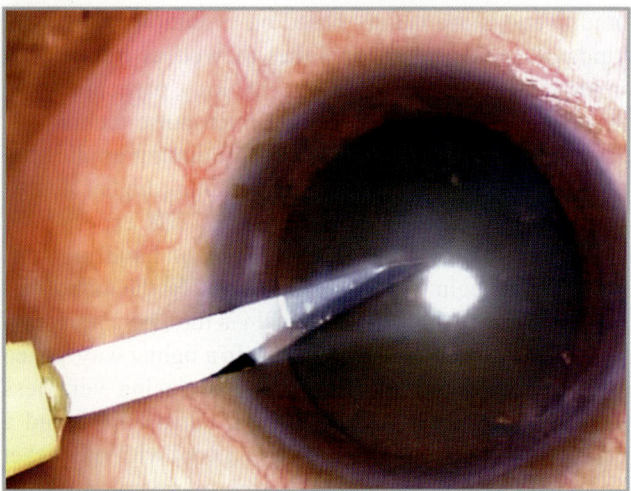

Fig. 13.2: DCN: Side port incision

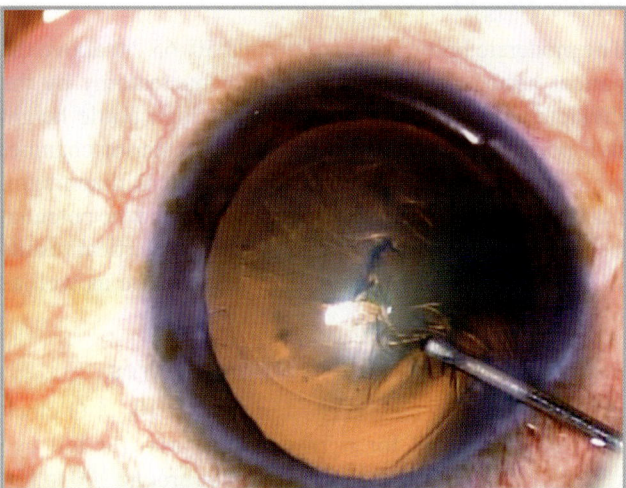

Fig. 13.3: DCN: Rhexis

Sequential and repeated hydro procedure is performed to achieve a smaller and soft nucleus with excellent rotation.

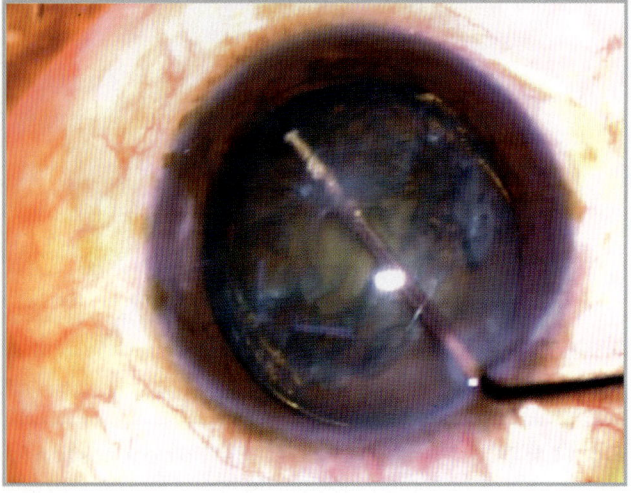

Fig. 13.4: Hydroprocedure for DCN

Such manoeuvres are essentially of immense benefit to reduce ultrasonic energy requirements as well as to enhance structural safety and ease during procedure.

Clearing of Superficial Cortex

A good clearing of superficial cortex extending right upto the periphery of the nucleus is preferred, since it provides quick and adequate rotation of nucleus as well as facilitates further softening of nucleus, thereby reduces US energy requirement during subsequent manipulations.

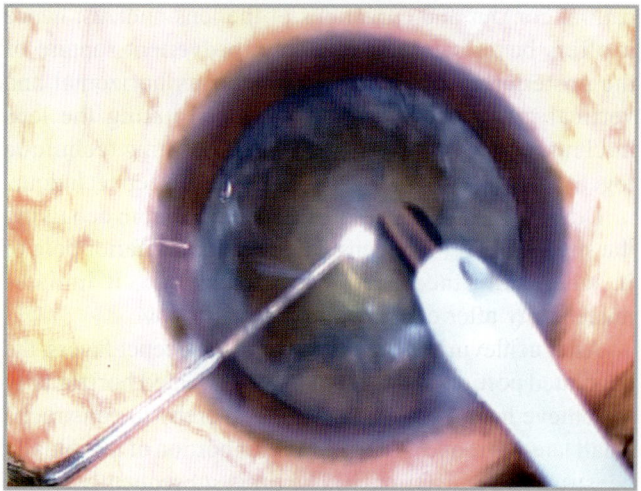

Fig. 13.5: DCN: Clearing of superficial cortex

Nucleotomy: Nucleus Sculpting/Trenching: An Ideal Trench

Size of the trench is invariably based on the hardness of the cataract and the size of the nucleus. The larger the nucleus, the wider and longer should the trench be. In the same way a deep trench will be essential for managing hard nucleus. An Ideal trench comprises of a length just short of rhexis margin, width should be about twice of the tip's diameter width so as to accommodate the tip along with a sleeve inside the trench.

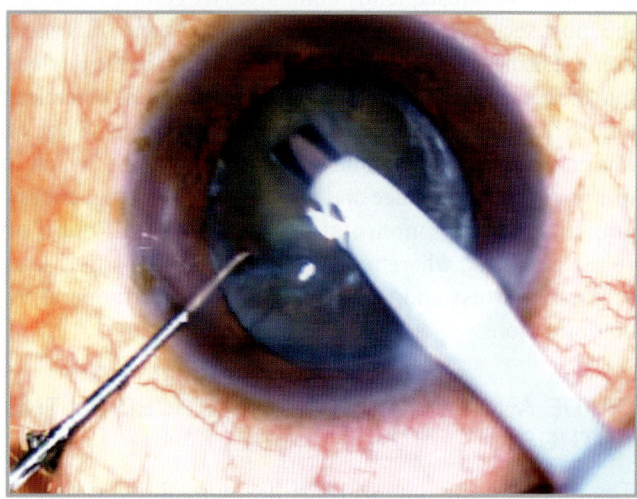

Fig. 13.6: DCN: Commencement of trenching

Depending upon the grading of nucleus and the surgical ease, nucleus can be divided into two or four segments. After the initial process of baring nucleus by cleaning of superficial cortical matter from nucleus by using phaco tip at irrigation mode, gradual trenching is made into nucleus by using US mode. Preferred settings of US power are 25–40%, Aspiration 60–100 mmHg with a low flow rate of 15–20 cc/mt on peristaltic system. (Details of settings for different grades of nucleus and types of machines are given in Tables 13.1 and 13.2). This trench should not be too wide or too long. A good trench should not be more than twice the diameter width of the phaco tip.

It is essential to have transient movements of tip while maintaining gradual angulations so as to have gradual down descend of the phaco tip to the nucleus. Trench should not exceed pupillary margins or towards the periphery of the nucleus. The key to achieve a good trench lies solely upon the depth of the trench rather than its own length. Every time the trench should be prepared at the 6 O'clock position by gradual rotation of the lens nucleus hence, directing the site of the next trench towards the 6 O'clock position on every occasion.

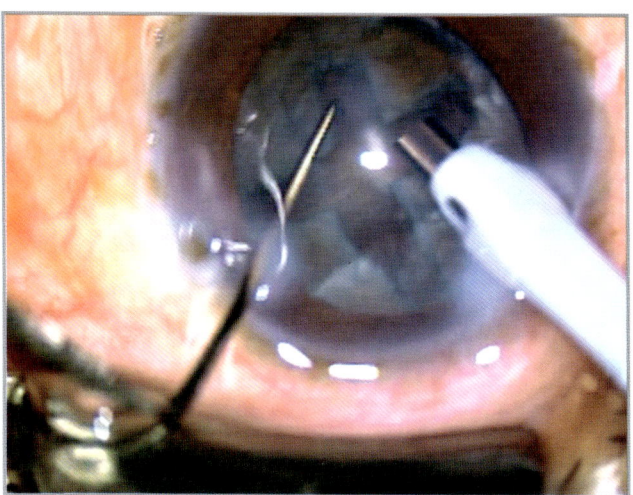

Fig. 13.9: DCN: Rotation of nucleus

A faintly visible red glow through the floor of the trench should suffice a satisfactory outcome. Most important is to have the posterior plate intact at this juncture so as to ensure an intact posterior capsule throughout the emulsification process.

Nuclear Fragmentation

Once adequate sculpting is being achieved, the next step is to have multiple nucleotomy. Best way to perform this, is to have gradual cracking by inserting two diallers deep into the trench right up to the floor of it and to have gentle movements of both dialler in opposite and criss-cross directions.

The direction of force is lateral and tangential. Slopping movements of this will facilitate further separation of nucleus into multiple pieces. The same can also be achieved by nudging a phaco tip into the nucleus in place of one dialler. The clockwise rotation of the nucleus during sculpting keeps the trench on the opposite side from the manipulator/phaco handpiece entry point, making further rotation comfortable and safe. It is most important to maintain intact posterior plate at this stage so as to avoid any threat to the posterior capsule during trenching and nucleus rotation.

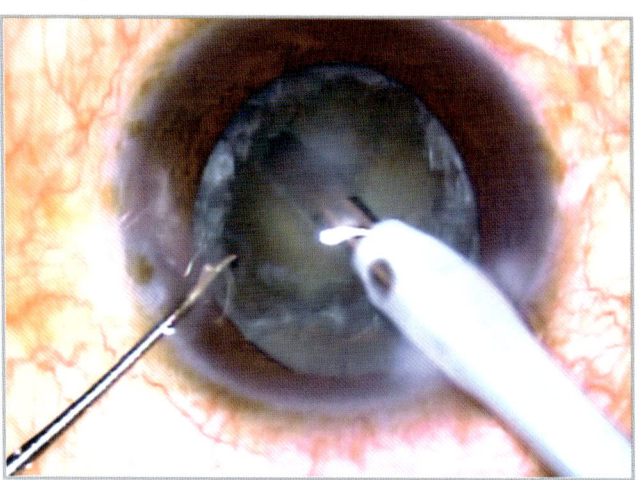

Fig. 13.7: DCN: Primary trenching

Removal of Lens Fragments

The nucleus requires to be broken into smaller fragments for being engaged into the phaco tip and emulsified. A satisfactory rotation of the nucleus during this process is very much essential. It is advisable to have anti-clockwise rotation of lens fragment and getting them every time in the inferior half of the capsular bag to ensure better safety and ease of procedure. Undoubtedly, presence of a posterior plate until removal of the last lens fragment is one of the most important tip to avoid a PC rent. A 30° to 40° phaco tip is ideal for this purpose since in manipulation mode, phaco is utilised to move the nuclear fragments or to crack the posterior plate. In this mode the footpedal is placed in position 1. Only irrigation is on and no vacuum or phaco power is used.

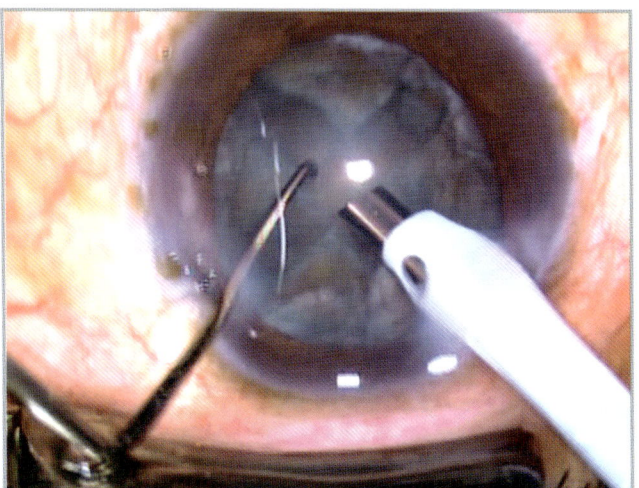

Fig. 13.8: DCN: Construction of four trench

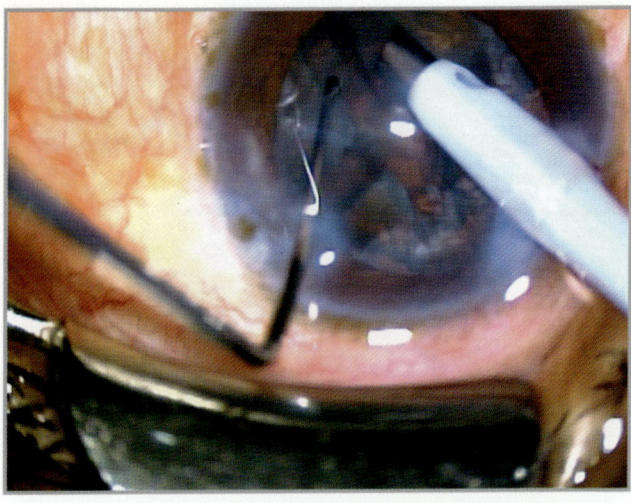

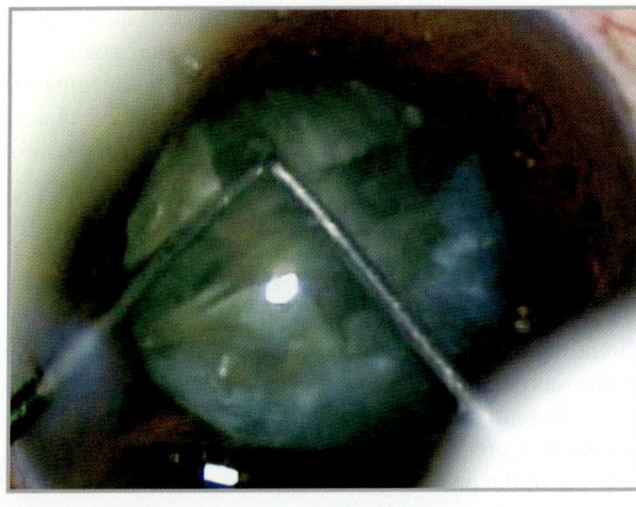

(a)   (b)

Fig. 13.10: (a) DCN: Gradual cracking by gentle pressure on the wall of the trench (adjacent to the floor of the trench) with the help of a phaco tip and a second instrument in the opposite direction, (b) DCN: Gradual cracking by inserting two diallers

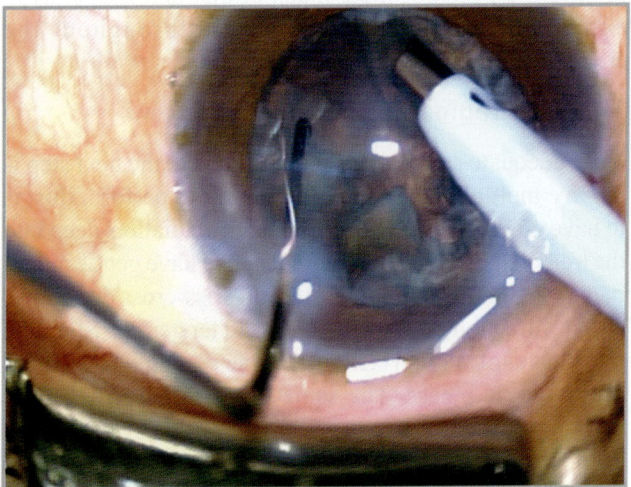

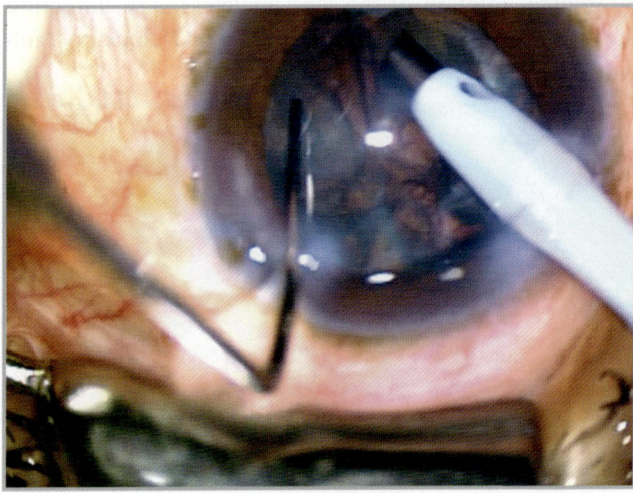

Fig. 13.11: DCN: Primary splitting of the nucleus (first quadrant)

Fig. 13.12: DCN: Multiple nucleotomy by sequential splitting of the nucleus

In the cutting mode, nuclear material is shaved away. A 45° tip is best for this procedure since the chances of tip occlusion are minimal in this particular type of tip. Here a moderate to high (20–30%) phaco power and vacuum and moderate flow rate are required.

In the suction mode the tip is occluded with the nuclear material. A short bevel tip either 30° or 15° is best for suction. A high vacuum and low phaco settings is required for this purpose. Removal of lens fragment is always preferred with pulse mode having 4–6 pulse rather than on continuous mode. While handling nuclear fragment to lift it away from the posterior of the capsular bag, nuclear fragment is always picked up from the base or centre of it rather than from apex of it. This again will provide a better grip of fragment and ultimate safety and minimal power utilisation.

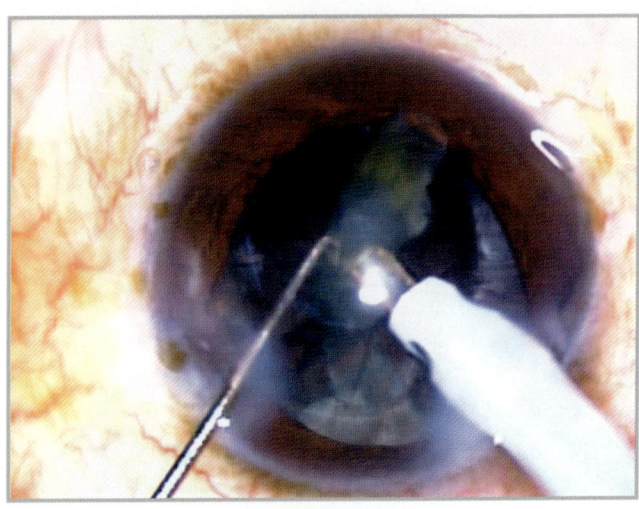

Fig. 13.13: DCN: Removal of lens fragments

Once the last or small lens fragment is being emulsified and aspirated away, phaco power and vacuum may further be lowered down. Repeated switching to position 1, 2 and small bursts of ultrasound at position three is the most beneficial step to maintain adequate AC depth, concave posterior capsule and proper contour of the corneal dome. All these have a significant role in maintaining intact posterior capsule and least postoperative reaction. Another important tip is to have fragment emulsification and aspiration in the capsular bag at the centre of the anterior chamber and just below the iris plane. This is advisable at all times, since lens has maximum thickness in the centre which amounts to be around 4 mm as well AC is also having maximum depth in the centre of it. Hence, this place provides maximum distance of phaco tip from corneal endothelium as well as from the posterior capsule; thus, enhancing more safety both intra and postoperative as far as results are concerned.

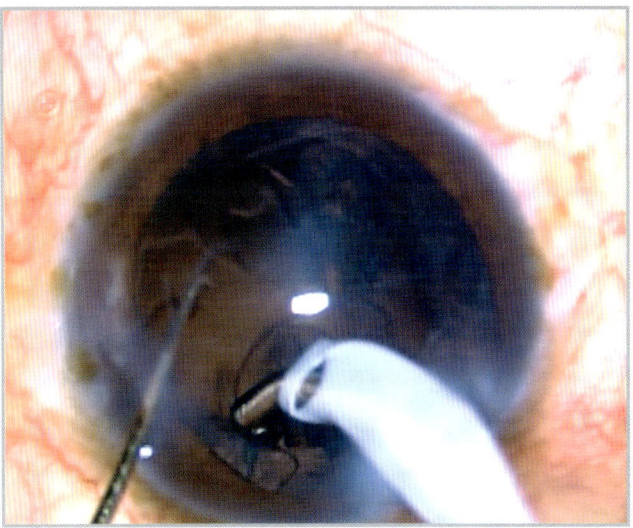

Fig. 13.14: DCN: Cortical removal

Removal of Posterior Plate

This will be dealt separately as management of residual cortex or cortical wash. Removal of the posterior plate can be done with the help of a phaco tip having position one with 'O' energy and high vacuum settings to lift a big chunk of plate in toto from the posterior capsule (Fig. 13.14)

This will reduce subsequent manoeuvres in I/A mode and will reduce surgical time as well, due to rapid aspiration of thick cortical plate (Figs 13.15 and 13.16).

CRATER DIVIDE AND CONQUER (CDC) TECHNIQUE

Crater Divide and Conquer (CDC) technique is a hybrid modification of the conventional divide and conquer (DCN) technique which was designed during prechopping era to suit the essential need of nucleofractis in cases of hard to very hard and even dense, brunescent cataract.

The genesis of crater and divide technique lies on the fact that in cases of very hard and dense nucleus, a conventional sculpting which is essential for nucleofractis may not be able to attain an adequate depth of trench without compromising safety.

The Crater Divide and Conquer (CDC) technique is more suitable for hard cataract along with small pupil or associated psuedoexfoliation. The chopping era has witnessed further innovations in the Crater Divide and Conquer (CDC) technique as a combination of central debulking of hard nucleus in the form of crater formation which is subsequently followed by a central chopping.

SURGICAL TECHNIQUE

Initial steps of incision and rhexis are essentially identical to conventional DCN technique. However, CDC can be undertaken with small pupils. The author prefers to apply

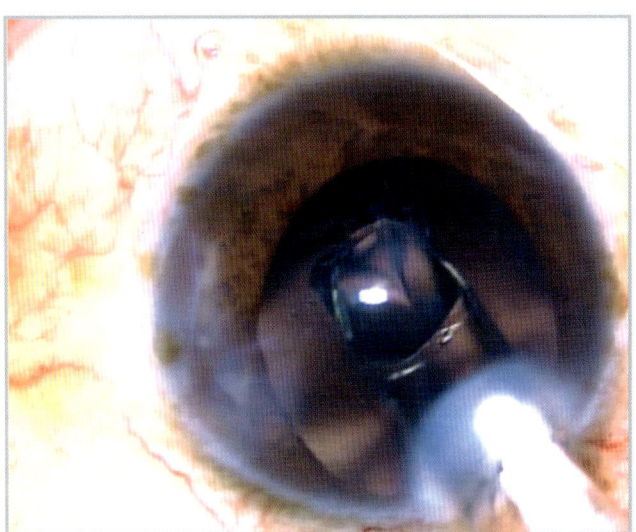

Fig. 13.15: DCN: IOL insertion

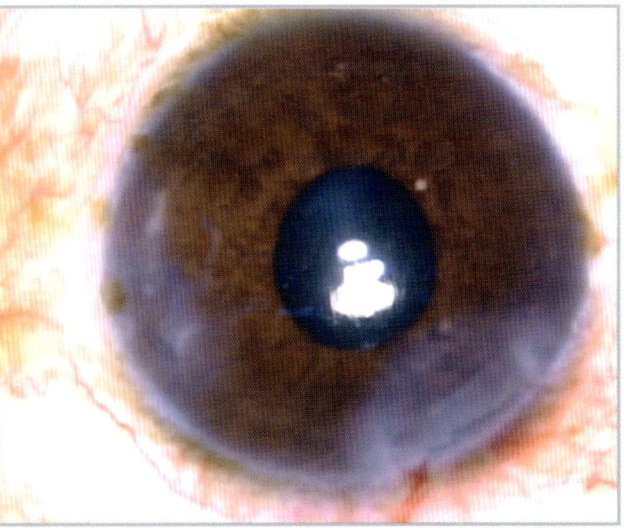

Fig. 13.16: DCN: Stromal hydration

Table 13.1: Phacoemulsification machine settings at different stages of Divide and Conquer technique (Peristaltic Pump)

Step/stage	Principle	Phaco settings	Flow (cc/min)	Vacuum	Continuous/Pulse
Baring nucleus	Low flow and vacuum	00–05%	10–15	60–100	Continuous
Trenching/sculpting	Low flow and vacuum	25–40	15–20	60–100	Continuous/micropulse
Subsequent multiple nucleotomy	Moderate vacuum	20–30	24–26	225–275	Continuous/micropulse
Fragment removal	High flow and vacuum	15–30	24–26	200–275	Continuous/micropulse
Removal of last fragment	Low flow and moderate vacuum	10–20	15–20	75–150	Continuous/micropulse
Removing posterior plate/epinucleus	Low flow and high vacuum A mode	00–05	10–15	100–125	Continuous/Pulse I
Residual cortical wash	Moderate flow and high vacuum	I/A mode	26–34	300–400	Continuous
Posterior capsule polishing	Low flow and vacuum	I/A mode/ Handpiece	5	10–20	Continuous

Table 13.2: Phacoemulsification machine settings at different stages of Divide and Conquer technique (Ventury Pump)

Step/stage	Principle	Phaco settings	Vacuum	Continuous/Pulse
Baring nucleus	Low vacuum	05%	45–60	Continuous/ micropulse
Trenching/sculpting	Low vacuum	25–50	15–30	Continuous/ micropulse
Subsequent multiple nucleotomy	Moderate vacuum	10–25	60–75	Continuous/ micropulse
Fragment removal	Moderate to high vacuum	05–20	80–100	Micropulse
Removal of the last fragment	Moderate vacuum	5–15	50–60	Micropulse
Removing the posterior plate/epinucleus	Moderate vacuum	0–05/ I/A mode	60–80	Continuous/ micropulse
Residual cortical wash	High vacuum	I/A mode	400–450	Continuous
Posterior capsule polishing	Low flow	I/A mode	0–5	Continuous

adequate yet guarded and repeated hydrodissection. One should not attempt to achieve repeated hydrodelineation since a large and hard nucleus carries a higher risk of posterior capsule rupture during repeated hydrodelineation.

To fashion a deep crater, a central sculpting is being performed by a gradual sloppy action of the tip into the nuclear substance. Dense nuclei essentially require relatively higher settings of ultrasonic energy (45 to 60% US energy with moderate to high flow and aspiration rate). A gentle and repeated nuclear rotation is mandatory to widen and deepen the crater right upto the posterior plate.

A peripheral rim of nucleus is being kept around the crater till the desired and adequate quantity of central core is removed so as to protect the capsular bag against any inadvertent injury to the bag while performing multiple nucleotomy as well as from sharp edges of small pieces of hard nucleus while performing removal of such fragments.

Sculpting becomes very difficult while negotiating within the deeper layers of the nucleus since the phaco tip attains a very obtuse angle of action. This acute angle is due to the fact that dense nucleus possess almost more than 90% of volume in hard brown cataracts, hence desired debulking upto the posterior pole of the nucleus will need very deep sculption of about 4 mm into the lens substance.

Angulated kelman tip is an ideal choice to handle dense hard cataract in this kind of situation.

The crater should be enough widened and gradually deepened before attempting splitting of the debulked core nucleus. As described earlier, a good cushion of peripheral rim of the nucleus is kept in the capsular bag around posterior plate so as to allow successful fracturing of the nucleus. Prior to the commencement of splitting of nucleus, a meticulous and judicious assessment of the depth of the crater is very essential. A gradual increase in the intraoperative brightness of the red reflex in the floor of the groove is a good yardstick. This intensity of brightness in the red reflex should further be correlated which will be possible in case of hard brown cataract unless a trench consisting of more than 75 to 80% thickness of the nucleus is being achieved. Once adequate depth is attained, multiple splitting of nuclear fragments is achieved by bimanual action of two instruments in a repeated manner and a continuous rotation of the nucleus. The highlight of good nucleofractis remains with the retaining of all the fragments in the bag until the desired number of fragments have been achieved. This action will enhance capsular bag, safety against inadvertent touch of a sharp fragment into the capsular bag, while performing nucleotomy as well. The distended capsular bag at this juncture further prevents risk of catching the posterior capsule by the phaco tip when conducting nuclear fragment removal. The next step is a gradual removal of lens fragments by engaging them with the help of a phaco tip, taking them out of the bag upto the pupillary plane and maintaining a deep and distended capsular bag by frequent application of irrigation mode and subsequent aspiration of lens substances. It is worth considering to lower down machine settings in respect of US energy, flow rate and vacuum as removal of fragments is going on. The stretched and debulked capsular bag due to the earlier presence of a hard brown nucleus becomes highly vulnerable to rupture of posterior capsule due to flutter and turbulence of the irrigating fluid. Hence, a surgeon must pay very cautious and deep attention towards distension of capsular bag and to maintain the chamber stability throughout the procedure specially while removing the last fragments.

V-SHAPED OR VICTORY TRENCH

The basic theme of divide and conquer remains multiple nuclear fragmentation and subsequent removal of these smaller fragments. The core nucleus happens to be the most thick and hard element of the nucleus. Hence, debulking of core nucleus remains the main issue to achieve desired nucleotomy. The four trench technique is an ideal and conventional way of gradual yet a very secured debulking of the central core nucleus. However, if multiple trenches can be made, then it should be better to produce small fragments even during primary splitting and cracking. Since now most of the phaco surgeons tend to keep the tip and the second instruments at around 110 to 120 degree or in case of true temporal or nasal incisions, "X" pattern, flower petal or "V" shaped trench appears to be more convenient. Rest of the steps are essentially identical to the conventional DCN technique.

CONCLUSION

Undoubtedly the basic theme of nucleofractis and subsequent ultrasonic emulsification remains, safety and no complication. Conventional divide and conquer enjoys the unique privilege of being a gold standard technique of ultrasonic phacoemulsification which has laid the foundation for all modern nucleotomy techniques including chopping. Various modifications in DCN like the Trench divide and conquer, crater divide and conquer, downslope sculpting, and phaco sweep are aiming towards effective and safe application of ultrasonic energy as per the need of different types and hardness of the nucleus. This can be achieved using nucleotomy by a method of the surgeon's choice. Safety is of utmost importance rather than surgeon's ego. Never mind to convert to conventional ECCE if required.

BIBLIOGRAPHY

1. Gimbel HV: Divide and Conquer. (Video) Presented at the European Intraocular Implant Lens Council meeting 1987.
2. Neuhann T: Theorie und operationstechnik der kapsulorhexis. Klin Monatsblc Augenheilkd 1987, 190: 542–45.
3. Hara T: Endocapsular phacoemulsification and aspiration (ECPEA—recent surgical technique and clinical results. Ophthalmic Surg 1989, 20: 469–75.
4. Gimbel HV, Neuhann T: Development, advantages, and methods of the continuous circular capsulorrhexis technique. Cataract Refract Surg 1990, 16: 31–37.
5. Gimbel HV. Continuous curvilinear capsulorrhexis and nucleus fracturing: Evolution, technique, and complications. Ophthalmol Clin North Am 1991; 4(2): 235–249.
6. Gimbel HV: CCC and nucleus fracturing. Ophthalmol Clin North Am 4: 235, 1991.
7. Gimbel HV. Divide and conquer nucleofractis phacoemulsification: Development and variations. J Cataract Refract Surg 1991; 17:281–291.
8. Gimbel HV. Evolving techniques of cataract surgery: Continuous curvilinear capsulorrhexis, Downslope sculpting and nucleofractis. Sem Ophthalmol 1992; 7:193–207.
9. Gimbel HV. Downslope sculpting. J Cataract Refract Surg 1992; 18:614–618.
10. Gimbel HV: Nuclear phacoemulsification—alternative methods. In: Steinert RF (Ed) Cataract Surgery: Technique, Complications, and Management Philadelphia: WB Saunders 1995, 148–81.
11. Gimbel HV, Ellant JP, Chin PK: Divide and conquer nucleofractis. Ophthalmol Clin North Am 1995, 8(3): 457–69.
12. Gimbel HV. Trough and crater divide and conquer nucleofractis techniques. Eur J Implant Ref Surg 1991; 3:123–126.
13. Gimbel HV, Chin PK. Phaco sweep. J Cataract Refract Surg 1995; 21:493–496.
14. Gimbel HV. Nucleofractis phacoemulsification through a small pupil. Can J Ophthalmol 1992; 27:115–119.
15. Gimbel HV: Challenges of topical anaesthesia in small incision cataract surgery. Ophthalmic Practice 1996, 14(3): 123–24.
16. Gimbel HV, Willerscheidt AB: What to do with limited view—the intumescent cataract. Cataract Refract Surg 1993, 19: 657–61.
17. Koch, P. New Techniques for Cataract Surgery. Current Opinion in Ophthalmology. 1995:6; 41–45.
18. Gimbel HV, Austin A: 'Polar expedition' technique expedites phaco. Ocular Surgery News 15(9): 27–32, 1997.
19. Koch, P. Simplifying Phacoemulsification: Safe and Efficient Methods for Cataract Surgery. Fifth Edition. SLACK Incorporated. Thorofare, NJ; 1997.
20. Buratto, L. Phacoemulsification: Principles and Techniques. SLACK Incorporated. Thorofare, NJ; 1998.
21. Buratto et al. Cataract Surgery in Complicated Cases. SLACK Incorporated. Thorofare, NJ; 2000.
22. Fishkind, William J. Complications in Phacoemulsification: Avoidance, Recognition, and Management. Thieme, NY, 2002.

14

Phaco Chop: Advanced Techniques of Nucleotomy and Emulsification

Col JKS Parihar SM, VSM

INTRODUCTION

There is no doubt that Divide and Conquer technique of trenching and sculpting is very safe and easy to learn; hence rightly and widely accepted all over the world. The emergence of newer techniques are essentially based on modifications in this basic technique. The author himself has practised these techniques for a long time at least in his initial 2000 or odd cases. It is always recommended to practice and master this technique before switching over to any advanced phaco technique like Chopping. However, there has been a great effort to reduce energy requirement to the least so as to enhance over all safety during entire course of intra and post operative period. Applications of mechanical force to crack the nucleus in the form of chopping and advanced fluid dynamics are essential components of this exercise.

The initial phase of phacoemulsification era in the early eighties witnessed effective utilisation of ultrasonic energy as a sheet anchor tool to emulsify the lens nucleus. Most phacoemulsifiers of that time were based on the cutting ability of the phaco tip. However, the present generation of modern phacotechniques rely upon the less utilisation of energy with more and more application of fluid dynamics, irrigation and aspiration. The concept of mechanical fragmentation of nucleus was conceived mainly with the aim to restrict the need of ultrasonic energy so as to enhance the safety of corneal endothelium and subsequently, reduce the risk of intraoperative complications that are mainly encountered with the sculpting technique while dealing with the hard nucleus.

The phaco chop technique is a unique and premium concept of nucleotomy which has transformed modern cataract surgery from a very small incision cataract surgery into an atraumatic keratorefractive surgery with enhanced intraoperative safety as well as excellent post operative outcomes.

HISTORICAL BACKGROUND

The phaco chop technique was derived by Dr Kunihiro Nagahara (Japan). This concept was presented for the first time in 1993 during the 3rd American–International Congress on Cataract, IOL, and Refractive Surgery in Seattle.

The genesis of this technique lies in the fact that sculpting takes more surgical time and ultrasound energy; hence may have adverse impact on corneal endothelium in the long term, particularly in certain selected cases like very hard cataract or patients having poor corneal reserves. The concept of chopping was derived from karate where, even a very hard object like a solid and a thick brick can be broken into multiple pieces by a proper and quick action of hand. As such, advancement in surgery is always with the zeal to achieve better than the best of the present at every attempt. Nagahara had applied mechanical energy of chopping movement into lens substance to produce multiple nuclear fragments in place of ultrasonic trenching, a step which enhances safety and reduces surgical and actual phaco energy application time.

The classic Nagahara chop enjoys nuclear fragmentation which is attained by mechanical manoeuvre of two instruments namely the phaco tip and a sharp metal needle in a horizontal plane in such a manner so as to produce nucleotomy when both instruments are directed towards each other. However, the Nagahara technique has witnessed numerous refinements and evolutions since its early days with more reliance on fluid dynamics and advanced applications of modulated energy systems.

APPLIED ASPECTS OF PHACO CHOP TECHNIQUE

Nagahara has adopted the concept of splitting a wood block by embedding chisel or axe in the wood piece exactly in the cleavage plane which gives a quick and smooth splitting of it with the application of least energy and efforts. Incidentally, the configuration of lens nucleus very much simulates the piece of wood which is derived from the stem where both structures have identical configuration of internal layers comprising of circular rings.

This internal lamellar orientation of lens fibres provides a natural plane of separation, hence any effort to separate lens fibers into multiple planes exactly as per the lamellar pattern of lens fibers will require the least energy and force to achieve intranuclear splitting of the lens substance which is very similar to splitting of wood by axe action. Thus, chopping at this particular anatomical plane will provide nuclear fragmentation with great ease yet least application of ultrasonic energy as compared to the classical sculpting technique.

Dr Nagahara's technique involves impaling the phaco tip into the lens nucleus with high vacuum so as to hold the nucleus whereas a second instrument is applied to hook the equator. The second instrument is directed to move forward with quick motion towards the centre of the nucleus in a horizontal plane so as to achieve the desired fragmentation of the nucleus along with the natural plane of configuration of lens fibres.

Merits of Phaco Chop

Phaco chop has several advantages:

1. Phaco chop is the most favoured technique by well experienced surgeons.
2. Consistency of surgical results.
3. Perfect blend of efficiency, safety, and reduced stress on the capsular bag—without the difficulty of prolapsing the entire nucleus out of the bag in one piece.
4. Minimal handling near the posterior capsule.
5. Very less surgical and Phaco energy application time. Total duration of surgery can be as less as 5 minutes from the construction of the incision. Total Phaco energy application time is also less than 30 seconds in most of the cases.
6. Handling nucleus in complicated cases like those associated with small pupil, uveitis, shallow chamber, zonulysis and traumatic/subluxated cataract or in cases of high myopia and post R/D, surgery can be safely managed with this technique by an expert with reliable and better results.
7. Minimises dependency on phaco tips, hence reducing the frequent change of tip as required in sculpting. A 0/15 Degree tip is preferred. However, other tips can also be used.
8. Can be performed through a scleral tunnel or a clear corneal incision, however clear corneal is always preferred.
9. An ideal technique for no anaesthesia or topical anaesthesia.
10. The author himself preferred this technique under topical anaesthesia in most cases including all types of cataracts with pre-existing preoperative complications or even in case of a one eyed individual.

Disadvantages

1. Master's technique.
2. Needs a good phaco machine with an excellent aspiration system.
3. Small or extended incomplete capsulorrhexis is not an ideal situation.
4. Soft cataract is not suitable for any kind of chopping methods.

TYPES AND SURGICAL TECHNIQUES OF CHOPPING

Most popular variations of Nagahara's chopping techniques are as follows:

1. Peripheral chop
2. Stop and chop
3. Central chop
4. Chopping with central deep bore digging
5. Phaco-pre chop
6. Phaco snap and split
7. Lateral chopping (my modification)
8. Chopping with cart wheel rotation

Peripheral Chop (Nagahara)

Peripheral Chop is the most basic and initial yet revolutionised technique of nucleotomy which was introduced by Dr Kunihiro Nagahara in 1993 at the annual meeting of the American Society of Cataract and Refractive Surgery (ASCRS) in Seattle, Washington.

Principle of Peripheral Chopping

The nucleus is chopped from the periphery. (Chopper is pushed from the periphery to the centre of the nucleus.) Hence, achieves outside to inside chopping action.

Technique

(i) **Side port incision:** Side port incision is kept at around 2 O'clock position away and left to the main incision. A relatively close proximity of the main and side port incisions are essentially required so as to attain an adequate transformation of mechanical energy to the nucleus, thus achieving desired and appropriate chopping action.

(ii) **Rhexis:** A large preferably 6.0 to 6.5 mm sized rhexis, more proximal inferiorly and oval vertically is an ideal choice (Fig. 14.1).

This kind of rhexis is more convenient to have easy prolapse of nucleus as well as to allow proper

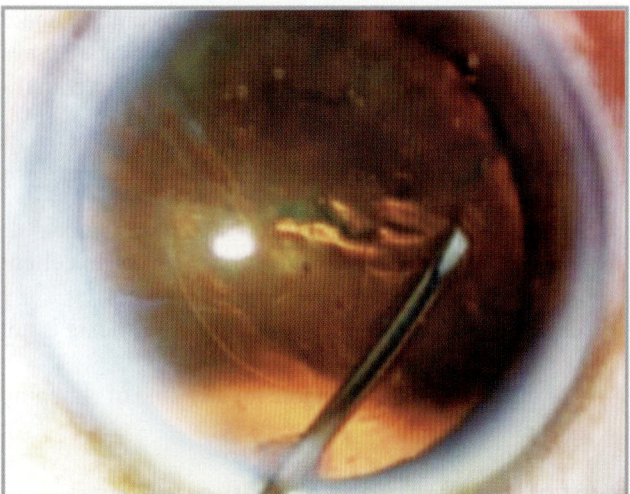

Fig. 14.1: Rhexis

karate chopping without compromising the integrity of the rhexis margins.

(iii) Hydroprocedure: A good hydroprocedure is of great value in the chopping technique as compared to the sculpting techniques. Multiple hydrodelamination separates the epinucleus from the nucleus; thereby reduces its size as well as provides an excellent cushion and a good rotation of nucleus. This will facilitate desired and appropriate intralenticular chopping.

(iv) Clearing of superficial cortex: Clearing of superficial cortex is done in a standard manner (Fig. 14.2).

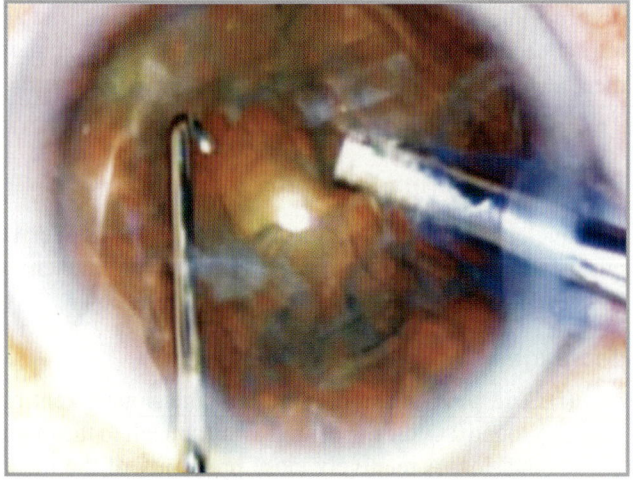

Fig. 14.2: Clearing of superficial cortex

(v) Nucleotomy: Once superficial cortex is cleared, the angulated (0 or 15 degree) phaco tip is introduced into the anterior chamber with bevel down and then rotated to make it bevel-up. The tip is subsequently placed on the centre of the anterior surface of the nucleus. The next step is to place the chopper over the nucleus just ahead of the phaco tip. While

maintaining position one (irrigation), the phaco tip has allowed to create a gentle pressure over the nucleus and pushing it down further in the bag so as to create a potential space between the under surface of the rhexis margin and the nucleus (Fig. 14.3).

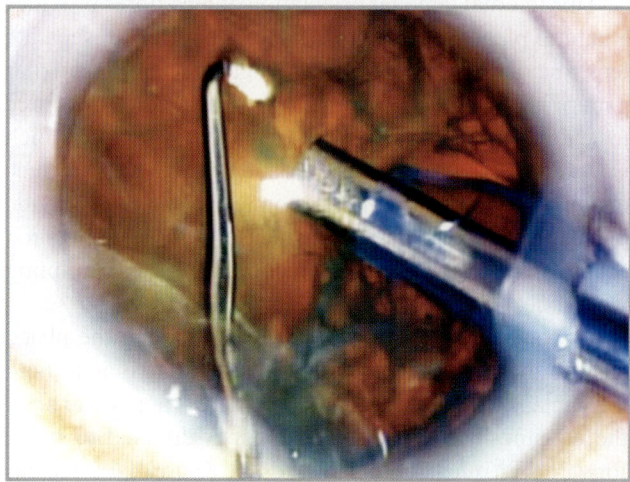

Fig. 14.3: Peripheral chopper is being placed under the rhexis margin

This intracapsular subluxation of nucleus facilitates subsequent chopping action inside the capsular bag. The chopper is being shifted towards the inferior pole of the nucleus and movement is arrested just short of the lens equator (Fig. 14.4).

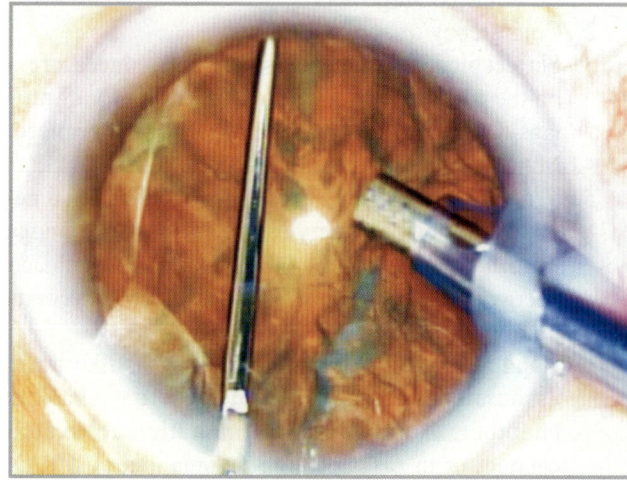

Fig. 14.4: Peripheral chopper is being placed at the equator of the nucleus under the rhexis margin

While retaining the chopper over the nucleus, under position 3, the phaco tip is embedded into the nucleus with the help of sliding movement. A positive grip is achieved over the nucleus by the action of vacuum (position 2). The nucleus is subsequently, partly pushed away from the bag, thus exposing the inferior pole of the nucleus from the fornices of the bag. The chopper is placed perpendicular to the phaco tip while retaining position 2 (irrigation and aspiration) and allowed to pierce into the nucleus substance by quick action which very much simulates a chopping action.

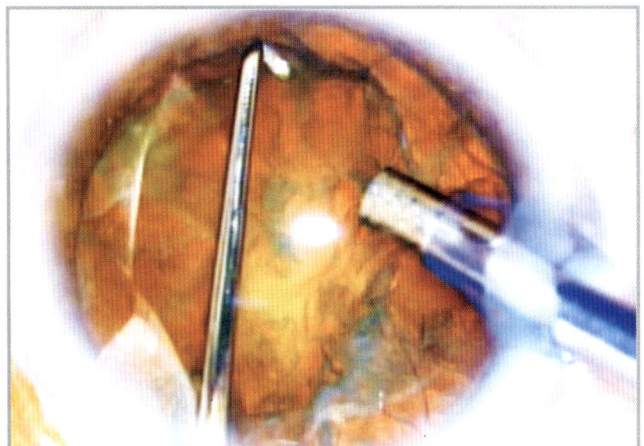

Fig. 14.5: Nucleus is being pulled with the help of a chopper a and tip under the rhexis margin

At this particular movement, the position 2 is shifted to three and simultaneously the phaco tip is pushed towards the moving chopper under a rapid transition of position two to three. Once chopper is very close to the oscillating phaco tip, the perpendicular action of the chopper towards the phaco tip is arrested within a fraction of a second and quick, tangential, lateral and divergent movements of the chopper from the phaco tip is achieved.

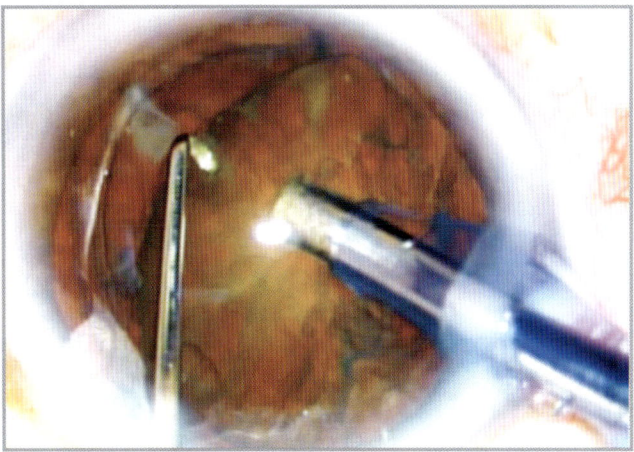

Fig. 14.6: Initiation of peripheral chopping

This lateral action along with pull and push of the phaco tip under ultrasonic oscillation creates nuclear fragmentation. This particular technique has dynamic and kinetic positions of both the phaco tip and the chopper since at the time of chopping, both the phaco tip and the chopper are moving simultaneously towards each other (Fig. 14.7).

Hence, providing more action force for better and safe chopping. Since in this particular procedure all the chopping actions are intranuclear; it may be called as intralenticular or intranuclear chopping (Fig. 14.8).

The author had enjoyed the merits of this technique in most cases with excellent and safe outcomes upto the switched over to the central chopping (Fig. 14.9).

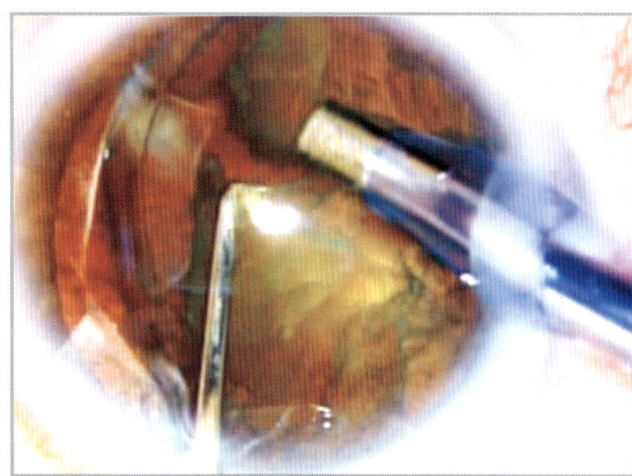

Fig. 14.7: Commencement of primary splitting of the nucleus in peripheral chopping

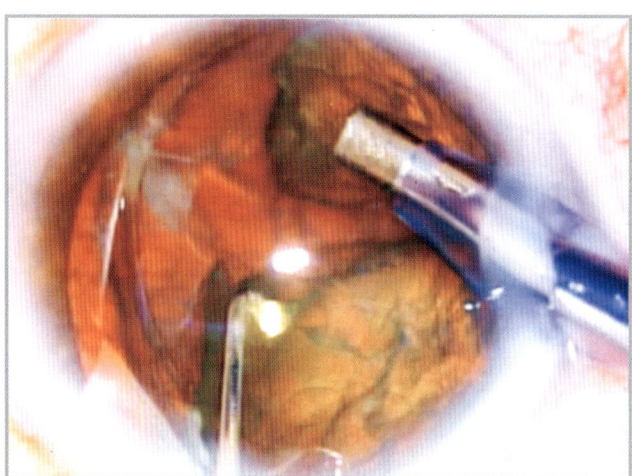

Fig. 14.8: Primary splitting of the nucleus in peripheral chopping

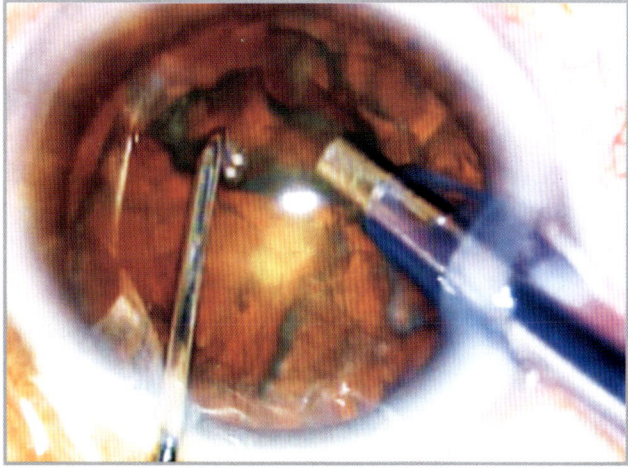

Fig. 14.9: Secondary splitting of the nucleus in peripheral chopping

The success of chopping lies exclusively on the excellent coordination of rapid movements of the chopper and the phaco tip (Fig. 14.10).

Subsequent multiple nuclear fragmentations are achieved by repeated chopping actions while creating sequential rotations of the nucleus (Fig. 14.11).

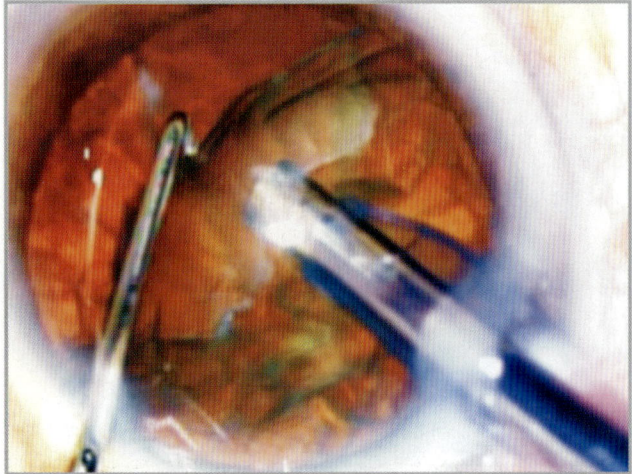

Fig. 14.10: Tertiary peripheral chopping

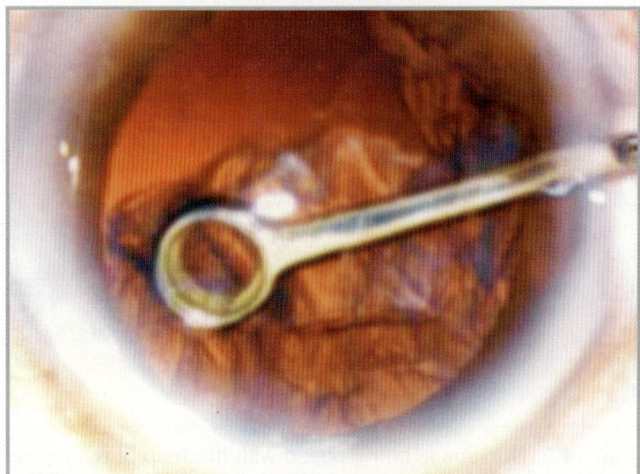

Fig. 14.13: Cortex is made free from the fornices of the capsular bag with the help of a polisher

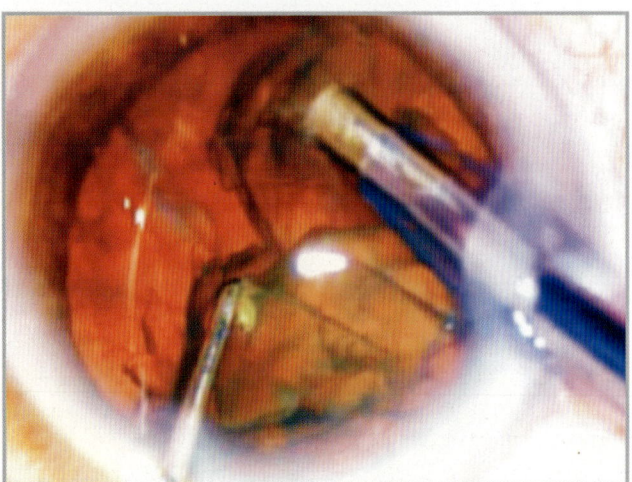

Fig. 14.11: Tertiary peripheral chopping: Splitting of the fragment

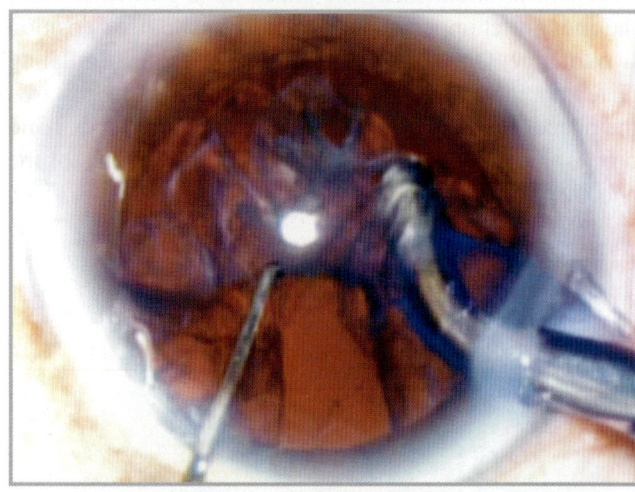

Fig. 14.14: Removal of the cortex and the posterior plate

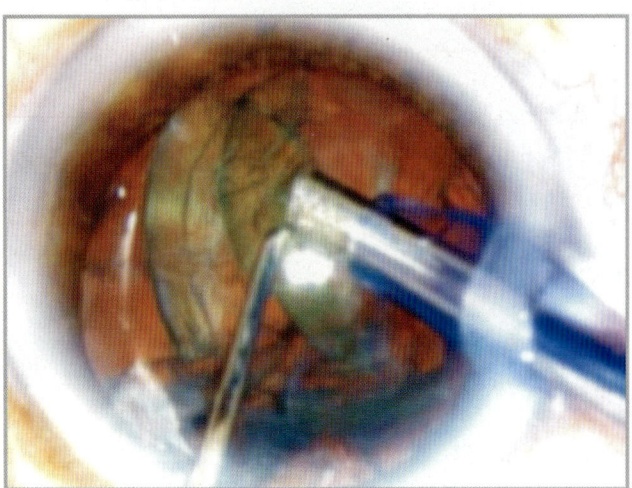

Fig. 14.12: Removal of nuclear fragments

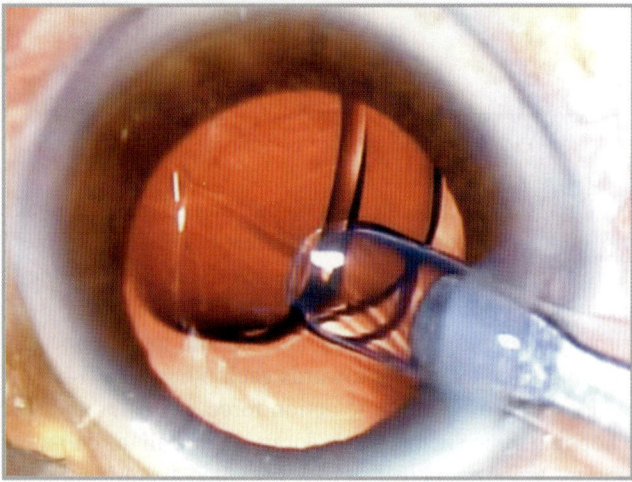

Fig. 14.15: Insertion of an IOL implant

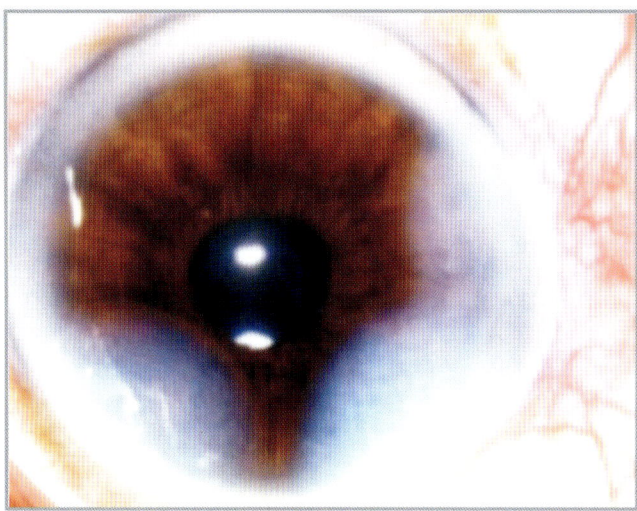

Fig. 14.16: Stromal hydration

The next step remains: removal of lens fragments under the guidance of titrated ultrasonic power.

Modified Peripheral Chop

Instead of sliding the chopper beneath the rhexis prior to the commencement of chopping, the nucleus can be pulled in the bag with the help of vacuum; thus exposing the peripheral rim visible in the inferior pole. Nucleofractis is performed by placing the chopper over the visible peripheral rim of the nucleus, thus without disturbing the rhexis margins. However, a good large rhexis is essentially required for the modified peripheral chop.

Merits of Peripheral Chopping

(i) Very effective for moderately hard cataract. (Grade III/IV).
(ii) Relatively safer for corneal endothelium as compared to sculpting, since nucleotomy is possible by applying less amount of energy.

Problems with Nagahara's Chop

(i) **Complex surgical technique:** Peripheral chopping appears to be a complex surgical procedure which demands a very high precision and accuracy particularly while performing chopping under the rhexis margins.
(ii) **Inadequate pupillary dilatation or a miotic pupil is a relative contraindication:** Inadequate mydriasis or a miotic pupil is a big hindrance to a successful peripheral chopping and involves a higher risk of intraoperative complications.
(iii) **High risk of rupture of the edges of the continuous curvilinear capsulorrhexis (CCC):** While performing chopping under the rhexis margin, great care has to be observed so as to avoid inadvertent rupture of the anterior capsule margin or even of the posterior capsule.

(iv) **Improper and inadequate grip of nucleus while performing horizontal chopping:** While rotating the chopper and piercing or performing chopping with an oscillating phaco tip into the nucleus, a groove fashioned by the tip may be widened improperly. This may lead to a loosened grip thereby chopping may be cumbersome and traumatic.

Stop and Chop

Phaco stop and chop technique is a combination of both the sculpting technique of Howard Gimbel and Phaco chop technique of Kunihiro Nagahara of Tokyo which has become popular in recent years. This hybrid technique of nucleotomy enjoys merits of both divide and conquer as well as of the direct chop.

Stop and chop appears to be much safer a procedure as compared to the conventional peripheral chopping, since the initial central trench produces central debulking of the nucleus as well as eliminates probable risks of inadvertent capsular margin tear. Subsequent chopping through the central trench or groove needs fewer efforts which are much more beneficial in cases of hard cataract.

Stop and chop has witnessed several modifications since its inceptions. Initially, stop and chop was a combination of central sculpting followed by peripheral chopping. Any kind of chopping technique, like peripheral chop or modified peripheral chop or central chop may be combined with sculpting or with the central groove.

Prerequisites

Essential prerequisites for stop and chop techniques are as follows:
(i) Grade II to IV cataract,
(ii) Good mydriasis,
(iii) Good rotation of nucleus and posterior cortical cushion are essential prerequisites for the stop and chop technique.

Surgical Steps

1. Initial deep central sculpting is performed same as with the case of the divide and conquer method.
2. Nucleus is divided into two equal halves with the help of a phaco tip and one or two diallers.
3. Posterior plate is cracked.
4. Subsequent nucleotomy by conventional chopping with the help of a chopper and repeated nucleus rotation.
5. Emulsification/aspiration of small nuclear fragments.
6. The posterior plate is mobilised with the help of a dialler and aspirated out exactly in the same fashion as in other techniques.

This technique appears to be safe and may be considered as a gradual transformation of chopping in toto.

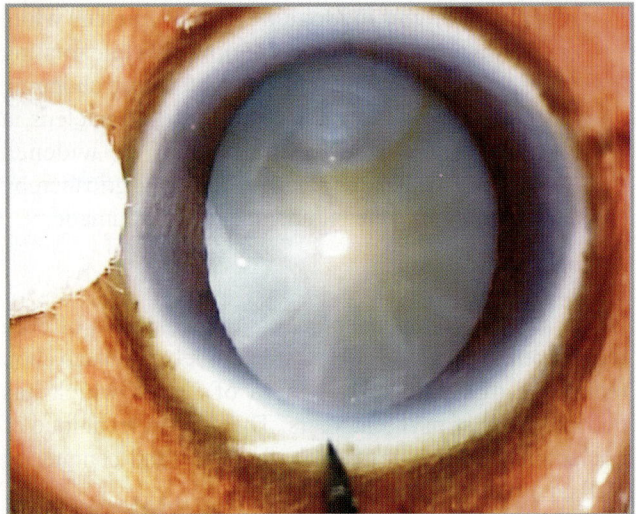

Fig. 14.17: Stop and Chop: Side port incision

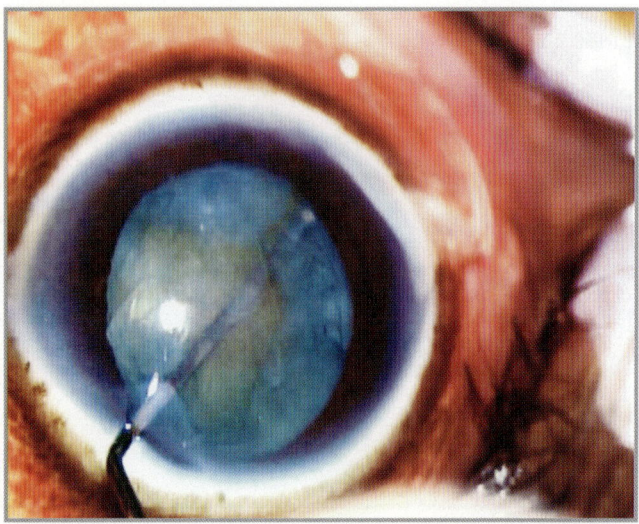

Fig. 14.20: : Hydroprocedure for stop and chop

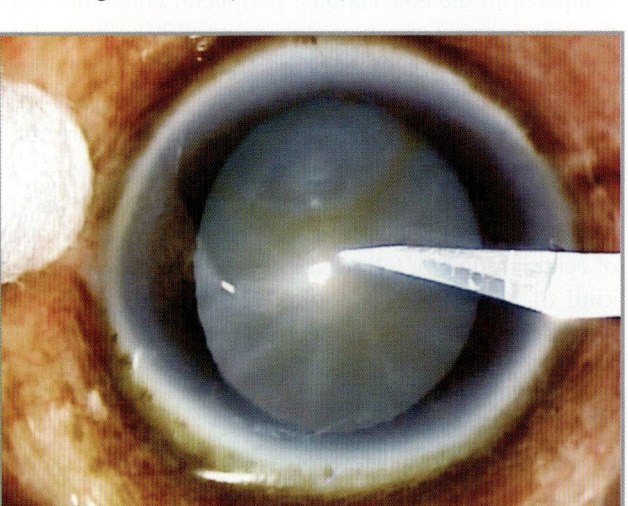

Fig. 14.18: Stop and chop: Primary Incision at 10–11 O' clock position for subsequent clear corneal incision, (temporal for the right eye and nasal for the left eye, respectively

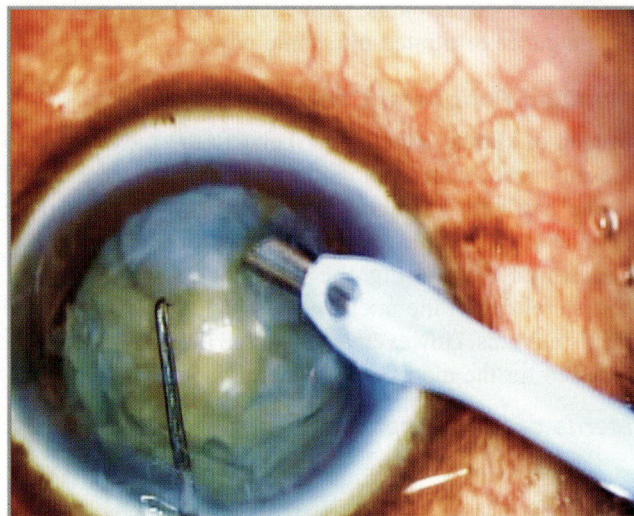

Fig. 14.21: Stop and chop: Clearing of superficial cortex

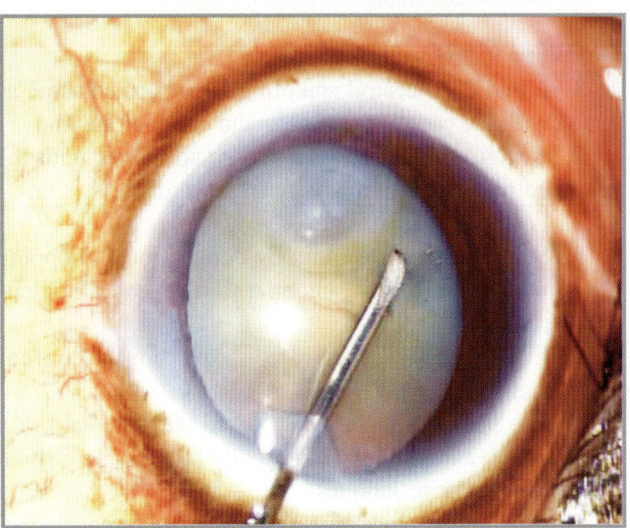

Fig. 14.19: Stop and chop: Rhexis

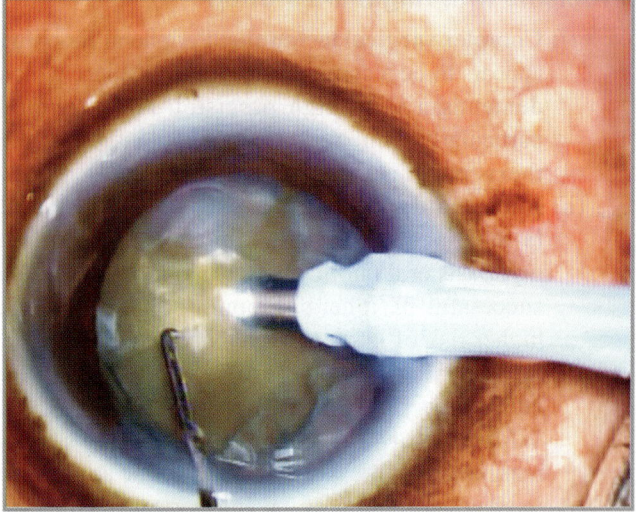

Fig. 14.22: Stop and chop: Commencement of trenching

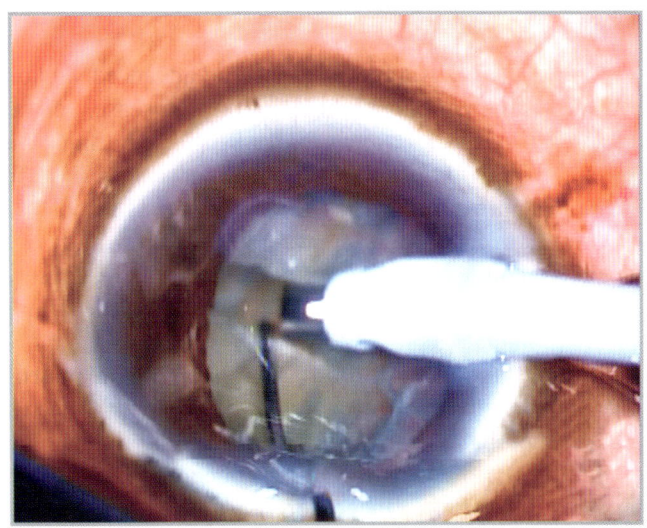

Fig. 14.23: Stop and chop: Initial trenching for heminucleotomy

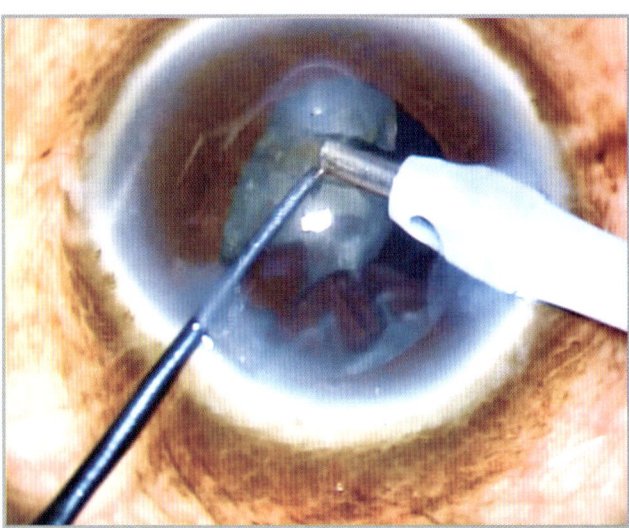

Fig. 14.26: Stop and chop: Removal of lens fragments

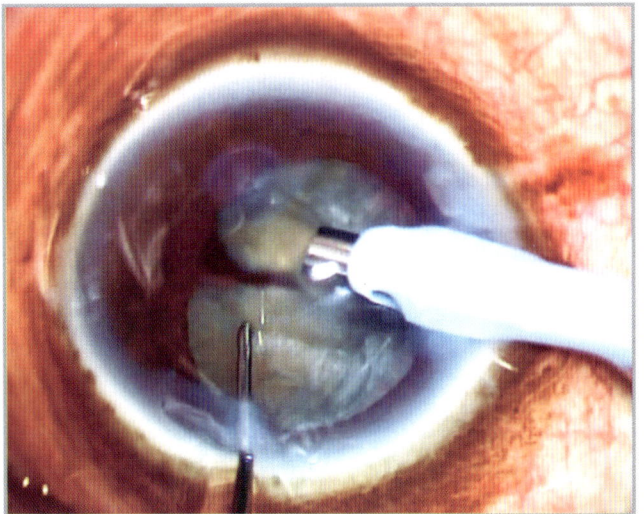

Fig. 14.24: Stop and chop: Primary splitting of the nucleus for heminucleotomy

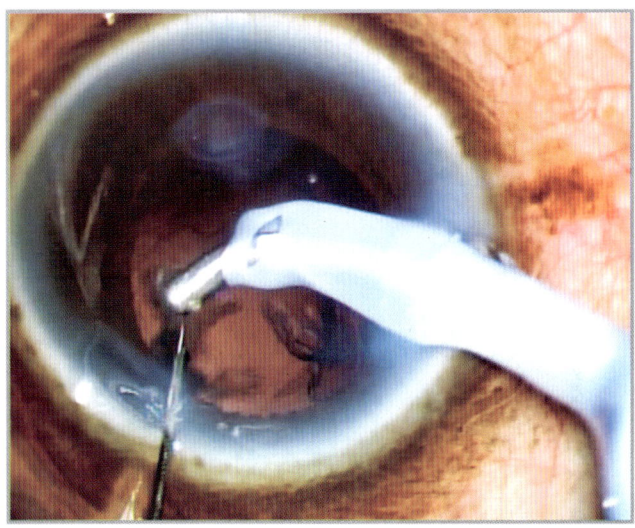

Fig. 14.27: Stop and Chop: Cortical removal

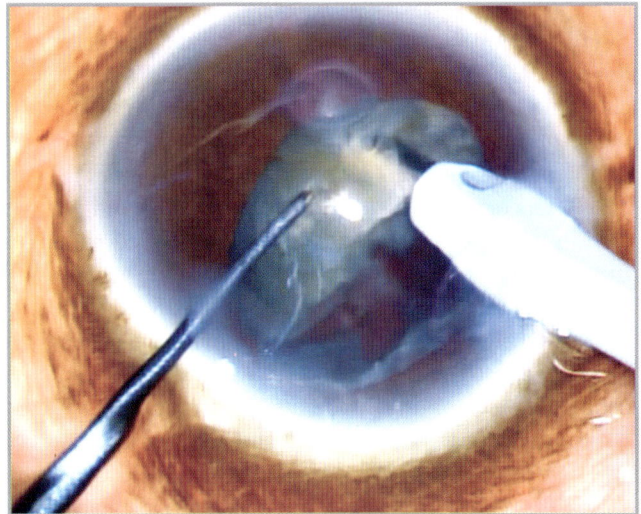

Fig. 14.25: Stop and chop: Multiple nucleotomy by sequential chopping

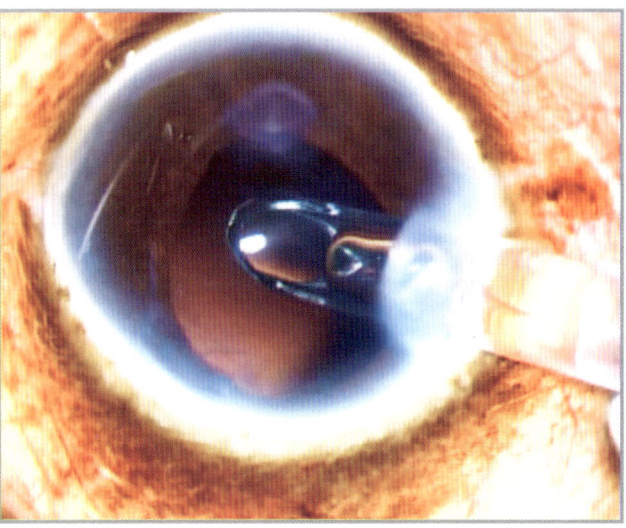

Fig. 14.28: Stop and chop: IOL insertion

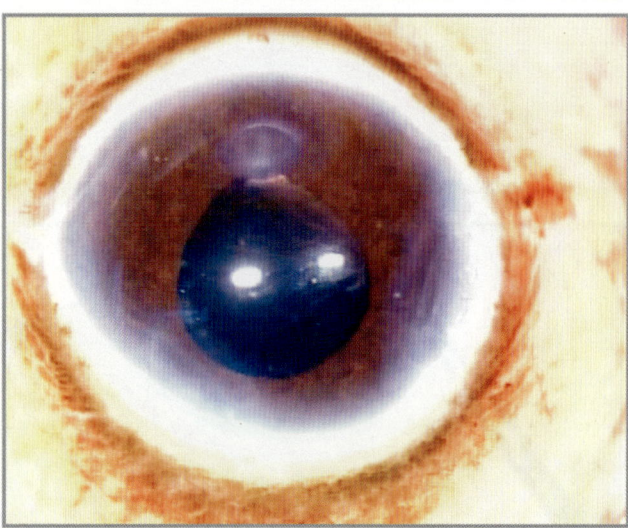

Fig. 14.29: Stop and chop: IOL is in situ

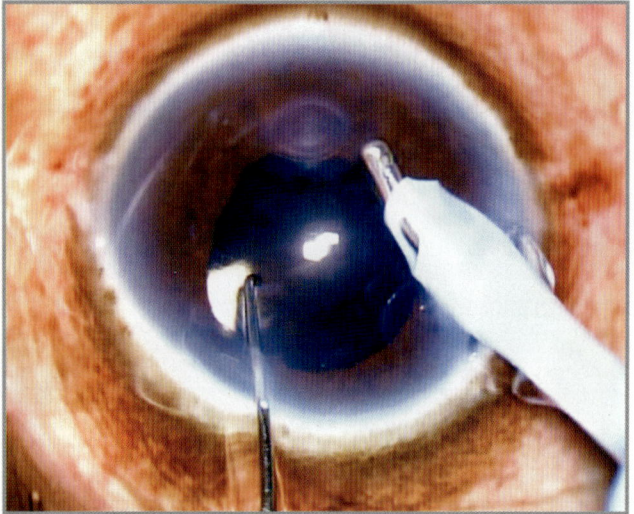

Fig. 14.30: Stop and Chop Post IOL implant wash insertion

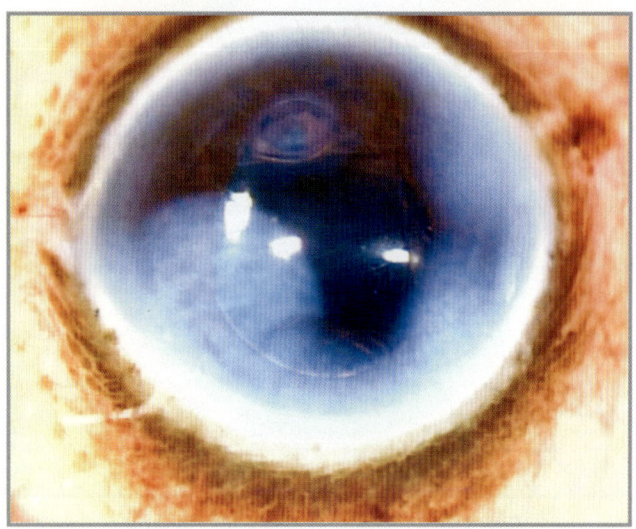

Fig. 14.31: Stop and Chop: Stromal Hydration

Central Chop

Central chopping is a more refined and advanced version of Nagahara's peripheral chopping. In true sense, central chop has opened up a new horizon of phacotechniques, safety, and revolution. It is very much possible to handle hard and supra hard nuclei without compromising corneal endothelium as well as creating severe intra and post operative complications. Central chopping has definitely made bimanual phacoemulsification technique more effective and surgeon-friendly.

Rapid transformation and advancement in instrumentations, fluid dynamics and energy delivery systems has resulted in several modifications in central chopping techniques. However, the basic concept of lifting the nucleus under the influence of vacuum, embedding the phaco tip into the core nucleus by using ultrasonic energy and creation of intranuclear mechanical cleavage by placing a sharp chopper into the mid-nucleus remains the same and applicable in all the variants.

The central chop carries several advantages over the peripheral chop.

(i) It can be performed through a miotic pupil or a small rhexis.

(ii) Least possibility of disintegration of capsulorrhexis, since chopping actions are carried out well away from the rhexis margins.

(iii) More safety to the posterior capsule since nucleus is slightly lifted in the bag; hence produces less mechanical stress on the capsule.

Principle of Central Chopping

The nucleus is chopped from the centre to the periphery. the (chopper is pushed into the centre of the nucleus and drawn away from the tip. Hence, achieves inside to outside chopping action).

Technique

(i) Incision and rhexis can be as per standard norms zero degree or 15 degree phaco tips are more suitable for chopping, since these tips provide a greater hold and stability while attempting chopping. The author has undoubted preference for the zero degree tip over any other tip.

(ii) Once, phaco tip and chopper is introduced into the anterior chamber, superficial cortex is removed under the irrigation mode of phaco handpiece. Moderate vacuum and a low flow rate are recommended settings for this step.

(iii) Once superficial cortex is removed, the phaco tip is embedded into the mid of nucleus just a little lower to the centre while applying moderate ultrasonic energy, high vacuum and flow rate settings. The high vacuum is very effective to attain a good hold and lift of the nucleus, thereby enhancing safety of the posterior capsule. The phaco tip is allowed to traverse into the nuclear substance till it crosses more than two third thickness of the core nucleus. It is

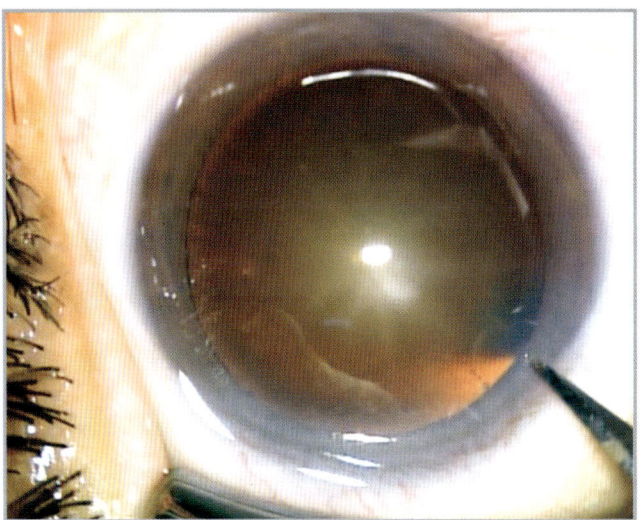

Fig. 14.32: Central chopping: Primary incision

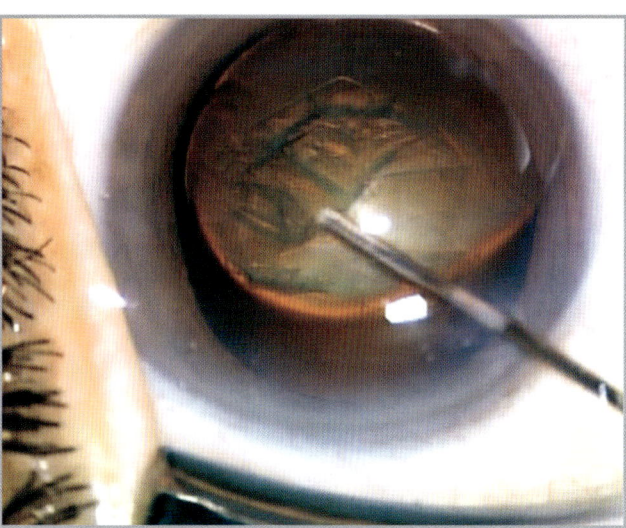

Fig. 14.35: Central chopping: Hydroprocedure

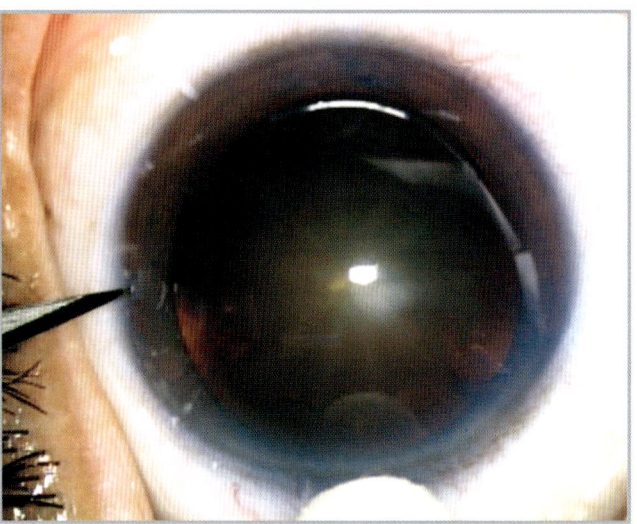

Fig. 14.33: Central chopping: Side port Incision

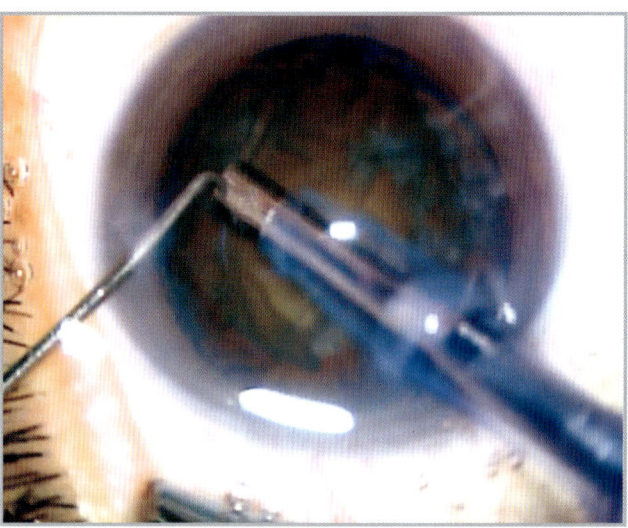

Fig. 14.36: Central chopping: Clearing of superficial cortex

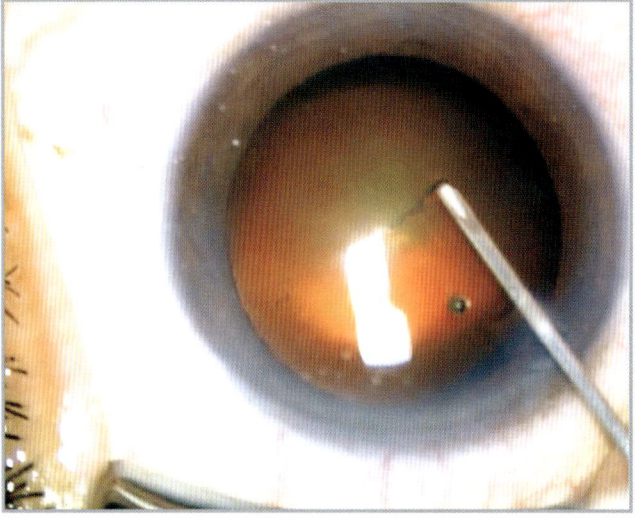

Fig. 14.34: Central chopping: Rhexis

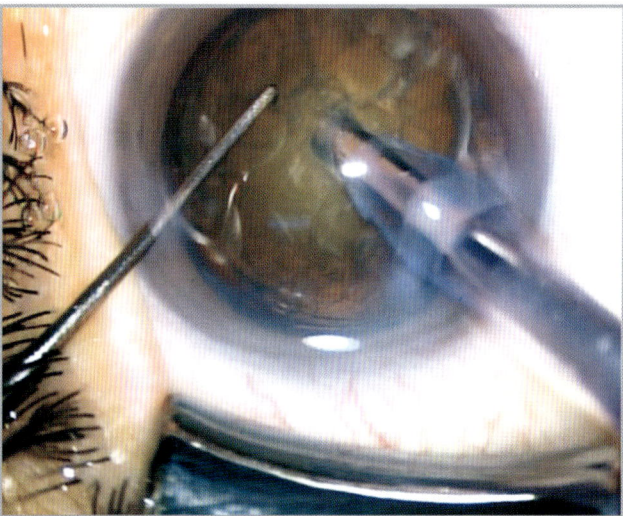

Fig. 14.37: Central chopping: Initiation of central chopping: Phaco tip is being embedded into the core nucleus

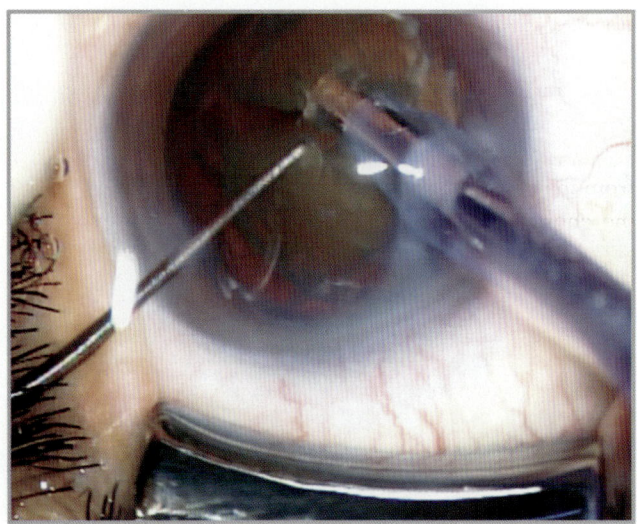

Fig. 14.38: Central chopping: Primary splitting of the nucleus

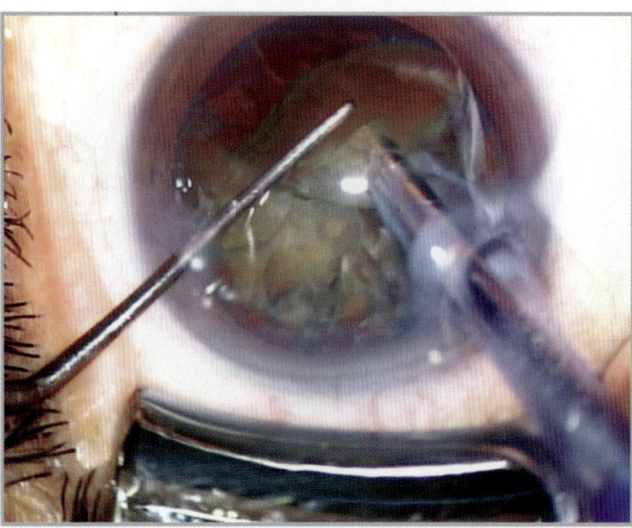

Fig. 14.41: Central chopping: Nuclear fragment removal

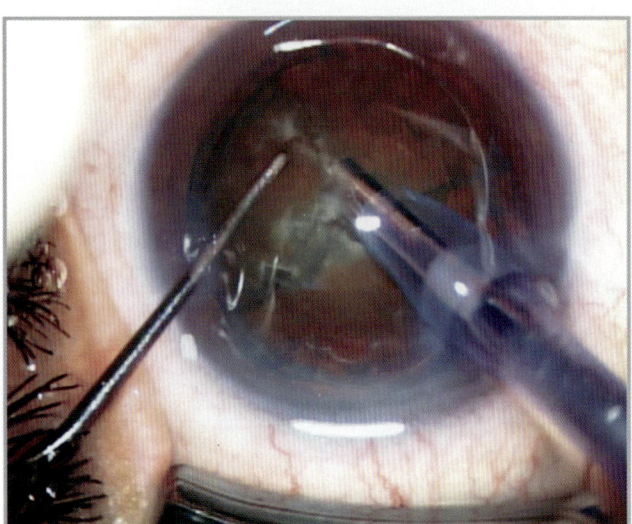

Fig. 14.39: Central chopping: Secondary splitting of the nucleus

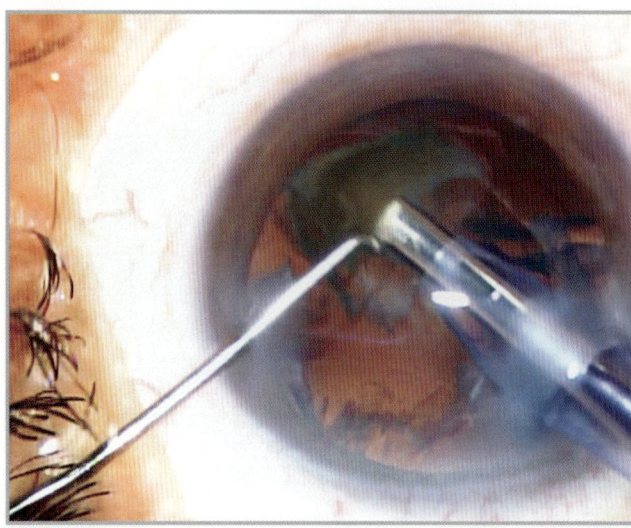

Fig. 14.42: Central chopping: Removal of the last fragment of nucleus

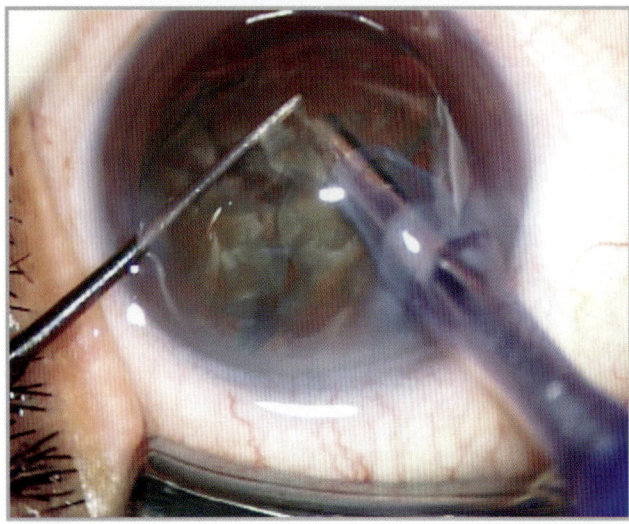

Fig. 14.40: Central chopping: Tertiary splitting of the nucleus

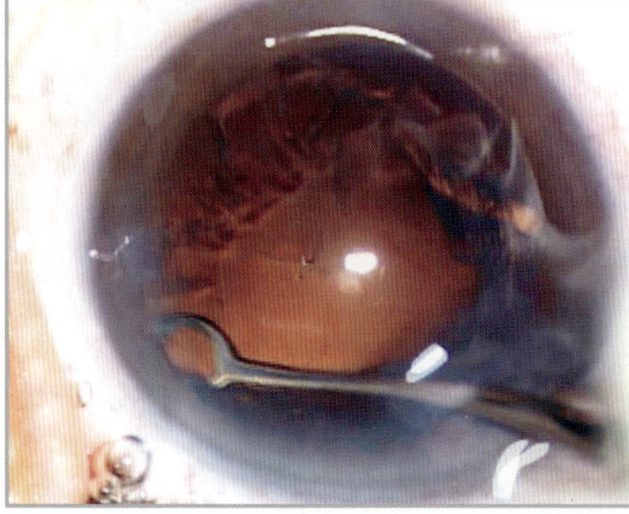

Fig. 14.43: Central chopping: Cortex is made free from the fornices of the capsular bag with the help of a polisher

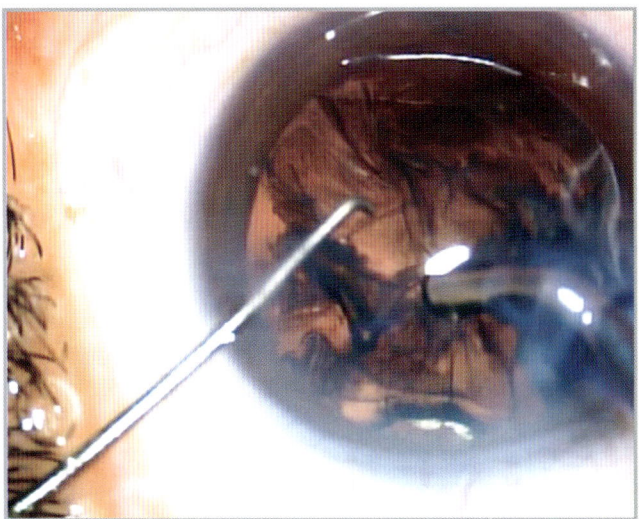

Fig. 14.44: Central chopping: Removal of cortex and posterior plate

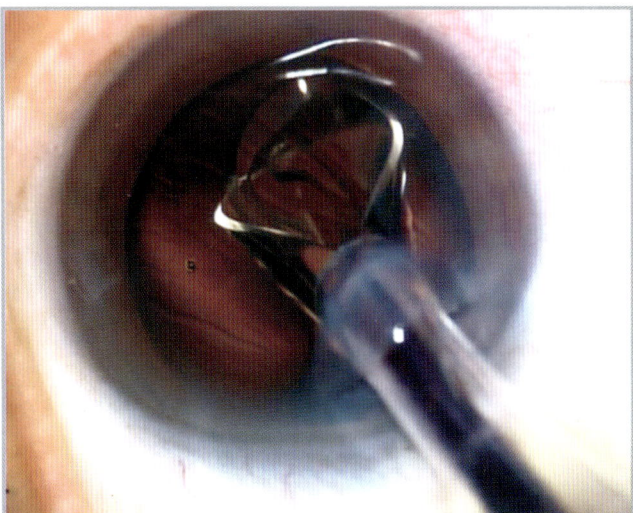

Fig. 14.45: Central chopping: Insertion of IOL implant

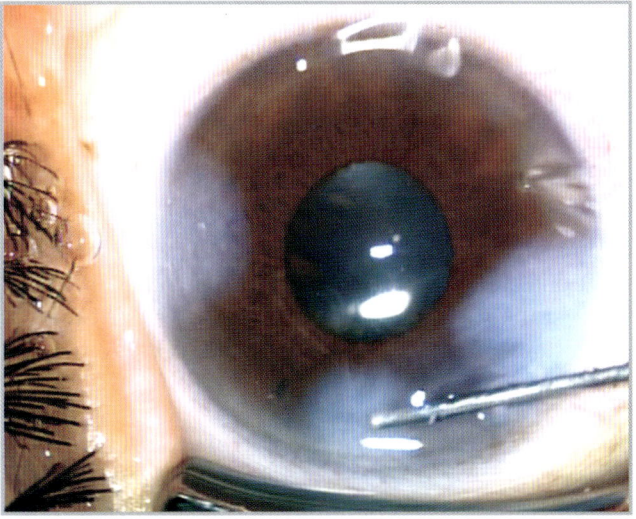

Fig. 14.46: Central chopping: Stromal Hydration

essential to ensure intact posterior cortical plate while performing this step so as to avoid any inadvertent injury to the posterior capsule. The next step is to place the cutting edge of chopper into the cleavage created by embedded phaco tip and just ahead of it. The chopper is quickly moved away from the phaco tip in a reverse L fashion so as to complete the chopping action. This particular stage requires least phaco energy, low flow rate and high vacuum so as to maintain a sustained and firm grip of the nucleus by the phaco tip throughout the entire duration of chopping action. Central chopping is also known as dynamic chopping, since both phaco tip and chopper are actively utilised to create nuclear fragmentation. Tangential chopping action will lead to primary hemi-sections of the nucleus. Multiple nuclear fragmentations are achieved by repeated chopping actions.

It is highly recommended to ensure completion of multiple nuclear fragmentation prior to the commencement of ultrasonic emulsification and removal of smaller nuclear fragments since it provides greater safety to the cortical plate and finally, reduces the risk of inadvertent posterior capsule rupture due to the oscillating phaco tip. It is a wise step to switch over to irrigation mode often during fragment removal so as to maintain an adequately distended capsular bag as well as to maintain the desired position of the posterior capsule in relation to the phaco tip.

Another important tip is to have a mobile foot on foot switch with continuous reshuffling of phaco settings between position one, two, three and then position two and one most of the time so as to have a constant and inflated capsular bag and anterior chamber all the time. Occasional and small burst of phaco energy from time-to-time will suffice. This resembles a good batsman who does not seem to exert while scoring and keeps on reshuffling himself with excellent foot work on the crease or else a fighter pilot who keeps on flying and intercepting all the time against enemy threat. Initially, phacomachine governs you, thus a surgeon tends to use more phaco power and that too for a longer duration. Gradually, the surgeon learns the technique to handle the machine; hence he relies less and less upon on Phaco energy and more and more on aspiration and irrigation mode. The author remembers his initial surgeries where surgical time used to be three to four minutes of 60–70% phaco power with sculpting which has touched to 65 to 75 seconds in sculpting and less than 20 seconds in chopping with much less energy settings. It is presumed that every phaco surgeon should be able to transform up to this stage with little effort but a consistent desire to improve all the time.

(iv) **Removal of cortical matter:** Removal of cortical matter is carried out in the usual manner.

Removal of Residual Cortex

As such, a large amount of cortical matter has already been removed prior to the nucleotomy, thus a very small amount

Table 14.1: Phacoemulsification machine settings at different stages of Central Chopping
(Zero degree tip on Peristaltic Pump)

Steps/stages	Principle	Phaco settings	Flow (cc/min)	Vacuum	Continuous/ micro pulse
Baring the nucleus	Low flow and vacuum	00–05 %	10–15	60–100	Continuous/micropulse
Nudging the phaco tip into the nucleus	Low flow and vacuum	10–30 (As per hardness of nucleus)	20–22	100–150	Continuous/micropulse
Lifting the nucleus	Moderate vacuum	00	22–28	200–275	Position two, no US energy
Central chopping	Moderate vacuum	00–10	22–28	225–275	Position two/three,
Subsequent multiple nucleotomy	Moderate vacuum	00–10	22–28	200–275	Position two/three,
Fragment removal	High flow and vacuum	15–30	24–26	200–275	Continuous/micropulse
Removal of the last fragment	Low flow and moderate vacuum	10–20	15–20	75–150	Continuous/micropulse
Removing the posterior plate/epinucleus	Low flow and high vacuum	00–05	10–15	100–125	Continuous/micropulse/ I/A mode
Residual cortical wash	Moderate flow and high vacuum	I/A mode	26–34	300–400	Continuous
Posterior capsule polishing	Low flow and vacuum	I/A mode/	5	10–20	Continuous

Table 14.2: Phacoemulsification machine settings at different stages of Central Chopping
(Zero degree tip on Ventury Pump)

Steps/stages	Principle	Phaco settings	Vacuum	Continuous/micropulse
Baring the nucleus	Low vacuum	05%	45–60	Continuous/micropulse
Nudging the phaco tip into the nucleus	Low vacuum	0–30 (As per hardness of nucleus)	100–125	Continuous/micropulse
Lifting the nucleus	Moderate vacuum	00	100–125	Position two, no US energy
Central chopping	Moderate vacuum	00–05	100–125	Position two, no US energy
Subsequent multiple nucleotomy	Moderate vacuum	00–05	60–75	Position two, no US energy
Fragment removal	Moderate to high vacuum	05–20	80–100	micro pulse
Removal of the last fragment	Moderate vacuum	5–15	50–60	micro pulse
Removing the posterior plate/epinucleus	Moderate vacuum	0–5/ US mode	60–80 on handpiece / 300–400 I/A	Continuous/micropulse
Residual cortical wash	High vacuum	I/A mode	400–450	Continuous
Posterior capsule polishing	Low flow	I/A mode	0–5	Continuous

of cortical matter is left following hydrofloat nucleotomy. Over and above, repeated irrigation results in an opening of capsular bag fornices as well as hydration of the leftover cortical fibres. Hence removal of such cortex demands much less a flow rate and vacuum as compared to the conventional chopping techniques. The zero degree tip can be employed to remove floating cortical matter under irrigation/aspiration position. It is wise to attempt removal of subincisional lens matter by clock and anticlock wise pull and push by I/A handpiece. This will facilitate a large chunk of cortex to be aspirated out in a single stroke.

Stromal Hydration

Stromal hydration by injecting BSS into the lip of corneal valve and the side port incision is a good option to achieve a self sealing wound. The whitish hue created at the site of incisions, generally disappears within six to seven hours.

Phaco-prechop

Since the advent of the ultrasonic phacoemulsification technique, there has been tremendous thrust on enhancing intraoperative safety, minimising the risk of corneal endothelial injury due to ultrasonic energy and subsequent thermal injuries due to heat generation from ultrasonic oscillations of the phaco tip. Divide and conquer and various the techniques of chopping and application of advanced fluidics system are glaring examples of this effort.

The concept of Prechopping was derived by Dr Takayuki Akahoshi, by keeping the need of reducing energy requirement during ultrasonic nuclear fragmentation. This concept originated from the surgical technique of manual nonphaco nuclear fragmentation, popularly performed during initial era of small incision cataract surgeries in the early nineties.

Principle of Prechopping

Phaco prechop is a technique of mechanical fragmentation of nucleus which is essentially carried out prior to the commencement of phacoemulsification. By this technique nucleus can be divided into fragments without carrying out sculpting or chopping. Prechopping significantly reduces the subsequent need of ultrasonic energy application. However, a specially designed metallic device called prechopper is mandatory for this purpose.

Specifications of a Prechopper

The prechopper comprises of two blades of different shapes and designs. Of these, one blade is relatively sharp and an angular configuration whereas, the other blade has blunt and smooth rounded surface. Sharpness of the surface varies according to the hardness of the nucleus. Sharp surface pierces into the nuclear substance while blunt surface ensures division of the nucleus.

Types of Prechoppers

(i) Smooth blade prechopper is the most suitable for the soft nucleus.
(ii) A sharp prechopper is ideal for grade two nucleus
(iii) Combo prechopper can be used for soft or grade two nucleus.
(iv) The universal prechopper is recommended for soft nuclei as a single device, where it can be applied in case of hard cataract once combined with nucleus manipulator.
(v) The conventional sharp prechopper is used in cases of hard cataract. However, it is recommended to restrict use of prechoppers upto the soft to moderate grade of nucleus only since prechopping in the case of hard nucleus may produce mechanical stress on zonules and the inadvertent rupture of the posterior capsule.
(vi) Use of the nucleus manipulator has been recommended in certain adverse situations like a very hard nucleus, small or improper rhexis, zonular weakness. However, the author strongly advices to refrain from prechopping in such adverse conditions and recommend to proceed with the conventional

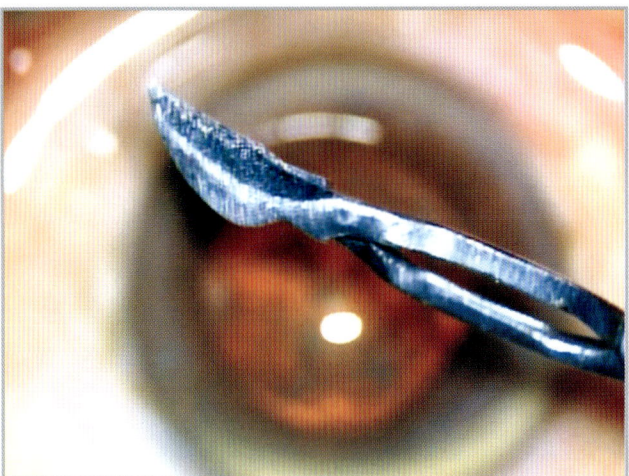

Fig. 14.47: The conventional sharp prechopper

central chopping technique so as to avoid an impending threat of intraoperative complications.

Technique

(i) **Choice of phacoemulsifier and machine settings:** Dr Takayuki Akahoshi had preferred high vacuum, high flow rate and increased bottle height on legacy phacoemulsifier system to emulsify prechopped nuclear fragments. However, it is not mandatory to continue on all high settings and any specific machine. The author had effectively utilised numerous phacoemulsifier systems on moderate settings and equipped with the zero degree tip so as to complete subsequent nucleotomy following prechopping.

(ii) **Initial steps of incisions, rhexis and hydroprocedures:** Initial steps of incisions, rhexis and hydroprocedures are same as in case of conventional chopping techniques. A good amount of high density viscoelastics are mandatory to protect corneal endothelium against any inadvertent insult to the endothelium while performing prechopping.

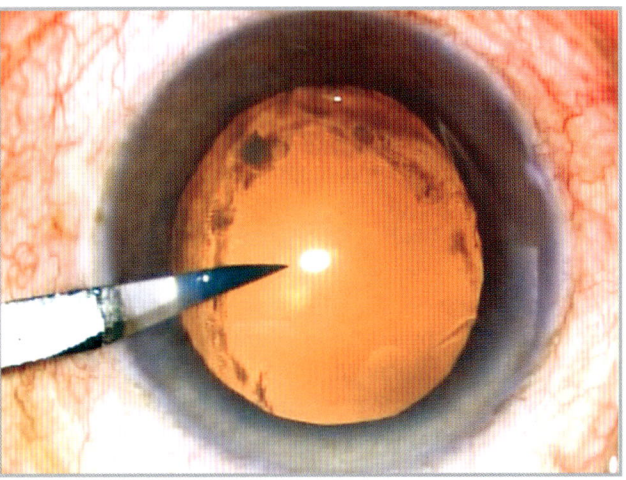

Fig. 14.48: Prechopping : Incision

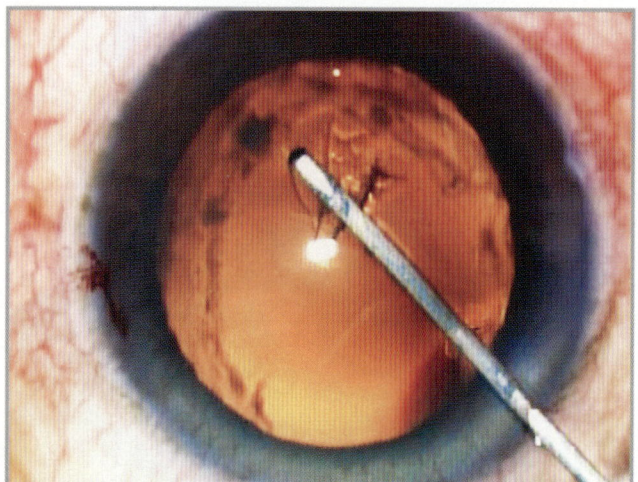

Fig. 14.49: Prechopping: Rhexis

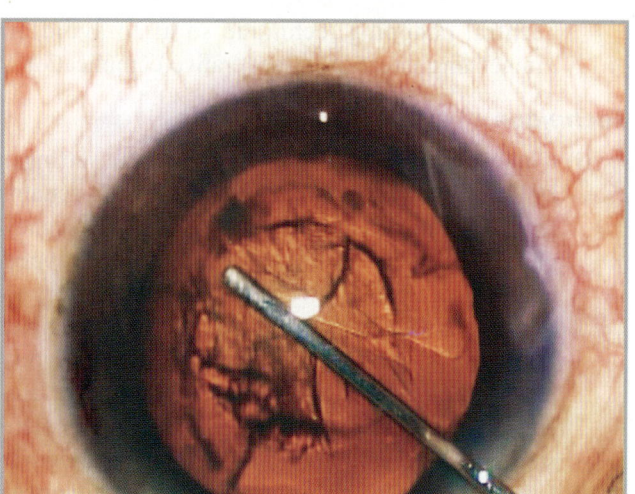

Fig. 14.50: Prechopping: Hydroprocedure

(iii) Removal of superficial cortical matter: Removal of superficial cortical matter is optional in case of prechopping. However, it is good to attempt nuclear fragmentation extending upto the posterior capsule. In certain peculiar conditions, prechopping may require assistance of the second instrument to facilitate counter traction as well as to provide additional support to the nucleus during procedure.

(iv) Prechopping: After completion of hydro-procedure, the prechopper tip is inserted towards the centre of the lens nucleus while retaining apposed blades. The prechopper blades are sub-sequently separated once pierced into the nucleus.

The next step is to attain initial cracks in the nucleus which is initiated by a gradual separation of the prechopper blades. It is recommended to maintain a sustained action of prechopper blades to pierce into the cracks until desired splitting of the nucleus is achieved. Multiple cracks can be obtained by rotating nucleus with the help of prechopper in perpendicular directions.

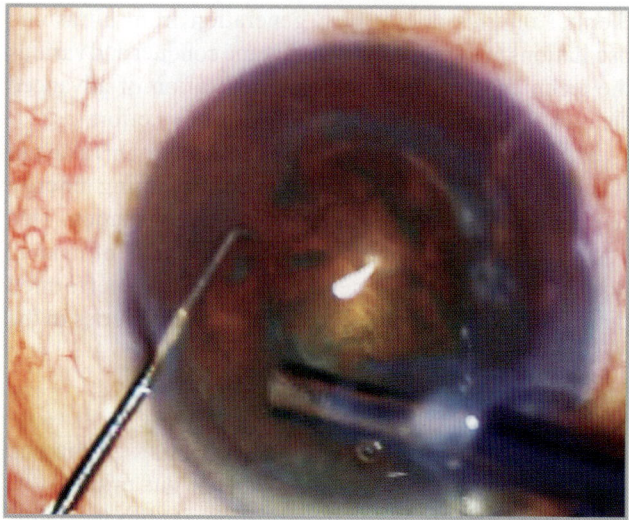

Fig. 14.51: Prechopping: Removal of superficial cortical matter

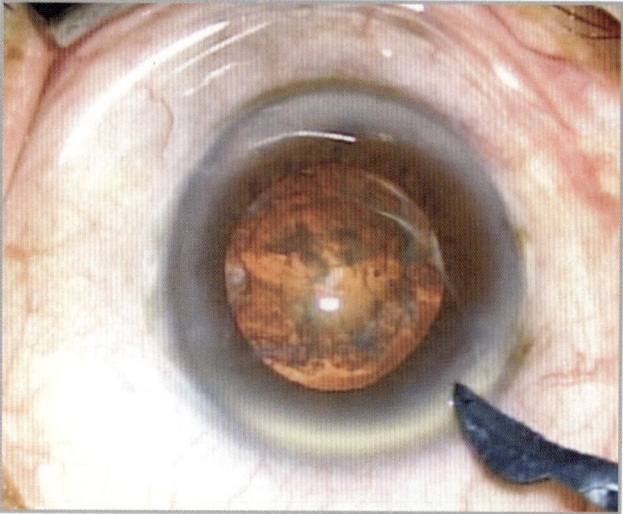

Fig. 14.52: Prechopping: Prechopper at the site of incision

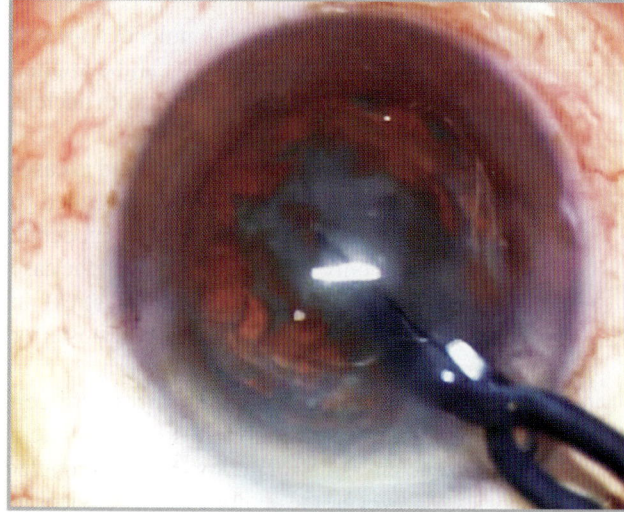

Fig. 14.53: Prechopping : Prechopper is being embedded into the nucleus while keeping blades closed

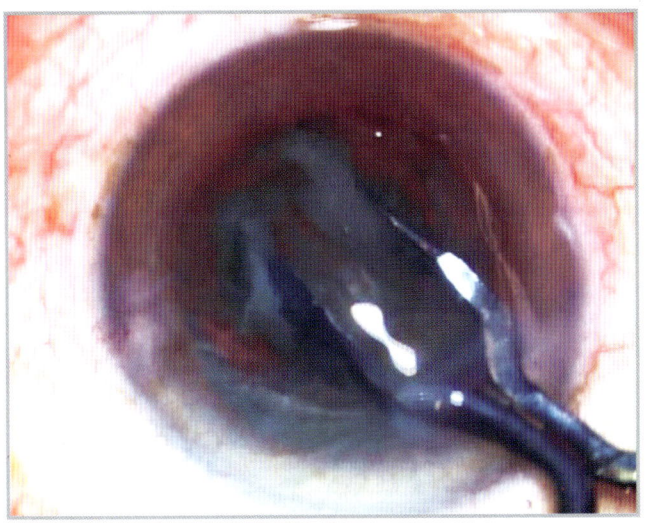

Fig. 14.54: Prechopping: Blades of embedded prechopper is being opened up to commence prechop splitting of nucleus

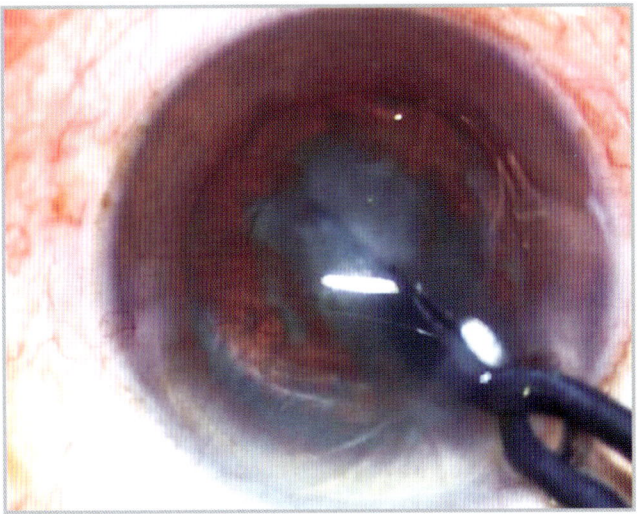

Fig. 14.55: Prechopping: Prechopper is being pushed into the crack in the nucleus

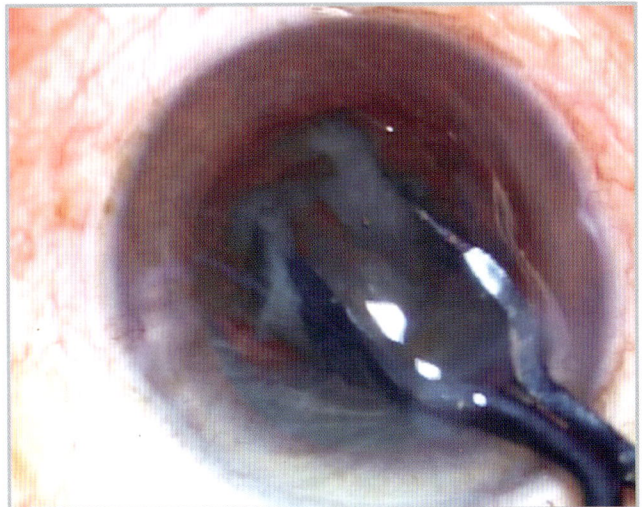

Fig. 14.56: Prechopping: Commencement of prechop nuclear splitting

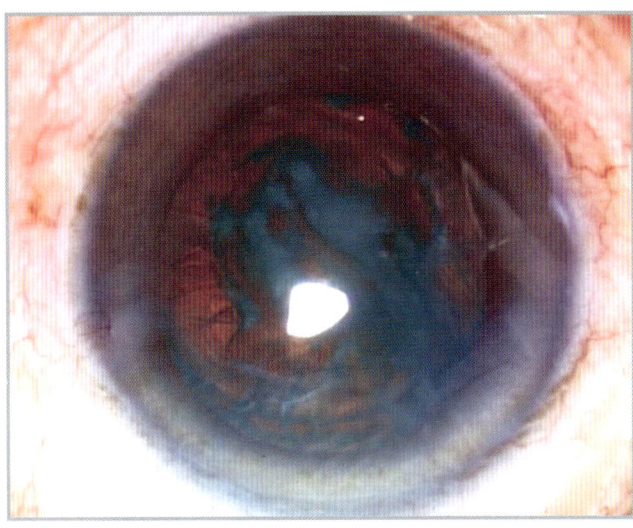

Fig. 14.57: Prechopping: Prechop nuclear splitting

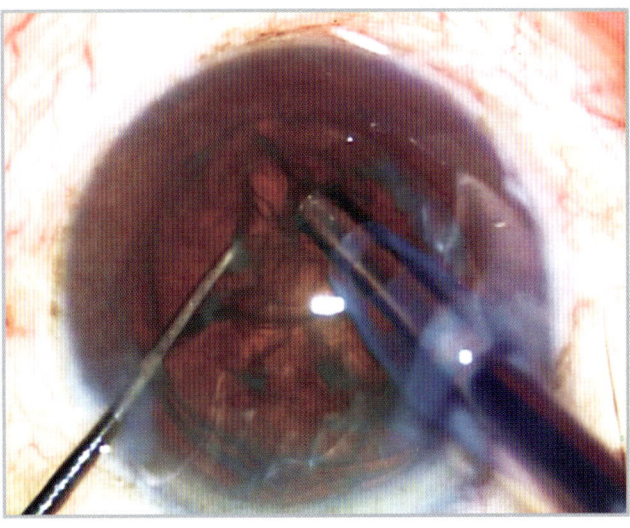

Fig. 14.58: Prechopping: Post prechop central chopping

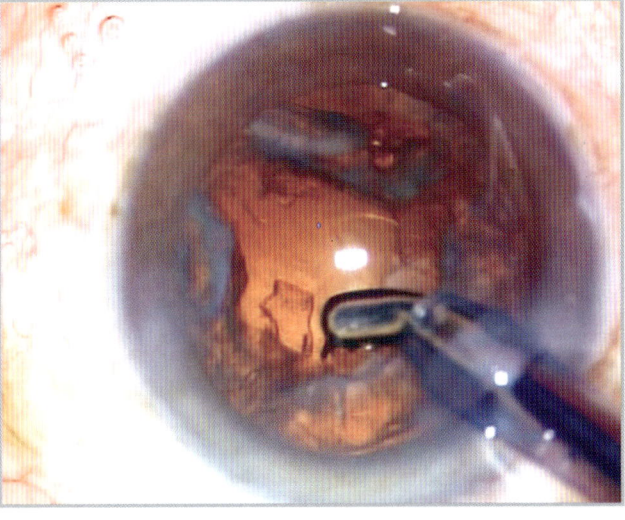

Fig. 14.59: Prechopping : Post prechop Irrigation/Aspiration

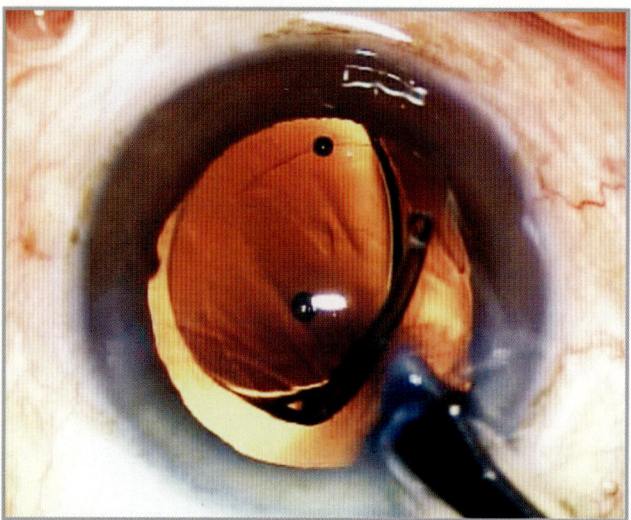

Fig. 14.60: Insertion of IOL implant

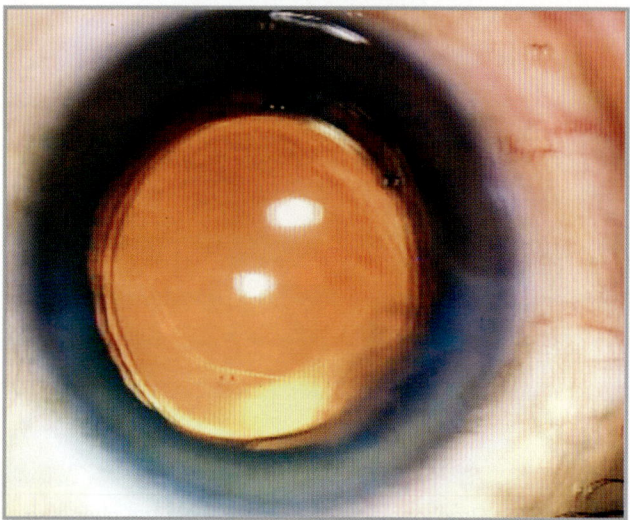

Fig. 14.61: Prechop: IOL implant is in situ

Remaining steps of nucleotomy and cortical wash are essentially same as for conventional sculpting or chopping techniques.

Merits

(i) Phacoemulsification can be completed without creating any sculpting or groove with the application of ultrasonic energy.

(ii) Very effective and significant reduction in ultrasonic energy requirement as well as in effective surgical time.

(ii) Minimises the risk of thermal corneal burns.

Demerits

(i) Pre-chopper is not an ideal technique in case of hard or dense nuclei, since pre chopper may not be able to pierce into the nuclear substance which is an essential pre-requisite for this technique.

(ii) Relatively higher risk of corneal endothelial insult due to inadvertent mechanical injury to the endothelium while manoeuvrng prechopping.

(iii) Additional care to be observed while attempting prechopping so as to avoid posterior capsule tear due to mechanical traction or direct injury to the capsule or zonules.

CONCLUSION

Phacoemulsification surgery has attained wide popularity and acknowledgement among both surgeons and patients. However, a complete transformation and adoption of a suitable technique depends not only on adequate practice and patience but also on the equipment and infrastructure as well as on the surgical experience and acumen of the surgeon himself.

Various techniques of Phaco chopping have minimised the need of ultrasonic energy to a great extent, resulting in overall safety and enhanced acceptability among surgeons and patients as well. Chopping techniques are going to enjoy the centre space in nucleotomy techniques in the form of some kind of modifications. Indeed the future of modern phacosurgeries lies, exclusively on application of fluidics and further refinement in various chopping techniques.

BIBLIOGRAPHY

1. Shepherd, J.R.In situ fracture.Journal of Cataract and Refractive Surgery1990, 16 (4), 436–440.

2. Ram, J., Wesendahl, T.A., Auffarth, G.U., Apple, D.J. Evaluation of in situ fracture versus phaco chop techniques. Journal of Cataract and Refractive Surgery 1998, 24 (11), 1464–1468.

3. Nagahara, K., Phaco-Chop, M.D.(1993) Technique Eliminates Central Sculpting and Allows Faster, Safer Phaco. Ocular Surgery News, 12–13.

4. Koch, P. New Techniques for Cataract Surgery. Current Opinion in Ophthalmology1995; 6:41–45.

5. Koch, P.S.Phaco chop. Simplifying Phacoemulsification; Safe and Efficient Methods for Cataract Surgery 1997, 123–129. (ed. Koch PS), Slack, Thorofare, NJ.

6. Ram, J., Wesendahl, T.A., Auffarth, G.U., Apple, D.J. Evaluation of in situ fracture versus phaco chop techniques. Journal of Cataract and Refractive Surgery 1998, 24 (11), 1464–1468.

7. Chang, D.F. Converting to phaco chop: Why? Which technique? How? Ophthalmic Practice 1999, 17 (4), 202–210.

8. DeBry, P., Olson, R.J., Crandall, A.S. Comparison of energy required for phaco-chop and divide and conquer phacoemulsification. Journal of Cataract and Refractive Surgery 1998, 24 (5), 689–692.

9. Davison, J.A. Phacoemulsification time and power requirements in phaco chop and divide and conquer nucleofractis techniques. Journal of Cataract and Refractive Surgery 2000, 26 (9), 1374–1378.

10. Gimbel, H.V.Divide and conquer nucleofractis phaco-emulsification: Development and variations. Journal of Cataract and Refractive Surgery 1991, 17 (3), 281–291.

11. Hayashi, K., Nakao, F., Hayashi, F. Corneal endothelial cell loss after phacoemulsification using nuclear cracking procedures. Journal of Cataract and Refractive Surgery 1994, 20 (1), 44–47.

12. Pirazzoli, G., D'Eliseo, D., Ziosi, M., Acciarri, R. Effects of phacoemulsification time on the corneal endothelium using phacofracture and phaco chop techniques. Journal of cataract and refractive surgery 1996, 22 (7), 967–969.

13. Bourne, R.R.A., Minassian, D.C., Dart, J.K.G., Rosen, P., Kaushal, S., Wingate, N. Effect of cataract surgery on the corneal endothelium: Modern phacoemulsification compared with extracapsular cataract surgery. Ophthalmology 2004, 111(4), 679–685.

14. Koch, P.S., Katzen, L.E. Stop and chop phacoemulsification. Journal of Cataract and Refractive Surgery 1994, 20 (5), 566–570.

15. Koch, P.S. Stop and chop phaco. Complications in Phaco-emulsification: Avoidance, Recognition, and Management 2002, 85–89. (ed. Fishkind, WJ), Thieme, New York.

16. Koch, P.S. Stop and chop. Simplifying Phacoemulsification; Safe and Efficient Methods for Cataract Surgery 1997, 131–145. (ed. Koch PS), Slack, Thorofare, NJ.

17. Davison, J.A. Phacoemulsification time and power require-ments in phaco chop and divide and conquer nucleofractis techniques. Journal of Cataract and Refractive Surgery 2000, 26 (9), 1374–1378.

18. Chang, D. Prevention pearls and damage control, Part 4 Complications in Phacoemulsification: Avoidance, Recognition, and Management 2002, 271–279. (ed. Fishkind WJ), Thieme, New York.

19. Steinert, R.F. Phaco chop. Cataract Surgery; Techniques, Complications, and Management, 2004 2nd Edn, 183–191. (ed. Steinert RF), Elsevier Science, Philadelphia

20. Nagahara, K.B. Phaco chop. Complications in Phacoemulsifi-cation: Avoidance, Recognition, and Management 2002, 94–99. (ed. Fishkind WJ), Thieme, New York

21. Leaming, D.V.Practice styles and preferences of ASCRS members – 2003. Journal of Cataract and Refractive Surgery 2004, 30(4), 892–900.

22. Fukasaku, H.The snap and split phacoemulsification technique.Tech Ophthalmol 2004, 2, 135–136.

23. Chang, D. Phaco-chop techniques: Comparing horizontal vs vertical chop. Highlights Ophthalmol 2004, 32, 11–13.

24. Vejarano, L.F., Tello, A.Vejarano's safe chop technique: A safer chopping. Tech Ophthalmol 2005, 3, 109–115.

25. Fine, et al. Optimising refractive lens exchange with bimanual microincision phacoemulsification. Journal of Cataract and Refractive Surgery 2004; 30:550–554.

26. Fishkind, William J. Complications in Phacoemulsification: Avoidance, Recognition, and Management. Thieme, NY, 2002.

27. Akahoshi, T. Phaco prechop: Manual nucleofracture prior to phacoemulsification. Operative Tech Cataract Refract Surg 1998, 1, 69–91.

28. Akahoshi, T. The karate prechop technique. Cataract Refract Surg Today 2002, 2, 63–64.

29. Charters, L. Chopping before phaco reduces ultrasound time Ophthalmology Times 2004.

15

Colonel Parihar's Hydro Floats Rapid Chop Technique: Advanced Techniques of Nucleotomy and Emulsification

Col JKS Parihar SM, VSM and Maj Jaya Kaushik

INTRODUCTION

Central chopping (karate chop) is the most significant innovation and an incredible refinement in the history of phacoemulsification in the recent past. Undoubtedly, central chopping has made phacoemulsification surgery safer, more secure and very quick and rapid depth applying less ultrasonic energy. Indeed, central chop has taken over centre stage among all techniques of nucleotomy. The author has further modified central chopping by modulating hydroprocedures and chopping actions in such a way that it minimises ultrasonic energy need up to the least level. It is possible now to emulsify even hard brown grade six nuclei with as low as 25 to 30% ultrasound energy settings, whereas grade three to grade four nucleus can be managed by 10 to 15% ultrasonic energy settings. In true sense, hydro floats rapid chop technique is a unique blend of applications of ball bearing cushion hydroprocedure and chopping under least cushion of minimal cortex and floating under continuous hydration yet applying least quantity of ultrasonic energy.

In a lighter vein, it can be said that modern and advanced phaco surgeons have attained the status of a powerless, toothless and least virulent paper tiger, yet very effective.

Principle of Central Chopping

The nucleus is chopped from the centre to the periphery. (chopper is pushed into the centre of the nucleus and drawn away from the tip, hence achieves inside to outside chopping action).

SURGICAL TECHNIQUE

Incisions (Figs 15.1 and 15.2)

The author prefers to make two small incisions like side port incisions. Out of these two incisions, the right-sided incision is converted into the main incision after completion of rhexis and subsequent hydroprocedures.

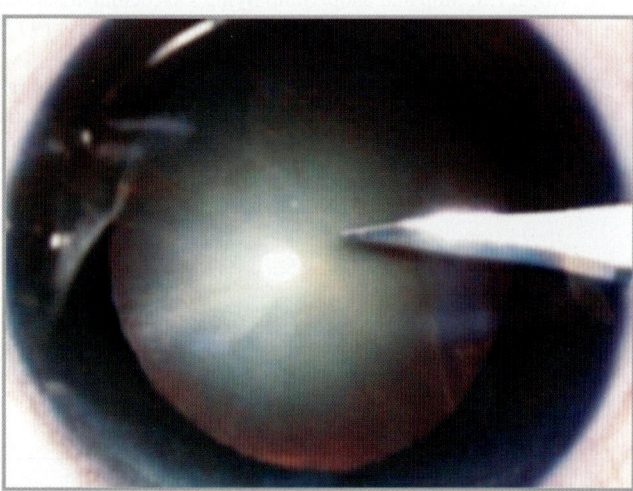

Fig. 15.1: Incision: This right-sided incision will be converted into the main incision after completion of rhexis and subsequent hydroprocedures

A temporal clear corneal incision is made for the right eye without shifting operating microscope or operation table, whereas the nasal incision is made for the left eye in the same fashion. In case of constructing left temporal incision, a slight shifting of operating microscope is required. The author tends to rely more on the position of elbow and extension of shoulder rather than shifting the microscope. Retrospective analysis of this habit seems to be influenced by the technique of 360 degree suturing performed in case of corneal transplant, that too, without shifting the operating microscope or rotating and self. Thankful to be a corneal surgeon primarily.

To achieve satisfactory hydro floats rapid chop, side port is kept around 120 to 130 degree apart from the main incision. This little wide angulation, facilitates adequate intranuclear instrumentation while performing central chopping, particularly through true temporal or nasal incision.

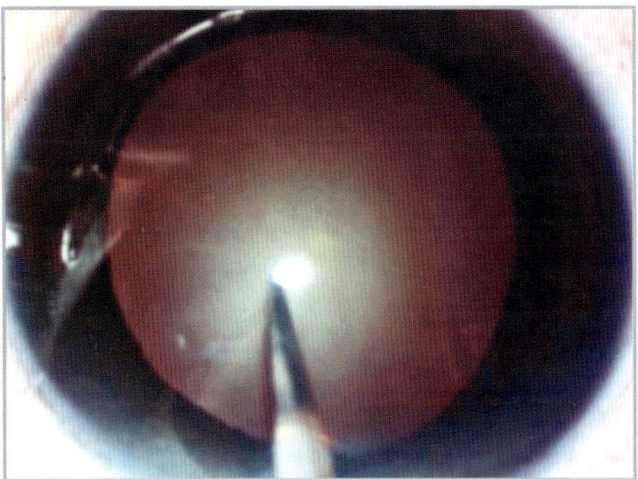

Fig. 15.2: Incision: Side port incision

Rhexis

An optimal size rhexis of around 5.5 to 6.0 mm is good enough for hydro floats rapid chop, which carries an advantage over the peripheral chop in terms of size of the rhexis, since hydro floats rapid chop can be performed even through small pupils. Capsulorrhexis is then performed anticlockwise through the second incision by using the 27 gauze bent needle cystitome.

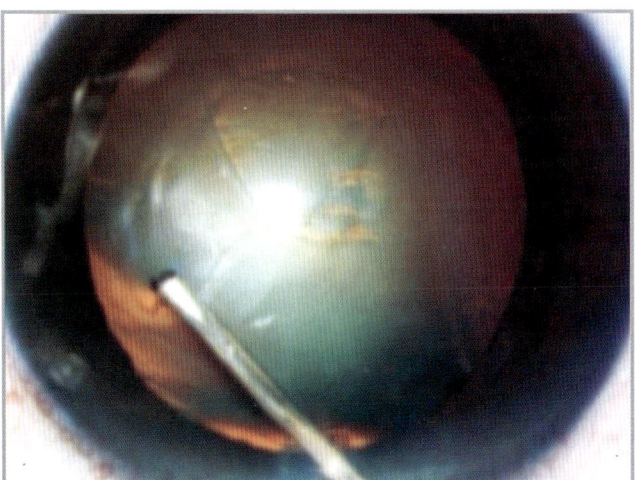

Fig. 15.3: An optimal size rhexis of around 5.5–6.0 mm is good enough for hydro floats rapid chop

Ball Bearing Cushion Hydroprocedure

An excellent hydroprocedure which is of immense significance in hydro floats rapid chop technique as compared to the conventional chopping or sculpting techniques. The key to success of hydro floats chopping, exclusively lies on gentle, repeated, sequential, and multilevel hydrodissection and hydrodelineation. Two small incisions are effectively used for 360 degree hydroprocedures. After

the initial hydrodissection, multilevel hydrodelineation is performed. After separation of epinucleus from peripheral cortex, inside out hydrodelineation is performed by achieving fluid wave cleavages.

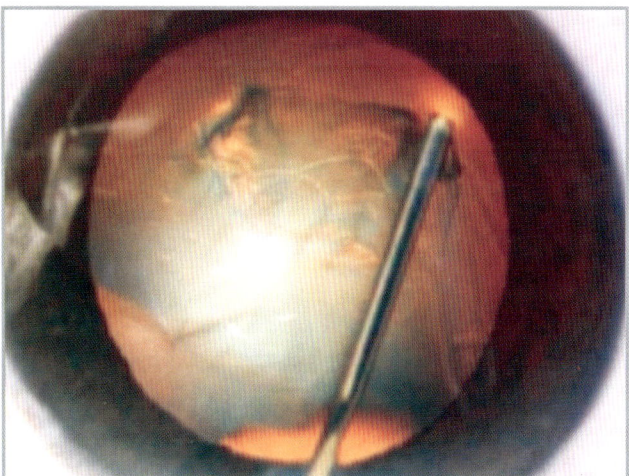

Fig. 15.4: Sequential hydrodissection

Once multiple intranuclear cleavages are achieved, the central core nucleus is gently pierced with hydrodelineation cannula to attain softening of the core nucleus.

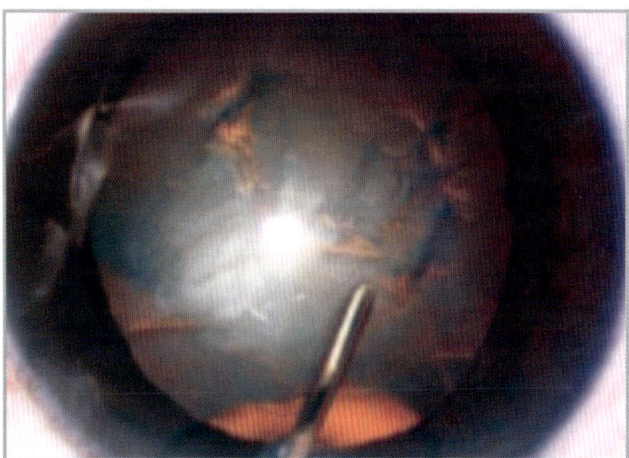

Fig. 15.5: Repeated and multilevel hydroids section and hydrodelineation

By this method we can achieve multiple rotating cushions around the central nucleus, thereby achieving ball bearing cushion effect around the central nucleus (Fig. 15.6).

During this process of hydrodissection–delineation, the lower lip of the second incision is repeatedly taped and depressed so as to allow debulking and secure the posterior capsule against any threat of inadvertent intrahydro-procedural rupture of the capsule.

Clearing of Superficial Cortex

The author has developed the technique of clearing a good amount of cortical matter not only from the superficial

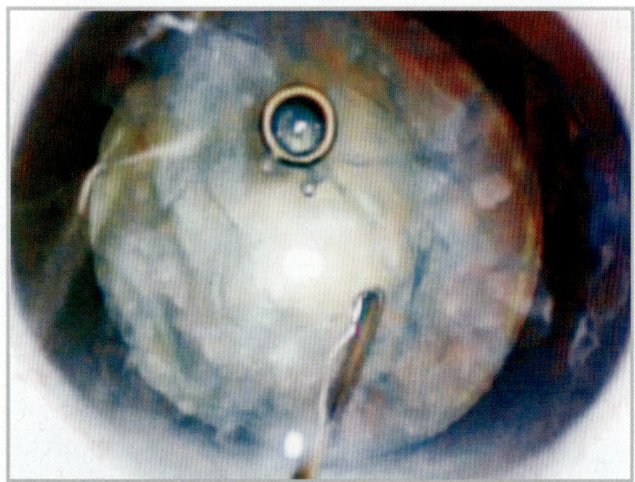

Fig. 15.6: Sequential, repeated and multilevel hydrodissection and hydrodelineation

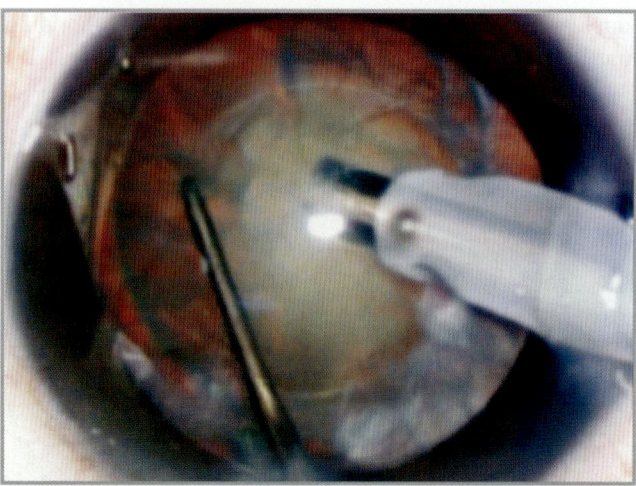

Fig. 15.7: Clearing of superficial cortex and the phaco tip is being embedded into the nucleus

surface of the nucleus but also from around the nucleus also. This allows the nucleus to float freely in the bag as well as facilitates subsequent removal of subincisional cortex with very less efforts.

The cortex is irrigated, initially with the help of continuous hydration under the rhexis margin while keeping settings of irrigation mode with moderate vacuum and flow rate. During the process of cortical hydration the nucleus is gently pressed downward with the help of Sinskey hook. Once secondary hydration is done, aspiration of superficial cortex is carried out. Occasionally, a small burst of US energy of less than 3% is delivered to dislodge sticky cortex from the anterior surface and the equator of the nucleus as well as a gentle stroke of Sinskey hook to dip the nucleus slightly in the bag allows to open up fornices of the bag and facilitates removal of cortex. To and fro clockwise and anticlockwise rotation of nucleus along with a slight pressure on the nucleus releases the cortex from all around the nucleus equator. At the same juncture, the foot pedal is repeatedly shuffled between irrigation and I/A (position one alone followed by position two). During position one, excessive fluid is allowed to egress out by a gentle pressure over the lower lip of second incision as well as a flick of position two in between. Key to success of hydro floats technique lies on this modulated and modified technique of hydroprocedures. A gentle and repeated hydration not only hydrates cortical matter but also softens the nucleus. This nuclear hydro float resembles very much a flying jet plane at a very high altitude where it consumes the least fuel, and without compromising the safety norms, attain a good velocity.

To initiate the process of removal of the superficial cortex, under the cushion of viscoelastics, Sinskey hook is introduced into the anterior chamber which is followed by introduction of a phaco tip into the anterior chamber while keeping the irrigation mode on.

The insertion of the Sinskey hook into the anterior chamber prior to the introduction of the phaco tip allows better stability of the eye during introduction of the phaco tip, particularly in performing the procedure under topical or no anaesthesia technique. Continuous irrigation mode during introduction of the phaco tip ensures an easy access of the tip into the anterior chamber. The use of the Sinskey hook in place of is chopper is of great help to avoid any inadvertent injury to the rhexis margin or the peripheral capsular rim while removing a large quantity of cortex prior to the initiation of chopping.

Nucleotomy by Hydro Floats Rapid Chop Technique

Nucleotomy technique in hydro floats rapid chop is a modification of the central chopping technique. Once a large amount of cortical matter is removed and nucleus is allowed to float under the cushion of viscoelastics and a continuous flow of irrigation, the process of chopping is initiated.

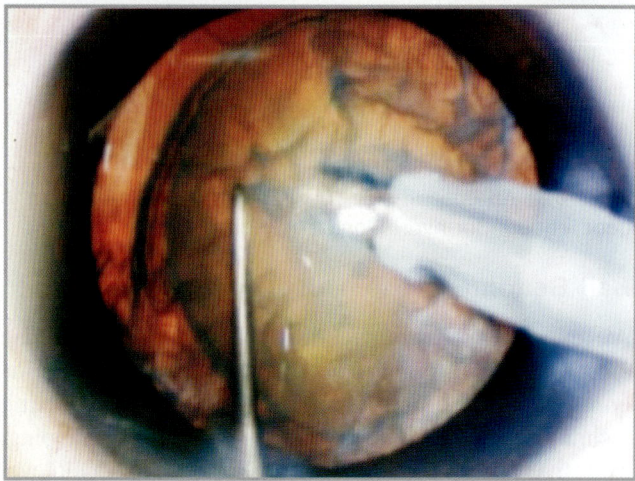

Fig. 15.8: Commencement of nucleotomy by hydro floats rapid chop technique

Under moderate vacuum and low ultrasound settings, nucleus is held with the help of a zero degree tip which is placed just below the central core nucleus as well as with the help of a chopper a little ahead of the phaco tip. Position one is maintained throughout this step. The next step is to achieve a good grip over nucleus by shifting to position two.

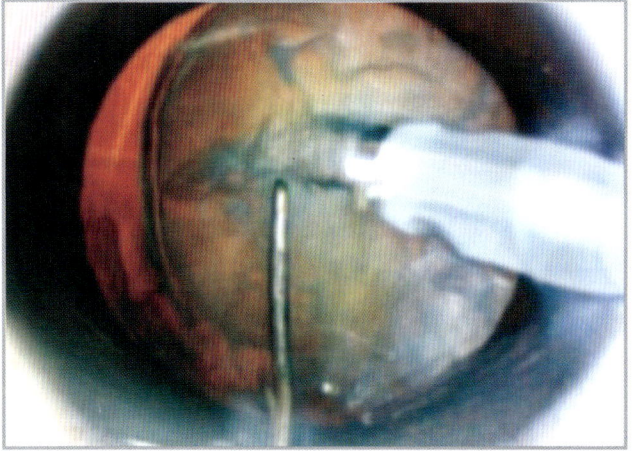

Fig. 15.9: Primary nucleotomy by hydro floats rapid chop technique is being initiated

Till this step, no ultrasonic energy is applied. Continuous and sustained irrigation not only softens the nucleus, but also hydrates the residual cortical matter and opens up fornices of the bag, thereby enhancing safety and ease of subsequent cortical wash. The next step is embedding the phaco tip in the nucleus under the influence of ultrasonic energy. The key to success lies upon the position of the phaco tip in the nucleus.

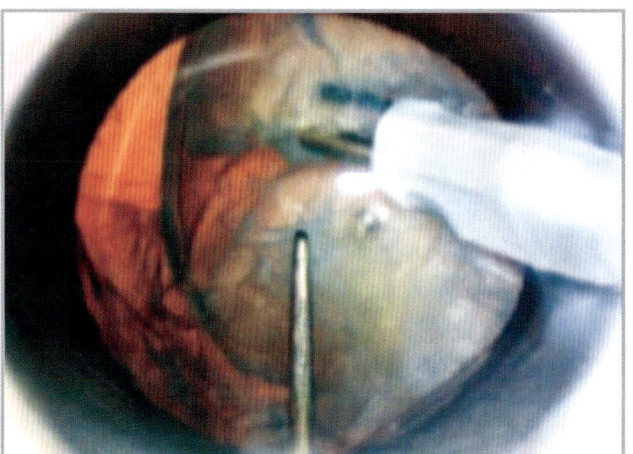

Fig. 15.10: Primary nucleotomy by hydro floats rapid chop technique

Splitting of Nucleus

The author prefers to pierce the tip into the nucleus just inferior and ahead of the central portion of core nucleus. This particular position allows the desired three fourth depth of the nucleus and a firm grip by phaco tip, despite application of least ultrasonic energy. The nucleus is slightly

lifted in the bag while switching over to position two (under moderate vacuum and no ultrasonic energy settings). While retaining nucleus grip, the chopper is placed vertically and ahead of the phaco tip under the cleavage in the nucleus created by the phaco tip. The next step is to draw the chopper away and perpendicular to the position of the phaco tip by quick, tangential and lateral actions. This particular manipulation results in nuclear fragmentation at the plane of natural intralamellar spaces with ease and that too without the application of any energy.

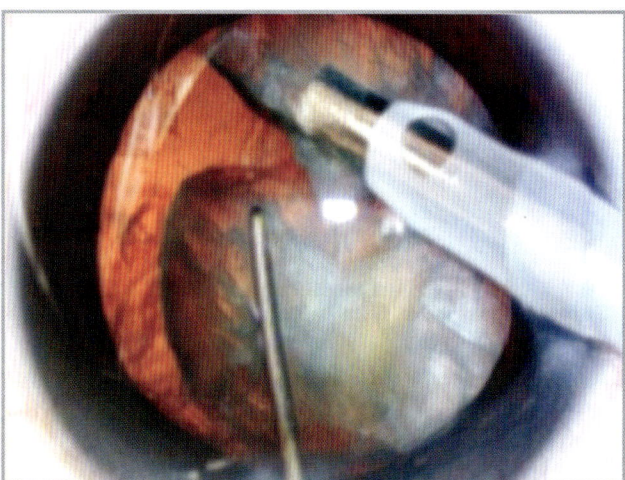

Fig. 15.11: Primary nucleotomy by hydro floats rapid chop technique

The author prefers to maintain a sustained irrigation mode for a couple of seconds prior to the commencement of secondary and subsequent tertiary chopping. This step is of immense value to hydrate intralamellar spaces, thereby minimising the need for ultrasonic energy while aspirating out small nuclear fragments. It is advisable to apply a small bolus of ultrasonic energy to commence aspiration of tertiary nuclear fragments followed by irrigation and ultimately aspirating it out.

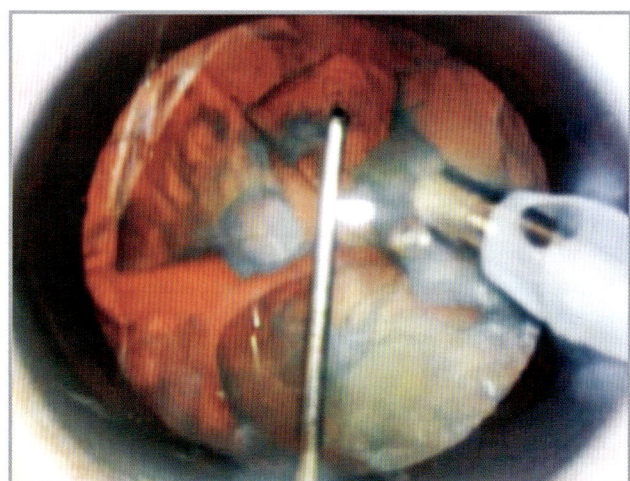

Fig. 15.12: Secondary nucleotomy by hydro floats rapid chop technique

In our view, hydro float rapid chop technique is an excellent example of clubbing the concept of modulation of advanced hydroprocedure, irrigation, aspiration and ultrasonic energy in relation to the understanding of applied anatomy of the lens fibre. Indeed, this has resulted in unbelievable reduction in the need of ultrasound energy in advanced phaco techniques. The author is very much convinced with the outcomes and has adopted this modification to the full extent.

Removal of Residual Cortex

As such, a large amount of cortical matter has already been removed prior to the nucleotomy; thus a very small amount of cortical matter is left following hydro float nucleotomy. Over and above, repeated irrigation results in opening of capsular bag fornices as well as hydration of

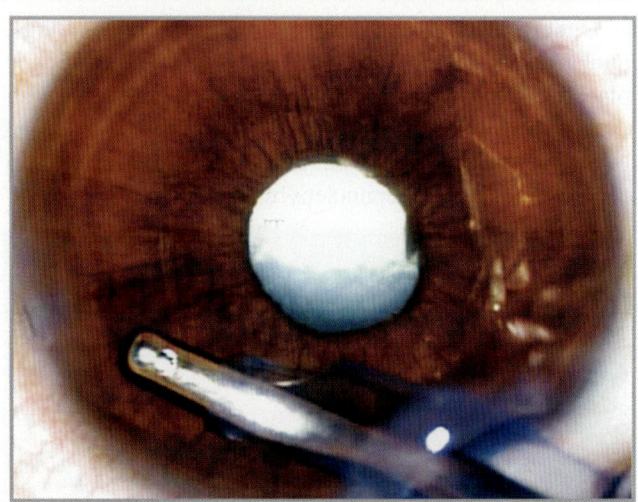

Fig. 15.13: Post IOL implantation wash

Table 15.1: Phacoemulsification machine settings at different stages of central chopping
(Zero degree tip on peristaltic pump)

Steps/stages	Principle	Phaco settings	Flow (cc/min)	Vacuum	Continuous/micropulse
Baring the nucleus	Low flow and vacuum	00–05 %	10–15	60–100	Continuous/micropulse
Nudging the phaco tip into the nucleus	Low flow and vacuum	10–30 (As per hardness of nucleus)	20–22	100–150	Continuous/micropulse
Lifting the nucleus	Moderate vacuum	00	22–28	200–275	Position two, no US energy
Central chopping	Moderate vacuum	00–10	22–28	225–275	Position two/three,
Subsequent multiple nucleotomy	Moderate vacuum	00–10	22–28	200–275	Position two/three,
Fragment removal	High flow and vacuum	15–30	24–26	200–275	Continuous/micropulse
Removal of the last fragment	Low flow and moderate vacuum	10–20	15–20	75–150	Continuous/micropulse
Removing the posterior plate/epinucleus	Low flow and high vacuum	00–05	10–15 I/A mode	100–125	Continuous/micropulse
Residual cortical wash	Moderate flow and high vacuum	I/A mode	26–34	300–400	Continuous
Posterior capsule polishing	Low flow and vacuum	I/A mode	5	10–20	Continuous

Table 15.2: Phacoemulsification machine settings at different stages of central chopping
(Zero degree tip on ventury pump)

Steps/stages	Principle	Phaco settings	Vacuum	Continuous/micropulse
Baring the nucleus	Low vacuum	05%	45–60	Continuous/micropulse
Nudging the phaco tip into the nucleus	Low vacuum	0–30 (As per hardness of nucleus)	100–125	Continuous/micropulse
Lifting the nucleus	Moderate vacuum	00	100–125	Position two, no US energy
Central chopping	Moderate vacuum	00–05	100–125	Position two, no US energy
Subsequent multiple nucleotomy	Moderate vacuum	00–05	60–75	Position two, no US energy
Fragment removal	Moderate to high vacuum	05–20	80–100	micropulse
Removal of the last fragment	Moderate vacuum	5–15	50–60	micropulse
Removing the posterior plate/epinucleus	Moderate vacuum	0–5/US mode	60–80 on handpiece / 300–400 I/A	Continuous/micropulse
Residual cortical wash	High vacuum	I/A mode	400–450	Continuous
Posterior capsule polishing	Low flow	I/A mode	0–5	Continuous

leftover cortical fibres. Hence, removal of such cortex demands much less flow rate and vacuum as compared to the conventional chopping techniques. A zero degree tip can be employed to remove floating cortical matter under irrigation/aspiration position. It is wise to attempt removal of subincisional lens matter by clock and anticlockwise pull and push by I/A handpiece. This will facilitate a large chunk of cortex to be aspirated out in a single stroke.

Stromal Hydration

Stromal hydration by injecting BSS into the lip of the corneal valve and the side port incision is a good option to achieve selfsealing wound.

The whitish hue created at the site of incisions, generally disappears within six to seven hours.

CONCLUSION

Phaco chop technique is a unique and premium concept of nucleotomy which has transformed modern cataract surgery from a very small incision cataract surgery to atraumatic keratorefrative surgery with enhanced intraoperative safety as well as excellent postoperative outcome. Hydro floats rapid chop technique is a new dimension of energy titration and the judicious application of fluidics which has transformed central chopping into a unique blend of application of ball bearing cushion hydroprocedure and chopping under least cushion of minimal cortex and floating under continuous hydration yet applying the least quantity of ultrasonic energy.

16

Flip and Chip Techniques of Nucleotomy and Emulsification

Col JKS Parihar SM, VSM and Maj SK Dhar

INTRODUCTION

During the last three decades of phacoemulsification era, the surgical technique has undergone significant transformation right from anterior chamber phacoemulsification to iris plane, mono manual technique to present bimanual handling of cataractous lens. There are several variants in bimanual phacoemulsification techniques.

Undoubtedly, DCN remains the basic and gold standard technique of nucleotomy, whereas chopping continues to enjoy the privilege of an advanced, widely accepted and modern technique of nucleotomy. However, the soft or sticky cortex or cataract associated with a miotic pupil poses significant constraints when handled with DCN or chopping techniques. A very hard cataract needs a hybrid technique where a combination of paracentral chopping, debulking of the central core nucleus and chipping of the perinucleus and hard posterior plate may be required. Hence the chip and flip technique offers an ideal option for such cataracts.

APPLIED ANATOMY OF THE SOFT CATARACTOUS LENS

Applied anatomy of the lens has already been described earlier in detail in a separate chapter. However, a crisp review of salient and important features of applied anatomy of soft lens or cataract with sticky cortex is worth considering.

From the surgeon's viewpoint, there are mainly two important points of relevance, which are to be kept in mind before attempting a nucleotomy: The soft lens consists of a small and central core nucleus surrounded by a comparatively softer epinucleus and the outermost layer of thin cortex. These types of cataracts are invariably associated with posterior subcapsular, posterior cortical or polar cataract. A sticky cortex further compounds

difficulty in nucleus rotation and lifting of it which is essential for chopping. Sculpting in a very soft nucleus carries an inherent risk of piercing the posterior plate despite low energy settings due to relatively less thickness of the nucleus, its high degree of softness as well as the very thin and adhered posterior plate. In authors view, a very soft or adhered nucleus is much more difficult, risky and tricky to handle as compared to the hard cataract.

HISTORICAL BACKGROUND

The present technique of chip and flip phacoemulsification was described by Sir Howard Fine in 1991. This technique was a modification of pre-existing Fines modification and the technique is based on the concept of lifting of the nucleus in the bag followed by dividing it circumferentially, removing the central core nucleus while retaining the protective epinuclear shell, until the peripheral portion of nucleus is being trimmed and tumbled. The residual shell is displaced subsequently from the posterior capsule and aspirated out. Howard Fine's technique is well suited for soft nucleus or cataract associated with sticky cortex

Earlier, Davison JA. described a technique of capsular bag phacoemulsification in 1988. Davison's technique is based on endocapsular bag phacoemulsification by applying minimal lift and multiple rotation of nucleus inside the capsular bag. The technique is very effective and provides adequate safety while performing endocapsular phacoemulsification in cases of both hard and soft type of cataract.

Arnold PN had described the technique flipping of nucleus in cases of small pupil phacoemulsification in 1991. This technique was based on an endocapsular flipping of nucleus and subsequent removal of it by floor of the nucleus bowl. Another peculiarity of this technique was the application of unconventional concept of one-handed phacoemulsification. This concept was initially described for small pupil cataract and was used in other cases also.

BASIC PRINCIPLES

Bottle Height

Flip and chip technique needs to have a moderate bottle height.

A too high bottle is known to have undue deepening of the chamber. This invariably pushes the lens diaphragm downward; hence may lead to have a steep and deep vertical position of the phaco tip resulting in a higher risk of posterior capsular tear, corneal burn and poor visibility. The author recommends a moderate bottle height of around 50–60 cm above the patient head level.

Ideal Ultrasonic Phaco Power

The basic principle of ideal power application remains based on the fact of equilibrium between optimal utilisation of energy, no undue under or over use of energy as well as good holding and no pushing of the nucleus. Too little power or quick and fast motions of the probe may lead to an undue forward push on the nucleus without compromising ultrasonic fragmentation of nucleus as well as undue stress on the zonules.

SURGICAL TECHNIQUE: AS PRACTICED BY THE AUTHOR

Position of Incisions

To achieve satisfactory flipping and chipping, the side port should be a kept little away and close to the 3 O'clock in case of superior incision and at the 12 O'clock in case of the temporal incision. This positioning provides better access to chipping thus ensures safety and easy mobility of soft nucleus during chip and flipping.

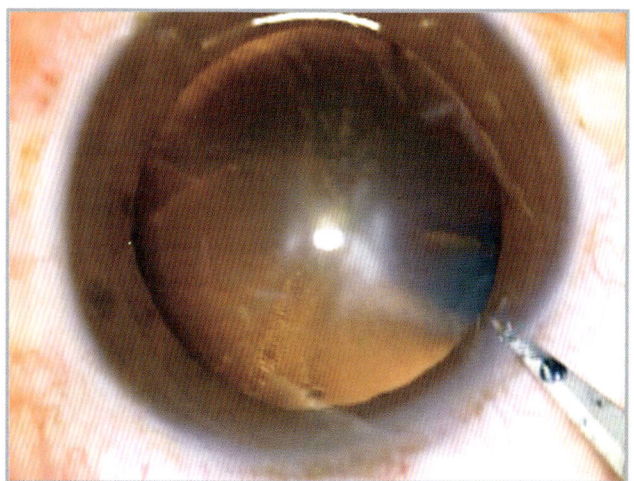

Fig. 16.1: Flip and chip: Primary incision for subsequent clear corneal valve incision

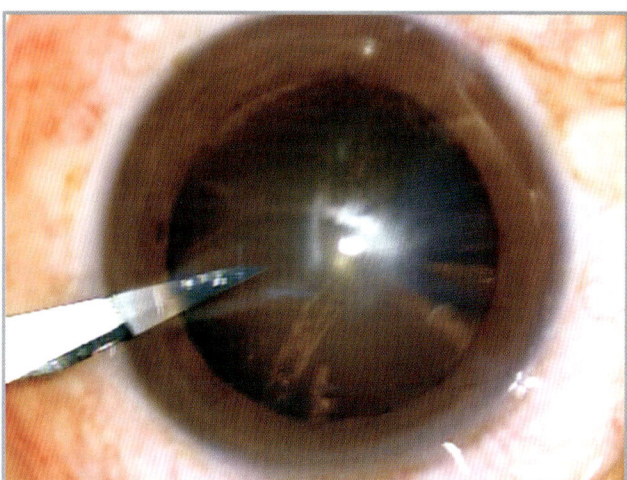

Fig. 16.2: Flip and chip: Side port incision

Rhexis

A preferably large 5.5 to 6 mm rhexis, more proximal superiorly and oval is an ideal choice. This kind of rhexis is more convenient to have an easy prolapse of nucleus following vacuum supported rotation as well as to allow proper chipping.

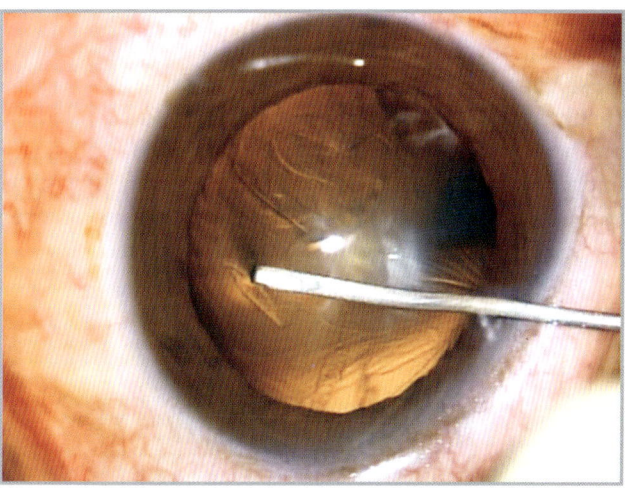

Fig. 16.3: Flip and chip: Rhexis

Hydroprocedure (Fig. 16.4)

An excellent hydroprocedure is of paramount importance in consideration to nucleotomy in modern techniques. Repeated, gradual and multiple hydrodelamination, significantly reduces the size of nucleus, releases adhesions from the sticky and adhered cortex as well as separates it from the epinucleus and hence facilitates proper intracapsular chipping of the nucleus.

Removal of Superficial Cortex

Initial steps of removing the epinucleus to expose and bare the nucleus are very much like trenching or chopping. The author prefers to use a zero degree tip with the least phaco

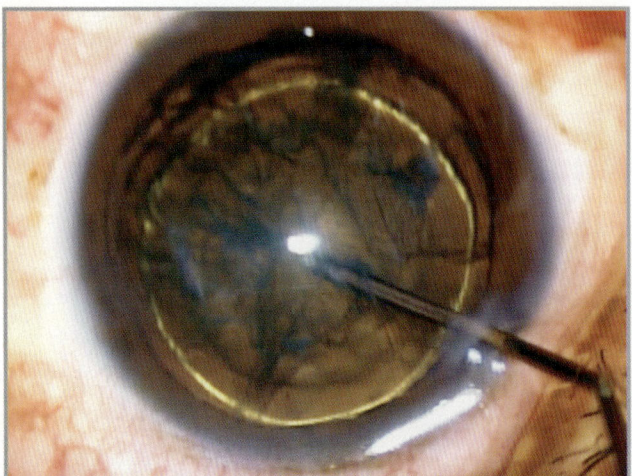

Fig. 16.4: Flip and chip: Hydroprocedure

energy accompanied by moderate vacuum settings, thus ensuring an excellent grip of nucleus as well as to avoid deep piercing into the nuclear substance. The phaco probe is gently moved above the nucleus to aspirate away the anterior cortical and epinucleus fibres up to the capsulorrhexis margin so as to expose the nucleus below. This will enhance the margins and the visibility of the nucleus; thus providing the desired intracapsular rotation and circumferential chipping and subsequent removal of the soft nucleus. A blunt tip Sinskey hook is being introduced simultaneously into the anterior chamber. The author himself prefers to introduce the Sinskey hook prior to the phaco tip into anterior chamber so as to achieve better stability of the eye during insertion of the phaco tip into anterior chamber particularly during topical or no anaesthesia technique.

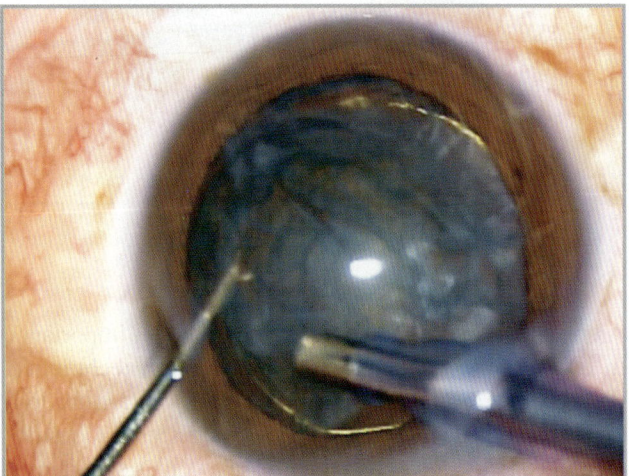

Fig. 16.5: Flip and chip: Removal of superficial cortex

Nucleotomy

Once adequate chipping is achieved, the next is have multiple nucleotomy done. The best way to perform this is to do gradual cracking by embedding the phaco tip into core of chipped nucleus while lifting it partly out of the

bag and up with the help of vacuum, thus exposing the inferior rim of nucleus. At this stage, the Sinskey hook is placed just at the nuclear rim having an alignment with the phaco tip to allow rotation of the nucleus.

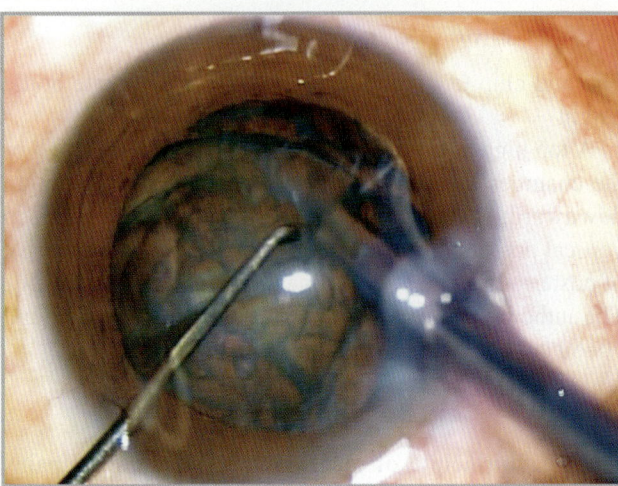

Fig. 16.6: Flip and chip: Peripheral chipping of the nucleus

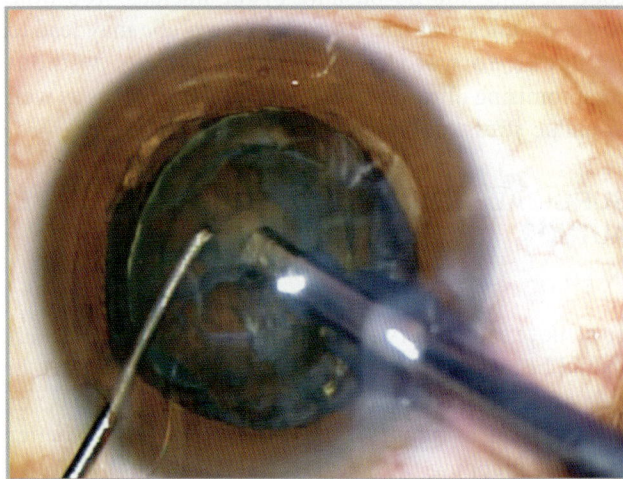

Fig. 16.7: Flip and chip: Hemi nucleotomy

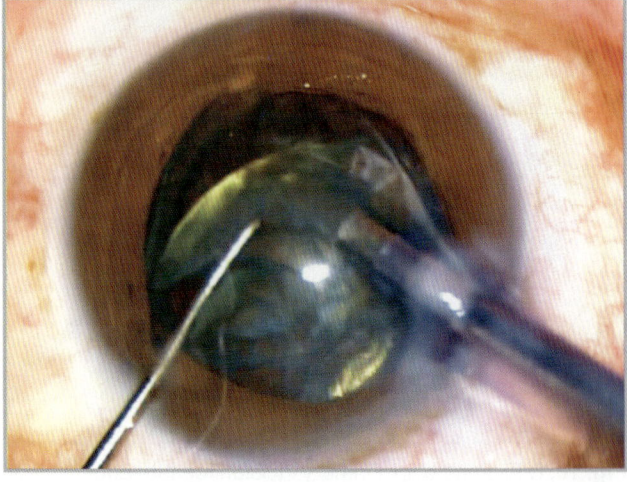

Fig. 16.8: Flip and chip: Nucleotomy and fragment removal

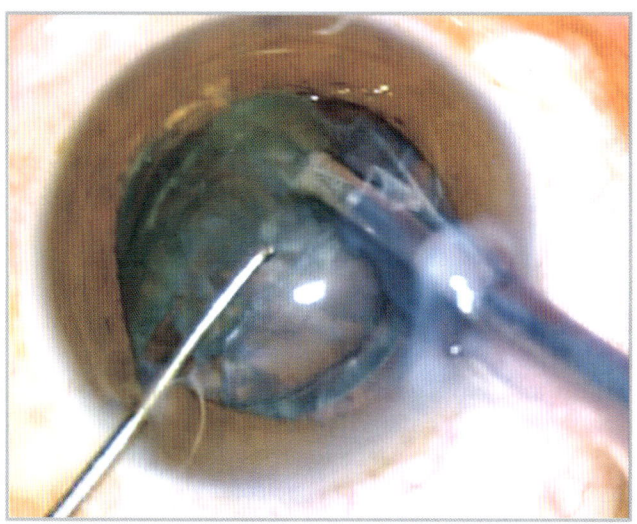

Fig. 16.9: Flip and chip: Tertiary chipping and fragment removal

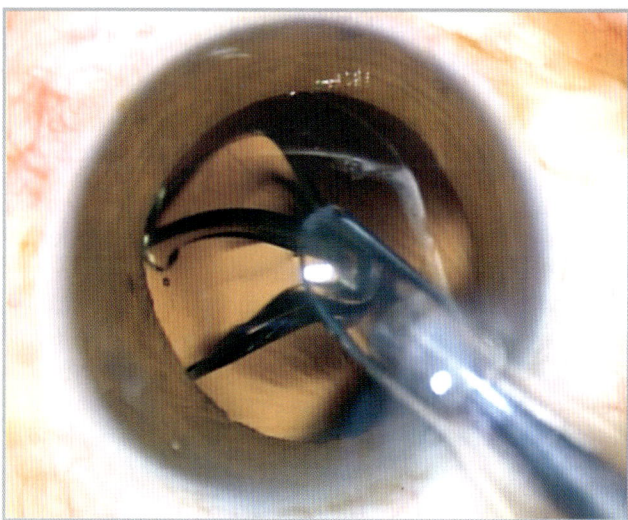

Fig. 16.12: Flip and chip: Insertion of IOL implant

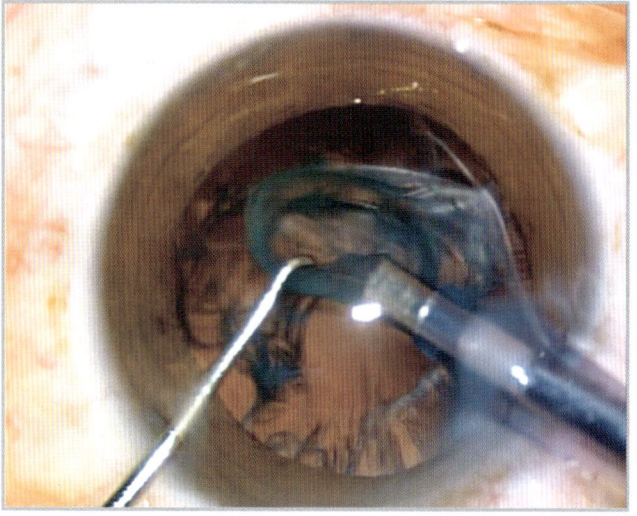

Fig. 16.10: Flip and chip: Removal of posterior plate

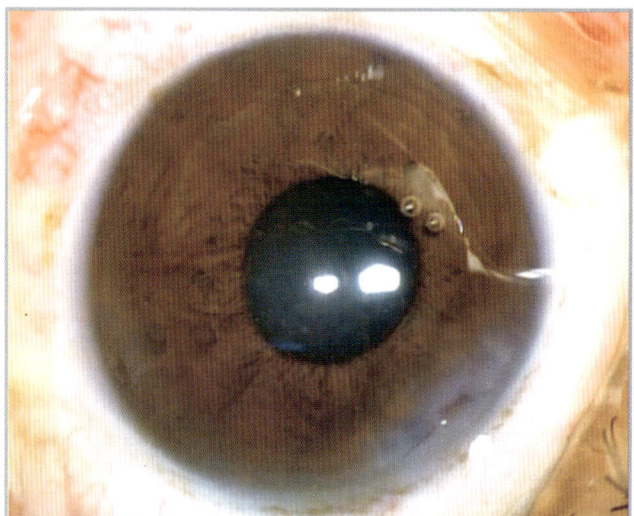

Fig. 16.13: Flip and chip: IOL implant is in situ

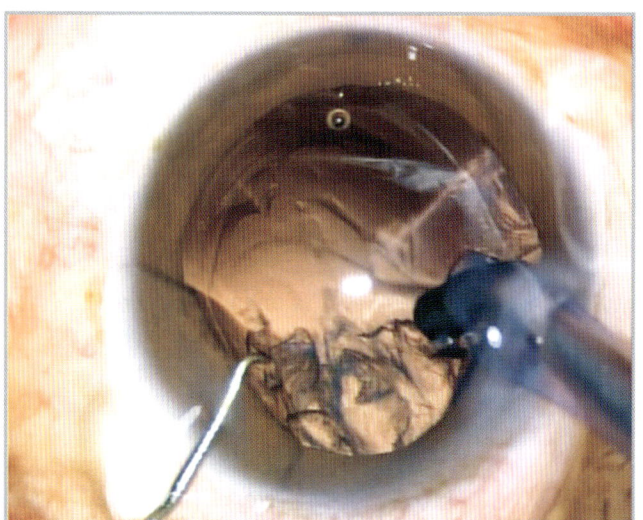

Fig. 16.11: Flip and chip: Removal of residual cortex (I/A mode)

The next step is to have peripheral chipping of the nucleus with simultaneous rotation and simultaneous chipping of the central core nucleus plate by using low energy settings like 05% to 10% US energy and 200 to 250 vacuum. A very gentle and extremely careful application of ultrasonic energy is essentially required at this stage, since soft and adhered nucleus may face inadvertent rupture of the thin posterior plate or posterior capsule. Hence, it is the most wise step is to release the nucleus from the bag by gradual debulking of peripheral margins under continuous and sustained application of vacuum and very low energy settings. A gentle stroke of the Sinskey hook beneath the released portion of nucleus and under the cushion of viscoelastics is highly beneficial to avoid injury to the posterior plate. Once nucleus is being freed from the bag, the chipped nucleus is broken into multiple pieces by ultrasonic fragmentation and subsequent aspiration of it is being carried out in a usual manner of I/A. Undoubtedly, the presence of posterior plate until removal of the last lens fragment is one of the most important tips to avoid a PC rent.

Removal of Posterior Plate

A word of caution while handling the posterior plate: Posterior plate is relatively thin yet densely adheres to the fornices of the bag as well to the posterior capsule. Hence, removal of the plate demands meticulous, gradual and repeated applications of I/A mode under moderate vacuum settings to lift a big chunk of plate in toto from the posterior capsule. The use of bimanual I/A is an ideal choice in this situation. This manoeuvre reduces surgical time as well as enhances safety of the posterior capsule against aspiration of a thick adhered cortical plate from the capsule.

COMPLICATIONS

The incidence of phacoemulsification related complications have shown significant decline in terms of severity and overall incidence. This is mainly due to cumulative experience gained by surgeons world over as well as availability of highly sophisticated machines, better quality of drugs, instrumentation and invention of modern surgical techniques. Flip and chip technique is not the exception to

it. Despite the fact that the procedure is very safe, meticulous attention is essentially required in consideration to the prevention of posterior capsular rent, particularly due to obvious proximity of adhered posterior capsule to the soft cataract or in the presence of sticky cortex. An excellent equilibrium between ultrasonic energy application and vacuum settings while chipping soft cataract, vigilant manipulation of sharp instruments like Sinskey hook to assist in lifting of the chipped plate from the posterior capsule is the most crucial step to minimise the risk of intraoperative complications.

Flip and chip as a part of the combined hybrid technique in cases of hard brown cataract: As described earlier, hard brown cataract carries significant technical constraints while performing nucleotomy even in cases of central chopping. These types of cataracts are invariably associated with a thick and very dense perinucleus and a sticky and thick posterior plate. Over and above, the problem is further compounded owing to the presence of a very thin and fragile posterior capsule which is adhered to the posterior plate. Such kind of peculiar anatomical configuration poses a big challenge and enhances the risks of intraoperative complications like the posterior capsular rent or even nucleus drop to a great extent.

Table 16.1: Phacoemulsification machine settings at different stages of flip and chip technique (ventury pump)

Steps/stages	Principle	Phaco settings	Vacuum mmHg	Continuous/micropulse
Baring the nucleus	Low vacuum	05%	45–60	Continuous/micropulse
Nudging the phaco tip into nucleus	Low vacuum	05–07	45–60	Continuous/micropulse
Lifting the nucleus	Moderate vacuum	00–05	125	Continuous/micropulse
Subsequent rotation of the nucleus and chipping	Moderate vacuum	05–10	100–125	Continuous/micropulse
Fragment removal	Moderate vacuum	05–10	80–100	Continuous/micropulse
Removal of the last fragment	Moderate vacuum	00–05	50–60	Continuous/micropulse
Removing posterior plate/epinucleus	Moderate vacuum	0–5	60–80	Continuous/pulse/I/A mode
Residual cortical wash	High vacuum	I/A mode	400–450	Continuous
Posterior capsule polishing	Low flow	I/A mode	0–5	Continuous

Table 16.2: Phacoemulsification machine settings at different stages of flip and chip technique (peristaltic pump)

Steps/stages	Principle	Phaco settings	Vacuum mmHg	Continuous/micro pulse
Baring the nucleus	Low vacuum	05%	125–150	Continuous/micropulse
Nudging the phaco tip into nucleus	Low vacuum	05–07	45–75	Continuous/micropulse
Lifting the nucleus	Moderate vacuum	00–05	175–225	Continuous/micropulse
Subsequent rotation of the nucleus and chipping	Moderate vacuum	05–10	175–225	Continuous
Fragment removal	Moderate vacuum	05–10	125–175	Pulse
Removal of the last fragment	Moderate vacuum	00–05	100–125	Pulse
Removing posterior plate/epinucleus	Moderate vacuum	0–5	100–125	Micropulse/I/amode
Residual cortical wash	High vacuum	I/A mode	400–450	Continuous
Posterior capsule polishing	Low flow	I/A mode	0–5	Continuous

A hybrid technique which comprises of a combination of paracentral chopping, debulking of central core nucleus and chipping of perinucleus and hard posterior plate appears to be a viable option.

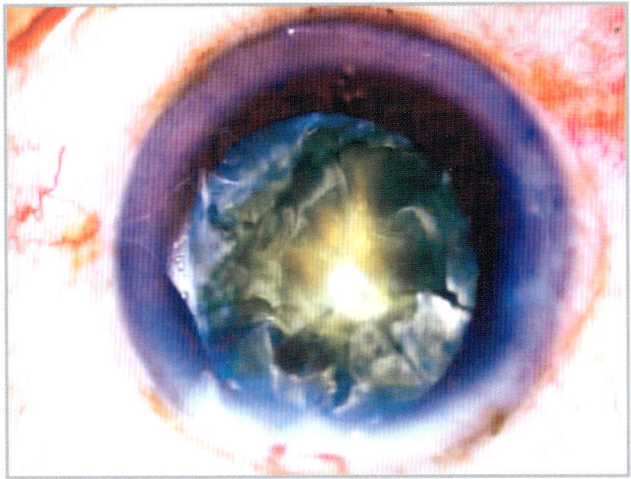

Fig. 16.14: Chipped posterior plate and paracentral nucleus

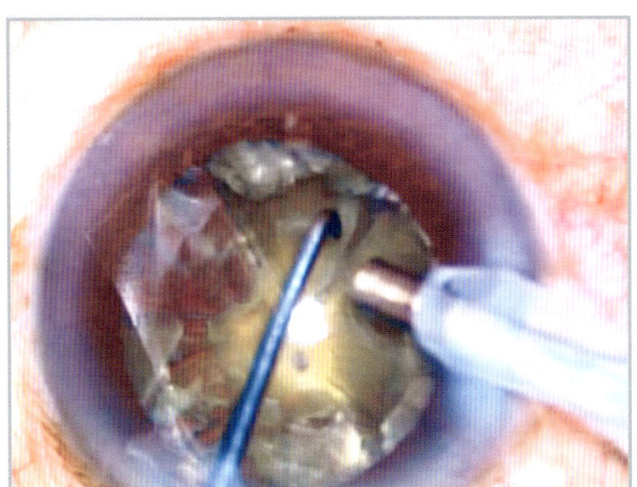

Fig. 16.15: Flipping, rotation and chipping of inner layers of the nucleus

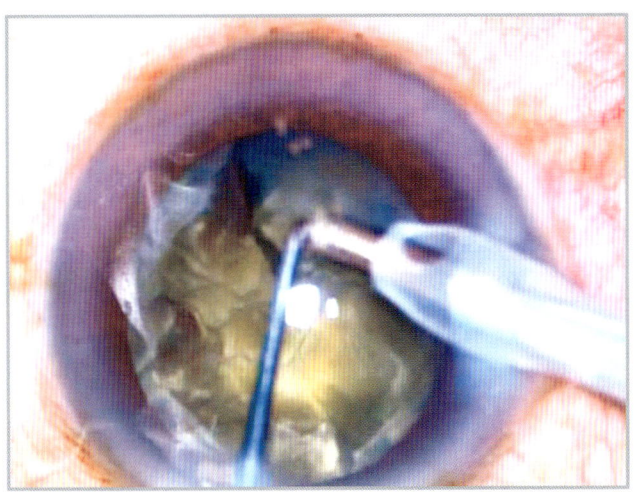

Fig. 16.16: Chip and break into nucleus plate

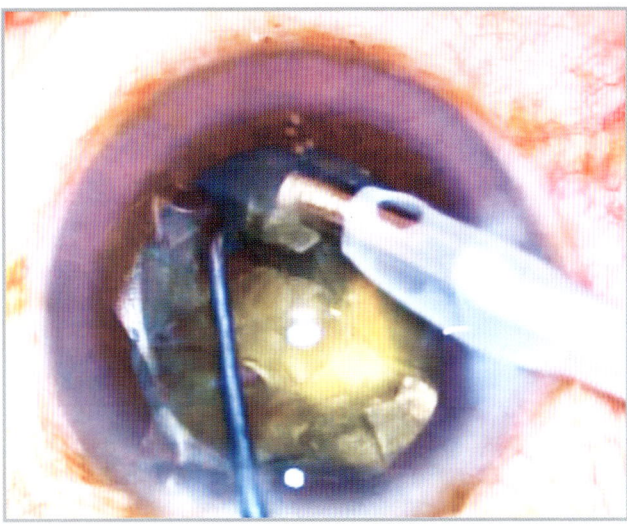

Fig. 16.17: Removal of chipped fragments

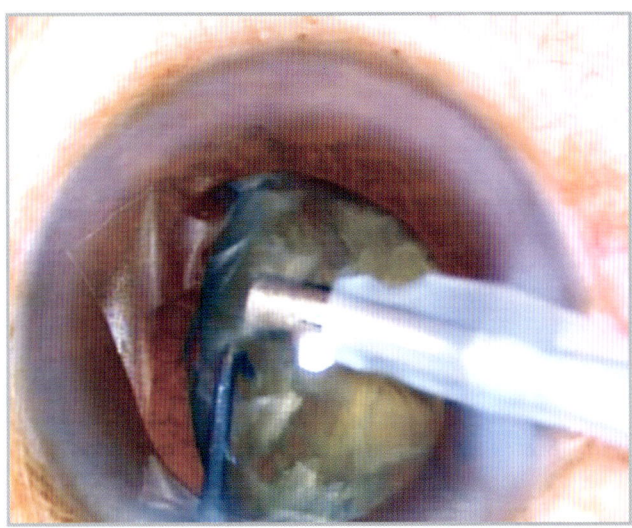

Fig. 16.18: Sequential flip and chip

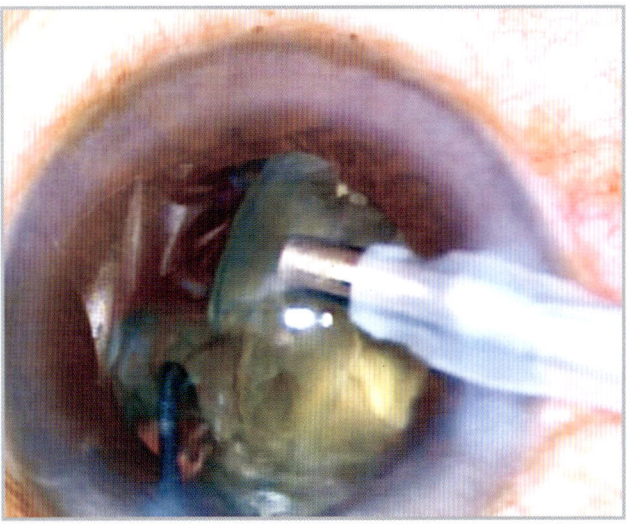

Fig. 16.19: Flip and break into adhered posterior plate

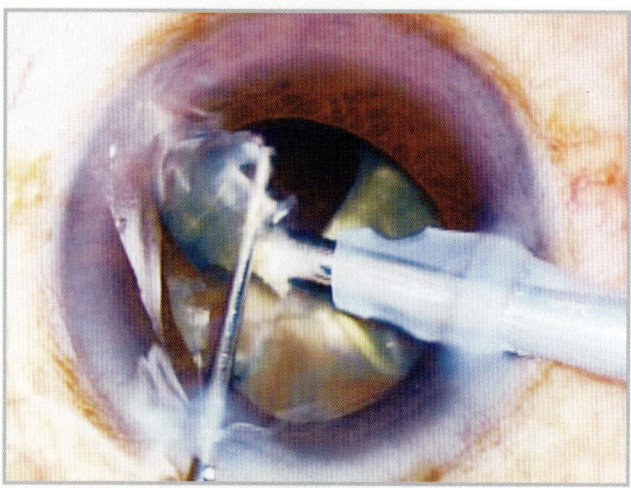

Fig. 16.20: Removal of chipped plate

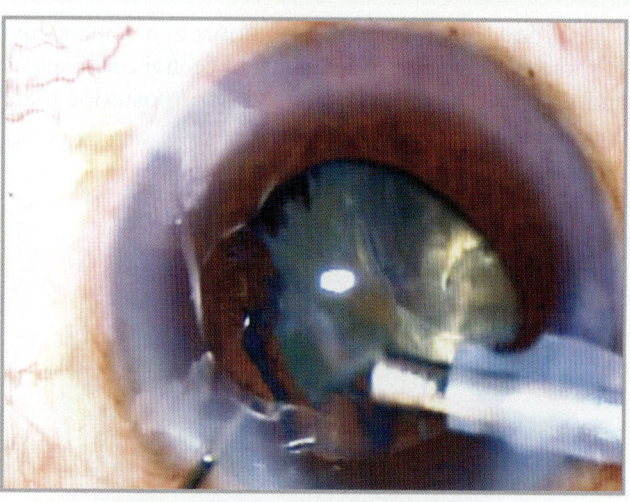

Fig. 16.22: Removal of chipped posterior plate

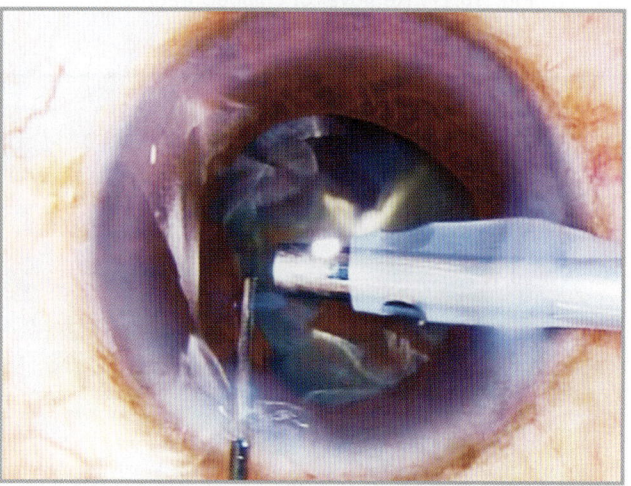

Fig. 16.21: Flip and sequential chipping of posterior plate

CONCLUSION

Since its inception by Howard Fine, the Flip and Chip technique of nucleotomy has undergone several transformations. The initial technique was of modifications in basic technique of sculpting which has undergone subsequent modifications as inclusion of stop and chop technique. The author has further modified flip and chip by applying a zero degree tip in collaboration with modern fluid dynamics, in coaxial MICS as well as in cases of bimanual MICS. The concept of flip and chip is very useful in cases of very soft nucleus particularly associated with sticky cortex.

BIBLIOGRAPHY

1. Gimbel HV, Neuhann T: Development, advantages and method of continuous circular capsulorrhexis technique. Cataract Refract Surg. 16: 31–37, 1990.
2. Gimbel HV: Evolving techniques of cataract surgery—continuous curvilinear capsulorrhexis, down-slope sculpting and nucleofractis. Setnin Ophthalmo/7: 193–207, 1992.
3. Gimbel HV: CCC and nucleus fracturing. Ophthalmol Clin North Am 4: 235, 1991.
4. Gimbel HV: Divide and conquer nucleofractis phacoemulsification—development and variations/Cataract Refract Surg 17: 281–91, 1991.
5. Gimbel HV, Ellant JP, Chin PK: Divide and conquer nucleofractis. Ophthalmo! Clin North Am 8(3): 457–69, 1995.
6. Gimbel HV: Down slope sculpting/Cataract Refract Surg 18: 614–18, 1992.
7. Gimbel HV, Chin PK: Phaco Sweep/Cataract Refract Surg 21: 493–96, 1995.
8. Gimbel HV: Divide and Conquer. (Video) Presented at the European Intraocular Implant Lens Council meeting 1987.
9. Gimbel HV: Nuclear phacoemulsification—alternative methods. In: Steinert RF (Ed) Cataract Surgery: Technique, Complications, and Management Philadelphia: WB Saunders 148–81, 1995.
10. Shepherd JR: In situ fracture/Cataract Refract Surg. 16:436–40, 1990.
11. Fine IH. the chip and flip phacoemulsification technique. J Cataract Refract Surg. 1991 May; 17(3):366–71. Comment in: J Cataract Refract Surg. 1991 May;17(3):267.
12. Arnold PN. Nuclear flip technique in small pupil phacoemulsification. J Cataract Refract Surg 1991; 17(2):225–7.
13. Hara T: Endocapsular phacoemulsification and aspiration (ECPEA—recent surgical technique and clinical results. Ophthalmic Surg 20:469–75, 1989.
14. Davison JA. Minimal lift-multiple rotation technique for capsular bag phacoemulsification and intraocular lens fixation. J Cataract Refract Surg. 1988 Jan; 14(1):25–34.
15. Nagahara K: Video presentation at ACRS meeting, Seattle, 1993.
16. Koch PS, Katzen LE: Stop and chop phacoemulsification/ Cataract Refract Surg 20:566–70, 1994.
17. Gimbel HV: Challenges of topical anesthesia in small incision cataract surgery. Ophthalmic Practice 14(3):123–24, 1996.

17

Cartwheel: Torsional Impact from Longitudinal Phaco

Col JKS Parihar SM, VSM and Maj Jaya Kaushik

INTRODUCTION

Torsional impact on phaco tip, delivers phacoenergy at 360° in a cyclic manner whereas linear phaco delivers energy only in one dimension; hence the same duration movements of the tip and will be less effective as compared to the torsional movement. In other words, the torsional system will require less energy and time for performing phacoemulsification for the same grade of nucleus as compared to the linear mode. However, logically, the same effect or better than that of a linear phaco can be achieved if the nucleus is being provided torsional movements by any means while performing phaco over the linear system. Hence, either the tip or the nucleus is being offered torsional impact; the modulation of ultrasonic energy and duration of delivery of it can be achieved effectively. Undoubtedly, torsional impact of the nucleus on conventional linear phaco will not be as good as with torsional phaco yet, it should be more effective and should have less dependency on US energy as compared to the classical linear phacoemulsification techniques. The author has effectively utilised this concept and offered a unique blend of mechanical torsional movement to the nucleus utilising conventional linear ultrasonic energy for nucleotomy simultaneously. The author was inspired by the torsional movement or cart wheel movement of a bullock cart wheel and the movement of a number of vessels arranged as a wheel with the system being pulled by cattle for drawing water from a well.

Application of the energy through a bent tip on the conventional linear phaco system in a cyclic manner will provide great opportunity to emulsify lens nuclei even without having sculpting or chopping. Once nucleus is made free from superficial cortical matter, the nucleus has access and is free to rotate in a cyclic manner. This free and cyclic spontaneous rotation will allow nucleus emulsification and aspiration even without breaking by sculpting or chopping. The energy required is more or less same as utilised in chopping settings. This particular method is very effective for grade two to three cataracts.

INDICATIONS

This method can be employed with any grade of nuclear density. However in our view, best results are obtained in grade two/three density nucleus. A very sticky cortex, inadequate pupillary dilatation, associated zonular dehiscence or any other ocular predisposing factors are relative contraindications for this technique.

TECHNIQUE

Modifications/Phacoemulsifier System

Any kind of conventional phacoemulsifier including basic ventury or peristaltic system can be used for torsional cart wheel technique yet an advanced system produces much superior outcomes due to their superior fluidics.

Phaco tip

A 30 degree bent Kelman tip is very effective and essentially required for this technique. Conventional phaco tips are not desirable and should not be considered, since effective grip and torsional impact is not possible with standard tips.

Bottle Height

To achieve effective torsional effect, a bottle height of more than 70 cm from the operating eye level is desirable.

Fluid Dynamics

To achieve adequate torsional impact, a free floating rotating nucleus is essential. Cart wheel torsional impact needs high flow and vacuum but moderate ultrasonic energy settings. Needless to stress, torsional and rotational impact is possible with stormy or aggressive fluidic settings. Despite high flow and vacuum settings, excellent chamber stability is an absolutely mandatory requirement.

Incision (Figs 17.1 and 17.2)

No specific preference for incision is required for this technique. The surgeon can opt for an incision of his choice. The author prefers to proceed with clear corneal temporal or nasal incisions which depends upon whether it is the right or left eye.

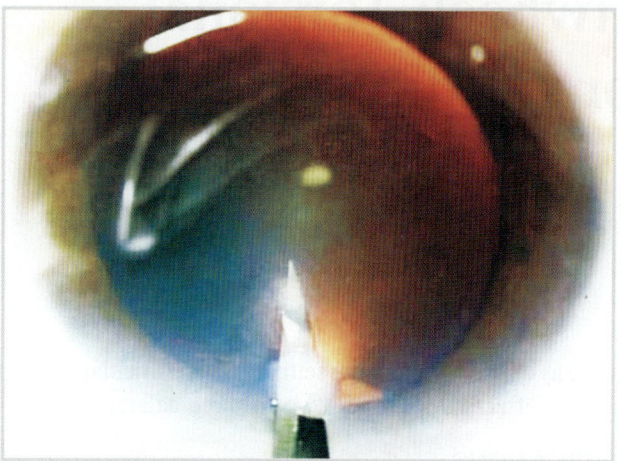

Fig. 17.1: Cart wheel phaco: Primary side port incision

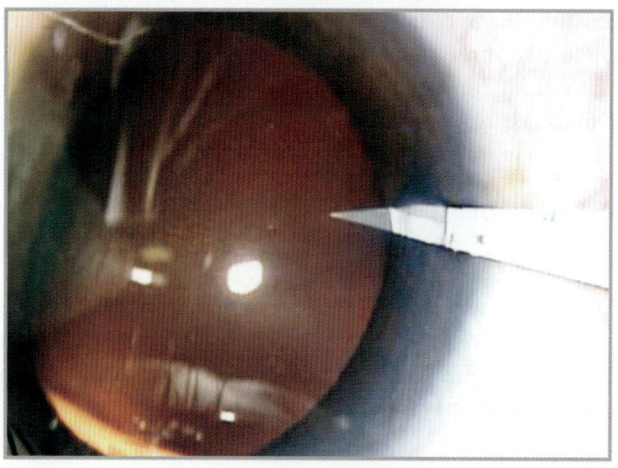

Fig. 17.2: Cart wheel phaco: Primary temporal incision

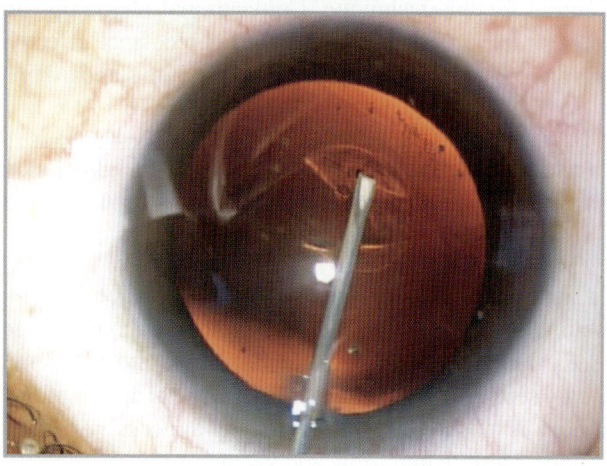

Fig. 17.3: Cart wheel phaco: Large rhexis

A relatively large size Rhexis of around six to six and a half mm is an ideal choice to attain good and free intracapsular in the bag cartwheel rotation of nucleus during nucleotomy as well as to have adequate torsional impact (Fig 17.3).

Hydroprocedure (Figs 17.4 to 17.6)

Multilevel and sequential hydroprocedure is of immense value to achieve excellent rotation of nucleus under the cushion of cortical matter and perinucleus. Cartwheel torsional rotation with the help of a bent tip is highly facilitated by an excellent hydroprocedure.

Nucleotomy (Figs 17.7 to 17.13)

Prior to the commencement of nucleotomy, a good amount of cortex is being removed from the superficial surface as well as from all around the nucleus. Good cortical clearing leads to excellent rotation of nucleus which is highly beneficial to achieve desired torsional impact.

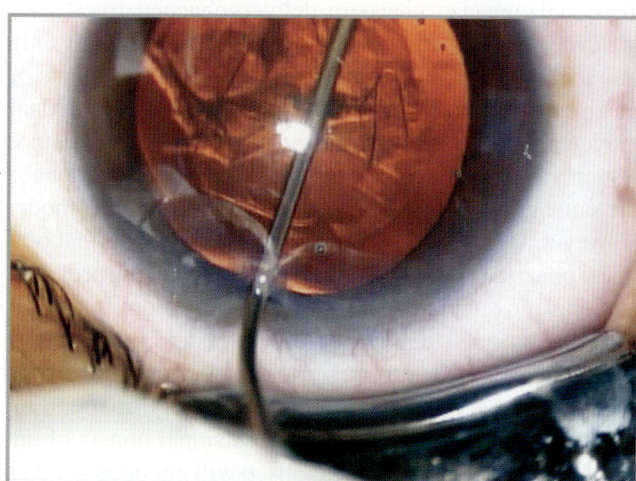

Fig. 17.4: Cart wheel phaco: Multilevel and sequential hydroprocedure

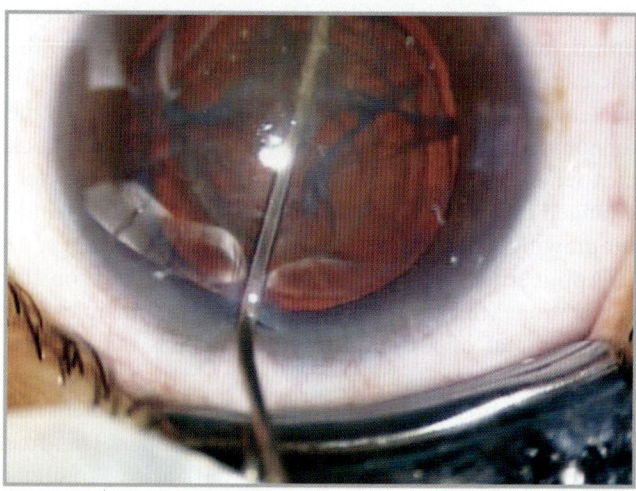

Fig. 17.5: Cart wheel phaco: Multilevel intranuclear hydroprocedure

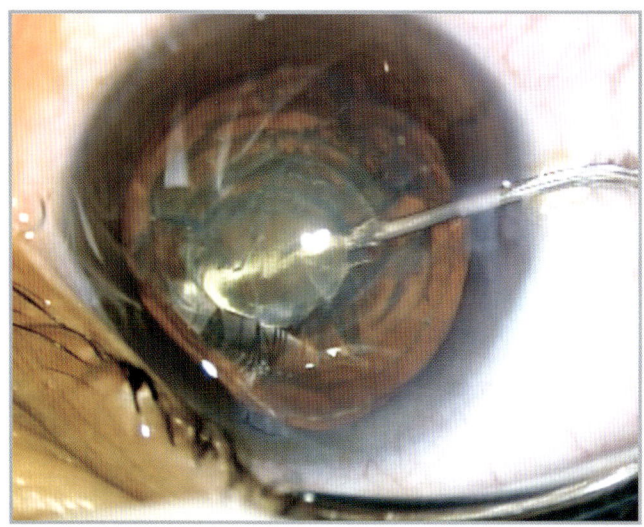

Fig. 17.6: Cart wheel phaco: Multilevel and sequential hydrodelineation

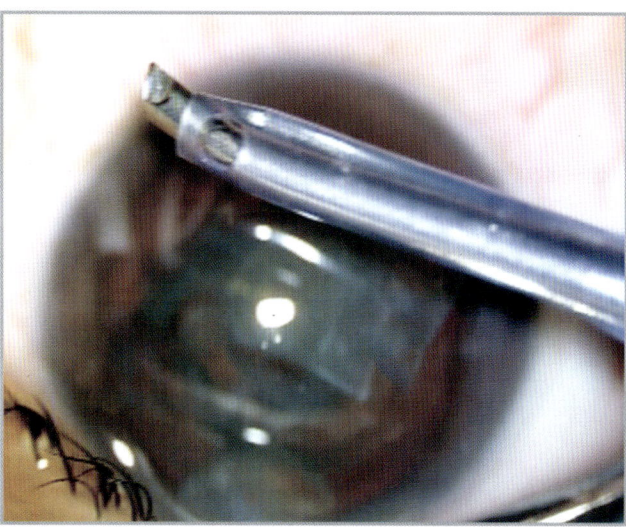

Fig. 17.7: Cart wheel phaco: Kelman tip

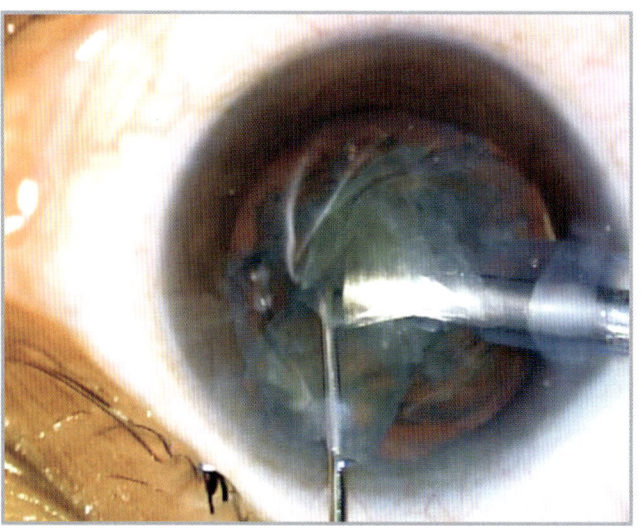

Fig. 17.8: Cart wheel phaco: Kelman tip is being impaled into the nucleus

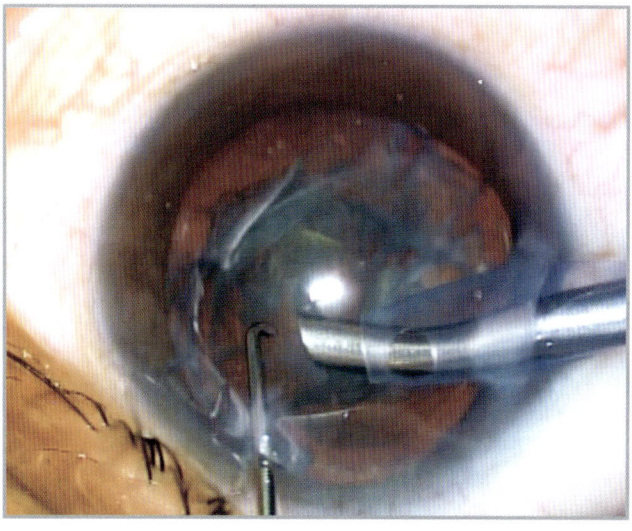

Fig. 17.9: Cart wheel phaco: Torsional rotational impact on nucleus by Kelman tip

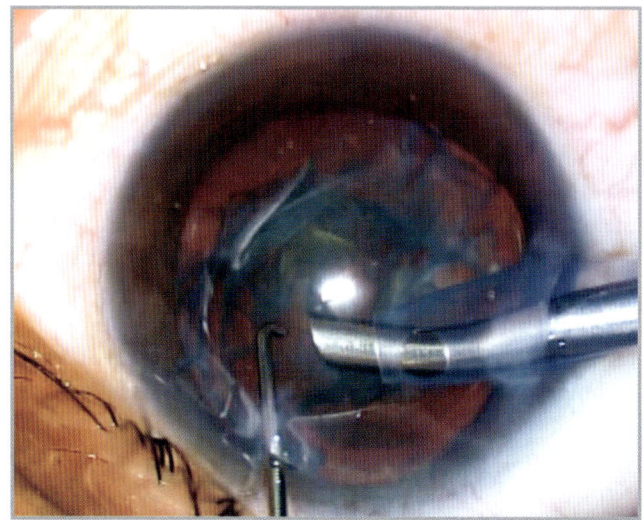

(a)

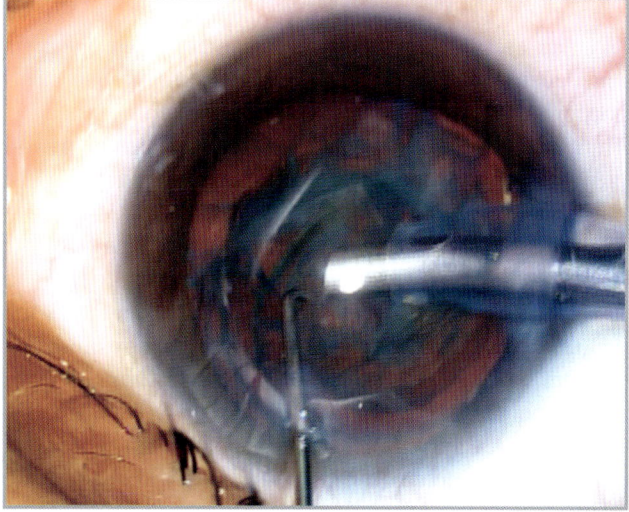

(b)

Fig. 17.10: (a) and (b) Cart wheel phaco: Torsional rotational impact on nucleus by Kelman tip

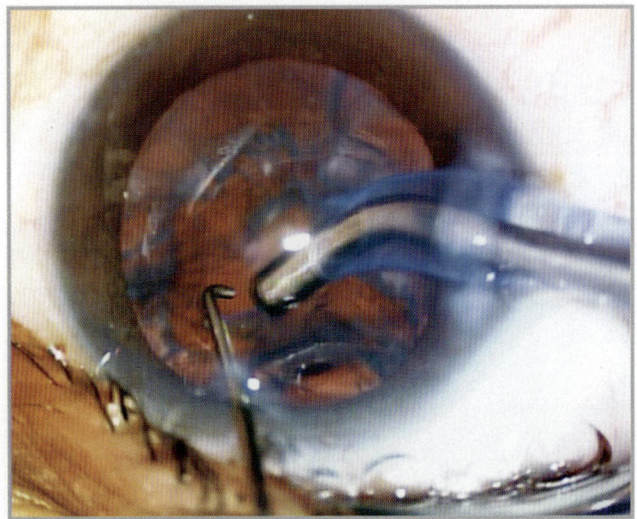

Fig. 17.11: Cart wheel phaco: Irrigation/Aspiration

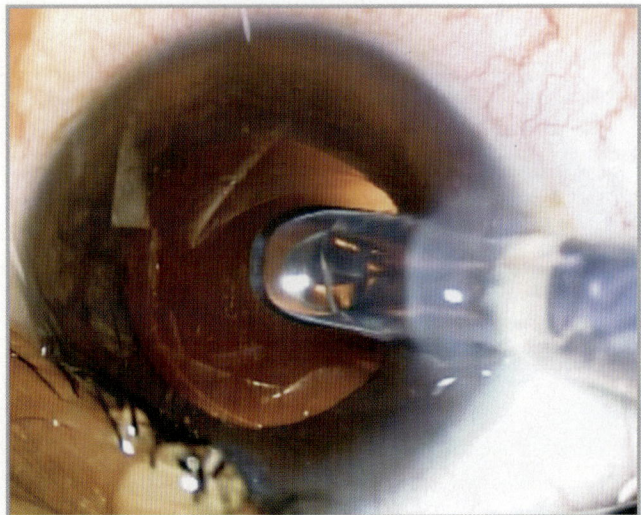

Fig. 17.12: Cart wheel phaco: Insertion of IOL

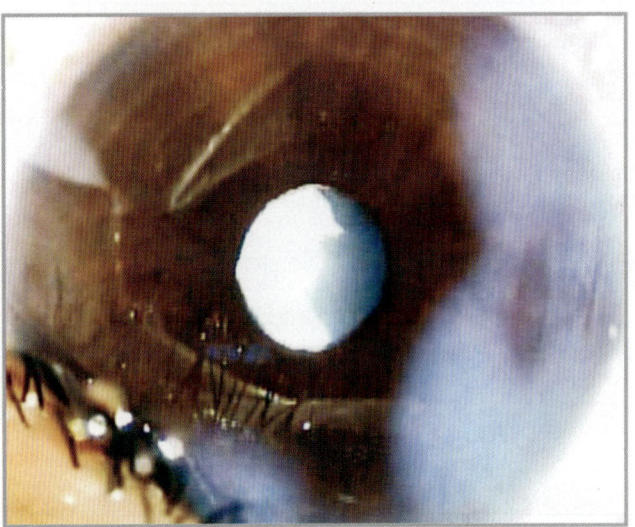

Fig. 17.13: Stromal hydration

Once cortical clearing is completed, Kelman tip is impaled into the core nucleus while directing the angulated portion of the Kelman tip laterally or facing inferiorly. Thus, the 30 degree angulated portion of the tip should provide a grip on the larger area of the core nucleus. The phacoenergy settings to hold the nucleus will vary from 5% to 20% US energy depending upon the density of the nucleus. Moderate flow rate and vacuum is required to have an adequate grip. In case of a very soft nucleus the central portion of the nucleus is just picked up by moderate vacuum, low flow rate and no US energy settings. A large sized nucleus will require two hemi sections to attain desired the cyclic motion on an angulated tip whereas a smaller sized nucleus can be emulsified without making

any fragmentation. Two hemi sections of the nucleus can be made by a gentle stroke of the chopper against the grip of a bent tip. In case of soft nucleus, no chopping is offered and the inner layer of soft nucleus is peeled off by an anticlockwise movement of the tip while retaining no power and only irrigation mode settings on an angulated phaco tip.

Once nucleus is allowed to move freely and in torsional action, the angulated portion of tip is impaled into the nuclear substance in a linear fashion so as to allow a good hold of the nucleus by the Kelman phaco tip. Moderate vacuum settings without application of US energy is good enough to hold on the nucleus. In case of soft nucleus, Sinskey hook is an ideal choice to perform nucleotomy.

The next step is to deliver a gentle stroke of US energy in such a fashion so as to make a break in the nucleus exactly in the manner of spokes in a cart wheel.

The combination of torsional movement of nucleus on irrigation mode, a stroke of position two to hold the nucleus in between and occasional pulse of US energy while engaging the equator of nucleus will facilitate quick emulsification of nucleus, despite applying less amount of energy. Angulated lumen of the Kelman tip is being used to hold the nucleus perpendicular to the main axis of the phaco tip; hence the tip will be able to provide a larger amount of acceleration lines, thereby higher quantum of ultrasonic energy will be available for nuclear emulsi-fication as compared to the conventional chopping techniques. In our view, the Cartwheel phacoemulsification technique on an angulated Kelman tip is an excellent way of effective utilisation and optimal titration of ultrasonic energy on the linear phacoemulsification system so as to achieve the best outcome.

Various Techniques of Irrigation and Aspiration in Phacoemulsification

▼ Irrigation and Aspiration Techniques
Lt Col S Mukherjee

18

Irrigation and Aspiration Techniques

Lt Col S Mukherjee

INTRODUCTION

The process of cortical aspiration is one of the most important steps in cataract surgery, as important as the immediately preceding step of nucleus extraction. Inadequate removal of cortical matter can render a poor visual outcome and the surgical effort, a total failure whatever the quality of surgery.

Cortical aspiration is defined as the removal of the lens cortical fibres piecemeal from the capsular bag. The basic principle revolves around a two way process namely, irrigation (inward flow) and vacuum aspiration (outward flow). This step has more or less remained unchanged whatever be the mode of surgery, i.e. phacoemulsification or conventional cataract extraction.

AIM

A complete cortex removal is absolutely essential for the following reasons:
- (a) To ensure a clear postoperative visual axis
- (b) To prevent early or late uveitis
- (c) To prevent posterior capsular opacification (PCO).

MODES AND INSTRUMENTATION

Irrigation and aspiration systems are basically of two types depending on the number of instruments used:
- (a) Coaxial I/A system
- (b) Bimanual I/A system.

Coaxial Irrigation/Aspiration System (Fig. 18.1a)

This system has a single probe or cannula in which the aspiration orifice is present at the anterior tip and the irrigation orifices are located slightly behind or at the sides. The tip may be straight or angulated at varying degrees. The gauge of the aspiration orifice varies from 0.2–0.8 mm diameter, wherein a smaller gauge is capable of creating a greater vacuum seal but the aspiration time is increased. Coaxial probes are to be used through the main port only.

Coaxial I/A probe (cannula) has a covering sleeve which may either be detachable or fixed (metallic). Detachable sleeves are made of silicon and the major advantage of soft silicon is that it provides a watertight compartment by fitting snugly in the entry wound. However, silicon sleeves have to be frequently replaced.

One must be careful while entering the eye because the irrigation sleeve might cause Descemet's stripping; therefore, it is wiser to start the irrigation (foot pedal-step 1) before entering the AC in order to maintain a formed chamber.

Bimanual I/A System (Fig. 18.1b)

This system has separate cannulae and tubing for irrigation and aspiration.

Bimanual system can be used through two separate ports for entry. Aspiration cannula is either curved or straight and is usually attached to a handle. The infusion cannula is usually thicker and can be used through either the main or side port. It is preferable to use infusion cannula with two side openings (180° apart) because it provides uniform infusion in the anterior chamber.

Technique

- The anterior chamber (AC) should be formed with viscoelastic; apart from preventing collapse of the AC, injecting viscoelastic has other advantages too, namely, it protects the corneal endothelium and opens up the capsular bag.
- It is ideal to start the infusion before entering the AC as it prevents collapse and Descemet's stripping, but on the other hand it may decrease visibility. The other alternative is to enter and then start infusion but this

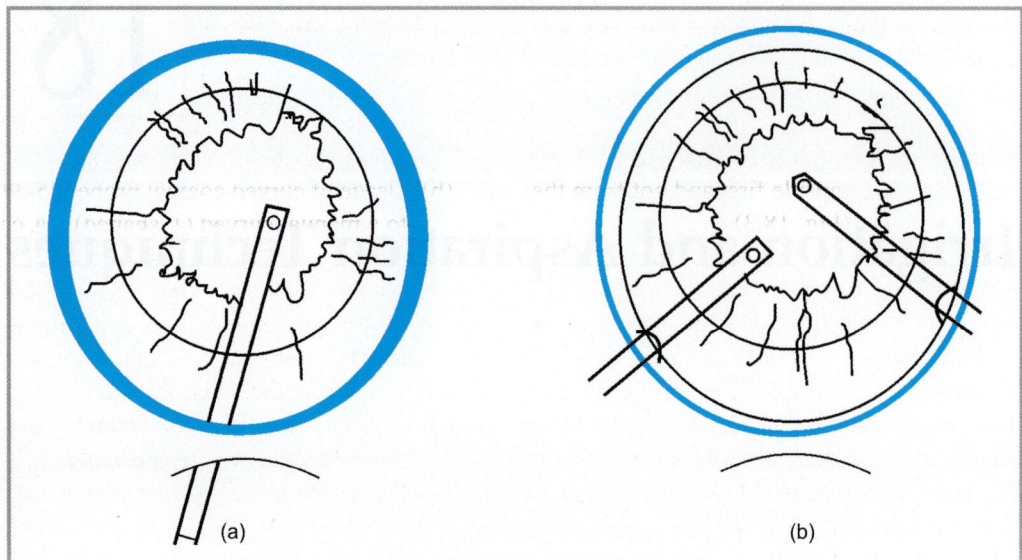

Fig. 18.1: (a) Coaxial I/A system (b) Bimanual I/A system

may introduce air bubbles in the AC (which have to be gobbled first before aspirating cortical material).

- The loose cortical matter floating in the AC should be *eaten up* before entering the capsular bag. Avoid disturbing the cortical fibres sticking to the endothelial surface of the cornea, because tackling them invariably leads to corneal haze (endothelial damage). These fibres eventually get dislodged during the process due to the turbulence in the AC; anyhow, mild retained cortical matter is a lesser evil than endothelial damage!

- The aspirator should enter the capsular bag (keep an eye on the CCC margin to be sure that one is beneath it); move to a particular sector (usually start from the diagonally opposite clock position to the incision site). Do not start aspirating (stay on the foot pedal step 1) till one reaches the periphery where one notices cortical fibres like 'jagged cliffs' against the fundal

glow. Engage the cortical fibres in one clock hour (foot pedal step 2) and pull towards the central safe area and then aspirate (Fig. 18.2).

- If the fibres do not 'follow' the probe tip or do not engage, then the probe is either not in the 'bag' (i.e. the tip is in a plane above, in the sulcus) or adequate vacuum has not built up for the probe to start sucking the fibres. Try and engage the fibres more by moving the probe deeper or to and fro. Increase the vacuum (foot pedal step 2) till the fibres peel off, then move to the adjacent clock hour position, engage cortex and repeat the procedure.

Few Practical Pearls for Beginners

- It is absolutely important to have the pupil dilated, otherwise it is impossible as well as dangerous to do a cortical clean up. In case the pupil has constricted due

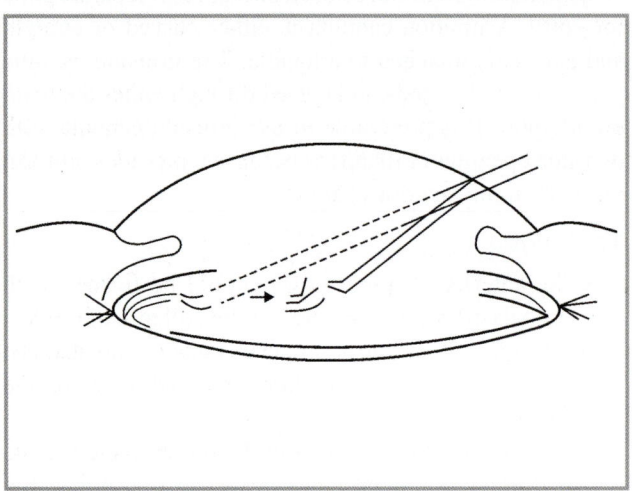

(a)

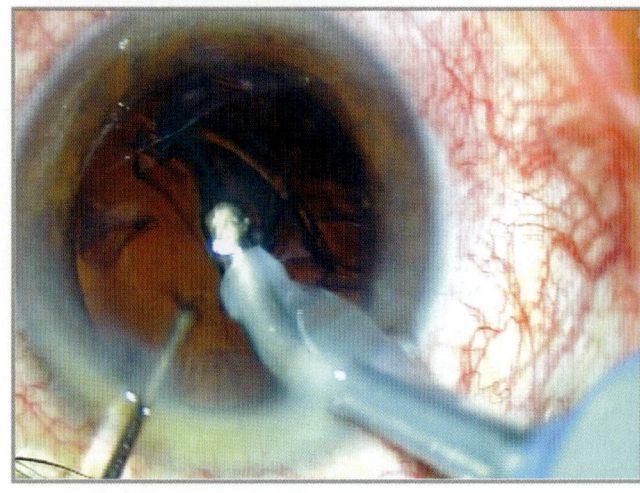

(b)

Fig. 18.2: (a) and (b) Always draw the cortical fibres from the periphery to the central safe zone before "eating them"

to the phaco procedure (due to excessive iris handling), it is always wise to spend a few extra minutes and dilate the pupil with viscoelastic or intraocular injection of adrenaline.

- Always face the aspirator orifice upward, peel the fibres from the anterior capsule first and not from the posterior cortical fibres (Fig. 18.3).
- Be absolutely gentle with the probe during cortex aspiration; remember the posterior capsule is only 0.4 mm thick and it doesn't take much effort to tear such a thin membrane.
- If one encounters 'sticky' cortex in one particular section, quit and move on to the adjacent part. The other alternative is to inject viscoelastic and try to dislodge/loosen the fibres. If it is still worse, it is always better to implant the IOL (in the bag) and rotate it. This will loosen the cortical matter for it to be eaten up (for this the eye should not be soft) postimplantation.
- Striae, radiating from the aspirator like 'sunrays' are a sure shot indicator of holding of the posterior capsule, if so, release the foot pedal, immediately (Fig. 18.4).

Subincision Cortex

Removal of subincision cortex remains a challenge even in the hands of an expert surgeon. The difficulty arises simply because this area lies immediately beneath the incision area, so getting underneath is relatively tougher more so in tunnel incision entries. Secondly, this area has decreased visibility, especially if it is a superior incision and an arcus is present. Using a straight coaxial I/A probe also adds to the difficulty. Hydrodissection of this area is invariably incomplete.

A typical situation is one in which the subincision cortex (especially in superior incision) becomes loose but does not get dislodged after repeated attempts, only to descend onto the pupillary area on the 1st postoperative day when the patient is ambulatory.

Suggested points to tackle this problem are:
(a) Create a large or superiorly decentred rhexis, it's always easier to tackle subincision cortex this way.
(b) Usage of curved coaxial probe (45–90°) or convert to a manual curved (J. shaped) I/A cannula.
(c) Bimanual I/A system is the ideal instrument to remove subincision cortex because this probe can be used through the side ports. Remember that the side ports should always be at least 2 clock hours away from the main port.
(d) Temporal incision is better and easier than superior incision in more ways than one.

Lastly, it is never too late to learn the fact that a little bit of retained cortical matter is always better than landing with a posterior capsular dehiscence in trying to achieve that perfect cortical clean up.

Coaxial vs Bimanual I/A Systems

Coaxial system has a shorter learning curve; therefore, beginners find it more convenient but it turns out that the bimanual system, though requiring good hand coordination, has various advantages to its credit.

The coaxial probe tip is generally thinner in calibre than the phaco tip; therefore the wound (created to fit the phaco probe) may be larger than the I/A probe leading to wound leak and poor vacuum build up. Secondly, the tip (with the sleeve) is too thick to enter through a side port.

The straight coaxial tip is highly unsuitable for removing subincision cortex (Fig. 18.5), whereas the bi-manual system requires two side port incisions, but is ideally suited for removing cortex from all quadrants. In fact, the concept of subincision cortex does not arise at all because the cannulae (irrigation and aspiration) can be interchanged through different ports (Fig. 18.6). Bimanual probe tips

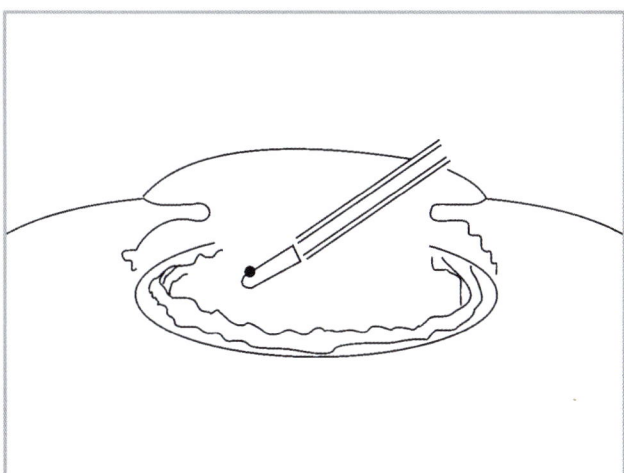

Fig. 18.3: Orifice of the aspirator should at all times face the surgeon and not towards the posterior capsule

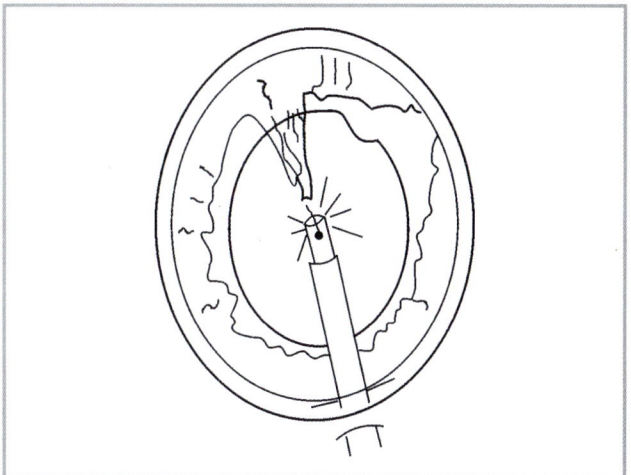

Fig. 18.4: 'Striae' radiating from the tip of aspirator: a sure sign of posterior capsule stress; release the foot pedal immediately

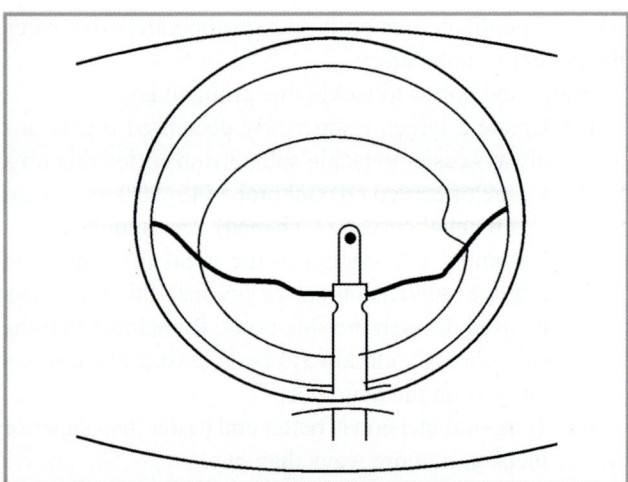

Fig. 18.5: Area covered by coaxial I/A system. Grey shaded area denotes the area reachable by this handpiece. Note that the subincisional area remains largely inaccessible

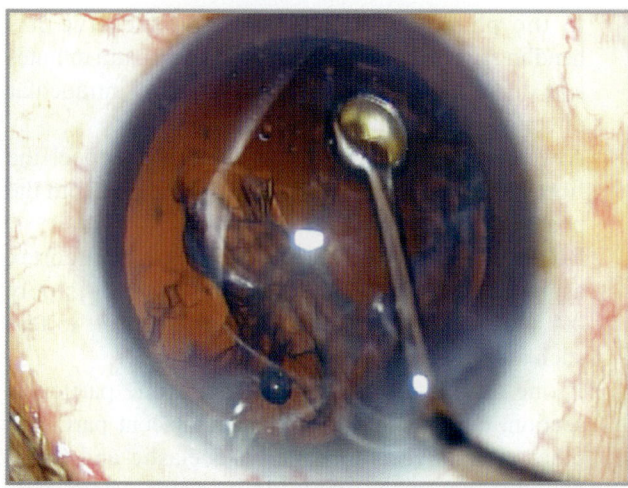

Fig. 18.6: Capsular polisher to dislodge the cortical plate from fornices of the bag

do not require any silicon sleeves. Overall the bimanual I/A is a smoother and safer procedure.

Mechanical I/A vs Manual I/A System

Even though the basic principle of irrigation and aspiration remains the same, there are a few differences that a cataract surgeon must know while graduating from the manual to the mechanical I/A system. Firstly, the irrigation flow rate in the manual I/A system is much lesser than in a mechanical I/A system. Secondly, the suction pressure generated at the aspiration tip is much higher in the mechanical system. Consequently, due to the higher volume transfer rate (the time taken for the fluid to travel into and out of the chamber), mechanical irrigation and aspiration is a faster procedure.

In small incision and microincision surgeries (including manual SICS), the anterior chamber is a water-tight compartment (in contradistinction to conventional ECCE), therefore the vacuum pressure built up at the aspirating tip is much higher.

In the mechanical I/A system, the flow rate is directly dependent on the vacuum pressure applied; therefore the chance of chamber collapse is much less.

However, mechanical I/A is a less forgiving procedure and in situations of poor visibility, it is better to use a manual I/A system.

Capsular Polishing

Capsular polishing is a procedure whereby the posterior capsule is scraped with a blunt instrument and cortical remnants are removed.

This is a procedure, which is not without risks and moreover not required in most cases. However there are a few situations where it may be helpful:

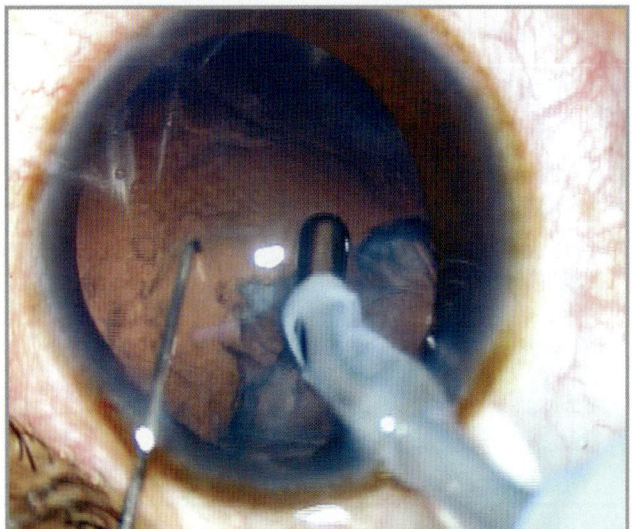

Fig. 18.7: Removal of subincision cortex by coaxial method

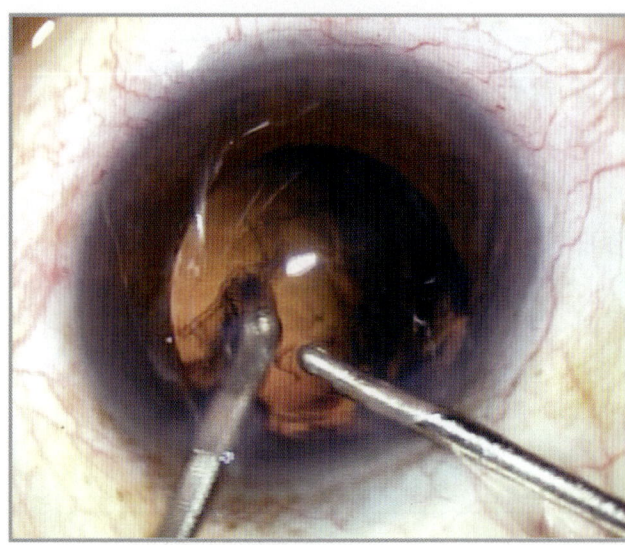

Fig. 18.8: Removal of subincision cortex by bimanual I/A

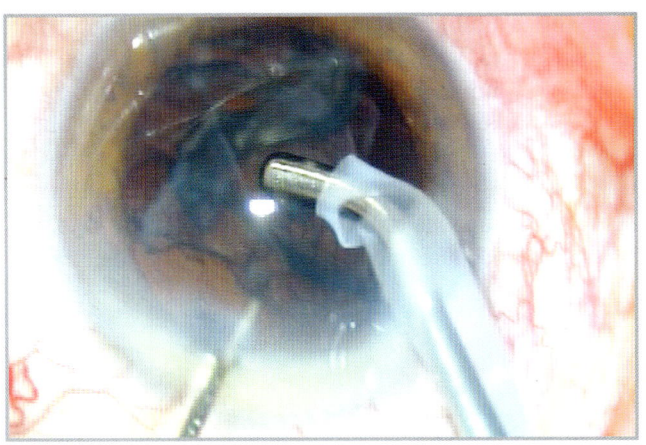

Fig. 18.9: Coaxial I/A systems

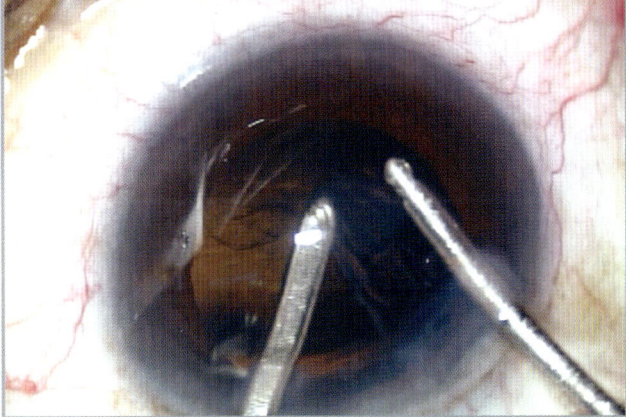

Fig. 18.10: Bimanual I/A systems

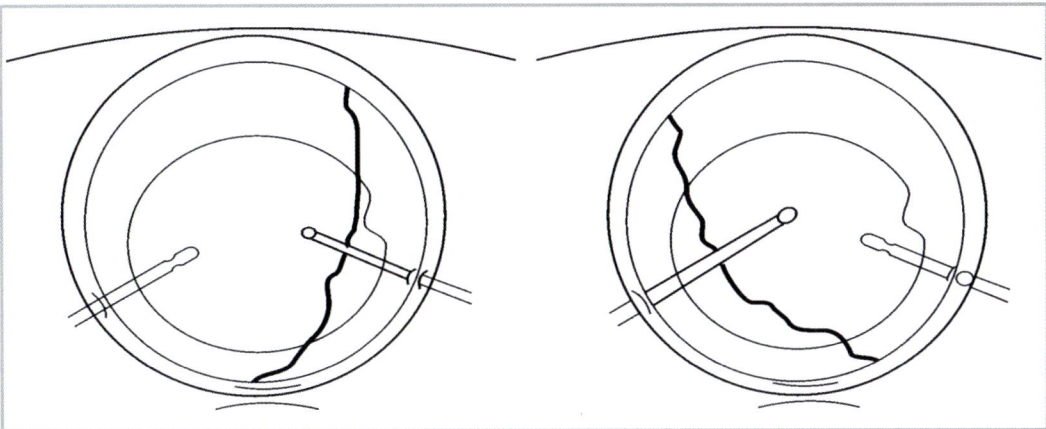

Fig. 18.11: Bimanual I/A system. Grey shade denotes the area covered by the aspirating handpiece (a) Aspirating handpiece through the 10 O'clock side port (b) Interchange the handpieces, now the aspirating probe passes through the 2 O'clock port and reaches areas that were inaccessible through the 10 O'clock port with the bimanual system, concept of subincision area ceases to exist

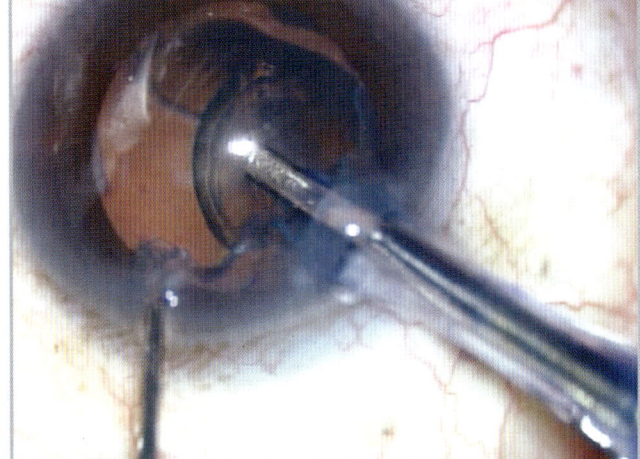

Fig. 18.12: Cortical removal by phaco handpiece

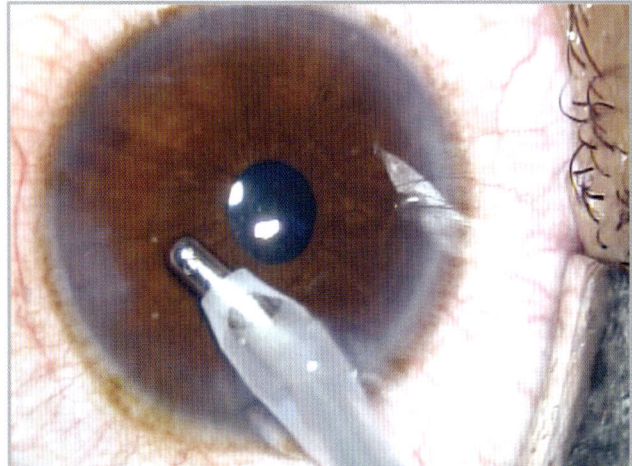

Fig. 18.13: Post IOL implant wash (coaxial method)

- Hypermature cataract with hydrated fibrils that tend to stick to the capsule.
- Complicated and traumatic cataract
- Cataract in the young
- Posterior subcapsular cataract with central plaque

TECHNIQUE

After cortical clean up has been done and before insertion of intraocular lens, the capsular bag is distended with viscoelastic in order to stretch the posterior capsule.

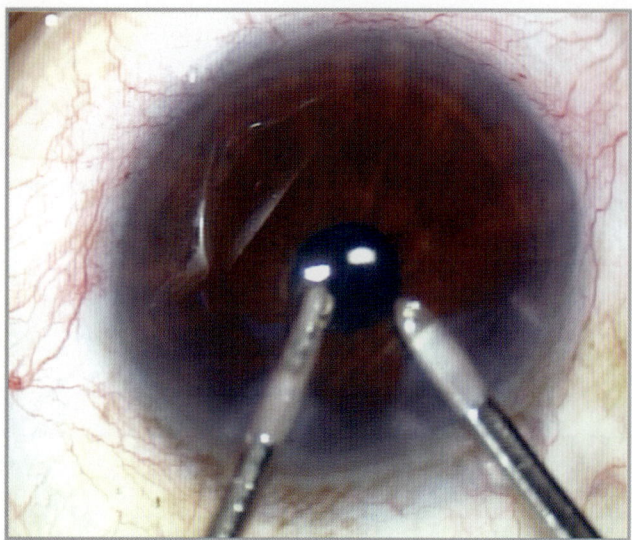

Fig. 18.14: Post IOL implant wash (bimanual method)

Magnification is raised to the maximum, posterior capsule level should be brought to focus and the eye should be perpendicular to the illuminating beam to get a good glow which provides a contrasting background.

Using a smooth rounded repositor or ring polisher, gently scrapes the capsule, preferably working only in the central 3–4 mm area.

Some higher end phaco machines have a 'cap vac' mode in which low vacuum is applied (upto 05 to 20 mm Hg max.) with the orifice facing downward, the force sufficient enough to scrape the capsule but not tear it. I reiterate, this is a risky procedure and not recommended for beginners.

CONCLUSION

Cortical irrigation and aspiration is a very important step in modern day extra capsular cataract surgery, whether it is conventional ECCE, small incision (SICS) or phacoemulsification. Mechanical I/A systems warrant the usage of probe/s incorporating high flow-rate irrigation and higher vacuum aspiration than manual I/A cannula system. A good cortical clean up ensures a smooth and uneventful postoperative period with lesser chances of increased IOP, uveitis and PCO formation thus, resulting in a good visual outcome.

BIBLIOGRAPHY

1. Schneider, Hanka .Changes of the accommodative amplitude and the anterior chamber depth after implantation of an accommodative intraocular lens. Graefe s Archive for Clinical and Experimental Ophthalmology, 2006; 244(3) 63:707–714.
2. Arthur HO.Theoretical Analysis of Accommodation Amplitude and Ametropia Correction by Varying Refractive Index in Phaco-Ersatz. Optometry and Vision Science (2001).
3. Parel, J. M. Endocapsular lavage with photofrin II as a photodynamic therapy for lens epithelial proliferation. Lasers in Medical Science, 1990: 5(1).
4. Stachs, Oliver. Three-dimensional ultrasound biomicroscopy, environmental and conventional scanning electron microscopy investigations of the human zonula ciliaris for numerical modelling of accommodation. Graefe s Archive for Clinical and Experimental Ophthalmology. 2005.
5. Glasser, Adrian (2001) International Ophthalmology Clinics, 2001; 41(2).
6. Koopmans, Steven A. Relation between injected volume and optical parameters in refilled isolated porcine lenses. Ophthalmic and Physiological Optics 2004, 24(6).
7. Charman, W. N. Restoring accommodation: a dream or an approaching reality? Ophthalmic and Physiological Optics, 2005, 25(1).
8. Barraquer, Joaquín .Cataract surgery and IOL implantation. Documenta Ophthalmologica. 1992: 81(3).
9. Dick, H. Burkhard (2005) Accommodative intraocular lenses: current status. Current Opinion in Ophthalmology 16(1) Atchoo PD. Double-barrel anterior chamber irrigating needle. Arch Ophthalmol. 1968 May; 79(5):580–581.
10. Bill A. The aqueous humor drainage mechanism in the cynomolgus monkey (Macaca irus) with evidence for unconventional routes. Invest Ophthalmol. 1965 Oct; 4(5): 911–919.
11. Bruun-Jensen J. Cataract aspiration-irrigation with twin-needle. Acta Ophthalmol (Copenh). 1969; 47(3):498–501.
12. Chandler PA. Surgery of congenital cataract. Am J Ophthalmol. 1968 May; 65(5):663–674.
13. FUCHS U. Uber den Nachweis von Anaesthetica im Urin nach perkutaner Applikation. Med Monatsschr. 1952 Sep; 6(9):590–592.
14. Girard LJ. Aspiration-irrigation of congenital and traumatic cataracts. Arch Ophthalmol. 1967 Mar; 77(3):387–391.
15. Harcourt B, Wybar K. Congenital cataract: surgical aspects. Proc R Soc Med. 1969 Jul; 62(7):689–693.
16. Hogan MJ. Congenital cataract surgery. Trans Am Ophthalmol Soc. 1966; 64:311–318.
17. Kelman CD. Phaco-emulsification and aspiration. A new technique of cataract removal. A preliminary report. Am J Ophthalmol. 1967 Jul; 64(1):23–35.
18. Maumenee AE, Goldberg MF. Push-Pull Cataract aspiration and franceschetti corepraxy . Arch Ophthalmol. 1965 Jul; 74:72–73.
19. Rice NS. Lens aspiration: a method of treatment for soft cataract. Trans Ophthalmol Soc U K. 1967; 87:491–498.
20. Ryan SJ, Blanton FM, von Noorden GK. Surgery of congenital cataract. Am J Ophthalmol. 1965 Oct; 60(4): 583–587.
21. Scheie HG. Aspiration of congenital or soft cataracts: a new technique. Am J Ophthalmol. 1960 Dec; 50:1048–1056.
22. Sears ML. Miosis and intraocular pressure changes during manometry: mechanically irritated rabbit eyes studied with improved manometric technique. Arch Ophthalmol. 1960 Apr.

Intraocular Lens Implants

19

Conventional Intraocular Lens Implants

Lt Col Anirudh Singh and Col JKS Parihar SM, VSM

INTRODUCTION

In the ever increasing market of intraocular lenses (IOL), the ophthalmic surgeon is posed by a challenge to give the best to his patients. The intraocular lenses are no more the surgeon's prerogative due to the increased patient's awareness about the lens and the vast information available on the Internet. What is required is a thorough knowledge about the types of lenses with the merits and demerits of the same so that the patient can be offered the best possible visual result, also keeping in mind the cost factor and the paying capacity of the patient.

IOL Materials

The **IOL materials** can be classified into the two following major groups:
1. Acrylate/methacrylate polymers, including polymethyl methacrylate (PMMA), hydrophobic acrylics and hydrophilic acrylics (hydrogels).
2. Silicone elastomers.

Types of IOL

During the last five decades, the IOL implantation has undergone a lot of changes and the entire concept of IOL implantation is still undergoing an evolution. The sixth generation of IOLs (foldable IOL) had come a few years ago and now it has been overtaken by the newer Rollable, Accommodative and the Phakic IOLs. Presently available IOLs can be grouped on the following bases:

Based on the Method of Fixation

(a) **Anterior Chamber IOL (ACIOL):** These lenses lie in front of the iris and are supported in the angle of anterior chamber. Kelman Multiplex is the more commonly used ACIOL. These IOLs are not very

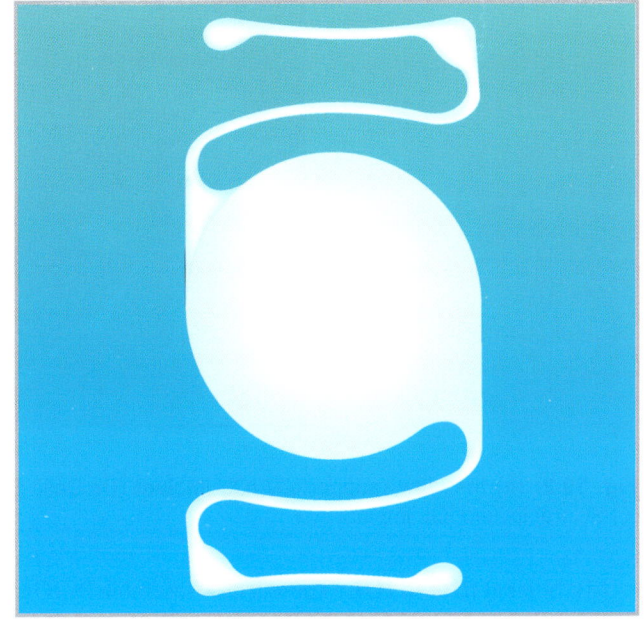

Fig. 19.1: Anterior chamber IOL

popular due to the high incidence of bullous keratopathy.

(b) **Iris supported lenses:** Theses lenses are fixed on the iris with the help of loops or claws.

Dr Daljit Singh and Worst iris claw lens is an example of iris claw lenses.

Iris claw lenses are not very popular and almost have become obsolete due to the high incidence of hyphaema and uveitis and the availability of excellent quality flexible posterior chamber IOL implants.

(c) **Posterior chamber IOL (PCIOL):** These lenses are placed either in the ciliary sulcus or more ideally in the capsular bag following the phacoemulsification of the lens. Nearly all the implantations nowadays are limited to PCIOL.

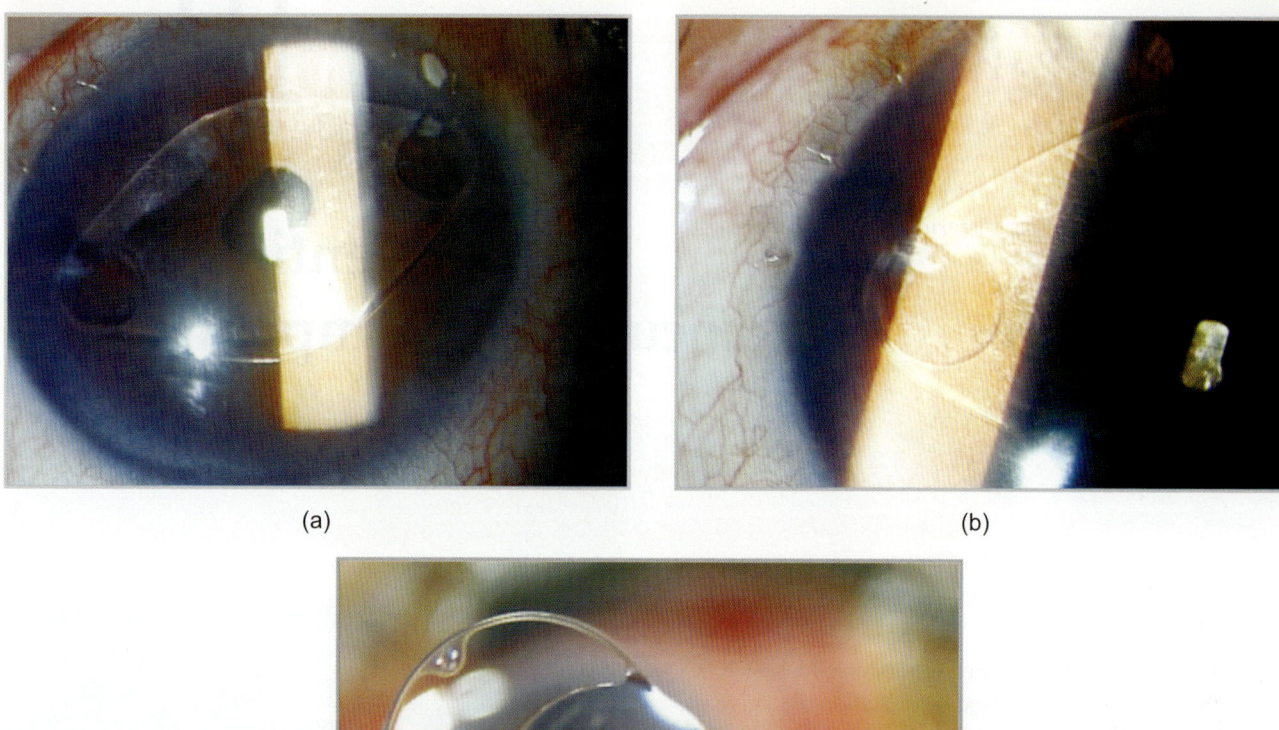

(a)

(b)

(c)

Fig. 19.2: (a) Iris claw (supported) IOL implant (Dr Daljit Singh), (b) Iris claw (supported) IOL implant is tucked into iris, (c) Scleral fixated IOL implant

(d) **Scleral fixated IOL:** These lenses resemble PCIOL with additional eyelets on the heptics to assist in fixing the lens in an aphakic eye with no capsular support.

(e) **Phakic IOL:** These lenses have been recently introduced and implanted over the normal lens in the ciliary sulcus to correct the refractive status of the eye.

Based on the Material of the Lens

(a) **Rigid lens:** They are made up of polymethyl methacrylate (PMMA) and its copolymers.

(b) **Foldable lens:** These lenses are made up of silicone or acrylic material and can be implanted through a smaller incision.

(c) **Rollable lens:** They are made up of acrylic material and can be rolled and implanted through an incision size of about 1 mm.

Based on the Refractive Status

(a) **Unifocal lens:** These lenses have a fixed refractive power for distance.

(b) **Multifocal lens:** These lenses have an additional component of near vision and can be of refractive or diffractive optics.

IOL Designs

The **broad design features** of the IOL can be:

(a) **Single piece or Three piece IOL:** The lens can have the optic and haptic of the same material or else the haptic can be made of a separate material. The point in favour of single piece lenses is that the incidence of posterior capsular opacification rates is lower. The point in favour for three piece lenses is enhanced lens centration and stability, and provides better resistance to postoperative contraction forces within the capsular bag.

(b) **Hole in the optic:** Helps in securing the lens due to the fibrosis that occurs through the hole. Few IOLs are made without the hole.

(c) **Square truncated optic edge:** To decrease the incidence of posterior capsule opacification by its enhanced barrier effect against cell migration/ proliferation on the posterior capsule towards the visual axis.

(d) **Multifocal lenses:** These are lenses with a component of near vision along with the distance correction. These lenses are either of the refractive type where concentric rings of different powers are combined or the diffractive type where both the near and distant corrections are put in each of the concentric rings.

(e) **Rollable lenses:** These lenses have a thickness of 150 μm and can be rolled and implanted through an incision size of about 1 mm.

(f) **Accommodative lenses:** The special design and mechanical properties of these IOLs enable the lens to change the power by a forward movement of the optic during the contraction of the ciliary muscle.

(g) **Light adjustable lens:** Three piece silicone-optic, PMMA-haptic lens with photosensitive silicone polymers, which move within the lens upon fine-tuning with a low intensity of laser light and thus, change the refractive power of the lens.

RIGID PMMA PC IOL

Rigid PMMA IOL forms the backbone of the IOL market today especially in the developing countries although the foldable IOL is slowly gaining a foothold. With the majority of clientele for cataract surgery coming from the less developed regions of the world, the cost factor of surgery is a major deterrent. In this respect, the rigid PMMA IOL proves to be a boon as the cost has been highly subsidised and lenses are available for as low as two-three hundred rupees.

Advantages

(a) Good optical quality due to better optics and reduced aberrations.

(b) Stable and less chances of decentration

(c) Stable in case of a partial loss of capsular integrity

(d) Rigid PMMA IOL has proved its efficacy in long term studies (still the most popular for paediatric cases).

Surface Modified PMMA IOL Implants

Surface modified PMMA IOL implants have been in practice for their better performance in various complicated or paediatric cataracts for the reason that they have less inflammatory reactions, cellular deposits and synechia formation.

Indications

(i) Paediatric population

(ii) Traumatic Cataract

(iii) Cataract associated with
    (a) Diabetes
    (b) Glaucoma
    (c) Chronic uveitis and
    (d) Pseudoexfoliation syndrome.

Types of Surface Modified PMMA IOL Implants

Two types of surface modified PMMA IOL implants are available:

(i) Heparin-surface-modified PMMA lenses

(ii) The fluorination process modified PMMA lenses

(i) Heparin-surface-modified PMMA lenses: Heparin-surface-modified PMMA lenses have successfully been used for the reason to have less inflammatory reactions, cellular deposits and synechia formation.

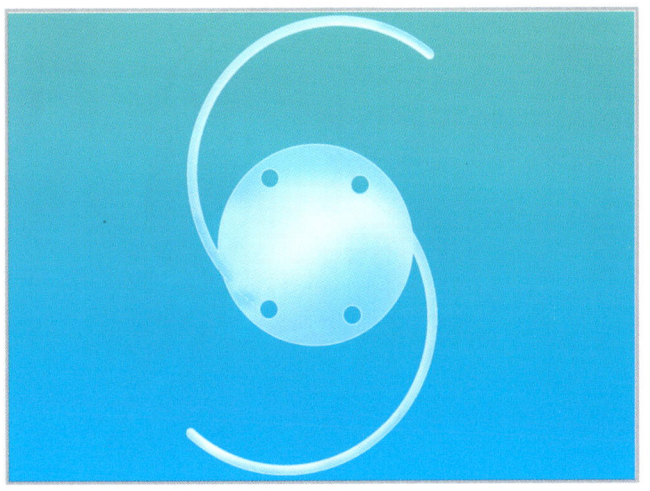
(a)

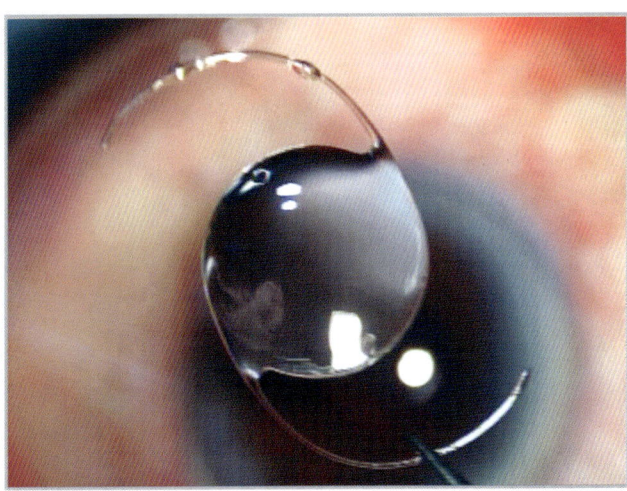
(b)

Fig. 19.3: (a) and (b) PMMA rigid (non foldable) posterior chamber IOL

(ii) The fluorination process modified PMMA lenses: The fluorine treatment process for IOL developed by Bausch and Lomb carries a permanent optimisation of PMMA biocompatibility as well as produces a stable and permanent surface coating thus guaranteeing long term clinical benefits.

PMMA implants are subjected to gaseous ion-rich plasma resulting in a substitution of hydrogen atoms by fluorine atoms along the outermost 0.01 m of the IOL PMMA surface. The resultant covalent binding of the fluorine atom layer is particularly stable ensuring a very durable coating.

Merits

(i) Enhancing surface smoothness as demonstrated in Atomic Force Microscopy (AFM); thus lowering surface energy and discouraging tissue interaction.

(ii) Diminishing cell adhesion leads to the following:
- Reduces adverse impact of surgical insult to the ocular tissue.
- Inhibits postoperative inflammation significantly by reduced granulocyte activation.
- Ensures better optical transparency of the IOL implant.

FOLDABLE IOL IMPLANTS

Commonly available foldable IOL implants are made up of following materials:

1. Hydrophobic acrylic lenses (single piece/multi piece)
2. Hydrophilic acrylic lenses (single piece/multi piece)
3. Silicon IOL implants.

Hydrophobic Acrylic Lenses (Prototype Single Piece AcrySof)

Hydrophobic acrylic IOL implant is made up of a copolymer of 2-phenylethyl acrylate and 2-phenylethyl methacrylate. These hydrophobic acrylic IOL implants possess very less water contents (less than 5%) as compared to hydrophilic IOL implants where the water content may be more than 10% and up to 38%. Hydrophobic acrylic IOL implant is known to have a high refractive index. They are biocompatible in nature, hence generate low inflammation. These IOLs have less elasticity and biomechanic properties which facilitate easier IOL implantation. Hydrophobic IOLs are preferred in pediatric and other complicated cases of cataracts.

Advantages

Hydrophobic single piece acrylic lenses are more biocompatible, hence generate low inflammation.

(i) Memory and flexibility of the AcrySof material: The haptics can be bent back on themselves, twisted and contorted to a much greater degree than PMMA haptics or even three piece IOLs.

(ii) Less incidence of PCO and ACO: The optic is biconvex with a fixed convexity of the posterior surface. The convexity of the anterior surface varies according to the IOL power. This is said to prevent epithelial proliferation under the IOL and thus low rates of Posterior Capsular Opacification (PCO). Single Piece AcrySof is a worldwide established IOL implant in this category.

The details of specifications are as follows:

(i) Refractive Index : 1.55 maintains thin lens even at high power
(ii) Water Content : 0.3 %

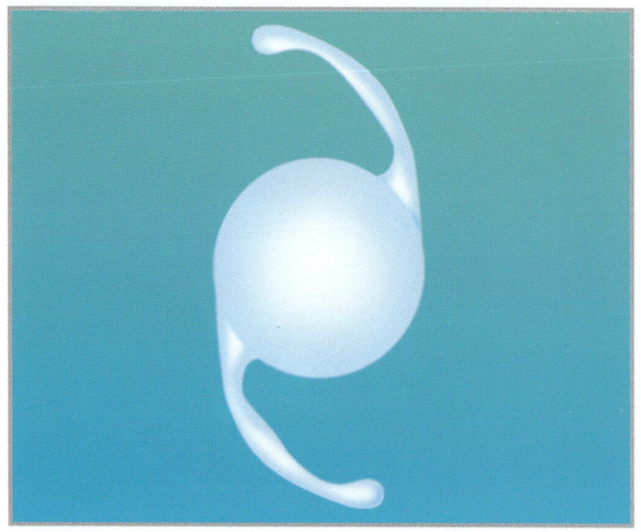

(a)

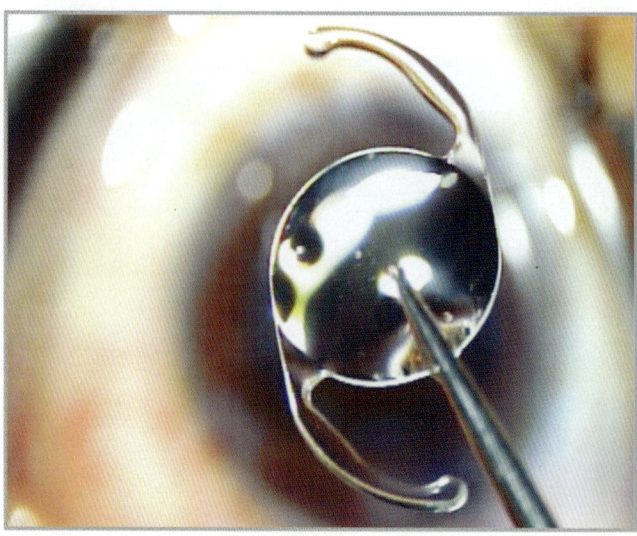

(b)

Fig. 19.4: (a) and (b) Single piece acrylic (hydrophobic) foldable posterior chamber IOL

(iii) Glass Transition: 11°C (+/–0.2°C)
(iv) Water Contact Angle: 72°
 (v) IOL is known to have less pitting against YAG capsulotomy procedure.
(vi) Bioadhesion mechanism:
  • Reduced PCO rate: AcrySof adheres firmly to the posterior as well as anterior capsule and stops the cell migration and proliferation.
  • Square profile of AcrySof edge acts as a physical barrier which prevents cells from migrating below the IOL optic.
  • Less anterior capsular movement
  • Better centration
  • Reduced phimosis and fibrosis.

Allergan Sensar Hydrophobic Acrylic IOL Implant

Sensar (AMO) AR-40/AR40E Hydrophobic Acrylic IOL implant is another very popular hydrophobic IOL implant. In fact, Sensar follows the IOPTEX ACR360, which was introduced back in 1986. Though Sensar claims to be a hydrophobic acrylic due to its low water contents, there is significant difference in the chemical properties between AcrySof and Sensar. The fluorinated chemical structure of the SENSAR IOL and the absence of aromatic chemical groups restricts the refractive index upto 1.47 as compared to the high refractive index of 1.55 in case of Acrysof IOL implant. However, clinical results are undoubtedly far superior to these of Acrylic Hydrophilic (HEMA Hydrogel) and Silicon IOL implants.

Material Specification

Material Structure: Terpolymer ethacrylate, Ethyl methacrylate and 2-2-2 trifluoroethyl methacrylate

    Optic Diameter   : 6 mm to 13.0 mm
    Haptics—   : Modified 'C' with 5 degree
    Extruded PMMA   angulation of haptics.
    Refractive Index : 1.47

Uniform Thickness across dioptres
Water Content   : 1.6 %
Glass Transition   : 10.6 +/– 0.2°C
Water Contact Angle : 88°
Incision Size   : 2.6 mm
                    (With the Emerald Unfolder)

Merits

 (i) Performance
 (ii) Consistent axial position
(iii) Excellent centration
(iv) Reduced risk of PCO due to specific design of optics. This exclusive optic edge design minimises the risk of PCO, edge glare and vacuoles. It is the first to offer both a squared posterior edge that minimises PCO and a rounded anterior edge that minimises glare.

Tecnis (AMO) IOL Implant

Tecnis acrylic IOLs have a patented wave front design based on corneal measurements of actual cataract patients.

Tecnis IOL incorporates the modified prolate anterior surface which induces negative spherical aberration in the lens which compensates for the positive spherical aberration of cornea thus resulting in safer, sharper vision for all patients as compared to other conventional monofocal IOLs.

Material-piece foldable UV absorbing polysiloxane material which is a proven biocompatible.

Optic design biconvex, with a modified prolate anterior surface and a square optic edge

Optic diameter: 6 mm, overall length: 13 mm

Blue, modified C PMMA haptics with haptic angulation of 6°

Refractive Index of 1.46 at 37°C
392–394 nm cut off.

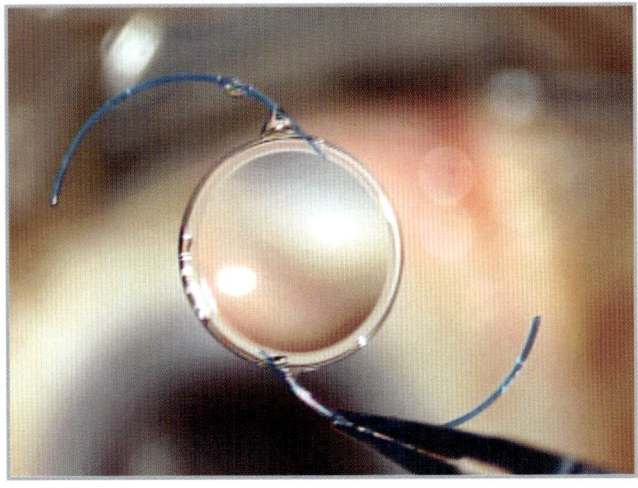

Fig. 19.5: Sensar (AMO) hydrophobic acrylic IOL implant

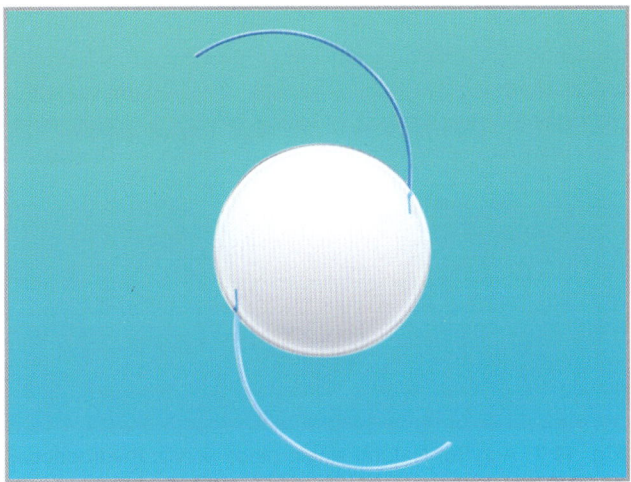

Fig. 19.6: Tecnis (AMO) IOL implant

Merits

(i) Proven biocompatibility.

(ii) Tecnis IOL can be implanted through an incision of 2.65 mm with the help of the AMO Emerald Series Unfolder System; thus chances of inducing astigmatism are further minimised.

(iii) Designed with patented Z-Sharp Optic Technology.

(iv) Wave front aberration analyses of human cornea led to its development. It significantly minimises spherical aberration.

(v) Specific OptiEdge designed optic reduces total ocular spherical aberration and improves functional vision. Anterior round optic edge minimises glares and halos, whereas sloping side edge of the optic further minimises halos and glares. Posterior 360° square edge minimises chances of PCO.

(vi) Provides better contrast sensitivity than a standard spherical IOL under mesopic and photopic conditions.

(vii) Provides good functional vision under varying light conditions by reducing glare, hence very effective in mesopic vision conditions and beneficial during night driving. Improves night driving by providing a 45-feet increase in identification distance.

(viii) Cap C heptics offer excellent centration with 98% rate of centration at 3 years postoperative.

AcrySof Natural

AcrySof Natural offers the benefits of AcrySof single piece with the addition of a 0.04% covalently bound yellow polymerise chromophore UV filter, which filters 61% more blue light than standard UV lenses. The optical quality of light filtration is designed to resemble the light filtering quality of the natural human crystalline lens.

This IOL claims to have adequate protections to the patients from damage caused by ultraviolet blue light (wavelengths from 400 nm up to 700 nm).

Filters the Harmful UV and IR Rays

It contains a proprietary, integrated polymer dye designed to filter both invisible infrared rays and visible blue rays of light, thus mimicking the protection provided by the natural human crystalline lens.

Restoration of normal adult precataract color vision

The features include 6.0 mm optic size and overall length of 13.0 mm and with anterior biconvexity at 0 degree angulation. High Refractive Index of 1.55 provides a thin Optic edge of 0.21 mm.

Since patients with advanced AMD had significantly higher blue light exposure. This might cause ocular damage, particularly in cases of AMD. Hence AcrySof Natural might be beneficial in cases of ARMD.

Hydrophilic Acrylic Lenses

One-piece, hydrophilic acrylic is made of a copolymer of hydrophilic and hydrophobic methacrylate (hydroxy ethyl methacrylate and/or poly hydroxy ethyl methacrylate) with a water content of 26%, (Ranging from 10% to 38%) namely, 2-hydroxyethyl methacrylate (HEMA) and methyl methacrylate, which is the main component of PMMA. The lens material also comprises ethylene glycol dimethacrylate (EDGMA) and a benzophenone ultraviolet absorbing agent.

Advantages

(i) It has a great resistance to damage.

(ii) **Refractive index: 1.44 to 1.46. IOL** unfolds in a controlled and safe manner, unlike silicone materials, which have the tendency to rapidly spring open.

(iii) This lens has a square edge to the optic and the haptics. The haptics have been designed to resist an asymmetrical capsular contraction, which provides the benefit of increasing support for the lens as the capsule contracts.

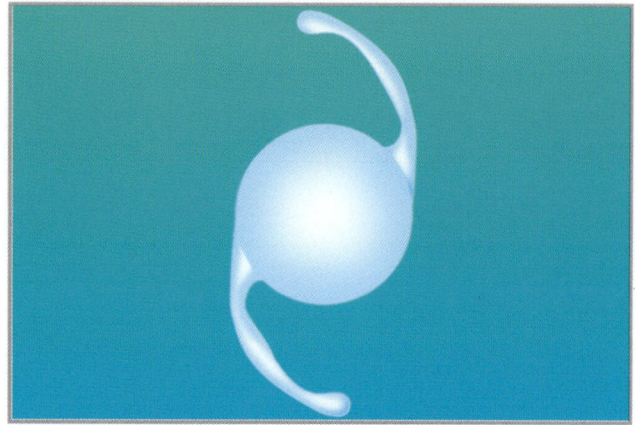

Fig. 19.7: AcrySof Natural single piece acrylic (hydrophobic) foldable posterior chamber IOL (addition of a 0.04 % covalently bound yellow polymerise chromophore UV filter)

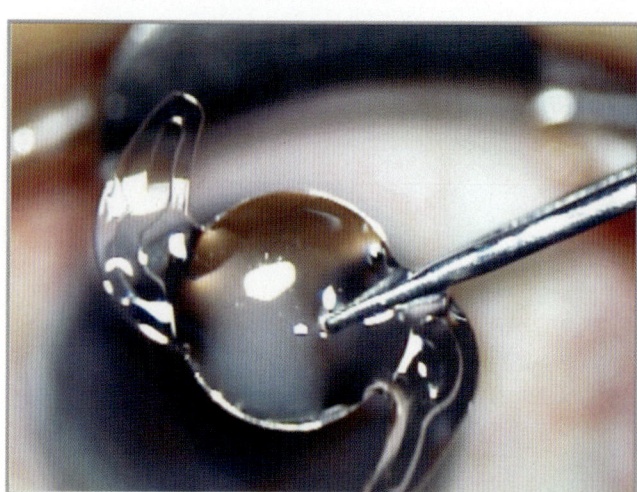

Fig. 19.8: Hydrophilic single piece acrylic IOL implant

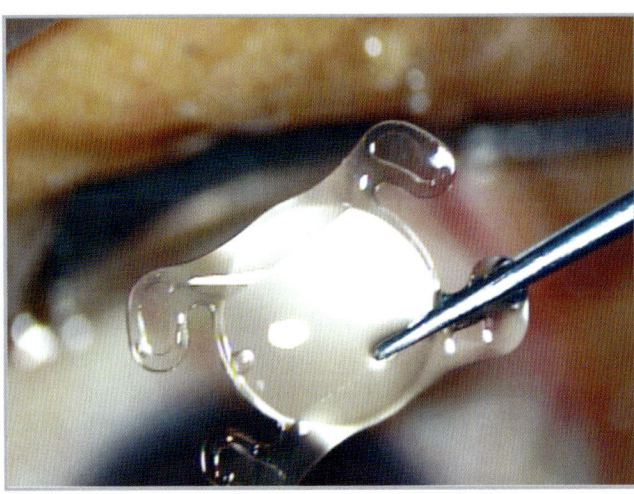

Fig. 19.9: Hydrophilic single piece acrylic IOL implant (advanced optic aspheric lens, square edge design foldable posterior chamber intraocular lens (Bausch and Lomb)

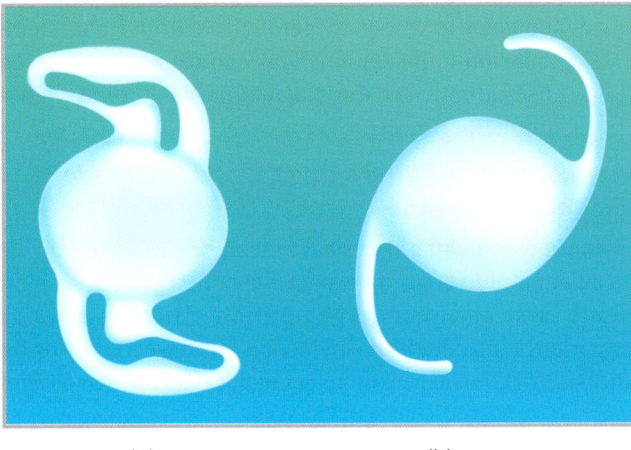

(a)   (b)

Fig. 19.10 (a) and (b): Hydrophilic single piece acrylic foldable posterior chamber intraocular lens (Appa Acryflex)

(iv) **UV blocker:** Acreos (B and L) IOL material has a built-in UV blocker that effectively blocks damaging UV radiation.

Disadvantages

(i) **Anterior capsule opacification:** Some surgeons have reported proliferation of anterior cell growth on hydrophilic acrylic lenses. There is a belief that the higher water content nature of these materials may contribute to a high degree of cell growth on this lens material.

(ii) **Opacification of IOL implantation:** Opacification of IOL implantation has been reported in cases of acrylic hydrophilic IOL implant. Author himself has explanted six acrylic IOL implants in the last six years.

(iii) **High Water content** may make this IOL prone to intraoperative contamination and theoretically carries a higher risk of endophthalmitis. However,

we could not correlate such an incidence in our experience.

There are several designs and brands globally available in acrylic hydrophilic series. Broad and Z-pattern design (Rayner) and square edge design (Bausch and Lomb) IOL implants are prototypes in this series. Appasamy, Auro labs, Acritec, Ocuflex are among a few other common and popular brands in India. Authors have used most of these IOL implants with good results; however, each and every IOL implant carries certain specific features in materials and design which are beyond the purview of this chapter due to diversity and paucity of space.

Technical Specifications of, Akreos (Adapt Acrylic Lens /Advanced Optic Aspheric Lens from Bausch and Lomb), Square Edge Design Foldable Posterior Chamber Intraocular Lens

Material optic and Haptics	Hydrophilic Acrylic copolymer with UV absorber
Overall length	Varying as per Diopteric power of IOLs
	11.0 mm (10 to 15.0 Dioptres)
	10.7 mm (15.5 to 22 Dioptres)
	10.5 mm (22.5 to 30 Dioptres)
Optic diameter	6.0 mm
Optic design	Biconvex, Aspheric anterior and posterior
A Constant	118.8
Haptic angulation	0°
Refractive Index When lens is in the eye (at 35° C):	1.458
Wet Lens at 20 degree	1.459

Technical Specifications of Appa Acryflex Foldable Posterior Chamber Intraocular Lens

Material optic and Haptics	Hydrophilic Acrylic copolymer with UV absorber
Overall length	Varying as per Diopteric power of IOLs
	11.0 mm (10 to 15.0 Dioptres)
	10.7 mm (15.5 to 22 Dioptres)
	10.5 mm (22.5 to 30 Dioptres)
Optic diameter	6.0 mm
Optic design	Biconvex, Aspheric anterior and posterior
A Constant	118.8
Haptic angulation	0°
Refractive Index When lens is in the eye (at 35° C):	1.458
Wet lens at 20 degree	1.459

Silicone Lenses

The silicone IOL enjoys the privilege of being first foldable IOL material which was approved by the FDA in 1989. The IOL was a three-piece silicone IOL having refractive indices of 1.41 (low as compared to 1.45 to 1.50 at present). The technique of IOL insertion had an inherent constrain of folding due to thick optics; hence a relatively large incision was mandatory. Second generation (SLM-2) lenses were introduced over ten years ago and developed to address those concerns. These second generation silicone lenses, with a slightly higher (1.46–1.47) refractive index, helped with foldability and implantation through a smaller incision.

The Cee On Edge model 911 is a foldable three-piece silicone optic-PVDF haptic design. The optic material has a refractive index of 1.46 and the optic rim has a square truncated edge to prevent PCO.

These lenses apply the Z-sharp technology to modify the surface of IOLs to produce a negative spherical aberration that would compensate the positive aberration of the cornea. This causes an improvement in contrast sensitivity to 100%.

Material Specifications

Material Structure	Polydimethyl siloxane (1st generation)
	Polydiphenyl siloxane (2nd generation)
Refractive Index 1.41	(1st generation)
1.47	(2nd generation)
Water Content	< 1.0 %

Sof Port (Silicone Lens /Advanced Optic Aspheric Lens from Bausch and Lomb), Foldable Posterior Chamber Intraocular Lens

Haptic angulation	0°
Material optic	Silicone Class I, copolymer with UV absorber
Haptics	Blue extruded PMMA, Modified C, 5 degree angulation
Overall length	13.0 mm
Optic diameter	6.0 mm
Optic design	Biconvex, Aspheric anterior and posterior

360 degree anterior/posterior square edge

A Constant	118.0
Refractive Index	
When lens is in the eye	
(at 35°C):	1.43

IOL is implanted through the Easy Load Lens Delivery System.

Demerits (Silicone IOL implants)

(a) **Incidence of PCO:** Silicone IOL are known to have a higher incidence of PCO as compared to hydrophobic IOL. Average incidence of PCO is around 25% after 30 months as compared to 12% to 14% after hydrophobic IOL implants of 36 months. Incidence of PCO is found to be 42–45% in cases of PMMA lenses.

(b) **Reduced usable optic:** Like other hydrophobic acrylics with lower refractive indices, some silicone lenses incorporate a controlled central thickness concept, in order to permit foldability and small incision implantation. This can result in a reduced useful optic for the patients particularly at higher diopteric powers.

Application of Square Edge Optic Design in Silicone IOLs

Some newer silicone lenses have incorporated square edges, in an attempt to control the significant cell growth seen on some first and second generation silicones. In our experience, no conclusive evidence was observed by us on the basis of clinical performances of this material and design.

Rollable /Ultra thin /Micro IOL

The rollable lens is an essential requirement of modern micro phaco surgery and microincision cataract surgery through a sub one mm incision. However, these IOLs need a little large incision for insertion. Rollable lenses can be inserted through a minimal incision ranging from 1.3–1.6 mm. The lens is placed on a special injector and rolled into a thin rod on inserting the plunger. When the lens is pushed through the injector it slides into the bag and slowly unfolds.

Various models of Ultra thin IOLs are available in the market. The specifications of commonly available thin IOLs are as in Table 19.1.

Table 19.1: Microincision IOLs

S.No.	Specification	Thinoptx	Micriol	Acrismart
1	Incision size	1.4–1.5	1.75–1.90	1.75–1.90
2	Optic zone	5.5 mm	5.5 mm	5.5mm
3	Total length	11.2 mm	11.0 mm	11.0 mm
4	Optic Geometry	Biconvex /Equiconvex	Biconvex/Equiconvex	Biconvex/Equiconvex
5	Profile	Plate haptic	Plate Haptic	Sharp-edged
6	Material	Hydrophilic acrylic18% WC	Hydrophilic acrylic 24%WC	Acrylic 25%WC
7	Insertion	Rollable	Foldable	Foldable

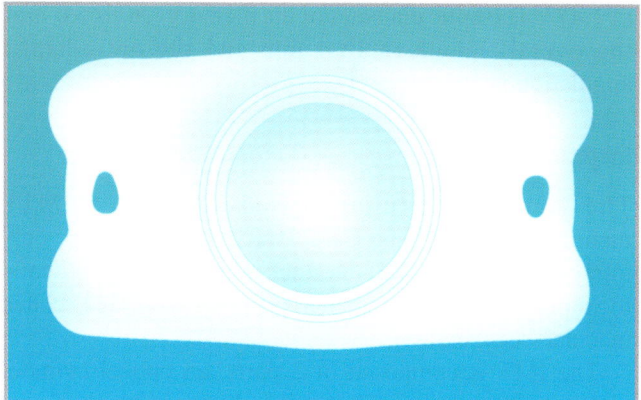

Fig. 19.11: Thinoptx Ultra thin Rollable IOL

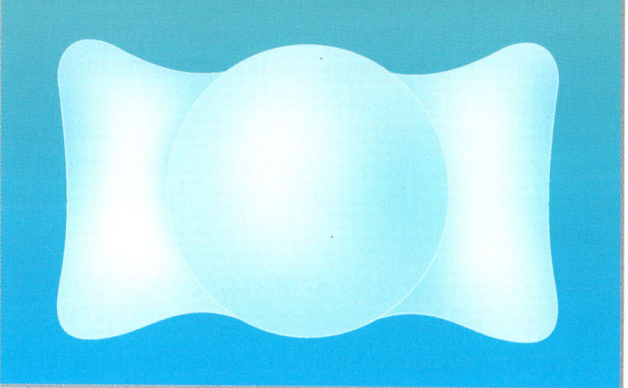

Fig. 19.12: Ultra thin IOL for MICS

The Ultra smart lens is a refractive design lens made up from 26% water content HEMA material, which had proven itself to be the calmest foldable IOL, inside the eye. The Benz HEMA is an ideal material for foldable IOLs for its proven records. The HEMA is more Biocompatible than the other material. The physical and chemical properties of the lens are stable than other materials.

The Design of the Lens

- The optics is Equibiconvex and the special haptic design with slots to prevent buckling or antero-posterior movement postoperatively.
- The haptics structure is stiff enough to withstand the forces of capsule contraction.
- The optical resolution is much better as compared to the Fresnel design.
- This design eliminates spherical aberration and improves the quality of vision.
- The nanotechnology lathe produces the finest part of the optics, free from astigmatic aberration.

- The lens can be injected through 1.8 mm incision. The smaller incision reduces the astigmatism. In case of the delivery of the trailing haptics, the lens swallow by itself because of the water content and settle in its original position in the bag without using any effort or instruments.

Specifications

- Optic Diameter : 6.00 mm
- Overall Length : 11.00 mm
- Positioning Holes : No
- Optic Design : Equibiconvex
- A Constant : 118.0
- Angulation : 0°

The lens is placed on a special injector and folded. The IOL is pushed gently through a plunger into the anterior chamber while maintaining only the injector's position at the site of incision only without placing the injector tip into the anterior chamber. When the lens is pushed through the injector it slides into the bag and slowly unfolds. Hence, the incision size can be restricted to sub 2 mm.

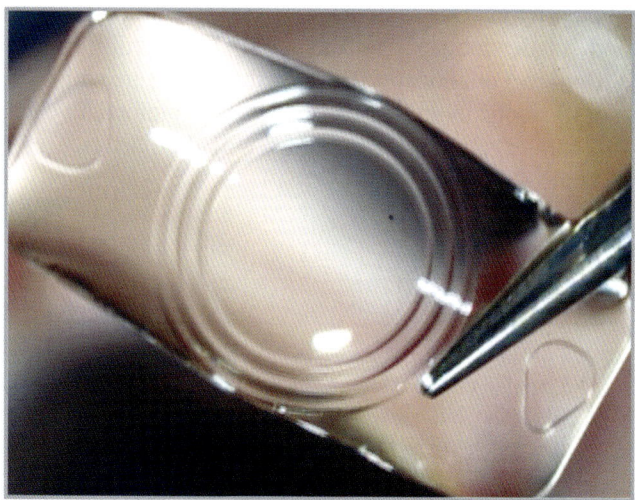

Fig. 19.13: Micriol thin IOL for MICS

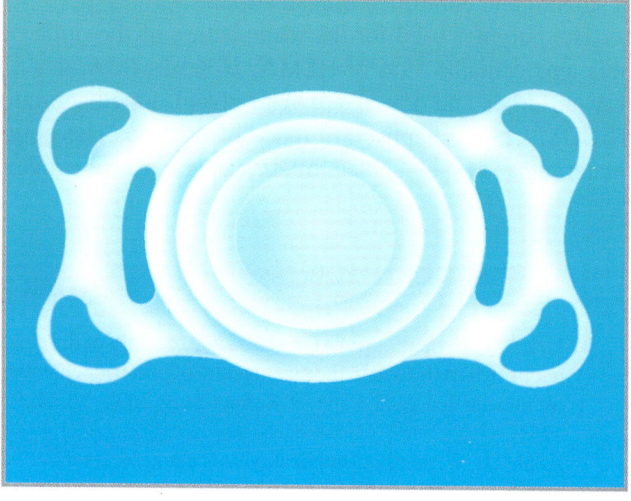

Fig. 19.14: Ultra smart (Appasamy) IOL for MICS

Reports are available of attempts to insert conventional hydrophobic IOLs like AcrySof through two mm incisions while using the same technique after certain modifications. In this technique, injector cartridge is cut at the tip and made like zero degree phaco tip. This modified cartridge is just kept at the site of incision and pushed through the two mm incision in the same manner as described for other thin IOLs.

Likely Disadvantages of Microincision/Rollable IOLs

(i) **Ring shadows/haloes:** Observed by a number of patients, particularly when they are exposed to glare and motor vehicle lights. However, most patients remain comfortable.

(ii) **YAG compatibility:** YAG capsulotomy is being considered difficult due to ultrathinness of IOLs and very close proximity to the posterior capsule. The incidence of PCO was found to be less than 10% after the follow-up period of more than three years. We did not notice any difficulty while performing YAG laser capsulotomy in these cases. Energy required for this procedure remained within 1.5 MJ. We have attempted to break the microincision IOL by direct exposure to YAG beam. However IOL remained unaffected up to 2 MJ except normal pitting. IOL sustained against tear up to direct exposure of 7 MJ. Hence, this may not be affected even during YAG iridotomy procedure in case of direct exposure.

Memory Lens

The memory lens manufactured by CIBA Vision is the prefolded acrylic IOL available in the market. The cartridge with the lens is kept at a temperature of 8°C. Following intraocular insertion the lens unfolds slowly under the affect of body temperature (approximately 15 minutes) providing a smooth and controlled implantation.

The polymer used for the manufacture of the optic of this lens contains 59% of HEMA, 16% of MMA, 4% of UV absorber and 1% of ethylene glycol dimethacrylate (EGDMA). The haptics are made of prolene. The optic material has a water content of 20% and a refractive index of 1.473. The optic diameter of the memory lens is 6.0 mm, the overall length is 13.4 mm and the optic-haptic angulation is 10°.

Implantable Miniaturised Telescope

The implantable miniaturised telescope (IMT), manufactured by Vision Care, Israel is at present the only intraocular device available that is designed specifically to improve vision of patients suffering from age-related macular degeneration.

The IMT is composed of 2 parts, an optical cylinder and a carrying device. The optic cylinder is made of pure glass and the carrying device which resembles a PC IOL is made of black PMMA. The anterior part of the optic extends anteriorly, for approximately 1 mm through the pupil.

Patients with bilateral ARMD and visual acuity below 6/60 are undergoing trials with these lenses.

Light Adjustable Lenses

A light adjustable lens is under development having photosensitive silicone subunits with unpolymerised silicone subunits (macromere) that polymerise under laser application upon fine-tuning with a low intensity of light laser (light adjustable lens). The refractive power of the lens can be adjusted after implantation to give the patient a definitive refraction. This changes the overall power of the lens.

SUMMARY

In spite of the fact that foldable lenses have captured the imagination and the market, the PMMA lenses are still maintaining a strong hold in developing countries with reasonable success. However, in the years to come the popularity of IOLs which can be injected through smaller and smaller incisions will increase. There will also be a stress on accommodative lenses in the near future with more modifications in the present models (Accommodative and full range vision IOL implants will be discussed in a separate chapter).

BIBLIOGRAPHY

1. Izak AM, Werner L, Apple DJ, et al. Loop memory of different haptic materials used in the manufacture of posterior chamber intraocular lenses. J Cataract Refract Surg 2002; 28:1229–1235.

2. Apple DJ, Werner L. Complications of cataract and refractive surgery: A clinicopathological documentation. Tr Am Ophth Soc 2001; 99:95–109.

3. Foldable Intraocular Lenses: Evolution, Clinicopathologic Correlations, and Complications. Apple DJ, Werner L, eds., Slack Inc. NJ, USA, 2002.

4. Nishi O, Nishi K. Preventing posterior capsule opacification by creating a discontinuous sharp bend in the capsule. J Cataract Refract Surg 1999; 25:521–526.

5. Werner L, Apple DJ, Pandey SK. Postoperative proliferation

of anterior and equatorial lens epithelial cells. In: Buratto L, Osher RH, Masket S, eds., Cataract Surgery in Complicated Cases. Slack Inc., Thorofare, NJ, USA, 2000; 26: 399–417.

6. Kent DG, Peng Q, Isaacs RT, et al: Security of capsular fixation: Small- versus large-hole plate-haptic lenses. J Cataract Refract Surg 1997; 23:1371–1375.

7. Werner L, Pandey SK, Escobar-Gomez M, et al. Anterior capsule opacification: A histopathological study comparing different IOL styles. Ophthalmology 2000; 107:463–471.

8. Werner L, Pandey SK, Apple DJ, et al. Anterior capsule opacification: correlation of pathological findings with clinical sequelae. Ophthalmology 2001; 108:1675–1681.

9. Werner L, Apple DJ, Pandey SK, et al. Analysis of elements of interlenticular opacification. Am J Ophthalmol 2002; 133:320–326.

10. Werner L, Apple DJ, Izak A, et al. Phakic anterior chamber intraocular lenses. Int Ophthalmol Clin 2001; 41:133–152.

11. Vargas LG, Peng Q, Apple DJ, et al. An evaluation of three modern single piece foldable intraocular lenses: A clinico-pathological study in a rabbit model with special reference to posterior capsule opacification. J Cataract Refract Surg 2002; 28:1241–1250.

12. Javitt J, Brauweiler HP, Jacobi KW, et al. Cataract extraction with multifocal intraocular lens implantation: clinical, functional, and quality-of-life outcomes. Multicentre clinical trial in Germany and Austria. J Cataract Refract Surg 2000; 26:1356–1366.

13. Schmitz S, Dick HB, Krummenauer F, et al. Contrast sensitivity and glare disability by halogen light after monofocal and multifocal lens implantation. Br J Ophthalmol 2000; 84:1109–1112.

14. Legeais JM, Werner L, Werner LP, Abenhaim A, Renard G. Pseudoaccommodation: BioComFold versus a foldable silicone intraocular lens. J Cataract Refract Surg 1999; 25:262–267.

15. Pandey SK, Werner 1, Apple DJ, et al. Evaluation of an accommodative intraocular lens in human and rabbit eyes. 1nvest Ophthalmol Vis Sci 2002; ARVO abstract S17.

16. Apple J D, Ram J, Foster A, Peng Q. Elimination of cataract blindness: A Global perspective entering the new millennium. Surv Ophthamol 2000; 45:21–24.

17. BenEzra D. Cataract surgery and intraocular lens implantation in children (letter). Am J Ophthalmol 1996; 121:224–225.

18. Chasset R., Legeay G., Touraine J, -C, Arzur B., Fluoration du polyethylene par plasma froid: mouillabilite indice limite d' oxygen, coefficient de frotterment, Eur, Polym. 1, 21, 1,1 1–7, 1985

19. Eloy R., Parrat D., Tranminh DUC, Legeay G., Bechetoille A.: CF-plasma induced surface modification of PMMA intraocular lenses : in vitro evaluation of the inflammatory cell response, in press.

20. Centre ESCA de Nano Analyse et Technologic de surface.

21. Legeay F., Epillard F., Brosse J.-C.: Surface modification of natural or synthetic polymers by cold plasma, Ed. H.U. Boeing technomic pub., Lancaster, 29 39, 1984.

20

Multifocal and Accommodative IOLs

Col JKS Parihar sm, vsm and Lt Col Anirudh Singh

INTRODUCTION

The ophthalmic surgeon is posed by a challenge to give the best to his patient in the ever increasing diversity and types of intraocular lenses (IOL) available. Despite excellent visual recovery following foldable IOL implantation, loss of accommodation remains to be the burning issue for any ophthalmic surgeon or the patient.

Each and every patient expects to have excellent visual acuity for all purposes following modern phacoemulsification surgery. The very same concept was first applied to design IOL implant which should have the capability to provide satisfactory visual acuity for distant as well as for near vision, hence eliminating the essentiality of spectacles for either near or distant vision which is a common need of everyone. The concept of bifocal IOL is based on this principle only. The second generation IOLs in this series cater for intermediate distance and are known as multifocal IOL implants. However, none of these IOLs possesses accommodation or accommodative efforts; hence in true sense, it cannot be effective for multiple focuses and can't attain full range of vision as available with normal human crystalline lens.

Classification of Multifocal/Accommodative IOL Implants

Bifocal IOL Implants

Multifocal/zonal refractive IOL implants full optic diffractive IOL

Accommodative IOL Implants

Full range apodised diffractive IOL implants.

Bifocal IOL Implants

With the concept of bifocal IOL to provide good vision for both near and distance, the following IOL implantation was,

for the first time applied in an IOL from IOLAB. This IOL was too simple for the two zone zonal refractive lens. However, this IOL was not very friendly due to sharp zones for both near and distance.

In the common bifocal intraocular lenses which are currently available, the light distribution in the two main foci is 50% each. The result is a strongly reduced light intensity which leads to a decrease in the contrast visual acuity by the factor compared to monofocal intraocular lenses of an equivalent design. In this way, the contrast decreases to half the value.

Multifocal IOL Implants

The optical performance of multifocal intraocular lenses has improved in the last few years. The clinical results have also improved due to the application of the astigmatism-neutral small incision surgery. However, the inherent system has characteristics of asymmetrical light distribution of refractive multifocal diffractive lenses which restricted the application of such IOLs in routine practice at a larger scale.

Concepts/Characteristics of Multifocal Lenses

Refractive multifocal lenses, concept-wise are very simple. Such IOLs have an annular ring that gives either a distant or a near image. However, such a concept is not free from inherent problems of optical quality and scattering and contrast sensitivity.

(i) The multifocal lenses have a zonal-progressive refractive multifocal optic with five concentric zones.

(ii) All of the optic zones have distance and near in different proportions.

- 50% of the available light is devoted to distant vision.
- 13% to intermediate vision and 37% to near vision.

- The addition for near is 3.5 dioptres.
- The IOL is available from 6.0 to 30.0 dioptres in 0.5 dioptre steps.

(iii) These lenses should be implanted only after a careful patient selection. There have been reports about reduced contrast sensitivity following multifocal implantation which have been disputed by studies by Javitt et al in 2000. However, affected contrast visual acuity needs due attention while considering multifocal IOL implants.

MERITS OF REFRACTIVE MULTIFOCAL LENSES

(i) Conceptually simple

(ii) Each annular zone contributes to either distance or near vision

(iii) Provides multifocal vision

(iv) Excellent visual outcomes for near and distant visions and a good intermediate vision in a good number of cases. The zonal progressive refractive multifocal IOL implants cater for sufficient functional vision to enable patients to refrain from using spectacles for various common day-to-day activities as compared to monofocal IOL implants.

(v) Following activities have been found to have less restrictions while performing near vision activities without glasses in a good number of patients:
- Casual reading or viewing telephone numbers
- Shaving or putting on makeup
- Playing cards or activities like painting

(vi) Distance vision activities without glasses
- Usual daily activities
- Recognising objects across the street or to be able to read bus numbers or street signs.
- Daytime driving

(vii) Social and routine activities without glasses
- Watching television
- Walking up or down the stairs
- Casual outing
- Viewing movies or common sport activities.
- Social cultural activities.

(viii) Relative freedom from spectacles in approximately 90% of patients, especially after bilateral implants with multifocals because of good binocular coordination of vision.

(ix) Refractive technology.

Problems/Constraints of Multifocal IOL Implants

(i) Severe loss in the contrast visual acuity.

(ii) Varying width of the pupil leads to further reduction in the contrast visual acuity.

(iii) Image quality is affected by annular apertures and pupil size restrictions, since the patient's ability to read under a normal photopic pupil is severely affected.

(iv) The visual acuity is limited by the diameter of one zone due to diffractive effects, leading to disturbing scattered light having persistent disturbances particularly at night.

(v) Rings visible at night from the second image. Multifocal IOL produces certain unwanted images which resemble multiple feathers over the cap and the patient may appreciate these images as different concentric images or shadows. Such multiple images are formed on each and every surface of the multifocal IOL as light waves discriminate refractive surfaces as separate lenses. Hence, their mesopic vision is also grossly affected due to wide open pupil in the dark, thereby exposing all refractive zones for maximising the opportunity for light scattering that creates a complex ghost image formation.

(vi) Ring images may adversely affect near visual acuity under normal photopic conditions.

(vii) Absolute centration is essential to achieve precise and accurate functional outcome.

(viii) Most multifocal IOLs are madeup on a silicone platform; thus with a higher incidence of PCO and subsequent YAG capsulotomies which invariably, adversely influence the quality of multifocal vision in these IOLs.

Selection of Cases

Following types of patients are ideally suitable for multifocal IOL implantations:

Preoperative Considerations

(i) **An intense desire and being highly motivated to be less spectacle dependent:** Highly motivated persons who are willing to become a patient with the process to recognises it, may take several months to adapt to their new visual system.

(ii) **Age:** The age group 35 to 70 years.

(iii) Patients with flexible, easy going personalities.

(iv) Strong desires to be less dependent on glasses.

(v) Best-corrected visual acuity should be 20/40 or better at distance and J3 at near.

(vi) Hyperopic, presbyopic or having astigmatism less than 1.5 D.

(vii) Type of Cataract: Unilateral traumatic cataract or congenital cataract.

Functional and Occupational Requirements

A detailed history on this point is most crucial. Does the patient have any of the hobbies like painting, playing the piano, playing cards or billiards or is he just the usual avid reader?

Patients often complain of the difficulty in multi-tasking post IOL surgery with monofocal lens implant. This category of patients is the one to target for.

EXCLUSION CRITERIA

Preexisting Ocular Diseases/Criteria

(i) Patients with best corrected visual acuity worse than 20/80.

(ii) Significant glaucoma, corneal dystrophy, dry eyes, uveitis, and posterior segment involvement like ARMD.

(iii) Irregular and high corneal astigmatism (more than 1.0 D) should be avoided as High astigmatism reduces near visual function as well as emmetropia may not be possible in this group.

(iv) Patients with abnormally long or short eyes due to more inaccuracy in IOL power calculations.

(v) Patients with pupils smaller than 2.5 mm.

(vi) The contralateral eye has a monofocal IOL implant. It is recommended to avoid this type of patients since binocular accommodative effort with uniocular monofocal IOL implant may not be effective or acceptable to the patient.

(vii) History of previous refractive surgery.

Relative Exclusion

(i) Hypersensitive patients to visual symptoms or those who have demanding lifestyles: should be avoided as minor visual disturbances with multifocal IOL implants may give annoying adjustment reactions.

(ii) Occupational night drivers: Glare, even for a transient period will be intolerable.

Intraoperative Exclusion Criteria

(i) Intraoperative complications, where foldable IOL implantation is not possible.

(ii) Injury to the pupillary sphincter.

(iii) Proper centring of the IOL is in question.

PECULIARITIES OF IOL POWER CALCULATION

Most precise IOL power calculation is an essential requirement for optimum desirable postoperative visual results. Precise preoperative measurements are essential factors to achieve IOL power accuracy. The ultimate key to success of multifocal IOL implantation is based on meticulous evaluation and determination of desired postoperative refraction, average K reading, axial length and measurement of anterior chamber depth in addition to excellent surgical skill and a highly motivated patient.

Power calculation by an IOL master is an ideal situation. However, in case of conventional biometry, following tips are highly beneficial:

(a) Periodic calibration of the biometry and keratometry instruments.

(b) Carefully review biometry and keratometry on the patient.

(c) Develop your own personalised surgeon constant. This consists of A-constant, anterior chamber depth and/or surgeon factor.

(d) Use a third generation IOL power formula that's based on the AC depth.

(e) For best results: put multifocal on both the eyes.

Intraoperative Peculiarities

Surgical Technique

Precision in a surgical technique, at each and every step is the most crucial factors which influences the success and final outcome of multifocal IOL implantation.

(i) Incision should be less than 2.4 mm.

(ii) A good circular and well-centreed capsulorrhexis ranging between 5 mm and 5.5 mm is most suitable.

(iii) Intact capsular bag and secure placement of the IOL within the bag.

Types of Common and Popular Multifocal IOLs

Few common and popular multifocal IOLs are as follows:

The Bifocal *Acri.Tech Twin Set

*Acri. Tech developed an absolutely new combination of diffractive ultrathin two foldable lenses with asymmetrical light distribution for bilateral implantation. IOLs are manufactured by Acritec (Berlin, Germany).

Acri. Tech twin set IOLs are based on the concept of asymmetrical light distribution in the far and near focus principle 70 : 30.

In the common multifocal or bifocal intraocular lenses which are currently available, the light distribution in the two main foci is 50% each. The result is a strongly reduced

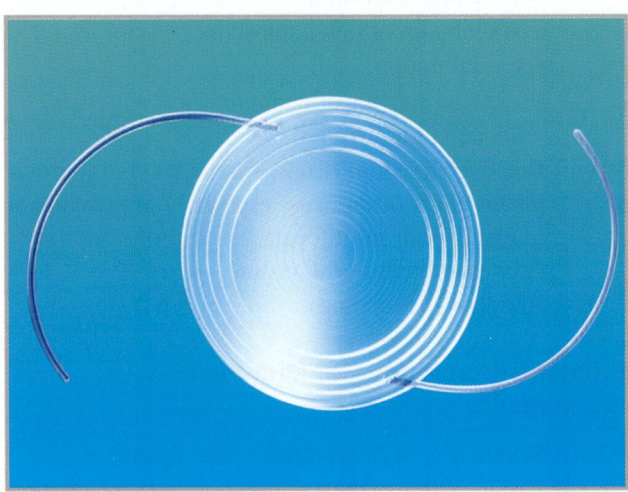

Fig. 20.1: Acri.Twin 737 D/733 D

light intensity which leads to a decrease in the contrast visual acuity by the factor 2 compared to monofocal intraocular lenses of an equivalent design. In this way, the contrast decreases to half the value.

Based on the concept of K Jacobi to allocate the light distribution in the near as well as in the far focus to one eye each and thus to considerably improve the contrast visual acuity and the visual acuity in the near and far focus compared to symmetrical multifocal lenses, the newly developed *Acri. Tech bifocal intraocular lenses, in contrast, are characterised by an asymmetrical light distribution. The dominant eye is implanted with a bifocal lens with a light distribution of 70% for the far focus and 30% for the near focus. The accompanying eye will receive an intraocular lens with a light distribution of 70% for the near focus and 30% for the far focus. As a result, a considerable improvement of the contrast can be achieved. The contrast visual acuity is only reduced by the factor 1.4 compared to monofocal lenses. This means that the contrast decreases only 28% compared to monofocal intraocular lenses. In this way, the asymmetrical light distribution results in an improvement of the contrast visual acuity of almost 50% in comparison to the symmetrical bifocal intraocular lenses.

Salient features of twin set bifocal IOL implants are as follows:

  (i) Two models, 737 and 733
  (ii) 737 distant centric, 733 near centric
  (iii) 737.70% for distance 30% near to be implanted in the dominant eye
  (iv) 733.70% near, 30% distance, to be implanted in the nondominant eye
  (v) Optic size: 6.0 mm, Overall length 12.5 mm
  (vi) Haptic angulations 5° to the front
  (vii) Haptic design helicoidal, madeup of Acri. Loop
  (viii) Optic design aspheric, biconvex, equiconvex, diffractive, bifocal madeup of Polydimethyl-siloxane + 4.0 D power addition, in the near focus. Asymmetrical distribution of near and distance focus.

Merits of bifocal *Acri. Tech Silicone Lenses

Addition of + 4 Dioptre for Independence of the Pupil Width

The bifocal *Acri. Tech lenses offer a supplementary addition of +4 D, so that a well-focused vision from infinite to a distance of 25 cm is made possible. These lenses are designed in such a way that in addition to the far focus obtained from the 6 mm diffractive/refractive optic the diffractive Fresnel structures create a supplementary "near focus" of +4 D. In contrast to the refractive bifocal lenses, no limitation due to the pupil width exists and the function of the lenses is independent of centration.

Ultra Thin lenses through Microstructuring of the Optical Margin

The bifocal *Acri. Tech silicone lenses include a microstructure of the optical margin which results in a significant increase in the refractive power. From the Fresnel lenses, the effect of focusing by diffraction has been known for a long time. By radial microstructures, light rays are diffracted within the quality of 10^{-3} mm. Each diffraction order of a Fresnel zone corresponds to one focus. The brightness of the foci is determined by the depth of the microstructures. The Fresnel structures can be calculated in such a way that in addition to several sub-foci, two main foci—one near focus and the other far focus—originate. For this reason, the simplified term for these lenses is bifocal, strictly speaking, even though they are multifocal lenses. However, the Fresnel structures can also be calculated in such a way that all rays are united in one focus. This principle is applied in the bifocal *Acri. Tech twinset lenses, thus reducing the central thickness of the lenses by at least 60% when compared to usual intraocular lenses. In this way, e.g. the central thickness of an intraocular lens with a refractive power of +35 D is reduced to 1 mm only. Due to the Fresnel structures, the single zones of the optical margin are designed in such a way that they have exactly the same focus as that of the central refractive area of the optic, so that a mutual image is created by all zones. (The principle of an optic construction without diffractive supplementary addition). The amount of scattered light produced by the microstructure of the margin is negligible. At a visual angle distance of 0.1° from the main focus, 1/10,000th of the light intensity is in the main focus, at a distance of 1° already only 1/10, 000th, and at a visual angle distance of 2° no scattered light can be observed any longer.

Completely Usable 6 mm Optic in Both Foci and over the Whole Diopteric Range

Disregarding the microstructure of the marginal area, the entire 6 mm optic can be fully used by the patient. The diffractive marginal zone is exactly adjusted to the refractive central portion, so that a far focus is created by the whole 6 mm optic. This is of vital significance, especially in the high diopteric range. Also, in this way, the juvenile patient, who is still capable of wider pupil opening, may have a full 6 mm optic available and is not disturbed by marginal phenomena. As it originates from diffraction, also the supplementary addition of +4 D is independent of the pupil width, so that the *Acri. Tec Twin Set lenses offer an optimum bifocal image in over the entire diopteric range of the bifocal lens 737 D with 22 D refractive power and +4 D near addition. The ideal curve results from the diffraction limit of a 6 mm optic. Both MTF curves demonstrate the excellent optical imaging quality.

Aspheric Geometry

Aspherical design of intraocular lens improves the optical imaging quality in terms of spherical aberrations and to obtain a sharper image. Aspherical design of intraocular lenses made up of silicone enhances contrast visual acuity due to minimal optical aberrations.

Stable Position in the Capsular Bag by New Helicoids Haptic

Helicoids haptic design of AcriTech IOL provides good stability inside the capsular bag despite thin optics. In addition, the haptics made up of PVDF, a biocompatible polymer claims to have adequate radial flexibility while offering axial stabilisation of the lens.

Ultrapurified Polydimethyl Siloxane

To increase the refractive index of silicone, modifications of the basic structure are required, usually phenylixation. However, the share of phenyl siloxane used in the *Acri. Tech silicone lens has a refractive index of 1.430. It offers a long-term tolerance and has been implanted as monofocal lenses internationally for a longer period of time.

Recommendation

The first implantation (in most cases into the leading eye) should be carried out with the IOL type 737 D with 70% of the light intensity in the distance focus. In the accompanying eye, the IOL type 733 D with 30% of the light intensity in the distance focus has to be implanted.

MF4 IOL

- Ioltech La Rochelle France
- Single piece, biconvex hydrophilic acrylic
- 3 point fixation: "tripod" design
- Optic dia. 6.00 mm, Total dia. 10.5 mm

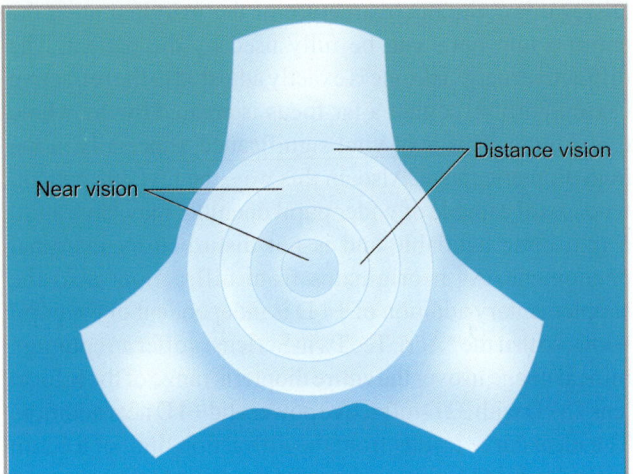

Fig. 20.2: MF4 IOL

- 4 refractive zones, alternating near and distance.
- Near centric: Add 4.00 D.

ZONAL REFRACTIVE LENSES

Array Multifocal IOL: Manufactured By AMO

How the Lens Works

The Array IOL is a zonal progressive refractive multifocal IOL implant with distant dominant design which provides patients a sustained range of variable focus at distance, intermediate and near vision need. The functional outcome is augmented with bilateral implantation of multifocal lens implant. The configuration and design is identical to AMD's existing foldable monofocal IOL(SI-40NB) but with multifocal technology on the anterior surface.

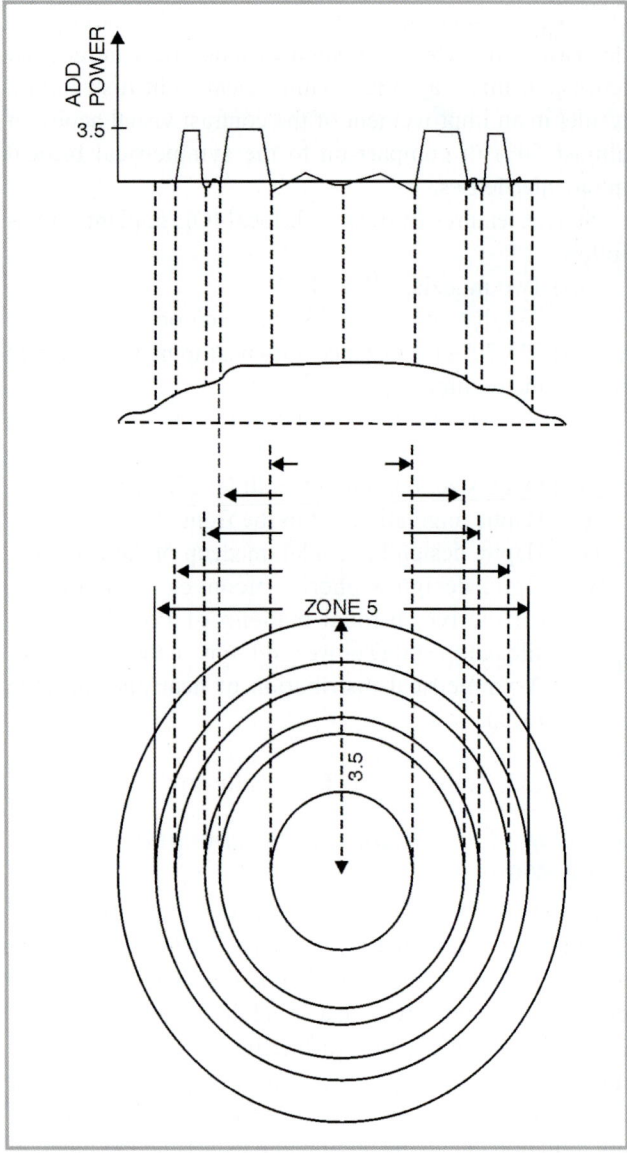

Fig. 20.3: Array multifocal IOL: Principle of optics

Other specifications are as follows:
- Silicone: SLM-2/UV Multifocal surface
- Angulated C haptic (extruded PMMA)
- Refractive index 1.46
- Zonal progressive multifocal optics with 5 concentric zones. Zones 1, 3 and 5 are weighted for distance, while zones 2 and 4 are weighted for near.
- Lens design is distance dominant
- 50% Distance: 13% Intermediate, 37% Near
- Addition for near distance is 3.5 D which translates to approximately 2.65 D at the spectacle plane.

TECNIS MULTIFOCAL (ZM 900/AMO)

Tecnis multifocal IOL offers a continuous range of high-quality, high-contrast distance and near vision in a range of light conditions.

The modified prolate anterior surface which induces negative spherical aberration in the lens compensates for the positive spherical aberration of cornea thus resulting in safer, sharper vision in all light conditions, especially in low light (5 mm pupil) condition.

Characteristic Features

- Based on the diffractive technology and wave front design based on corneal measurements of actual cataract patients.
- 3-piece foldable, UV absorbing polysiloxane material
- Refractive index of 1.46
- 12.0 mm overall length
- Biconvex 6 mm monofocal optic
- Square edge designed optic
- PVDF Hepatics with Cap-C design
- +4D is the near add power.

Merits

- Can be implanted through microincisions of 2.8 mm; thus chances of inducing astigmatism become minimal.

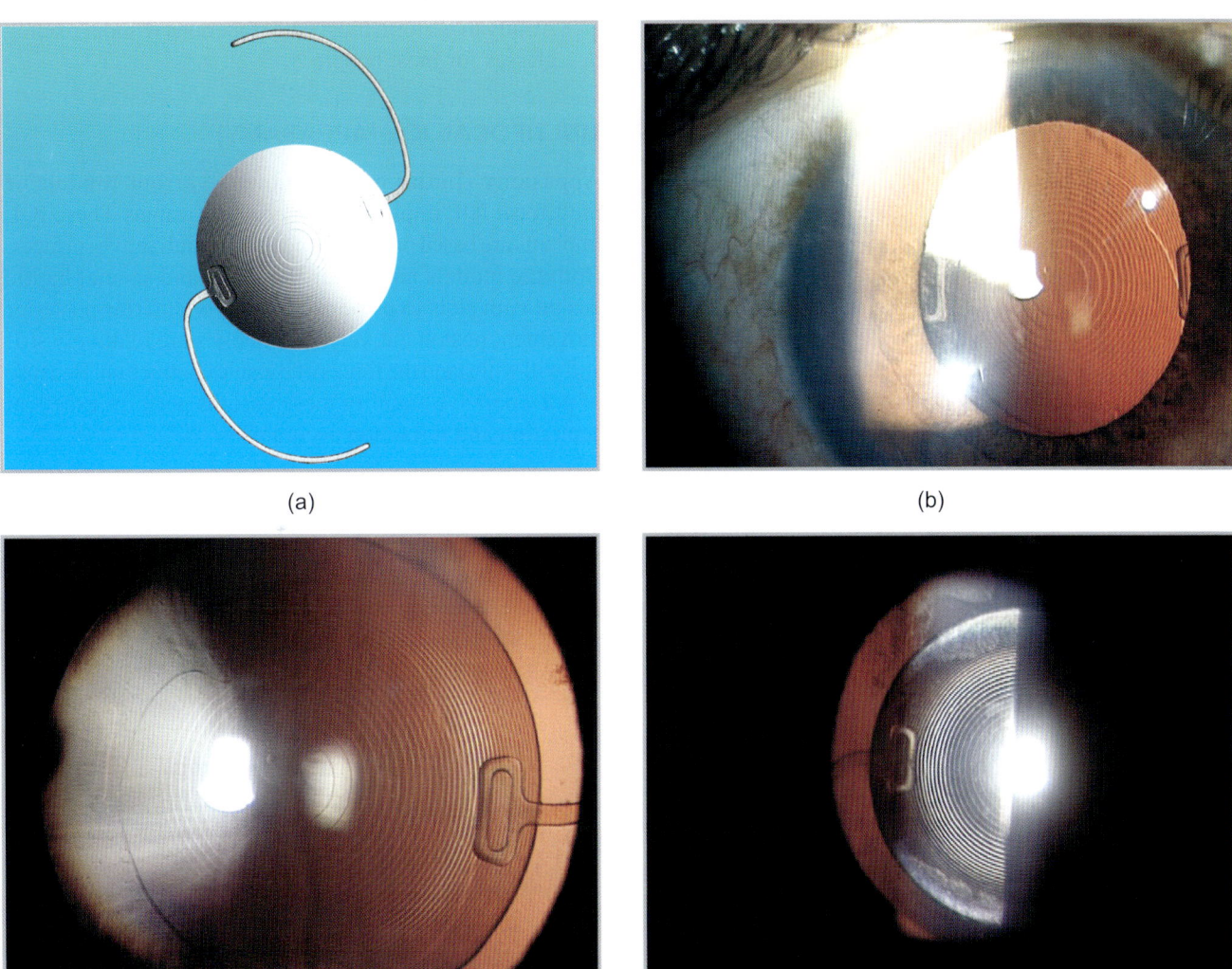

(a) (b)

(c) (d)

Figs 20.4: (a), (b), (c) and (d) Tecnis multifocal (ZM 900/AMO)

- Reducing total ocular spherical aberration.
- Improves functional vision.
- Improves night driving simulator performance, providing a 45 feet increase in identification distance.
- Less chances of PCO due to posterior 360 degree square edge of the optics.

REZOOM LENS (AMO)

The ReZoom (AMO) multifocal IOL with balanced view optics is a second-generation refractive multifocal acrylic IOL that provides excellent multifunctional vision for qualified hyperopes—especially those with cataracts and a loss of accommodation, hyperopic cataract patients with greater independence from glasses than monofocal IOLs.

Characteristics Features of ReZoom Multifocal IOL Implant

(i) 3-piece multifocal hydrophobic acrylic material.
(ii) 6.0 mm optic, 13 mm Overall length.
(iii) Second-generation balanced view optics triple edge PC IOL design provides expanded distance-dominant zones and light distribution needed for good vision under a range of light conditions.
(iv) Angulated C haptic (extruded PMMA capsule fit haptics)
(v) Refractive index 1.46
(vi) Based on zonal progressive diffractive technology multifocal optics with 5 concentric zones proportioned to provide good visual function across a range of distances in varying light conditions. Certain modifications in the 4th ring as compared to array multifocal IOL.

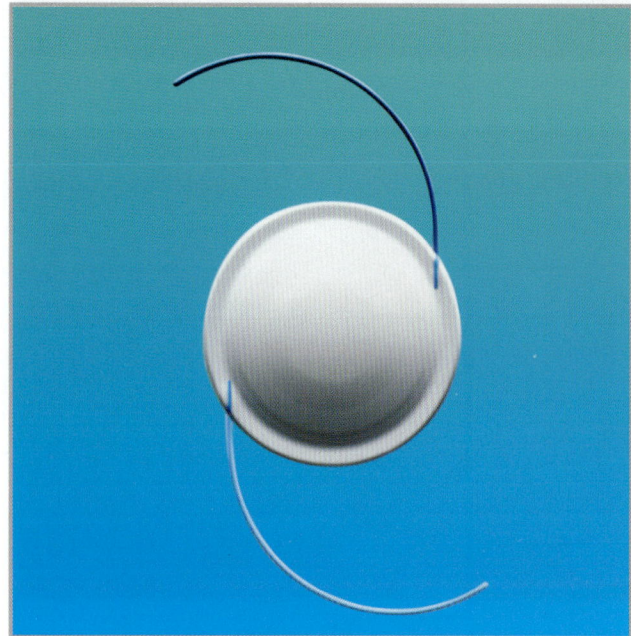

Fig. 20.5: ReZoom multifocal IOL implant

- Lens design is distant dominant. 50% Distance, 13% Intermediate, 37% Near
- Zones 1, 3 and 5 are distance dominant
- Zones 2 and 4 are near dominant
- Near add greater than crystalline
- Near-dominant zones provide +3.5 D near add power at the IOL plane which ultimately provides near add greater than the 2.0 D needed by most adults over 50*.

(vii) Aspheric transition between zones provides balanced intermediate vision.
(viii) Specific design minimises PCO as compared to those associated with double-square edge barrier designs.

Merits of ReZoom IOL Implantation

- Excellent distance vision during the day
- Independence from glasses for most activities
- "Natural" transition from seeing distance objects to near objects
- Ability to perform most daily functions without reading glasses for most people.

MULTIFOCAL IOL (APPASAMY)

Appasamy (India) has introduced various models of multifocal IOL implants in an economy range. These IOL implants are based on three zone variable refractive surfaces. Both the models have equi-biconvex and special haptic design with slots to prevent buckling or anterior-posterior movement postoperatively. The haptics are relatively stiff and will withstand the forces of capsule contraction. Because of postoperative stability these designs perform excellent centration and refraction accuracy.

Characteristics of Appasamy Multifocal Lenses

(a) **Lens design**
   (i) Refractive design
   (ii) Distance dominated
   (iii) + 4.5 diopter add
   (iv) Three zone
   - First zone: Distance dominant (Dia. 1.9 mm)
   - Second zone: Near dominant (Dia. 1.9 to Dia. 2.8 mm)
   - Third zone: Distance dominant (Dia. 2.8 to Dia. 6.0 mm).
(b) **Material:** Hema 26% water content, stable and more biocompatible than the other material. While IOL insertion, the delivery of the trailing haptics, the lens swallows by itself because of the water content and settles in its original position in the bag without using any effort or instruments.

(c) The perfect centration multifocal.

(d) The square edge designs of these models reduce PCO.

(e) These lenses may be injected through an unenlarged 2.2 mm wound even when of high power (up to +34.0 D).

Multifocal IOL (Appasamy)

- Optic Diameter: 6.00 mm
- Overall Length: 11.00 m
- Positioning Holes: No
- Optic Design: Equibiconvex
- A-Constant: 118.0
- Angulation: 0°

Constraints of Zonal Refractive IOL Implants

Multiple Refractive Surfaces without Slopping Optical Interface

(i) This is the kind of optical surface under normal photopic conditions, which will be somewhere about 2¼ 2.3, 2.4 millimetre pupil, zonal refractive lens (ReZoom IOL implants) acts exactly as it is designed to act as a monofocal distance lens. However, near visual acuity under normal photopic conditions may be grossly affected consequently. It's an inherent problem with zonal refractive lenses. Under normal photopic conditions, no energy is going to form the near image. It is all going to form the distance image.

(ii) Optical discontinuity of zonal refractive lens gives rise to a jagged appearance (again indicating area on slide). When light traverses through five zones of zonal refractive lenses, the surfaces do not act as a single optic surface but as five lenses superimposed upon itself making a very complex wave front equation. This results in an appreciation of "got to jump over" by the observer before he readjusts himself from distance visual acuity to near vision objects.

(iii) Energy system designed in zonal refractive IOL implants is inefficient to have ideal distribution of light under normal mesopic conditions. Approximately, 50% of the energy is consumed to form a near image. Since most of us are more comfortable in photopic light conditions as compared to mesopic conditions, this inadequate distribution of light energy for near and distance objects simulates working conditions into mesopic-like vision. Hence, five zones of optics may simulate like a jagged appearance of multiple secondary images. Over and above, frequent change in visual focus from distance to near and intermediate distances in variable sequences will simulate several unwanted images like piggy bag images; or slice to the belly of the image.

Adverse Effect on Mesopic Vision

Under normal mesopic conditions at night time, the pupil opens up. When the pupil opens up, the light now encounters all the 5 zones, maximising the opportunity for light scattering and maximising the opportunity for inefficiency of the light usage.

In this particular situation, starburst and glare particularly with oncoming traffic while driving at night is a problem.

FULL OPTIC DIFFRACTIVE IOL 3M OR PHARMACIA (PFIZER) 811 E

Diffractive Diffractive (28 Diffractive Zones)

Light goes into both distance and near powers from all zones.

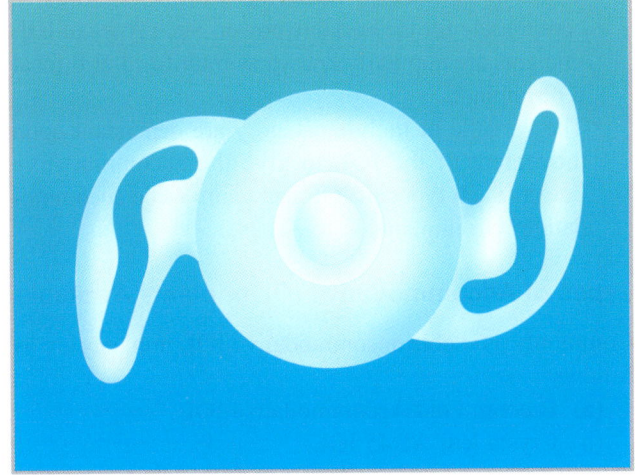 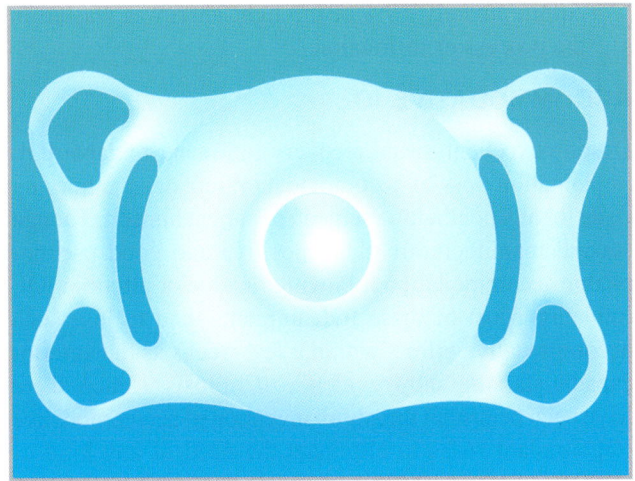

(a)   (b)

Fig. 20.6: (a) and (b) Appasamy multifocal IOL implant

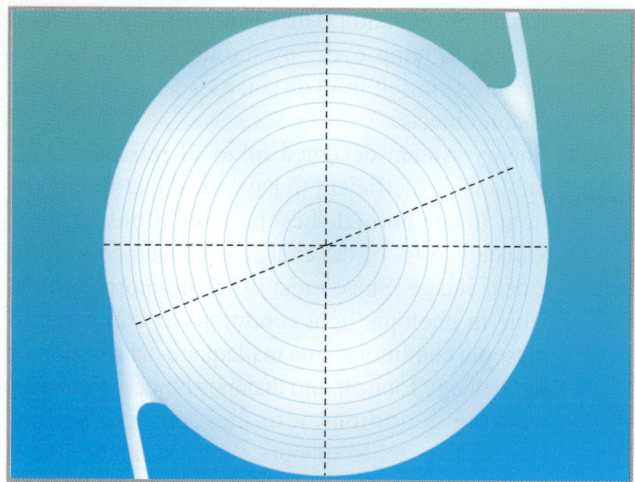

Fig. 20.7: Full optic diffractive IOL (3M or pharmacia (Pfizer) 811 E)

Advantages

(i) *Provides Multifocal Vision*

- It represents a technological advancement towards multifocality with less optical distraction in frequently varying light conditions.
- Acts as a full optic diffractive IOL implant.
- Provides better opportunity to have simultaneous vision, (near and distance objects) in different light conditions as compared to traditional multifocal IOLs which can provide either near or distance in one given point of light conditions. Hence, patient can read under normal light conditions.

(ii) *Reduced Pupil Dependency*

- Quality of vision is not adversely affected by the size of pupil in different light conditions.

Disadvantages

- Equal distribution of light energy for all pupils
- Potential for glare and halos at night
- Approximately 18% of the light energy is wasted in the process of diffraction.

ACCOMMODATIVE IOL

Despite excellent visual recovery following foldable IOL implantation, loss of accommodation remains the burning issue for any ophthalmic surgeon or patient himself. Though several manufacturers claim positive and good pseudophakic accommodation following flexible or ultrathin IOL implants. Most of these IOL implants tend to lose such accommodative efforts within a few weeks as the anterior capsule starts to show evidence of fibrosis. Hence, there have been persistent thrusts on invention of accommodative IOL implant so as to eliminate the need of any kind of refractive correction following cataract surgery. In other words emmetropia can be achieved in true sense and spirit for both near, distance or any intermediate distance.

Accommodative IOL implants involve special technology of manufacturing as well as of implantation technique.

Mechanism of Accommodative Action in Accommodative IOL Implants

The special design and mechanical properties of this IOL are stated to enable the lens to change power by a forward movement of the optic during the contraction of the ciliary muscle. However, such action has been provided by different mechanism and actions in different types of accommodative IOL implants as described with each type of IOL implants.

Merits of Accommodative IOLs

Accommodative IOL implant may eliminate the need for any kind of refractive correction following cataract surgery for multiple distances required for routine purposes. In other words, emmetropia can be achieved in true sense and spirit, for both near, distance or any intermediate distance.

Demerits/Constraints with Accommodative IOLs

(a) Essentially static lenses, whereas the entire concept of accommodation is a dynamic and active process.

(b) The present concept is based on a single plate IOL. Capsular collapse of the anterior on the posterior is inevitable with a resultant freeze of function.

(c) None of the present crop of IOL really fill a bag, leaving it lax. For a relax contact zonular concept to work, a partial bag which is loose and thus laxness leads to poor zonular tug relax functioning.

Classification of Accommodative IOL Implants

Accommodative lenses can be categorised into two categories: (a) Fixed and (b) Variable.

- Fixed categories of IOLs have multiple rings to compensate for the variable power. Such types of IOL implants are popularly known as multifocal or bifocal IOL implants.
- The variable or mobile category are dependant upon movement of the IOL to give the accommodative power. Such types of IOL can claim to be accommodative IOL implants in true sense.

Types of Accommodative IOL Implants Available

Commonly available accommodative IOL implants are as follows:

(a) Biocom Fold Accommodative IOL.

(b) Crysta lens AT 45 IOL.

(c) Visiogen Accommodative IOL System.

(d) Clamshell Variable Accommodating IOL.

(e) Accommodative 1 CU.

BIOCOM FOLD ACCOMMODATIVE IOL

The Biocom Fold, manufactured by Morcher Stuttgart, Germany.

  (i) It is composed of a hydrophilic copolymer of PMMA and polyHEMA with a water content of 28%.
 (ii) The circular haptic ring design of IOL prevents PCO formation.
(iii) Refractive index of 1.46.
 (iv) Its overall length is 10.0 mm and its biconvex optic, 5.8 mm. A peripheral bulging ring is connected to the optic via an intermediate, forward angled (10°) perforated ring section.
  (v) For near vision the accommodation efforts cause the centripetal force of the elastic hollow ring of the equator to narrow the peripheral ring, thereby steepening the intermediate ring section of the lens, which pushes the optical part forward.
 (vi) For distance vision, the elastic properties of the bulging ring and of the intermediate ring section of the lens return the optic to its primary position.

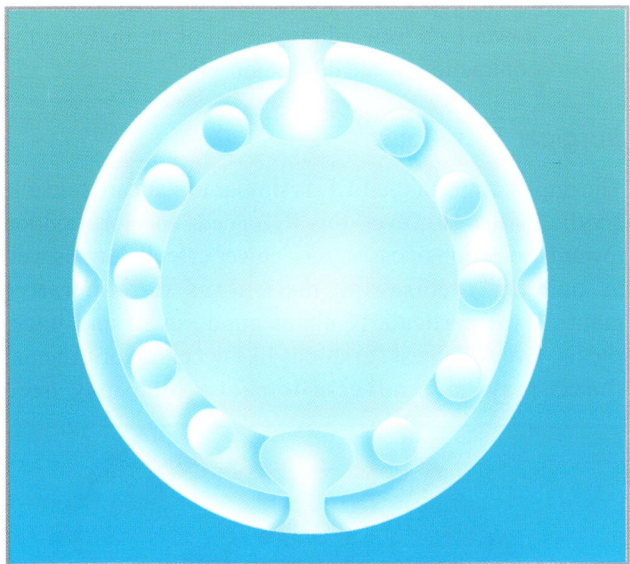

Fig. 20.8: Biocom fold accommodative IOL

CRYSTA LENS AT 45 IOL

Crysta lens AT 45 IOL is a modified plate haptic accommodative IOL implant which is manufactured by CandC Vision CA USA.

Specific Features

  (i) Modified plate haptic lens made from silicone polymer dimethylsiloxane (Biosil) material.
 (ii) The lens is hinged next to the optic and has small polyamide haptic which fixates firmly in the capsular bag. The grooves across the plates adjacent to the optic provides flexibility to the lens.

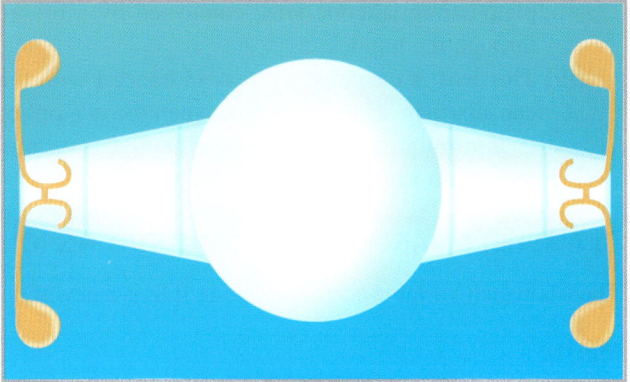

Fig. 20.9 : Crysta lens AT-45

(iii) Optic 4.5 mm
 (iv) Length 11.5 mm, loop to loop
  (v) Refractive index 1.432

Mechanism of Action

  (i) With pseudophakic accommodative effort, redistribution of the ciliary body mass ensues, resulting in increased vitreous pressure which will move the optic forwards anteriorly.
 (ii) Hinge incorporated to permit forward movement of the optic by minimising possible resistance.

VISIOGEN ACCOMMODATIVE IOL SYSTEM

  (i) The Visiogen, USA accommodating IOL system is a one-piece lens made from silicone.
 (ii) The lens has two major components (anterior and posterior), each having the general design of a

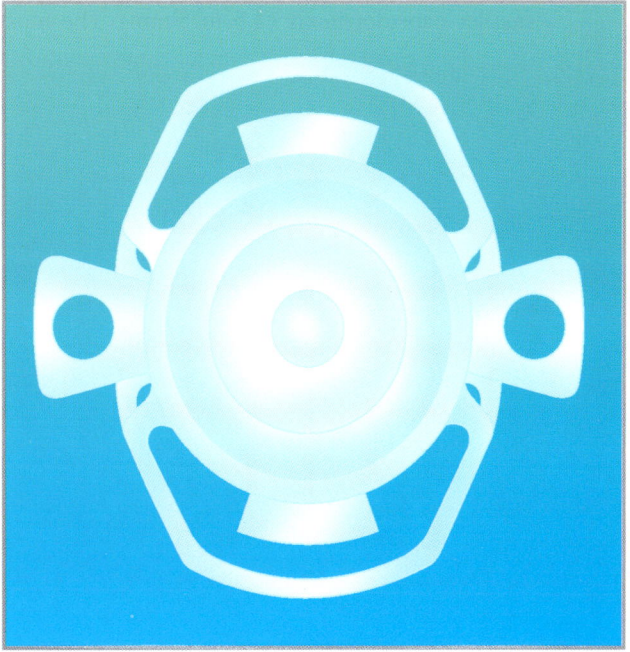

Fig. 20.10: VISIOGEN Accommodative IOL system

plate-haptic silicone lens, connected by a bridge through the haptics.

(iii) This lens is designed to work in concert with the capsular bag. The distance between the two optics is minimum in the unaccommodated state and maximum in the accommodated state.

CLAMSHELL VARIABLE ACCOMMODATING IOL

The Clamshell variable accommodating IOL is a new IOL.

Merits

(i) This IOL meets with the basic need of filling the bag fully so as to achieve effective and full accommodative efforts.

(ii) Simple to insert, simple to position.

(iii) Variable accommodating IOL can be implanted through an injective device through a standard 2.8 mm incision.

(iv) Functional: Unlikely to lead to any fibrosis in future.

(v) Most patients are 20/20 or better and they are very happy with the fact that they have no need for glasses.

(vi) An ideal IOL implant for clear lens extraction, correcting not only high myopia and high hyperopia but also of retaining accommodation.

Demerits/Constraints

(i) Significant PCO or subsequent YAG capsulotomy may adversely influence the pseudophakic accommodating mechanism.

(ii) Zero error phacoemulsification surgery through a smaller capsulorrhexis (4.5 to 5 mm). The most

difficult task remains to maintain an intact capsular bag. A capsule tear may compromise the intact capsular bag which may lead to loss of accommodative efforts.

ACCOMMODATIVE 1 CU

The Accommodative 1 CU, by Human Optics, Germany is manufactured from a hydrophilic acrylic material.

The author has adequate experience of this particular accommodative IOL. The technique of application of Human Optics Accommodative 1 CU IOL implant will be discussed in detail in the subsequent paragraph.

Special Characteristic Features of Accommodative 1 CU IOL Implant

(i) IOL is madeup of acrylic material.

(ii) The optical diameter of this lens is 5.5 mm with an overall diameter of 9.8 mm.

(iii) The refractive index of the lens material is 1.46.

(iv) The special design and mechanical properties of this IOL are stated to enable the lens to change power by a forward movement of the optic during contraction of the ciliary muscle.

Surgical Technique

The implantation of the 1 CU is similar to standard foldable acrylic lenses. However, this IOL needs special attention towards selection of cases, IOL power calculations as well as on very precise and meticulous intraoperative manoeuvres particularly about good, small and intact rhexis. Even slightest variations like eccentric or irregular rhexis may have adverse impact which may need

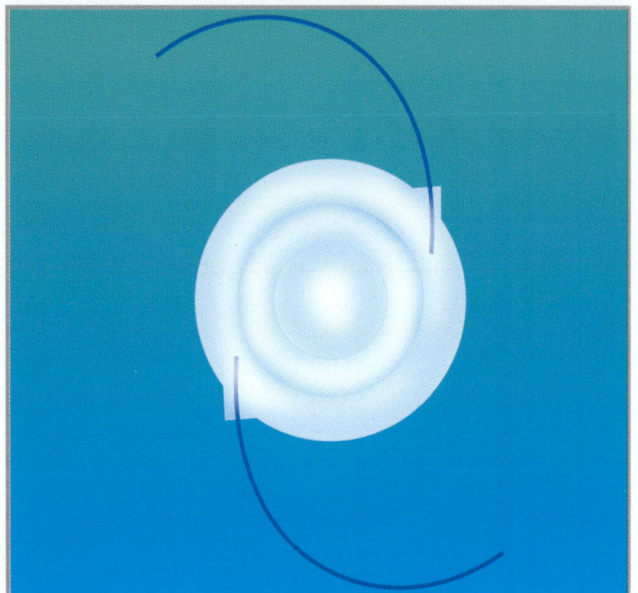

Fig. 20.11: The Clamshell variable accommodating IOL

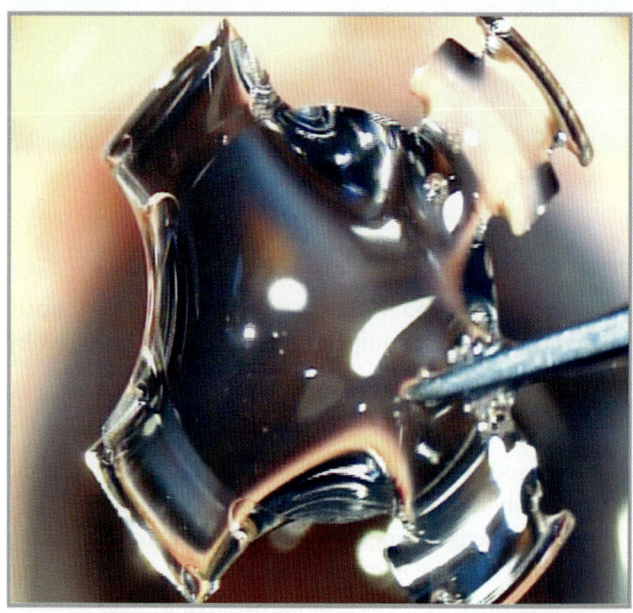

Fig. 20.12: Accommodative 1 CU IOL implant

abandoning of implantation of accommodative IOL implant and use of conventional foldable IOL implant.

Preoperative Evaluation for Accommodative IOL implantation

Patient Selection

All cases of cataract are not suitable for implantation of 1 CU, Human Optics Accommodative IOL implant. However, the following types of cases are being considered ideal for accommodative IOL implantation.

(i) Uncomplicated grade two to three cataract
(ii) Motivated and with a desire to accommodate
(iii) Good preoperative ability to accommodate
(iv) Myopic contralateral eye.

Excluding Criteria

Patient specific

• Mature or hard cataract.
• Conventional IOL including foldable IOL in the fellow eye.
• Any kind of prior surgery on the selected eye including laser treatment.
• Too high hyperopic or myopic eye with the axial length shorter than 22.0 mm and longer than 25.0 mm
• Preexisting glaucoma, pseudoexfoliation syndrome, uveitis, retinal involvements or any other ocular disease.
• Preexisting central corneal astigmatism greater than 1.0 diopter.
• Poor endothelial cell count.
• Large pupil: More than 6 mm of size.
• Phacodonesis and damaged zonules.
• Amblyopia.
• Preexisting diabetes or significant systemic involvement which may adversely influence visual acuity subsequently.

Relative Contraindications due to Intraoperative Constraints or Complications

• Capsulorrhexis larger than 5.0 mm.
• Eccentric, extended, or torn rhexis.
• Significant intraoperative complications rendering in the bag foldable IOL implant impossible.
• IOL implantation along with any other implant or device like with capsular tension ring.
• Damaged IOL.

IOL POWER CALCULATION

Accommodative IOL implants desire very accurate and high precision in IOL power calculation. The target refraction for the Accommodative 1 CU IOL implant should always be between 0.0 D and –0.5 D. Any significant variation from this deviation is likely to affect the final outcome. Viewing above, certain modifications in

estimated A constant are required for the different formula's and need to be incorporated.

The Manufacturer Recommends Special Attention towards Following Specifications

(i) Meticulous cross check on each lens power calculation. Biometry and keratometry data should be consistent with lens power calculation. Precisely large eyes tend to require a lower dioptre and short eyes need higher dioptres on the same manner, flatten corneal curvature will require a higher dioptre of IOL implant as compared to steeper corneal curvature which will require a lower dioptre due to higher corneal power.

(ii) Simultaneous IOL power calculation of both eyes even though only one eye is being considered for IOL implantation at that time. This will help to analyse variations and the possible outcome.

Selection of Mode of IOL Power Calculations

Non-Contact Optical Measurement Method by Zeiss IOLMaster™

Undoubtedly, optical measurement method by Zeiss IOLMaster™ provides excellent prediction of presumptive IOL power, since this method is based on non-contact evaluation of both corneal curvature and axial length, hence human error from both the patient and surgeon factors is practically eliminated. However, a meticulous database of the surgeon's own variation in A constant should be programmed in IOL master for precision in results.

Conventional Biometry

The technique of conventional biometry is affected by several factors related to indentation, human factors of the surgeon and patient both, as well as, data processing which is based on median of stored data. Such data may not produce satisfactory results as it may be based on data of different races and populations of western countries displaying genuine variations as well as in the readings obtained on either ends of the spectrum of refractive errors.

Multiple readings minimise extent of errors. Minimum 5 consecutive A-scan measurements per patient should be performed in each and every case. Of these five readings, extreme values on either ends of the readings should be discarded and the mean of the remaining axial length (AL) measurements should be considered. Needless to specify the essentiality of calibration of the A-scan on a regular basis to avoid unexpected and unpleasant results.

(a) **Axial length measurements by direct contact method:** In A-scan biometry, the value of the axial length measurement may be smaller due to induced contact pressure. Hence, an average correction contact factor of 0.2 mm to the measured axial length is to be added in readings. However, certain A-scan like OcuScan™ of Alcon does not require such modifications as it has already been incorporated in the program. Hence, it is advisable to study the user's manual of respective A scan before making any corrections in the axial length readings.

(b) Axial length measurements by immersion method: In immersion procedure, the ultrasonic probe and the cornea remain away from direct contact or indentation pressure by a fluid (gel of saline) as a transition medium. Hence, the contact factor corrections as applicable to direct contact applanation is not required in this technique.

PECULIARITIES IN KERATOMETRY

It is worth considering that different keratometry devices use special different refractive indices which need special attention.

Human optics recommends using the K-reading in millimetre and not in dioptre for the lens power calculation.

As per the manufacturer this carries significant impact on the presumptive IOL power.

Modifications in Different Formula's of IOL Power Calculations

The manufacturers recommend certain modifications in different formula's for IOL power calculations and suggest to add the surgeon's factor. In our view, such modifications and requirements necessitate further self introspective analysis, and results can accordingly be customised.

Surgical Technique for Implantation of the Accommodative 1 CU IOL Implant

Incision, Rhexis and Hydroprocedures

Quality outcome is always based on quality performance. This is equally applicable on accommodative IOL implant technique which demands a very high order of accuracy and precision.

The most important aspect is an ideal and relatively smaller rhexis preferably less than 5 mm. It is essential to have adequate and sustained accommodative action

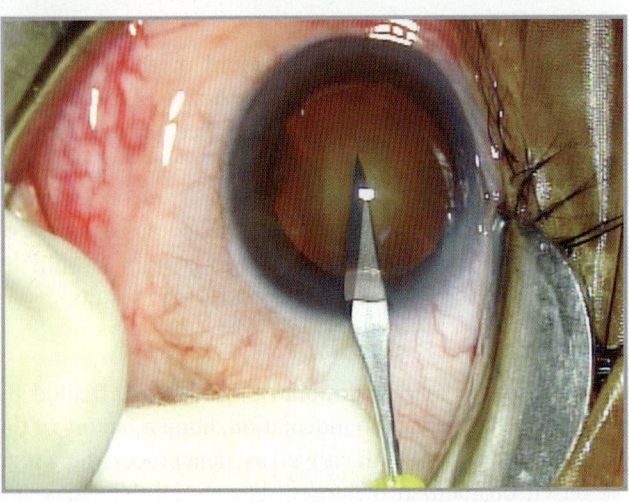

(a)

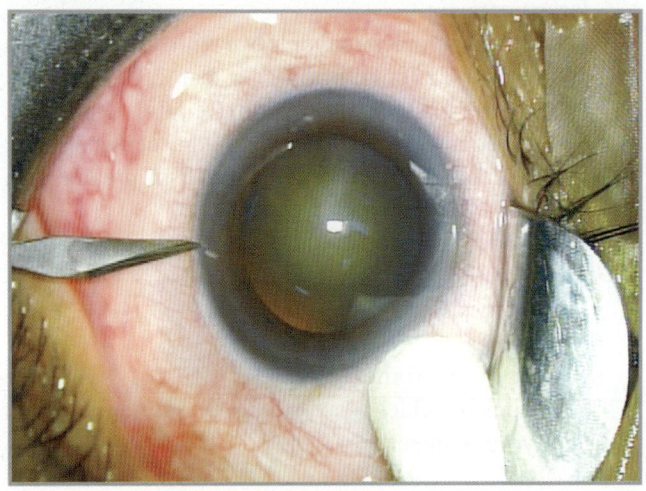

(b)

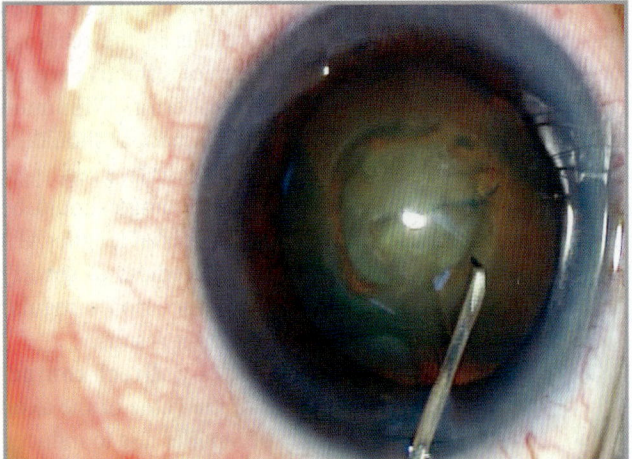

(c)

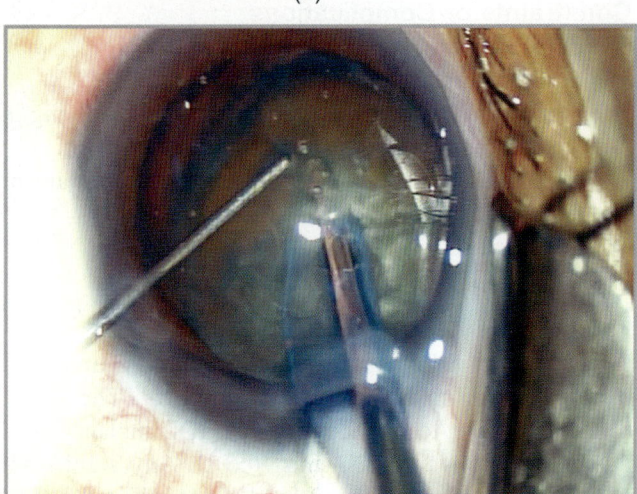

(d)

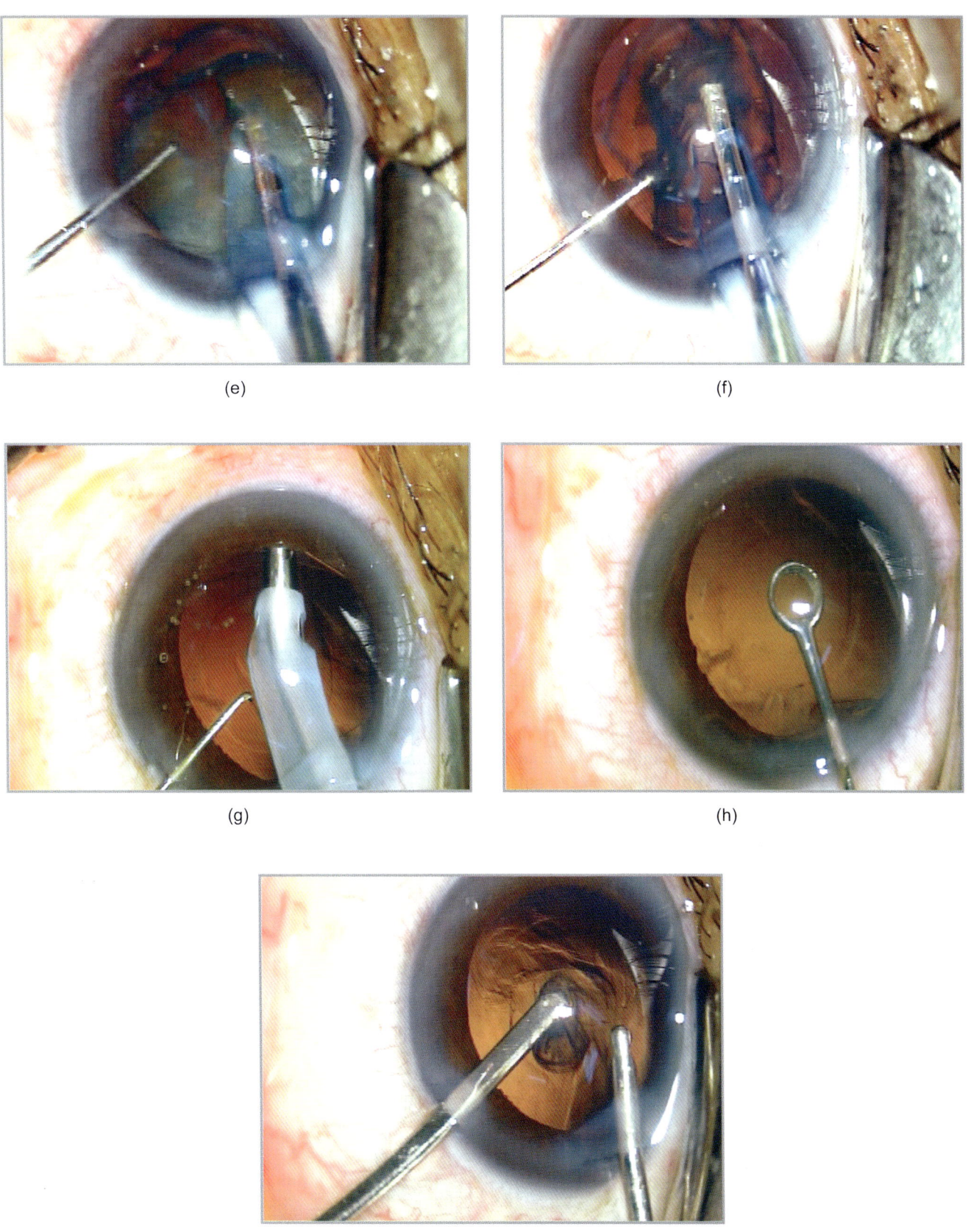

Fig. 20.13: (a) Incision for Accommodative 1 CU IOL implant, (b) Side port incision, (c) Rhexis for implantation of Accommodative 1 CU IOL implant, (d) and (e) Nucleotomy by direct chopping, (f) and (g) Cortical washing, (h) Posterior capsule polishing, (i) Bimanual I/A

Modifications in different formula's of IOL power calculations						
Formula	Est. A-constant	ACD	Optimised constant	Formula	Surgeon factor	PACD
Haigis	118.1	5.03	A0 :1.08A1 :0.40A2 :0.10	Holladay 1	1.56	-
SRK/T	118.6	5.03	-	Holladay 2	-	5.39
SRK/II	118.7	5.03	-	Hoffer Q	-	5.39

following accommodative IOL implantations. Hence, one should attempt to make a rhexis of 4 to 4.5 mm so as to get maximum of 5 mm diameter. Meticulous attention is the basic need to have a well-centred continuous curvilinear capsulorrhexis.

The author prefers to initiate two-valve incisions of 1 mm size with the help of the side port blade itself. The advantage of these initial incisions is to maintain good anterior chamber depth during rhexis and hydroprocedures as well as second incisions may be utilised to inject viscoelastic simultaneously or else to debulk the AC immediately through the second incision during hydroprocedures if warranted to release undue pressure exerted by fluid waves. Once the hydroprocedure is completed, the main incision is readily extended with the help of a 2.8 mm keratome for good phacoemulsification without compromising the tunnel and valve configuration. However, a 3.2 mm incision will finally be required for implantation of accommodative IOL.

Technique of Nucleotomy and I/A

Nucleotomy technique remains the surgeon's preference for any procedure. The basic aim is an uncomplicated successful outcome. The technique which is good in one case may not be that effective in another. The most important fact is to maintain integrity of rhexis and capsular bag till the IOL implantation is over.

Author prefers to use the flip and chip technique for soft cataract, whereas direct phaco chop by peripheral or central chopping in remaining grades of the nucleus.

Needless to specify, we prefer to have low US power settings with a high flow rate and high vacuum, to make the procedure fast and precise.

Nuclear fragment aspiration is invariably performed over the iris plane to avoid any adverse impact on rhexis. We prefer to perform I/A with high flow and vacuum of 450 to 500 mmHg under continuous and repeated hydration of cortical matter by position one. In other words, it is something like stop, irrigate, open fornices and aspirate subsequently.

One should not hesitate to use capsule polisher to push thick cortex into the centre from the periphery so as to minimise stress on the capsular bag during I/A. A neat and clean capsular bag will reduce incidence of PCO, which may adversely affect the outcome of accommodative IOL implantation, and hence, final polishing of anterior and posterior capsule should be undertaken as routine practice.

Implantation of Accommodative IOL

The basic technique of IOL implantation technique through the injector system remains the same. However, special attention and certain modifications are required with accommodative IOL implants while loading and delivering IOL through this system.

- **The injector system:** The injector (model RS 310 from Human Optics) and the cartridge (model RS 420) are exclusively designed for implantation of 1 CU IOL implant.

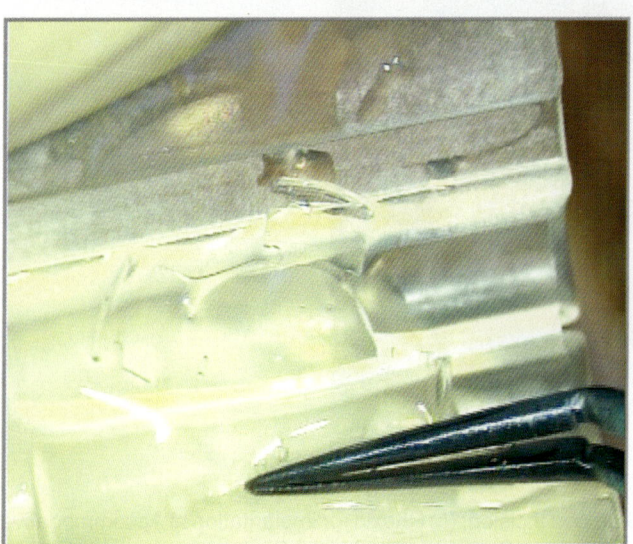

(a)

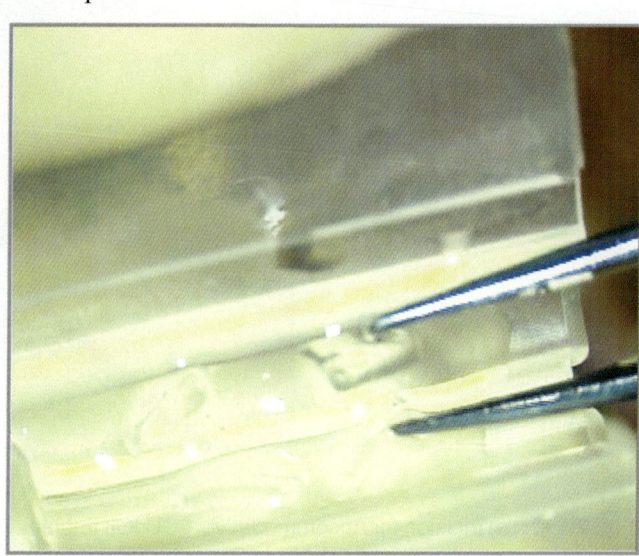

(b)

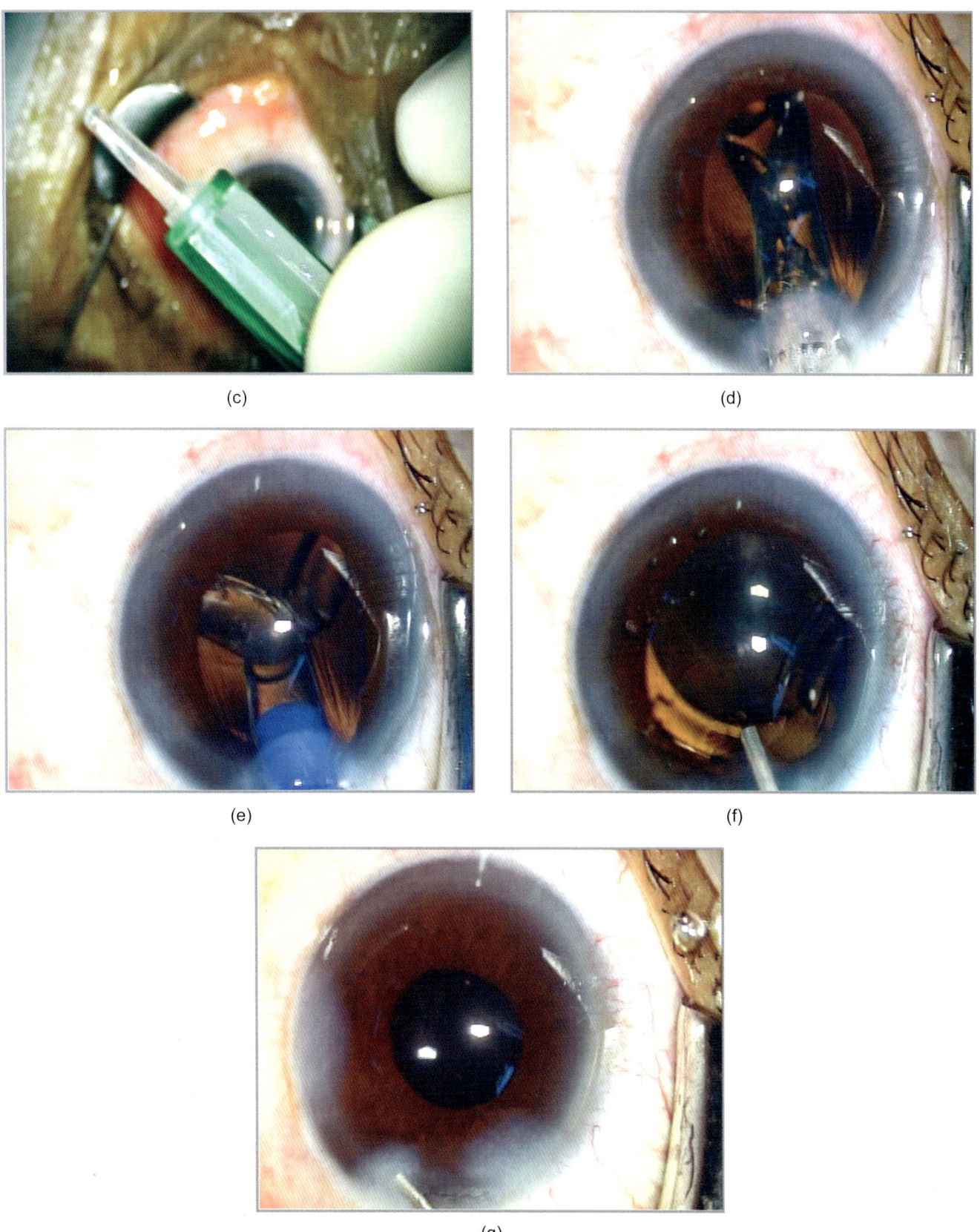

Fig. 20.14: (a) and (b) Loading of accommodative IOL into cartridge, (c) Injector system is loaded with accommodative IOL implant, (d) and (e) Delivery of Accommodative IOL implant into anterior chamber, (f) Accommodative IOL implant is being positioned into the capsular bag, (g) Accommodative IOL implant is positioned into the capsular bag and stromal hydration is in progress

- **Implantation technique:** Being hydrophilic in nature, 1 CU IOL is placed in BSS and rinsed thoroughly prior to implantation. Needless to specify, the prerequisite demand to maintain IOL hydrated prior to the implantation due to its obvious hydrophilic property. Once the 1 CU IOL implant lens is being removed from the primary container with the handling forceps (model RS 211 from Human Optics) or McPherson's forceps, small quantity of Viscoelastic is beneficial and essential for a smooth delivery of the IOL implant.

- **Loading of the IOL implant:** Specific design of the accommodative IOL implant demands little modification in these particular steps as compared to other acrylic IOL implants.

  The open fringes or hook type ends of the distal ends of haptics should be placed facing up in the cartridge. The IOL implant should not be engaged in between the folded wings of the cartridge and should rightly be placed into the tunnel so as to ascertain the desired and uninterrupted delivery of the implant into the capsular bag.

  The next step is to place the IOL implant into the channel with the help of the special lens loader (Human Optics RS 211 or equivalent). The lens loader should be inserted right up to the distal end of the loading chamber until the IOL implant is placed at the desired position so as to avoid any injury to the lens during procedure.

- **Loading of the cartridge into the injector system:** Loading of the cartridge into the injector system is more or less same as with other injector and IOL delivery systems. The cartridge is placed down in the positioning slot. The tunnel of cartridge should remain in parallel to the tip of the injector for smooth conduct of lens delivery.

- **Delivery of IOL implant into the capsular bag:** Once the IOL implant is properly loaded into the injector system, it is deemed appropriate to be implanted into the capsular bag.

  After inserting the injector into the AC, the leading end of cartridge should remain under the rhexis margins at least for 2 mm. This will ensure proper delivery of IOL haptics into the bag. Now the IOL implant is gradually and gently pushed into the bag until it is positioned. The optics will unfold gradually, however the peculiar haptics of 1 CU IOL implant may remain unfolded for some time which may require mechanical assistance to unfold the haptics.

  Great care is essentially required to ensure proper positioning of the IOL implant in the bag.

- **Intraoperative complications:** In addition to routine complications, accommodative IOLs are prone to have certain specific complications as under mentioned. Very soft and different configuration of haptics of accommodative IOL poses the specific problem of unfolding or reverse defolding. It is very difficult to re-open inverted haptics under the posterior surface of IOL implant. One has to be very careful while unfolding IOL through the injector system. Haptics needs to be everted gradually and one by one. Great care is demanded against injury to the posterior capsule while readjusting accommodative IOL in the bag.

Postoperative Management

Postoperative care and management is more or less identical as with any other IOL implantation surgery. However, use of mydriatics and cycloplegics require some modifications.

(i) **Evaluation of accommodation:** Evaluation of accommodation cannot be done unless and until cycloplegic drops are discontinued. Hence, short course of such drugs is being recommended.

(ii) **Prescription of glasses:** A useful recovery of vision for distant and near vision is expected to be attained following accommodative IOL implantation. However, the patient should be cautioned against need of spectacle corrections for specific purposes like working on very fine focus or reading small prints.

The changes in the capsular bag in due course of time, like bag shrinkage, directly influence the accommodative potential. These changes may prolong the final and complete recovery of accommodative efforts and the prescription of glasses. Most of these cases are likely to have over-refraction, particularly hypermetropia immediately after implantation. It is also observed that early spectacle correction may adversely influence the stimulus of accommodation and the final outcome. The unoperated contralateral eye should be corrected, even if a prescription of spectacles, which is generally given after some time, is being provided to the operated eye. This is more so with myopes, since full correction in the contralateral eye is likely to provide positive accommodative stimulus to the operated eye.

CONCLUSION

In spite of the fact that foldable lenses have captured the imagination and the market, the concept of accommodative IOL implants is gradually being accepted widely. The increasing demands and expectations of both the patient and the surgeon is posing a greater challenge towards achieving the most ideal full range vision following cataract surgery, which is now no longer being considered as cataract extraction but keratorefractive surgery in the true sense. We are confident to see better types of full range IOLs in the near future.

BIBLIOGRAPHY

1. Foldable Intraocular Lenses: Evolution, Clinicopathologic Correlations, and Complications. Apple DJ, Werner L, eds., Slack Inc. NJ, USA, 2002.

2. Apple DJ, Werner L, eds., Slack Inc. NJ, USA, 2002 Foldable Intraocular Lenses: Evolution, Clinicopathologic Correlations, and Complications.

3. Sparrow JR, Miller AS, Zhou J. Blue light –absorbing IOL and Retinal pigment epithelium protection in vitro. J Cataract Refract Surg.2004; 30; 873–878.

4. Javitt J, Brauweiler HP, Jacobi KW, et aI. Cataract extraction with multifocal intraocular lens implantation: clinical, functional, and quality-of-life outcomes. Multicentre clinical trial in Germany and Austria. J Cataract Refract Surg 2000; 26:1356–1366.

5. Schmitz S, Dick HB, Krummenauer F, et aI. Contrast sensitivity and glare disability by halogen light after monofocal and multifocal lens implantation. Br J Ophthalmol 2000; 84:1109–1112.

6. Pandey SK, Werner 1, Apple DJ, et al. Evaluation of an accommodative intraocular lens in human and rabbit eyes. Invest Ophthalmol Vis Sci 2002; ARVO abstract S17.

7. Chaim PJT, Chan JH, Aggarwal RK, et al. acrysof ReStore IOL in cataract surgery; quality of vision. J Cataract Refract Surg.2006; 321459incision–1463.

8. Chwiegerling J, Ye X, Choi J, et al. Night time visual quality with different multifocal IOL. Poster presented at;XXIV Congress of the ESCRS Exhibition, September, 9–13, 2006; London.

9. Seyland M, Zinicola E., Multifocal versus monofocal intraocular lenses in cataract surgery: a systematic review. Ophthalmology. 2003 Sep; 110(9):1789–98

10. Ingolo EM, Grenga P, Iacobelli L, Grenga R, Visual acuity and contrast sensitivity: AcrySof ReSTOR apodised diffractive versus AcrySof SA60AT monofocal intraocular lenses.;J Cataract Refract Surg. 2007 Jul; 33(7):12447.

11. Souza CE, Muccioli C, Soriano ES, Chalita MR, Oliveira F, Freitas LL, Meire LP, Tamaki C, Belfort R Jr., Visual performance of AcrySof ReSTOR apodised diffractive IOL: a prospective comparative trial. Am J Ophthalmol. 2006 May; 141(5):827–832. Epub 2006 Mar 20.

12. Petermeier K, Szurman P, Subjective and objective outcome following implantation of the apodised diffractive AcrySof ReSTOR, Ophthalmologe. 2007 May; 104(5):399–404, 406–8.

13. Glasser A, Kaufman PL. The mechanism of accommodation in primates. Ophthalmology. 1999; 106:863–872.

14. Bito LZ, Miranda OC. Accommodation and presbyopia. In: Reinecke RD, ed. Ophthalmology Annual. New York: Raven Press; 1989:103–128.

15. Fisher RF. The elastic constants of the human lens. J Physiol. 1971;212:1:147–180.

16. Fisher RF. Presbyopia and the changes with age in the human crystalline lens. J Physiol. 1973; 228:3:765–779.

17. Krag S, Olsen T, Andreassen TT. Biomechanical characteristics of the human anterior lens capsule in relation to age. Invest Ophthalmol Vis Sci. 1997; 38:357–363.

18. Lutjen-Drecoll E, Tamm E, Kaufman PL. Age changes in rhesus monkey ciliary muscle: light and electron microscopy. Exp Eye Res. 1988; 47:885–899.

19. Neider MW, Crawford K, Kaufman PL, Bito LZ. In vivo videography of the rhesus monkey accommodative apparatus: Age-related loss of ciliary muscle response to central stimulation. Arch Ophthalmol. 1990; 108:69–74.

20. Croft MA, Kaufman PL, Crawford KS, et al. Accommodation dynamics in aging rhesus monkeys. Am J Physiol. 1998; 275: 6 Pt 2:R1885–1897.

21

Recent Advances in IOLs: Full Range Vision Apodised Diffractive IOL

Col JKS Parihar SM, VSM

INTRODUCTION

There has been tremendous change in the concept of cataract surgery and IOL implants in the recent past. Phacoemulsification with conventional foldable IOL implantation is no more the method of choice for the management of cataract only. The present concept demands keratorefractive surgery in true sense which should provide emmetropia for full range and all types of vision. Each and every aware patient dreams of complete freedom from spectacles. Bimanual micro phaco, ultrathin, multifocal or accommodative IOL implants are a step toward the ultimate goal for full range, all purpose emmetropia. However, results are still far away from finality.

Recent introduction of apodised diffractive intraocular lenses by Alcon international may leap one step forward towards full range vision. However, final results are yet to be critically analysed against all types of cataract operations particularly in long term follow ups.

THE EVOLUTION OF ZONAL AND DIFFRACTIVE IOLs

Monofocal IOL implants possess uniform refractive status all around the optics which provides a fixed range of vision at all the foci and distances. Hence, such kind of IOL implants require spectacle corrections for different purposes and distances.

Bifocal IOL implants have two zones in optics with different dioptres; hence can be useful for both near and distance vision. However, bifocal IOLs do not cater for intermediate vision. As such two fixed focuses produce several discomforts to the patient including reduced contrast sensitivity and glare. The next generation multifocal IOL implants have multiple concentric rings of different dioptres so as to provide multiple foci for different distances. Despite such modifications, these IOL implants are still not free from

problems and constraints like reduced contrast sensitivity and compromised vision. Zonal refractive lenses like bifocal and multifocal IOLs do not possess continuous lens surface. The boundaries between zones have optical discontinuities resulting either in a distance or a near image at a given point. This kind of surface spreads out light at the inner and outer boundaries when light hits an optical discontinuity. This spreading of light leads to deflection of light energy in some other direction which creates unwanted images around the point source as glare and disturbed vision. Over and above, annular (ring-shaped) multifocal lens regions have reduced image quality.

The technology of apodised diffractive intraocular lenses may provide a promising direction towards sharp single image full range vision at all distances.

CONCEPTS/CHARACTERISTICS OF APODISED DIFFRACTIVE IOL IMPLANTS

Diffraction

As the waves spread out and bump into each other, crest to crest and trough to trough collisions will cause areas of intense light. Crest to trough collisions will cancel each other, and no light will appear.

However, in case of multifocal or bifocal IOLs, the optics simulates the situation of two overlapping light surfaces or semicircular waves of water. Once, these two surfaces interact simultaneously, a single sharp image is formed in contrast to the second image, in case of two different surfaces refracting light at variable points. In case of multifocal IOLs with five or more concentric zones, each and every zone will produce several images due to multiple diffractive rings of focus of variable dioptres. Theoretically, this phenomena of light diffraction through multiple interfaces can only be eliminated by repositioning light rays of variable intensity and dioptre in such a fashion

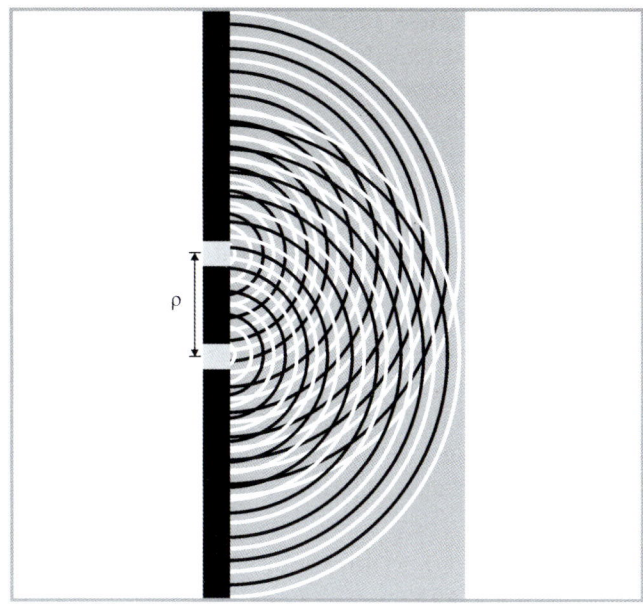

Fig. 21.1: Principle of diffraction

so as the interface junction should have a difference of just one wavelength of light, i.e. 500 nanometres. Apodised diffractive IOL implants are based on the same principle.

Apodisation

The term apodisation defines gradual modifications in the optical properties of a lens from its centre to its edge. Apodisation is the gradual decrease of the height of these optical surfaces extending from the centre to the periphery.

The essential feature of apodised diffractive design is to maintain equilibrium in image quality and light energy. The height of the step, basically directs the light waves to travel in one particular direction. The width of the slope determines the separation of the two foci. Apodisation is not a new concept in physics and optics since it has been in practice to improve quality of optics in microscopy and astronomy to improve image quality for several years. The classic example is a telescope that could visualise objects clearly and deeper into space due to the inherent quality of apodisation which inhibits and controls the diffusion of excessive or undue light.

In the same way, the quality of images has been improved in microscopes used in cellular studies by anatomists by using aspheric and apodised optics. In normal optics there is significant distortion of images due to diffusion of excessive light and optical aberrations leading to bleaching of finer details, whereas aspheric apodised optics undoubtedly minimise aberrations and improve the quality of images.

However, the same principle has been effectively applied recently to improve the optical performance of newer apodised diffractive IOL implants.

Apodised Diffractive IOL

Apodised diffractive IOLs possess a unique triad of apodisation, diffraction and refraction.

These IOLs can titrate appropriate light energies as per the need of the activity and light levels irrespective of the pupillary size, in contrast to other diffractive IOLs which are dependent on variations of the pupillary diameter.

In case of multifocal IOLs with five or more concentric zones, each and every zone will produce several images due to multiple diffractive rings of focus of variable dioptres. Theoretically, this phenomenon of light diffraction through multiple interfaces can only be eliminated by repositioning light rays of variable intensity and dioptre in such a fashion so that the interface junction should have a difference of just one wavelength of light, i.e. 500 nanometres. Apodised diffractive IOL implants are based on the same principle.

This particular quality makes apodised IOLs more responsive to remain effective in various light conditions, both mesopic and photopic visions.

Hence, classical characteristics of apodised diffractive IOLs are as follows:
- Optical surface has concentric diffractive steps or grating patterns.
- Steps create advancing waves of light energy that are allocated to multiple focal points by the diffractive design.
- Utilises the wave theory of light to form an image.

Gradual sloping interface of less than 500 nanometres separates images by 4 dioptres which provides intermediate, variable focuses for different distances which is essentially beneficial for full range vision and minimises optical aberrations to a great extent as well. The height of the step basically directs the light waves to travel in one particular direction. The width of the slope determines the separation of the two foci.

Concepts of Sloping Optics/Interface of 500 nm

The significance of optical interfaces of 500 to 550 nanometres is based on the fact that the wavelength of green light is 550 nanometres in which one expects to have good

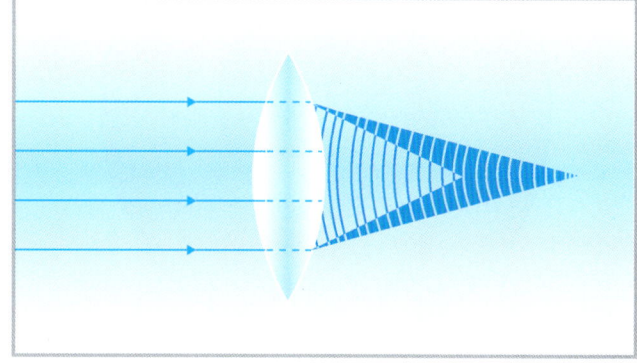

Fig. 21.2 : Principle of apodised diffractive pattern

distance or photopic visual acuity. In the same fashion, the apodised optical slope in optics provides add plus four dioptre power and hence, the same can be effectively utilised for near vision under photopic conditions.

Concepts of Defocus Curves and Sloping Optics Add Power 4 Dioptres at the IOL Plane

Defocus curves at the separation between two images add power to the optics. In the case of apodised diffractive IOL, it is separated by roughly 4 dioptres at the IOL plane or 3.2 dioptres at the corneal plane. This is a very crucial quality which provides separation from near foci to distance foci. The concept of the defocus curve is based on the amplitude of accommodation at various ages and its correlation with functional near vision. The maximum amplitude of accommodation is found in a child right up to 30 to 40 dioptres. However, there is a gradual and progressive decline in the accommodative capabilities which reduces to 4.5 to 5 dioptres at the age of 25 and further declines up to zero to one dioptre by the age of 40–45. Hence, restoring an amplitude of accommodation and functional near vision of over 4 dioptres following IOL implantation will provide good near visual acuity as for 25 years old patients.

APODISED DIFFRACTIVE IOL DESCRIPTION (RESTOR ALCON LENS™ (PATENTED DESIGN OF ALCON)

Optics

(i) Overall optic size is 6 millimetre.
(ii) Central 3.6 millimetres possess diffractive and apodised characters. Beyond the 3.6 millimetre zone is an optical zone.
(iii) Zone boundary is placed whenever optical path length increases by one wavelength.
(iv) Characteristic zone boundary pattern.

(v) Optics possess surface like an annular ring and zonal refractive, however, it differs from conventional multifocal, since surfaces do not have power curves but act in conjunction with this curve, so that all the wavelengths of light that hit on optical surface are separated by only one wavelength.
(vi) Steps yield phase discontinuity
(vii) Zones are shaped to direct light
(viii) Adjacent zones have similar effects
(ix) Light from all zones goes to both primary images
(x) Optical phase discontinuities at gradual slope in surface produce two images. Hence, manipulated light will produce two images; one on the fovea and one just in front of the fovea. This will form distinct images at near as well as at distance.

Merits of Apodised Diffractive IOL

The very first IOL implant has combinations of three optical systems namely apodisation, diffraction and refraction.
(i) Apodised diffractive design controls both image quality and energy balance.
(ii) Optics engineered to provide quality near-to-distance performance with no pupil size restrictions. Plus 4 dioptre add power to achieve optimal separation of near and distant images.
(iii) Optics with apodised diffractive central zone possesses unique optical design which matches performance to vision needs. Combination of apodisation and diffraction is crucial to provide a full range of vision under all lighting conditions like photopic and mesopic, or low light conditions.
(iv) Central 3.6 mm zone acts as the diffractive and apodised zone to provide full range vision at all distances in photopic vision light conditions, whereas after this 3.6 mm zone, the remaining outer and peripheral portions of optics transforms the

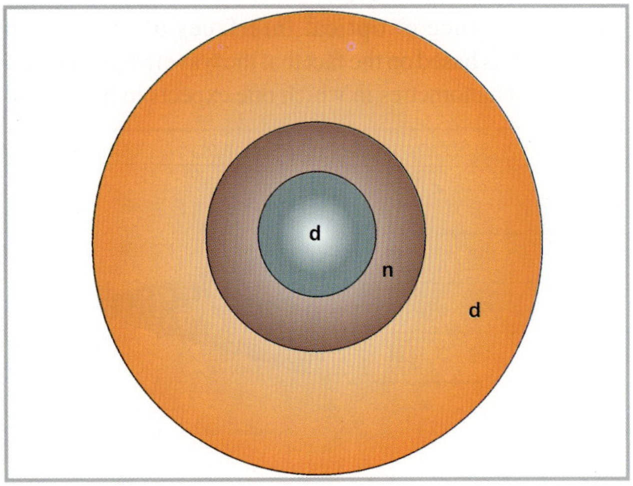

Fig. 21.3: Concepts of defocus curves and sloping optics

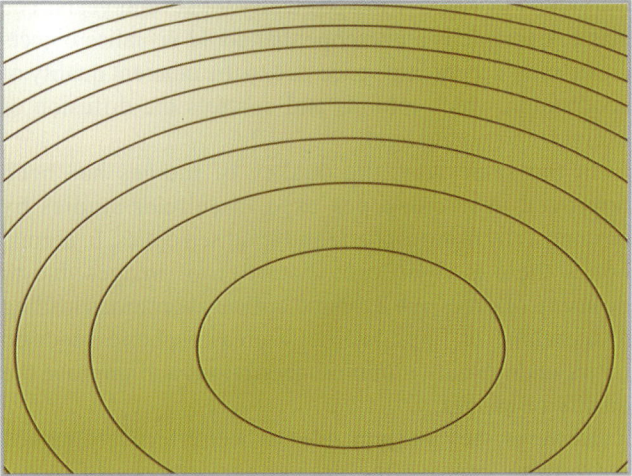

Fig. 21.4: Optics of apodised diffractive IOL implants

apodised diffractive surface to the refractive surface which is not affected by pupillary size; hence under mesopic conditions when the pupil is wide open the IOL is still able to provide near and distance vision with the help of the sloping optic surface (add plus 4 dioptre interface). This combines all the benefits of apodisation, refraction and diffraction all together.

(v) Simple to insert through a standard 2.8 mm incision.

(vi) Simple to position.

(vii) Functional: Unlikely to lead to any fibrosis in future.

(viii) Most patients are 20/20 or better and they are very happy with the fact that they have no need for glasses.

(ix) An ideal IOL implant for clear lens extraction, correcting not only high myopia and high hyperopia but also for retaining accommodation.

Problems/Constraints of Apodised Diffractive IOL Implants

(i) Any probable adverse impact of significant PCO or subsequent YAG capsulotomy on pseudophakic accommodating mechanism is yet to be evaluated since the lens is recently introduced.

(ii) It is not recommended to use it contralaterally with other multifocal lenses. This is a complex optical system. It is designed to work best when implanted binocularly.

COMPARISON OF LIGHT SCATTERING AND MESOPIC VISION (LEADING TO PUPILLARY SIZE OF 5 MM OR LARGER) IN DIFFERENT TYPES OF IOL IMPLANTS

(i) **Monofocal single piece PMMA IOL implants:** Monofocal single piece PMMA IOL implants

deliver excellent mesopic vision in terms of ability and quality since there is no scattering of light as most of the light that's going through the lens is effectively utilised.

(ii) **Zonal refractive multifocal:** A common zonal refractive multifocal IOL possesses five refractive zones. Each and every zone represents as a separate optical surface in true sense against mesopic light conditions (pupillary size of 4.5 to 5 mm). These multiple zones face light scattering; leading to formation of surrounding unwanted images like concentric circles or shadows around a main image.

(iii) **Apodised diffractive optics:** Efficacy of night vision is of excellent order and at par with the performance of the monofocal IOL implants.

The apodised diffractive optics has two sloping zones, the central 3.6 millimetres of the lens and the remaining part of a 6 millimetre optic. The central 3.6 millimetres zone acts as a diffractive region and is apodised. The remaining zone is a refractive region. The combination of these two zones are critical to produce a full range of vision under all lighting conditions, both photopic, or light conditions, and mesopic, or low light conditions.

Zonal Refractive (5 Zones) IOL Implants

Light energy dramatically varies with the number of zones exposed by pupil, contributing to halos at nights.

Full Optic Diffractive IOL Implants

Light energy equally shared over a broad range of pupils/ lighting conditions, contributes to halos at nights. Light energy when equally shared for bright to moderate pupils/ lighting conditions. Apodisation gradually increases distance energy with larger pupils, reducing halos at night.

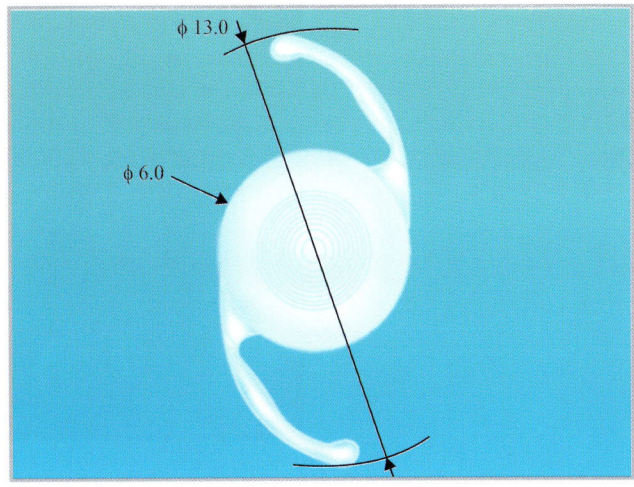

(a) (b)

Fig. 21.5: (a) and (b) Apodised diffractive IOL

TECHNIQUE OF IMPLANTATION OF APODISED DIFFRACTIVE IOL IMPLANTS (RESTOR ALCON LENS TM PATENTED DESIGN OF ALCON)

Implantation technique including IOL delivery injector system and methods is exactly identical to the Single piece hydrophobic acrylic IOL implants. Keys for Successful IOL implantation of Apodised Diffractive IOL is exclusively based on following factors

    (i) Patient Selection
  (ii) Accurate biometry
 (iii) IOL power calculation
 (iv) Surgical technique.

Selection of Patient: Preoperative Considerations

• Patients who no longer desire to wear glasses
• Age
• Functional and occupational requirements

• Degree of general alertness
• Ocular pathology
• Patients visual demands
• Expectations for near vision needs
• Qualify for bilateral implants.

Patient Selection: Preoperative Exclusion Criteria

Subjective Exclusion

• Hypercritical patients
• Patients with unrealistic expectations
• Occupational night drivers.

Medical Exclusion

• >1.0 D of corneal astigmatism
• Preexisting ocular pathology
• Previously refractive patients
• Individuals with a monofocal lens.

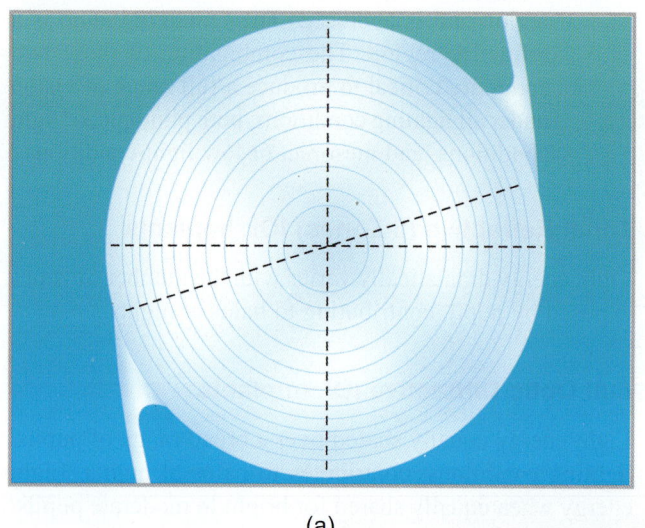

(a)

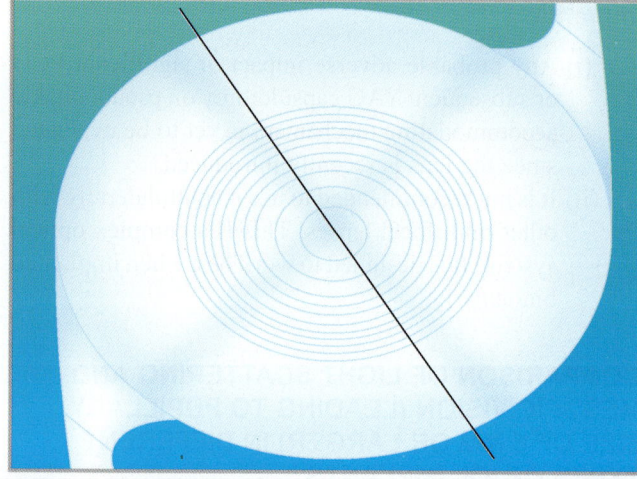

(b)

(c)

Fig. 21.6: (a) and (b) Apodised diffractive IOL implant, (c) Apodised diffractive IOL implant placed in situ: Multiple concentric rings of apodised surface are visible

Patient Selection Intraoperative Exclusion Criteria

Exclusion during Surgery

- Significant vitreous loss
- Pupil trauma
- Factors that impact long-term IOL performance
- Zonular damage
- Capsulorrhexis tear
- Capsular rupture

Role of Accurate Biometry and Various Methods of IOL Power Calculation

Accurate biometry and selection of an appropriate method of IOL power calculation has an immense role in the ultimate outcome of any IOL implantation. Such variants in calculation have tremendous impact on the outcome of apodised diffractive IOL implantation. The stacking effects are:

- Various small errors result in a large error
- Inaccurate keratometry + contact biometry + wrong formula selection = unexpected postoperative refraction.

Target IOL Power Calculations for Apodised Diffractive IOL Implantation

Maximise visual outcomes by calculating a postoperative refractive spherical equivalent from plano to <+0.25

Instrumentation

Standard immersion A-scan ultrasound or optical biometry by IOL Master™ is recommended to avoid axial malalignment, corneal compressions, or tear bridge.

Biometry at its Best

- Have readings that differ >0.20 mm between the two eyes confirmed by a second technician or physician.

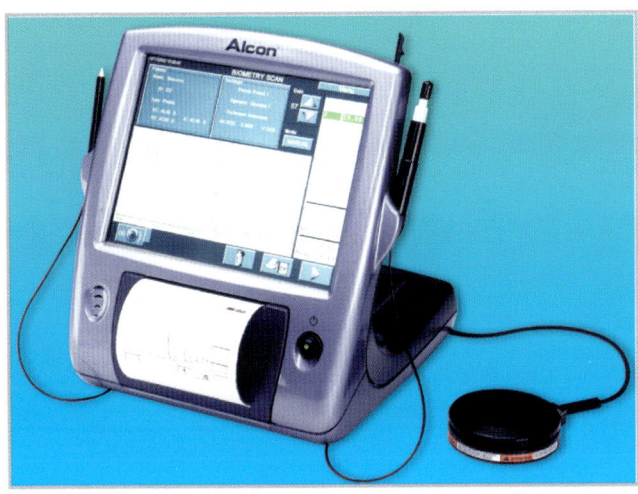

Fig. 21.7: Optical biometry by IOL master

- When possible, compare the precataract refractive error with bilateral IOL calculations for consistency.
- Use the average of multiple consistent measurements in your calculations, delete outliers.

Keratometric Considerations

- Avoid taking measurements immediately after corneal contact or use of drops that dry the ocular surface.
- Discontinue wearing contact lens until stable (recurring) corneal values are obtained.

Lens Position and How it Relates to the Postop Refraction

- In a myopic eye, a 0.1 mm error could change the postoperative refraction by 0.1 D.
- In an emmetropic eye, a 0.1 mm error could change the postoperative refraction by 0.15 D.
- In a hyperopic eye, a 0.1 mm error could change the postoperative refraction by 0.25 D. Therefore, in a hyperopic eye, a 1 mm error could change the postoperative refraction by 2.50 D.

Formulation and Customisation

- Use a new generation IOL calculation formula, i.e. SRK/T, Holladay 2 or Haigis.
- Customise the A-constant (118.2), ACD (5.08), and the surgeon factor (1.34) with postoperative data obtained from at least 30 patient outcomes.
- To successfully customise, outcomes should be of the same direction and magnitude.

Pearls to Summarise Calculation of IOL Power

- Calibrate the instrumentation.
- Compare bilateral measurements.
- Calculate using modern formula's.
- Customise A-constant, ACD, and surgeon factor.

Surgical Technique

Basic technique of phacoemulsification and implantation of IOL through an IOL delivery injector system designed for a single piece hydrophobic IOL implantation is very much suitable for implantation of apodised diffractive IOL implants. However, following surgical tips are very useful:

- Round centred capsulorrhexis, slightly smaller than optic.
- Remove all viscoelastic from behind the lens.
- Seat the lens.

PATIENT'S RESPONSE ON APODISED DIFFRACTIVE IOLS

It has been observed that following activities can be performed without using additional spectacle correction

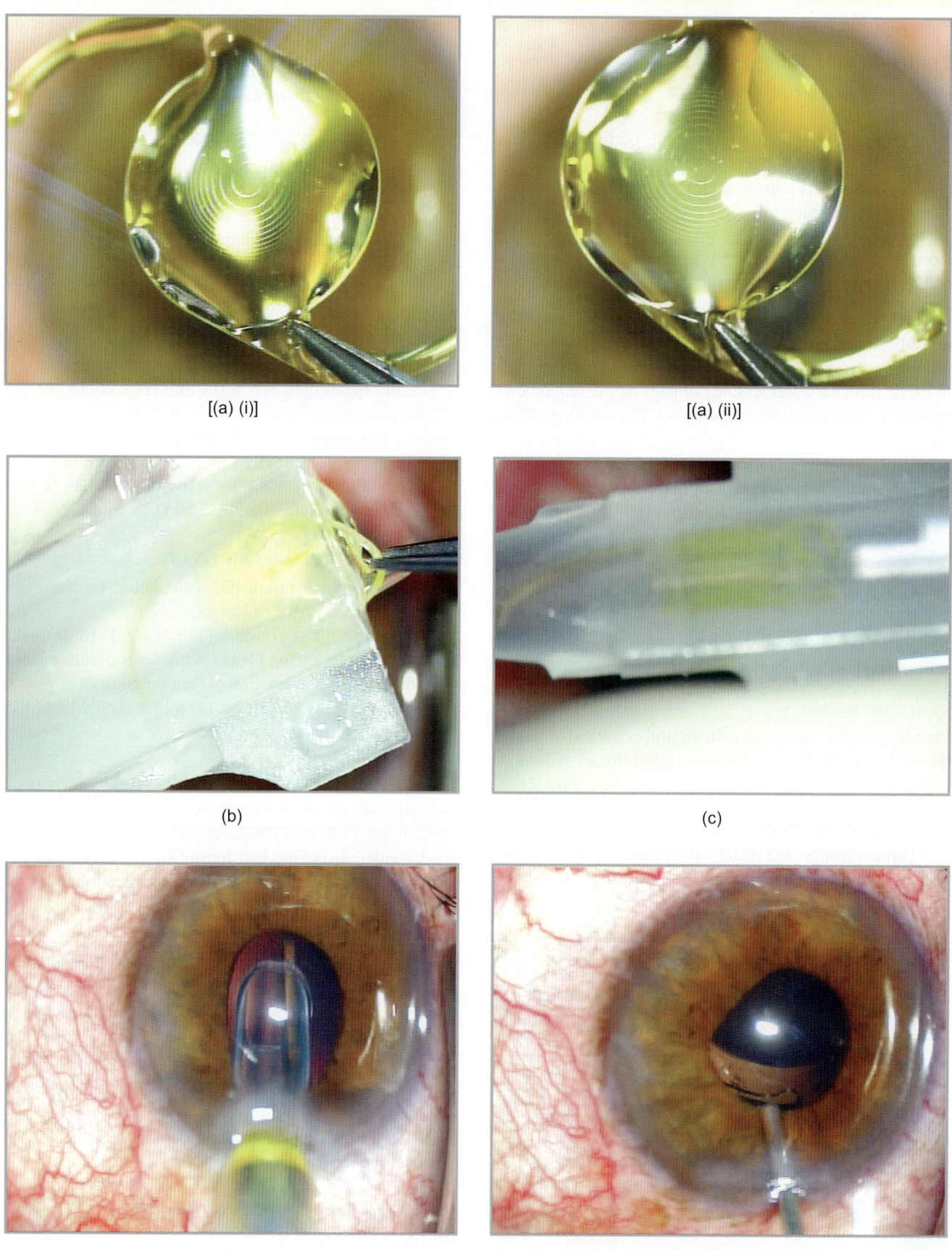

Fig. 21.8: (a) Apodised diffractive IOL implants, (b) and (c) Loading of apodised diffractive IOL into the cartridge, (d) Gradual release of apodised diffractive IOL into the capsular bag, (e) Apodised diffractive IOL is being positioned into the capsular bag

(a) (b) (c)

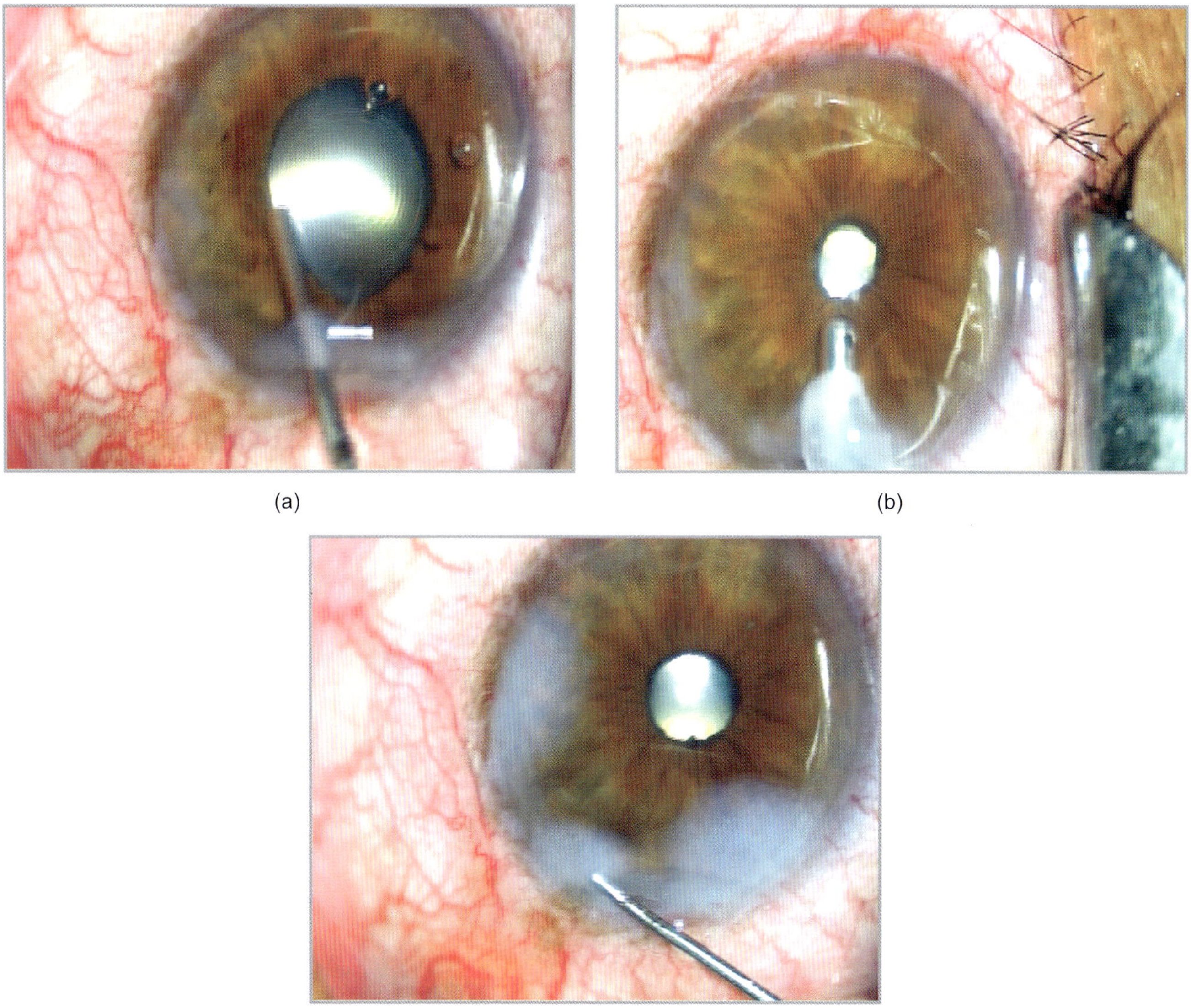

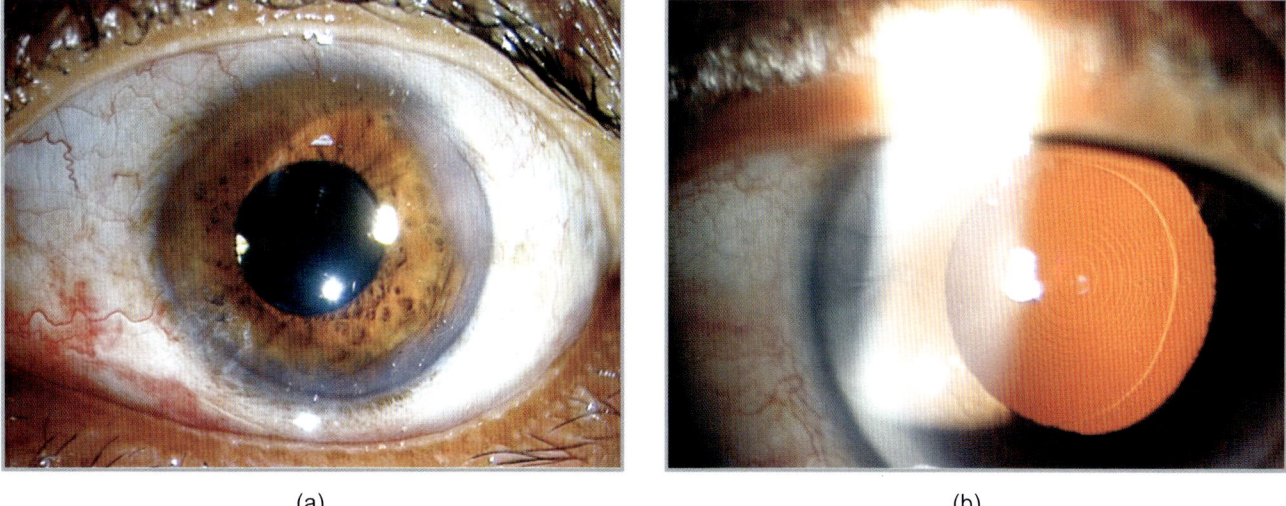

Fig. 21.9: (a) A well-placed apodised diffractive IOL, (b) Postapodised diffractive IOL implant wash, (c) Stromal hydration

(a) (b)

Fig. 21.10: (a) and (b) Apodised diffractive IOL implants: Ist postoperative day

in case of cataract patients following apodised diffractive IOL implantation.

Activities Involving Good Distance Vision and Simultaneous Frequent use of Accommodation

• Driving: Comfortable driving in day and night both.
• TV viewing: This is an important issue of life quality for modern living especially in the case of elderly patients. Most patients are comfortable viewing TV without wearing their glasses.
• Walking up or down the stairs: This particular activity involves good depth perception and frequent accommodation and adjustment.
• Playing golf, table tennis.

Activities Involving Good Intermediate Vision and Simultaneous frequent Change in Focus/ Accommodation

• Activities involving intermediate vision: Like working on computers, playing cards, viewing objects, labels on the mall.
• Shaving or putting (intermediate vision) and applying makeup (near vision). Most patients can manage the above tasks without any need for spectacles.
• Playing video games.

Activities involving Good Near Vision and Simultaneous Frequent Change in Focus/ Accommodation

• A classic near vision task like reading, threading, cutting papers, nails, sewing or sketching or painting is possible without additional glass corrections.
• Any other activity requiring very rapid alteration in range of vision, light intensity and other factors.

CONCLUSION

Theoretically, apodised diffractive IOL implant appears to be most effective to attain full range vision in all light conditions for the rehabilitation of postcataract surgery patients. A spectacle-free life is possible throughout full range of vision: near, intermediate and distance. However, its long term efficacy in terms of various professional requirements and the follow-up period is yet to be established.

22

Crystalens: Birth of a New Generation Accommodative IOL

Col JKS Parihar SM, VSM, Surg Cdr T Choudhary, Lt Col Shantanu Mukherjee
Maj Jaya Kaushik and Surg Lt Cdr AS Parihar

INTRODUCTION

Intraocular lens implants have made a significant landmark in terms of quality of material, design and precision in visual rehabilitation. This has provided a new dimension to kerato-refractive lenticular surgery by modulating the refractive status to the extent of providing emmetropia at all range of vision including distance, intermediate as well as near. Undoubtedly, the newer generation multifocal IOL implants have set a benchmark for qualitative visual rehabilitation and yet issues like compromised mesopic vision, ring halos and the status of intermediate vision continue to remain points of debate and controversy.

Accommodative IOL implants claim to provide multi range vision without influencing mesopic vision, intermediate range of visual acuity as well as contrast the sensitivity. Such IOL implants function by the virtue of synchronised action of haptics, the mechanism of accommodation being induced by the ciliary body. However altered integrity of the capsular bag and subsequent intra capsular fibrosis remains the major issue that reduces the efficacy of accommodative IOL implants.

The introduction of the newer generation premium intraocular lens has made it possible to give accommodation faculty to patients post surgery—thus imparting a 'spectacle free' vision for distance, intermediate as well as for near. Crystalens revolutionises the premium IOL category and significantly improves on the vision quality of accommodative lenses. The lens utilises a proprietary optic design and material that is optimised to increase the depth of focus and as a result it is designed to improve near vision without compromising intermediate or distance visual acuity. Crystalens delivers this near vision benefit while maintaining contrast sensitivity, amplitude of accommodation and low risk of halos and glare which are commonly encountered in multifocal IOL's. However the long term outcome and efficacy of this newer generation accommodative IOL implant is yet to be established.

APPLIED ANATOMY AND PHYSIOLOGY OF ACCOMMODATION

Accommodation

A normal individual is not only able to clearly see distant objects but is also able to focus and see near ones with clarity. When an object is located near the eye as during reading, the rays are diverging to such an extent that in normal circumstances they would not come to a focus at the retina. The phenomenon of accommodation is that the inherent ability of the crystalline lens to change its shape, thereby increasing its curvature and convergence power, to bring the divergent rays to a focus.

The curvature of the lens at rest is spherical with the anterior radius of curvature 10 mm and the posterior radius of curvature 6 mm. During accommodation, there is an increase in the anteroposterior thickness, decrease in the equatorial diameter and a forward displacement of the lens-iris diaphragm. This convergent state of the eye is known as dynamic refraction.

The mechanism of change in the curvature of the lens is not clearly known. However, an accepted theory is that during accommodation, the ciliary muscle contracts leading to approximation of the ciliary body, relaxation of the zonules and thereby reshaping of the lenticular bag into its accommodated form. In short, the shape of the lens at any time is the balance product of the elasticity of itself and that of the lenticular capsule.

The nearest point of clear focus is the 'punctum proximum,' wherein the accommodation is at its maximum. The punctum remotum or far point is dependent on the static refraction. With age, the lens becomes less flexible and is unable to increase its curvature. The near point recedes gradually with age.

Usage of presbyopic spectacles is a bothersome experience for a vast majority of the middle aged population and therefore, a need has been felt to come up with solutions for getting rid of or avoiding glasses altogether.

Theories of Mechanism of Accommodation

(i) **Helmholtz Theory:** The most widely held theory of accommodation is the one that was proposed by Hermann von Helmholtz in 1855. During accommodation, the circular fibers of the ciliary muscle contract, thereby decreasing the equatorial perilenticular space which reduces zonular tension and allows the lens to round up and increase in optical power. The increase in zonular tension causes the surface of the lens to flatten and the optical power of the lens to decrease. Helmholtz's theory of accommodation is inconsistent with the documented flattening of the anterior peripheral surface of the lens and negative shift of spherical aberration that occurs during human in vivo accommodation.

(ii) **Schachar Theory:** Ronald Schachar has developed a hypothesis whereby the focus by the human lens is associated with increased tension on the lens via the equatorial zonules. Moreover, the evidence supporting the Schachar hypothesis disproves the older theory concerning the mechanism of accommodation of von Helmholtz. Schachar found that when the ciliary muscle contracts, equatorial zonular tension is increased. The increase in equatorial zonular tension causes the central surface of the crystalline lens to steepen, the central thickness of the lens to increase (anterior-posterior diameter), and the peripheral surface of the lens to flatten. While the tension on equatorial zonules is increased during accommodation, the anterior and posterior zonules are simultaneously relaxing. As a consequence of the changes in the lens shape during human *in vivo* accommodation, the central optical power of the lens increases and spherical aberration of the lens shifts in the negative direction. Because of the increased equatorial zonular tension on the lens during accommodation, the stress on the lens capsule is increased and the lens remains stable and unaffected by gravity. The same shape changes that occur to the crystalline lens during accommodation are observed when equatorial tension is applied to any encapsulated biconvex object that encloses a minimally compressible material (volume change less than approximately 3%) and has an elliptical profile with an aspect ratio d" 0.6 (minor axis/major axis ratio). Equatorial tension is very efficient when applied to biconvex objects that have a profile with an aspect ratio ≤ 0.6. Minimal equatorial tension and only a small increase in equatorial diameter causes a large increase in the central curvature. This explains why the aspect ratio of a vertebrate crystalline lens can be used to predict the qualitative amplitude of accommodation of the vertebrate eye. Vertebrates that have lenses with aspect ratios ≤ 0.6 have high amplitudes of accommodation, e.g. primates and falcons, while those vertebrates with lenticular aspect ratios > 0.6 have low amplitudes of accommodation, e.g. owls and antelopes. The decline in the amplitude of accommodation eventually results in the clinical manifestation of presbyopia, i.e. when the near focal point of the eye is more remote than the near reading distance. It has been widely suggested that the age-related decline in accommodation that leads to presbyopia occurs as a consequence of sclerosis (hardening) of the lens. However, the lens does not become sclerotic until after 40 years of age. In fact, the greatest decline in the amplitude of accommodation occurs during childhood, prior to the time that any change in hardness of the lens has been found. The decline in accommodative amplitude is rapid in childhood and slow thereafter, following a logarithmic pattern that is similar to that of the increase in the equatorial diameter of the lens, which is the most likely basis for the accommodative loss. As the equatorial diameter of the lens continuously increases over life, baseline zonular tension simultaneously declines. This results in a reduction in baseline ciliary muscle length that is associated with both lens growth and increasing age. Since the ciliary muscle, like all muscles, has a length-tension relationship, the maximum force the ciliary muscle can apply decreases, as its length shortens with increasing age. This is the etiology of the age-related decline in accommodative amplitude that results in presbyopia. Any procedure that can prevent equatorial lens growth or increase the effective distance between the lens equator and the ciliary muscle can potentially increase the amplitude of accommodation.

(iii) **Catenary - D. Jackson Coleman Theory:** D. Jackson Coleman proposed that the lens, zonules and anterior vitreous comprise a diaphragm between the anterior and vitreous chambers of the eye. Ciliary muscle contraction initiates a pressure gradient between the vitreous and aqueous compartments that support the anterior lens shape in the mechanically reproducible state of a steep radius of curvature in the centre of the lens with slight flattening of the peripheral anterior lens, i.e. the shape, in cross section, of a catenary. The anterior capsule and the zonules form a trampoline shape or a hammock-shaped surface that is totally reproducible depending on the circular dimensions, i.e. the diameter of the ciliary body (Müeller's muscle). The ciliary body thus directs the shape like the pylons of a suspension bridge; but does not need to support an equatorial traction force to flatten the lens.

Objective Measures of Accommodation

(i) **Dynamic retinoscopy:** This method was originally devised by Edward Jackson in 1895. Using a Smith-prestley retinoscope, the examiner observes the retinoscopic reflex of a distance-corrected eye without additional lenses, a "with" movement is observed. Then the patient fixes at the retinoscope, this will lead to accommodation- the beam broadens to neutralisation. Nearer fixation (in front of the retinoscope) will lead to an "against" movement. Dynamic retinoscopy readily detects the degree of accommodation as well as the presence of irregular light reflexes due to corneal or lens aberrations' inducing multifocality.

(ii) **Infrared optometres (using Scheiner's principle):** Since infrared optometres provide refractive measurement through only a small portion of the eye's optics, the alignment of the various measuring apertures with the patient's pupil is critical. Newer versions of infrared optometres use photoretinoscopy. They offer the advantage of rapidly measuring the refraction at distance. These instruments calculate an average refraction for the entire pupil, however, they do not provide any information on multifocality. Because devices are calibrated for the smaller amount of aberrations present when the lens is in a relaxed state, they underestimate the degree to which accommodation increases aberrations.

(iii) **Wave front analysis:** Technology based on the principle of Hartmann-Shack aberrometry is now available for clinical use. This measures the shape of the wavefront of light as it leaves the optical system of the eye from an effective point source on the retina. These aberrometres determine multifocal refractive states across the pupil, both before and during accommodation, and the difference in these values is the exact measure of true accommodation. Fully dilated pupils give the best result which is achieved after instilling phenylephrine. Using Hartmann-Shack aberrometry, researchers have demonstrated small but significant degrees of accommodation in patients who recently received the hinged accommodative lens.

Mechanism of Action of Accommodative IOL

There has been a considerable amount of discussion and deliberation about the exact mechanism of action of the Crystalens. Till date, all methods claiming to deliver clear vision at multi-distances have done so by pseudo-accommodation. Whether it be multifocal and diffractive IOLs, contact lenses, progressive additions or corneal refractive procedures—they have all utilised pseudo-accommodation for presbyopia.

Various objectives and subjective mechanisms have been used to determine true pseudophakic accommodative changes in the eye.

Forward Lens Movement

This is the primary mechanism of action in accommodation. Upon the concentric contraction of the ciliary muscle— there is redistribution of the muscle mass posteriorly, thereby leading to increase in anterior vitreous pressure. This pressure change moves the optics forward. This has been documented by MRI and UBM. This movement is adequate to explain the change in accommodation.

Dell, Burrato and Di Chiara in separate studies have analysed the forward movement of the crystalens. Dell used the immersion A scan to determine the ACD change and came to the conclusion that the optics moves forward by 0.84 mm (SD 0.16, range 0.53 to 1.11 mm), corresponding to a power increase of 1.79 diopters. The study by Di Chiara is significant because it shows that the forward movement recorded by the IOL master (Carl Zeiss Meditec) (which was based on the average of 5 AC depth measurements at each of two distances—15 cm and 3 m) was achieved without the benefit of chemical stimulants.

Optic Flexure or Forward Arching of IOL

This has been postulated as the secondary mechanism of action of accommodation of the crystalens. Optic flexure or forward arching may explain as to why patients implanted with the crystalens have better near vision than can be explained by the change in dioptric power due to forward lens movement.

(i) **Assessment of optic flexure by wavefront aberrometry:** Waltz first used the wavefront aberrometry to objectively show forward arching of the Crystalens optic—a process which has been named as accommodative arching. His theory states that the crystalens most likely changes shape as well as moves back and forth to produce accommodation. These wavefront aberration changes were demonstrated by Dr. Waltz using Tracey wavefront images and were found to be similar to those observed in a natural crystalline lens·

(ii) **Assessment of optic flexure by dynamic retinoscopy:** As on date, dynamic retinoscopy is the most practical and reliable method of assessing amplitude of accommodation. In the study conducted by Dell, five patients after crystalens implantation were subjected to dynamic retinoscopy. The patients were made to read 'J3' letters with the reading card being stuck above the retinoscope. Patients were made to look at a distance with the required correction ('with movement' reflex was obtained). Then the patients were made to switch fixation to the card above the retinoscope ('neutralisation' reflex was obtained on full accommodation). The testing was started at a distance of 25 inches (and gradually drawing closer) and the patients were instructed to read aloud the letters. The mean amplitude of accommodation measured by dynamic retinoscopy was 3.14 D (range = 2.16 D to 4.44D).

In a larger, masked randomised evaluation, Dr. Marian Macsai compared accommodation in the crystalens to that of a standard monofocal IOL in 224 eyes of 112 patients. Measurements were performed by a single observer, again using a variety of methods, including dynamic retinoscopy, which in this study was categorised as an objective method of measuring power changes in the eye. The examiner did not know which eye had been implanted with the crystalens or standard monofocal IOL. Half of the eyes (112 eyes in 56 patients) had received the crystalens and the other half (112 eyes in 56 patients) had received standard monofocal IOLs. The crystalens demonstrated a significantly greater power change than the standard monofocal (2.42 D vs. 0.91 D).

Evolution of Accommodative IOL Implants

Accommodative IOL implants have gone through significant evolution in last two decades since its inception. The first generation accommodative IOL implants of 1989 were based on the principle of plate haptics IOL's. Seven lens designs have been implanted during the initial period of over 9 years. These IOL implants had provided mixed results in terms of quality of visual acuity. Various studies on the accommodative functions had revealed corneal curvature steepening at 90 degrees and residual myopia in a significant number of cases. Average lens movement was restricted upto 0.7 mm during the early period and has shown a gradual decay in the subsequent period. Professor Kammann had observed anterior dislocation of IOL implant in few cases of different designs of accommodative IOL implants.

Second and Third Generations of Accommodative IOL Implants are as follows:
(a) Biocom dold accommodative IOL
(b) VISIOGEN accommodative IOL system
(c) The Clamshell variable accommodating IOL
(d) Accommodative 1 CU IOL
(e) Crystalens at 45 IOL

Accommodative 1 CU IOL
Special characteristic features of accommodative 1 CU IOL implant are as follows:
(i) The IOL is made-up of hydrophilic acrylic material.
(ii) The refractive index of the IOL is 1.46.
(iii) The overall diameter of IOL is 9.8 mm including the optical diameter of 5.5 mm.

Mechanism of Action
The pseudophakic accommodative effort of this IOL is produced by a change in dioptric power of the central axis

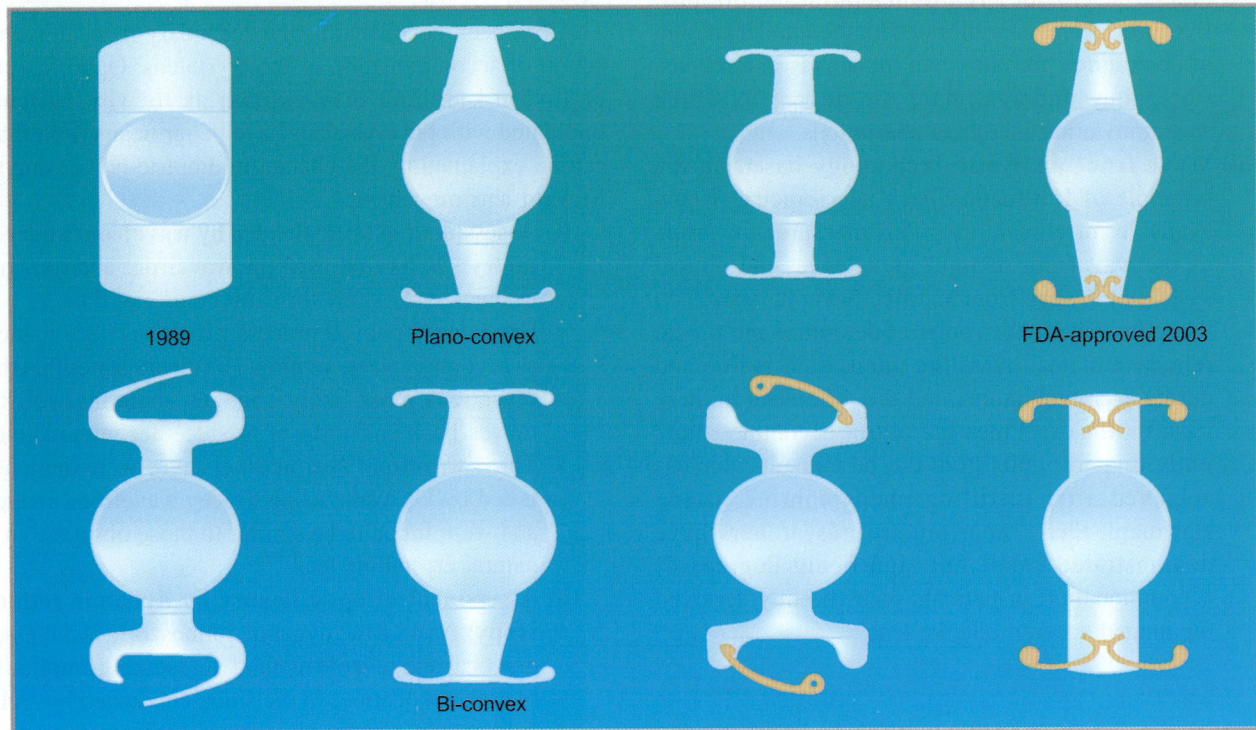

1989   Plano-convex   FDA-approved 2003

Bi-convex

Fig. 22.1: Early (1989) Crystalens evolution—1989 to Present (*Courtesy:* Bausch and Lomb)

of the IOL by a forward movement of the optic by the virtue of action of the ciliary muscle.

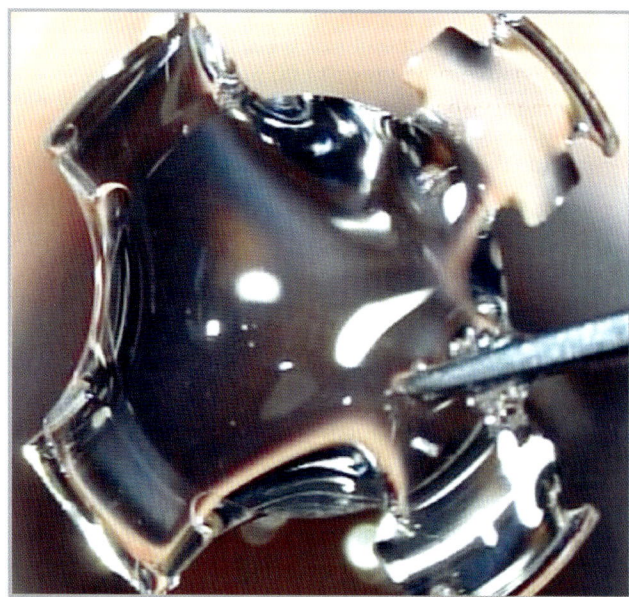

Fig. 22.2: Human optic Accommodative 1 CU IOL implant

Small and soft haptics are prone to loose accommodative efforts due to subsequent fibrosis of anterior capsular rim. This has restricted its employability and efficacy in the long term particularly in the younger age group patients.

Evolution of Crystalens

Initial models of Crystalens accommodative IOL implant were manufactured by C&C Vision CA USA. However, the newer generation Crystalens IOL has been launched by Bausch and Lomb. Crystalens accommodative IOL implant is made up of silicone polymer Dimethylsiloxane (Biosil) material. The IOL implant possesses the basic concept of modified plate haptic lens design. The peculiarity in the design of IOL optics is the presence of hinges next to the optic along with adjoining small polyamide haptics which secure the IOL implant in the capsular bag. The contraction of the ciliary muscles facilitates the vaulting of IOL optics by virtue of the presence of the grooves adjoining the optics. However, relatively smaller sized optic of 4.5 mm as well as over all loop to loop length of 11.5mm restricted efficacy of accommodative mechanism of Crystalens AT 45 IOL in the long term. HD-500 is latest version of Crystalens which has received the FDA approval in 2008 for its design and mechanism of action of accommodative actions. HD-500 is available in the range of + 17.0 to 33.0 Dioptres where as HD-520 is available in the range of+10.0 to 16.75 Dioptres.

Other models of Crystalens are as follows:
  (i) AT 50 SE
  (ii) AT 52 SE
  (iii) HD 520

A comparative evaluation of the features of different generations of Crystalens is as follows:

Table 22.1: Comparative evaluation of features of different generations of Crystalens (Courtesy Bausch and Lomb)

	AT50SE	HD500
Optic diameter	5.0 mm	5.0 mm
Overall length	11.5 mm	11.5 mm
Material	Biosil	Biosil
A-constant	119.0	119.0
Refractive index	1.427	1.427
Diopters available	17.0 to 33.0 D	17.0 to 33.0 D
Optic Design	Spherical, square-edged design	Spherical, square-edged design with an enhanced optic

	AT50SE	HD500
Optic diameter	5.0 mm	5.0 mm
Overall length	12 mm	12 mm
Material	Biosil	Biosil
A-constant	119.0	119.0
Refractive index	1.427	1.427
Diopters available	4.0 to 16.75 D	10.0 to 16.75 D
Optic Design	Spherical, square-edged design	Spherical, square-edged design with an enhanced optic

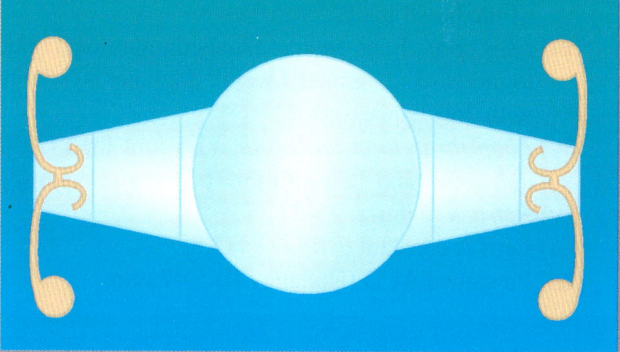

Fig. 22.3 : Crystalens AT-45

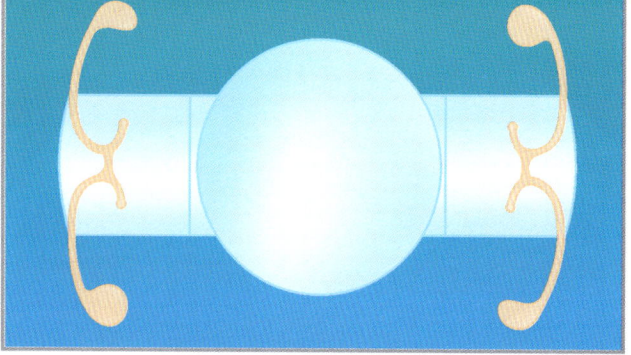

Fig. 22.4: Crystalens HD 500

How the Present Generation Crystalens Differs from Previous Generation Accommodative Crystalens IOL Implants

Lens Design

The crystalens HD is a modified plate haptic monofocal lens that exercises ciliary muscle contractions to induce natural accommodative efforts to provide variable focus on objects at all distances for near, distance and intermediate vision while retaining the quality of vision at all times. The surface has been shaped to enhance the depth of focus with an optical modification.

The 1.5 mm diameter modification to the centre of the lens provides a 3 micron increase in the centre thickness relative to the Five-O. This configuration results in negative spherical aberration in the central 1.5 mm zone of the optics. The aberration pattern then gradually reduces and shifts to the positive towards the periphery of the lens. The negative spherical aberration centrally provides an increased depth of focus which is designed to improve near vision without compromising intermediate or distance vision. An improved contrast sensitivity is also achieved, that too without inducing undesirable dysphotopsia or night vision symptoms.

Lens Parametres

(i) Made up of Biosil (Dimethylsiloxane), a third generation silicone elastomer.
(ii) *Haptic material:* Flexible coloured polyamide (Kapton) loops are attached to each distal extremity of the biosil plates.
(iii) *Lens optic:* Lens optic is a hinged monofocal optic to increase movement. Overall diameter is 5.0 mm with 360° square-edge.
(iv) *Loop tip to loop tip length:* 11.5 mm for 17.00D and above and 12.0 mm for 16.75D and below.
(v) *Refractive index:* 1.427
(vi) Lens A constant (SRK-T) 118.8
(vii) Presumed ACD (Holladay II) 5.47 mm

(viii) Available lens powers:
   HD : +10.00 to 33.00 in ½ D steps
   Five-O: +4.00 to 10.00 in 1 D steps
      +10.00 to 16.00 in ½ D steps
      +16.00 to 27.00 in ¼ D steps
      +27.00 to 33.00 in ½ D steps

Mechanism of Action

(i) With psuedophakic accommodative effort, there is redistribution of the ciliary body mass resulting in an increased vitreous pressure which will move the optic forwards anteriorly.
(ii) The hinge incorporated permits optic flexure or forward movement of the optic by minimising possible resistance. Various studies have shown average anterior movement of 1.44 mm in this action. This has been postulated as the secondary mechanism of action of accommodation of the crystalens. Optic flexure or forward arching may explain as to why patients implanted with the crystalens have better near vision than can be explained by the change in dioptric power of the forward lens movement.
(iii) Crystalens HD possesses a single point of focus. The central 1.5 mm zone of the lens adds approximately 1.00 dioptre of power which helps for reading, particularly during miotic status of the pupil. This configuration very much simulates the status of lens pupillary diaphragm during physiological accommodative mechanism observed in a normal phakic eye.

Merits of Crystalens

(i) The peculiar design of the optics and high grade biosil lens material produces increased depth of focus which in turn delivers excellent all range visual functions.
(ii) The patient possesses useful accommodative faculty, hence casual work at distance, intermediate as well as at close range is possible without spectacles.

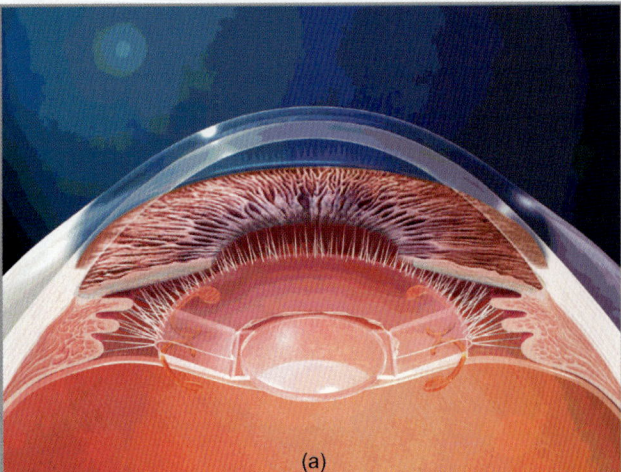
(a)

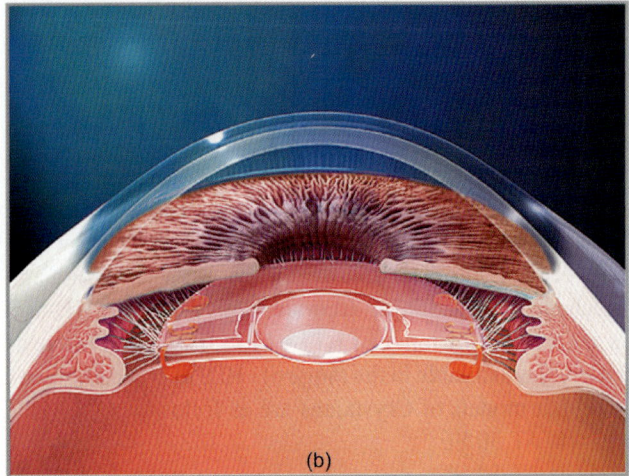
(b)

Fig. 22.5: Mechanism of accommodative action of crystalens: (a) Disaccommodated, (b) Accommodated

(iii) Identical good vision and sustained depth of focus in both mesopic and photopic conditions.

(iv) Visual acuity and contrast is independent of pupil size. Minimised glare and halos due to proximity to the nodal point.

(v) Uniform contrast sensitivity at all range of vision.

Demerits and Constraints of Crystalens

(i) Complete freedom from spectacles may not be possible for very fine quality of vision or in cases of aberrations in IOL power calculations (15 to 20% cases.)

(ii) Optical aberrations and glare may be seen in 10 to 15 % cases, particularly in high myopic eyes due to the narrow or small optic (< 5.5 mm) of crystalens or slight decentration of small optics in a large sized pupil.

(iii) Crystalens is a white transparent lens and its efficacy to absorb ultraviolet light is debatable. Hence its utility in cases of posterior segment disorders or bright sunlight exposure needs due consideration. A proper UV400 protection is essential while exposed to bright sunlight.

(iv) Accommodative action may be affected in due course of time due to impending and inevitable delayed changes in the capsular bag such as fibrosis of the anterior Capsulorrhexis margins and posterior capsular opacification. Over and above, long term impact on accommodative efforts of ciliary body in the presence of alerted capsular bag in terms of open bag due to Capsulorrhexis and presence of smaller sized artificial IOL as contents of the bag are yet to be evaluated.

(v) Meticulous follow-up is mandatory to monitor mechanical and biological integrity and stability of hinges.

(vi) The efficacy of the accommodative action of crystalens may be adversely influenced in a vitrectomised eye due to the fact that pseudophakic accommodative effort generated by crystalens has direct correlation with the combined action of movement of ciliary body mass and the vitreous thrust.

(vii) Smaller size of IOL and rigid haptics refrain ciliary sulcus insertion of crystalens.

(viii) The safety and efficacy of crystalens is not known in younger patients.

(ix) Viewing smaller diameter of optics, meticulous evaluation of size and time of YAG-laser posterior capsulotomy is very crucial. Early capsulotomy or larger opening increases the risk of IOL dislocation. Hence, the posterior capsulotomy osteum should be less than 4 mm of diameter and should not be attempted before 12 weeks of the postoperative period.

Preop Work-up

The pre-operative work-up, as for any intraocular surgery, involves immaculate and precision driven preoperative evaluation. Crystalens can be implanted in most of the cataract, however considering peculiarities in lens design as well as the patient's expectations of very high quality full range visual outcome, all patients must be thoroughly counselled in detail about all the pros and cons of procedures and the final outcome.

It is worth considering excluding under mentioned associated conditions for accommodative IOL implants.

Relative Contraindications

(i) Corneal astigmatism of more than 1 dioptre.

(ii) Amblyopia

(iii) Associated congenital anomalies

(iv) Congenital bilateral cataracts

(v) Recurrent anterior or posterior uveitis

(vi) Significant posterior segment involvement like Diabetic retinopathy. CNVM and history of retinal detachment.

(vii) Rigid and miotic pupil which may interfere with the surgical manoeuvres.

(viii) High Myopia or large pupillary aperture where small optic of IOL may produce annoying symptoms of glare and halos

(ix) Long standing Glaucoma

(x) Poor status of Cornea or Corneal endothelial dystrophy

(xi) Post corneal transplant cases

(xii) Post traumatic cataract with associated anterior segment derangements like zonulolysis or angle recession.

(xiii) Intraoperative constraints or complications

(xiv) Any evidence of Abnormal retinal correspondence

Patient Selection

All types of cataracts can be considered for Crystalens implantation except the above mentioned contraindications. However, the final onus and decision of patient selection rests with the operating surgeon. The following guidelines are recommended to achieve best functional outcome, particularly in initial cases:

(i) Bilateral Presenile or senile cataract (Paediatric and traumatic cataract may face surgical constraints especially while attempting an ideal capsulorhexis, hence should be ruled out.)

(ii) Uncomplicated ocular status. (Intact binocular vision with normal optical, anterior and posterior segment configuration without any retinal or optic nerve involvement.)

(iii) A moderate grade of Nucleus density (Grade two to three) Too soft or too hard cataract may not be an ideal cataract to achieve excellent surgical outcome

(iv) Avoid extremes of refractive error. (Ideal IOL powers from +16.0-27.5 D (0.25D steps)

(v) Corneal astigmatism should be less than 1.0 dioptre.

(vi) Adequate depth of the anterior chamber

(vii) Realistic expectations.

Assessment of IOL Power Calculation

Undoubtedly, precise and meticulous IOL power calculation is one of the most crucial aspects of an excellent and desired visual outcome following any IOL implantation procedure. This is more important while considering premium IOL implantation. Manual keratometry and application of self titrated A-constant on an excellent A-scan is of utmost important. The authors recommend using IOL Master(Carl Zeiss Meditec) for this purpose.

Various IOL power calculation formula's are required in specific and peculiar structural and optical conditions of the eye. To achieve the desired post IOL implantation and the desired refractive visual, the following guidelines are important.

Selection of which Eye to be First: Dominant or Non-dominant

Dominant eye first: According to this concept, it is advisable to operate the dominant eye first so as to observe the refractive outcome for near and subsequently readjust the IOL power in the non-dominant eye. However, the author prefers to take up the non-dominant eye first and fine tune the IOL power in the dominating eye subsequently, so as to achieve best full range vision. Most patients remained much more comfortable and satisfied with this situation. This is akin to performing a dry run or a full dress rehearsal for any important event. It is a better option to smoothen out all wrinkles and shortcomings in the surgery on the non-dominant eye and be fully prepared with individualistic corrections for the all important dominant eye.

Target Refraction for Crystalens

A slight myopic shift or myopic astigmatism is a standard concept in the monofocal IOL implantation procedure. This provides some degree of pseudophakic accommodation. However, it is recommended to target a Plano to slightly hyperopic shift for the dominant eye when implanting crystalens. This shift provides a better range of uncorrected vision for near and intermediate range following accommodative and multifocal IOL implantation.

Assessment of Corneal Curvature

Assessment of corneal curvature is the critical first step in calculating the IOL power to be implanted in order to give the patient a near perfect vision. There are a multitude of methods employed for calculating the corneal curvature, or the K readings. In this regard, the latest is not necessarily the best. We recommend calculation of the corneal curvature ideally by the IOL Master(Carl Zeiss Meditec). This is based on the same principle as the age old placido disc, but takes five individual accurate keratometry readings within 0.5 seconds. It is a good idea to have the patient blink his eyes just before taking the keratometry readings, so as to have a fresh and uniformly distributed tear film as the ideal reflecting surface. In case of non availability of IOL Master (Carl Zeiss Meditec), K readings can be taken with the manual Bausch and Lomb or the Javal-Schiotz keratometre. It is strongly recommended that the K readings from the automated kerato-refractometres should not be used for the purpose of calculating IOL power, more so when a sensitive and precise outcome is desired, as while implanting an accommodative IOL. The standard protocol is to take the Keratometry readings before instilling any drops into the eyes, especially topical anaesthetics, as the epithelial damage and derangement caused by them causes a less than perfect reflection from the corneal surface.

Ideally, all patients wearing contact lenses should abstain from wearing their contact lenses in order to get the correct keratometric values of the cornea without ortho-keratological factors coming into play. At our centre we recommend stoppage of wearing contact lens two weeks prior to IOL power calculation for soft contact lenses and four to six weeks of abstinence from the lenses in case of RGP lenses.

Measurement of the Axial Length (Biometry)

The second and equally important step in ideal IOL power calculation is the measurement of the Axial length of the eye. Only non-contact methods of IOL power calculation are employed for calculating the IOL power when accommodative IOLs are being planned to be implanted. The technique and accuracy of Axial length measurement has been taken to newer heights by the IOL Master (Carl Zeiss Meditec) which is based on the principle of optical biometry vis-à-vis earlier A-scan machines which were based on the principle of ultrasonic measurements. The IOL Master (Carl Zeiss Meditec) measures the distance from the anterior surface of the cornea (actually the anterior surface of the tear film) to the retinal pigment epithelium, whereas the ultrasonic A-scan biometres measure the distance from the front of the cornea to the Internal limiting membrane of the retina. Also, there is an inevitable compression of the cornea by about 300 microns due to the pressure of the probe or the coupling agent while performing ultrasonic biometry. The IOL Master (Carl Zeiss Meditec) measures the exact distance existing in the viewing process, whereas ultrasound instruments determine only the approximated distance. With the IOL master (Carl Zeiss Meditec) the measured lengths are operator-independent. Needless to say then, that IOL master (Carl Zeiss Meditec) offers a much more accurate and precise method of IOL power calculation and must necessarily be employed for IOL power calculation when implanting accommodative IOLs.

Mode of IOL Power Calculation

The required data for IOL power having been ascertained satisfactorily, the next question to be addressed is the IOL power calculation and the formula that needs to be employed to calculate it. The following principles need to be kept in mind while calculating IOL power for the crystalens:

(i) SRK-T formula is ideal for all eyes with axial lengths over 22.0 mm and the targeted refraction should be emmetropia to minimal hypermetropia.

(ii) The Holladay II is more ideal for eyes with mean K's flatter than 42.00 D or steeper than 47.00 D independent of the axial length. The Holladay II is more beneficial for all eyes 22.0 mm or shorter and the targeted postoperative refraction in both these cases should be -0.5DS.

(iii) Best results in our hands have been obtained when the A-constant employed is 118.8 for SRK(T) and 119.0 for Holladay II

(iv) The predicted Anterior Chamber Depth for all calculations is 5.47 mm

(v) The final power selection of the crystalens in the second eye is also influenced by the refractive outcome of the eye operated earlier.

Preoperative Counselling

The importance of pre-operative counselling cannot be overemphasised. The deluge of advertisements and the colossal amount of data available on the subject delivers a very educated, intelligent and demanding patient with high, almost unrealistic aspirations. It is our duty to bring these expectations to realistic and achievable levels with counselling. Our patients are explained in detail all the known complications of surgery. In addition, more stress is laid on the fact that although the patient will have good vision for all distances; for precise fine work, the aid of spectacles may still be required. The vagaries of IOL power calculations are also discussed and the possibility of a refractive surprise mentioned. A pre-informed patient yields happier outcomes for the surgeon, the patient and the relatives.

Preoperative Medications

We do not recommend any variations in the regimen of preoperative medications as compared to the protocol used for standard Phacoemulsification and Foldable IOL implantation procedures. Use of preoperative antibiotics in the form of topical and systemic medications is as per the surgeon's own choice. As a routine, we do not advocate preoperative use of antibiotics in any form, including topical or systemic administration. However topical application of NSAIDs is definitely beneficial to maintain a good and sustained preoperative mydriasis.

Surgical Technique

There are a very few deviations from the standard phaco-emulsification procedures in surgeries where accommodative IOLs are being planned. The general rule of thumb is that everything has to be done better, more precisely and more accurately. This said, there are however some deviations from the conventional steps which are peculiar to surgeries with the accommodative IOL implantation. They are enumerated below as a guideline to be practiced in amalgamation with the procedure discussed in the earlier chapters.

Incisions

The incisions, both the side port and the main tunnel need to be of the exact dimensions and adequately beveled and stepped so as to be water tight. Any main tunnel larger than 2.8 mm or not adequately stepped can lead to an

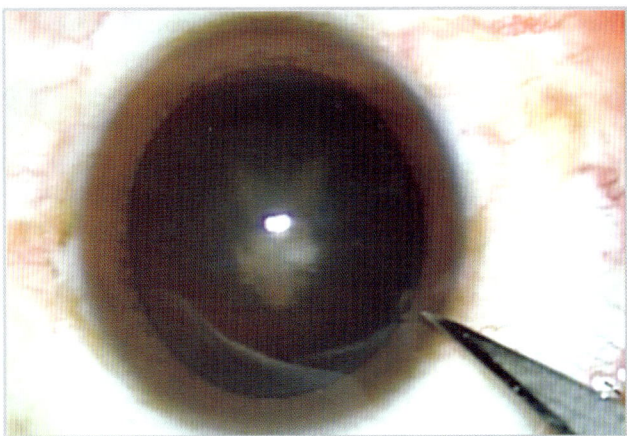

Fig. 22.6(a): 2.8mm clear corneal tunnel

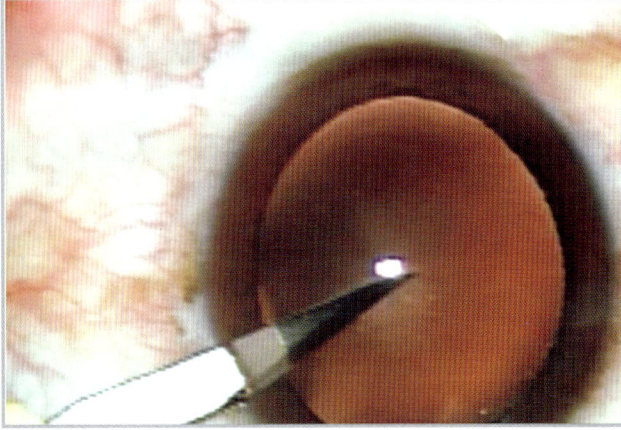

Fig. 22.6(b): Side-port incision

immediate postoperative leak in the incision which might cause a forward displacement of the accommodative lens. It might have minimal influence in the case of monofocal IOL implantation, but makes the whole postoperative refractive calculation go awry and negates all the good done by using an accommodative IOL.

Rhexis

The execution of an ideal controlled rhexis needs to be perfected as an art and not just a scientific technique. The accommodative effect of the IOL and the incidence of post/operative contracture and opacification are not influenced as much by any other step of the surgery as it is by the rhexis. In cases where accommodative IOL implantation is being planned, we prefer to make a slightly smaller rhexis. A rhexis of 5.5 to 6 mm is ideal (as the IOL optic of crystalens is 5 mm). This ensures that there is no overlap of the anterior capsular frill over the anterior optic surface. In case of such an overlap, the anterior movement of the lens during the process of accommodation is physically restricted by the anterior capsular frill, causing a decrease in the amplitude of the available accommodation. The rhexis needs to be absolutely smooth to prevent migration and vaulting of the lens and absolutely central as the optic of the lens is small. In case of a perceivably subnormal rhexis, it is better to revert to the implantation of a monofocal IOL. In the beginning, at our centre we use a 6.0 mm OZ optical marker to mark a rough template on the cornea. This makes sure that the rhexis does not become abnormally large and also ensures perfect centration of the rhexis (6 mm because of the corneal curvature, a rhexis collinear with a 6 mm corneal mark will only be 5.6–5.75 mm on the anterior capsule of the lens).

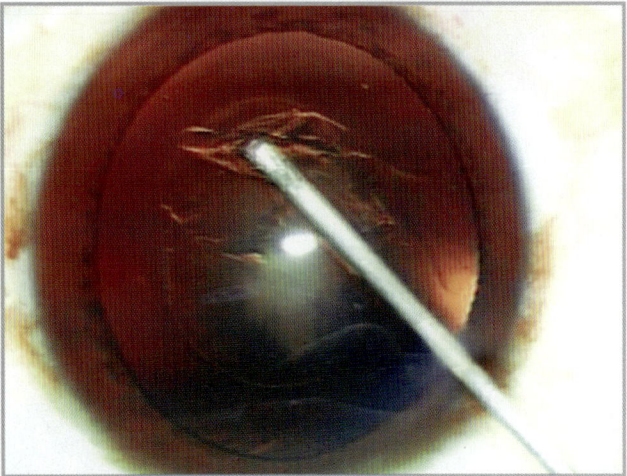

Fig. 22.7: Capsulorrhexis

Phacoemulsification

There is no deviation in the steps of phacoemulsification except that care is taken to make sure that the chopper does not damage any part of the CCC, nor does the process of phacoemulsification cause excessive stress on the zonules. Needless to say, any complication warrants an implantation of a monofocal IOL.

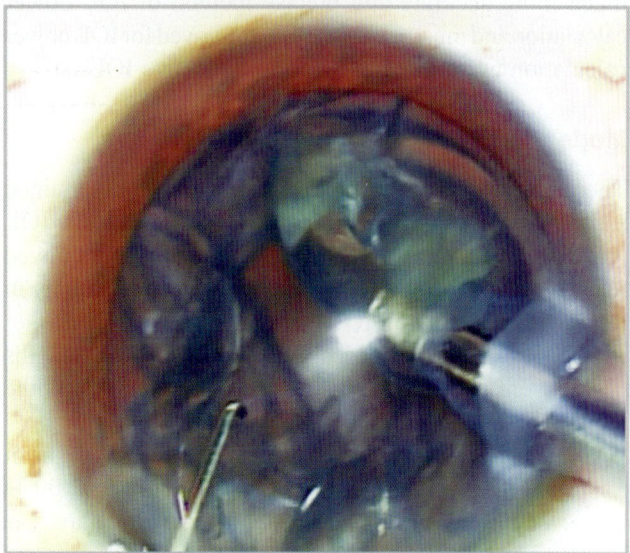

Fig. 22.8: Nucleotomy and phacoemulsification

Cortical Clean-up

The clearance of the cortex needs to be meticulous and thorough. Any cortex left behind is a harbinger of future troubles like capsular phimosis, lens decentration and capsular opacification. At our centre, sheppard capsular polisher (momentum medical) is routinely used for all surgeries with the accommodative IOL. It also is a good practice to employ the cap-vac mode for removing the epithelial cells from the undersurface of the anterior capsular frill and the posterior capsule.

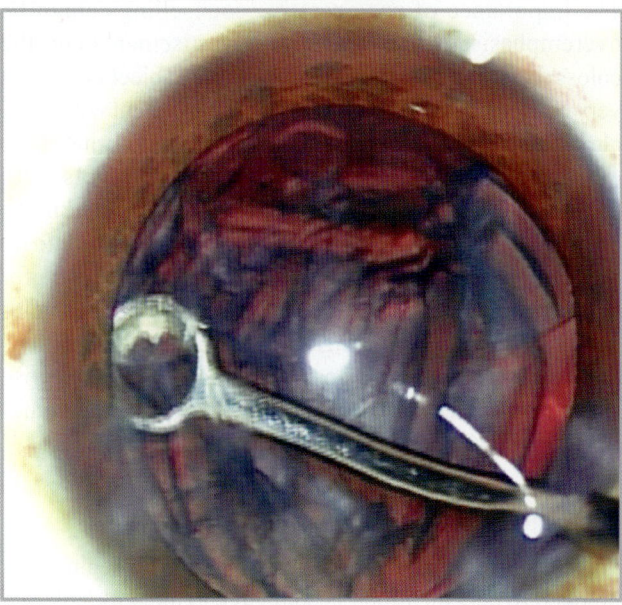

Fig. 22.9: Thick capsular plate being dislodged from the capsular fornices

Insertion of Accommodative Crystalens IOL

The crystalens is easily inserted with the already available crystalsert inserters and delivery system introduced by Bausch & Lomb. Crystalsert inserters and delivery system is a disposable plastic device comprising of a syringe shaped body and tip with a plunger and a drawer. Crystalens can be inserted into capsular bag with a single continuous forward motion. To begin loading crystalens into the injector system, the IOL is placed in the load area with optic in contact with the body floor and ensuring that the leading circular haptic is under the IOL track edge and the leading plate haptic is tangential to the body of the edge. The trailing haptic should be in contact with the track. It is very important to ensure that the plate haptics are in contact with the body floor. The trailing circular haptic lobe must be positioned for correct lens orientation.

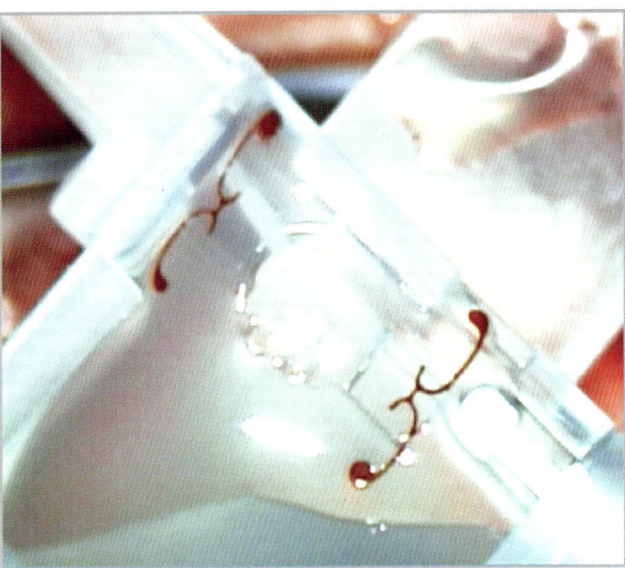

Fig. 22.12: Loading of Crystalens HD 500

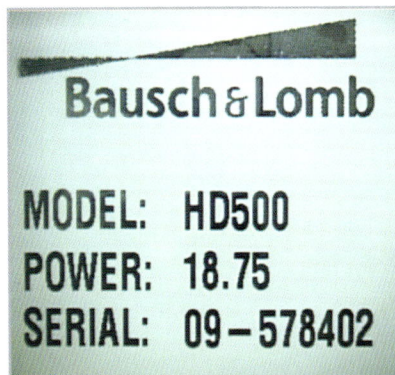

Fig. 22.10: Crystalens HD 500 specifications

It is advisable to place the lens in the bag in one go with all the four haptics below the anterior capsular frill. But in case this cannot be achieved, gentle manipulation with a ball dialler or a Y hook does the trick.

A cohesive viscoelastic like Amvisc Plus (Bausch & Lomb) should be used for lubrication of the injector when injecting the lens as this ensures smooth insertion and prevents lens slippage which is common with silicon material. Visual confirmation that both the plates and the four haptics are in the bag is imperative. Place the lens posteriorly in the bag.

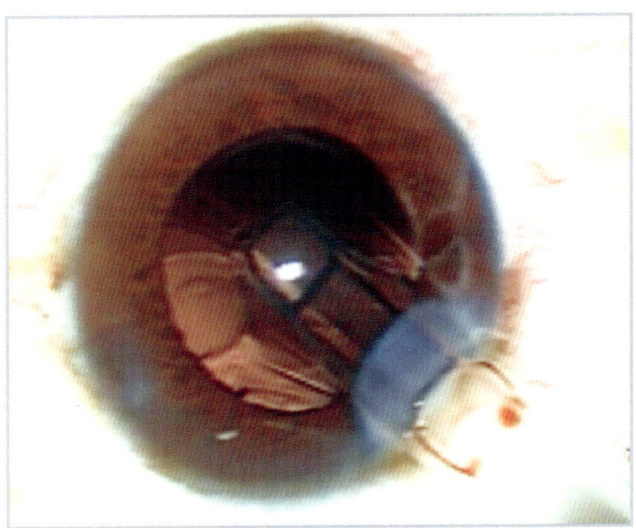

Fig. 22.13: Insertion of Crystalens HD 500

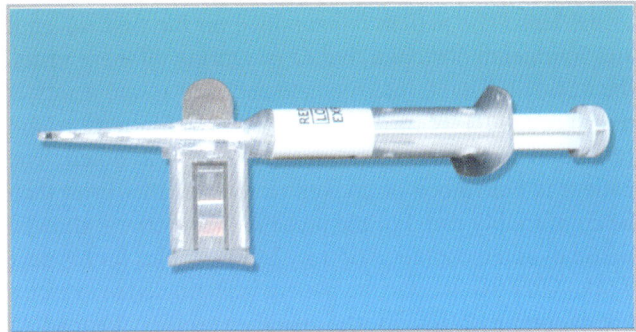

Fig. 22.11: Crystalsert inserters and delivery system (Bausch & Lomb)

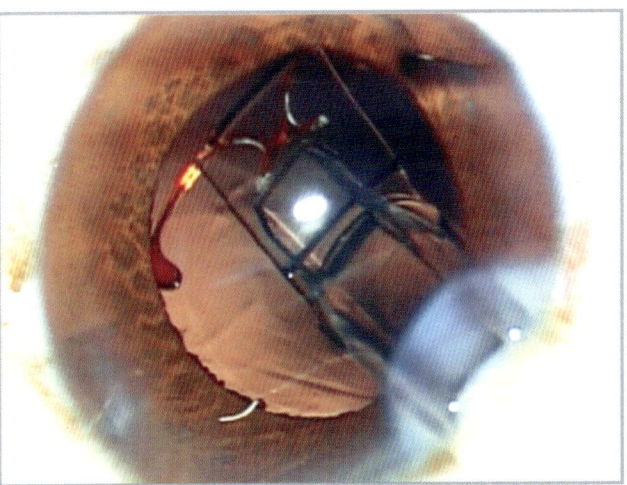

Fig. 22.14: Crystalens HD 500 being released in the capsular bag

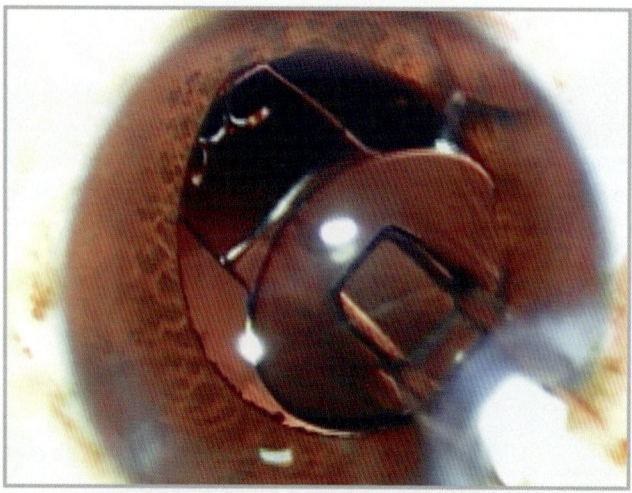

Fig. 22.15: Crystalens HD 500 unfolding in the capsular bag

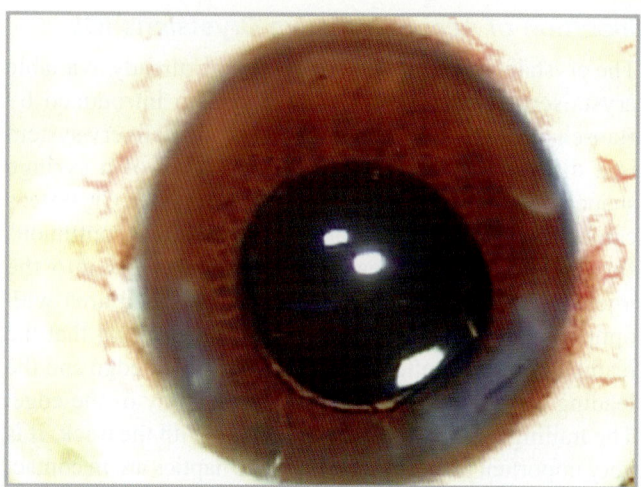

Fig. 22.16: Crystalens HD 500 well placed in the capsular bag

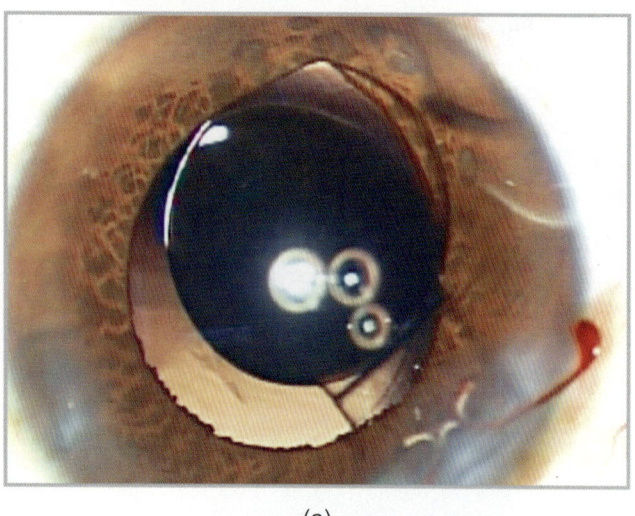

(a)

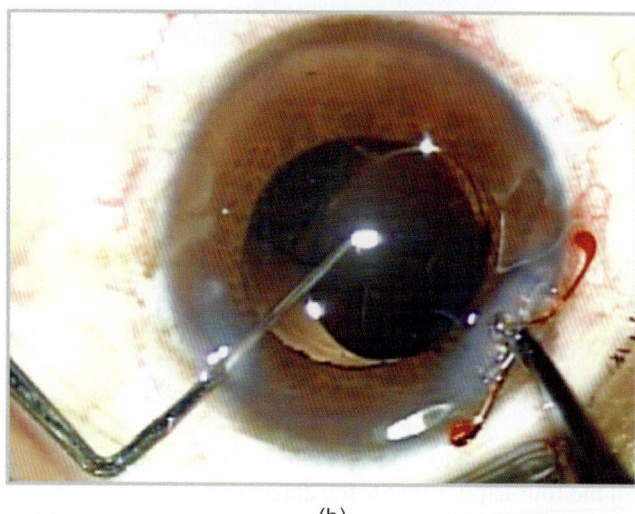

(b)

Fig. 22.17: (a) Improper opening of an IOL outside of the capsular bag and over the capsulorhexis margins, (b) Crystalens is being dialled for positioning into the capsular bag

Post-IOL Insertion Irrigation-aspiration (I-A)

To ensure an ideal placement of the lens, it is necessary to do an adequate post-insertion irrigation-aspiration. Rocking the lens sideways generally ensures that there is no viscoelastic trapped behind the lens, and here the small optic acts to our advantage. The authors generally do hydration of the corneal wounds prior to the I-A, to prevent forward vaulting of the IOL during the procedure.

Completion of Surgery

At the completion of surgery, the corneal wounds are again hydrated and their integrity checked. In case of any doubt, applying one suture, though not too tightly is not a bad practice. At the end of surgery, we routinely instill a drop of a cycloplegics, preferably Gt. Atropine 1%. This ensures a quiet postoperative eye, and also ensures a posteriorly nestled IOL in the immediate postoperative period.

Postoperative Care

The postoperative care does not vary from that of a normal patient after phacoemulsification and foldable IOL implantation. Only that the use of cycloplegics is advisable for the first one week to ensure proper posterior positioning of the lens. The patient is examined on the first, seventh and fourteenth postoperative days. During all these visits, the unaided distant, intermediate and near visual acuity is measured, IOT recording, Slit lamp examination and refraction for distance and near add are also noted. The patient is not forced or coaxed to read smaller print than he comfortably can. For the present, the patient is allowed to use over the counter +1.5 to +2.0 spectacles for his near work. After two weeks, the patient is instructed to exercise his accommodation by the usual exercises. Instead of focusing on an approaching pencil or rod, he is told to concentrate on J3 print and bring it closer and closer to his face. This is not just a pacifier or placebo and really helps in the accommodation adjusting to the new environment of an open anterior capsule and a silicone lens in contrast to the normal environment. At 10 days postoperative and two weeks postoperatively, refraction is carried out. Cycloplegic refraction and keratometry is also carried out and analysed. It is preferred to do a cycloplegics refraction when visual acuity and refraction do not correlate or if near visual acuity is less than J3.

Cause for any deviations from the expected is looked into. Generally there can be an unexpected myopic shift. This commonly occurs due to:

  (i) Micro incision leaks causing micro anterior movements of the lens
  (ii) Retained cortical matter tilting or pushing the lens
  (iii) A hypotonous postoperative eye.

Surgical intervention is contemplated as appropriate in scenarios (i) and (ii) but eyes in which the cause of myopic shift is a relative hypotony are best left alone to regress with time.

One point which needs consideration is the inertia of accommodation with crystalens. The speed of change in the accommodative power is not as fast as with natural accommodation. This means, we might get a falsely myopic distant refraction in case the patient has indulged in some near work just before entering the consultation chamber. This needs to be kept in mind. A good practice to follow is to do cycloplegics refraction in all patients after two weeks of surgery.

Accommodative IOLs can deliver their potential outcomes only if the postoperative refraction meets the pre operative calculations. This is generally a -0.75 DS and/or a -0.5DC. Studies have shown that this is achievable only in one third of the patients postoperatively despite using the most advanced techniques. This lack of consistency and predictability is the limiting factor in use of these accommodative IOLs as of today.

CONCLUSION

The Crystalens accommodating IOL implants have revealed excellent uncorrected near, intermediate, and distance vision in pseudophakic eyes. There is no deterioration in contrast sensitivity with these IOL implants in comparisons to the standard monofocal IOLs. The accommodative lenses have opened a new realm of opportunities and possibilities. No doubt, we are still to hear the last word and see the last innovation in this field, but looking back at the milestones we have crossed, the future is indeed rosy. The only thing which we need to guard against is that the patient's expectations are always one step ahead of what we can deliver. A judicious mix of technological advances and patient counselling is the only way forward to make the two ends meet.

REFERENCES

1. Devgan U, Lindstrom Richard L., Jack A Singer, Jeffrey Whitman. First Impressions of the Crystalens HD. Cataract and Refractive Surgery Today, November 2008, 17
2. I. Howard Fine, Richard S. Hoffman, Mark Packer, Avoiding Complications with Refractive Lens Exchange. The steps we take to minimise problems with this procedure. Cataract and Refractive Surgery Today July 2004, 24
3. Schachar RA. The mechanism of accommodation and presbyopia. International Ophthalmology Clinics. 46(3): 39–61, 2006
4. Coleman DJ. On the hydraulic suspension theory of accommodation. Trans Am Ophthalmol Soc 1986, 84:846–68.
5. Coleman DJ, Fish SK. Presbyopia, Accommodation, and the Mature Catenary. Ophthalmol 2001; 108(9):1544–51.
6. Abolmaali A, Schachar RA, Le T. "Sensitivity study of human crystalline lens accommodation." Computer Methods and Programs in Biomedicine. 85(1):77–90, 2007
7. Schachar RA. The lens is stable during accommodation. Ophthalmic Physiological Optics. In press, 2007.
8. Schachar RA, Davila C, Pierscionek BK, Chen W, Ward WW. The effect of human in vivo accommodation on crystalline lens stability. British Journal of Ophthalmology. 91(6): 790–793, 2007.
9. Schachar RA, Pierscionek BK, Abolmaali A, Le, T. The relationship between accommodative amplitude and the ratio of central lens thickness to its equatorial diametre in vertebrate eyes. British Journal of Ophthalmology. 91(6):812–817, 2007.
10. Schachar RA, Fygenson DK. Topographical changes of biconvex objects during equatorial traction: An analogy for accommodation of the human lens. British Journal of Ophthalmology. In press, 2007.
11. Schachar RA. Equatorial lens growth predicts the age-related decline in accommodative amplitude that results in presbyopia and the increase in intraocular pressure that occurs with age. International Ophthalmology Clinics. 48(1): In press, 2008.
12. Schachar RA, Abolmaali A, Le T. Insights into the etiology of the age related decline in the amplitude of accommodation using a nonlinear finite element model of the accommodating human lens. British Journal of Ophthalmology. 90: 1304–1309, 2006.
13. Coleman DJ. Unified model for the accommodative mechanism. Am J Ophthalmol 1970, 69:1063–79.
14. Alió JL, Ben-nun J, Rodríguez-Prats JL, Plaza AB. Visual and accommodative outcomes 1 year after implantation of an accommodating intraocular lens based on a new concept.J Cataract Refract Surg. 2009 Oct, 35(10):1671–8.
15. Li XR, Zhao L, Hu BJ. Clinical research of accommodating intraocular lens. Zhonghua Yan Ke Za Zhi. 2009 Apr., 45(4): 328–31. Chinese.
16. Tang X, Song H. Matching and selection of two different types of pseudo-accommodative intraocular lens in two eyes

after cataract phacoemulsification. Zhonghua Yan Ke Za Zhi. 2008 Dec, 44(12):1060–2. Chinese.

17. Yu AY, Wang QM, Zhuge J, Jin WQ, Jiang J, Zhao YE.Enhanced near stereopsis after phacoemulsification and implantation of posterior chamber intraocular lens by prescribing addition properly. Zhonghua Yan Ke Za Zhi. 2008 Aug, 44(8):711–4. Chinese.

18. Hermans EA, Dubbelman M, Van der Heijde R, Heethaar RM. Equivalent refractive index of the human lens upon accommodative response.Optom Vis Sci. 2008 Dec, 85(12): 1179–84.

19. Schor CM, Bharadwaj SR. Adaptive calibration of dynamic accommodation—implications for accommodating intraocular lenses. J Refract Surg. 2008 Nov., 24(9):984–90.

20. Hermans EA, Terwee TT, Koopmans SA, Dubbelman M, van der Heijde RG, Heethaar RM. Development of a ciliary muscle-driven accommodating intraocular lens. J Cataract Refract Surg. 2008 Dec, 34(12):2133–8.

21. Ehmer A, Mannsfeld A, Auffarth GU, Holzer MP. Dynamic stimulation of accommodation. J Cataract Refract Surg. 2008 Dec, 34(12):2024–9.

22. Missotten T, Verhamme T, Blanckaert J, Missotten G.Optical formula to predict outcomes after implantation of accommodating intraocular lenses. J Cataract Refract Surg. 2004 Oct, 30(10):2084–7.

23. Gupta N, Wolffsohn JS, Naroo SA, Davies LN, Gibson GA, Shah S. Development of a near activity visual questionnaire to assess accommodating intraocular lenses. Cont Lens Anterior Eye. 2007 May, 30(2):134–43. Epub 2007 Feb 26.

24. Li XM, Wang W. To observe clinical effect of accommodative IOL on different age patients. Zhonghua Yan Ke Za Zhi. 2008 Jan, 44(1):30–2. Chinese.

25. Heatley CJ, Spalton DJ, Boyce JF, Marshall J. A mathematical model of factors that influence the performance of accommodative intraocular lenses. Ophthalmic Physiol Opt. 2004 Mar, 24(2):111–8.

26. Strenk SA, Strenk LM, Guo S. Magnetic resonance imaging of aging, accommodating, phakic, and pseudophakic ciliary muscle diametres. J Cataract Refract Surg. 2006 Nov, 32(11): 1792–8.

27. Hancox J, Spalton D, Heatley C, Jayaram H, Marshall J. Objective measurement of intraocular lens movement and dioptric change with a focus shift accommodating intraocular lens. J Cataract Refract Surg. 2006 Jul., 32(7):1098–103.

28. Langenbucher A, Jakob C, Reese S, Seitz B. Determination of pseudophakic accommodation with translation lenses using Purkinje image analysis. Ophthalmic Physiol Opt. 2005 Mar, 25(2):87–96.

29. Auffarth GU, Schmidbauer J, Becker KA, Rabsilber TM, Apple DJ. Miyake-Apple video analysis of movement patterns of an accommodative intraocular lens implant. Ophthal-mologe. 2002 Nov, 99(11):811–4. German.

30. Marchini G, Pedrotti E, Sartori P, Tosi R. Ultrasound biomicroscopic changes during accommodation in eyes with accommodating intraocular lenses: pilot study and hypothesis for the mechanism of accommodation. J Cataract Refract Surg. 2004 Dec., 30(12):2476–82.

31. Stachs O, Schneider H, Stave J, Beck R, Guthoff RF. Three-dimensional ultrasound biomicroscopic examinations for haptic differentiation of potentially accommodative intraocular lenses. Ophthalmologe. 2005 Mar, 102(3):265–71. German.

32. Stachs O, Schneider H, Stave J, Guthoff R. Potentially accommodating intraocular lenses—an in vitro and in vivo study using three-dimensional high-frequency ultrasound. J Refract Surg. 2005 Jan-Feb, 21(1):37–45.

33. Marchini G, Pedrotti E, Modesti M, Visentin S, Tosi R. Anterior segment changes during accommodation in eyes with a monofocal intraocular lens: high-frequency ultrasound study. J Cataract Refract Surg. 2008 Jun, 34(6):949–56.

34. Schneider H, Stachs O, Göbel K, Guthoff R. Changes of the accommodative amplitude and the anterior chamber depth after implantation of an accommodative intraocular lens. Graefes Arch Clin Exp Ophthalmol. 2006 Mar, 244(3): 322–9. Epub 2005 Aug 17.

35. Stachs O, Schneider H, Beck R, Guthoff R. Pharmacological-induced haptic changes and the accommodative performance in patients with the AT-45 accommodative IOL. J Refract Surg. 2006 Feb, 22(2):145–50.

36. Koeppl C, Findl O, Menapace R, Kriechbaum K, Wirtitsch M, Buehl W, Sacu S, Drexler W. Pilocarpine-induced shift of an accommodating intraocular lens: AT-45 Crystalens.J Cataract Refract Surg. 2005 Jul, 31(7):1290–7.

37. Koeppl C, Findl O, Kriechbaum K, Drexler W. Comparison of pilocarpine-induced and stimulus-driven accommodation in phakic eyes. Exp Eye Res. 2005 Jun, 80(6):795–800. Epub 2005 Jan 4.

38. Findl O, Kriechbaum K, Menapace R, Koeppl C, Sacu S, Wirtitsch M, Buehl W, Drexler W. Laserinterferometric assessment of pilocarpine-induced movement of an accommodating intraocular lens: a randomised trial. Ophthalmology. 2004 Aug, 111(8):1515–21.

39. Kriechbaum K, Findl O, Koeppl C, Menapace R, Drexler W. Stimulus-driven versus pilocarpine-induced biometric changes in pseudophakic eyes. Ophthalmology. 2005 Mar, 112(3):453–9.

40. Patel S, Alió JL, Feinbaum C.Comparison of Acri. Smart multifocal IOL, crystalens AT-45 accommodative IOL, and technovision pres by LASIK for correcting presbyopia. J Refract Surg. 2008 Mar, 24(3):294–9.

41. Alessio G, L'Abbate M, Boscia F, La Tegola MG. Capsular block syndrome after implantation of an accommodating intra-ocular lens. J Cataract Refract Surg. 2008 Apr, 34(4):703–6.

42. Harman FE, Maling S, Kampougeris G, Langan L, Khan I, Lee N, Bloom PA. Comparing the 1CU accommodative, multifocal, and monofocal intraocular lenses: a randomised trial. Ophthalmology. 2008 Jun., 115(6):993–1001.e2. Epub 2007 Nov 26.

43. Strobel J, Müller M, Soa B. Intact accommodation in pseudophakic eyes. Strobel J, Müller M, Soa B. Klin Monatsbl Augenheilkd. 2007 Sep, 224(9):716–21. German.

44. Dong Z, Wang NL, Zhu SQ, Wang J, Wang KJ, Jia LY, Zhao SQ, Wang XB. Relationship between ciliary muscle contraction and the pseudo-accommodation after the implantation of foldable intraocular lenses' Zhonghua Yan Ke Za Zhi. 2007 Feb, 43(2):99–103. Chinese.

45. Marchini G, Mora P, Pedrotti E, Manzotti F, Aldigeri R, Gandolfi SA.Functional assessment of two different accommodative intraocular lenses compared with a monofocal intraocular lens.Ophthalmology. 2007 Nov;114(11):2038-43. Epub 2007 Jun 6.

46. Mastropasqua L, Toto L, Falconio G, Nubile M, Carpineto P, Ciancaglini M, Di Nicola M, Ballone E.Longterm results of

1 CU accommodative intraocular lens implantation: 2-year follow-up study. Acta Ophthalmol Scand. 2007 Jun, 85(4): 409–14. Epub 2007 Apr 2.

47. Sanders DR, Sanders ML. Visual performance results after Tetraflex accommodating intraocular lens implantation. Ophthalmology. 2007 Sep, 114(9):1679–84. Epub 2007 Mar 21.

48. Uthoff D, Gulati A, Hepper D, Holland D. Potentially accommodating 1CU intraocular lens: 1-year results in 553 eyes and literature review. J Refract Surg. 2007 Feb, 23(2): 159–71. Review.

49. Ossma IL, Galvis A, Vargas LG, Trager MJ, Vagefi MR, McLeod SD. Synchrony dual-optic accommodating intraocular lens. Part 2: pilot clinical evaluation. J Cataract Refract Surg. 2007 Jan, 33(1):47–52.

50. McLeod SD, Vargas LG, Portney V, Ting A. Synchrony dual-optic accommodating intraocular lens. Part 1: optical and biomechanical principles and design considerations. J Cataract Refract Surg. 2007 Jan, 33(1):37–46.

51. McLeod SD. Optical principles, biomechanics, and initial clinical performance of a dual-optic accommodating intraocular lens (an American Ophthalmological Society thesis). Trans Am Ophthalmol Soc. 2006, 104:437–52.

52. Subjective and objective performance of the Lenstec KH-3500 "accommodative" intraocular lens. Br J Ophthalmol. 2006 Jun, 90(6):693–6. Epub 2006 Mar 10.

53. Wolffsohn JS, Hunt OA, Naroo S, Gilmartin B, Shah S, Cunliffe IA, Benson MT, Mantry S. Objective accommodative amplitude and dynamics with the 1CU accommodative intraocular lens. Invest Ophthalmol Vis Sci. 2006 Mar, 47(3): 1230–5.

54. Ben-Nun J. The NuLens accommodating intraocular lens. Ophthalmol Clin North Am. 2006 Mar, 19(1):12–34, vii. Review.

55. Wang J, Fu J, Wang NL, Kang HJ, Yang WL. Accommodation in pseudophakic eyes with the 1CU accommodative intraocular lens. Zhonghua Yan Ke Za Zhi. 2005 Sep, 1(9): 807–11. Chinese.

56. Dogru M, Honda R, Omoto M, Toda I, Fujishima H, Arai H, Matsuyama M, Nishijima S, Hida Y, Yagi Y, Tsubota K. Early visual results with the 1CU accommodating intraocular lens. J Cataract Refract Surg. 2005 May, 31(5):895–902.

57. Claoué C. Functional vision after cataract removal with multifocal and accommodating intraocular lens implantation: prospective comparative evaluation of Array multifocal and 1CU accommodating lenses. J Cataract Refract Surg. 2004 Oct, 30(10):2088–91.

58. Alió JL, Ben-nun J, Rodríguez-Prats JL, Plaza AB. Visual and accommodative outcomes 1 year after implantation of an accommodating intraocular lens based on a new concept. J Cataract Refract Surg. 2009 Oct, 35(10):1671–8

59. Küchle M, Seitz B, Langenbucher A, Martus P, Nguyen NX; Erlangen Accommodative Intraocular Lens Study Group. Stability of refraction, accommodation, and lens position after implantation of the 1CU accommodating posterior chamber intraocular lens. J Cataract Refract Surg. 2003 Dec, 29(12):2324–9.

60. Findl O, Kiss B, Petternel V, Menapace R, Georgopoulos M, Rainer G, Drexler W. Intraocular lens movement caused by ciliary muscle contraction. J Cataract Refract Surg. 2003 Apr, 29(4):669–76.

61. Auffarth GU, Martin M, Fuchs HA, Rabsilber TM, Becker KA, Schmack I. Validity of anterior chamber depth measurements for the evaluation of accommodation after implantation of an accommodative Humanoptics 1CU intraocular lens. Ophthalmologe. 2002 Nov, 99(11):815–9. German.

23

IOL Implantation Techniques and Injector Systems

Col JKS Parihar SM, VSM and Col Vijay Mathur

INTRODUCTION

In the concept of cataract surgery and intraocular lens (IOL) implants, there has been tremendous change particularly in the recent past. For the management of cataract alone phacoemulsification with conventional foldable IOL implantation is no longer the method of choice. The present concept demands keratorefractive surgery in true sense and it should provide emmetropia for full range and all types of vision.

The selection of intraocular lenses is no longer the surgeon's prerogative. Increased patient awareness about the IOLs has made the patient a consumer who wants to know the details of what is being implanted. What is required is a thorough knowledge about the types of lenses with the merits and demerits of the same so that the patient can be offered the best possible visual result.

The role of injector system cannot be undermined in respect of the size of incision, precise, atraumatic and contamination-free placement of the IOL in the bag as well as its impact on final structural and the functional outcome.

An attempt is being made to evaluate delivery system and IOL implantation techniques pertaining to different types of IOL including their merits, constraints as well as their historical and applied aspects.

IMPLANTATION TECHNIQUES

Implantation techniques can be grouped as per the type and material of intraocular lens implant.

Implantation of Anterior Chamber IOLs

Kelman Type AC IOL

This anterior chamber intraocular lens (AC IOL) has multiflex type of haptics and optic measuring 6.5 mm.

The haptics are so designed that they provide four points of contact. The aim was to provide minimum contact with the trabecular meshwork, thereby minimising chances of secondary glaucoma as well as to provide a stable fixation within the eye. Kelman type of AC IOL is of universal size and due to 'Z' shape of its haptics with multiflex design it can be placed inside any size of eyeball. Prior to inserting this IOL, the surgeon should ensure that corneal endothelium is healthy and the anterior chamber is adequately deep. Pre-existing glaucoma and uveitis are contraindications. The anterior chamber should be thoroughly cleared off any vitreous and the pupil should be constricted using intra-cameral Pilocarpine. Adequate viscoelastic should be injected into the anterior chamber to push the vitreous face back and protect the endothelium. A lens glide made of PMMA or silicon is inserted up to the angle of anterior chamber from the incision. This prevents the AC IOL from going behind the pupil and from engaging the iris during insertion. Once the inferior haptic is in the angle, the glide can be removed and the superior haptic inserted. The superior haptic is placed under the scleral lip. Alternatively, the AC IOL can be inserted without using a glide by simply holding with a McPherson forceps and guiding the haptics into the angle of anterior chamber. Once placed inside the chamber, the AC IOL can be gently dialled such that the superior haptic moves away from the section. It is mandatory to create at least one surgical iridectomy to prevent pupillary block glaucoma. The section can be sutured after ensuring that there is no vitreous in the anterior chamber.

Iris Claw IOL

The initial steps are similar to those as in insertion of the Kelman AC IOL. The iris is enclaved within the haptics of the IOL (Fig. 23.1).

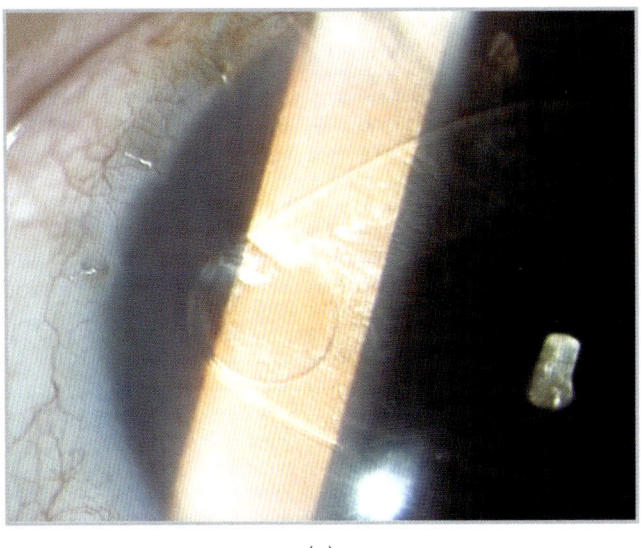

(a)

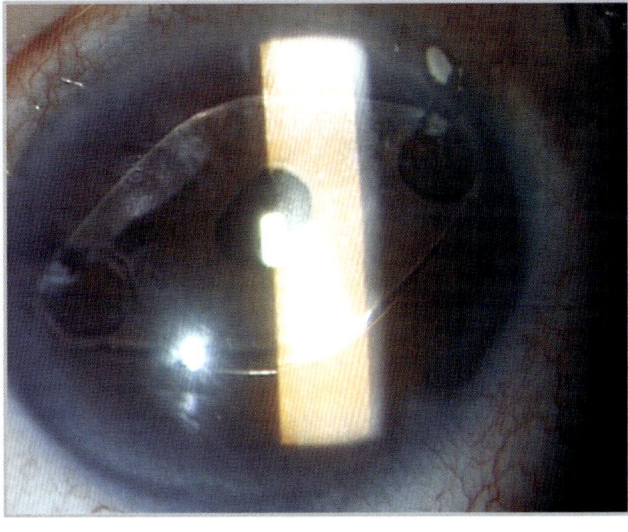

(b)

Fig. 23.1: (a) Iris claw IOL (haptics of iris claw lens is showing claw having enclaved iris. Multiple steel sutures are also visible at the limbus, (b) Iris claw IOL is positioned in the anterior chamber

Sputnik IOL

Once popularised by ophthalmic surgeons from Russia, this IOL is no longer in use and is confined to the annals of history. This was an iris supported IOL having four haptics projecting out, giving an appearance of the Sputnik satellite. After initial steps of cataract extraction like in AC IOL or iris claw lens, the iris was tucked in between its four haptics. The optic of the IOL came to rest in the pupillary area. This was followed by at least two iridectomies. Numerous adverse effects like pupillary block glaucoma, persistent iritis, dislocation into the vitreous cavity, interference with retinal examination and corneal endothelial decompensation did not allow this lens to have widespread acceptance.

Implantation of All PMMA Rigid Posterior Chamber IOLs

Conventional (6–6.5 mm × 13 /13.5 mm) PC IOL Implants

Conventional rigid posterior chamber intraocular lenses (PC IOL) have revolutionised the outcome following cataract surgery. There are many methods to implant rigid 6–6.5 mm PMMA lenses with 13–13.5 mm overall length.

(a) **McPherson forceps:** The implant is simply held from its optic and introduced into the anterior chamber. The inferior haptic is guided behind the inferior pupillary margin into the ciliary sulcus. Then the superior haptic is supported by using another forceps and is held again by changing the

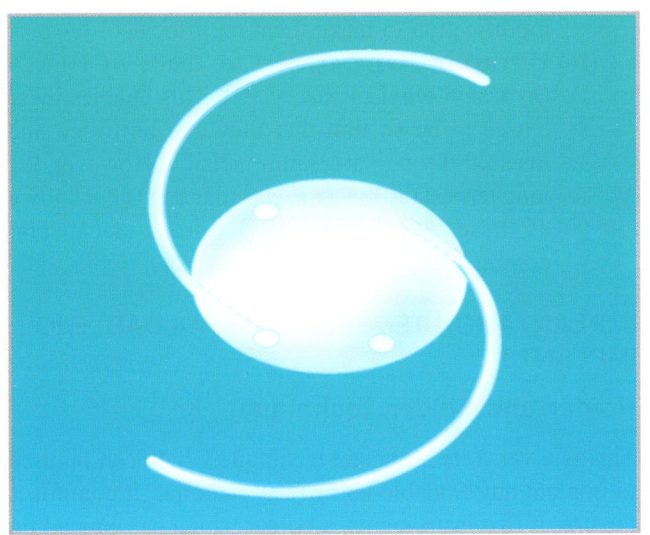

(a)

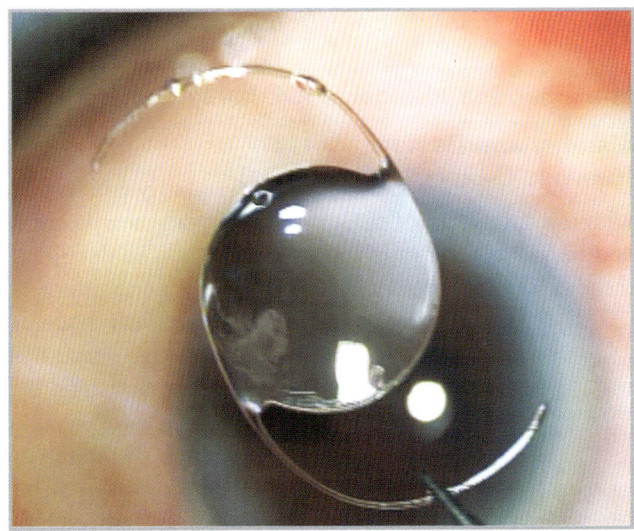

(b)

Fig. 23.2: (a) and (b) PMMA rigid (nonfoldable) posterior chamber IOL implant

grip of the McPherson forceps. The superior haptic is now pushed into the anterior chamber so as to clear the superior pupillary margin. The haptic is now dipped below the pupillary margin and released to occupy its place in the ciliary sulcus.

(b) **Sinskey hook:** The inferior haptic is introduced using a McPhersons forceps as mentioned above. A Sinskey hook or a dialler is engaged into the superior dialling hole and the superior haptic is dialled in clockwise manner behind the iris by exerting a mildposterior pressure.

(c) **Clayman forceps:** This is a spring action forceps with a vertically curved spatulated holding surface. The PC IOL is held by its optic and introduced into the posterior chamber. Once the inferior haptic and optic are in place, McPherson forceps can be used to place the superior haptic in the ciliary sulcus as described above.

Phacoprofile all PMMA IOL

This IOL has a 5 mm optic and 12 mm overall length. Prior to its insertion one must ensure that the capsular bag is intact; placing this IOL in the sulcus causes it to decentre. Another difference from a standard PMMA PC IOL is that this lens does not have any dialling holes. The incision is enlarged to 5 mm using a blunt tip implantation keratome. Care is taken to maintain the integrity and the plane of initial entry tunnel as this will enable the tunnel to be self sealing. Anterior chamber is reformed with viscoelastic. The IOL is held with McPherson forceps from its optic and introduced into the anterior chamber such that the inferior haptic enters the capsular bag. The dialler is engaged at hapticoptic junction and dialled towards the 3 o'clock position while exerting a slight posterior pressure to introduce the superior haptic into the capsular bag. It is mandatory to have the capsular bag distended with viscoelastic while inserting this IOL.

Implantation of Foldable IOL Implants

Material and Design

Foldable intraocular lenses have evolved fairly rapidly and within a few years of their inception many new designs and materials are available in the market. The details of these IOLs have been discussed in a separate chapter.

(i) **Silicon:** The earliest foldable IOL was made of silicon. Silicon has excellent refractive properties and is a durable material which can withstand the rigorous of folding and unfolding. However, it is associated with a high incidence of posterior capsular opacification (PCO) and capsular contraction syndrome. The unfolding of silicon IOL is very rapid leading to the damage of the capsular bag, if compromised. Initially, IOLs manufactured

from silicon had plate haptics which made them liable to dislocation following YAG laser capsulotomy. These IOLs also created an opaque interface with silicon oil used for vitreoretinal surgeries. Now, IOLs manufactured from second and third generation silicon materials are coming (siloxanes) which claim to have lesser incidence of capsular reaction and fibrosis. Silicon IOLs should not be rinsed into BSS since it may lead to hydration of the IOL and its insertion may become difficult.

(ii) **Acrylic hydrophilic:** Most complications of silicon were overcome by the use of foldable acrylic material to manufacture IOLs. They have excellent optical properties and are biocompatible. These IOLs are packed in BSS to retain their properties and pliability. Incidence of posterior capsular opacification was much less as compared to silicon IOLs and they could remain stable in the bag after YAG capsulotomy. Initially, three-piece IOLs with prolene haptics were manufactured. Now single piece IOLs with various haptic designs and additional features like square edge, biconvex optic, UV absorbing optic, aspheric and multifocal optic are available.

(iii) **Acrylic hydrophobic:** To reduce the incidence of PCO and capsular reaction even further, hydrophobic acrylic material was invented. This material has proved to incite minimal postoperative reaction. It has been widely used in eyes with paediatric cataracts, postuveitis complicated cataracts and post traumatic cataracts with good results. These lenses are dry packed and their optics are less pliable as compared to hydrophilic IOLs. They have been noted to be good in the bag stability even in the presence of posterior capsular tear. They are now also available with apodized surface modification to make them multifocal.

(iv) **Ultrathin IOLs:** These are made of HEMA (hydroxyl ethyl methacrylate). This enables these lenses to be so thin that they can be rolled and inserted through a 1.9 mm incision. However, the long term stability in the capsular bag is not known as these IOLs cannot resist forces of capsular contraction.

IMPLANTATION TECHNIQUE OF FOLDABLE IOL IMPLANTS

Holder and Folder Technique

This is a versatile bimanual technique which can be used to implant any foldable lens of any material. It comprises the use of two instruments, a holder which has cupped tip with a cross action handle and a folder which has two plate-like tip. Initially, the IOL is held from its optic using

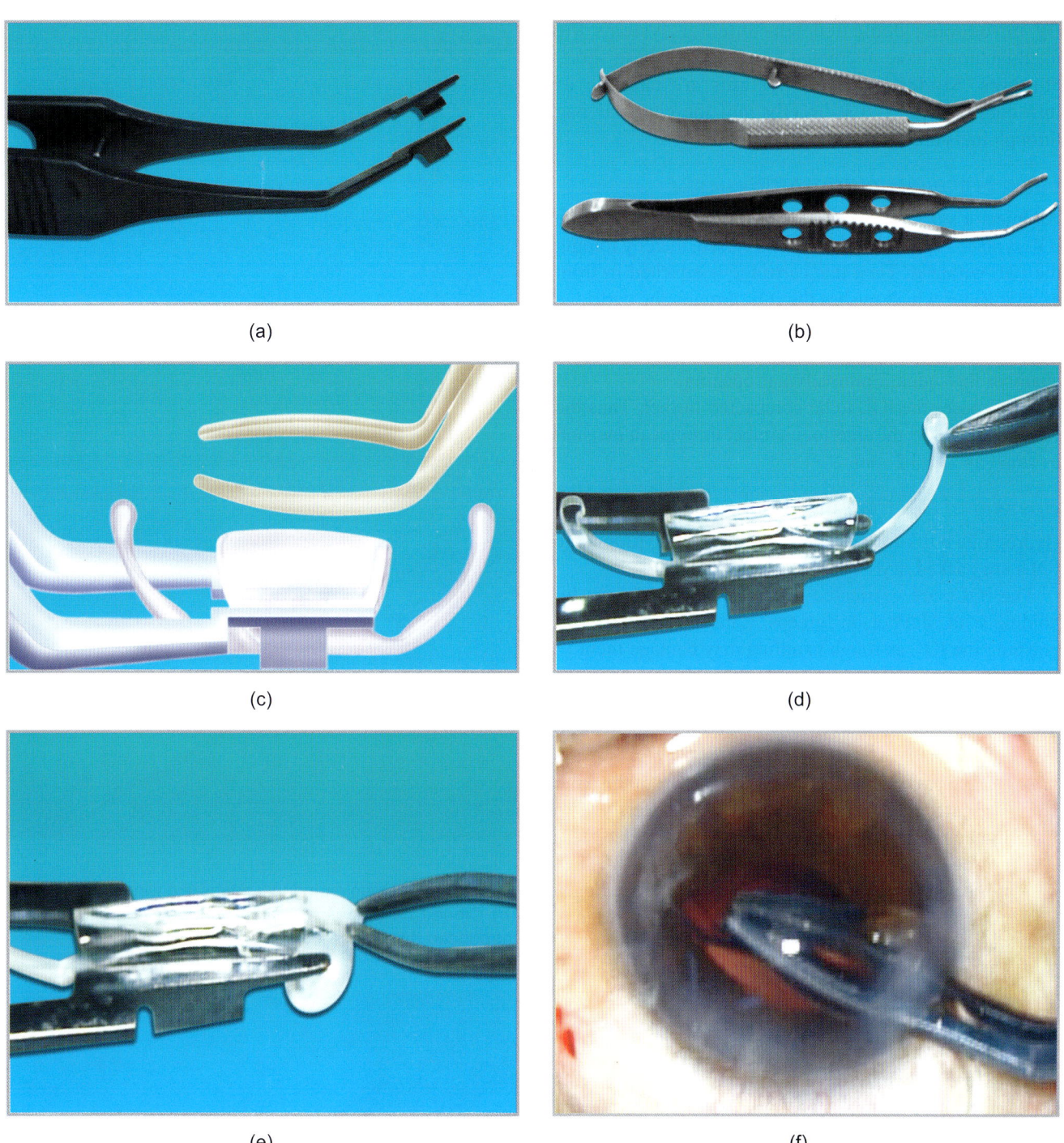

Fig. 23.3: (a) Holder and folder technique: IOL folder, (b) Various types of folder, (c) Holder and Folder technique, (d) and (e) Foldable IOL is being folded, (f) Insertion of foldable IOL

the holder; its cupped tip prevent any damage to the IOL surface. Using the tip of holder with IOL as fulcrum, the folder is used to fold the IOL from its middle between its plates.

The holder is now released from its original grip and the IOL is held again in the folded state. In this position, it can be inserted into the anterior chamber through a 3–3.5 mm incision.

Injector Delivery Systems

The basic flaw in using holderfolder system is the collapse of anterior chamber while inserting the lens. Another problem is that there is excessive handling of IOLs which predisposes the delicate foldable lens to mechanical trauma and damage. The incision needs to be enlarged to 3.5–4.0 lmm for comfortable insertion using holder-folder.

By introducing dedicated lens injector systems the manufacturers have attempted to overcome these shortcomings. Modern injector systems are capable of introducing these IOLs directly into the capsular bag through incisions as small as 2–2.5 mm.

Basic Technique of Injector System

All injector systems follow a common principle where the IOL is placed in a cartridge which is closed, thereby folding the IOL within it. Then this cartridge is attached in front of an injector which pushes the IOL through the cartridge which has a smaller opening. This further compresses the foldable IOL which can be introduced into the anterior chamber through a 3 mm valvular opening.

This causes the IOL to be compacted further. Thus the IOL finally enters the anterior chamber through an incision as small as 2.8–3.2 mm.

Opening of IOL from the Bottle/Case

Hydrophilic IOLs are packed in BSS, whereas hydrophobic IOLs are packed dry.

The IOLs are extricated from their bottles/cases by holding with McPherson forceps. Care must be taken in grasping the IOL as rough handling may damage them.

Loading of IOL into Cartridges

There are various types of cartridges into which these lenses are loaded:

(a) **Open cartridges:** The loading chamber of this kind of cartridge opens like wings of a butterfly. The injecting nozzle and the chamber are filled with viscoelastic and the IOL is placed.

The optic of the IOL is pressed below the side ridges and the wings are closed. This loaded cartridge is attached to the injector and snapped into position. The plunger is pushed once outside the eye to check that the IOL is being correctly pushed. All these manoeuvres should be performed under the microscope.

(b) **Closed cartridges:** The loading chamber of this type of cartridge is closed and the IOL is introduced through an opening at the rear. After filling the cartridge with viscoelastic, the IOL is pushed into the front part of the cartridge with the help of a blunt-tipped pusher. This part of the cartridge is narrower and this forces the IOL to fold. The loaded cartridge is now mounted on a disposable or a reusable injector and injected into the anterior chamber through a 3–3.2 mm incision.

(c) **Preloaded IOL implants:** The latest versions of few IOLs available in the market are coming pre- loaded into the injector cartridge. The Memory lens manufactured by CIBA Vision is a prefolded acrylic IOL, whereas Staar is a prefolded silicon IOL implant. This

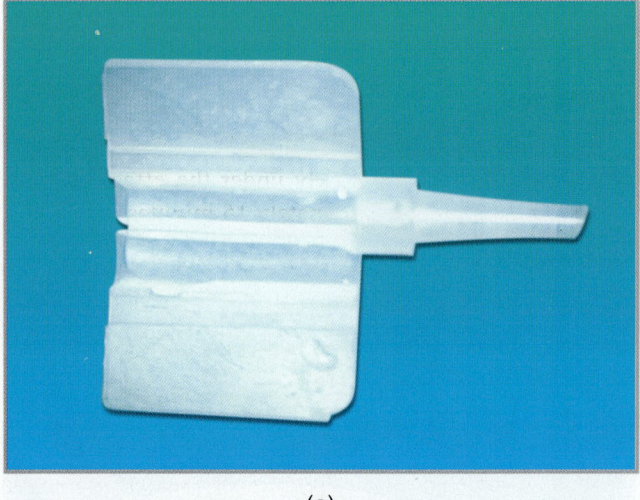

(a)

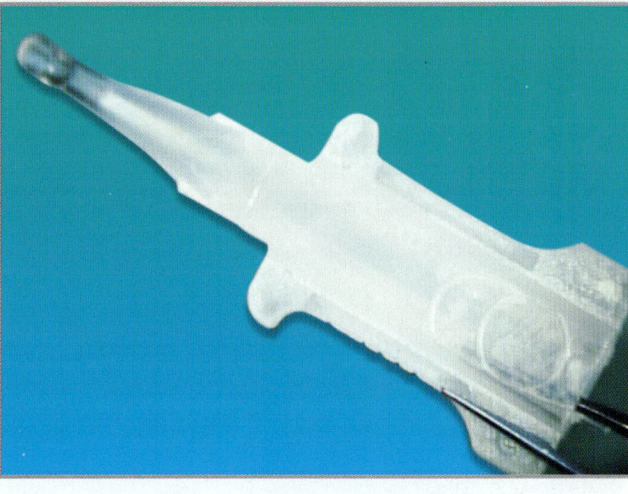

(b)

Fig. 23.4: (a) Open cartridges: opens like wings of a butterfly (b) Closed cartridges: cartridge is closed and the IOL is introduced through an opening at the rear

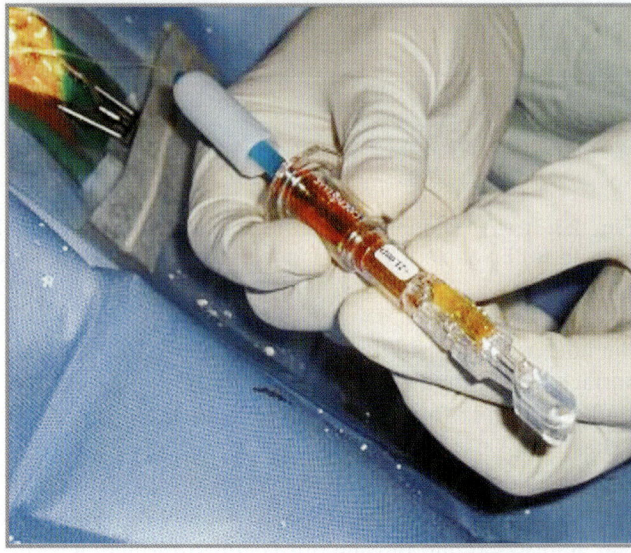

Fig. 23.5: Preloaded IOL implants

avoids any kind of handling of the implant and associated complications like risk of contamination, damage or incorrect placement in the cartridge.

The cartridge with the Memory lens is kept at a temperature of 8°C. Following intraocular insertion the lens unfolds slowly under the effect of body temperature (approximately 15 minutes) providing a smooth and controlled implantation.

Types of Injector Systems

Injectors can be either disposable or reusable made of steel or titanium. Disposable injectors are light weight, safer and carry a lesser risk of contamination. The tip of their plungers are made of soft silicon or plastic and do not damage the posterior capsule. Reusable injectors have metallic plunger tip which can damage the posterior capsule if it touches the posterior capsule.

1. **Direct pushing type:** The plunger moves by forward push of the plunger. In this type of injector,

the control of the plunger movement is more with the surgeon.

Movement of plunger should be delicately controlled during final stages of IOL insertion as posterior capsule can be damaged by rough movement.

2. **Screw type:** In this injector, the plunger moves forwards by rotatory movements with the help of screw mechanism. The forward movement is very slow and controlled but the 'feel' during IOL insertion is lost. They are more cumbersome to use and require use of both hands.

Basic Method of Insertion

Once loaded into the cartridge, the injector is inspected prior to its insertion into the anterior chamber. The plunger is pushed and the lens movement within the cartridge is observed under the microscope. If this movement is appearing to be normal, the anterior chamber is reformed and the tip of the injector introduced into the anterior

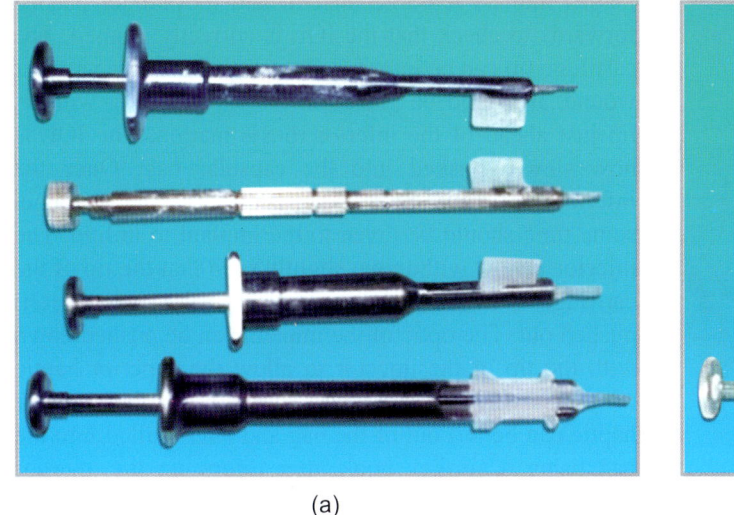

(a)

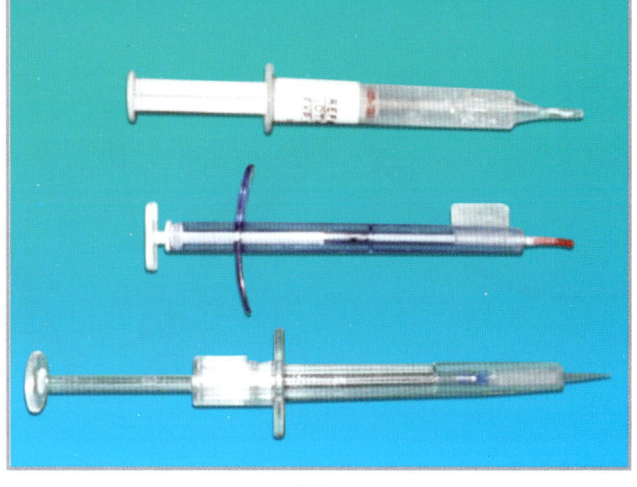

(b)

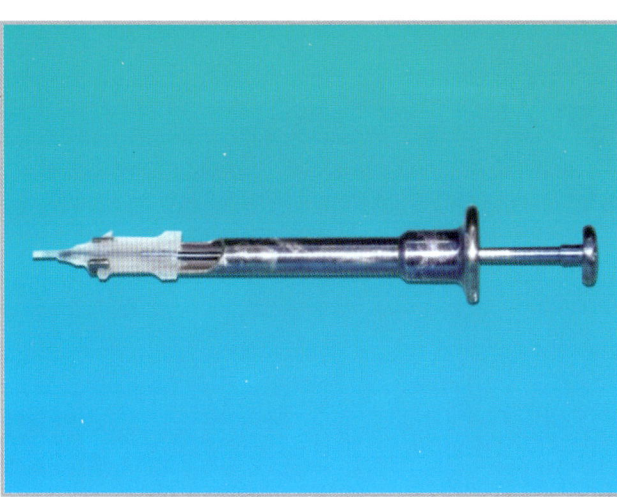

(c)

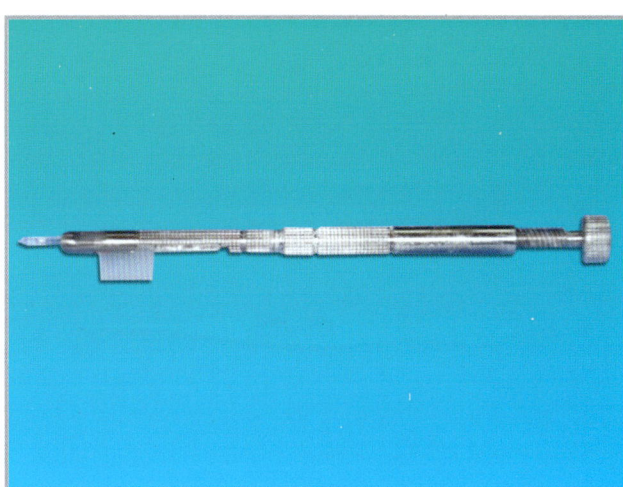

(d)

Fig. 23.6: (a) Reusable injectors, (b) Disposable injectors, (c) Direct pushing type injector system, (d) Screw type injector system

chamber. One should be careful during this step as forceful insertion might cause Descmet's stripping or tearing of the section. In case the section is appearing to be small for the injector tip, it is better to extend it using a keratome. Inside the anterior chamber, the injector tip is positioned inside the capsular bag ahead of the anterior capsular margin. The IOL is now pushed out of the injector slowly.

Time should be given to the implant to gradually unfold on its own. The injector can be rotated to counter the rotatory movement of the IOL if any. Traction or pressure on the posterior capsule or zonules should be avoided. Once the inferior haptic and the optic are in the bag, the injector is withdrawn into the anterior chamber and the superior haptic is slowly pushed out. The injector can be withdrawn and the superior haptic positioned inside the bag with the help of a dialler or sinskey hook. With practice, the superior haptic can be directly placed into the bag using sliding movement of the plunger of the injector itself.

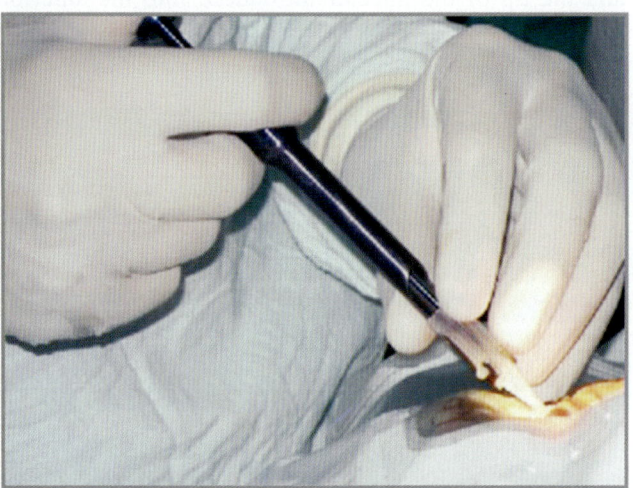

Fig. 23.7: Basic method of IOL insertion: Direct pushing type injector system

INSERTION TECHNIQUES OF COMMONLY AVAILABLE IOL IMPLANTS

AcrySof Single Piece Acrylic (Hydrophobic) Foldable Posterior Chamber IOL

This is perhaps the most commonly used foldable implant. The IOL is made of relatively tougher material which is not as pliable as hydrophilic material. This makes this IOL suitable for implantation even in the presence of posterior capsular tear. It is loaded into a closed type of disposable cartridge. The cartridge has an upper slot and a lower slot. The IOL should be introduced into the upper slot such that it is aligned with the tip of the plunger. After filling the cartridge with dispersive type of viscoelastic like 2% hydroxy propyl methyl cellulose, the leading haptic is tucked under the optic and introduced into the cartridge. The trailing haptic should be placed above the optic and the IOL is pushed into the front part of the injector using a blunt pusher. The cartridge is now loaded into its reusable injector and its plunger pushed forwards to check that the IOL is correctly aligned. The cartridge tip can be introduced through a 3.0 mm valvular wound. It should be placed in the capsular bag with its tip just ahead of the inferior rhexis margin. The IOL is now slowly pushed into the capsular bag. Once the inferior haptic with optic is partially out of the cartridge, some time should be given to the implant to unfold. The injector is now withdrawn slightly such that the tip of the cartridge is in the iris plane and the other half of IOL pushed out. The optic of the implant can be pushed down with the tip of the injector to allow the superior haptic to go into the capsular bag. Alternatively, the superior haptic can be left out of the bag and later dialled into the bag using a sinskey hook after reforming the anterior chamber with viscoelastic.

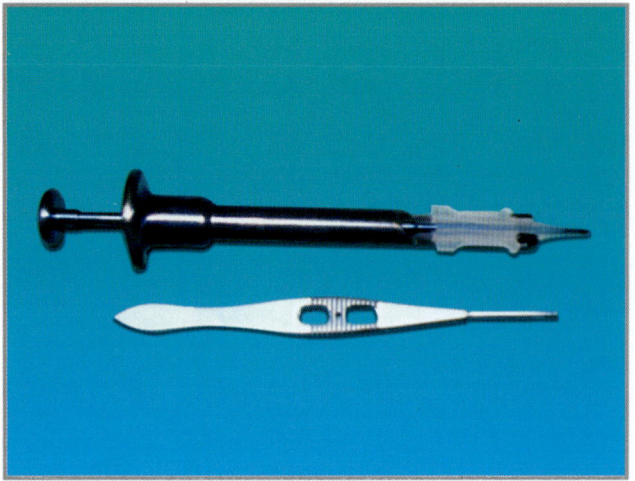

(a)

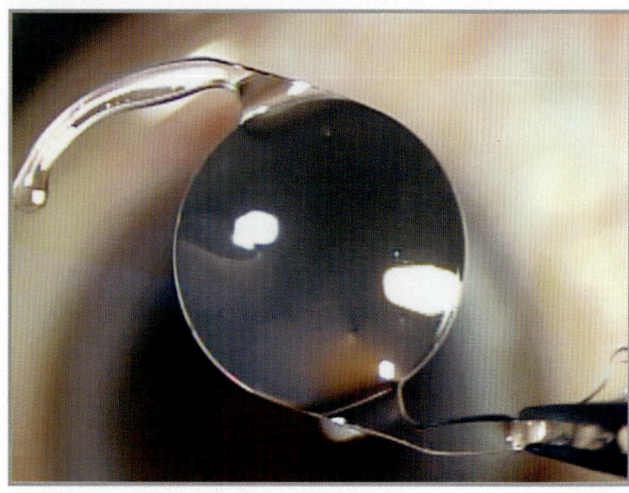

(b)

Fig. 23.8: (a) Direct pushing type injector system with IOL pusher, (b) Single piece acrylic (hydrophobic) foldable posterior chamber IOL

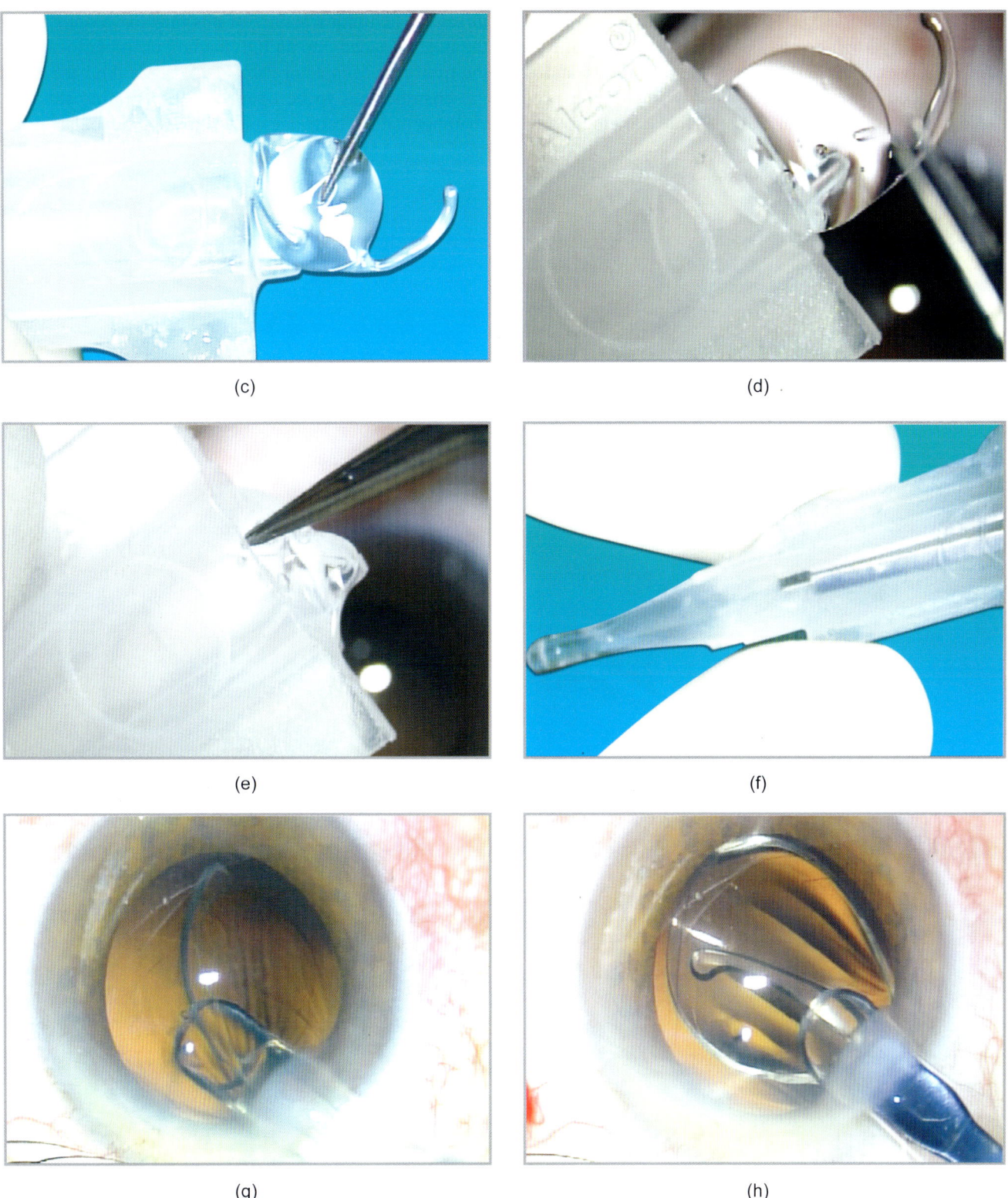

Fig. 23.8: (c) The leading haptics of single piece acrylic (hydrophobic) foldable posterior chamber IOL is being pushed over the optics prior to its insertion into the closed cartridges through an opening at the rear, (d) Loading of single piece acrylic (hydrophobic) foldable posterior chamber IOL into cartridge of injector system, (e) The trailing haptics of single piece acrylic (hydrophobic) foldable posterior chamber IOL is being pushed over the optics prior to its insertion into the closed cartridges through an opening at the rear, (f) The single piece acrylic (hydrophobic) foldable posterior chamber IOL is being pushed up to the tip of the closed cartridges through an opening at the rear, (g) The single piece acrylic (hydrophobic) foldable posterior chamber IOL is being introduced into the anterior chamber, (h) The single piece acrylic (hydrophobic) foldable posterior chamber IOL is being introduced into the capsular bag

Hydroport (B and L) Disposable Injector System

This IOL is hydrophilic and has a square edge with four haptic designs. This IOL is very easy to insert and it achieves good centration with a slightly smaller rhexis of 5–5.5 mm. It comes with a disposable cartridge with injector. The unique feature of this injector system is that the IOL is loaded into an IOL loading chamber located in the front part of injector itself. To load the IOL, the lid of the chamber has to be opened. After priming the IOL chamber and the cartridge with dispersive viscoelastic, the

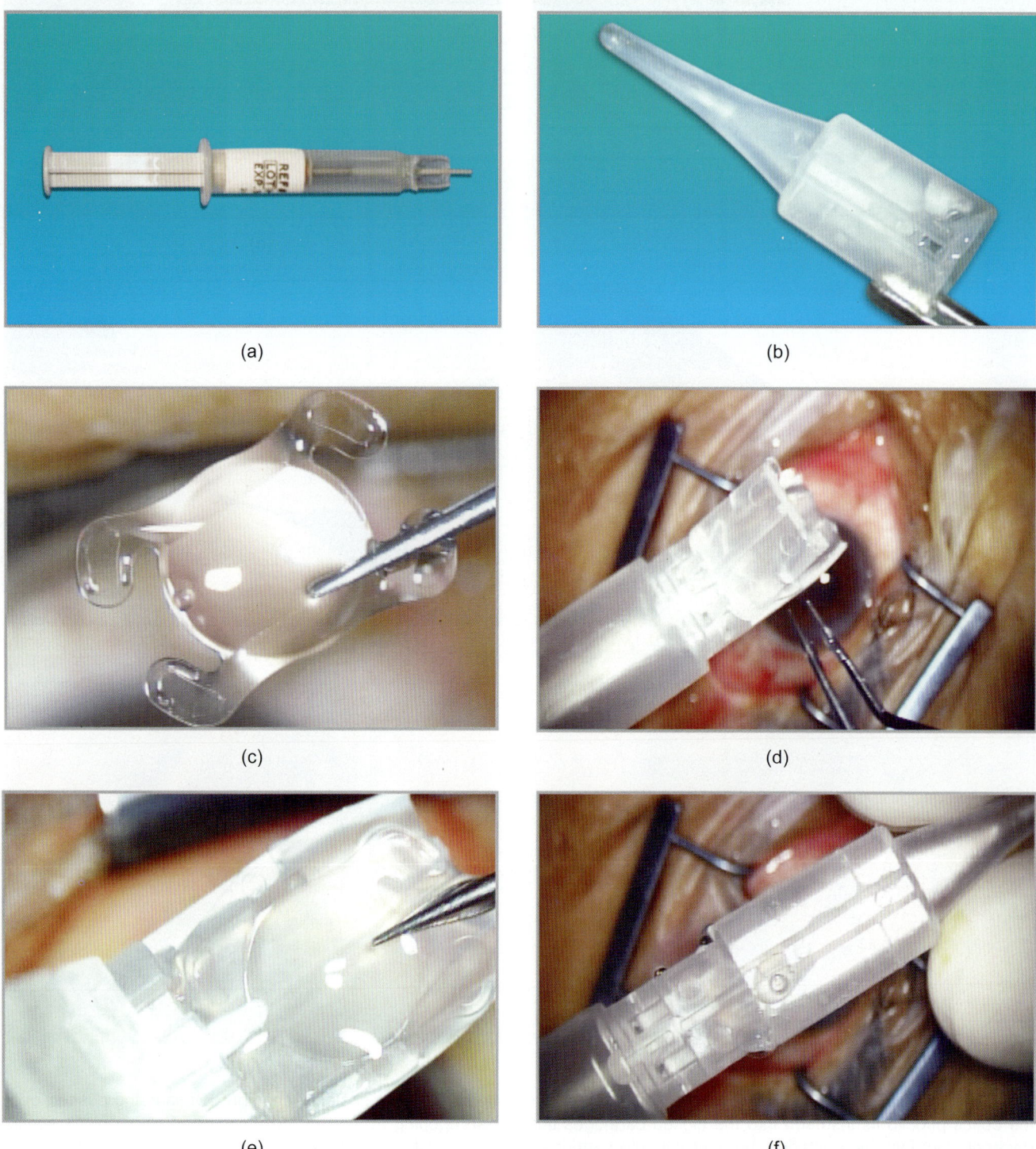

Fig. 23.9: (a) Hydroport (B and L) disposable injector system, (b) Closed cartridges: cartridge is placed over the loaded leading edge of the injector system, (c) Square edge acrylic akreos IOL implant, (d) hydroport (B and L) Disposable injector system is being prepared for the placement of IOL implant, (e) Akreos IOL implant is being placed on the socket of hydroport (B and L) disposable injector system, (f) Closed cartridge is placed over the loaded leading edge of the hydroport (B and L) Disposable injector system

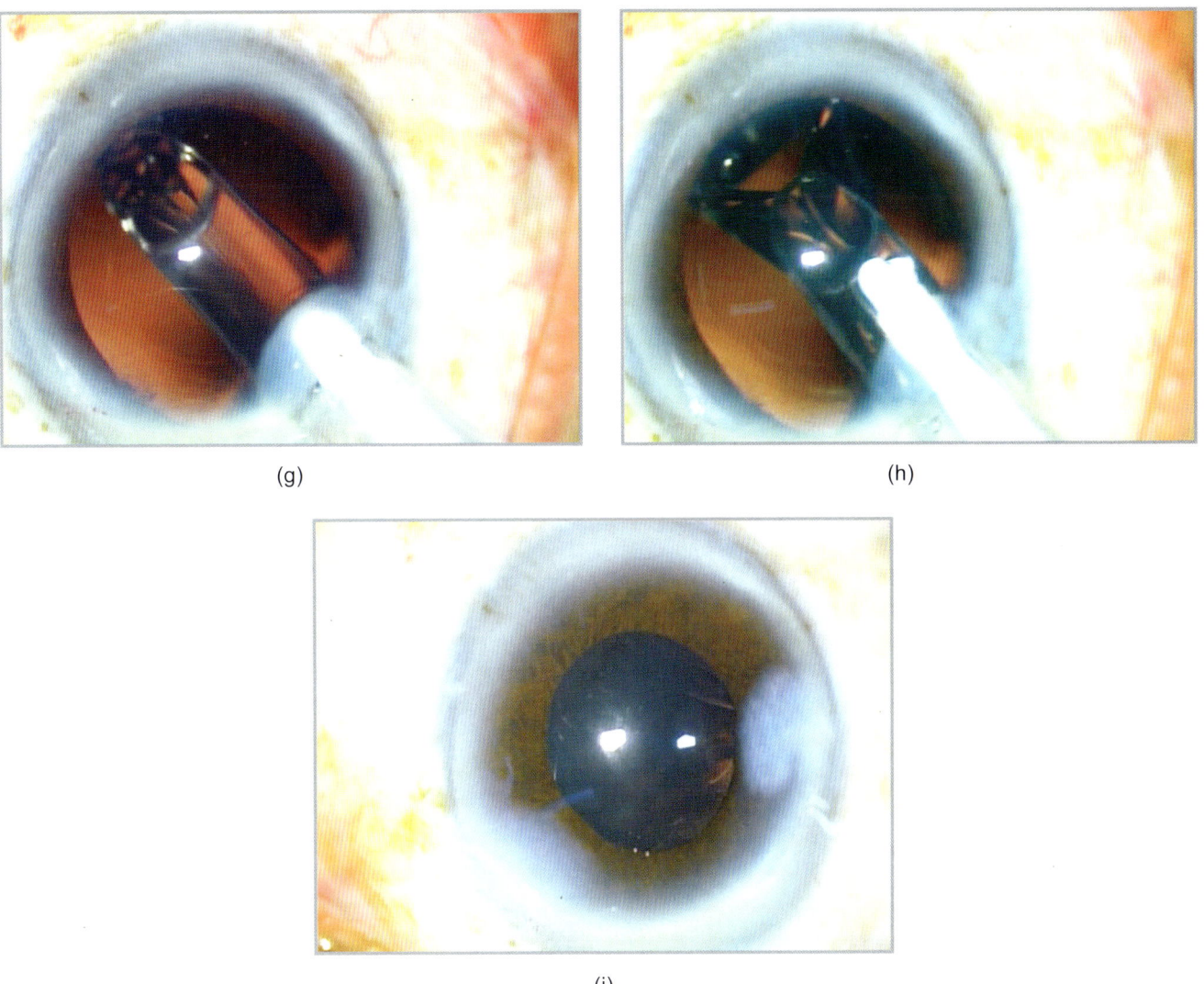

(g) (h)

(i)

Fig. 23.9: (g) Insertion of akreos IOL implant, (h) Insertion of akreos IOL implant into AC, (i) Akreos IOL implant is well placed

IOL is removed from its bottle and placed into the IOL chamber. Its leading haptics should project just ahead of the loading chamber and the plunger tip has a bifurcation which should engage the posterior edge of the IOL. The lid of the IOL loading chamber is now closed and the cartridge attached to it. When the cartridge is appropriately placed, a 'click' is heard. The plunger is pushed to ensure that it is engaging the implant. The cartridge tip of this injector system requires a 3.5 mm incision. The cartridge tip should be placed in the capsular bag ahead of the inferior capsular margin. The IOL is injected into the bag.

Rayner's Centre Flex Design

Rayner introduced a design which had the modified 'C' loop type of haptics with square edged optic. This ensured good centration and stability to the IOL. This IOL can be implanted in the presence of tear in the rhexis margin or a large irregular rhexis. It can be placed in the sulcus. The

IOL is placed in the open type cartridge after filling it with viscoelastic. The IOL is placed in the chamber and its edges are tucked below a ridge present on the cartridge wall. The cartridge is now closed thereby folding the IOL. The two wings of the cartridge should be well opposed. The cartridge is mounted on the injector and its plunger pushed forwards to ensure that the IOL is engaged properly (Fig. 23.10).

Appasamy and Other Indian IOLs

Most of the Indian made foldable hydrophilic IOLs use injector systems and techniques which are similar to that of the Rayner centre flex injector systems.

IOL Implantation Technique through Screw Pattern Injector System (AMO)

Aspheric hydrophobic single or three-piece IOLs are now coming with reusable metallic screw type injector. The IOL

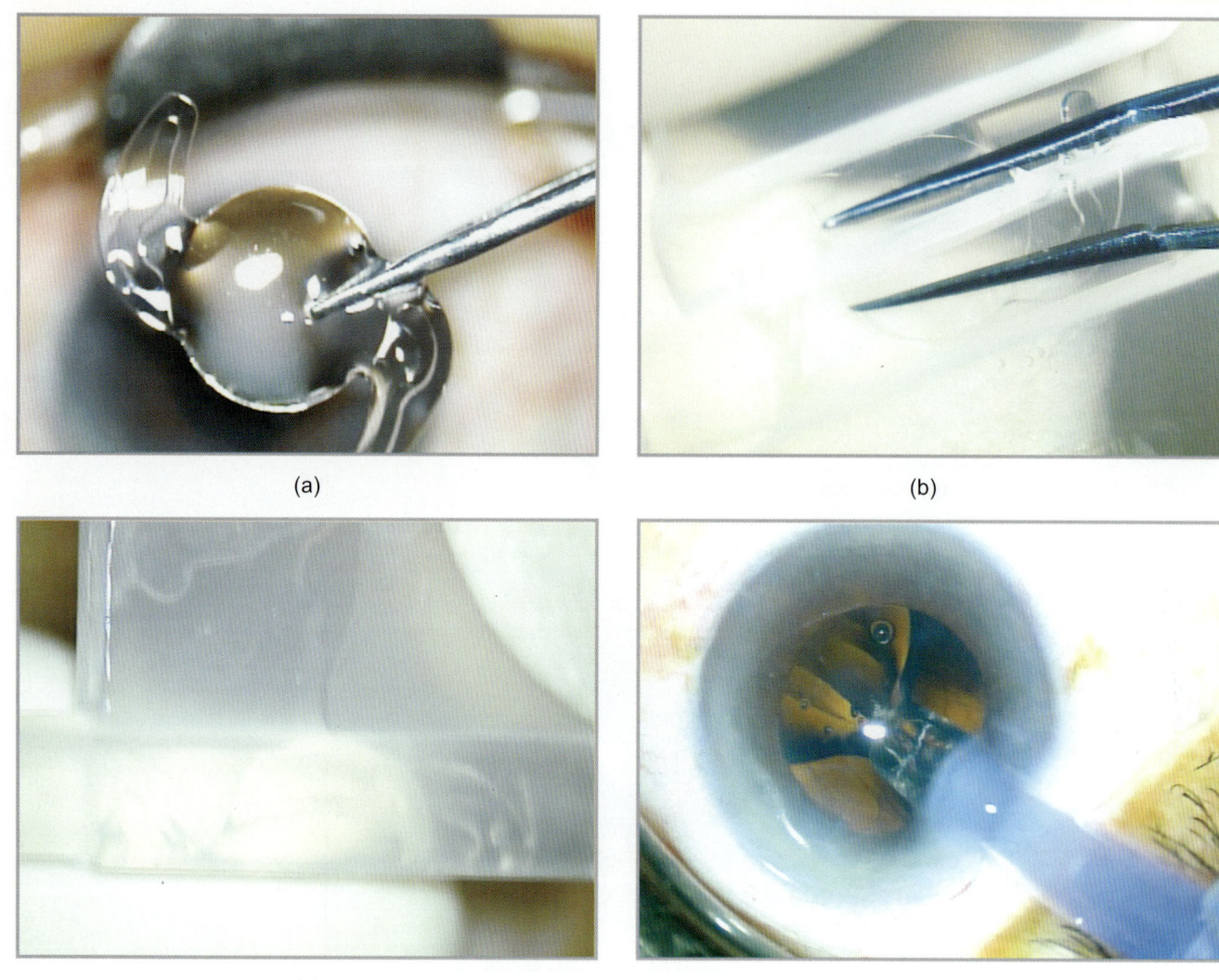

(a)

(b)

(c)

(d)

Fig. 23.10: (a) Centre flex design with modified 'C' loop type haptics and square edge optic, (b) Centre flex design IOL is placed into the cartridge and being folded with the help of McPherson's forceps, (c) Centre flex design IOL is well placed into the cartridge, (d) Centre flex design IOL is being pushed into the AC

is loaded into a disposable cartridge in which the IOL chamber is open. Once in its correct place, the cartridge is closed and the cartridge is placed into the injector. This type of injector has a metallic plunger. The plunger is advanced by turning the screw clockwise till it touches the IOL. The anterior chamber is filled with viscoelastic and the tip of the injector cartridge is just under the inferior rhexis margin. Once the inferior haptic and IOL optic are injected out, the injector is withdrawn into the iris plane. The superior haptic is now pushed out by turning the screw clockwise. Gliding movement of the plunger tip can be used to position the superior haptic in the bag (Fig. 23.11).

Insertion of Multifocal/Accommodative IOLs

Insertion of multifocal IOLs is essentially the same as that of hydrophobic IOLs except that the capsulorrhexis needs to be of correct size (5.5 mm) and well centred.

Accommodative IOLs with four pliable haptics have a different technique. The rhexis in this IOL needs to be 5.5 mm in size and well centred. The haptics are narrow at the point where they join the optic. There is a tendency for the rhexis margin to get trapped in the narrow portion of the haptic. This type of IOL has a disposable open cartridge and pushing type disposable injector. While loading the IOL into the cartridge, care should be taken to orient the four haptics along the walls of the cartridge. The haptics should be pressed beneath the side ridges of the cartridge and the cartridge closed.

Constraints and Complications

(i) IOL haptic entrapped into the incision/Out of incision: This is the result of improper loading of the IOL in the cartridge. Proper loading under the microscope and checking the movement of the IOL

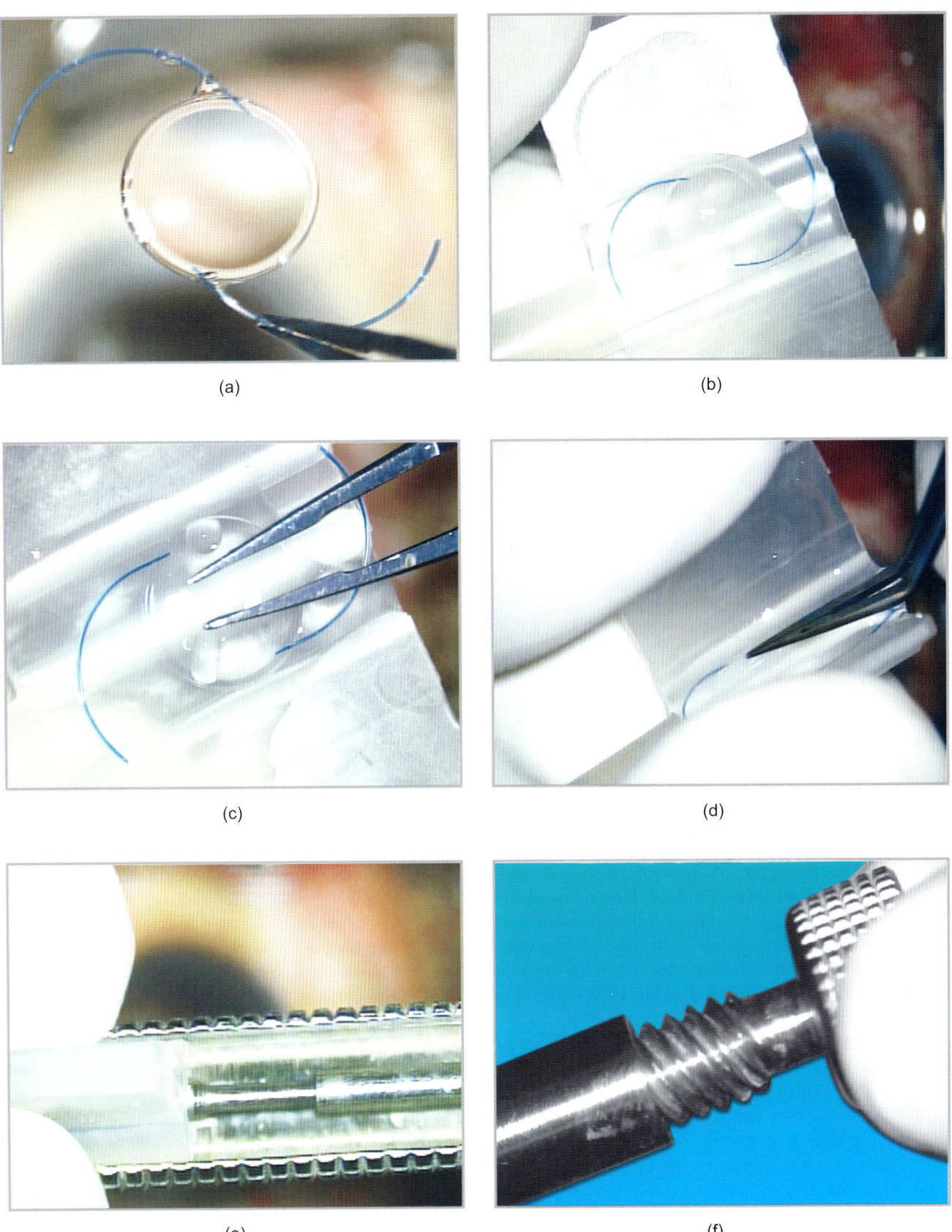

Fig. 23.11: (a) Aspheric hydrophobic three-piece IOLs (sensar/AMO), (b), (c) and (d) Aspheric hydrophobic three-piece IOLs (sensar/AMO) is being placed into the cartridge, (e) Cartridge is being placed into the socket of screw pattern injector, (f) Screw pattern injector is being pushed

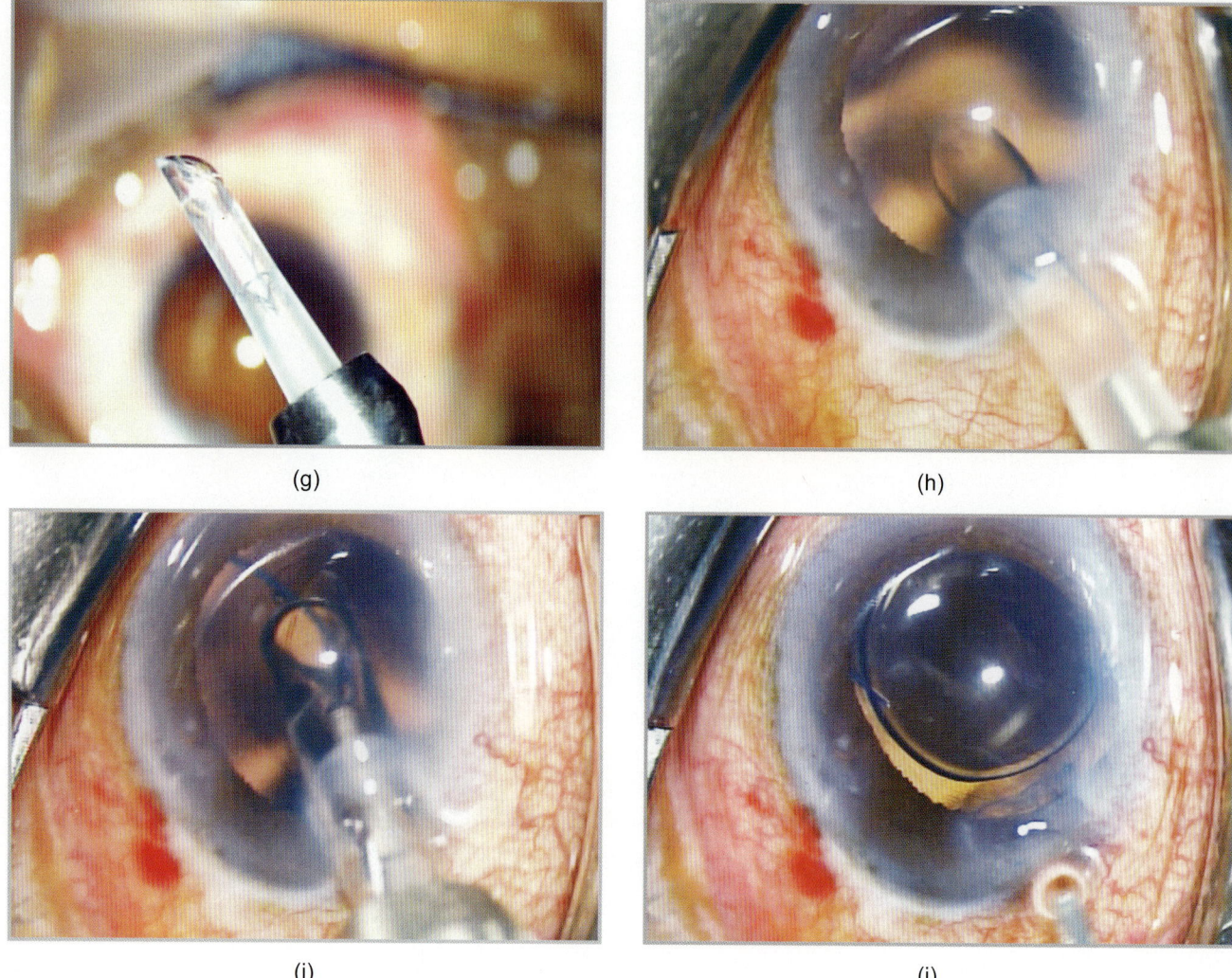

(g)   (h)

(i)   (j)

Fig. 23.11: (g) Sensar IOL is well placed into the cartridge, (h) Sensar IOL is being inserted into the AC, (i) Sensar IOL is being inserted into the capsular bag, (j) Sensar IOL is well placed into the capsular bag

prior to its insertion will prevent this complication. Once stuck within the cartridge, the IOL invariably gets damaged and torn. Fresh IOL with new cartridge needs to be loaded. If the IOL is moving smoothly within the cartridge, the incision could be small in size. Extending the incision using a keratome will resolve this problem.

(ii) Twisting of haptics outside/inside the bag: At times, the IOL haptics get unduly strained during the process of loading and injecting. This causes loss of memory and they do not regain their shape. This leads to an unstable lens within the capsular bag. The IOL haptics should be gently coaxed to open up. Any fracture or a tear in the haptics is an indication for explanting the damaged IOL. Minor tears can be left if the IOL is well centred and they are not encroaching upon the visual axis.

(iii) IOL opening out of the bag: The IOL can open in the anterior chamber. This can create some anxious moments for a beginner. The anterior chamber should be formed with viscoelastic; the viscus should be injected anterior to the IOL so as to push it into the capsular bag. Tip of the visco cannula can also be used to push the inferior haptic and optic of the IOL into the bag. Otherwise, a dialler can be used to place the IOL inside the bag.

(iv) Vitreous disturbance

This can occur during IOL insertion by:

(a) Inadvertent tear in capsulorrhexis margin with the dialler tip or at a point where the rhexis is not continuous.

(b) Zonular dehiscence following excessive pressure on zonules during IOL insertion or dialling.

(c) Posterior capsular rent during IOL delivery can occur with the tip of the plunger or during rapid IOL insertion. Pre-existing weakness of the posterior capsule, as in posterior polar cataract, also predisposes to PCR during IOL insertion.

(v) Subluxation/Posterior dislocation of IOL: A foldable IOL has greater incidence of subluxation/dislocation if implanted in the presence of a rent as compared to the rigid IOL. The incidence is higher with hydrophilic IOLs as compared to hydrophobic IOLs, probably due to the soft and pliable nature of its optic. Once this happens, IOL removal and replacing it with a rigid 6.5 mm PMMA IOL should be done.

(vi) Descemet's disinsertion: This can occur when forced entry is being made through a smaller section. The blunt tip of injector cartridge can strip off the Descemet's membrane or it can aggravate an existing Descemet's strip. If not recognised and treated in time this can lead to severe striate keratitis and corneal decompensation depending upon its extent and position.

Conditions Warranting IOL Explantation

(i) Broken haptics: Haptics of foldable IOLs often get damaged during injection. If this is discovered before the IOL goes into the bag, the lens can easily be explanted. If the IOL is already in the bag when damage to haptic is noted, centration should be seen. A well-centred IOL in the bag with clear visual axis can be left as such.

(ii) Cracks in the IOL optic: This defect causes more visual disturbances than damage to the IOL haptic. In such cases, the IOL should invariably be explanted.

(iii) Severe reaction to IOL: Severe reaction to IOL is rare. Poorly manufactured IOLs can incite severe reactions. Toxic anterior segment syndrome and endophthalmitis are the other conditions which should be differentiated.

(iv) Dislocation and subluxation of IOL: These have already been discussed before.

Methods of Explantation of Broken/Cracked IOL

(i) Through 3 mm incision: The IOL is first prolapsed into the anterior chamber using visco-elastic. Using a vannas scissors, the IOL optic is cut into two parts. Each part can now be removed separately through a 3 mm incision. The choice of implanting the new IOL depends upon the indication for IOL explantation. If explantation was carried out due to a defect in the IOL, any suitable foldable IOL can be implanted.

(ii) Through 6 mm incision: In cases of IOL decentration/dislocation, the foldable IOL should be exchanged with a 6 mm rigid IOL. In case implantation of a rigid 6 mm IOL is being contemplated, the incision can be enlarged to 6 mm using a 5 mm blunt-tipped keratome. The anterior chamber should be formed with viscoelastic and the IOL gently prolapsed into the anterior chamber. Care should be taken to preserve as much of the capsular bag as possible. If vitreous comes into the anterior chamber, limited anterior vitrectomy using low vacuum settings should be carried out. IOL can be visco expressed throughout the enlarged section. A 6mm IOL can be implanted over the capsular frill in the sulcus. If the integrity of capsular bag is adequate, a 6 mm IOL can be implanted in the bag. Wound integrity should be ensured at the end of the procedure.

CONCLUSION

Implanting the intraocular lens is an important part of cataract surgery. Incorrectly implanted IOL can negate the benefits accrued from a good cataract surgery. The techniques of IOL implantation have undergone changes that have kept pace with the advances in cataract surgery. Correct loading of the implant is a prelude to its correct injection into the bag.

BIBLIOGRAPHY

1. Lindstrom R. Foldable Intraocular Lenses. Steinert F (ed): Cataract Surgery: Technique, Complication and Management. W B Saunders Co, 2004, pp 279–294.
2. Hoffman RS, Fine IH. New techniques and instruments for lens implantation. Curr Qpin Ophthalmol. 1999 Feb; 10(1):16–21, Review.
3. Baldeschi L, Rizzo S. Damage of Foldable Intraocular Lenses by Incorrect Foldable Forceps. Am J Ophthalmol, 1997 Aug; 124 (2): 245–247.
4. Fabian E:Injector Systems for Foldable Intraocular Lens Implantation. Kohnen, T (ed): Modern Cataract Surgery.Dev Ophthalmol. Basel, Karger, 2002, vol 34, pp 147–154.
5. A. Coombes.Silicone plate-haptic lens injection without prior incision enlargement. Journal of Cataract and Refractive Surgery, Volume 27, Issue 10, Pages 1542–1544.
6. B. Shingleton. Anterior chamber maintainer versus viscoelastic material for intraocular lens implantation: case-control study. Journal of Cataract and Refractive Surgery, Volume 27, Issue 5, Pages 711–714.
7. Kohnen T:Incisions for Implantation of Foldable Intraocular Lenses.Kohnen, T (ed): Modern Cataract Surgery.Dev Ophthalmol. Basel, Karger, 2002, vol 34, pp 155–186.
8. Kohnen T, Kasper T. Incision sizes before and after implantataion of 6 mm optic foldable intraocular lenses using Monarch and Unfolder injector systems. Ophthalmology 2005 Jan; 112(1): 58–66. Review.

9. N. Mamalis. Incision width after phacoemulsification with foldable intraocular lens implantation. Journal of Cataract and Refractive Surgery, Volume 26, Issue 2, Pages 5237–241.

10. Faschinger CW. Surface abnormalities on hydrophilic acrylic intraocular lenses implanted by an injector. J Cataract Refract Surgery. 2001 Jun; 27 (6):845–9.

11. G. Kleinmann and D. J Apple. Evaluation of a new soft tipped injector for the implantation of foldable intraocular lenses: Br. J. Ophthalmol., August 1, 2007; 91(8):1070–1072.

12. Mencucci R, Dei R,Danielli D, Susini M, Menchini U. Folding procedure for acrylic intraocular lenses:Effect on optic surgaces and bacterial adhesion. J Cataract Refract Surg. 2004 Feb; 30(2):457–63.

13. A L Marcovich, G Kleinmann, D Epstein, and A Pollack :The course of surface deposits on a hydrophilic acrylic intraocular lens after implantation through a hexagonal cartridge. Br. J. Ophthalmol., October 1, 2006; 90(10):1249–1251.

14. Pfister D, Stress Fractures after Folding an Acrylic Intraocular lens. AmJ Ophthalmol. 1996 May; 121(5):572–574.

15. Kohnen T, Magdowski G, Koch D. Scanning electron microscopic analysis of foldable acrylic and hydrogel intraocular lenses. J Cataract Refract Surg. 1996 (22): 1342–1350.

16. Haring G, Winter M, Behrendt S. Effects of Folding on the Multifocal silicone intraocular lenses: Scanning electron microscopic study. J Cataract Refract Surg. 1999 Nov; (25): 1505–1509.

17. Milazzo S, Turut P, Blin H. Alterations to the Acrysof intraocular lens during folding. J Cataract Refract Surg. 1996; (220): 1351–1354.

18. Gunenc U, Oner F, Tongal S,Ferliel M. Effects on visual function of glistenings and folding marks in AcrySof intraocular lenses. J Cataract Refract Surg.2001 Oct; (27): 1611–1614.

19. Schmidbauer J, PengQ, Apple D, Pandey S, Escobar –Gomez M, Auffarth G, Werner L, Vargas L, Rates and causes of Intraoperative removal of foldable and rigid intraocular lenses: Clinicopathological analysis of 100 cases. J Cataract Refract Surg.2002 July; 28(7): 1223–1228.

20. Mamalis N, Davis B, Nilson CD, Hickman MS, Leboyer RM. Complications of foldable intraocular lenses requiring explantation or secondary intervention 2003 survey update, J Cataract Refract Surgery. 2004 Oct; 30(10): 2209–18.

21. Altmann GE, Nichamin LD, Lane S S, Pepose JS, Optical performance of 3 intra ocular lens designs in the presence of decentration. J Cataract refract surg 2005 Mar, 31(3):574–85.

24

Phaco Pandora: Complications of Phacoemulsification Surgery

Lt Col Anirudh Singh and Col JKS Parihar SM, VSM

INTRODUCTION

Phacoemulsification is fast becoming a common surgery for the ophthalmic surgeon but it is like a double-edged weapon with superb results on the one hand to visually devastating complications on the other hand. A few complications are mainly due to the steep learning curve for the phaco-surgeon in transition. But complications can occur in seemingly simplest of cases in any step during the surgery. What is required from a phaco surgeon is a thorough knowledge of the possible complications and how to deal with them in a methodical and precise surgical manner. In this chapter, we will examine the various possible complications that can occur in each phase of surgery, how to reduce them, how to avoid them, and how to treat them.

Specific complications like endophthalmitis, nucleus and IOL implant drop posterior capsule and IOL implant opacification will be discussed in detail elsewhere as separate chapter.

COMPLICATIONS RELATED WITH SURGICAL DRAPING AND CLEANING

Allergy to Povidone Iodine

Cleaning with povidone iodine of the surgical area of interest (face, eyelids, conjunctiva and cornea) is the most initial step in the commencement of any ocular surgery. Some patients are allergic to povidone iodine solution with this procedure during postoperative period.

Allergic Manifestations of Povidone Iodine

(a) **Manifestations in the form of**
   - Irritation
   - Scratching
   - Burning sensation
   - Redness, erythema, hives on skin and eyelids

- Mild to severe degree of conjunctival chemosis, and haziness of cornea and increased swelling.

(b) **Management:** Repeated cleaning of the area with clear fluids/BSS/normal saline should be done immediately. Local and systemic use of antihistaminic should be considered.

The patient may experience severe degree of burning pain sensation in the eye when poor anaesthesia of the eyeball is achieved.

ANAESTHESIA DRUGS AND PROCEDURE RELATED COMPLICATIONS

Complications due to Infiltration of Anaesthetic Drugs

Ocular anaesthesia is almost free of side effects. However, toxicity can be seen following accidental intravenous injection or following an overdose. This is more common when the injections have been given more rapidly. In very occasional circumstance, one may develop anaphylactic drug reactions to anaesthetic agents.

(a) Local Toxicity

Local toxicity is manifested in the form of:

- Redness • Swelling and • Necrosis.

There may be episodes of localised damage to nerve with routine clinical concentration. Micronecrosis can be seen inside the muscle.

(b) Hypersensitivity Reaction

There may be appearance of weals, intense itching, asthmatic breathing and hypotension. Hence, skin sensitivity test should be done prior to the injection of the drug. Adequate equipment should be there to treat any toxic reaction. A source of oxygen with rebreathing bag, laryngoscope, ambubag, endotracheal intubations facility should be ready beforehand. Ideally, an intravenous cannula or atleast a needle should be in position in the peripheral vein before injecting the drug. An emergency tray containing essential drugs, such as thiopentone, diazepam, adrenaline, antihistaminic, aminophylline and hydrocortisone 100 mg ampoule should be available to treat the patient in emergency situations.

(c) Early Signs of Toxicity

Patient may experience:
- Numbness of the tongue and mouth
- Tinnitus
- Visual disturbances, e.g. objects moving from side to side.
- These signs appear within 2–3 minutes of injection.

(d) Late Signs

- Later there may be:
- Mental confusion
- Amaurosis or extraocular paresis/paralysis of the fellow eye
- Slurring of speech
- Muscle tremor, twitching, irrational conversation Nausea, vomiting, dysphagia
- Sudden cardiovascular alteration
- Grandmal epilepsy
- Dyspnea or respiratory depression
- Comma, apnea.

(e) Management

These signs can progress very rapidly, within 10–20 minutes. If any of these signs are present, the surgeon must be able to tackle the progression of the symptoms by taking the necessary therapeutic actions.

   (i) **Discontinue administration of the anaesthetic agent:** Discontinue administration of the anaesthetic agent, if signs of toxicity appear immediately. The injection must be stopped at once.

   (ii) **Oxygenation:** Oxygen is administered by a face mask and manual inflation of lungs may be necessary in apnea.

   (iii) **Treatment of convulsions:** If convulsions are prolonged beyond 30 seconds 2.5% thiopentone 150–200 mg or diazepam 5–10 mg is injected intravenously.

   (iv) **Bronchospasm:** Bronchospasm is treated by a slow intravenous injection of aminophylline 250–500 mg.

   (v) **Management of local allergic reactions:** Intense itching, urticaria is treated by 10–20 mg of chlorpheniramine.

   (vi) **Hypotension:** Hypotension is treated by rapid infusion of normal saline or plasma expander haemaccel 500 ml. Bupivacaine has got serious adverse effects on cardiovascular function.

(f) Oculo Cardiac Reflex

This is the bradycardia which may follow traction on the eye. An effective block ablates the oculocardiac reflex by providing an afferent block of the reflex pathway. However, the institution of the block and especially rapid distension of the tissues by the solution or by haemorrhage might occasionally push the eyeball.

Complications of Topical Anaesthesia Administration

Epithelial Erosion

This is more commonly encountered when cocaine drops are used. But this can also be seen in the use of other anaesthetic drugs.

Clinical presentation: Topical anaesthesia can cause following problems:
- Burning sensation in eye and blepharospasm
- Cloudiness
- Desquamation
- Sloughing of the cornea.

After the block is given, the cornea is exposed for some time owing to paralysis of lids, especially seen in the facial block. When the cornea is anaesthetised, the protective blink reflex is lost. As the eye remains exposed and the cornea becomes dry, it becomes vulnerable to accidental damage. To prevent this complication, the eye is firmly covered with a pad over the closed lids and it is left in place for a few hours until corneal sensation has returned back.

Procedure related Complications

(a) Penetration

It is due to entrance of the needle tip inside the eyeball. This follows retrobulbar and peribulbar injection. Perforation provokes acute pain, which is exacerbated by the injection of a local anaesthetic drug inside the eye. This is suspected when there is marked hypotony of eye, flattening of anterior chamber, alteration of fundal reflex and vitreous haemorrhage. It eventually may result in detachment of retina.

(b) Nerve Damage

Deeper injection can cause direct damage to the optic nerve. This damage may also be indirect, due to compression of its blood supply following retrobulbar haemorrhage. There may also be injury to the ciliary ganglion in retrobulbar injection which leads to a postoperative atonic pupil.

(c) Retrobulbar Haemorrhage

The severity of retrobulbar haemorrhage is variable. It may result from injury to vortex vein, and posterior ciliary arteries. Injury to veins provokes slow bleeding with a gradual increase in intraocular pressure. Lesions of arteries provoke rapid swelling of the orbit, protrusion of eyeballs and immobility, haemorrhagic chemosis of the eyelids and conjunctiva. Close observation of the orbit immediately after withdrawing the needle can minimise the bleeding. The use of blunt 23G needle can reduce the risk of injury to the blood vessels and eye ball. This catastrophe is managed by measurement of IOP, use of osmotic diuretics, lateral canthotomy or the surgical decompression of orbit. To avoid this complication, injection should be given in the least vascularised insertion area and a fine, blunt needle should be used.

(d) Subconjunctival Haemorrhage

This is undesirable as it may interfere with suturing. It can be minimised by slowing the rate of injection. It rapidly disappears when gentle pressure is applied to the closed eye.

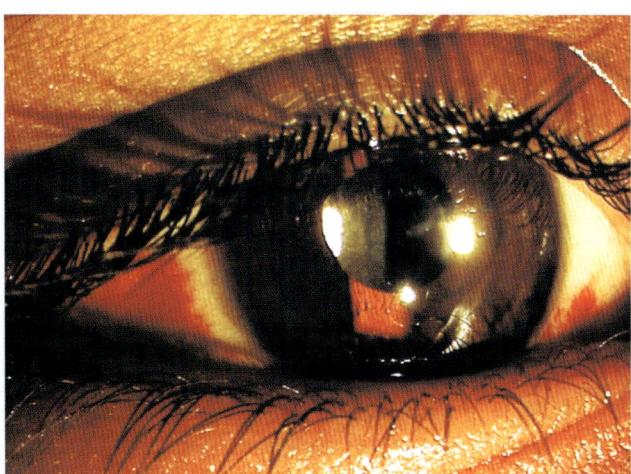

Fig. 24.1: Subconjunctival haemorrhage

COMPLICATIONS DUE TO DRAPE

Hard drapes are particularly more inconvenient both to the surgeon and patients. Whenever the skin is not dry enough of betadine paint, it does not adhere to it and it obstructs the operative field and produces glare because it is not retained by the lid guard of the speculum. Moreover, the sharp cut ends cause abrasion injury of the cornea, conjunctiva and lids.

The drape cutting scissors may also injure the cornea and conjunctiva while cutting the drape over the exposed eye.

Prevention of Drape related Complications

(a) To prevent drape related complications, the skin should be made dry of the betadine paint and a soft drape is always preferable.

(b) The unattached free portion should be excised liberally to prevent it from obscuring the operative field. It is also advisable to give multiple relaxing incisions in the free cut ends of the drape.

(c) To prevent injury to cornea and conjunctiva, the drape should be lifted from the eye and the limb of the scissors is inserted beneath the drape taking due care and maintaining distance from cornea.

COMPLICATIONS DURING SPECULUM INSERTION

Adjustable speculum with proper lid guards to retract the eyelashes is preferred. Wire speculums are not preferred in cases of topical anaesthesia because they don't provide adequate exposure of the eye. The speculum can injure the cornea if there is difficulty in inserting the speculum, particularly when the patient is resisting in cases of topical anaesthesia. It can also injure the cornea when it is rusted or it is not cleared of hard particles attached to it. Tight speculums can also lead to rise in intraocular pressure of the eye.

ASSISTANT'S HAND

The patient may feel uncomfortable if the assistant puts the weight of his hand on patient's unoperated eye or face or chin. The patient will try to resist in the form of forceful closure of the eyelids to get rid of the discomfort. He might also try to move his head and chin during surgery. Hence, it is mandatory for the assistant to take note of this point.

ECCHYMOSIS OF LIDS

This happens in most cases due to injury to small blood vessels of the lids and periorbita by the sharp cutting edge of the needle. The lid becomes slightly swollen and gives an angry looking colour. It never becomes catastrophic unlike expulsive haemorrhage. At times, only slight digital pressure suffices to control it. The colour passes off gradually within a couple of weeks like any other haematoma or ecchymosis in the body.

INCISION RELATED COMPLICATIONS

The incisions commonly used for phacoemulsification surgery are scleral, corneal and limbal.

Scleral Tunnel related Complications

(a) **Thin flap:** A flap which is too thin can tear while an instrument is being introduced. Extra suture has to be given to close the incision.

(b) **Tearing of the flap:** The edge of the incision can be damaged by the tip of the phaco probe or other instruments which means the incision is not watertight and must be sutured.

(c) **Deep incision/perforation of the globe:** An incision which is too deep particularly in myopic/ elderly patients, or when the surgeon has used excessive superficial diathermy can damage the ciliary body or even perforate the globe.

(d) **Wrong shaped incision:** It can result in astigmatism.

(e) **Premature entry to the anterior chamber:** It will mainly cause prolapse of the iris and the pupil may contract, leading to difficulty with the surgery and consequent iris damage. Even the introduction of the phacoemulsifier tip or frequent rubbing of the instrument sleeve during surgery can provoke tearing or disinsertion of the iris base. It can also damage the trabecular meshwork or cause formation of postoperative synechia.

(f) **Short tunnel:** Corneal valve will not be self-sealing. A suture may be needed which may lead to excessive induced astigmatism..

(g) **Long tunnel:** This may create folds on the cornea and cause difficulty in manoeuvring the instruments, particularly the phaco probe through the incision. An acute angulation of the phaco probe will cause difficulty in visualising the sculpting, irrigation and aspiration causing an imminent risk to the posterior capsule.

(h) **Haemorrhage:** Bleeding can occur from the edges of the scleral tunnel leading to hyphaema in the first postoperative days. Hyphaema can be prevented by creating a tamponade effect with an air bubble injected into the anterior chamber.

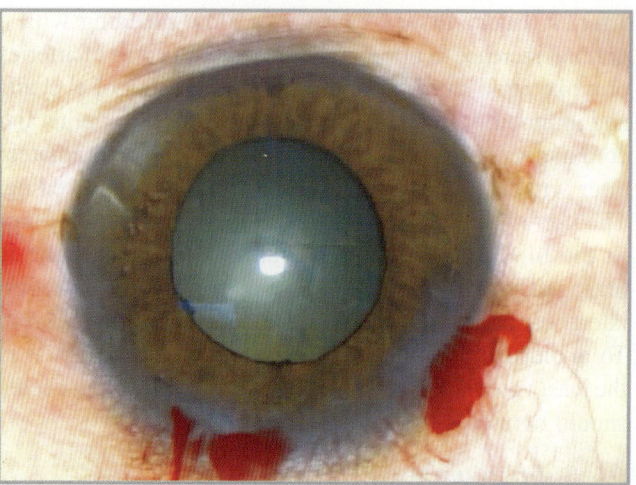

Fig. 24.2: Bleeding from the edges of the limbal tunnel

Corneal or Limbal Tunnel related Complications

(a) **Superficial incision:** Has a chance of perforating the roof of the tunnel so either a separate incision is made or the existing incision is deepened.

(b) **Deep incision:** The probable premature entry may compromise the integrity of tunnel, hence either a separate incision is made or if the surgeon is confident and very experienced, phaco can still be attempted.

(c) **Short tunnel:** Requires one or more sutures to the secure the incision.

(d) **Detachment of Descemet's membrane:** Due to the use of blunt instruments or even the phaco probe. The detached membrane can be reattached with either viscoelastic or air bubble.

(f) **Haemorrhage:** Bleeding can occur from the edges of the limbal tunnel or from conjunctiva just adjacent to the incision.

This may lead to hyphaema in the first postoperative days. Hyphaema can be prevented by creating a tamponade effect with an air bubble injected into the anterior chamber.

Side Port related Complications

(a) **Site of the incision:** The site of side port incision can affect the phacoemulsification procedure and make subsequent manoeuvres too difficult.

An incision that is either too close or too far from the entry site will make the phaco manoeuvres, like cracking or chopping, very difficult. The ideal incision site of the side port incision should be around 45–60 degrees to the initial entry site in case of the sculpting technique, whereas up to 75 degrees in case of the chopping technique.

(b) **Wide incision**: Will cause excessive loss of infusion fluid from the anterior chamber resulting in chamber instability which is the major cause of posterior capsular rupture. This site should be closed with a suture and another side port incision should be made.

VISCOELASTIC SUBSTANCES/INJECTION TECHNIQUE RELATED COMPLICATIONS

Viscoelastic substances are a great boon for safe and smooth phacoemulsification surgery. However, visco-elastics may lead to certain complications, either due to the procedure itself which is mainly mechanical in nature or due to the improper wash of residual visco which may lead to immediate or delayed problems.

Common complications with this procedure are as follows:

1. **Inadvertent capsulotomy or extension of capsulotomy:** May take place in any situation, however, this is more common with hypermature cataract.

2. **Hyphaema:** Due to accidental injury to the iris due to cannula.

3. **Dislocation of nucleus in toto or its fragment:** Due to the mechanical push being more common in cases of very hard, high myopia and traumatic/subluxated cataract. Hence, a gentle and cautious manoeuvre is desirable.

4. **Secondary glaucoma (early/transient):** Most common during early postoperative periods, particularly within two-three days are invariably associated with blockage of trabecular meshwork due to viscoelastics itself or additional adhesions of blood components along with this. Sodium hyaluronate is more prone to have such complications due to its chemical properties. These complications are preventable and can be avoided by meticulous and adequate washing of viscoelastics. This can be confirmed by watching iris movements during I/A. The iris tends to have iridodonesis once adequate wash is being completed. A uniform and large air bubble occupying the anterior chamber right up to the periphery is also suggested for a good visco wash. It is advisable to use antiglaucoma medication during immediate and subsequent days to combat transient/early postoperative glaucoma.

5. **Corneal striate:** Seen during early postoperative days may be associated with inadequate wash of viscoelastics.

ANTERIOR CAPSULOTOMY RELATED COMPLICATIONS

Capsulorrhexis is one of the basic and the most important steps in phacoemulsification surgery as all the subsequent steps are dependent on a successful completion of this step. Any deviation from the standard capsulorrhexis spells trouble in all the following steps. The safety of the capsular bag is such that it allows many learning manoeuvres without compromising either the corneal endothelium or the integrity of the posterior capsule.

While the conventional technique can open capsulotomy because its multiple edge tears are most likely to result in a posterior capsular rupture. Hence, at least the learning phaco surgeon should not proceed any further with the phaco probe manipulations if there is any break in the integrity of the capsulorrhexis.

The complications that are often seen are loss of integrity of the capsulorrhexis and less problematic is inappropriate size.

Loss of Integrity of Capsulorrhexis

During the Capsulorrhexis

In case of a break in capsulorrhexis, the surgeon has to assess the probability of its extension to the equator and then proceed ahead.

For a beginner without any back up of a senior surgeon, it is advisable to convert to the conventional small incision cataract extraction. But if the surgeon has the requisite back up, he can attempt to chop the nucleus or rotate the nucleus out of the bag and then proceed ahead with either sculpting or still better chopping.

During the Phacoemulsification

Loss of integrity of the capsulorrhexis can happen due to either the phaco probe, dialler or chopper in the left hand or the I/A probe if it catches the edge of the capsular rim especially if there is any irregularity.

The probe and even the dialler or iris repository should be kept away from the edge of the capsular rim. The I/A probe can be used to keep the edge of the capsular rim away. If the capsulorrhexis is torn at one end during the sculpting phase, keep the probe away from the torn end as there is a high chance of the tear extending towards the equator. Try and bring the nucleus out of the bag and do a supracapsular phaco. If torn during the I/A phase, it is better to put a large diameter (6.5 mm) optic lens in the bag or in the sulcus depending on the capsular support.

Inappropriate Size of Capsulorrhexis

The optimal diameter of the capsulorrhexis should be just 0.5 mm smaller than the size of the optic, i.e. just cover the edge of the optic of the lens.

(a) **Small capsulorrhexis:** There is a risk of damage to the edge during the phaco manoeuvres. However it can still be managed with experience and the diameter can be increased if desired with the help of the capsulotomy needle and capsulorrhexis forceps.

(b) **Large diameter capsulorrhexis:** Tends to cause prolapse of the nucleus into the anterior chamber. The trick is to use less fluid for hydrodissection and use a good viscoelastic to push the nucleus back into the bag. Again—while IOL insertion—the optic size of the lens has to be borne in mind or else the optic capture of the IOL can occur. You may have to consider inserting a rigid lens with a 6.5 mm optic if the capsulorrhexis is too large or if it is eccentric.

RUPTURE OF THE ZONULES

Zonular rupture or capsular dehiscence is again a very important point which should be dealt with as soon as recognised otherwise it can lead to a devastating nucleus drop. Such a complication is anticipated in case of the elderly, pseudoexfoliation or those with brown or hypermature cataracts where the zonules are already weakened.

The surgeon has to be vigilant and aware of this complication to detect it in time. A sudden deepening of the chamber, an uneven depth of the chamber during the phacoemulsification, a sudden tilting of the lens or vitreous in the anterior chamber before phacoemulsification has started, signifies a zonular or capsular dehiscence. For a beginner and especially if no senior colleague is available, it is advised to convert to small incision and prevent a lens drop. Depending on the experience of the surgeon, he can attempt to stabilise the capsular bag with iris hooks or the endocapsular ring and then attempt the phaco chop as this puts less stress on the zonules than the 4-quadrant nuclear sculpting.

HYDRODISSECTION/DELINEATION RELATED COMPLICATIONS

Hydrodissection

It is again a very important step for successful phacoemulsification with both the endocapsular and supracapsular techniques. A good hydrodissection is also one of the most important steps in phacoemulsification surgery. Inadequate or incomplete hydrodissection can make all the difference between a comfortable phacoemulsification manoeuvre and a struggling surgeon trying to rotate the nucleus and in turn causing zonular stress.

One should be very careful if capsulorrhexis is torn or incomplete as the pressure of fluid can extend the tear. Avoid injecting more than 1 ml fluid in one go as the pressure of fluid itself can cause a posterior capsular rent.

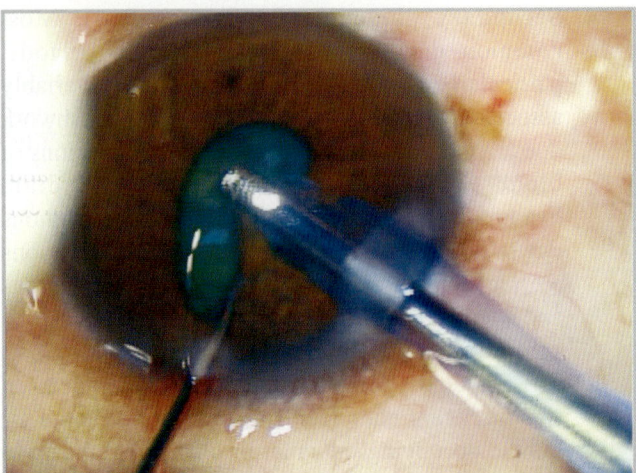

Fig. 24.3: Inadvertent touch of the phaco tip resulting mechanical injury to the iris

Nucleus Rotation

Nucleus rotation against improper hydroprocedures particularly in cases of soft cataract or in cases of posterior subcapsular cataract may lead to disastrous situations like zonulysis, posterior capsular break or even nucleus drop and vitreous prolapse.

PHACOEMULSIFICATION RELATED COMPLICATIONS

A variety of complications can occur during the actual phacoemulsification especially during the learning curve. A proper case selection for a beginner is essential not only for the patient's benefit but also for possible medicolegal problems, if they arise.

Complications can occur during any stage during phaco-emulsification. The surgeon's patience and presence of mind coupled with some experience is the only saving grace in a few odd circumstances. Of course there are certain problems anticipated in difficult cases which one will be able to handle only with experience and there is no shortcut to that. Cases with high myopia, small pupil, hard nuclei or pseudoexfoliation need separate discussions altogether. We shall consider commonly encountered problems during phacoemulsification, especially during the learning phase.

The technique used for phacoemulsification does matter to some extent. Problems can occur with either "divide and conquer" or "phaco chop", but it is easier to manage with the latter technique, especially if the capsulorrhexis has a break or if the hydrodissection is incomplete one can still manage with the phaco chop technique.

Iris Prolapse

Repeated Iris prolapse through the main or side port incision may be an annoying situation for any phaco surgeon.

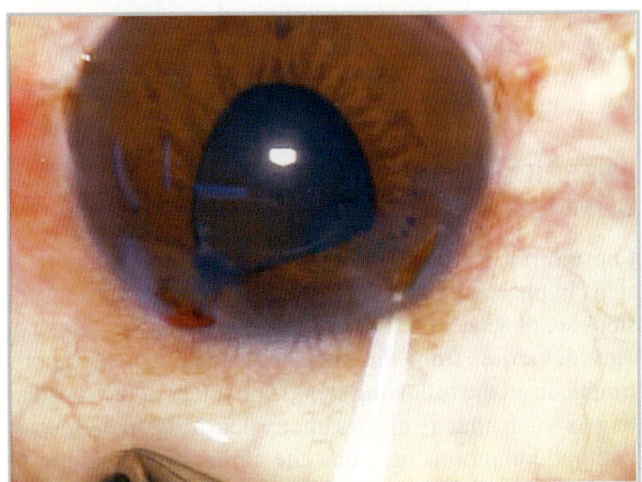

Fig. 24.4: Iris prolapse from the incisions

Repeated iris prolapse may lead to iris chaffing, iridodialysis or even posterior capsule rupture. This may arise due to following reasons associated with phaconucleotomy.

(a) **Improper posterior incision**

(b) **Improper machine settings** like inappropriate settings of US energy, flow rate and vacuum depending upon the hardness of nucleus as well as of surgical technique of chopping/sculpting.

(c) **More ominous rise in IOP due to choroidal effusion or impending expulsive haemorrhage:** Immediately use a cotton bud to assess for IOP and see the depth of anterior chamber. If IOP is apparently normal and depth of the AC is regular, there is no need for concern and the surgeon can proceed through the same incision after repositing the iris or closing the incision with a suture and making another entry. However, if the IOP appears to be high on palpation or the depth of anterior chamber is reducing, immediately close the incision with multiple 8'0' or 10'0' and start IV mannitol.

Miosis

Intraoperative miosis is another factor which requires a great deal of experience and skill. For a beginner such cases are better avoided till considerable experience is attained in phaco. There are many ways to tackle these cases and careful planning is required to handle this in the correct manner. First of all an injection of high dispersive viscoelastic should be tried to cause a viscodilatation, and if that fails then an intraocular injection of adrenaline 3–5 ml of (1:1000) should be injected ruling out any cardiac/ respiratory ailment prior to this injection. In case no response is seen to this, use either of these methods depending on the availability of equipment or experience:

(a) **Sphincterotomies** with angled vanna's scissors at 3, 6 and 9 O'clock positions.
(b) **Stretching of the iris using mobile/fixed iris hooks:** Four nylon hooks (Grieshaber) are inserted through 0.5 mm limbal incisions through four quadrants. They can be adjusted with a silicone button which prevents them from sliding along the incision.
(c) **Implantable devices** like "the perfect pupil", can be inserted to hold the pupil open, while the operation is being carried out, and then removed after the IOL has been inserted.

Sphincter/Iris Injury

Most commonly seen with a miotic pupil, particularly after mechanical stretching which may lead to atonic pupillary aperture.

Iris chaffing is invariably associated with an inadvertent touch of the phaco tip over iris due to accidental touch, mechanical friction over thin iris, miotic pupil, hard cataract or abnormal fluid and phaco dynamics. Repeated iris stroking with the help of sinskey hook to attain miotic and central pupil may lead to localised iris atrophy.

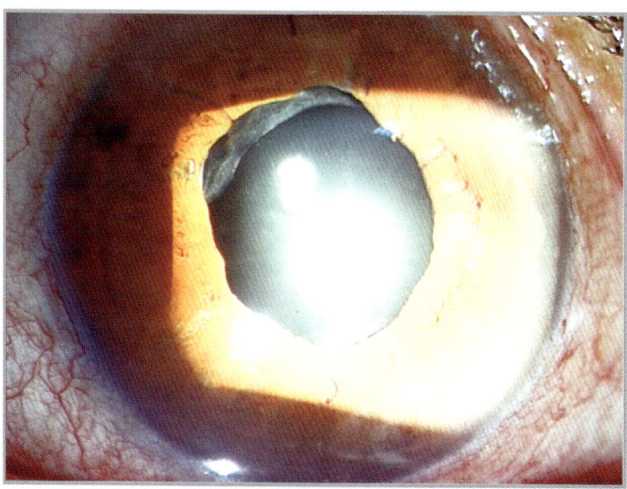

Fig. 24.5: Sphincter injury

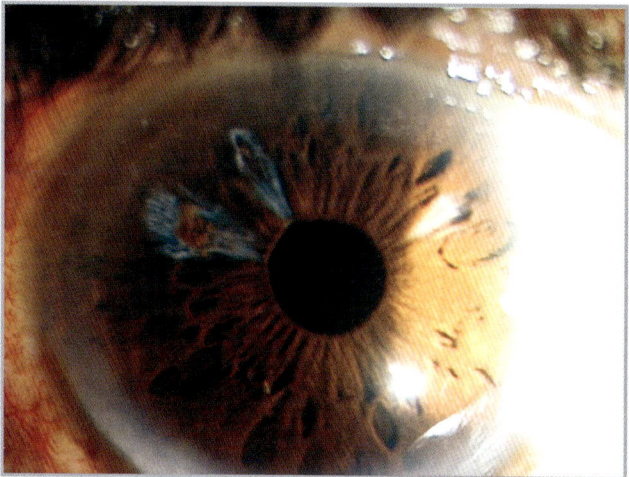

Fig. 24.6: Localised iris atrophy due to repeated iris stroking with the help of sinskey hook resulting in mechanical injury

Subluxation of Lens/Zonular Dehiscence

The earliest sign is tilting of the lens or phacodonesis during the surgery. Inject viscoelastic under the lens and carefully attempt the capsulorrhexis, secure the edges of capsulorrhexis with iris hooks inserted through separate side port incisions or insert endocapsular tension ring before proceeding for phacoemulsification through the phaco chop technique.

Rupture of the Posterior Capsule

This can occur either due to the vacuum surge, inadvertent deep phacoemulsification, damage by dialler/chopper or due to its being sucked up during the irrigation or aspiration as occlusion breaks after a piece of nucleus has been phacoemulsified into the tip and subsequently ruptures. It can be avoided by maintaining a balance between the vacuum and the flow rate in the peristaltic machine and balancing the vacuum in the Ventury machine.

The management varies with the stage of phacoemulsification.

(a) **In the initial stage:** When most of the nuclear material is left, the prime concern is to save the nucleus from falling into the vitreous. Inject highly dispersive viscoelastic under the lens but this may not always be possible due to its non-availability. In such a case the management depends on the experience of the surgeon. The safer and easier option for the novice surgeon is to increase the incision size and remove the nucleus with the help of wire vectis or viscoexpression. If the surgeon is confident then the nucleus can be impaled with the Phaco probe and phaco chopping can be done in the anterior segment. A large (6.5 mm optic) rigid lens can be implanted over the frill.

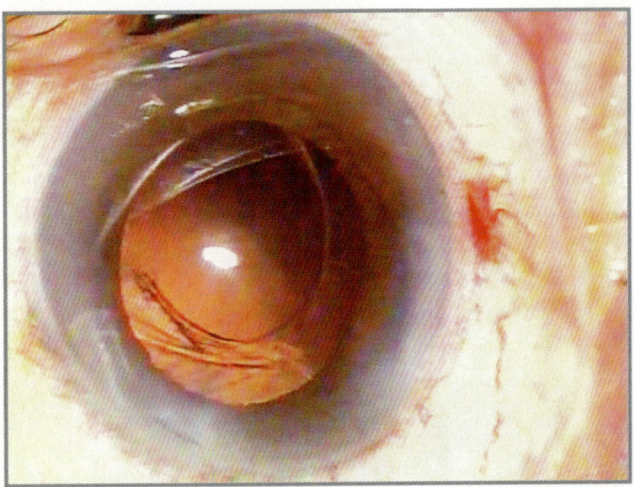

Fig. 24.7: Posterior capsule ruptures during irrigation and aspiration

(b) **During the cortical plate removal:** If the posterior capsule ruptures, the phaco aspiration can be done while the second hand is used with an iris repositor to prevent the cortical plate from falling into the vitreous.

(c) **During irrigation and aspiration if the posterior capsule ruptures**, the irrigation is continued with the probe directed away from the rupture site.

If the rupture is extending, the I/A cannula (Simcoe) is used to aspirate the epinuclear material. A rigid lens can be implanted over the frill.

Dropped Nucleus

Rupture of the posterior capsule and loss of the nucleus into the vitreous which may occur at any stage of the cataract removal, i.e. during hydrodissection, rotation, sculpting, cracking or chopping and emulsification of the nuclear quadrants.

The surgeon should be aware of the early signs of dropped nucleus like sudden deepening of the anterior chamber, decentration of the nucleus or loss of aspiration of nuclear fragments due to occlusion with the vitreous. If dropped nucleus is anticipated then manage as explained above in the last paragraph to prevent it from dropping.

Dropped nucleus and IOL will be discussed in length subsequently as a separate chapter.

When the Nucleus has Dropped

Depending on the experience of the surgeon, the surgeon can proceed to do a thorough anterior vitrectomy and refer the patient to a vitreoretinal surgeon. But if the surgeon has no access to the same or if the psychosocial and medical factors preclude the referral or better still the surgeon is ready to take the plunge literally, then he can do a thorough vitrectomy and use his phacoprobe with zero power, moderate vacuum (250–300 mmHg) to directly visualise

and impale the nucleus and bring it to the anterior chamber and remove it through another large limbal incision or use the phaco energy to emulsify it over the iris tissue. This technique resembles phacovit, however in our view, the appropriate approach remains a proper three port pars plana vitrectomy to avoid delayed complications like retinal detachment.

With slightly more experience one can attempt to remove the dislocated lens or even PC IOL with PFCL. Inject PFCL with a syringe directly over the optic disc (about 2.5–3 ml) after doing anterior and posterior vitrectomy, the lens will float up and it can be stabilised with a dialler/iris repository before doing phaco chopping with a high power (30–45%) and high vacuum (250–350 mmHg). All the infusion liquid (PFCL) contained in the vitreous cavity is aspirated through a cannula mounted on a syringe.

Intraocular Haemorrhage

This complication occurs more commonly when the incision is placed in a more temporal, more posterior, or deeper position than usual. This is managed by injecting viscoelastic substances which serves to tamponade the bleeding site. Alternatively, elevating the IOP by overfilling the chamber with balanced salt solution with added epinephrine is also advantageous with smaller self-sealing wounds. Point cautery to the feeder vessel away from the wound itself is also useful.

It is best for the surgeon to evacuate intraocular blood before clot formation occurs by simply depressing the posterior lip of the wound with a cannula at the site where blood has entered the eye. Alternatively, blood can be aspirated and exchanged for balanced salt solution.

Expulsive Haemorrhage

This catastrophic complication is more commonly seen in patients with brunescent lenses, preexisting uveitis,

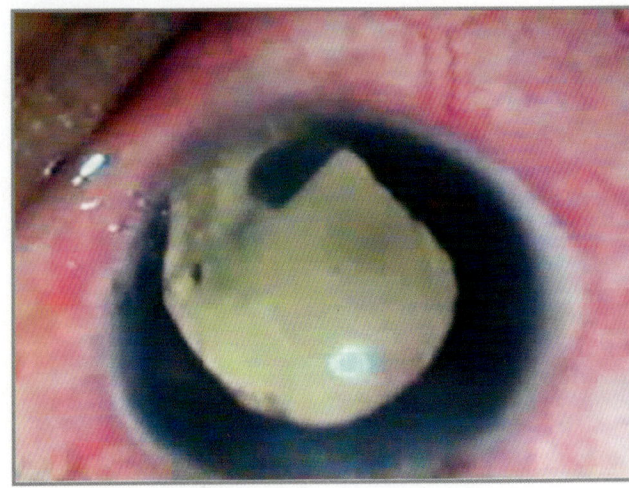

Fig. 24.8: Dislocated IOL implant

glaucoma, high myopia, or systemic hypertension or in those receiving anticoagulation therapy. Early recognition prevents subsequent catastrophe and better management of this complication. Anterior chamber shallowing with positive pressure may be the first sign of choroidal haemorrhage. The surgeon may notice a loss of the red reflex, and the patient may complain of pain despite adequate anaesthesia. The surgeon must do immediate indirect ophthalmoscopy in the slightest degree of suspicion.

Management is done by immediate closure of the eye. If the surgeon is not able to close the wound immediately, because of extensive pressure, he should tamponade the wound with a finger while infusing intravenous mannitol. After the incision is closed, the uveal tissue is repositioned back and the anterior chamber is deepened with air, balanced salt solution, or a viscoelastic. If the anterior chamber fails to deepen or the closure of the wound is unsuccessful, drainage of choroidal haemorrhage should be attempted via a posterior sclerotomy 3.5 to 4 mm posterior to the limbus.

Serous or Haemorrhagic Choroidal Effusion/Detachment

This complication is seen in case of any decompression procedure performed in the eye. This complication is more commonly found in people who are elderly or have arteriosclerosis, hypertension, diabetes mellitus, blood dyscrasias, glaucoma, or severe myopia. The detachment appears as a dark curved elevated line with the convexity towards the disc. This is usually peripheral and found in the inferior quadrants. The resulting mass may create a force sufficient to compress the vitreous to a dangerous degree. Three forces have been proved to be the contributing factors in its pathogenesis. First is the intraocular pressure, which tends to prevent transudation from the choroidal vessels. This falls to zero as soon as the globe is opened. The second is the intravascular pressure. Since transudation occurs chiefly at the capillary

level, the blood pressure within the choroidal capillaries is considered. According to Best and Taylor, the blood pressure at the arterial end is about 32 mmHg and that at the venous end is 12 mmHg. This force favours transudation into the tissue fluids. The third force is offsetting the intravascular pressure, the oncotic pressure exerted by the protein colloids of the plasma, which tends to draw fluids from the tissues into the vascular tree. The most important factor is how long the globe remains open. The possible fact is that the longer the ciliary vessels are exposed to an intraocular pressure of zero, the greater the likelihood of choroidal detachment. A sudden precipitous fall in intraocular pressure favours more massive transudation, which compresses the vitreous at the time of surgery. The fall in intraocular pressure can be prevented by reducing the intraocular pressure to hypotension before making the incision.

Immediate management is done by closure of the incision and administration of a hyperosmotic agent. Posterior sclerotomy, if performed can exacerbate the bleeding and result in a vicious cycle leading to a loss of the eye. Postoperatively the patient should be treated with topical and systemic steroids to reduce intraocular inflammation. Subsequent treatment is between 7 and 14 days later when liquefaction of blood clot allows better drainage of the haemorrhage. It involves drainage of blood followed by pars plana vitrectomy and air-fluid exchange. Although the visual prognosis is grave, useful vision may be salvaged in some cases.

In some rare occasions there may be occurrence of massive choroidal detachment where there may be no signs of vitreous pressure during surgery. This may primarily be due to massive serious transudates in the choroid. This is treated by immediately suturing the wound at the 12 O'clock position and performing a subchoroidal tap in the region of choroidal detachment. This entity is called as 'Expulsive Choroidal Effusion.'

Ciliochoroidal detachment presents as a convex brownish mass in the involved quadrant with a shallow anterior chamber. In most cases, choroidal detachment is cured within 4 days with pressure bandage and the use of oral acetazolamide. If the condition persists, suprachoroidal drainage with injection of air into the anterior chamber is indicated.

Subconjunctival or Corneal Emphysema

This is a very rare complication seen during any type of cataract surgery. This usually happens when the surgeon attempts to introduce air (into the anterior chamber in order to form the anterior chamber before staining the anterior capsule with Trypan blue) with a cannula which either makes its way into the subconjunctival region at the entry site or into the corneal stroma in a case of improper incision. Air bubbles are seen under the elevated conjunctiva in a case of subjunctival emphysema. Similarly, tiny air bubbles

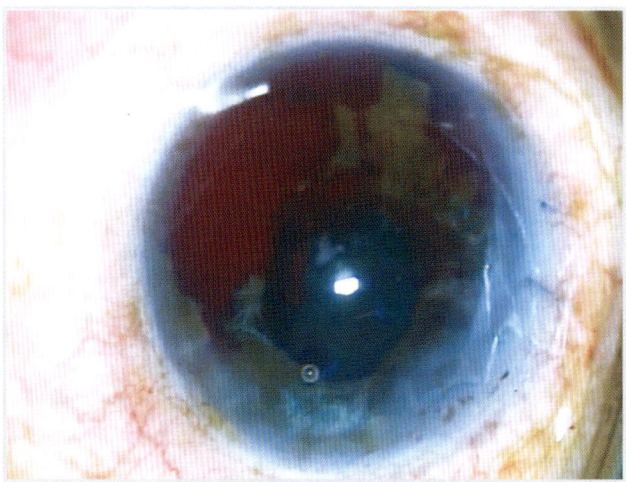

Fig. 24.9: Hyphaema

are seen in the corneal stromal substances near and around the entry site. The good thing about this complication is that this gets absorbed within a day or two without leaving behind any permanent sequel which would affect the final outcome of a surgery.

COMPLICATIONS RELATED TO THE IOL

IOL Decentration

The IOL can get decentred either upwards, downwards or sideways with a tilt. Such a condition is generally encountered if the IOL is placed over the capsular frill following the posterior capsular rent. It can also occur due to a small lens (optic size 5.25 mm) placed in a large capsular bag or due to capsular bag contraction. Foldable IOL may also be decentred due to improper position of one of the haptics outside the bag, abnormal position of IOL particularly seen with large or irregular rhexis. Contraction of capsular bag can also lead to subluxation of the IOL implant.

In such a condition lens exchange has to be done and a larger lens (6.5 mm optic) implanted over the frill in case the capsular support is lacking then a scleral fixated lens is considered.

IOL Power Miscalculation

Any IOL which is differing from refractive status by 2 dioptres or more in the postoperative period should be exchanged.

CONVERSION TO ECCE

Once the decision to convert has been made it is important to stabilise the intraocular structures. The further mode of action depends on the integrity of capsulorrhexis. A cohesive viscoelastic with an intact capsule can be injected to keep the fragments from falling into the vitreous and a wire vectis is used to remove the fragments from the anterior chamber. The next step is to extend the incision; it becomes difficult in case of a corneal incision than in case of a scleral incision. In such a situation the experience of the surgeon is taken into account and if the surgeon feels that he cannot tackle the case, a senior surgeon should be consulted. It is best not to let the ego come in between the surgery.

CORNEAL COMPLICATIONS

Phacoemulsification surgery may face several corneal complications which may be encountered at any stage including intra or postoperative period.

Predisposing Factors

(a) Preexisting corneal pathology
   (i) Postinfective/traumatic corneal opacities, Trachoma or corneal inflammation due to any other chronic disorders.
   (ii) Corneal dystrophies/degenerations
   (iii) Poor endothelial cell reserve.
(b) Preexisting glaucoma, pseudoexfoliation and uveitis.
(c) Intraoperative surgical complications/Excessive tissue handling, excessive use of US energy/thermal burn.

Descemet's Membrane Detachment

Descemet's membrane detachment can occur either due to the dialler, phaco probe or the I/A tip any time during the surgery. All it requires is an injection of air at the end of surgery to oppose the two layers together; although sometimes if the detachment is large, one or two 10 'O' sutures may be required.

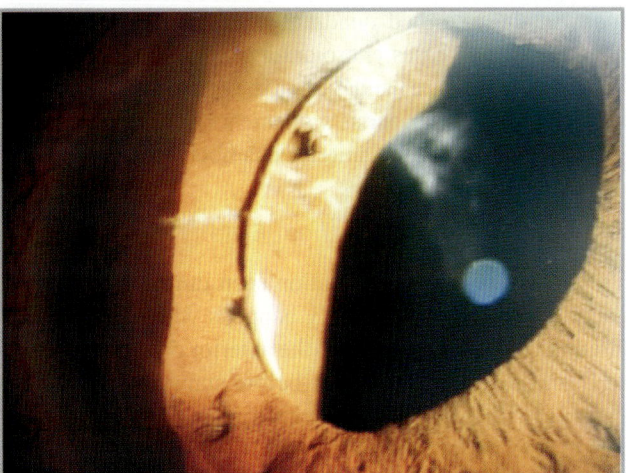

Fig. 24.10: Pupillary capture (IOL margin is over riding on the pupillary margin)

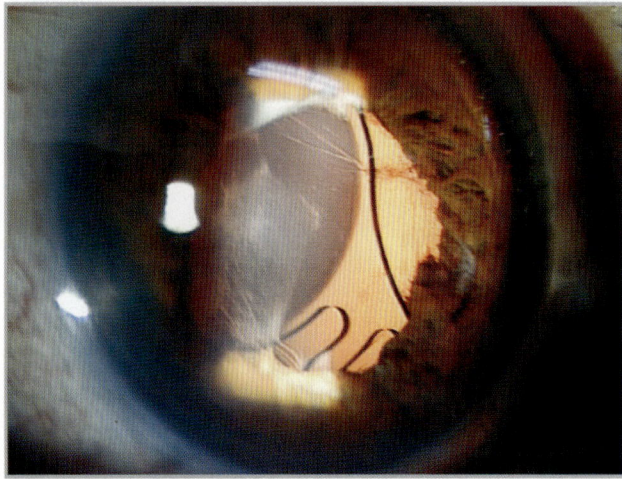

Fig. 24.11: IOL decentration

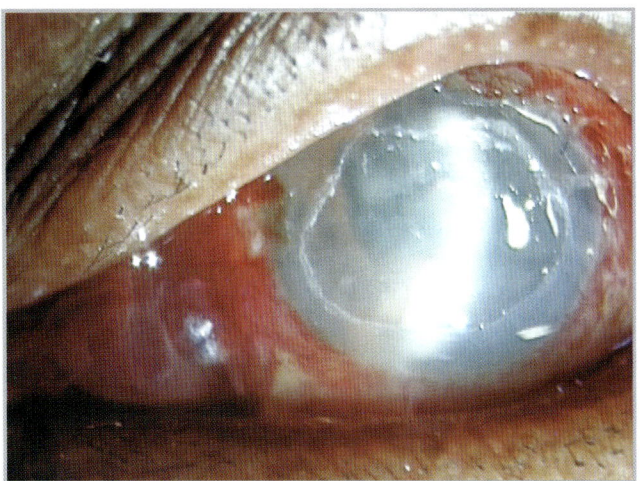

Fig. 24.12: Large persistent epithelial defects

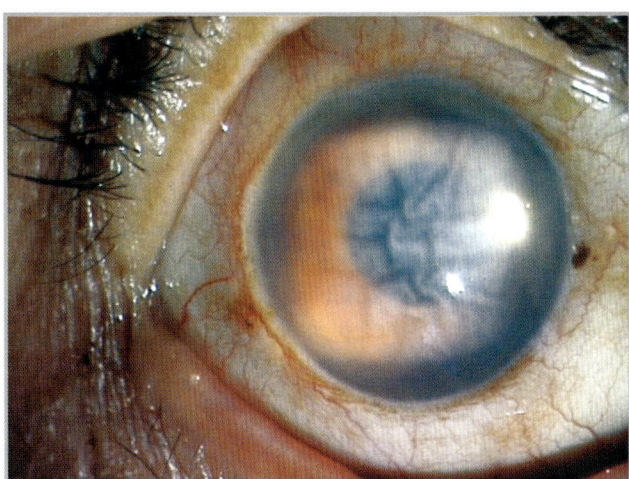

Fig. 24.13: Corneal decompensation

Thermal Burns

Due to the heat dissipated by the phaco tip during phaco-emulsification if either the wound is too tight, flow is inadequate or more phacoenergy is used. An appropriate wound size which is not too tight is formed. Attention towards the flow through the phaco tip and the use of pulsed mode and frequent injections of viscoelastic will prevent such complications

Corneal Decompensation

Cornea can decompensate and have persistent epithelial and stromal oedema if the cornea has a low endothelial cell count preoperatively or there was intraoperative endothelial trauma or prolonged postoperative inflammation.

Such cases should be aggressively managed in the initial stage with topical steroids, topical hypertonic sodium chloride eye drops along with topical NSAIDs. It generally takes from a few days to even 3–4 months in few cases to resolve. If the corneal oedema has not resolved even after 4 months, penetrating keratoplasty has to be considered.

SECONDARY GLAUCOMA

Transient Rise in IOP due to Viscoelastic Substances

Transient rise of IOP due to viscoelastic substances does occur with the use of all viscoelastics. The peak pressure usually occurs within 6–8 hrs after surgery. The mechanism responsible for the increase in pressure is probably related to a decrease in outflow facility. Sodium hyaluronate and possibly all other viscous solutions are eliminated from the anterior chamber primarily through the trabecular meshwork. Benson and associates found a 65% decrease in aqueous outflow facility after anterior chamber injection of 1% sodium hyaluronate into enucleated human eyes. Anterior chamber washout doesn't eliminate the decrease in outflow

facility, but it does decrease the level and duration of postoperative pressure rise. So a washout or aspiration of viscoelastics at the end of surgery is recommended. Viscoat requires more meticulous aspiration in all quadrants of the anterior chamber than other viscous solutions. This is because Viscoat contains chondroitin sulphate which retains its viscosity during aspiration and irrigation. Removal of viscous will not prevent the pressure rise in all cases. So, the use of intraocular carbachol (miostat) or topical apraclonidine or a systemic carbonic anhydrase inhibitor for pressure control during the first 24 hours after surgery is needed.

Glaucoma due to Hyphaema/Intraocular Haemorrhage

During early postoperative period, fresh blood appears in the anterior chamber, typically from the cataract incision site, or from papillary sphincter tears. IOP can rise from any amount of bleeding, but larger hyphaema usually cause higher IOPs. An endocapsular location is an unusual type of postoperative haemorrhage.

Postoperative hyphaemas and glaucoma are generally limited and resolve without complications. A healthy optic nerve can withstand a moderate rise of pressure without damage and doesn't require antiglaucoma therapy. Medical treatment is favoured if the IOP is acutely elevated to greater than 30 mmHg for 2 weeks. In the presence of pre-existing glaucomatous optic nerve damage or sickle cell disease, earlier and more aggressive management is required.

Despite medical therapy, surgical intervention may be required. Indications of surgical intervention include IOP criteria, corneal blood staining, and a clot of prolonged duration. Traditional criteria for surgical intervention to avoid optic nerve damage in hyphaemas are an IOP greater than 50 mmHg for 5 days or greater than 35 mmHg for 7 days. Surgical intervention is indicated when any sign of corneal blood staining appears. Patients with compromised corneal endothelial function may require earlier intervention. Stagnant, large clots that persist longer than 10 days or total hyphaemas lasting more than 5 days are often evacuated because they may lead to peripheral anterior synechiae.

Surgical techniques for hyphaema evacuation include anterior chamber washout with or without coaxial irrigation-aspiration, automated cutting, aspiration of clot material, or clot expression. Simple removal of circulating RBCs and debris often suffices for IOP control, but visual rehabilitation is hastened by clot removal.

Glaucoma due to Excessive Inflammation (Uveitis)

This rarely results from the mild postoperative inflammation that routinely occurs after cataract surgery. Usually glaucoma occurs in eyes with severe inflammatory response. Uveitic glaucoma can be an open angle or a closed- angle, or a combination of both. Open angle glaucoma results from inflammation related alteration in the trabecular meshwork structure. These changes include swelling of the trabecular matrix, endothelial cells dysfunction, or accumulation of inflammatory cells and debris. Angle closure glaucoma can occur from peripheral anterior synechiae, posterior synechia, or rubeosis iridis.

Postoperative glaucoma may be managed medically by controlling inflammation with frequent use of corticosteroids. Cycloplegic and sympathomimetic agents are given to prevent or break posterior synechiae. Periocular or systemic antiinflammatory medication may be needed for severe intraocular inflammation. IOP is regulated as needed with topical beta blockers, systemic carbonic anhydrase inhibitors, and hyperosmotic agents. Miotics are avoided. Iridectomies are indicated to relieve the pupillary block.

Glaucoma due to Residual Lens Matter

Residual cortical material after cataract extraction can cause significant IOP elevation by either open or closed angle

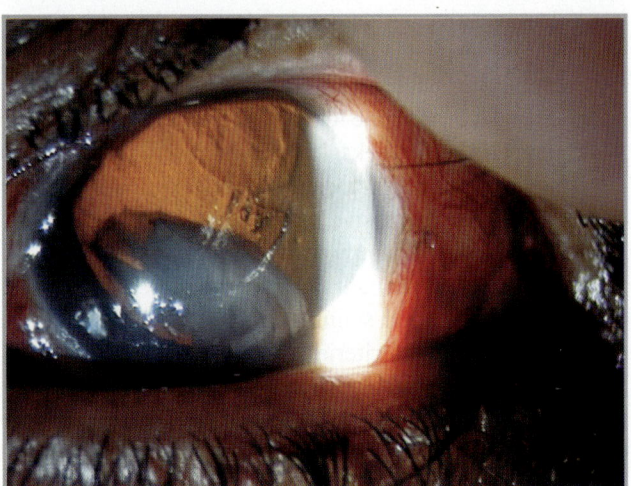

Fig. 24.14: Residual lens matter

mechanism. Typically this occurs early in the postoperative period, although it can occur after years if a soemmering ring cataract suddenly opens. The patient presents with a painful red eye. Lens material causes severe obstruction of the trabecular meshwork and outflow channels. Obstruction may also result from lens material filled with macrophages inflammatory cells or persistent inflammation. Treatment with topical corticosteroids and antiglaucoma medication, excluding miotic agents, is usually sufficient until IOP normalises. Surgery may be required in cases of severe inflammation or persistent pressure elevation, with removal of residual lens material.

Glaucoma due to Lens Drop

This is most commonly encountered in beginners who are in their learning curve of phacoemulsification surgery. Here the lens dislocates into the vitreous cavity through the posterior capsular rent. The patient present with reduced vision, uveitis, secondary glaucoma, corneal oedema and retinal detachment. The glaucoma is often refractory to medical management; and surgical removal of the fragment is required. This is done either by the anterior segment approach or a three port pars plana vitrectomy lensectomy by an experienced vitreoretinal surgeon. The procedure is not without complications. Despite the procedure, the patient attains the final visual acuity of 6/24 or worse in more than 50% of cases in one study.

Glaucoma due to Vitreous Disturbances

This particular complication appears when a posterior capsular rent occurs during the surgery. As a result vitreous cavity is disturbed and it finds its way into the anterior chamber. If the vitreous is not cleared with proper anterior vitrectomy and irrigation/aspiration, it remains stuck in the angles of AC and blocks the trabecular meshwork and the aqueous outflow tract. This is prevented with thorough anterior vitrectomy using vitrectomy cutter and aspiration from the AC and the angles intraoperatively. Postoperatively, this is managed medically by putting topical corticosteroid drops, topical antiglaucoma measures, and systemic corticosteroid administration for a longer period.

ENDOPHTHALMITIS

This is a potentially devastating complication both for the patient and the surgeon; hence every minute detail should be looked into while going in for phacoemulsification surgery. Although, the incidence is even lower (0.9%) with phacoemulsification as compared to the extracapsular cataract extraction (1.6%) yet, due to the enormity of complications involved, it is better to take all precautions to avoid infection and to recognise and treat endophthalmitis with aggressive management protocol.

Endophthalmitis and its prevention will be discussed in length subsequently as a separate chapter.

The safety precautions in general and in particular to phacoemulsification are summarised as below:

(a) Use of standard quality topical eye drops preoperatively.

(b) Meticulous scrubbing both by the surgeon and assistant.

(c) Using autoclaved balanced salt solution as irrigating fluid.

(d) Aseptic painting with betadine (a single drop of betadine instilled just before the surgery is known to reduce the incidence of endophthalmitis to a great extent).

(e) Ensuring that the phaco tubing and the tip have been cleaned and autoclaved before starting of the surgery in the morning.

(f) Ensuring that the suction cassette is empty and cleaned before the surgery.

(g) Autoclaved instruments only.

(h) Meticulous patient preparation to rule out any foci of infection beforehand.

(i) Most important, ensuring to see that **consent form should be signed beforehand** (a detailed consent form highlighting the possibility of infection can save the surgeon from medicolegal hassles if misfortune does strike). A copy of the consent form is given in the previous chapter on general information on cataract surgery.

The clinical characteristics of endophthalmitis are ciliary injection, conjunctival chemosis, hypopyon, decreased visual acuity and ocular pain. It may develop as acute or chronic form. The acute form develops in 2–3 days and the chronic form may take a few weeks to a few months also. Once the diagnosis has been confirmed, straight away give intravitreal Vancomycin 1 mg in 0.1 ml + Ceftazidime

2.25 mg in 0.1 ml. Just before giving the intravitreal injection, aspirate using the tuberculin syringe attached to the 26 gauge needle and send the vitreous specimen for culture and ABST. However, a vitreous biopsy is preferred to obtain a better vitreous sample. Along with this systemic third generation cephalosporin, fortified antibiotic drops, systemic and topical NSAIDs, topical cycloplegics and antiglaucoma medication are also given. Vitrectomy is generally required in case the response to the above regimen is not seen in 24–48 hrs.

RETINAL DETACHMENT

The incidence is lower with phacoemulsification cataract surgery than extracapsular cataract surgery.

Predisposing Factors Include

(a) Axial length more than 24.5 mm (myopia)

(b) Retinal degenerations: lattice degeneration

(c) Intraoperative vitreous loss

(d) Postoperative ocular trauma

(e) History of retinal detachment in the fellow eye.

The Management

Management of retinal detachment is in the purview of the vitreoretinal surgeon, which will involve vitrectomy followed by intraocular gas tamponade or injection of PFCL and endolaser photocoagulation to seal the tear or conventional retinal detachment surgery depending upon the merits of the case.

Subconjunctival Injection Related Complications

Subconjunctival haemorrhage following subconjunctival injection of antibiotics and steroids is not an unusual occurrence. However, it may not lead to any postoperative complications except for an annoying appearance. Subcon-

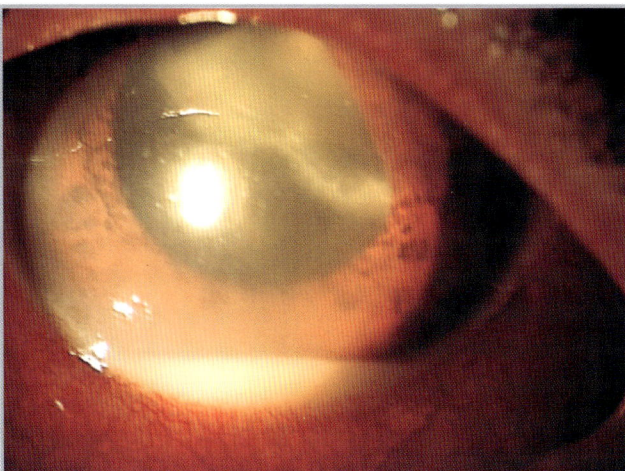

Fig. 24.15: Endophthalmitis

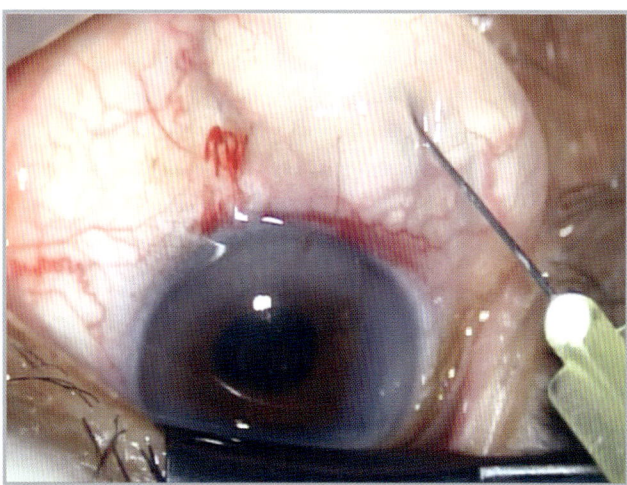

Fig. 24.16: Subconjunctival haemorrhage following subconjunctival injection

junctival haemorrhage is a self-resolving condition that resolves within a two weeks' period.

Intraocular penetration of subconjunctival needle is a very rare occurrence which may be seen in cases of high myopia or thin sclera. Such eventuality is very serious and may lead to intraocular haemorrhage or even endophthalmitis.

CONCLUSION

Phacoemulsification is undoubtedly the technique which gives the best results in cataract surgery. Although, the skills are needed to be learnt, with adequate training this should not result in adverse results for the patient along the way.

It is to be hoped that the foregoing will encourage both the training surgeon and those with more experience to take an analytical view of the likely problems which may arise in phacoemulsification. By this means, anticipation will replace surprise when difficulties arise and a suitable plan will have been formulated by both the surgeon and just as importantly, the nursing staff.

In the vast majority of cases it is a simple, rapid, and safe procedure, yet complications may arise in a small proportion of cases, however, much expert the surgeon might be. Every phase of the operation can bring about its own set of problems and a failure to deal with these adequately can have profound effects on the anatomical and functional outcome.

BIBLIOGRAPHY

1. Cionni R, Osher R. Complications of phacoemulsification. In: Weinstock F, ed. Management and Care of the Cataract Patient. Cambridge, Mass: Blackwell Scientific Publications; 1992:198–211.
2. Cionni R, Osher R. Complications of phacoemulsification surgery. In: Steinert R, ed. Cataract Surgery: Techniques, Complications and Management. Philadelphia, Pa: WB Saunders; 1995:327–340.
3. Osher R, Cionni R. The torn posterior capsule: Its intra-operative behavior, surgical management and long-term consequences. J Cataract Refract Surg. 1990; 16: 157–162.
4. Cionni R, Osher R. Management of zonular dialysis with the endocapsular ring. J Cataract Refract Surg. 1995; 21: 245–249.
5. Osher R. New approach: Synthetic zonules. In: Osher R, ed. Video Journal Cataract Refract Surg. 1997; 13:1.
6. Cionni R, Osher R. Management of profound zonular dialysis or weakness with a new endocapsular ring designed for scleral fixation. J Cataract Refract Surg. 1998; 24:1299–1306.
7. Eller A, Barad R. Miyake analysis of anterior vitrectomy techniques. J Cataract Refract Surg. 1996; 22:213–217.
8. Pfeifer V. Suturing the ring. In: Osher R, ed. Video Journal Cataract Refract Surg. 1998; 14:4.
9. Novak J. Flexible iris hooks for phacoemulsification. J Cataract Refract Surg. 1997; 23:828–831.

25

Management of Dropped Nucleus and IOL Implants

Col RP Gupta and Col JKS Parihar SM, VSM

INTRODUCTION

Cataract surgery has undergone rapid changes in the recent past and almost parallelling in the field of medicine too. Evolving from the days of ICCE, graduating to ECCE with conventional methods and finally to its peak, phaco-emulsification, cataract surgery has become the most frequently performed surgery worldwide. As expected, with the refinement in the technique and availability of sophisticated machines and modern intraocular implants, the complication rates have gone down. But as every coin has two faces, phacoemulsification on one hand has done away with most of the complications of conventional surgery, but on the other hand has presented its own dreaded complications, out of which posterior dislocation of the lens or the intraocular implant is the most important.

Various studies quote the incidence of approximately 0.3% in the US and 1.1% in the UK. The incidence of dislocated intraocular implants has not been mentioned in any study. There is no structured study to reveal incidence of this complication in India. But the authors with their vast experience in the field of phacoemulsification have found that the incidence of posterior dislocation of lens was 0.4% and posterior dislocation of intraocular lens was 0.1% among 4800 cases operated by this technique in the last 5 years.

NUCLEUS DROP

Causes

(a) Elderly person with hard nucleus.
(b) Pseudoexfoliation and its inherent zonular weakness and dehiscence.
(c) History of trauma with zonular dehiscence.
(d) Phacoemulsification in beginners is supposed to have a long learning curve because of need for bimanual control, better hand-foot coordination and more reliability on machine controls than on manual control.
(e) Chronic glaucoma.
(f) Inherently weak zonules—Marfan's syndrome, Weil Machesney's syndrome.

Clinical Presentations of Dropped Nucleus

Posterior dislocation of lens—In a case of posterior dislocation of lens the presentation can be an intraoperative realisation of the dislocation or at a later date due to complications caused due to retained lens fragments or the lens as a whole in the form of:

(a) Phacolytic glaucoma caused due to blockage of the trabecular meshwork by macrophages and lens material.
(b) Severe uveitis leading to formation of pupillary membrane.
    (Dislocated lens with intact capsule rarely causes intraocular inflammation).
(c) Cystoid macular edema due to chronic inflammation
(d) Retinal detachment due to traction caused by the retained lens material or attempts to remove it.

How to Minimise the Incidence of Intraoperative dropped Lens

When a lens drops it sends a chill down the spine of the operating surgeon, but the need of the hour is not to panic and do hasty and heroic procedures but to keep a cool composure which is actually not very easy to achieve. Going by the known dictum that prevention is better than cure, the following measures should be taken intraoperative to minimise the incidence of dropped lens:

(a) Vigorous hydrodissection should be avoided. It should be gentle at all times in one's surgical career. It is suggested that gentle tapping of the nucleus to release any fluid pockets should be done if a fluid wave is not seen during hydrodissection. It prevents hydrodistension of the posterior capsule and avoids posterior capsular rupture.

(b) Use of the endocapsular tension ring in cases of cataract associated with zonular dialysis stabilises a loose lens and allows phacoemulsification and in-the-bag implantation of intraocular implant.

(c) Prompt detection of signs of posterior capsular dehiscence in the form of shallowing of the AC, stretching of capsulorrhexis and presence of vitreous in AC and taking preventive measures so that there is no nuclear drop.

(d) Forceful sculpting without adequate power causes more stress on zonules and may cause zonular dehiscence and accordingly should be avoided.

(e) When a capsular dehiscence is detected, a barrier by means of a viscoelastic (preferably Healon-5 or Viscoat) injected may be helpful.

Management

Management of a dislocated lens or lens material depends on when the dislocation is recognised intraoperatively:

(a) Actions to be taken by anterior segment surgeon

(b) Availability of a VR surgeon to tackle the situation immediately.

(a) Actions to be taken by Anterior Segment Surgeon

Refrain chasing the dropping fragment with phacoemulsification probe through anterior approach: If the lens is dropping, the anterior segment surgeon should resist any heroic attempts to chase the dropping fragment with phacoemulsification probe as it will lead to traction on the formed vitreous leading to multiple retinal tears and retinal detachment. Once the drop of lens has occurred, further management depends on the availability of a VR surgeon. The anterior segment surgeon should keep his composure and do a thorough cortical clean up. He can proceed with an anterior vitrectomy to prevent vitreous incarceration in the corneoscleral wound. In panic he should not follow the dropping fragments with his phacoemulsification probe or a wire vectis or else will find himself swimming in a pool filled with algae, the more he struggles, the more he is entangled and the lens fragment will continue to fall down. It is preferable that, the anterior segment surgeon should not put any IOL if he is sure of the drop of fragments as it will impair adequate visualisation during subsequent surgery. An IOL can always be inserted after vitrectomy.

A prompt referral to a VR surgeon is needed after properly apprising the patient about the event. Interaction with the patient is the most important issue. Truth coupled with assurance is the best method. The VR surgeon should be informed about the size of the dropped fragment, the amount of fishing attempted and how the matter was communicated to the patient. It is the author's experience that patients are more satisfied when they are better informed. If the VR surgeon is available in the same complex, the dropped lens can be removed immediately after suturing the wound.

(b) Availability of a VR Surgeon to Tackle the Situation Immediately

For a VR surgeon, the management of a posterior dislocation of lens falls into two categories

(i) Intraoperative management.

(ii) A planned VR surgery.

(i) Intraoperative Management

There is a high incidence of lens dislocation during hydrodissection and sculpting in phacoemulsification especially in cases done by the clear corneal route.

Immediate measure that can be undertaken when a lens is dropping are:

(a) Support the falling nucleus by two MVR blades passed through the pars plana route by the 'crossed spear technique'. According to the author, this is the quickest method to tackle this emergency situation.

(b) Injecting viscoelastic behind the floating lens.

(ii) Planned VR Surgery

A proper preoperative workup is necessary for the success of any surgery. In this case this includes

(a) DVA

(b) Intraocular pressure.

(c) Signs of uveitis: presence of pupillary membrane, vitreous haze which will impair the visibility of lens fragments during surgery.

(d) Corneal edema.

(e) Presence of capsular rim.

(f) Status of surgical wound of previous surgery.

(g) Indirect ophthalmoscopy for size and characteristics of dropped lens matter and any signs of retinal break/ retinal detachment.

(h) USG A/B scan, in cases of hazy media to rule out any retinal detachment and to know about the characteristics of the dropped lens matter, i.e. whether the whole lens has dropped or only fragments are present.

The decision of when to operate postoperatively after the initial posterior dislocation of lens depends on various factors including:

(a) Size of lens fragment-small lens fragments (< 25% of lens or < 2 mm in size) can be tolerated in the vitreous cavity. The author has found that keeping the patient on systemic steroids was sufficient to keep the inflammation under control and the patient is asymptomatic with the treatment.

(b) Residual cortical matter in vitreous cavity is also treated with only systemic steroids in cases less than 2 mm in size.

(c) Intraocular inflammation: If it has not subsided even after 2 weeks of steroids, surgery should be undertaken, however small the fragment be.

(d) Level of intraocular pressure: If IOP is not controlled with steroids and antiglaucoma medications, surgery should be undertaken.

(e) Associated RD, retinal tear, sterile endophthalmitis warrant immediate surgery.

VR Surgery

A standard three port pars plana vitrectomy with phacofragmentation is the surgery of choice. If there is an associated retinal detachment, an encircling scleral buckle is given prior to the pars plana vitrectomy.

The cataract surgery wound is examined and if found weak is reinforced with additional sutures.

First, clearing up of anterior chamber is necessary to have a clear view of the posterior segment. Any retained cortical matter in AC is promptly removed with a vitrectomy probe. Pupillary membrane if present is peeled off with a small needle. Author usually uses a cystitome with a 26G needle to create an opening in the pupillary membrane which is then peeled off and chewed up by a vitrectomy probe. Any herniated vitreous in the AC is removed.

Pupillary dilatation is a prerequisite for any VR surgery. It is done by topical medications and, if needed, intracameral adrenaline or iris hooks in cases where refractory pupil is used. Author usually uses translimbal flexible hooks introduced through 26 G needle perforations. A proper three port pars plana vitrectomy is done leaving a layer of vitreous under the lens fragments to serve as cushion.

Various surgical techniques of removal of lens fragments are described. Out of all these, the author feels the most useful and safe is the use of phacofragmentation. Small amounts of perfluorocarbon liquid is injected behind the lens/fragment which will raise it into midvitreous. This will also help to keep the phacofragmatome away from the retina. In cases of associated retinal detachment, the PFCL also helps in keeping the retina attached.

Large amounts of PFCL injection should be avoided as it will form a convex meniscus which can cause the fragments to move to the periphery.

Keeping the power at 5–10% and aspiration at 150–200 mmHg, the lens fragments are aspirated by a phacofragmatome. This allows more efficient extraction by continuous occlusion of suction port, thus minimising trauma to the retina by projectile fragments.

If the whole hard nucleus is dropped, many a times a fragmatome fails to aspirate the nucleus. Higher power cannot be used as it may cause damage to the retina. In such situations, PFCL alone can be used to raise the nucleus to just beneath the iris. Then a light pipe or any other soft tipped cannula can be used to manipulate the lens into the AC, after which it can be removed by a limbal incision. Lens should not be taken into the AC with PFCL alone as it will cause damage to the corneal endothelium by contact of nucleus and PFCL.

Various techniques are used to support the lens fragment during aspiration. A lighted pick can be used to spear the fragment and stabilise it. The author has always used the 'light pipe like a chopstick' to support the lens during fragmentation. After the removal of lens fragments, the posterior segment is visualised for any evidence of retinal tear/ detachment. If present, endolaser treatment is applied around the retinal break. PFCL is removed and long acting gas tamponade is given.

An IOL if not inserted during the initial procedure can be inserted through the previous limbal/corneal incision. In case

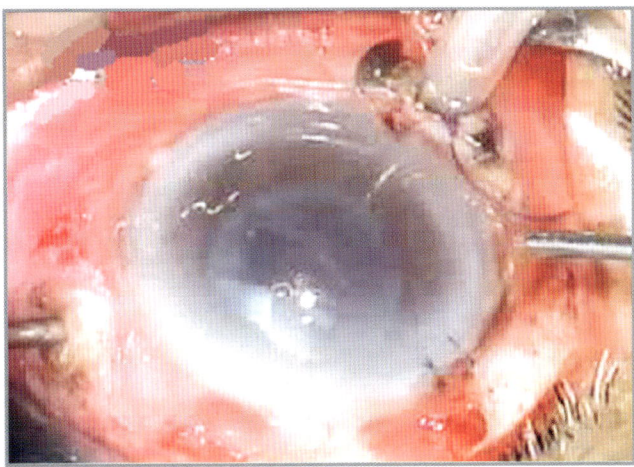

Fig. 25.1: Management of dropped nucleus: Pars plana approach

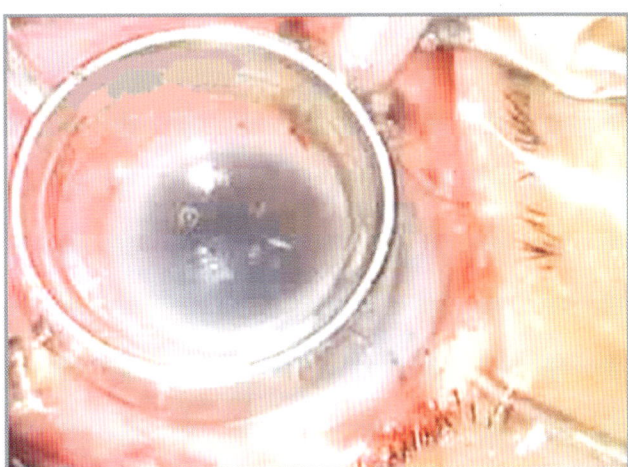

Fig. 25.2: Fragmatome removal of dropped nucleus: Pars plana approach

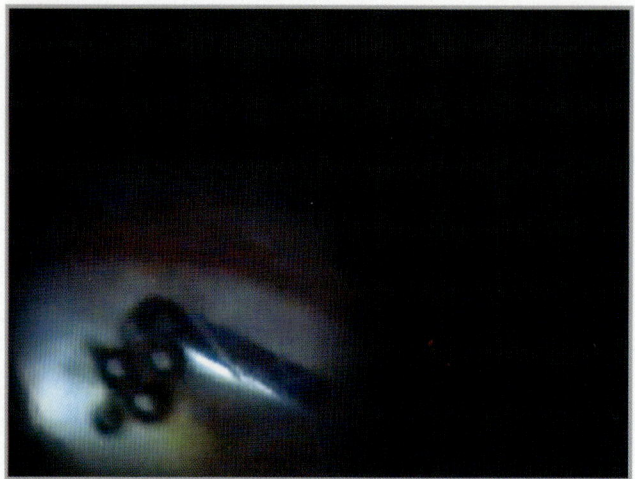

Fig. 25.3: Cortical plate removal by vitreous cutter

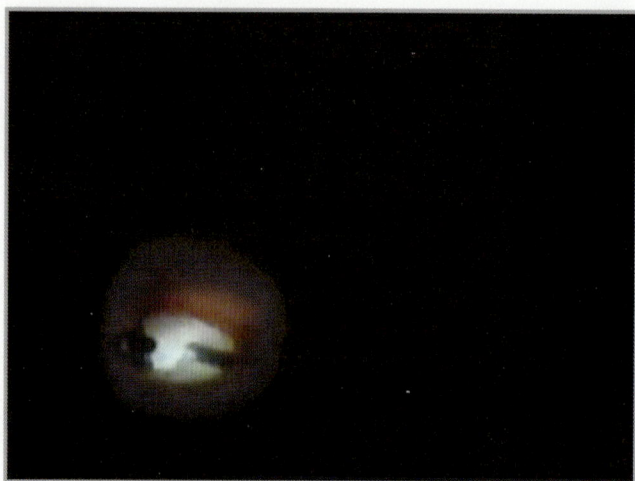

Fig. 25.4: Cortical plate removal by fragmatome

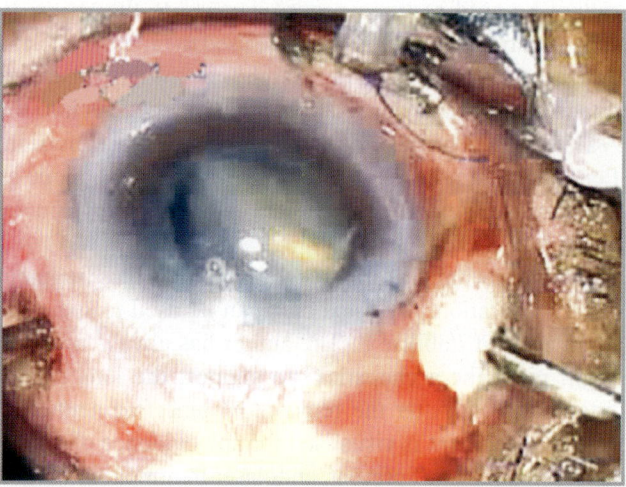

Fig. 25.5: Fragmatome removal of dropped Nucleus: Posterior to iris plane

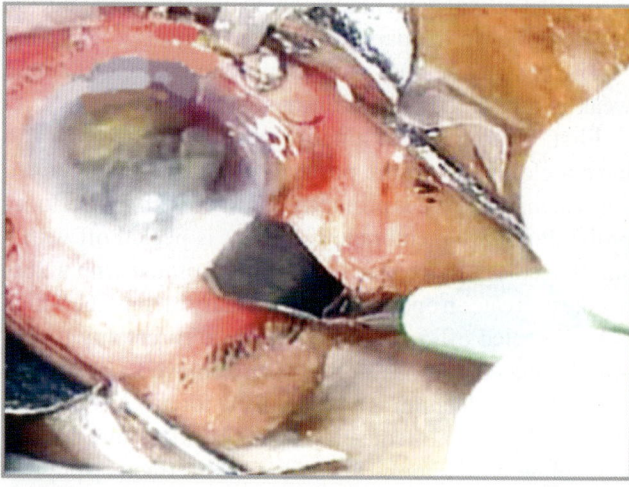

Fig. 25.6: Removal of dislocated lens fragments through anterior approach

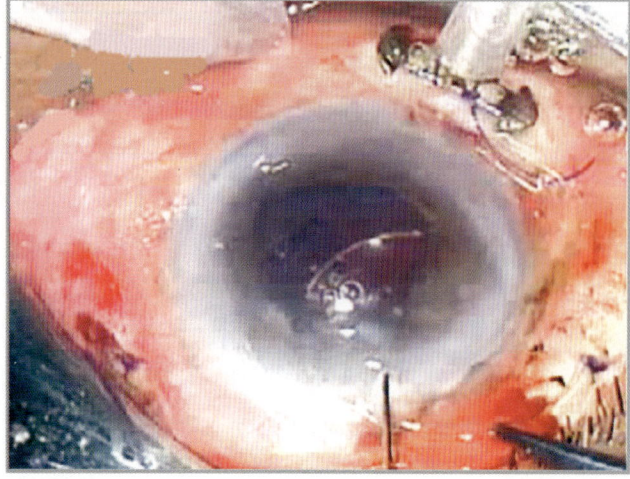

Fig. 25.7: Dropped Nucleus: Implantation of PC IOL implant over frill

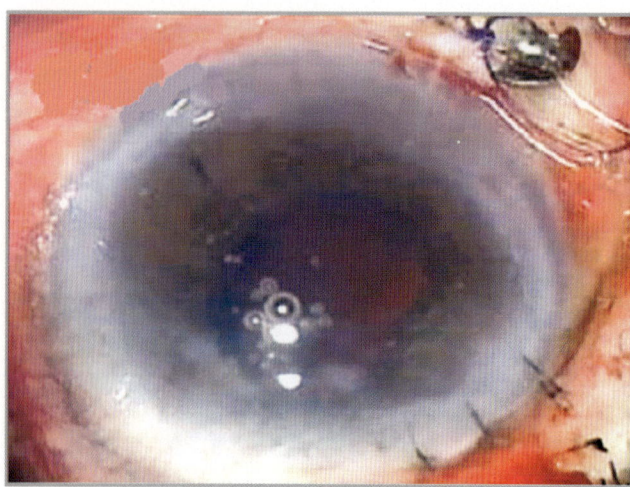

Fig. 25.8: PC IOL is placed over frill

adequate capsular rim is available, a PCIOL is inserted over it in the sulcus. In cases without adequate capsular support, either a sulcus fixed or an ACIOL is implanted. In case a retinal detachment is detected and repaired, the patient is left aphakic and is planned for a secondary IOL implantation.

Sclerotomies are closed and the patient is treated with antibiotics and steroids in the postoperative period.

Newer Modalities

Favit is a new technique of removal of dislocated lens. Here, a vitrectomy probe connected to a peristaltic pump is used. Here all the three modes, i.e. cutter, aspiration and infusion are present in a single port used from the initial corneal incision. Endoilluminator is passed through the side port entry and an adequate vitrectomy is done. Once the lens is free of all vitreous attachments, a phacoprobe is passed via the corneal incision. At settings of 50% power, 50 mmHg suction and 18 ml/min flow rate, lens material is engaged by the probe by means of suction alone. Initially a small burst of phacoenergy is used to embed the probe into the lens, which is then lifted to the iris plane supported by an Endoilluminator. It is finally nibbled by the phacoprobe. In case of a hard nucleus, it is removed via the corneoscleral incision.

The advantage of this procedure is that there is no need for creating separate ports because all the instruments enter through the phacoincisions and the side port incision. Whether the ultrasonic power will damage the retina is a matter of debate and will require long term follow ups and controlled studies to quantify. Certainly visualisation of the posterior segment is compromised in this procedure.

Endoscopic removal of lens fragments is useful in the presence of corneal edema, miosis and media opacities which will impair adequate visualisation.

An endoscopic probe incorporated with a video monitor, fiberoptic light source and a Diode laser are used. Under direct visualisation the lens fragments are emulsified or removed via the limbal route.

Advantages: are better visualisation and localisation of lens fragments, detection of anterior retinal breaks and features of the capsular rim. The major disadvantages of the technique are the absence of stereopsis, a long and steep learning curve and the high cost of the equipment.

Visual Prognosis

Encouraging results after pars plana vitrectomy has given hope to hundreds of budding phaco surgeons all over the world who were otherwise desperate after a long and steep learning curve for mastering the technique. Postoperative visual acuity of 20/40 or better has been achieved in the majority of patients after pars plana vitrectomy. But all the inherent complications of pars plana vitrectomy are also applicable in this setting.

INTRAOCULAR LENS DROP

ACIOL dislocation is extremely uncommon; hence this discussion will be restricted to more commonly encountered dislocation of posterior chamber intraocular lens implants.

A common factor in all PCIOL dislocations is the subnormal posterior capsular support. Because of an increasing trend to implant a PCIOL even in the presence of a posterior capsular rent, there is an increase in the incidence of posterior dislocation of IOL.

The causes of posterior dislocation of IOL are:
- (i) Large posterior capsular rent.
- (ii) Zonular dehiscence esp. in pseudoexfoliation syndrome
- (iii) Small PCIOL implanted over a large PC rent
- (iv) Trauma.

The patient may present with mild decentration of lens or total posterior dislocation of IOL. In decentration, the patient may present with a decreased visual acuity or glare due to the exposed edge of the IOL. A mobile PCIOL generates a unique floater like sensation and may lead to a pupillary block causing raised intraocular tension.

Decentration is a mild malposition with the optic still covering more than half of pupillary area. Decentration may increase with progressive capsular fibrosis and subsequent capsular contraction. A luxated IOL is one that is completely dislocated into the vitreous cavity, these patients are usually present within one week after the surgery. A subluxated IOL remains at least partially attached to anterior segment structures.

Preoperative Workup

- (i) Distant visual acuity with aphakic correction should be assessed in complete dislocation of IOL. Usually it is good in the absence of any posterior segment pathology.
- (ii) Posterior segment evaluation to assess the mobility or fixation points of the IOL is essential.
- (iii) Any underlying retinal pathology like CME, retinal detachment or tears are ruled out.
- (iv) Residual capsular components are assessed. At least 6 clock hours of well defined peripheral capsule, 2/3rd of which is located inferiorly is necessary for reliable support of IOL without sutures.

Management is described under following headings.
- **(a) Observation:** This is usually done in cases with decentred IOL, patients unwilling to go for a second surgery and in presence of an intraocular inflammation.

  In decentred IOL, miotics may sometimes be useful. But patient usually develops cystoid macular oedema.

Even a completely dislocated IOL can be left undisturbed, but according to the author, it is always better to remove the IOL to prevent sight threatening retinal involvement.

(b) IOL removal/ exchange: Exchange is usually done if the IOL is damaged during surgical manipulation. Injury to the lens is more commonly seen in silicone IOL's.

A three port pars plana vitrectomy is done with ports 3 mm from the limbus (aphakic eye). Dislocated IOL is made to float over the PFCL injected beneath it (Figs 24.7 and 24.8). This is more useful in cases of underlying retinal detachment. The IOL can also be lifted using the two hand technique by a lighted pick and an intraocular forceps, by which it is brought to the anterior vitreous and removed by a limbal route. The IOL can be removed and exchanged by a scleral fixed IOL or an ACIOL. A scleral fixed IOL is preferred over an ACIOL.

(c) IOL reposition: It is the most commonly preferred approach. The IOL can be repositioned without sutures on the remnants of anterior or posterior capsule, by iris fixation or scleral suture fixation.

It is best to place the IOL over the capsular support; hence after a pars plana vitrectomy, using an intravitreal forceps, the IOL is lifted up and one haptic is brought anterior to the iris thus capturing the IOL anteriorly. The front haptic is placed into the sulcus with the intravitreal forceps still holding the optic. Then the second haptic is placed into the sulcus. This is useful as most surgeons do a capsulorrhexis so that anterior capsular remnants are present.

Grieshaber Snare method consists of a 20 G tube and a handle with a movable spring loaded finger slide for adjusting the size of a protruding polypropylene loop. The distal portion of the tube with polypropylene loop is inserted through an anterior sclerotomy for engaging a dislocated haptic in the vitreous cavity. Once the looped haptic is pulled up against the anterior sclerotomy, the external portion of the polypropylene loop is cut free and guided by a 30G needle for anchoring by the anterior sclerotomy.

In scleral fixation of IOL, after standard three port pars plana Vitrectomy and mobilisation of IOL, partial thickness limbus based scleral flap are made at 1 O' clock and 7 O' clock. A 5/8th inch 25G needle prethreaded with 9-0 prolene suture is introduced into the eye 1 mm posterior to the limbus in the beds of scleral flap. A loop is made by slightly withdrawing the needle. IOL haptic is guided into the loop using an intraocular forceps and the needle is withdrawn capturing the haptic in the loop and the IOL is fixed with a scleral suture in the partial thickness scleral bed. Similar procedure is done on the other side.

One piece silicone plate IOL presents unique problems. The slippery nature of the surface makes the IOL mobile even long after it is implanted. It can extrude into the vitreous cavity even after a small capsular rent or a Nd: YAG capsulotomy opening. It's retrieval from the vitreous is also difficult. The best method is to hook the IOL with a lighted pick after a pars plana vitrectomy and then engage the elevated edge with forceps. The author feels it is better to explant the silicone IOL than to reposit it. It is also useful if individual developing rhegmatogenous retinal detachment is tackled by silicone oil tamponade.

Uniqueness of Two Intraocular Implants

It is a difficult situation in which the surgeon inserts a second IOL after the first IOL has dislocated in the vitreous cavity. If the dislocated IOL is of inert material it can always be watched, but should be promptly removed if it is causing any complications. The dislocated IOL is considered as an intraocular foreign body and removed by a pars plana vitrectomy by an extended sclerectomy or the already positioned lens can be explanted and the dislocated lens can be removed. The second option remains the best proposition. The author has seen a case in which 3 IOL's were placed inside the eye, with two in the vitreous and one scleral fixed with patients having a good visual acuity without any adverse symptoms. However, this kind of situation is very unusual and rarely provide good or useful outcome in the long run. One should not attempt placing another IOL in the case of an existing dislocated IOL in the posterior segment. We have seen four cases of two intraocular implants in the same eye. Out of these four cases, two cases were found to have dropped acrylic flexible IOL and having sulcus fixated all PMMA IOL implants over frill. Both the cases were found to have retinal detachment with giant tear. Whereas out of the remaining two cases, one case had revealed AC IOL and dropped multi piece PMMA IOL into the posterior segment resulting in total retinal detachment with incarcerated haptics into retina. The remaining case was detected to have AC IOL and dropped PC IOL placed vertically into vitreous cavity with one haptic lodged into ciliary body. This case continues to have chronic uveitis.

CONCLUSION

Vitreoretinal surgery, though a highly advanced surgical procedure, has provided relief to phaco surgeons all over the world and is readily available now. Though it has helped to regain vision in many complicated cases of dislocated lens or IOL, yet it is not without its own inherent complications. Hence, the dictum—prevention is better than cure—is highly applicable in such a scenario. This can be achieved by a careful and detailed preoperative evaluation of cases and then tailoring the surgical technique to suit the individual eye.

26

Post Phacoemulsification Endophthalmitis: Prevention and Management

Dr S Natarajan DO and Dr Arif Adenwala MS, DNB, FRCS, ICO (UK)

DEFINITION

Postoperative endophthalmitis (POE) is defined as severe inflammation involving both the anterior and posterior segments of the eye after intraocular surgery.

Typically, postoperative endophthalmitis is caused by preoperative induction of microbial organisms into the eye either from the patient's normal conjunctiva and skin flora, from air or from contaminated instruments. It is a catastrophic complication of intraocular surgery.

INCIDENCE

The incidence of POE has been reducing recently due to extreme vigilance during sterilisation and improved surgical skills. After cataract surgery, the incidence is between 0.07–0.12%, where as, after secondary IOL implant, the incidence is 0.4%.

CLASSIFICATION

Postsurgical endophthalmitis can be classified as under:

(a) Clinical Classification

  (i) Fulminant (< 4 days): Gram negative bacteria like Pseudomonas, etc.
     Streptococci
     Staphylococcus aureus

  (ii) Acute (5–7, days):
     Staphylococcus epidermides
     Coagulase negative cocci

 (iii) Chronic (> 4 weeks):
    (a) Delayed entry (bleb related).
    (b) Delayed Onset—Propionibacterium acnes
      — Fungi
      — *Staphylococcus epidermides*

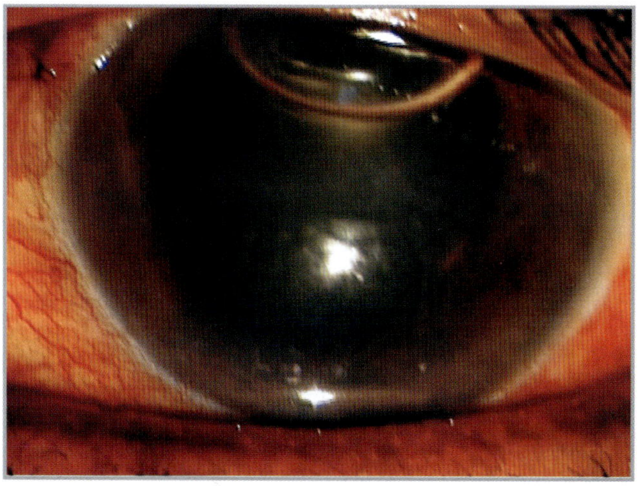

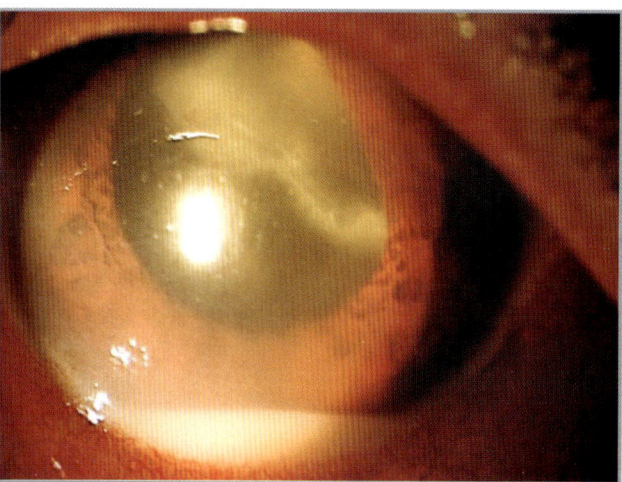

Fig. 26.1: Acute postoperative endophthalmitis with minimal hypopyon

Fig. 26.2: Acute postoperative endophthalmitis with severe hypopyon

(b) According to the Mode of Entry

Exogenous	Endogenous
Microorganism introduced direct from environment Commonly seen after surgery (phaco) or trauma. i.e. structural defect in layers of eye Commonly bacterial	Hematogenous spread from organisms No structural defect of eyes is seen
	Common predisposing factor are seen like immune compromised, IV drug abuse, septicaaemia, mainly fungal

(Ref Indian J Med Micro 1999; 17(3) 108–115)

(c) According to Etiological Agents

  (i) Bacterial
 (ii) Fungal
(iii) Viral

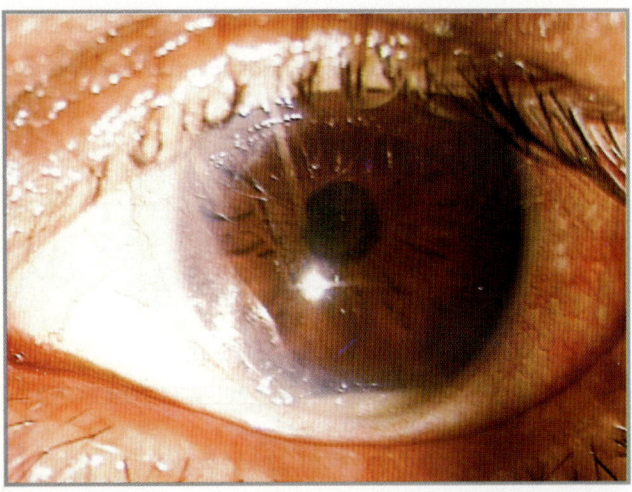

Fig. 26.3: Acute postoperative endophthalmitis

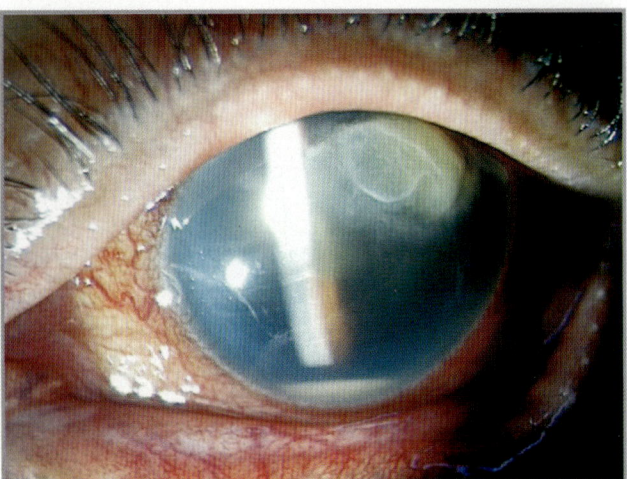

Fig. 26.4: Delayed severe postoperative endophthalmitis (Fungal) in a diabetic patient with corneal involvement

RISK FACTORS

The ocular surface and the adnexa are the primary source of bacteria in culture positive cases of endophthalmitis. The possible risk factors can be divided into:

  (a) Preoperative: Blepharitis, conjunctivitis, dacryo-cystitis, immunosuppression, diabetes mellitus, etc. We have to rule out these infections before surgery.
  (b) Intraoperative: Prolonged surgical time, vitreous loss, inadequate draping of the lids and lashes away from the surgical site has also been mentioned as possible risk factors for the infection.
  (c) Postoperative: Wound leak or dehiscence, inadequately buried sutures, sutural removal, vitreous incarceration in the wound or the presence of filtering bleb.

PROPHYLAXIS

The ocular surface and adnexa are the primary source of bacteria in case of POE.

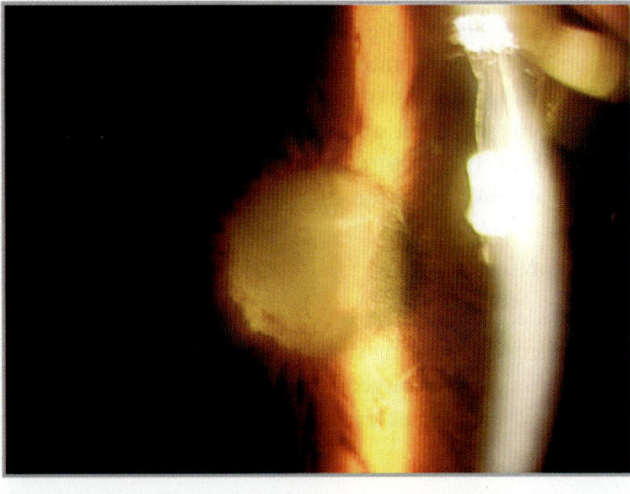

(a)

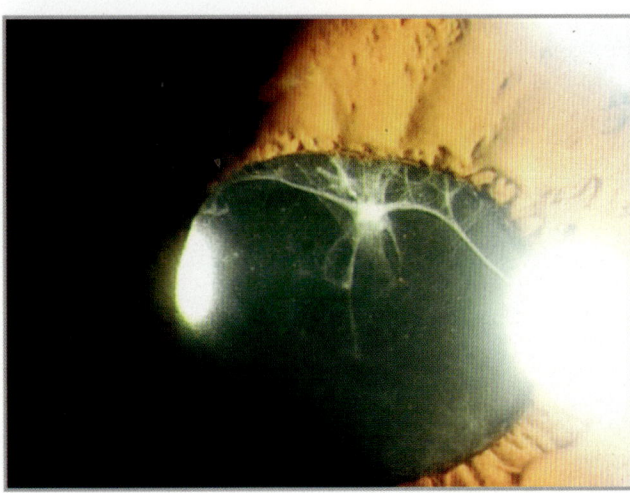

(b)

Fig. 26.5: Delayed postoperative endophthalmitis (Fungal)

(a) Use of Povidone: Iodine solution: It is an excellent antiseptic in use. It is available in two forms: Skin 10% solution and Conjunctiva (5%). Nowadays, eye drops are available. It is instilled prior to the surgery. It is effective against bacteria, fungi, viruses, protozoa and spores. The solution has to be washed from the conjunctival surface to avoid endothelial toxicity.

(b) Use of antibiotics: Antibiotics can be used pre-operatively or intraoperatively as a prophylactic agent.

(i) Topical: The use of prophylactic preoperative topical antibiotics in all patients has been recommended by some doctors. If used it should be bactericidal and effective against both gram positive and gram negative organism. Treatment should start about 2–3 days prior to the surgery.

(ii) Topical fluoroquinolones are the commonly used prophylactic agents because of their broad spectrum of activity covering the majority of these pathogens found in endophthalmitis.
Commonly used drugs are ciprofloxacin, ofloxacin and gatifloxacin.

(iii) Infusion fluid: Antibiotic injections can be infused in the irrigating fluid which is used during phacoemulsification. But powerful agents like vancomycin should not be used due to emergence of vancomycin resistant stains of staphylococci.

Preoperative contamination of the anterior chamber as a common source of infection has also been reported. In these cases, prompt anterior chamber irrigation with anterior chamber drug injection is one of the effective treatment.

The decision regarding use of antibiotics is left to the operating surgeon due to its side effects like macular infarction and endothelial toxicity.

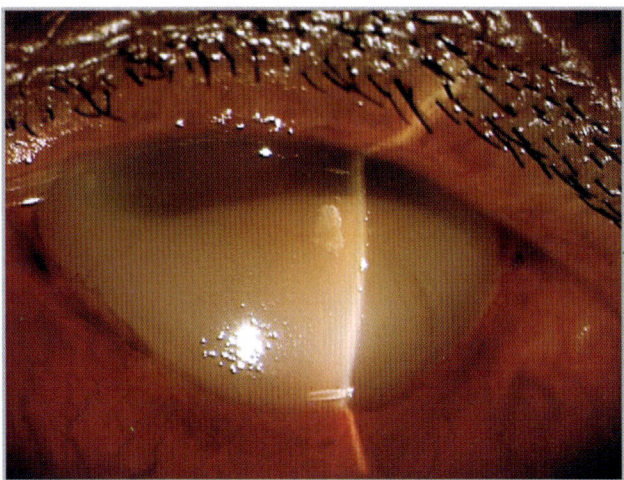

Fig. 26.6: Severe endophthalmitis

CLINICAL FEATURES

Within a few hours to six weeks of intraocular surgery, patients usually present with the following complaints except in chronic cases where it takes longer time.

Common signs and symptoms in endophthalmitis are:
(i) Pain
(ii) Decreased visual acuity
(iii) Red eye
(iv) Hazy cornea
(v) Disproportionate anterior chamber reaction
(vi) Pupillary membrane
(vii) Hypopyon
(viii) Poor or absent fungal glow
(ix) Relative afferent papillary defect (RAPD)

If these signs cannot be explained or if there is any doubt, the eyes should be treated as if they were infected.

Clarity of the media can be graded by using indirect ophthalmoscope depending on the visibility of retinal details as:

Grade I – more than 6/12 (20/40) view of retina
Grade II – second order retinal vessels visible
Grade III – some vessels visible but not second order
Grade IV – no retinal vessels visible
Grade V – no red reflex seen.

PATHOPHYSIOLOGY

The Endophthalmitis Vitrectomy Study (EVS) showed that most isolates causing clinical endophthalmitis were introduced into the eyes from the patient's conjunctival flora.

(a) **Important risk factors** for the development of postoperative endophthalmitis are:
(i) Increased operative time
(ii) Posterior capsule rupture/vitreous loss
(iii) Retained lens fragments
(iv) Inadequate sterilisation of the operative field or poor OT hygiene
(v) Contamination of the surgical instruments, irrigating solutions, IOL's or contamination of tap water.

(b) Once the clinical infection occurs, damage to ocular tissues occurs due to direct effect of bacterial replication and due to inflammatory mediators.

(c) Endotoxin and other bacterial products cause direct cellular injury while eliciting cytokines that attract neutrophils, which enhance the inflammation.

MANAGEMENT

Microbiological diagnosis plays an important role in the confirmation of diagnosis of POE.

(i) Micro-organism commonly responsible for acute endophthalmitis are:

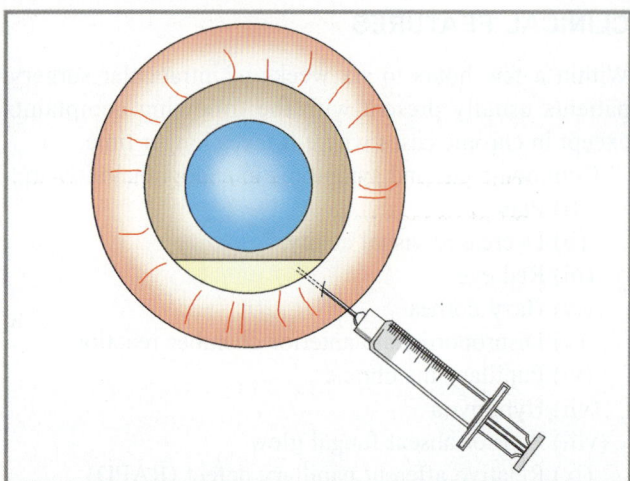

Fig. 26.7: Paracentesis for aqueous tap. (*Courtesy:* Vitreoretinal Surgical Techniques, First Pub: 2001: Dr. Gholam A Peyman and Dr. Mandi D. Conway)

 (a) Gram positive organisms, most common being coagulase negative staphylococcus 70%, *Staph. aureus* in 9.9% cases, streptococci species in 9% cases.

 (b) Gram negative organisms were involved in 6% of cases,

 (c) Fungi, e.g. Candida, *Aspergillus fusarium,* etc.

(ii) In cases of other surgery like trabeculectomy the common species is coagulase negative staphylococcus.

(iii) In chronic cases of POE, commonest causative organism is propionobacterium acne, a slow growing gram positive bacillus that is associated with characteristic white intracapsular plaque that develops weeks or months after cataract surgery. Coagulase negative staphylococcus, fungal species have also been reported to cause chronic POE. Most common fungal species includes Candida, Aspergillus, Cephalosporium and Fusarium.

Confirmation of the diagnosis: Diagnosis is confirmed by culture of the organism and the samples are taken from aqueous cavity and vitreous cavity. In recent past, the samples from conjunctival sac and lid margin were taken for culture. This is no longer useful because of poor yield and culture of unrelated organism. The possibility of isolating an organism from vitreous is 50–70% and from aqueous 30–40%, respectively.

(iv) **Aqueous Tap:** It is obtained by paracentesis using 27 or 30 gauge needle mounted on a tuberculin syringe. Topical anaesthetic agent is instilled and about 0.1 ml of aqueous fluid is aspirated in a controlled manner by gently withdrawing the plunger. The sample is sent for culture sensitivity, gram staining and KOH preparation.

(v) **Vitreous tap:** Vitreous approach is done through pars plana approach – 3.5 mm behind the limbus. A 23 guage needle attached to 2 cc syringe is injected; the direction of needle should be towards the centre of the eyeball. The vitreous sample is obtained just before injecting the intravitreal antibiotics. This provides a undiluted specimen and creates space for intravitreal drug to be injected. About 0.1–0.2 cc of the vitreous sample is aspirated.

(vi) **Vitreous biopsy:** Is another technique of taking vitreous sample. The main advantage that it provides adequate volume of sample to be obtained.

Ideal recommended handling of sample obtained:

 (a) Place one drop of sample on two separate slides for Gram and KOH stain. Smear is allowed to dry for gram stains. 1drop of KOH is put over the slide and then it is covered with a cover slip and sent for examination.

 (b) Place one drop of fluid on blood agar plate with careful stream of sample and incubating at 37ºC.

 (c) Place one drop of fluid on chocolate agar and incubate at 37ºC in 4–10% CO_2 enriched environment.

 (d) Inoculate one drop into Sabourauds medium without any inhibitors and maintain that at room temperature.

 (e) Inoculate one drop onto Thioglycolate broth and inoculate at 37ºC for anaerobic and microphilic organisms.

(vii) **A/B Scan Ultrasonography:** In patients with suspected endophthalmitis and cases where retinal pathology is not visible Ultrasonography is indicated.

It helps in the confirmation of the diagnosis although it is not done in all cases of POE.

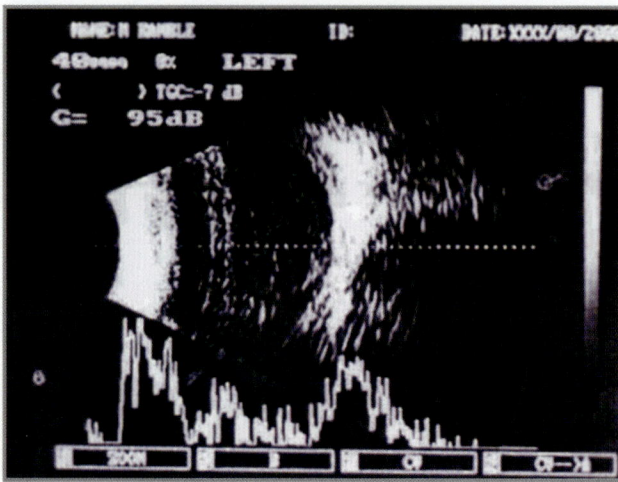

Fig. 26.8: A-B scan showing multiple exudates in the vitreous

TREATMENT

Treatment is started on the suspicion of diagnosis and if required modified after confirmation and culture sensitivity. The patient is explained about the diagnosis, the therapeutic intervention that may be required and also visual prognosis in some cases. Everything should be explained to the patient.

Objectives in Endophthalmitis Treatment

  (i) Primary objectives:
- Control/eradicate the infection
- Manage complications
- Restoration of vision.

 (ii) Secondary objectives:
- Symptomatic relief
- Prevent panophthalmitis
- Maintain globe integrity to prevent cosmetic disfigurement.

The mainstay of treatment of POE is antibiotics that can be used in many forms like intravitreal, topical subconjunctival or rarely systemically.

Acute Postoperative Endophthalmitis

Intraocular Antibiotics

(a) **Intravitreal injection:** It is at present the mainstay of treatment for postcataract surgery endophthalmitis.

Recommended drugs used intravitreally for treatment of acute POE after cataract surgeries are:
- **Vancomycin:** It is a macrolide antibiotic, which is highly effective against most gram positive organism.
  Dose: Intravitreal = 1000 μg/0.1 ml
  Subconjunctival = 25 mg.
  Topical = 50 mg/ml.
- **Ceftazidime:** It is a third generation cephalosporin with broad spectrum gram negative activity. It is very effective against resistant organism.
  Dose: Intravitreal = 2.25 mg/0.1 ml.
  Renal toxicity is not seen at this dosage
  Subconjunctival = 100 mg
  Topical = 50 mg/ml.
- **Amikacin:** It belongs to the aminoglycoside group of antibiotics. It is effective against gram negative organisms.
  It has fewer side effects like scleral toxicity, compared to the other agents of this group like gentamycin.
  Dose: Intravitreal = 400 μg/0.1ml
  Usually a combination of vancomycin and Ceftazidime is preferred as it covers both gram positive and gram negative organisms (EVS Study).

- Preparation of an antibiotic solution for intravitreal injection:
- **Vancomycin:** (vial of 500 mg in powder form).
  Step I: Inject 10 ml of saline in a vial of 500 mg of vancomycin.
  This gives a solution of 500 mg/10 ml = 50 mg/ml of vancomycin
  Step II: Remove 0.2 ml of this solution to a syringe.
  Step III: Take 0.8 ml of saline to this syringe to make it 1 ml
  This will contain 10 mg of vancomycin.
  Step IV: Take 0.1 ml from this which is equivalent to 1 mg or 1000 μg of vancomycin.
- **Ceftazidime:** (vial of 500 mg/1000 mg – powder form).
  Step I   : Inject 2cc of saline in a vial of 500 mg of Ceftazidime.
             This gives a solution of 500 mg/2 ml or 250 mg/ml.
  Step II : Remove 0.1ml of this solution in syringe.
  Step III : Take 0.9 ml of sterile saline or water in the syringe to make it 1 ml.
             This syringe will contain 25 mg/1 ml.
  Step IV : Take 0.1 ml of solution from the syringe which is equivalent to 2.5 mg (2.25 mg of active ingredient) and is used for intravitreal injection.
- **Amikacin:** (vial solution 500 mg/2 ml)
  Step I   : Take 0.1 ml of Amikacin solution from the vial.
             This will contain 25 mg of Amikacin.
  Step II : Add 6.15 ml of sterile water to the syringe, i.e. 25 mg in 6.25 ml of water.
  Step III : Take 0.1 ml of this solution for intravitreal injection.
  It will contain 0.4 mg or 400 μg of Amikacin solution.
  Nowadays, this dosage is not recommended as it is very toxic to the macula.
- **Procedure: Anaesthesia**: Usually performed under topical anaesthesia. Facial block can be given in some cases. Peribulbar anaesthesia is usually avoided. No digital massage is given, acetazolamide tablets can be given to decrease intraocular pressure.

(b) **Periocular region**: Painted with povidine iodine solution. Eye drape is then put In order to obtain good stability of globe, a cotton tipped applicator is placed at the opposite quadrant.

The 26–30 gauge needle attached to tuberculin syringe containing the drug is inserted through the pars plana approach. Site of puncture is about

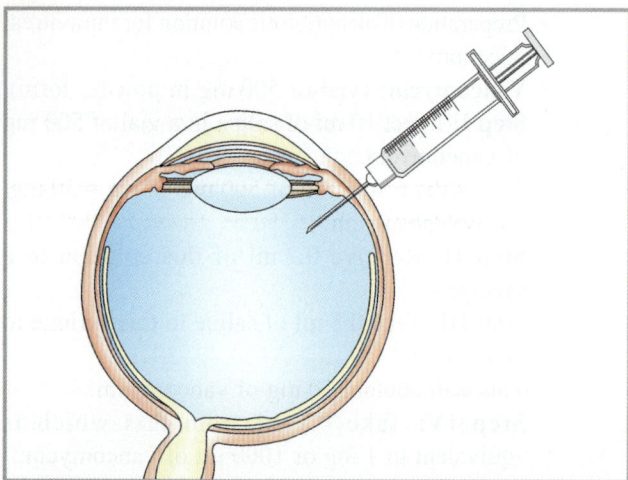

Fig. 26.9: Diagrammatic picture showing proper technique of giving intravitreal injection (*Courtesy:* Vitreoretinal Surgical Techniques, First Pub: 2001: Dr. Gholam A Peyman and Dr. Mandi D. Conway)

3.5 to 4 mm behind the limbus. The tip of the needle should be directed towards the centre of the globe.

(c) **Topical and Subconjunctival antibiotics:** For topical medication, usually fortified preparations are used. A combination of two antibiotics is used; one with predominant effect on gram positive organisms and the other on gram negative organism. Preparation of the commonly used fortified eye drops are:

- Tobramycin (15 mg/ml): Add 2 ml of parentral tobramycin containing 80 mg of the drug to 5 ml vial of tobramycin eye drops. (0.3%)
- Gentamycin (15 mg/ml): Add 2 ml of parentral gentamycin containing 80 mg of the drug to 5 ml vial of gentamycin eye drops. (0.3%)
- Cefuroxime (15 mg/ml): An injection vial of 1000 mg cefuroxime is first diluted with 2.5 ml of sterile water. This is then added to 12.5 ml of artificial tears. This is stable at room temperature for 24 hrs and in a refrigerator for 96 hours.

Subconjunctival injections: Subconjunctival injections are not routinely used by us in our practice. Commonly used drugs with their dosages are given below:

— Vancomycin: 25 mg/0.5 ml
— Ceftazidime: 100 mg/0.5 ml
— Gentamycin: 20 mg/0.5 ml

(d) **Systemic antibiotics:** Systemic antibiotics have no role to play in the treatment of postoperative endophthalmitis. This was proved by the endophthalmitis vitrectomy study (EVS).

Anti-inflammatory Agents

Role of Corticosteroids: One of the major causes of damage in POE is due to release of inflammatory mediators.

These agents have chemotactic properties that attract polymorph nuclear leucocytes and macrophages into the vitreous cavity. They also release enzymes, which are harmful to the intraocular tissues.

Corticosteroids: Corticosteroids are the most potent anti-inflammatory agents. They can be used in any forms like oral, intravitreal, topical or subconjunctival provided there are no contraindications for its use.

The uses of intravitreal steroids are controversial. The decision is left to the discretion of the ophthalmologist.

The recommended dosages are given below:

- Intravitreal dexamethasone: 400 mg in 0.1 ml
- Systemic: Prednisolone: 1mg/kg/day orally.
- Subconjunctival Dexamethasone: 1mg/0.5ml

Surgical

Vitrectomy

Vitrectomy for endophthalmitis may be necessary at two stages. Primary during acute infection (according to guidelines of EVS) and secondary in reserved phase for removal of the organised vitreous membranes.

According to EVS, Vitrectomy should be done when visual acuity is reduced to perception of light. But nowadays it is left to clinical experience and the surgical skill of operating surgeon to decide about surgical interventions.

(a) **The advantages of vitrectomy:** The advantages of Vitrectomy are that it helps in removing the infecting organism and associated toxins, removes vitreous membranes that could lead to retinal detachment and also helps in improved intraocular distribution of antibiotics.

(b) **Surgical steps:** Usually the 3-port pars plana vitrectomy (PPV) is preferred using a long infusion cannula.

- Important principles which should be remembered in case of postoperative endophthalmitis (POE) are:

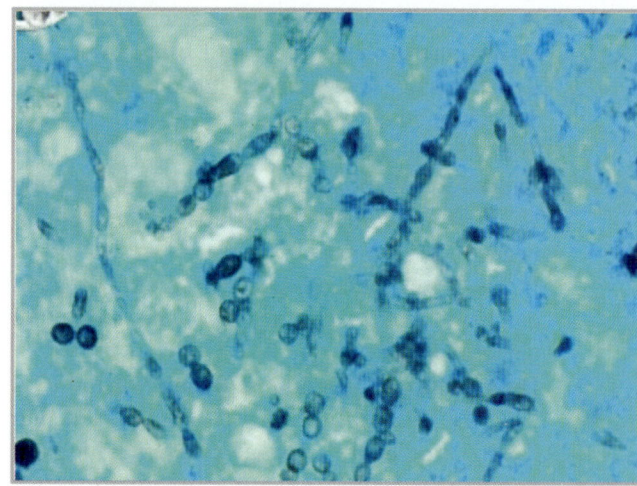

Fig. 26.10: Slide showing *Candida albicans*

- To use maximum cutting rate with less suction rate and not to attempt PVD or a complete Vitrectomy.
- Retina is very friable and so the chances of retinal detachment are very high. PPV plus intravitreal antibiotic injection is more effective in sterilising the eye than the vitreous tap and intravitreal injection.

- **Endophthalmitis Vitrectomy Study (EVS):** EVS was a multicentric study undertaken in the USA involving 120 patients who had developed bacterial endophthalmitis within 6 weeks of cataract surgery or secondary IOL implantation. The main aim of the study was to evaluate the role of early PPV versus intraocular antibiotic injection (TAP) and systemic antibiotics as treatment of POE. Patients included had visual acuity between 20/50 and light perception and a view good enough to perform vitrectomy.

The patients were randomly divided into 4 groups:
  (i) PPV with systemic antibiotics,
  (ii) PPV without systemic antibiotics,
  (iii) TAP with systemic antibiotics and
  (iv) TAP without systemic antibiotics.

The results demonstrate no difference in final visual outcome in patients who underwent initial TAP or Vitrectomy if the visual acuity was better than light perception. But in patients presenting with only light perception vision and who underwent initial vitrectomy had a nearly 50% reduction in risk of severe visual loss compared to patients who underwent TAP. No long-term difference occurred in media clarity between treatment groups. Intravenous Antibiotics has no effect on either treatment outcome.

(c) **Chronic postoperative endophthalmitis:** The treatment of the chronic variety depends on the causative agent. The commonest ones are given below:

- **Fungal endophthalmitis:** Fungal infection usually exhibits a white "string of pearls" infiltrate in the anterior chambers and vitreous. Hypopyon is usually fixed. Vitreous shows snowball and fluffy opacities.

  (i) **Common fungi involved are:** Candida, Aspergillus, and Cephalosporium species.

  (ii) **Management:** The main objective of treatment on fungal endophthalmitis is same as that in bacterial endophthalmitis.

  (a) **Antifungal agents required included:**
  - **Amphotericin B:** It is a usually very effective antifungal agent. Amphotericin B is both fungistatic and fungicidal depending on the concentration of the drug inside the tissues.

Dose: Sow IV infusion: 0.7 mg/kg in 500 ml of 5% dextrose

Treatment should be continued until the inflammation or any chorioretinal lesion shows complete resolution.

- **Adverse effects:** Anaphylaxes, convulsion, phlebitis, chills, fever, anaemia, thrombocytopenia. They are normally seen after intravenous use.

  Intravitreal – commonest mode which is used.

- **Intravitreal injection:**
  Dose: 5–10 μg/0.1 ml

- **Azoles derivatives:** The drugs included in this group have good systemic absorption and better penetration with fewer side effects.

Common oral agents used are:
- **Fluconazole** 200 mg twice daily
- **Ketoconazole** 400–600 mg daily.

  Oral fluconazole is very effective in endogenous fungal endophthalmitis.

  Intravitreal dose: Fluconazole 25 mg / 0.1 ml

- **Flucytosine:** This drug is not used routinely. It is used in a combination with amphotericin B when intraocular inflammation is quite severe and is resistant to routine treatment.

  Dose: Orally 5–100 mg/kg/day in four divided doses.

(b) **Vitrectomy:** In case of fungal endophthalmitis, early vitrectomy with intravitreal injection is recommended.

- Propionobacterium acnes endophthalmitis (PAE): *P. acnes* is an anaerobic gram positive bacillus which is normal commensal of conjunctival sac.

P. acnes stimulates the immune system but is resistant to killing by the polymorph and monocytes. It stimulates immune response against the soft lens matter remaining after cataract surgery.

The incidence of *P. acne* endophthalmitis after phaco surgery is quite less than conventional extracapsular cataract extraction.

PAE is characterised by white intercapsular plaques that develop weeks to months after cataract surgery.

Important technique of diagnosis of *P. acne* is by polymerase chain reaction (PCR) directed at 16S rDNA.[12]

Treatment: After the confirmation of diagnosis, all areas of the involved lens capsule and the retained lens cortex are excised. This is done with good pars plana vitrectomy.

If capsular fibrosis is very high, intraocular lens has to be removed as well. It is performed mainly when patients do not respond to the conservative approach.

- Antibiotic of choice in these cases is vancomycin. Intravitreal dosage is 1 mg/0.1 ml or 1000 µg/0.1 ml Vancomycin is very effective against *P.acnes*.

STERILISATION

It is a process used to achieve complete sterility, i.e. absence of the entire viable microorganism. The complete description won't be covered in the chapter and only important precautions related to the phacomachine are described.

In order to prevent postphacoemulsification endophthalmitis extreme importance should be given to the sterilisation of phacomachines.

We take good care of operating theatres including all the instruments in test of sterility. But the phacomachine as a source of infection had been neglected till recently.

The part that should be given importance is phaco tubing. When the tubing enters the phacomachines and exits into the drainage bag, it goes through a channel inside the phacomachine. The parts of tubing are not properly sterilised before the cataract surgery. This part of tubing is attached to two manometres that gauge the pressure in the tubing. A vent can release the pressure in the tubing to atmospheric levels as soon as the other foot switch goes from position 3 to 2 to 1. When we do this, air from the operating room goes into the tubing. In case if air contains bacteria, it goes directly inside the eye.

Pseudomonas is the commonest organism which is isolated.

PREVENTION

- This can be prevented either by changing the internal tubing after every case which cannot be done as it is not practical.

- To keep the air totally sterile and make sure no infection goes into tubing through the vent. This can be achieved with the ozone generator for the total operation room area.
- The next important thing which should be done is proper cleaning of the phacomachine and air filters placed on the vent.
- The tubings have to be changed every week. Culture sensitivity test has to be done preferably before and after every case. Samples should be collected from ringer lactate solution and from the aspiration tube both before and after the operation.
- The ringer lactate solution should also be taken from the front end of the internal tubing. This tedious measure has to be undertaken in order to reduce the incidence of postoperative endophthalmitis after phacoemulsification.

CONCLUSION AND PERSPECTIVES

A more detailed understanding of the interactions between offending organism and the intraocular host response is needed to treat postoperative endophthalmitis and improve visual outcome.

As more information becomes available with respect to the natural course of different varieties of endophthalmitis, several steps in the evolution of infection may emerge on new therapeutic opportunities.

Therapeutic targets of the bacteria may include global regulation of virulence factor, including specific retinal focus, blocking bacterial motility or blocking bacterial tissue attachment and colonisation

Further research in the field of treatment will help in prevention and reduction in the incidence of postoperative endophthalmitis.

REFERENCES AND BIBLIOGRAPHY

1. Brandon L. Davis, MD · Laura Kearsley MD · Nick Mamalis, MD Postoperative Endophthalmitis vs. Toxic Anterior Segment Syndrome (TASS).
2. Busbee, Brandon G Advances in knowledge and treatment: an update on endophthalmitis. Current Opinion in Ophthalmology 2004; 15(3):232–237, June, 2004.
3. Clark WL, Kaiser PK, Flynn HW Jr, et al: Treatment strategies and visual acuity outcomes in chronic postoperative Propionibacterium acnes endophthalmitis. Ophthalmology 1999 Sep; 106(9): 1665–70.
4. Colleaux KM, Hamilton WK. Effect of prophylactic antibiotics and incision type on the incidence of endophthalmitis after cataract surgery. Can J Ophthalmol 2000; 35:373–378.
5. Das T, Sharma S; Hyderabad Endophthalmitis Research Group. Current management strategies of acute postoperative endophthalmitis Semin Ophthalmol 2003 Sep; 18(3):109–
15. LV Prasad Eye Institute, LV Prasad Marg, Banjara Hills, Hyderabad, India.
6. Deramo, Vincent A. MD; Ting, T. Daniel MD, PhD Treatment of Propionibacterium acnes endophthalmitis. Current Opinion in Ophthalmology 2001; 12(3):225–229, June.
7. Driebe WT, Mandelbaum S, Forster RK, et al. Pseudophakic endophthalmitis. Ophthalmology 1986; 93:442–448.
8. Endophthalmitis Vitrectomy Study Group: Results of the Endophthalmitis Vitrectomy Study. A randomised trial of immediate vitrectomy and of intravenous antibiotics for the treatment of postoperative bacterial endophthalmitis.
9. Endophthalmitis Vitrectomy Study Group. Arch Ophthalmol 1995 Dec; 113(12): 1479–96.
10. Endophthalmitis Vitrectomy Study Group: Microbiologic factors and visual outcome in the endophthalmitis vitrectomy study. Am J Ophthalmol 1996 Dec; 122(6): 830–46.

11. Endophthalmitis Vitrectomy Study Group: Results of the Endophthalmitis Vitrectomy Study. A randomised trial of immediate vitrectomy and of intravenous antibiotics for the treatment of postoperative bacterial endophthalmitis.

12. Hykin PG, Tobal K, McIntyre G, Matheson MM, Towler HM, Lightman SL. The diagnosis of delayed postoperative endophthalmitis by polymerase chain reaction of bacterial DNA in vitreous samples J Med Microbial. 1994; 40(6):408–15.

13. Johnson MW, Doft BH, Kelsey SF, et al: The Endophthalmitis Vitrectomy Study. Relationship between clinical presentation and microbiologic spectrum. Ophthalmology 1997; 104(2): 261–72.

14. John T, Sims M, Hoffmann C. Intraocular bacterial contamination during sutureless, small incision, single-port phacoemulsification. Department of Ophthalmology, Loyola University Medical Centre, Maywood, Illinois, USA.

15. Jaffe NS: Cataract Surgery and its Complications. St Louis, CV Mosby.

16. Lalit Verma, Pradeeep Venkatesh, H.K.Tiwari. Management of Endophthalmitis, CME Series No.4 AIOS India.

17. Leong JK, Shah R, McCluskey PJ, Benn RA, Taylor RF. Bacterial contamination of the anterior chamber during phacoemulsification cataract surgery. Department of Ophthalmology, Royal Prince Alfred Hospital, Sydney, Australia.

18. Montan PG, Koranyi G, Setterquist HE, et al. Endophthalmitis after cataract surgery: risk factors relating to technique and events of the operation and patient history. Ophthalmology. 1998; 105:1271–1277.

19. Mandelbaum S, Meisler DM: Postoperative chronic microbial endophthalmitis. Int Ophthalmol Clin 1993 Winter; 33(1): 71–9.

20. Michael Kresloff MD; Alessandra A Castellarin, MD and Marco A. Zarbin, MD. Endophthalmitis. Department of Ophthalmology New Jersey Medical School, Newark, New Jersey, USA.

21. Michelle C. Callegan, Michael Engelbert David W. Parke II, Bradley D. Jettand Michael S. Gilmore. Clinical Microbiology Reviews, January 2002, p. 111–124, Vol. 15, No. 1 Bacterial Endophthalmitis: Epidemiology, Therapeutics, and Bacterium-Host Interactions

22. Montan, Per MD, PhD. Endophthalmitis. Current Opinion in Ophthalmology. 2001; 12(1):75–81.

23. Mamalis, Nick MD; Kearsley, Laura MD; Brinton, Eric BA. Postoperative endophthalmitis. Current Opinion in Ophthalmology. 2002; 13(1):14–18, February.

24. Masket S. Preventing, diagnosing, and treating endophthalmitis (Guest editorial). J Cataract Refract Surg. 1998; 24:725–726.

25. Meinkoff JA, Speaker MG, Marmor M, et al. A case-control study of risk factors for postoperative endophthalmitis. Ophthalmology. 1991; 98:1761–1768.

26. Sunita Agarwal, Amar Agarwal, Ashok Garg: Sterilisation. Clinical Practice in Small Incision Cataract Surgery (Phaco Manual).

27. Sternberg P, Martin D. Management of endophthalmitis in the post-endophthalmitis vitrectomy study era. Arch Ophthalmol. 2001; 119:254–255.

28. Shah G, Stein J, Sharma S, et al. Visual outcomes following the use of intravitreal steroids in the treatment of postoperative endophthalmitis. Ophthalmology. 2000; 107:486–489

29. Soriano, Eduardo S.; Nishi, Mauro Endophthalmitis: incidence and prevention. Current Opinion in Ophthalmology. 2005; 16(1):65–70, February.

30. Schmitz S, Dick HB, Krummenauer, et al. Endophthalmitis in cataract surgery: results of a German survey. Ophthalmology. 1999; 106:1869–1877.

31. Weber DJ, Hoffman KL, Thoft RA, Baker AS. Endophthalmitis following intraocular lens implantation: Report of 30 cases. Rev of Infect Dis 1986; 8:12–20.

32. Yan Ke Xue Bao. Management of infectious endophthalmitis following phacoemulsification] Zhongshan Ophthalmic Centre, Sun Yat-sen University of Medical Sciences, Guangzhou 510060, China.1999 Jun; 15(2):124–6.

33. Jay S. Duker, MD and Carmen A Puliafito MD: Management of Acute Postoperative endophthalmitis.

27

Posterior Capsule Opacification: Prevention and Management

Dr VK Saini and Col JKS Parihar SM, VSM

INTRODUCTION

The field of cataract surgery has been the focal point of exciting mutations during the past two decades and the resurgence of extracapsular cataract surgery as the most effective and least traumatic way of treating cataracts is one major phase in this process.

The most common complication secondary to ECCE is after cataract. Amongst the various types, posterior capsular opacification is the most common. This has a detrimental effect on vision, necessitating secondary capsulotomy for visual rehabilitation.

Surgical capsulotomy has decreased in popularity during the past several years because of the higher incidence of vitreous disturbance, CME, RD and technical difficulties. With the advent of Nd: YAG laser, the necessity for surgical capsulotomy has been obviated.

Duke Elder in 1976 defined "after cataract", also known as "secondary cataract" as the term applied to the opacified remnants of the lens, left behind after extra capsular cataract extraction, discission or spontaneous reabsorption of lens matter following trauma.

MORPHOLOGICAL FORMS OF PCO

Fibrosis

(a) **Early:** Presents in the first few days to weeks postoperative. It is due to leftover cortical lamellae during surgery.

(b) **Late:** Residual lens epithelial cells still attached to the anterior capsule differentiate into fibroblast-like cells. These cells proliferate and migrate to the posterior capsule. They secrete extracellular matrix component—collagen, usually type I, III and IV fibrillar collagen which leads to opacification. Further contraction of collagen fibers results in the formation of numerous folds and wrinkles on the posterior capsule. This can cause decentration of the IOL apart from visual distortion. This occurs months to years postoperatively.

(c) **Membrane formation:** A new mode of cellular proliferation has been observed leading to membrane formation. In cases where the cut edge of the anterior capsule rests on the IOL optic, residual anterior capsular cells may proliferate and extend from this cut edge onto the surface of IOL resulting in the formation of a membranous outgrowth. This appears approximately 1 week postoperatively. It could also form from the left over lens matter.

Elsching's Pearl Type

Clinically, cases of pearl formation occurs somewhat later than fibrosis (upto 5 years postoperatively). Pearls formed in this type of PCO are identical to Wedl cells (Bladder cells) involved in the formation of posterior subcapsular cataracts.

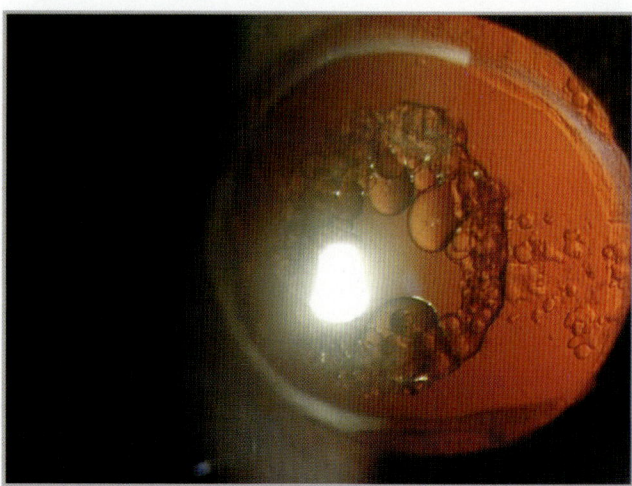

Fig. 27.1: Elsching's pearl type PCO

These cells originate from equatorial epithelial cells. It consists of swollen, bloated epithelial cells which give the appearance of a pearl or soap bubble.

Soemmering's Ring

The remains of the anterior capsule (cut edge) may adhere to the posterior capsule within 4 weeks postoperatively and the equatorial epithelial cells proliferate and continue forming new lens fibers which remain trapped between the anterior and posterior capsules which results in the formation of a ring. Vision is usually not affected as it is located in the periphery behind the iris.

PREVENTION

Many factors have to be considered to decrease the incidence of PCO of which immaculate surgery and proper choice of IOL design are the prime factors.

The following guidelines would help to decrease the incidence of PCO.
(a) Surgical technique
(b) IOL design
(c) Pharmacological and immunological inhibitors.

Surgical Technique

(i) **Atraumatic surgery:** This is the first priority at all stages. By minimising intraoperative and postoperative breakdown of blood aqueous barrier and inflammation some of the stimuli for cellular responses and PCO are decreased. Use of heparin in the irrigating solution may decrease incidence.

(ii) **Thorough removal of lens material:** Thorough surgical removal of lens epithelial cells and cortical remnants, especially in the equatorial region is very necessary. This is best accomplished after rhexis and with adequate hydrodissection.

(iii) **Anterior capsulotomy:** The continuous curvilinear capsulorrhexis is the best modality for prevention of PCO. It secures long term in-the-bag IOL fixation, which decreases the incidence of PCO and IOL decentration. It also enhances the efficiency of hydrodissection and subsequent cortical clean up.

(iv) The adhesion between the cut anterior capsular flap and the posterior capsule may prevent ingrowth of retained epithelial cells into the visual axis.

(v) Presence of visible anterior capsular rim helps in polishing of anterior subcapsular epithelial cells and thus prevents PCO.

The secure in-the-bag IOL fixation creates a radial stretch or tautness of the posterior capsule. This increases the contact between the posterior surface of IOL optic and the posterior capsule, thus creating a mechanical barrier effect between the two, thus reducing incidence of PCO.

It is also advantageous in decreasing the chronic breakdown of blood aqueous barrier and/or inflammation that results from chaffing both of which may represent a stimulus for PCO.

IOL Design

(i) Optic design
(ii) In-the-bag fixation
(iii) IOL biomaterial
(iv) Surface modification
(v) Down sized IOLs
(vi) Three piece versus single piece IOLs.

(i) Optic Design

The relationship between the posterior aspect of IOL optic and adjacent posterior capsule plays an important role in the occurrence of PCO.

(a) **Disc IOLs:** Completely fills the lens capsular bag and so retards migration, thus theoretically leaves no spaces for cell growth and movement.

(b) **Barrier ridge optics:** They have a rim on the posterior surface of an IOL, which acts as a barrier to inhibit migration of residual lens epithelium into the central visual axis behind the IOL optic. Another advantage is that they create a laser-friendly space between posterior surface of IOL and the posterior capsule.

(c) **Posterior convex or biconvex optics:** The IOL is snugly apposed to the posterior capsule, thus decreases PCO.

(d) **Posterior angulation of IOL Optics:** With respect to loop the IOL optic is angulated upto 10° posteriorly. This enhances the optic capsule contact and decreases PCO.

(ii) In-the-Bag Placement of IOL

Placement of the optics and both the haptics into the bag decreases PCO due to close contact.

(iii) IOL Biomaterial

Polyacetic implants have a decreased incidence of PCO as compared to PMMA or silicon implants.

(iv) Surface Modifications

Modifications of the surface of IOL, by coating with heparin, indomethacin or fibroblast growth factor reduces the postoperative inflammation and thus decreases PCO.

(v) Down sized/Capsular IOLs

These days down sized in-the-bag IOLs (12–12.5 mm) are preferred because they ensure contact between the IOL and the posterior capsule.

Since the average diameter of human capsular bag is 10.5 mm, the IOL specifically designed for capsular bag implantation should have a diameter of approximately 12 to 12.5 mm, just large enough to provide a snug fit.

(vi) Three Piece vs. Single Piece IOLs

Incidence of PCO depends on the material being used. Basic difference lies in compressibility, rigidity and 'memory'.

Flexible loops (e.g. polypropylene) as in the three-piece IOL have a lesser retention of memory, thus less likely to provide the desired reexpansion or reopening of loops in the capsular bag.

On the other hand, because the loops of one piece, all PMMA, retain their memory, they greatly expand the posterior capsule in the radial direction, thereby maintaining an even continuous stretch on the posterior capsule, and hence, less or no space, between the posterior surface of IOL and the posterior capsule and thus decreases the PCO.

Pharmacologic and Immunologic Inhibitors

Various pharmacological agents have been tried to reduce the incidence of PCO. These compounds must be administered directly into the posterior chamber so that high concentration is reached and toxicity reduced.

The injection of sterile water into the capsular bag during cataract surgery destroys the epithelial cells by hypo-osmolar effect.

Antimiotic drugs inhibit the rapidly dividing mitotic lens epithelial cells, while avoiding toxic effects on non-mitotic cells. e.g. 5 FU, daunorubicin, methotrexate, colchicines, mitomycin C.

Transfer of suicide or growth-inhibiting genes into lens epithelial cells using viral vectors is under trial.

TREATMENT OF AFTER CATARACT

1. Surgical
2. Non-surgical.

Initially before the advent of Nd:YAG laser or even today in parts of the world where Nd:YAG laser is not available or there is thickness after cataract which is not amenable to laser capsulotomy, the surgical option is chosen.

Surgical Technique

(a) Anterior or Limbal Approach

(i) **Discission of after cataract:** Applicable in cases in which the after cataract consists of a delicate membrane. Capsulotomy can be done with a 26 gauge needle which is introduced through the limbal route to give a nick in the posterior capsule.

(ii) **Extraction after cataract:** Dense membranes which are either non-adherent to the iris or are adherent by delicate posterior synechiae are extracted with forceps.

(iii) **Complications:**
   (a) Vitreous loss.
   (b) Vitreous incarceration in wound.
   (c) Flat anterior chamber.

(b) Pars Plana Approach

In cases in which the posterior capsule is very thick, especially in badly done cataract surgery with retained lens matter, membranectomy and anterior vitrectomy has to be done with the help of a vitrectomy cutter via pars plana approach. 20 gauge MVR blade, vitreous scissors or even a capsulotomy punch may have to be used.

Complications

(a) Corneal oedema, striate keratopathy, bullous keratopathy.
(b) Transient elevation of IOP.
(c) Retinal detachment.
(d) Irreversible corneal endothelial damage with permanent clouding and fibrous proliferation in patients who underwent vitrectomy.
(e) Eye may become phthisical if trauma to the eye is severe during the pars plana vitrectomy.

Since all the surgical techniques for the management after cataract are associated with high risk for complications, there was a constant search for a non-invasive technique. The introduction of Neodymium: YAG laser has given a new dimension in the management of after cataract.

Nd:YAG Laser Capsulotomy

Nd:YAG laser is an infrared laser and has a wavelength of 1064 nm.

Principle

It works on the principle of photo-disruption. An intense electromagnetic radiation is focused into a small area during a brief period of time. The electromagnetic field of the laser pulse strips electrons from atoms and molecules creating plasma. A plasma is a mixture of ions and free electrons rarely existing in nature outside the atmosphere of sun or other stars. The rapid expansion produces shock and pressure waves which creates mechanical damage at the target. The shock wave is followed by cavitation and bubble formation. The cavitation is however, too rapid to be visible.

The head of the Nd: YAG laser is made in such a way that a He-Ne aiming laser due to its red continuous beam provides a precise visible marking for the invisible pulsed Nd:YAG laser beam. The two laser beams (He-Ne and Nd:YAG) should be perfectly co-axial and focused at a single point by means of the main objective through which they pass.

Two Techniques

(i) Q-switched technique – maximum output 10–20 mJ.

(ii) Mode Locked technique – maximum output 4.5 mJ. Adequate visualisation of the posterior capsule has to be there for its cutting by Nd:YAG laser. Conditions like corneal opacity or edema preclude adequate visualisation and hence, Nd:YAG laser cannot be used in such patients.

Pre-Laser Assessment

Direct ophthalmoscopy is the single most reliable technique to assess the severity of PCO. If the PCO is dense enough, fundus details will be obscured. If the ophthalmologist can see the retinal details clearly, but the patient is not able to see clearly through the same media, it should arouse suspicion and other causes should be looked for, e.g. CME, ARMD, etc.

Procedure

(i) Informed consent.

(ii) Pressure lowering drops (Apraclonidine or B-blockers) are administered 1 hour prior to and also immediately upon completion of Nd:YAG procedure so as to prevent the rise of IOP.

(iii) Topical anaesthetic (e.g. Lignocaine hydrochloride 4%) is instilled.

(iv) Use of Contact Lens: Peyman and Abraham contact lens can be used for Nd:YAG laser. It should be of high quality glass and provided with an anti-reflective coating.

Advantages of Contact Lens

(i) Helps in focusing the beam onto the posterior capsule.

(ii) Controls eye movements.

(iii) Separates the eyelids, thus increasing the size of the aperture.

General Principles

(i) The opening must be centred around the visual axis.

(ii) The capsular opening should be around 2–3 mm in size.

(iii) In order to avoid lesions over the intraocular lens, the spots must be placed 0.6 mm behind the capsule so that the opening results from the return of the shock wave and by post mechanical action.

(iv) Tissue ionisation occurs at the point of focus and the tissue is converted into ionised gas (Plasma).

(v) Minimal energy is used at first (1 mJ / pulse) and it may be increased according to the kind of capsule and opacity level.

(vi) Usually we start superiorly at the 12 O'clock position and progress inferiorly towards the 6 O'clock position. The aim is to produce a cruciate opening with flaps based inferiorly.

Complications of Nd:YAG Laser Capsulotomy

(i) **Rise of IOP:** This is the most common complication. It can be avoided by the use of anti-glaucoma medications like β blocker (Timolol), acetazolamide (Diamox) or Apraclonidine drops before the procedure and topical steroids and topical β-blockers after the procedure for 1 week.

(ii) **Uveal reaction:** Dispersion of uveal pigments is seen over the lens. It usually disappears in a few days with topical drugs.

(iii) **Retinal detachment:** Incidence of retinal detachment secondary to Nd:YAG laser posterior capsulotomy is quite low (0.08–3.6%). Retinal detachment is a serious complication, usually seen in eyes with thickened capsules, without an implant in which the vitreous tends to move forward.

(iv) **CME:** CME is a common complication, occurs in 10–15% of Pseudophakics undergoing laser capsulotomy. Treatment with steroids and NSAIDs is doubtful. There is some evidence that low doses of Diamox (1–2 tablet/day) may be effective. CME may even preexist before the capsulotomy and may be exacerbated following it.

(v) **Damage to the intraocular lens:** In YAG laser capsulotomy, the most common complication is pitting in the implant optic. These pits do not affect visual acuity but longer pits or cracks indicate severe damage to the optics. PMMA lens usually sustains cracks on exposure to YAG laser. Lathe cut high molecular weight PMMA lens are more resistant than moulded PMMA lens.

(vi) **Posterior IOL subluxation or dislocation:** This is a rare complication, but may occur with plate haptic silicone and hydrogel IOLs.

(vii) **Chronic endophthalmitis:** Propionobacterium acnes endophthalmitis can occur following Nd:YAG laser capsulotomy. Most probably the bacteria are sequestrated in the capsule and following capsulotomy, the bacteria are released and get an opportunity to reach the vitreous and cause endophthalmitis.

(viii) **Macular holes:** Rarely, macular holes could occur following capsulotomy. However, the complications can be very well prevented with adequate prophylaxis and can also be controlled efficiently, if timely managed.

Advantages of Nd: YAG Capsulotomy

(i) Non-invasive, hence lesser chances of hemorrhage and infection

(ii) Less time consuming

(iii) Safer

(iv) Performed as an OPD procedure.

Thus, the Nd: YAG laser plays a very important role in the management of PCO. With advancing technology, we hope to soon have a yet better alternative to Nd: YAG laser, which would be absolutely free of any complications, for the management of PCO.

BIBLIOGRAPHY

1. Davison J. Neodymium:YAG laser posterior capsulotomy after implantation of AcrySof intraocular lenses. J Cataract Refract Surg 2004; 30:1492–1500.

2. Daynes T, Spencer TS, Doan K, et al. Three-year clinical comparison of 3-piece AcrySof and SI-40 silicone intraocular lenses. J Cataract Refract Surg 2002; 28:1124–1129.

3. Apple DJ, Peng Q, Visessook N, et al. Eradication of posterior capsule opacification: documentation of a marked decrease in Nd:YAG laser posterior capsulotomy rates noted in an analysis of 5416 pseudophakic human eyes obtained postmortem. Ophthalmology 2001; 108:505–518.

4. Vasavada A, Raj S. Anterior capsule relationship of the AcrySof intraocular lens optic and posterior capsule opacification. Ophthalmology 2004; 111:886–94.

5. Smith S, Daynes T, Hinckley M, et al. The effect of lens edge design versus anterior capsule overlap on posterior capsule opacification. Am J Ophthalmol 2004; 138:521–526.

6. Auffarth GU, Golescu A, Becker KA, Volker HE. Quantification of posterior capsule opacification with round and sharp edge intraocular lenses. Ophthalmology 2003; 110:772–780.

7. Nagamoto T, Fujiwara T. Inhibition of lens epithelial cell migration at the interaocular lens optic edge; role of capsule bending and contact pressure. J Cataract Refract Surg 2003; 29:1605–1612,

8. Buehl W, Findl O, Menapace R, et al. Effect of an acrylic intraocular lens with a sharp posterior optic edge on posterior capsule opacification. J Cat aract Refract Surg 2002; 28:1105–1111.

9. Nishi O, Nishi K. Preventing lens epithelial cell migration using intraocular lenses with sharp rectangular edges. J Cataract Refract Surg 2000; 26: 1543–1549.

10. Nishi O, Nishi K, Osakabe Y. Effect of intraocular lenses on preventing posterior capsule opacification: Design vs. Material. J Cataract Refract Surg2004; 30:2170–2176.

11. Buehl W, Menapace R, Sacu S, et al. Effect of a silicone intraocular lens with a sharp posterior optic edge on posterior capsule opacification. J Cataract Redact Surg 2004; 30: 1661–1667.

12. Buehl W, Findl O, Menapace R, et al. Long-term effect of optic edge design in an acrylic intraocular lens on posterior capsule opacification. J Cataract Refract Surg 2005; 31:954–961.

13. Hayashi K, Hayashi H. Posterior capsule opacification in the presence of an intraocular lens with a sharp versus rounded optic edge. Ophthalmology 2005; 112:1550–1556.

14. Wren SM, Spalton DJ, Jose R, et al. Factors that influence the development of posterior capsule opacification with a polyacrylic intraocular lens. Am J Ophthalmol 2005; 139:691–695.

15. Sacu S, Menapace R, Buehl W, et al. Effect of intraocular lens optic edge design and material on fibrotic capsule opacification and capsulorhexis contraction. J Cataract Refract Surg 2004; 30:1875–1882.

16. Sacu S, Findl O, Menapace R, et al. Comparison of posterior capsule opacification between the 1-piece and 3-pieceAcrysof intraocular lenses: two-year results of a randomised trial. Ophthalmology 2004; 111:1840–1846.

28

Opacification of IOL

Col JKS Parihar SM,VSM

INTRODUCTION

The most common types of IOL used for implantation after cataract surgeries are PMMA, Silicone and Acrylic. Of these, in the recent past, acrylic intraocular lenses (IOLs) of hydrophilic and/or hydrophobic types have been widely accepted and are extensively used in phacoemulsification cataract surgery. It is claimed that chemical materials commonly used in IOL are inert and biocompatible. Hence, IOL is claimed to remain transparent for optical purposes as well as nonreactive forever. The first PMMA IOL was implanted in Nov 1949. There is no report available in the literature world so far claiming any alteration in the optical clarity of the lens. However, the same does not hold true with silicone or Acrylic flexible IOL implant. The intraocular environment, although considered as a privileged site, is not immune to the opacification phenomenon. Opacification of Silicone IOLs have been reported.

Acrylic IOL opacification after cataract surgery is a rare entity and a recently recognised phenomenon. Yu and Shek have very recently reported late postoperative opacifications of Hydro view, a modern foldable hydrophilic acrylic IOL. The author has experienced opacification of six IOL implants belonging to different makes and manufacturers since 2001.

In this chapter an attempt is made to cover various aspects related with this unusual and very complex phenomenon.

PATHOGENESIS

The exact pathogenesis of IOL opacification is not known though various concepts have been proposed. Two important concepts are degeneration of the UV filtration material and calcium deposits within the optic biomaterial. Werner et. al. analysed nine-explanted hydrophilic acrylic

IOLs and demonstrated the presence of calcium deposits within the optics of IOL responsible for its opacification. Kim et. al. describes opacification of Hydrophilic acrylic IOL with exacerbation of uveitis. Ramani et. al. demonstrated presence of calcium, oxygen and carbon in a different type of hydrophilic acrylic IOL, viz., AQUA Sense, a copolymer of PHEMA and Poly ethoxy ethyl methacrylate (PEOEMA). Additionally, traces of sodium and chlorine were also found and were perhaps due to the contribution from the saline preservative. However, a separate EDAX spectrum on a control IOL did not show any evidence of calcium in it. This confirms that the dense opacification is mainly due to calcification.

Bucher and co-authors reported clinical observations of opacification due to calcification in IOGEL 1103, made of polyhydroxyethyl methacrylate (PHEMA). Nowadays, hydrogel lenses are generally manufactured from PHEMA and other copolymers of hydrophilic acrylic. There also are reports of opacification of a few different types of acrylic IOLs. Opacification of hydrophilic acrylic lens SC 60B – OUV, a copolymer of hydrophobic poly methyl methacrylate (PMMA) and hydrophilic PHEMA has been found. Yu et.al. reported opacification in Hydroview, another copolymer of HEMA with hydroxy hexyl methacrylate (HOHEXMA). Thus the potential of an IOL material to opacify must be taken into consideration when evaluating the long-term bio-compatibility of the material.

The ability of a material to imbibe macromolecules such as proteins and lipids from the extracellular matrix is thought to play a significant role in calcification. Normal aqueous humour contains calcium and the continuous supply of minerals is a more convincing explanation for the delayed and progressive calcification in our patient. Additionally, postopacification after cataract surgery in diabetic patients is generally not uncommon. Few reports are recently available in literature citing the permanent blue discolouration of a Hydrogel IOL due to use of intracameral Trypan blue for performing capsulorrhexis. The most common cause of opacification remains calcification in the IOL implant itself. In our view, the affinity of the hydrogel copolymer to calcium is responsible for this dystrophic calcification. Although, the mechanism of calcification is not fully understood, it is not seen to be directly related to substances used during surgery as it occurs in the late postoperative period. However, further research work is most essential which can throw more light on the mechanism of calcification as this involves multiple factors such as irregularities in the IOL manufacturing, interactions with intraoperative materials as well as patient factors such as metabolic imbalance, etc. It is also important to follow the clinical outcomes of this lens in order to determine if this phenomenon is rare and sporadic or may be more widespread as this involves multiple factors such as irregularities in the IOL manufacturing, interactions with intraoperative materials as well as patient factors such as metabolic imbalance, etc.

CLINICAL PRESENTATION

Most of the cases with opacification of IOL experienced progressive and gradual diminution of vision of the operated eye in due course of time. The onset of IOL opacification was generally reported after 14 to 20 months after initial phacoemulsification surgery.

This phenomenon is generally considered as the most common occurrence of posterior capsular opacification (PCO) by the patient or even by ophthalmic surgeons.

These patients have invariably been subjected to or have undergone YAG laser capsulotomy, obviously without any positive improvement in visual acuity. In this situation, the possibility of a dense PCO not responding to YAG is invariably kept under consideration.

On a slit lamp examination, opaque lens may exactly look like mature cataract in a very advanced stage of opacification. At the beginning of opacification, IOL may reveal evidence of opacities in the peripheral and in the outer portion of the IOL.

The posterior capsule opacification may or may not be present. The remaining ocular examination including the posterior segment may remain normal.

MANAGEMENT

Once the IOL has become opaque, the treatment remains an explanation of the opaque IOL followed by an IOL exchange. However, the technique of IOL exchange may pose certain challenges during the procedure itself. Over and above, the probable risk of intra and postoperative complications of additional intraocular surgery including infection should be explained to the patient.

The choice of the IOL for exchange itself is debatable. Undoubtedly, theoretically one can choose another foldable IOL as the exchanged one. However, in our opinion, it is better to opt for all PMMA IOL since there is no report available in literature world regarding opacification of rigid PMMA IOL.

Surgical Technique

Though the procedure can be completed under topical anaesthesia, since maneuver for IOL explant are different and needs precise control on surgical steps, it is preferred to perform surgery under Peribulbar anaesthesia.

Incisions

The surgeon may opt for an incision of his own choice. The author has great preference for Limbal-Corneal self sealing incision in all types of cataract surgery including coaxial or bimanual phacoemulsification. Hence, by habit

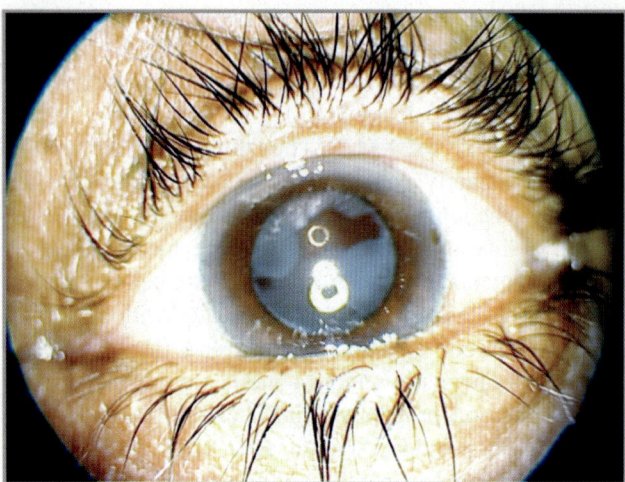

Fig. 28.1: Opacification of acrylic foldable PC IOL implant

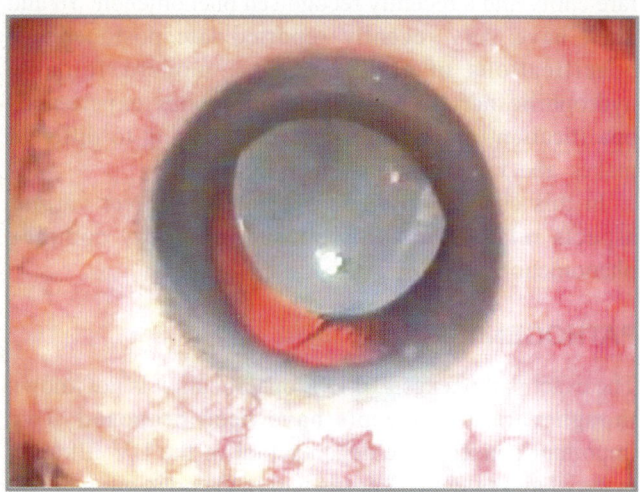

Fig. 28.2: Opacification of acrylic foldable PC IOL implant

the same incision has been used by him in explantation of opaque IOL. It also is advisable to have the side port incision in this procedure since, it will facilitate bimanual manipulations while rotating and explanting opaque IOL out of bag.

A self-sealing semitemporal 11 or 1 O'clock in the right or left eye, respectively. Clear corneal incision of 0.9 mm was made with the help of a specially designed 0.9 mm corneal Keratome. Another side port incision was made around 105–120 degree from the main incision.

Removal of Opaque IOL from Capsular Bag

After reforming the anterior chamber with an injection of Sodium Hyaluronate, an Iris repositor was introduced under the inner surface of the anterior capsule and above the opaque IOL to fashion gentle and very slow, progressive, through and through sliding movements right up to the fornices of the bag. This will relieve any adhesion between the inner surface of anterior capsule. Capsular phimosis may also be taken due care of by this maneuver. Capsular phimosis and adhesions are expected more with opaque silicon IOL as compared to acrylic IOL implant.

Once opaque IOL is made free from the anterior capsule, one of the haptic, preferably the lower haptic is dialled with the help of Synskey's hook and attempted to get it out of the bag. This particular manoeuver is very crucial and needs great attention, since this may involve zonular dialysis or a posterior capsular rent. Another dialler through the side port is beneficial and enhances bag security during dialling of the haptics. Lower haptic can also be rotated in the same manner. Repeated administration of viscoelastics in the capsular bag is recommended during the entire procedure.

Explanation of Opaque IOL from the Anterior Chamber

Once Opaque IOL is released from the capsular bag, subsequent maneuver is relatively simple. Corneal incision

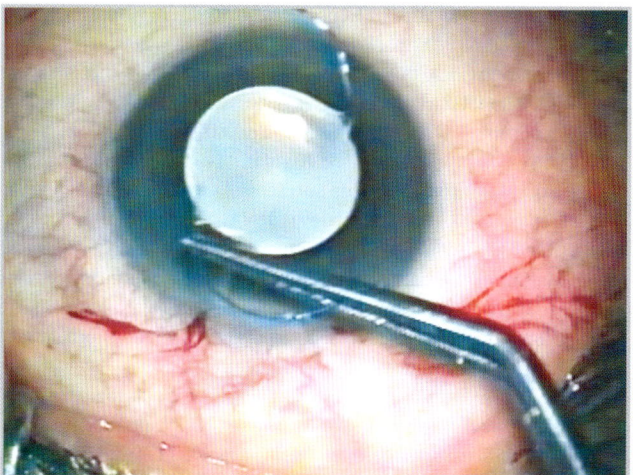

Fig. 28.3: Explantation of opaque acrylic foldable PC IOL implant

is extended with the help of a 5.5 mm Keratome/incision extender. Opaque IOL can be explanted under viscocushion with the help of Mc Pherson's forceps.

IOL Exchange

Once opaque IOL is being removed, implantation of another IOL implant can be considered. The choice of IOL depends upon the integrity of capsular bag and the surgeon's own preference. Theoretically, one can consider foldable IOL implant as a replacement. However, in our view, All PMMA IOL implants should be preferred over acrylic IOLs due to the following reasons:

(i) The exact mechanism of opacification of the IOL is not yet known. Process of calcification may be associated with manufacturing defects in the IOL or polymer compatibility. The possibility of intrinsic mechanism related with body immune system or metabolism cannot be excluded.

(ii) PMMA IOL carries more than 50 years of track record of intraocular inert status except evidence of PCO. However, not a single report is available in literature regarding opacification of rigid PMMA lens.

Depending upon the situation in the bag, IOL (5.5 × 12 mm) or Sulcus fixated (6 mm × 13 mm) PMMA IOL can be implanted in the usual manner.

Closure of Incision

Closure of incision is made with the help of one or two sutures of 10 "O" monofilament suture.

Subconjunctival injection of dexamethasone, 4 mg and gentamycin, 20 mg was given. Eye pad was given and removed after 3–5 hours of the surgery.

Postoperative Management

Postoperative management is essentially on the same guidelines as being observed for phacoemulsification surgery.

INTRAOPERATIVE OBSERVATIONS

Opaque IOL may be associated with following changes

(a) **Anterior capsular phimosis:** More common with silicon IOL/associated systemic diseases like diabetes or ocular diseases like uveitis or Glaucoma.

(b) **Adhesions between anterior capsule and Opaque IOL:**
(i) More common with silicon IOL implants.
(ii) Multi-piece IOL carry more risk than single piece IOL implants.

(c) **Opacification of posterior capsule:** Not a regular feature.

INTRAOPERATIVE COMPLICATIONS

Incidence of intraoperative complications remains high in IOL exchange as compared to primary IOL implantation. This procedure may reveal any of the complications as observed in other intraocular surgery. However, risk of PC rent and zonulysis is much higher due the fact that the explantation procedure put posterior capsule under more stress and stretch compare to primary IOL implantation.

POSTOPERATIVE COMPLICATIONS

Incidence of postoperative complications remains high in IOL exchange as compared to primary IOL implantation. Common problems are as follows:

(i) Moderate to significant corneal striates which lasts for longer duration.

(ii) Postoperative uveitis.

(iii) Secondary glaucoma

(iv) Decentration of IOL implant.

(v) CME.

(vii) Higher incidence of PCO.

Management of above mentioned complications follows the same standard regimen as practiced in any other intraocular surgery.

CONCLUSION

Use caution on implantation of hydrophilic acrylic IOLs because late opacification is a serious complication and requires further surgery.

The most common cause of opacification remains calcification in the IOL implant itself. In our view, the affinity of the hydrogel copolymer to calcium is responsible for this dystrophic calcification. Although the mechanism of calcification is not fully understood, it is not seen to be directly related to substances used during surgery as it occurs in the late postoperative period. However, further research work is most essential which can throw more light on the mechanism of calcification. It is also important to follow the clinical outcome of this lens in order to determine if this phenomenon is rare and sporadic or may be more widespread.

REFERENCES AND BIBLIOGRAPHY

1. Christ FR, Buchen SY, Deacon J, et al. Biomaterials used for intraocular lenses. In: Wise DL, Trantolo DJ, Aliobelli DE, et al., eds, Encyclopedic Handbook of Biomaterials and Bioengineering. Part B: applications, vol 2. New York, NY, Marcel Dekker, Inc, 1995; 1261–1313.

2. Apple DJ, Werner L, Pandey SK and Charleston SC. Newly recognised complications of posterior chamber intraocular lenses. Arch Ophthalmol 2001; 119: 581–2.

3. Mamalis N. Hydrophilic acrylic intraocular lenses (Editorial). J Cataract Refract Surg 2001; 27:1339–1340.

4. Tognetto D, Toto L, Ballone E, Ravalico G. Biocompatability of hydrophilic intraocular lenses. J. Cat and Ref Surg 2002; 28: 644–651.

5. Buchen SY, Cunanam CM, Gwon A, Weinschenk JI, Gruber L and Knight PM. Assessing intraocular lens calcification in an animal model. J Cat and Ref Surg 2001; 27: 1474–1484.

6. Yu AKF, Kwan KYW, Chan DHY and Fong DYT. Clinical features of forty six eyes with calcified hydrogel intraocular lenses. J. Cat and Ref Surg 2001; 27: 1596–1606.

7. Olson RJ, Caldwell KD, Crandall AS, Jensen MK, Huang SC. Intraoperative crystallisation on the intraocular lens surface. Amer J Ophthalmol 1998; 126: 177–184.

8. Schauersberger J, Krugcr A, Abela C, et al. Course of postoperative inflammation after implantation of 4 types of foldable intraocular lenses. J Cataract RefracL Surg 1999, 25:1116–1120.

9. Hayashi K, Hayashi H, Nakao F and Hayashi F. Changes in posterior capsule opacification after poly(methyl methacrylate), silicone and acrylic intraocular lens implantation. J. Cat and Ref Surg. 2001; 27:817–824.

10. Oner HF, Durak I, Saatci OA. Late postoperative opacification of hydrophilic acrylic Intraocular lenses. Ophthal Surg and Lasers 2002; 33: 304–308.

11. Sharma TK, Chawdhary S. The opaiescence of hydro-gel intraocular lens. Eye 2001; 15:97–98

12. Apple DJ, Werner L, Pandey SK. Opalescence of hydrophilic acrylic lenses (letter). Eye, 2001; 15:817–19).

13. Apple D.J, Werner L, Escobar-Gomez, M, Pandey SK: Deposits on the optical surfaces of Hydroview intraocular lenses (letter). J Cataract Refract Surg 2000; 26:796–97.

14. Werner L, Apple D J.I, Escobar-Gomez, M, et al. Postoperative deposition of calcium on the surfaces of a Hydrogel intraocular lens. Ophthalmology 2000; 107:2179–85.

15. Izak A, Werner L, Pandey SK et al :Calcification on the surface of the Bausch & Lomb Hydroview " Intraocular lens". In: Werner L, Apple DJ, eds. Complications of Aphakic and Refractive Intraocular Lenses. Int Ophthalmol Clin. Lippincott Williams & Wilkins, Philadelphia, PA, USA, 2001; 41:62–78.

16. Fernando GT, Crayford BB. Visually significant calcification of hydrogel intraocular lenses necessitating explantation. Clin Experiment Ophthalmol 2000; 28:280–286.

17. Jensen MK, Crandall AS, Mamalis N, Olson RJ. Crystallisation on intraocular lens surfaces associated with the use of Healon GV. Arch Ophthalmol 1994; 112:1037–1042.

18. Ramani R, Parihar JKS, Ranganthan C, Awasthi P, Alam S, Mathur GN. Free volume study on calcification process in an intraocular lens after cataract surgery: Journal of Biomedical Materials Research - Part B: Applied Biomaterials John Wiley Publications 2005, 222–226.

19. Hollick E.J, Spalton DJ, Ursell P(J. Surface cytologic features on intraocular lenses: can increased biocompatibility have disadvantages? Arch, Ophthalmol 1999; 117:872–878.

20. Pavlovic S, Magdowski G, Brueckel B, Pavlovic S. Ultra-structural analysis of opacities seen in a hydrophilic acrylic intraocular lens. Eye 2001; 15:657–659.

21. Werner L, Apple DJ, Kaskaloglu M, Pandey SK. Dense Opacification of the optical component of a hydrophilic intraocular lens: A clinicopathological analysis of 9 explanted lenses. J Cataract Refract Surg 2001; 27:1485–1492.

22. Yu AKF and Shek TWH. Hydroxyapatite formation on implanted hydrogel intraocular lenses. Arch Ophthalmol 2001; 119: 611–614.

23. Macky TA, Trivedi RH, Werner L, et al. Degeneration of UV absorber material and calcium deposits within the optic of a hydrophilic IOL lens (manufactured by Medical Developmental Research). In: Werner L, Apple DJ, eds. Complications of Aphakic and Refractive Intraocular Lenses, hit Ophthalmol Clin. Lippincott Willinmx & Wilkins, Philadelphia, PA, USA, 2001; 41:79–90.

24. Bucher PJM, Buchi ER, Daicker BC. Dystophic calcification of an implanted hydroxyethylmethacrylate intraocular lens. Arch Ophthalmol 1995; 113: 1431–1435.

25. Yu AKF, Kwan KYW, Chan DHY, Fong UYT. Clinical features of 46 eyes with calcified hydrogel intraocular lenses. J Cataract Refract Surg 2001; 27.1596–1606.

26. Groh JMM, Schlotzer-Schrehardt U, Rummelt C.et al. Postoperative Kunstlinsen-Eintrubungen bei 12 Hydrogel-Intraokularlinsen (Hydroview). Klin Munalnbl Augenheilkd 2001; 218:645648.

27. Kim CY, Kang SJ, Lee SJ, Park SH, Koh HJ. Opacification of a hydrophilic acrylic intraocular lens with exacerbation of Behcet's Uveitis. J Cat and Ref Surg 2002; 28: 1276–1278.

28. Frohn A, Dick HB, Augustin AJ and Grus FH. Late opacification of the foldable hydrophilic acrylic lens SC 60 BOUV. Ophthalmol 2001; 108: 1999–2004.

29. Sharma A, Ram J, Gupta A. Late clouding of an acrylic intraocular lens following routine phacoemulsification (letter). Eye 2001; 15:361.

30. Chang BYP, Davey KG, Gupta M, Hutchinson C. Late clouding of an acrylic intraocular lens following routine phacoemulsification. Eye 1999; 13:807–808.

31. Pandey SK, Werner L, Apple DJ and Kaskaloglu M. Hydrophilic acrylic intraocular lens optics and haptics opacification in a diabetic patient: Bilateral case report and clinicopathologic correlation. Ophthalmol 2002; 109: 2042–2051.

Phacoemulsification in Challenging Situations

29

Phacoemulsification Surgery in a very Hard Supra Brown Cataract

Col JKS Parihar SM,VSM, Surg Cdr T Choudhary, Maj Jaya Kaushik and
Surg Lt Cdr AS Parihar

INTRODUCTION

A couple of decades ago, there was a constant tug of war between the advocates and critics of phacoemulsification, but today we have reached a stage of finesse in terms of techniques, machines and materials to an extent that the gold standard of cataract extraction surgery, as of now, is phacoemulsification. With each passing day one sees improvements and advancements to such an extent that there is a paradigm shift in the attitude of the patients towards cataract surgery.

The patient today is well aware of the merits of stitchless surgery and the intricacies and benefits of phaco-emulsification over conventional surgery. He comes demanding a stitchless, prick-less, pad-less cataract surgery. His queries centre around two basic parametres—the machine that will be used and the lens that would be implanted.

Coupled with this is the fact that in India, a large population is still at a fair distance from comprehensive health care. Due to the peculiar cultural, social, economic and demographic characteristics of our country, it is not uncommon to find a patient, generally a lady, with rock brown grade VI cataract and a vision in both eyes of projection of rays or hand movements at the most. And to top it all, once a successful surgery is performed on one eye and the patient visually rehabilitated, the patient does not find it necessary to get the other eye operated, and nurtures the cataract in the other eye, to lead some poor ophthalmologist to difficulty, disaster or doom at a later date. Today, it is possible to channelise the advances in technology and consumables and couple them with scientifically sound refinement in techniques to tackle even the hardest cataracts with relative ease and safety.

The basic aim of this chapter is to direct the thought process of the receptive reader so that he can ponder over the techniques described herein, and use his own finer modifications to handle the supra-hard brown cataracts with reasonable confidence.

APPLIED ANATOMY

The task of understanding the modifications described will become even simpler if it is based on anatomical inputs. There are certain peculiarities which occur in the anatomy of the eye with a supra-hard brown cataract. These anatomical transgressions are as follows:

Lid Laxity and Tear Film Instability

At the advanced age at which these supra-hard cataracts present themselves, other physiological and senile changes might co-exist and compromise the result of the surgery. Though unrelated to the aetiology and management of cataract per se, it is better to tackle them beforehand, than to repent later. These patients generally have a lax lower lid and it is not uncommon to find an involutional entropion. This in-turned lid with eyelashes is an ominous sign and needs to be tackled before attempting the cataract surgery. Coupled with the tear film instability which is also a common finding at that advanced age, the author has seen perfectly performed surgeries landing up with sight compromising complications like persistent epithelial defects, corneal vascularisation and opacities and infective keratitis.

Cornea

The changes which occur in the cornea with age are well known. The senile changes in the tear film, epithelium and the stromal collagen lead to a cornea with an arcus and peripheral haze hindering visualisation. The most important factor is the decreasing endothelial cell count and the polymegathism encountered in the patients of this age. There is very little room for error while performing phacoemulsification, lest the critical count be breached and the patient should land up with PBK. This makes it imperative to do a thorough corneal assessment preoperatively, in order to anticipate and preempt any complications or difficulties. It is absolutely essential to perform a specular microscopy and corneal pachymetry in these patients. Use of suitable Ophthalmic Viscoelastic Devices (OVD) can also help decrease the endothelial cell loss during surgery.

Anterior Chamber

As age progresses, the lens increases in size and girth. Thus, it stands to logic that these patients with supra-hard cataracts have a relatively shallow anterior chamber. The corneo-lenticular distance, even in the central deepest part is never more than 2 mm. This leaves very little space to maneuver the instruments. The line between in-the-bag and pupillary plane in phacoemulsification becomes blurred, resulting in an increased collateral energy transmission to the surrounding tissues during phacoemulsification.

Lens

The lens tissue is the one which affects the surgical technique maximally and therefore as this is the tissue whose anatomical and physical characteristics have ensured that a full chapter in this monograph be dedicated to it. The supra-hard brown lens has a thicker girth and a larger overall diameter. The increased girth means decreased endothelio-lenticular distance and decreased radius of curvature of the anterior and posterior surfaces of the lens. The decreased radius of curvature makes the CCC much more difficult to perform.

The anterior capsule is thin, papery, stretched out and brittle. It is not uncommon to find a run-off of the CCC by an innocuous and simple maneuver of removing an instrument from the anterior chamber. Also, the posterior capsule is stretched out, making it thin and friable. In addition, when the major part of the cataract has been removed, this stretched out posterior capsule does not have any scaffolding and wrinkles, and writhes eagerly to find its way into the phaco tip. It requires additional care to ensure that this loose and floppy posterior capsule does not follow the lenticular material into the phaco tip while dealing with the last piece.

Also, the main change is the consistency of the cataract. The supra-hard brown cataract has a rock hard central core. The core is surrounded by a hard peri-nucleus (less harder than the core) and a softer and less dense epi-nucleus. The peculiarity is that these three parts of the nucleus are not easily separable or discernable. They are adhered to each. The nucleus forms the major bulk and there is very little, if any cortex. All this requires a modification in our approach in tackling these cataracts.

The large bulk of the cataract creates a situation where the edge of the CCC is snugly encompassed by the thin lens cortex and the epi-nucleus from behind. Thus, there is not enough spongy area of cortex or free space to allow the egress of the fluid returning after hydro dissecting the nucleus. This can easily result in the entrapment of the fluid behind the nucleus and a "blow out" of the posterior capsule, which might go undetected till the heart-sinking sight of a sinking nucleus as soon as the first phaco stroke is applied.

Since the cataract is hard, the pieces of the nucleus once created are rigid and do not mould to occlude the phaco tip. This causes a partial occlusion and egress of phaco energy to undesirable locations.

The hard cataractous material from the nucleus mixes with the viscoelastic to create a putty of such consistency that blocks the aspiration port of the phacoemulsification handpiece. With the blockage of the aspiration, there is very little, if any, inflow of fluid into the eye. This lack of flow rate causes US energy heat transmission to the corneal incision, increasing the likelihood of corneal burns. Another peculiarity of such cataracts is the presence and persistence of a thick posterior plate which is actually a part of the peri-nucleus and is very difficult to manage in case of not being separated into the relevant pieces with each chop in the end.

Zonules

Needless to say, these cataracts are invariably accompanied by weak and loose zonules. Any excessive downward pressure or outward pressure on the nucleus with the probe when trying to separate the pieces may lead to a zonular dehiscence. The loose zonules also fail to give enough countertraction for easy CCC and the whole bag moves while performing a CCC, especially if the cystitome is blunt.

Vitreous

As age progresses, the vitreous humor becomes more fluid in consistency from the gel-like consistency it had in youth and middle age. This alters the dynamics of surgery, as the posterior capsule does not have a firm posterior support and is more likely to balloon forward during the last stages of nucleus removal due to the absence of anterior and posterior support. However, to our advantage, the fluid vitreous is much more easier to manage in the case of a posterior capsular rent and vitreous loss. This fluid vitreous is cleared easily and rarely leaves behind a traction band or residual vitreous in the incision, pupillary area or the angle.

Retina

As the cataract is dense and opaque, it is not a bad idea to routinely do a screening USG A-B scan in all such patients before they are accepted for surgery. This will leave us in a better position to prognosticate our results. Also, it is a better idea to counsel the patients regarding the unpredictable visual prognosis as most of these patients have some element of ARMD in their eyes.

General Condition

Old age is in itself the biggest morbidity. These patients are generally suffering from diabetes, hypertension, COPD, IHD etc. These need to be factored in for the surgery.

CLINICAL EVALUATION OF LENS

It is of utmost importance that the evaluation of two structures in the eye viz. the Lens and the Cornea be done in detail. It is being re-emphasised in this monograph again and again at the cost of repetition because it has a critical bearing on the outcome. The lens needs to be graded, seen in detail on a slit and features of subluxation or pseudo-exfoliation actively searched for. Details of corneal assessment and lens assessment have already been dealt with earlier.

SURGICAL TECHNIQUE

This book has in various appropriate places enumerated in detail the steps encountered or recommended in normal phacoemulsification. Relevant chapters on special situations encountered in phacoemulsification have highlighted the deviations from these standard steps involved in the concerned special situations. So also, this section of this chapter will deal with only the differences, deviations and special precautions required for tackling Supra-hard brown cataracts and is not intended to be a step by step guide for the basic learner.

Anaesthesia

The golden rule of choosing the anaesthesia according to the comfort of the surgeon and the patient holds good here. Though the author prefers topical anaesthesia augmented by intracameral 0.5% preservative free Xylocaine where required, the choice of anaesthesia is left to the individual surgeon. There is no harm in peribulbar anaesthesia for the first few cases when the surgeon's heart is aflutter, the fingers trembling and the operating time slightly more.

Position and General Care

It is always a good idea to communicate the initial steps of cleaning and draping to the patient to have a relation going. Make sure that all co-existing morbidities have been dealt with. Cater for the spinal deformities of the old age by cushioning the appropriate parts of the body. Then the patient's cooperation and immobility can be solicited and the surgery started.

Incisions

The initial incisions are the same as in any other case depending on the surgeon's preferred technique. Only care that should be taken that the tunnel is of adequate length to

prevent shallowing of the already shallow anterior chamber. It is not a bad idea to keep cooling the incision site with chilled BSS to prevent corneal burns.

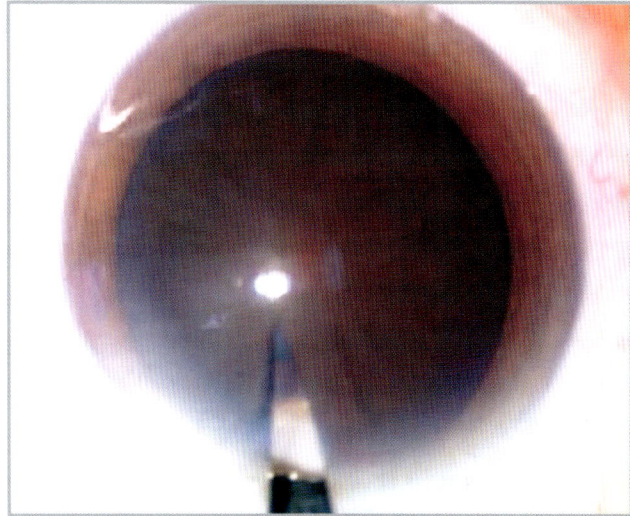

Fig. 29.1: Supra hard brown cataract: Side port incision

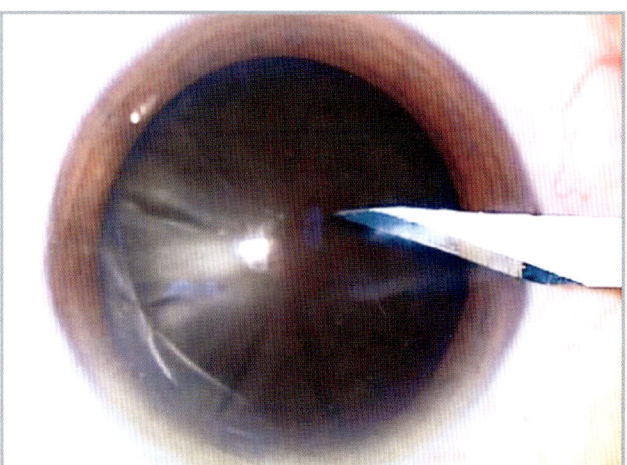

Fig. 29.2: Supra hard brown cataract: Temporal clear corneal incision

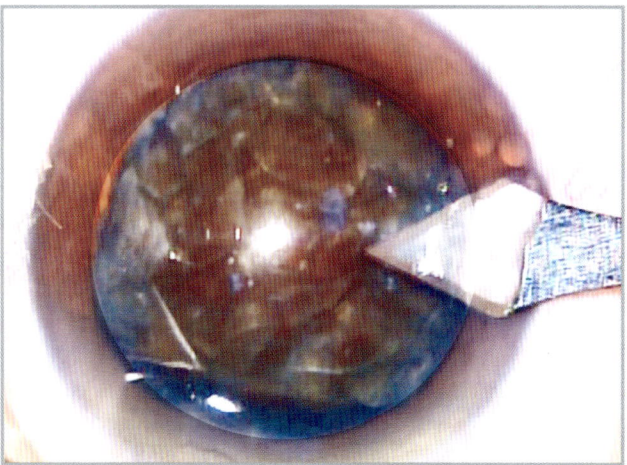

Fig. 29.3: Supra hard brown cataract: Temporal clear corneal incision

Rhexis

The rhexis is slightly tricky in these supra-hard brown cataracts due to the following factors:
  (i) No Glow
  (ii) Shallow anterior chamber
  (iii) Thin, stretched, friable anterior capsule
  (iv) Decreased anterior radius of curvature of the lens (more convex anterior capsule)
  (v) Loose or lax zonules, not providing sufficient counter traction for the capsulotomy to proceed easily

Once we know the anticipated problems, it becomes very easy to preempt them. Use of trypan blue is recommended, especially so in the initial or more difficult cases. Remember, rhexis is the third hand of the surgeon in phaco, and a good rhexis done is half the battle won. The author, due to the number of cases performed, has now given up the use of anterior capsular staining adjuncts.

Ideally, the rhexis should be done before the full entry with the 2.8 or 3.2 mm keratome, through the side port or after a partial entry with the phaco incision keratome. Also, sufficient good quality viscoelastic will ensure that the convexity of the anterior capsule is reduced and so are the chances of run-off of the rhexis. It is recommended that at least in the beginning the surgeons perform the rhexis with the micro-capsulorrhexis forceps. This is a wonderful instrument which combines the advantage of good control as offered by the utrata capsulorrhexis forceps and entry through a small incision plus a formed anterior chamber as seen in a 26 gauge needle cystitome. This cross action 23 gauge instrument enables the surgeon to perform rhexis even in the most difficult situations and also to retrieve a rhexis which is threatening to run out.

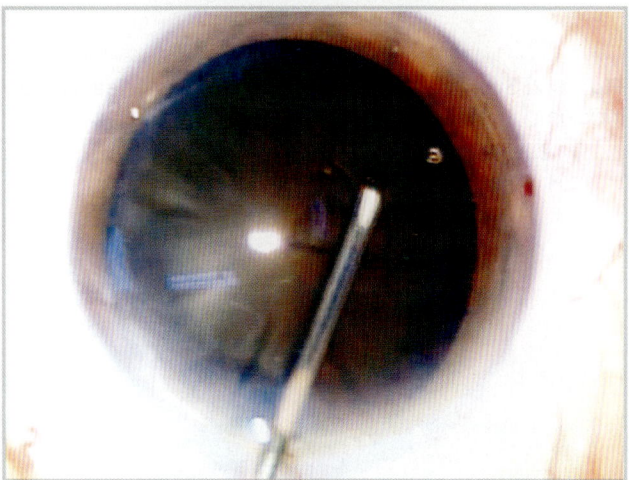

Fig. 29.4: Supra hard brown cataract: Rhexis

The rhexis should be of a size slightly larger than in normal cases due to the large size of the nucleus, but aim for a normal sized rhexis and invariably you will end up with a larger rhexis. Make sure that the rhexis does not

encompass the most central zonules as tearing these zonules may be the last straw on the camel's back.

Hydrodissection and Hydrodelineation

As cited earlier, gentle hydro dissection is recommended as the lips of the rhexis are tightly closed by the underlying bulging lenticular material and there is every chance of entrapment of fluid above the posterior capsule and a subsequent "blow out" of the posterior capsule. Small fluid spurts in multiple quadrants with frequent decompression of the nucleus by slight posterior and sideways push are the magic mantras.

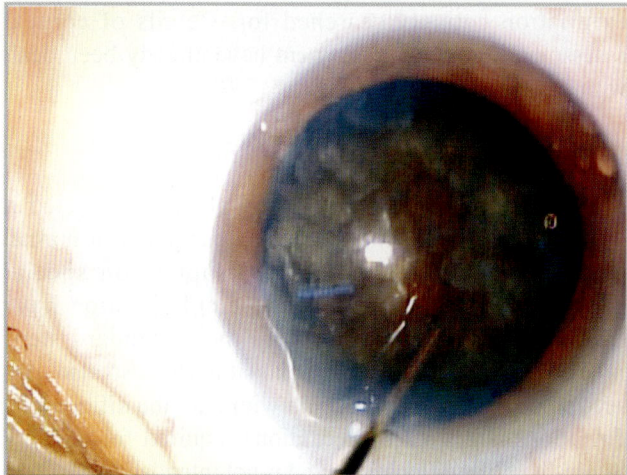

Fig. 29.5: Supra hard brown cataract: Hydroprocedure

Choice of Nucleotomy Techniques

Various nucleotomy techniques have been described in detail in earlier chapters. Their relevance to these supra-hard brown cataracts will be dealt with here.

Divide and Conquer (DCN)

It is well known that this particular technique involves the maximum posterior pressure and consequent stress on the zonules. Also the energy used in creating the two trenches is added to the total energy and does not help matters much. More often than not we are so conscious of the energy being used that in an effort to minimise the energy usage, we use less energy and more physical push inferiorly and posteriorly while trenching. This causes traction on the already aged superior zonules and such repetitive strokes invariably lead to zonulolysis. On the other extreme, seeing the hardness of the cataract if we employ greater energy, there is that sword of corneal decompensation hanging over our heads. Also, not reducing the energy voluntarily in the last few strokes and not following the physiological curve of the lens can result in the posterior plate being breached and a posterior capsular rent being created in the mid-peripheral posterior capsule. Needless to say, the large and hard nucleus requires dangerously high energy to tackle the cataract, making this technique redundant for tackling supra-hard cataracts.

Stop and Chop

This technique again entails making one initial trench and then switching over to the more energy efficient chopping. Thus, it carries all the demerits of DCN.

Direct Chop

Logically, a direct chop would be the most ideal technique to emulsify these hard nuclei. But due to their rock hard nature and large volumes, certain factors have to be taken into consideration. Firstly, if employing the peripheral chop, displacement of the large hard nucleus to allow the chopper to gain access to the peripheral nucleus entails severe stress transmission to the zonules and the capsular bag. In contrast, the central chop causes the same zonulocapsular stress at the time of physically separating the two halves of the big nucleus during the first chop. It would be clear to the reader that out of all the techniques described herein, the central chop, with a few modifications, is best suited in cases of supra-hard brown cataracts. These modifications in instrumentation and technique will be discussed in the next paragraph.

Colonel Parihar's Paracentral chopping and hydrofloat Nucleotomy

The basis of this technique is in the anatomical fact that the paracentral part of these supra-hard nuclei is relatively less bulky and lass hard. Thus they are more amenable to chopping. The chopper we employ as a routine is a 2 mm long ice-axe chopper which is sharp at both the surfaces. This allows us to move both centrally and peripherally once the chopper is buried in the paracentral area.

The preferred phaco tip is a 0° tip which provides maximal and strongest hold (we do not require any cutting here). Add to this the benefit of less chance of puncturing the posterior plate while emulsifying it (described below), zero degree scores over the 30° or the 15° tip as these tip do not have as good a hold until more power is used to bury their full bevels into the nuclear material, thus spending more energy.

In the initial step of this technique, whatever little cortical matter there is, must be removed to provide space for maneuverability which is at a premium in such cases. This makes the central, hard, bulky nucleus float on a cushion of water between the posterior capsule and the posterior surface of the nucleus.

The phaco probe with the 0° tip is buried into the central nucleus with a burst of US energy. Thereafter, the direction of the probe is made tangential to the nuclear surface. In this manner, after getting an initial good hold, the central dense nucleus is circumvented and the paracentral less dense nucleus is invaded. After moving the tip in this

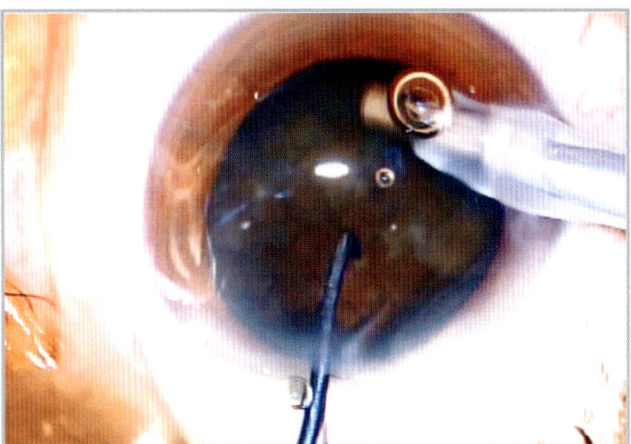

Fig. 29.6: Supra hard brown cataract: Superficial cortical clearing

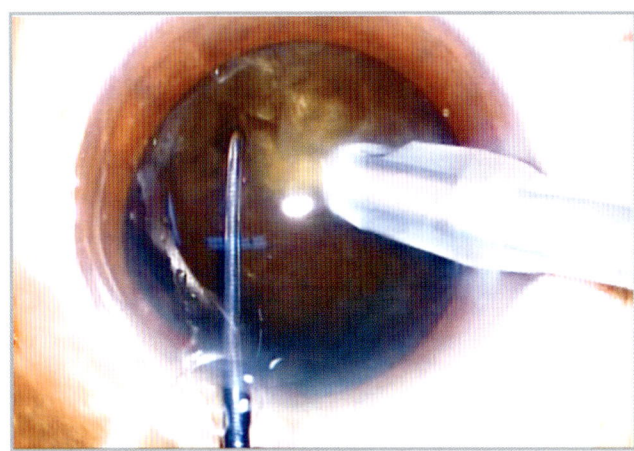

Fig. 29.7: Supra hard brown cataract: Embedded phaco tip to commence para central chopping

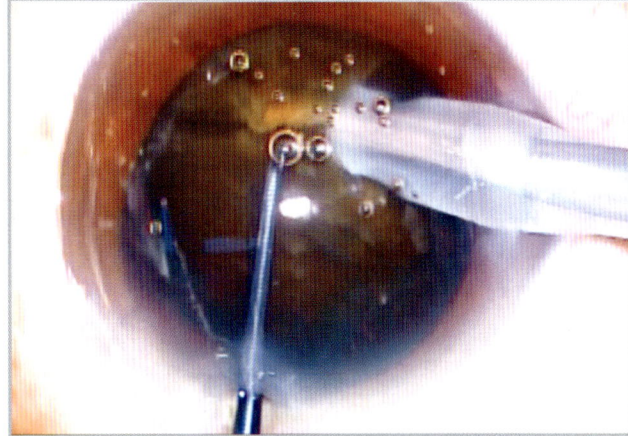

Fig. 29.8: Supra hard brown cataract: Commencement of para central chopping

paracentral direction for about 2 mm, foot pedal is brought to step II. Now the ice-axe chopper is placed in the paracentral nucleus, buried there, moved peripherally for 1 mm, when the outer cutting edge separates the outer (peripheral) perinucleus and then brought centrally towards the buried phaco tip in order to cut the inner (central) perinucleus. In this way, the rock hard central core is circumvented. This is the step to create a nucleotomy in the paranucleus.

This paracentral chop is repeated over to execute multiple nucleotomies and divide the paracentral nucleus into 6–10 parts.

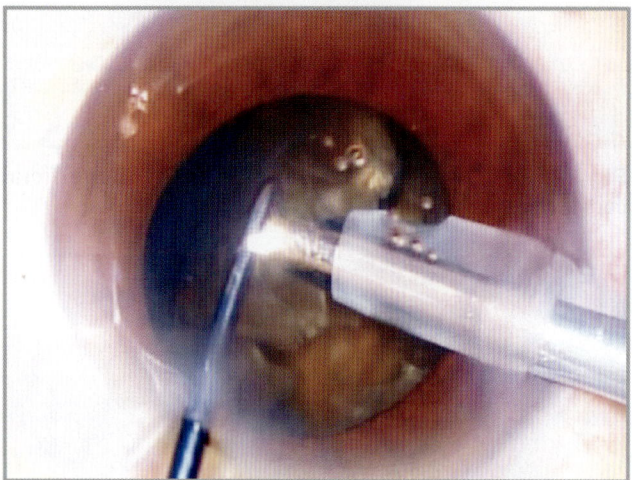

Fig. 29.9: Supra hard brown cataract: Tertiary nucleotomy

It is pertinent to point out that till this stage the central hard core has been left untouched. This is akin to tackling and attacking the weak and poorly defended areas of your adversary in a battle, rather than exhausting yourself tackling a strong line of defence. As the strong line of defence becomes restless in anticipation of the attack and careless with the passage of time, so also the supra-hard nucleus sheds some of its previous hardness due to being bathed continuously in the irrigating fluid. Now that the paranucleus has been divided, the central hard core is tackled by repeated chops and phacoemulsification.

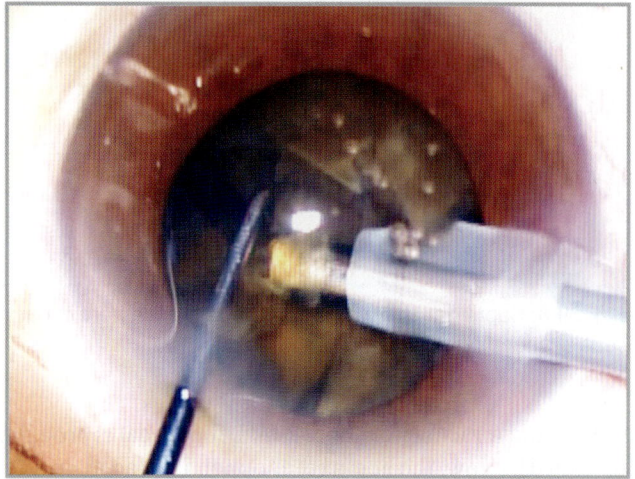

Fig. 29.10: Supra hard brown cataract: Debulking of core nucleus

Once the central core is gone, we are left with multiple paranuclear pieces, all joined at the posterior plate. At this stage, these paranuclear fragments are emulsified one by one in the bag after bringing them to the centre. Here, first the inner fibers of the paranucleus are emulsified in order to debulk the paranuclear piece without disturbing the smooth outer surface of the piece. Doing otherwise would cause the creation of sharp edges in pieces which because of their hardness and sharpness would pose a threat to the integrity of the posterior capsule. One by one these paranuclear pieces are tackled till we are left with a thick posterior plate.

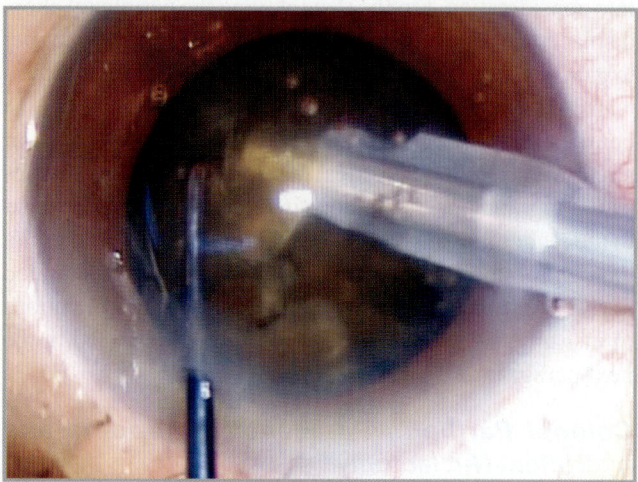

Fig. 29.11: Supra hard brown cataract: Fragment removal

This posterior plate requires special care as we have already removed the cortical matter and the posterior plate is separated from the posterior capsule and is floating over it on a thin cushion of fluid. For this, the posterior plate is held only with aspiration without any US energy and lifted up towards the cornea. This allows even more fluid to course posteriorly and push the posterior capsule (remember, it was already lax and floppy) back. Once the posterior plate is lifted, the central part is first emulsified with a burst of energy and once the central thick part is gone, the peripheral plate just crumples into the phaco tip. Maximal finesse and experience is required to tackle the last piece of this posterior plate. It is here, after putting in so much effort to remove the whole nucleus, that we have seen many surgeons lose their patience, resulting in complications. Readers are best advised to now discard the ice axe chopper and switch over to a Sinskey hook instead. Spend a few seconds in step I of the foot pedal (only irrigation) before venturing to step II. Your non dominant hand holding the Sinskey hook should always be in the centre. Use short minimal excursions of the foot pedal during step II and III to achieve the annihilation of the last piece.

The settings that are recommended to be employed with various machines for various steps described herein are appended in Tables 29.1 and 29.2.

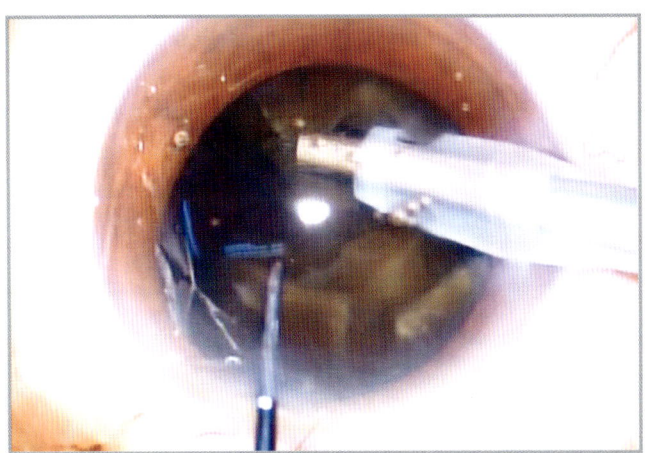

Fig. 29.12 : Supra hard brown cataract: Splitting of posterior plate

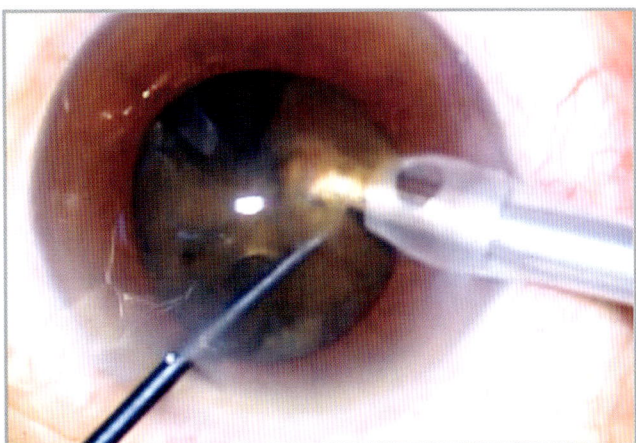

Fig. 29.13: Supra hard brown cataract : Posterior nuclear plate removal

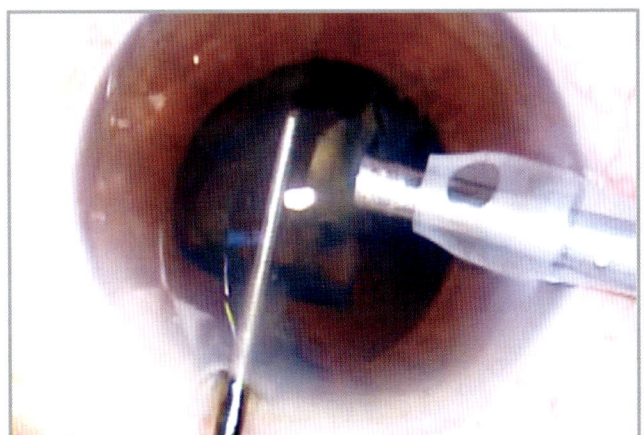

Fig. 29.14: Supra hard brown cataract: Removal of last fragment

IOL Implantation and Subsequent Steps

Once these preceding maneuvers have been executed perfectly, there is no variation in the following steps. As such a large amount of cortical matter has already been removed prior to the nucleotomy; thus a very small amount of cortical matter is left following hydrofloat nucleotomy. Hence, removal of such cortex demands a much less flow rate and vacuum as compared to the conventional chopping techniques. A zero degree tip can be employed to remove floating cortical matter under the irrigation/aspiration position. It is wise to attempt the removal of sub incisional lens matter by clockwise and anticlockwise pull and push by an I/A handpiece. This will facilitate a large chunk of cortex to be aspirated out in a single stroke. Stromal hydration by injecting BSS into the lip of corneal valve and the side port incision is a good option to achieve a self sealing wound. The whitish hue created at the sites of incisions generally disappears within six to seven hours.

The IOL implantation is done in the usual manner.

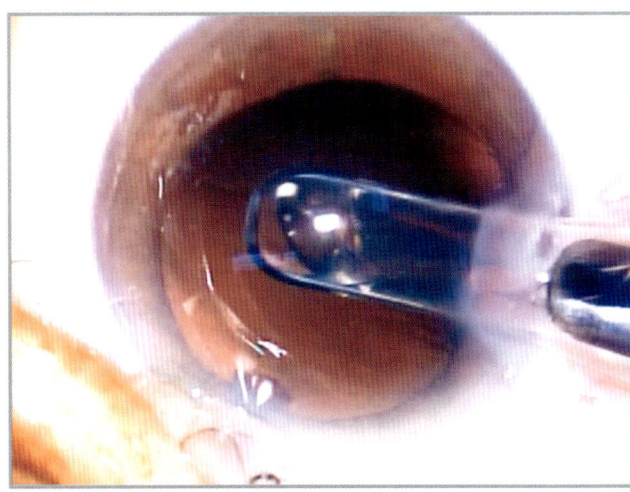

Fig. 29.15: Insertion of IOL implant

The post implant I/A has to be more meticulous in view of the copious amount of viscoelastic that would have invariably been employed.

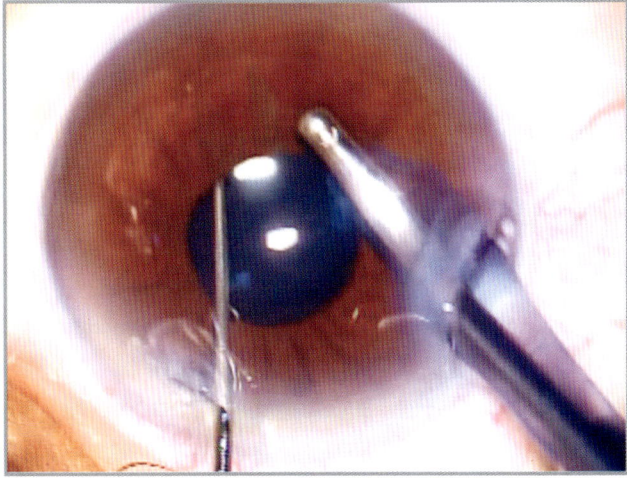

Fig. 29.16: Supra hard brown cataract: Post IOL implant wash

Table 29.1: Supra Hard Brown Cataract: Phacoemulsification machine settings at different stages of Colonel Parihar's Hydro floats rapid Chop technique: (Zero degree tip on Peristaltic Pump)

Steps/stages	Principal	Phaco settings	Flow (cc/min)	Vacuum	Continuous/ micro pulse
Baring Nucleus	Low flow and vacuum	00–05 %	10–15	60–100	Continuous/micro pulse
Nudging phaco tip into nucleus	Low flow and vacuum	25–35 (As per the density and size of core nucleus)	20–22	100–150	Continuous/micro pulse
Lifting nucleus	Moderate Vacuum	00	22–28	200–275	Position two, no US energy
Para Central Chopping	Moderate Vacuum	00–10	22–28	225–275	Position Two/Three,
Subsequent Multiple nucleotomy	Moderate Vacuum	00–10	22–28	200–275	Position Two/Three,
Debulking of core nucleus	Moderate Vacuum	25–30	22–28	200–275	Position Two/Three
Debulking of perinucleus and inner contents of nuclear fragments	Moderate Vacuum	20–30	22–28	200–275	Position Two/Three
Fragment removal	High flow and vacuum	20–30	24–26	200–275	Continuous/micro pulse
Removal of last fragment plate/epinucleus	Low flow and moderate vacuum	10–20	15–20	75–150	Continuous/micro pulse
Removing posterior	Low flow and high vacuum	00–05	10–15	100–125	Continuous/micro pulse/I/A Mode
Residual cortical wash	Moderate flow and high vacuum	I/A mode	26–34		300 – 400 Continuous
Posterior capsule polishing	Low flow and vacuum	I/A mode	5	10–20	Continuous

Table 29.2: Phacoemulsification machine settings at different stages of Colonel Parihar's Hydro floats rapid Chop technique: (Zero degree tip on Ventury Pump)

Steps/stages	Principal	Phaco settings	Vacuum	Continuous/Pulse
Baring Nucleus	Low vacuum	05%	45–60	Continuous/ micropulse
Nudging phaco tip into nucleus	Low vacuum	0–30 (As per hardness of nucleus)	100–125	Continuous/ micro pulse
Lifting nucleus	Moderate Vacuum	00	100–125	Position two, no US energy
Central Chopping	Moderate Vacuum	00–05	100–125	Position two, no US energy
Subsequent Multiple nucleotomy	Moderate Vacuum	00–05	60–75	Position two, no US energy
Fragment removal	Moderate to High vacuum	05–20	80–100	micro pulse
Removal of last fragment	Moderate vacuum	5–15	50–60	micro pulse
Removing posterior plate/	Moderate vacuum epinucleus	0–5/ US mode	60–80 on handpiece / 300–400 I/A	Continuous/ micro pulse
Residual cortical wash	High vacuum I/A mode	I/A mode	400-450	Continuous
Posterior capsule polishing	Low flow	I/A mode	0-5	Continuous

Other Pearls

(i) Use of Kelman tip or other bent tip is beneficial due to their energy transmission characteristics, but these are more liable to get blocked due to the consistency of the nuclear material. In addition, manipulating these bent tip to reach the paranucleus requires good manual dexterity and experience.

(ii) Torsional phacoemulsification offers a definite advantage in tackling such hard cataracts due to the multidimensional movement of the phaco tip. This and other non conventional movements of modern phaco machine tips have been dealt in detail elsewhere.

(iii) High vacuum and burst mode—While advantageous under ordinary circumstances, these phacodynamic parametres become particularly important in managing the dense cataract. The burst mode and high vacuum combine to provide a maximal grip. Inadequate holding power makes it more likely that the vertical chopper will dislodge pieces from the phaco tip, and make it more difficult to elevate large fragments out of the bag. Particularly with a brunescent lens, continuous mode cavitations core out the firm material surrounding the phaco tip. This facilitates sculpting but prevents the total tip occlusion by eroding the seal. Because high vacuum levels require a well-occluded phaco tip, the burst mode is particularly advantageous for the dense lens.

CONCLUSION

Ophthalmologists practicing in our country are routinely encountered with supra-hard brown black cataracts. In the past the viable options included extra-capsular cataract extraction or small incision manual cataract extraction in such cases. It has been the endeavour of the author to initiate the general ophthalmologist to move in graded and measured steps towards tackling these cases with phacoemulsification with the use of modern technology and a few modifications and variations from the conventional phacoemulsification techniques as we all have been taught. Col. Parihar's paracentral chop with hydrofloat offers a means to effectively tackle these cases with minimal energy and capsule-zonular stress. The basic principle is to first tackle the perinucleus with multiple nucleotomies, leaving the hard central core for later, by this time it sheds some of its hardness due to constant hydration, then debulking the central core, followed by emulsification of the paranuclear pieces. Last of all, it involves lifting the posterior plate away from the posterior capsule and emulsifying it. This technique if broken into the above described steps when implemented can make this complex surgery into an amalgamation of small simple steps, enabling each one of us to tackle these monsters with ease.

REFERENCES

1. Heyworth P, Thompson GM, Tabandeh H, McGuigan S. The relationship between clinical classification of cataract and lens hardness. Eye. 1993, 7 (Pt 6):726–30.

2. Hu C, Zhang X, Hui Y. The nuclear hardness and associated factors of age-related cataract. Zhonghua Yan Ke Za Zhi. 2000 Sep, 36(5):337–40. Chinese.

3. Huang CC, Ameri H, Deboer C, Rowley AP, Xu X, Sun L, Wang SH, Humayun MS, Shung KK. Evaluation of lens hardness in cataract surgery using high-frequency ultrasonic parametres in vitro. Ultrasound Med Biol. 2007 Oct, 33(10): 1609–16. Epub 2007 Jul 6.

4. Huang CC, Chen R, Tsui PH, Zhou Q, Humayun MS, Shung K. Measurements of attenuation coefficient for evaluating the hardness of a cataract lens by a high-frequency ultrasonic needle transducer. Phys Med Biol. 2009 Oct 7; 54(19): 5981–94. Epub 2009 Sep 17.

5. Huang CC, Zhou Q, Ameri H, Wu da W, Sun L, Wang SH, Humayun MS, Shung KK. Determining the acoustic properties of the lens using a high-frequency ultrasonic needle transducer. Ultrasound Med Biol. 2007 Dec, 33(12):1971–7. Epub 2007 Jul 30.

6. Laudañska-Olszewska I, Synder A, Wesotek-Czernik A, Omulecki W. Comparison of efficacy and safety of cataract phacoemulsification in patients with different degree of nuclear sclerosis. Klin Oczna. 2008, 110(4–6):172–5. Polish.

7. Wang X, Zhou L, Huang Y. Clinical significance of accumulated energy complex parametre in phacoemulsification. Zhonghua Yan Ke Za Zhi. 2002 Oct, 38(10):610–3. Chinese.

8. Chercotã V. 20 rules for hard nucleus phacoemulsification. Oftalmologia. 2005, 49(1):6–7. Review. Romanian.

9. Kim HK. Decrease and conquer: Phacoemulsification technique for hard nucleus cataracts. J Cataract Refract Surg. 2009 Oct, 35(10):1665–70

10. Vanathi M, Vajpayee RB, Tandon R, Titiyal JS, Gupta V. Crater-and-chop technique for phacoemulsification of hard cataracts. J Cataract Refract Surg. 2001 May, 27(5):659–61

11. Li SW, Xie LX, Song ZH, Meng L, Jiang J. Peripheral radial chop technique for phacoemulsification of hard cataracts. Chin Med J (Engl). 2007 Feb 20, 120(4):284–6

12. Cataract phacoemulsification techniques: "divide and conquer" versus "stop and chop"—comparative evaluation of operation course and early results. Mierzejewski A, Kałuzny JJ, B, Eliks I.Klin Oczna. 2004, 106(4–5): 612–7. Polish.

13. Zeng M, Liu X, Zhang X, Xia Y, Liu Y, Yuan Z, Liu Y.A comparative study of non-chopping rotation and axial rotation versus quick chop phacoemulsification techniques. Ophthalmic Surg Lasers Imaging. 2009 May-Jun, 40(3): 222–31.

14. Ma S, Liang N, Wang S. Combining application burst and occlude mode in the treatment of hard nucleus cataract during phacoemulsification. Yan Ke Xue Bao. 2003 Jun,19(2): 101–3. Chinese.

15. Zeng M, Liu X, Liu Y, Xia Y, Luo L, Yuan Z, Zeng Y, Liu Y. Torsional ultrasound modality for hard nucleus phacoemulsification cataract extraction. Br J Ophthalmol. 2008 Aug, 92(8):1092–6. Epub 2008 Jun 20

16. Akaishi L, Silva RV. Performance evaluation of NeoSoniX technology in cataract surgery. Arq Bras Oftalmol. 2006 May-Jun, 69(3):389–93. Portuguese.

17. Vasavada AR, Raj SM, Lee YC. NeoSoniX ultrasound versus ultrasound alone for phacoemulsification: randomised clinical trial. J Cataract Refract Surg. 2004 Nov, 30(11):2332–5.

18. Jirásková N, Kadlecová J, Rozsíval P, Nekolová J, Pozlerova J, Dúbravská Z. Comparison of the effect of AquaLase and NeoSoniX phacoemulsification on the corneal endothelium. J Cataract Refract Surg. 2008 Mar, 34(3):377–82.

19. Assaf A, El-Moatassem Kotb AM. Feasibility of bimanual microincision phacoemulsification in hard cataracts. Eye. 2007 Jun, 21(6):807–11. Epub 2006 May 5.

20. Baykara M, Ercan I, Ozcetin H. Microincisional cataract surgery (MICS) with pulse and burst modes. Eur J Ophthalmol. 2006 Nov-Dec, 16(6):804–8.

21. Liu Y, Jiang Y, Wu M, Liu Y, Zhang T. Bimanual microincision phacoemulsification in treating hard cataracts using different power modes. Clin Experiment Ophthalmol. 2008 Jul, 36(5): 426–30.

23. Pong JC, Lai JS. Managing the hard posterior polar cataract. J Cataract Refract Surg. 2008 Apr, 34(4):530, author reply 530–1.

24. Chee SP. Management of the hard posterior polar cataract. J Cataract Refract Surg. 2007 Sep; 33(9):1509–14.

25. Kaushik S, Ram J, Brar GS, Bandyopadhyay S. Comparison of the thermal effect on clear corneal incisions during phacoemulsification with different generation machines. Ophthalmic Surg Lasers Imaging. 2004 Sep-Oct, 35(5): 364–70.

26. Stumpf S, Nosé W. Endothelial damage after planned extracapsular cataract extraction and phacoemulsification of hard cataracts. Arq Bras Oftalmol. 2006 Jul-Aug, 69(4): 491–6. Portuguese.

27. Chiotoroiu S, Pandelescu M, Epure C, Stefaniu I. Comparative study of endothelial changes in cataract surgery with phacoemulsification technique. Oftalmologia. 2008; 52(1): 95–9. Romanian.

28. Tajunisah I, Reddy SC. Dropped nucleus following phacoemulsification cataract surgery. Med J Malaysia. 2007 Dec, 62(5):364–7.

29. Lai TY, Kwok AK, Yeung YS, Kwan KY, Woo DC, Yuen KS, Loo AV. Immediate pars plana vitrectomy for dislocated intravitreal lens fragments during cataract surgery. Eye. 2005 Nov, 19(11):1157–62.

30. Liu YZ, Jiang YZ, Liu YH, Wu MX. A preliminary report on bimanual microphacoemulsification. Zhonghua Yan Ke Za Zhi. 2004 May, 40(5):302–5. Chinese.

31. Bu J, Zou Y. Hard nucleus chopping technique for non-phacoemulsification in small-incision cataract surgery: two-knife chopping. Yan Ke Xue Bao. 2001 Jun, 17(2):93–5. Chinese.

32. Miyata K, Nagamoto T, Maruoka S, Tanabe T, Nakahara M, Amano S. Nucleus's Cataract Refract Surg. 2002 Sep, 28(9):1546–50.

33. Zhu S, Wu X, Xu B. Hard nucleus cataract extraction by phacoemulsification with intraocular lens implantation. Zhonghua Yan Ke Za Zhi. 1998 Mar, 34(2):90–2. Chinese.

34. Li Z, He S, Wang F. Effect of high-vacuum-manual-chop technique in phacoemulsification. Zhonghua Yan Ke Za Zhi. 2001 May, 37(3):185–7. Chinese.

35. Song X, Shi Y, Zhu X, Chai J.The application of chopping method for phacoemulsification of hard nucleus cataract. Zhonghua Yan Ke Za Zhi. 1999 Mar, 35(2):88–90. Chinese.

36. Dada VK, Sharma N, Dada T, Vajpayee RB Sinus fracture—phacoemulsification technique for dense cataracts. Ophthalmic Surg Lasers. 2001 Nov-Dec, 32(6):503–4.

37. Shastri L, Vasavada A. Phacoemulsification in Indian eyes with pseudoexfoliation syndrome. J Cataract Refract Surg. 2001 Oct, 27(10):1629–37.

38. Vanathi M, Vajpayee RB, Tandon R, Titiyal JS, Gupta V. Crater-and-chop technique for phacoemulsification of hard cataracts. J Cataract Refract Surg. 2001 May, 27(5):659–61.

39. Zetterström C, Laurell CG. Comparison of endothelial cell loss and phacoemulsification energy during endocapsular phacoemulsification surgery. J Cataract Refract Surg. 1995 Jan, 21(1):55–8.

30

Phacoemulsification Surgery in a very Soft Cataract

Col JKS Parihar SM, VSM and Surg Lt Cdr AS Parihar

INTRODUCTION

Surgical management of cataract has witnessed unbelievable transformation and revolution both in terms of the surgical technique as well as in respect to the time frame for surgical intervention in the recent past. Even modern phaco surgeons and patients advocate early surgical intervention. In true sense, modern cataract surgical techniques have been considered as a Kerato lenticular refractive procedure rather than management of cataract alone. This changing pattern is also responsible for the rising occurrence of handling soft cataract in general.

The management of a very soft cataract is a much more difficult proposition as compared to the management of hard cataract due to constraints of nucleotomy, an obvious risk of higher incidence of Intraoperative complications as well as of posterior capsular thickening.

We have analysed various aspects of management of very soft cataract to minimise intraoperative risk, complications and improve the ultimate outcome.

CLASSIFICATION

Lens opacities classification system (LOCS III), 1993 is used for grading the cataract. It grades the lens opacity in steps of 0.1 degree from 0.1 to 5.9. However soft cataract may have a wide spectrum of clinical presentations and morphological patterns owing to the age of the patient as well as based on the aetiology of cataract. An early cataract due to the presence of lenticular opacities which involve the posterior pole is likely to produce much more visual symptoms. Hence, such cataract may require surgical intervention at an early stage of cataract. Common occurrences of soft cataract are as follows:

(i) Congenital and developmental cataract
(ii) Rosette-shaped traumatic cataract
(iii) Posterior subcapsular cataract
(iv) Lenticular sclerosis (Grade One/Two)
(v) Early onset complicated cataract
(vi) Clear lens extraction for high refractive errors

Posterior Subcapsular cataracts (PSC), early lenticular sclerosis and complicated cataracts in a relatively younger age group of patients are the leading causes of soft cataract.

APPLIED ANATOMY OF VERY SOFT CATARACT

Anatomical configuration of a very soft cataract will vary in accordance to the aetiology of cataract. Posterior Subcapsular opacities reveal features, like sheets of vacuoles, water clefts, coronary flakes, focal dots, retro dots, or fibre folds. Traumatic cataract will have intra lamellar rosette pattern whereas soft sclerotic cataract will have a central circular well-circumscribed pale amber coloured core nucleus. Early onset and juvenile cataract are invariably associated with thin, fragile, and adhered posterior capsule and hence, the surgeon needs to be highly vigilant while performing a rhexis and hydroprocedure so as to avoid tear or extension of rhexis. Association of posterior polar cataract has been seen in around 10–15% of the cases of posterior subcapsular cataract. Hence, extreme care and a meticulous approach is an essential need while conducting hydroprocedures in these cases to avoid inadvertent posterior capsular rupture during hydroprocedure.

Very soft cataract in a pre senile or senile age group is associated with a small nucleus surrounded with a thick and well-adhered perinuclear cortical sheet. Peripheral cortex is also, by and large, found to be sticky and that to without any demarcation and desired cleavage plane during Hydroprocedure. Such anatomical configuration poses significant intraoperative constraints while handling very soft cataract. A clearly visible red glow, softness of nucleus and presence of a sticky cortex invariably lead to inadvertent and an undesirable deep pierce by the phaco tip into the lens substance that may result in an unpleasant consequence of posterior capsular rent.

The exact grading of nuclear density should be assessed after hydroprocdeure since most of nucleus except the very soft and the nonsclerotic type in consistency appear much harder after the hydroprocedure.

PREOPERATIVE EVALUATION OF SOFT CATARACT

Needless to stress the significance of a meticulous and thorough slit lamp evaluation, both pre and post mydriasis status is of immense value in planning the surgical technique as well as helps to predict and to be prepared to combat intraoperative constraints. Post mydriasis pupillary diameter, configuration of cortex, size, and consistency of nucleus and last but not the least the status of posterior capsule can be ascertained by a slit lamp examination. Hence, a meticulous pre and per-operative evaluation of the core nucleus is very crucial and essential.

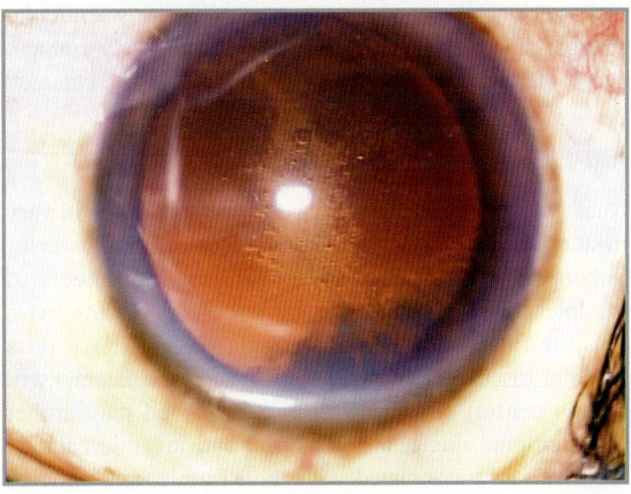

Fig. 30.1: Soft cataract: Thin yet dense sheet of post sub-capsular cataract produces significant visual disturbances due to its proximity to the nodal point

SURGICAL MANAGEMENT OF ULTRA SOFT (VERY SOFT) CATARACT

Selection of Phacoemulsifier System

1. **Aqualase system:** Theoretically, aqualase system is the best option to handle an ultra soft cataract. A hybrid pre-chop on this system is a much more efficient, rapid and a very safe procedure particularly in cases of soft nuclei. However, limited access to the system and its limitations to use in any other type of cataract other than soft cataract remains a practical hurdle.
2. **Torsional or linear system:** Though newer generation advanced linear phacoemulsifier system

enjoys excellent control on fluid dynamics, surge control and solid rock chamber stability, torsional system continues to carry unparalleled precedence over any other kind of phacoemulsifier system irrespective of the type of cataract. However, every surgeon will have his own settings and techniques.

Selection of Nucleotomy Technique for Soft Cataract

As stated earlier, conventional DCN or chopping techniques are not suitable for a very soft cataract. The titration of ultrasonic energy corresponding to the density of lens nucleus as well as precise assessment of the depth of the sculpting is very difficult and unpredictable in the presence of a very soft cataract. It is not possible to attain classical chopping due to an inability to achieve intra nuclear cleavage within the core of the nucleus due to its soft configuration. Hence, flip chip, hybrid nucleotomy technique, phacoaspiration methods or torsional cart wheel method adopted by author may be a suitable option.

Author's Technique

Anaesthesia

Modern phacoemulsification surgery techniques are precise, quick, and much safer as compared to the conventional phacotechniques. It is better to choose peribulbar or topical anaesthesia technique, which should be based on the surgeon's own preference and the ultimate surgical comfort at both the recipient and the surgeon's end. An experienced surgeon can handle any cataract under topical anaesthesia. We prefer to manage any kind of soft cataract under topical anaesthesia.

Incision

Classical phaco incisions like scleral tunnel or clear corneal incisions may be adopted. Author prefers to go ahead with

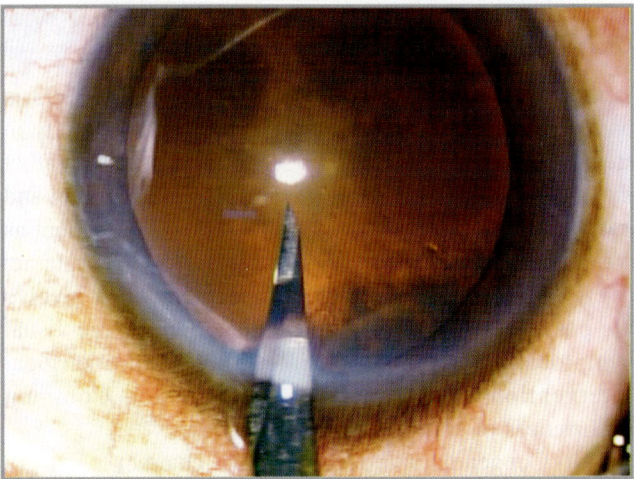

Fig. 30.2: Thin post subcapsular ultra soft cataract: Side port incision

a clear corneal temporal incision for its precision, safety, and quicker application. We recommend constructing two identical incisions as side ports and one of them can be converted into the main incision once the initial steps like Rhexis and hydroprocedures are complete. These two side port incisions provide an excellent water tight chamber while performing rhexis and hydroprocedures. In case bimanual phacoaspiration is being considered while relying upon the softness of the nucleus, it may be continued with these identical incisions.

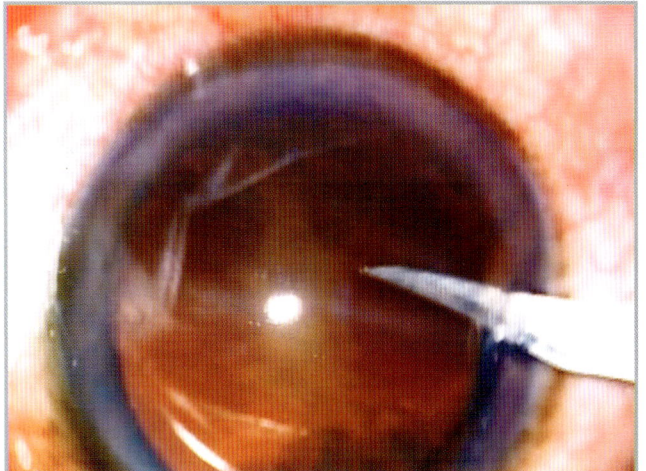

Fig. 30.3: Soft cataract: Initial entry for subsequent temporal incision

Capsulorrhexis

A large rhexis of around 6 mm provides an adequate access to desired nucleus manipulation in cases of soft cataract where nucleus needs to be pulled out of the bag with the help of vacuum assistance, rotated, fragmented, and aspirated. Ideally, the capsulorrhexis should not be larger than 5 to 5.5 mm in size. The use of needle cystitome or rhexis forceps is exclusively a surgeon's own preference. In our view, rhexis forceps enjoy a

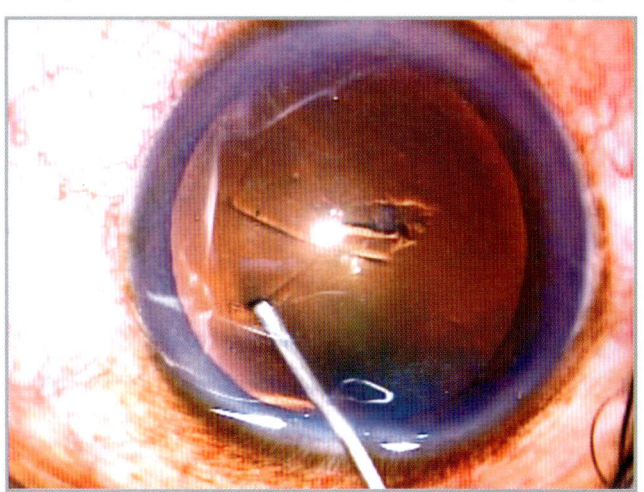

Fig. 30.4: Ultra soft cataract: Rhexis

superiority over needles in certain situations like a thin and fragile capsule especially in younger patients where forceps provide a better control as compared to the linear movements by a needle.

Hydroprocedures

(a) **Hydrodissection:** Meticulous hydroprocedures with utmost care remain the single most and crucial steps in cases of soft cataracts associated with posterior capsular pathologies like posterior polar cataract, posterior subcapsular, rosette-shaped traumatic cataract or early nuclear sclerotic type cataracts. Multisequential, repeated, and very slow cortical cleaving hydrodissection extending just ahead of the periphery of posterior capsule is very much desirable until the inside out reverse hydro-delineation is not completed. A very small quantity of just 0.5–1 ml of fluid should be introduced in two quadrants to separate the capsule from the cortex. Rapid injection of fluid should be avoided

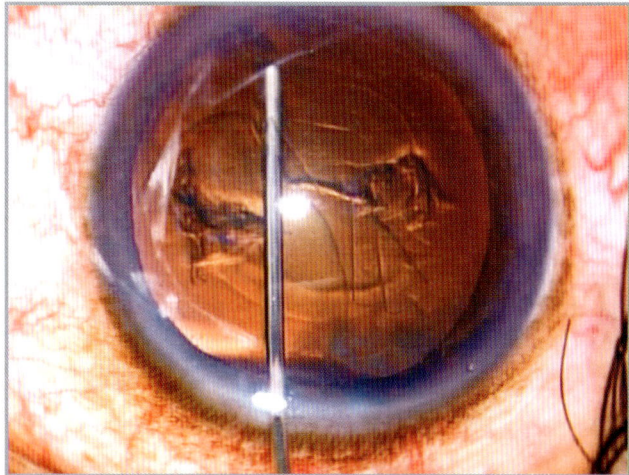

Fig. 30.5: Hydrodissection in cases of very soft posterior subcapsular cataract

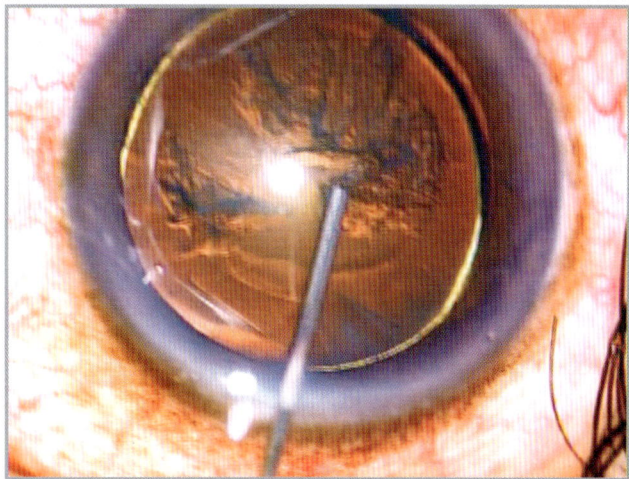

Fig. 30.6: Hydrodissection in cases of posterior subcapsular cataract: Golden ring appearance

since it may trigger off a hydraulic rupture of the posterior capsule. An ideal and complete delineation especially in cases of soft cataract will terminate with the appearance of multiple golden rings.

Subsequent injection of fluid will provide multiple peri and epinuclear bowl or cushions that will act as a mechanical cushion to protect the posterior capsule during subsequent manoeuvres. Once hydroprocedure is being completed, infiltration of sodium hyaluranate at the same plane into the cortex will augment the cushion effect around the core nucleus and provide better access to the intraoperative site and protection to the posterior capsule.

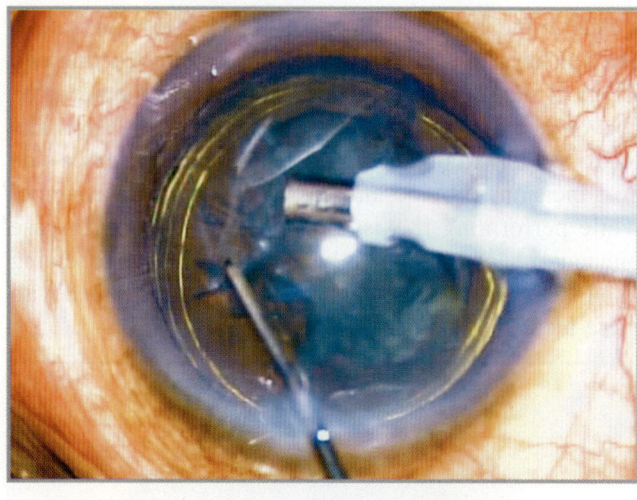

(a)

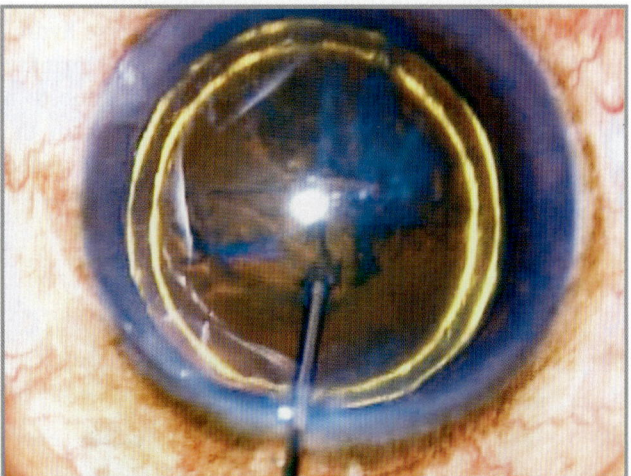

Fig. 30.7: Sequential hydrodelineation in cases of posterior subcapsular cataract: Multiple golden ring appearance

Nucleus Management (Figs 30.9a to g)

Excellent hydroprocedures is the backbone of subsequent nuclear management. Conventional nucleotomy techniques like DCN, different chopping methods and Flip and Chip are based on the principle of nuclear fragmentation under the cushion of epinucleus and cortical matter. Classical Divide and Conquer or Central Chopping is practically impossible to perform in case of a soft nucleus of less than Grade two in consistency. In our view, the ideal approach would remain Phacoaspiration, Cartwheel, or hybrid technique in these situations. Application of the least energy along with moderate flow and vacuum settings are an ideal combination to handle very soft or Ultra soft cataract. A word of extreme caution should be kept in mind of a higher risk of posterior capsular rent or direct injury to the capsule due to ultrasonic energy in soft cataracts.

While dealing with specific situations like a posterior plaque, dense posterior subcapsular sheet or fibrosed capsule in traumatic, yet soft cataract, is being managed so as to minimise the risk of posterior capsular rent or direct injury to the capsule due to ultrasonic energy in soft cataracts.

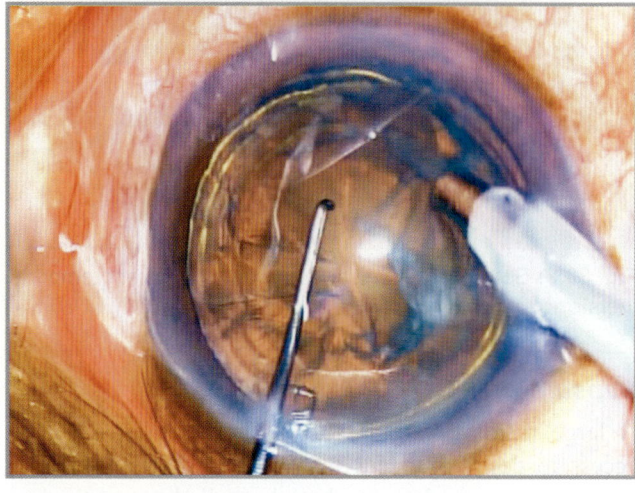

(b)

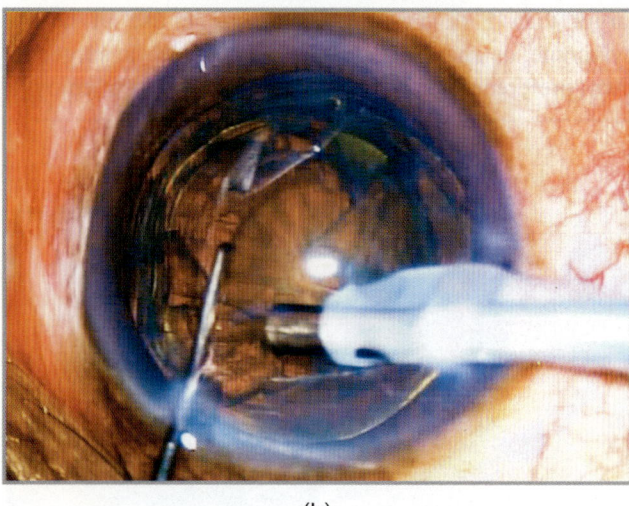

(b)

Fig. 30.8: (a) Post subcapsular cataract: Cortical clearing, (b) Post subcapsular cataract: Cortical clearing and (c) Post subcapsular cataract: Cortical clearing

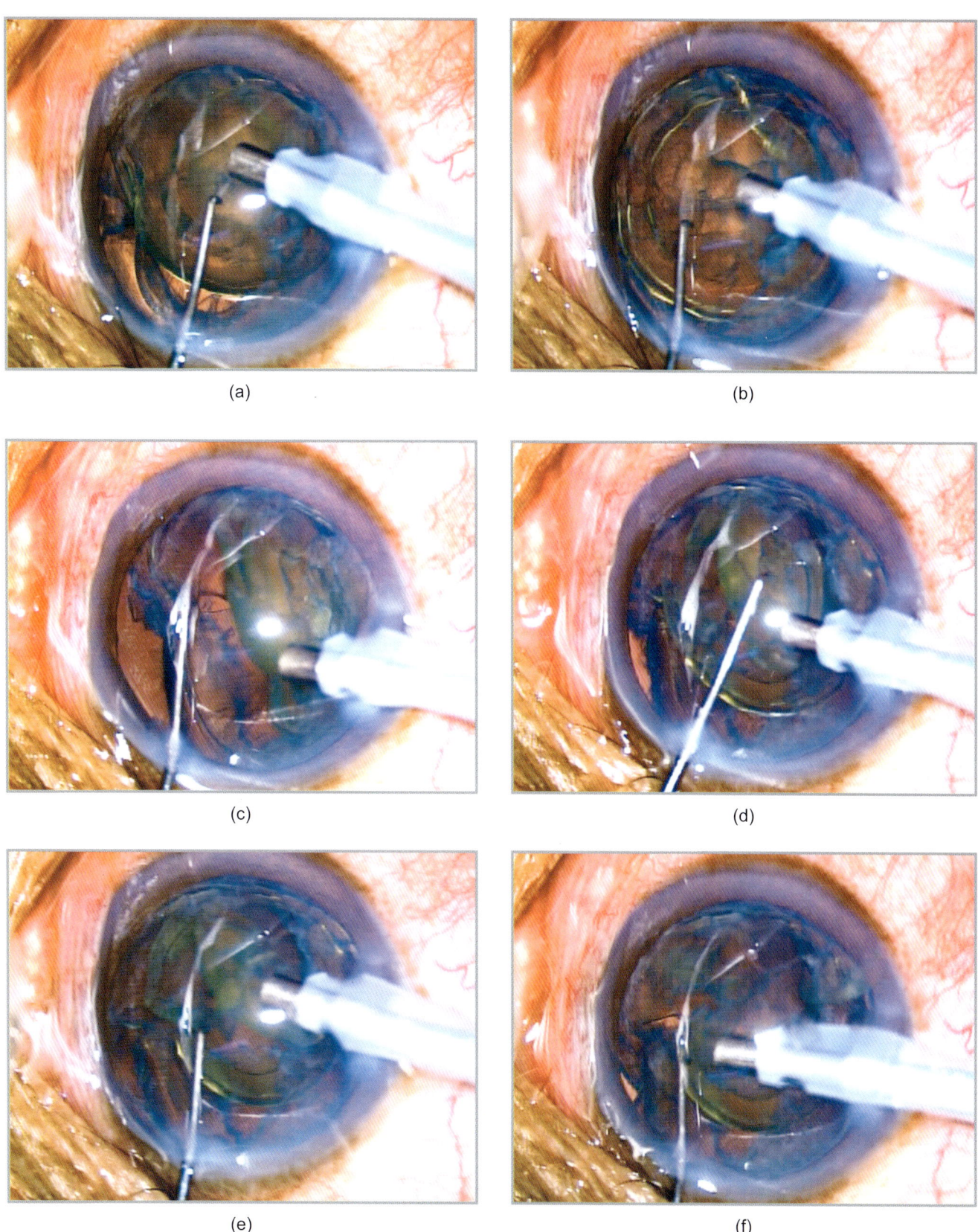

Fig. 30.9: (a) Post subcapsular cataract: Vacuum assisted pulling of the nucleus, (b) Post subcapsular cataract: Vacuum assisted pulling of the nucleus, (c) Nucleus management in posterior subcapsular cataract (Removal of central core nucleus), (d) Nucleus management in posterior subcapsular cataract (Removal of central core nucleus), (e) Nucleus management in posterior subcapsular cataract (Removal of central core nucleus) and (f) Nucleus management in posterior subcapsular cataract (Removal of central core nucleus)

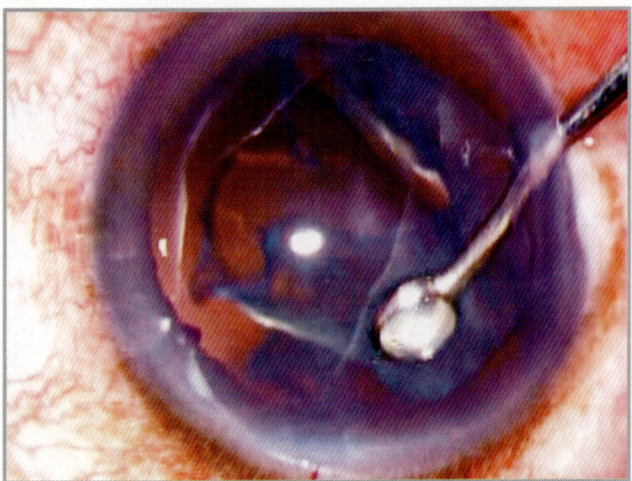

Fig. 30.9(g): Separation of posterior plate from the fornices of the capsular bag

We prefer to use zero degree tip in case of soft cataracts since they carry least risk of an inadvertent mechanical injury to the posterior capsule. Most of the ultra soft cataracts can be managed comfortably by Phacoaspiration on bimanual or co axial irrigation aspiration mode while maintaining 250 to 350 mmHG aspiration and 28 to 30ml/mt flow rate on peristaltic system or 150 to 200 mmHg for a Ventury system.

In case of more than grade one and less than grade two of nucleus, 0 to 5 % US energy on a zero degree tip with moderate vacuum settings of 150 to 225 mmHG is an ideal setting to hold and pull the nucleus out of the bag to be fragmented and aspirated out, subsequently.

Management of Epinuclear Shell (Fig. 30.9h to j)

Posterior plate along with residual cortical matter is protected until core nucleus is removed to ensure complete safety of the posterior capsule against any inadvertent mechanical injury. Author recommends low flow rate and aspiration rate at this stage.

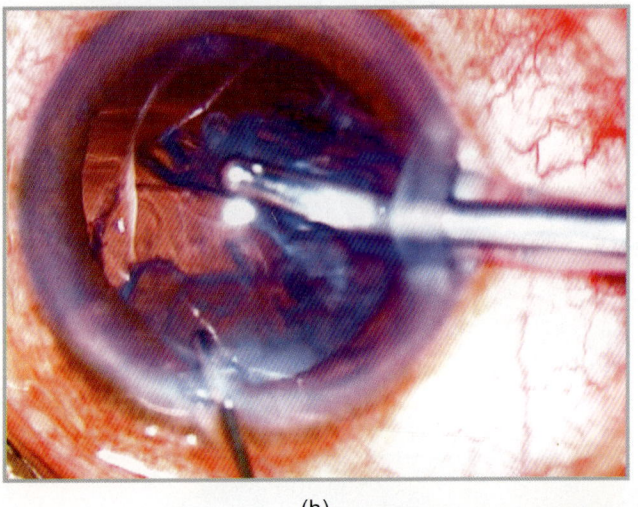

(h)

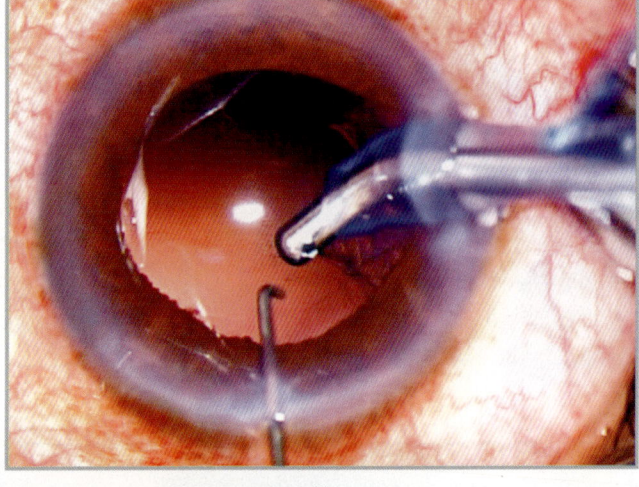

(i)

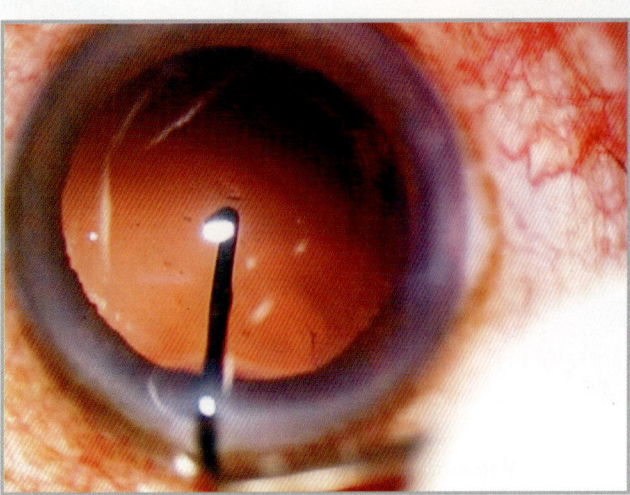

(j)

Fig. 30.9: (h) Post subcapsular cataract: I/A aspiration, (i) Post subcapsular cataract: Removal of sub-incisional cortex, (j) Post subcapsular cataract: Removal of densely adhered thin plaques on the posterior capsule

IOL Implantation

Single piece hydrophobic acrylic IOL implant remains our first preference for any kind of cataract. We have switched over to multifocal IOL implants in the recent past in all suitable soft cataracts since most of these cases belong to a younger age group and have shown gratifying results. However, if a PC tear is noticed, every effort is made to prevent the extension of the tear to minimise vitreous loss. Depending upon the site and extend of the rent, All PMMA IOL implantation in the ciliary sulcus or multi piece /Single piece acrylic IOL implantation over CTR may be considered following adequate vitrectomy to clear vitreous from the site of IOL insertion.

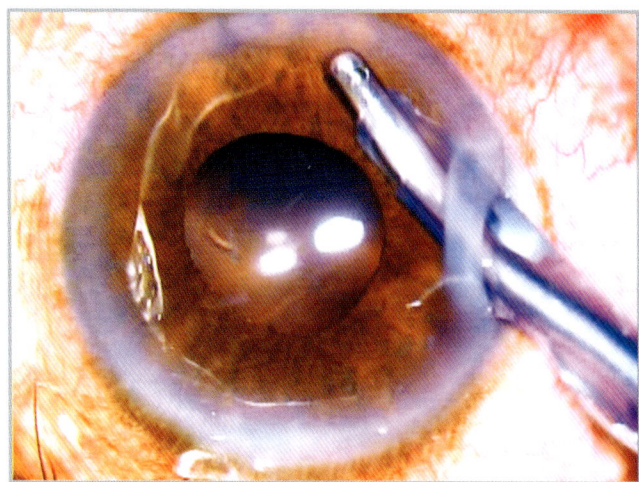

(a)

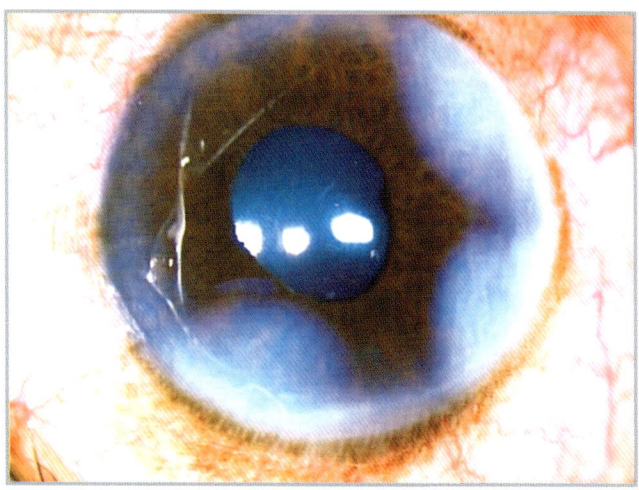

(b)

Fig. 30.10: (a) Post subcapsular cataract: Post IOL implant wash, (b) Post subcapsular cataract: Stromal hydration

PHACOASPIRATION

As described earlier, bimanual or coaxial Aspiration of ultrasoft cataract on I/A mode is the safest method to handle soft cataracts in younger individuals of less than 45 years of age. The author advocates bimanual Phacoaspiration

for its dexterity to irrigate cortical matter in any direction, flexibility to aspirate lens matter while maintaining a water tight chamber throughout the procedure.

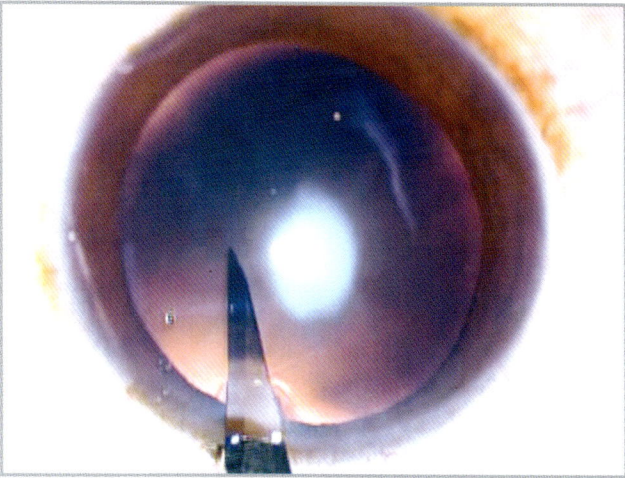

Fig. 30.11: Side port incision: Phacoaspiration

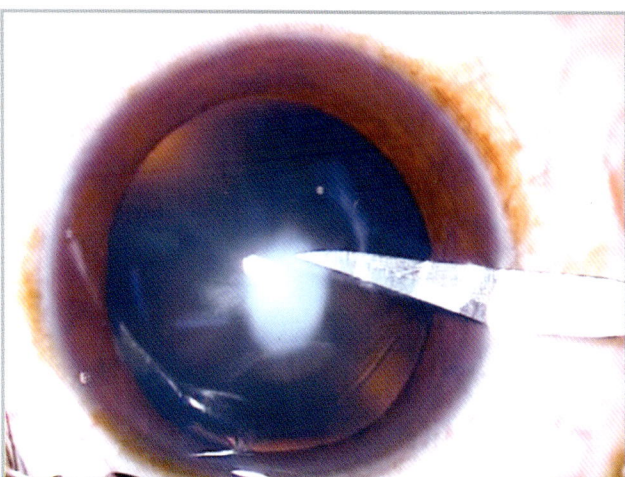

Fig. 30.12: Temporal incision: Phacoaspiration

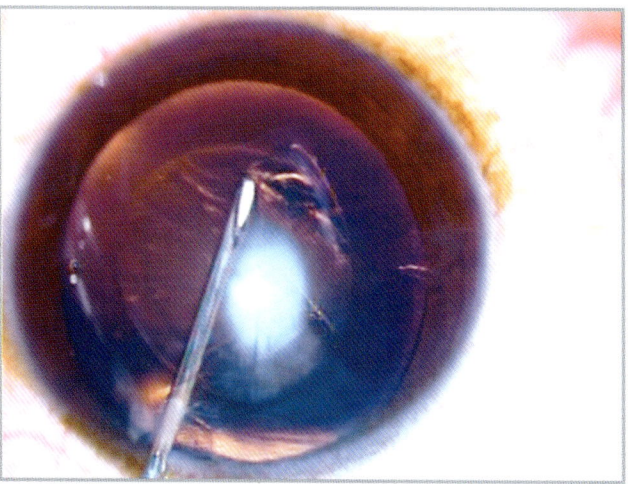

Fig. 30.13: Capsulorrhexis: Phacoaspiration

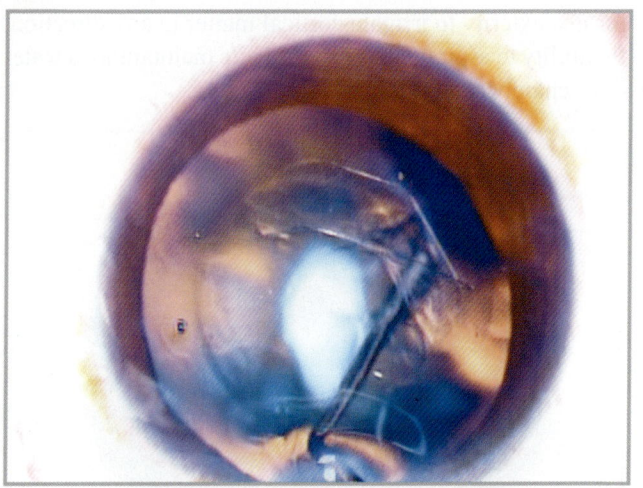

Fig. 30.14: Hydroprocedure: Phacoaspiration

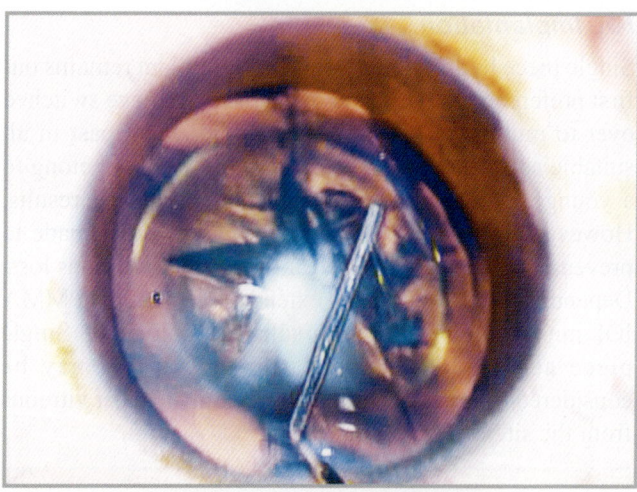

Fig. 30.15: Sequential hydrodelineation: Phacoaspiration

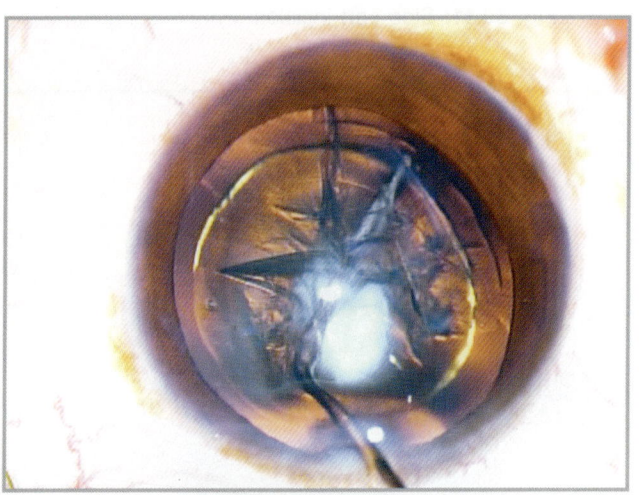

Fig. 30.16: Hydrodelineation of core nucleus: Phacoaspiration

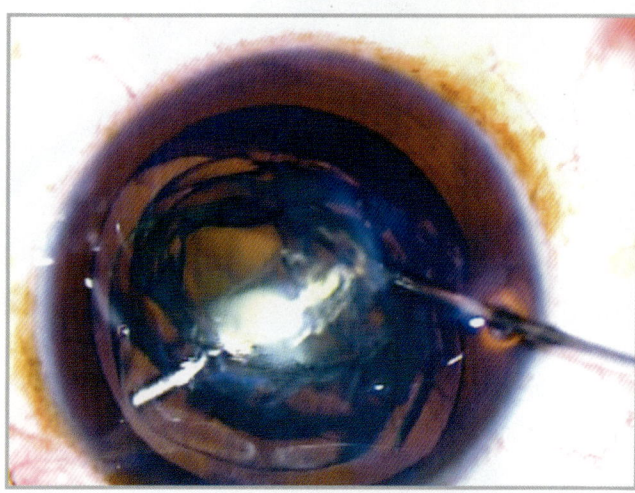

Fig. 30.17: Floating core nucleus following hydroprocedure: Phacoaspiration

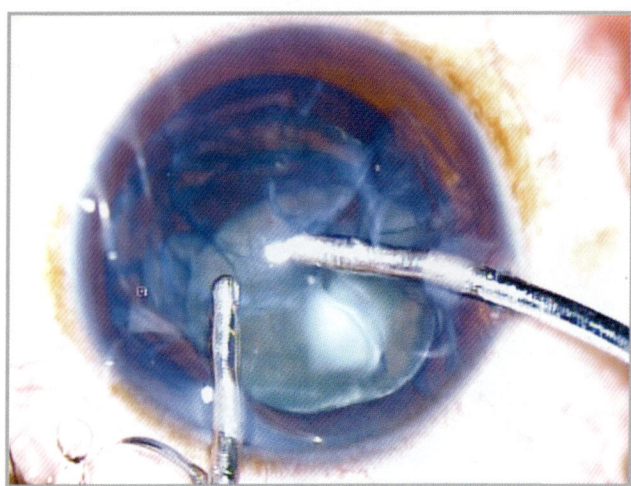

Fig. 30.18: Commencement of bimanual phacoaspiration of floating core nucleus

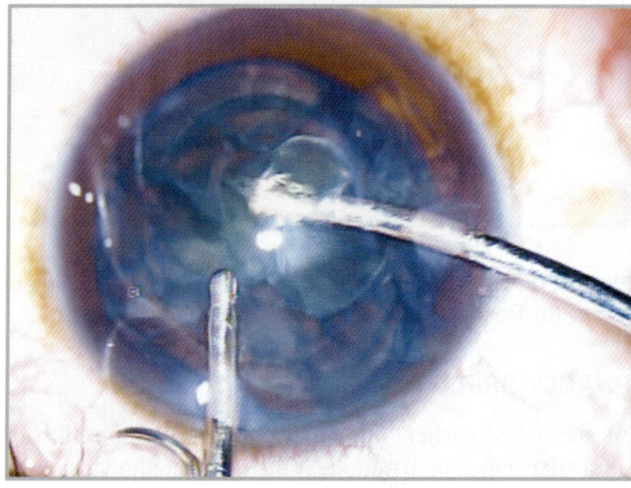

Fig. 30.19: Bimanual phacoaspiration is in progress

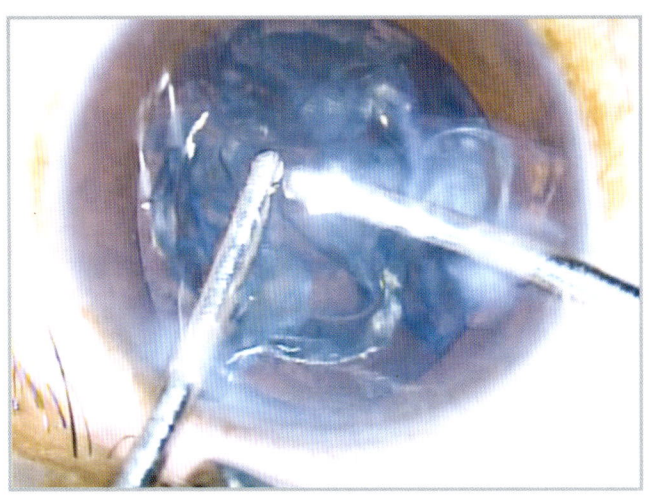

Fig. 30.20: Phacoaspiration of perinucleus and cortical plate

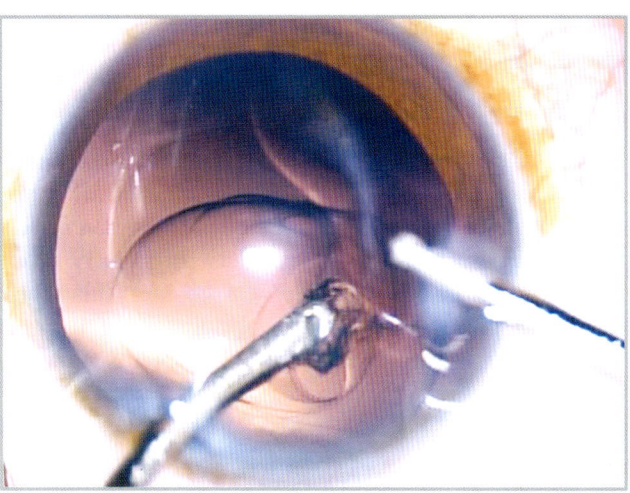

Fig. 30.21: Removal of subincisional cortex: Phacoaspiration

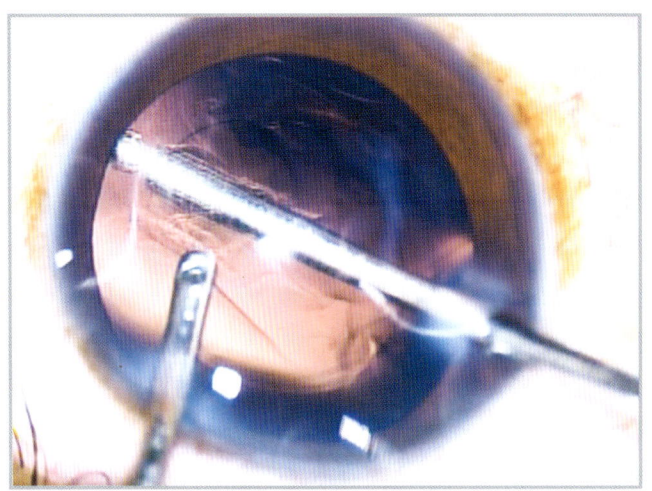

Fig. 30.22: Anterior capsular polishing: Phacoaspiration

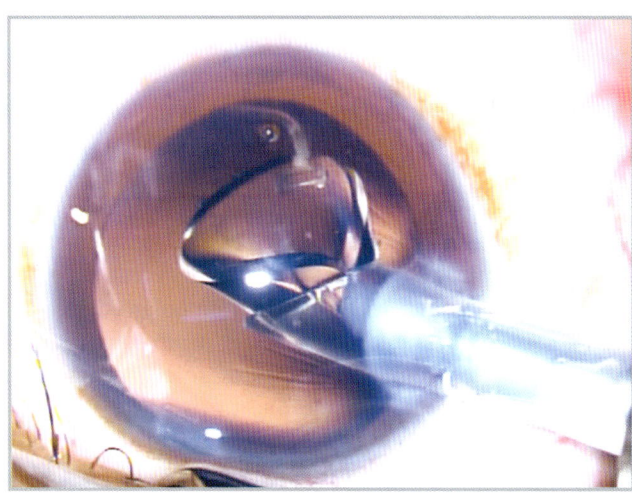

Fig. 30.23: Insertion of multifocal IOL implant in case of soft traumatic cataract

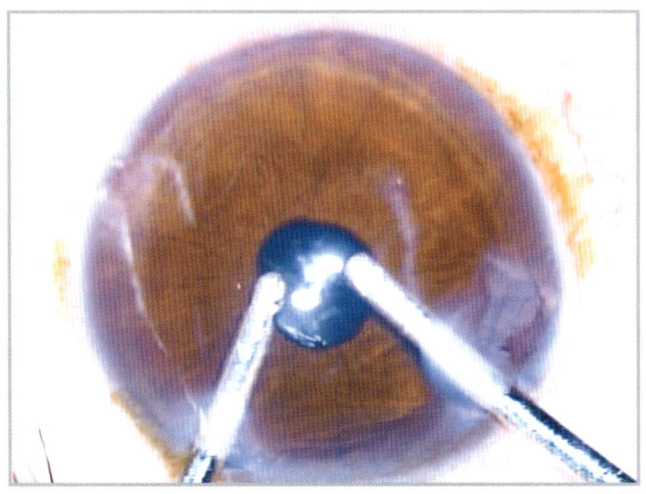

Fig. 30.24: Post IOL implant wash: Soft cataract

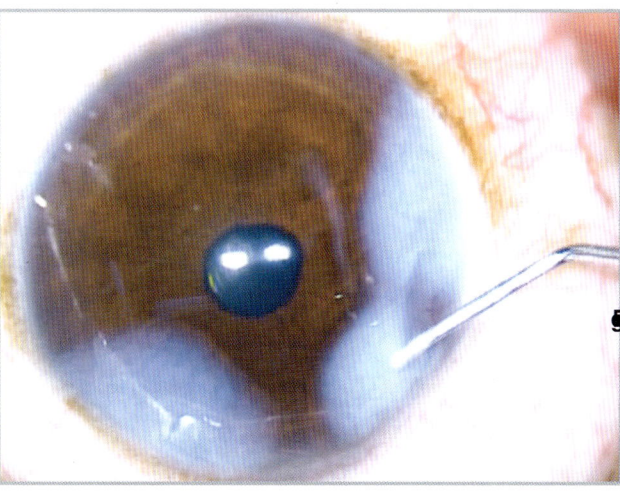

Fig. 30.25: Stromal hydration: In soft traumatic cataract

And above all, the risk of injury to the posterior capsule due to a vibrating phaco tip, which is inadvertently proximal in the presence of very soft cataract, can also be minimised. We recommend moderate machine settings like aspiration on 250 to 350 mmHG and flow Rate of 28 to 30 ml/mt on a peristaltic system or 150 to 200 mm for a Ventury system. In our view, slow and guarded aspiration is very crucial in cases of ultrasoft cataracts particularly in the presence of a posterior plaque, a thin subcapsular sheet or in cases of traumatic subcapsular cataract due to higher probabilities of inherent cortico posterior capsular adhesions.

INTRAOPERATIVE COMPLICATIONS/ OBSERVATIONS

Incidence of PCR in Ultra Soft Cataract

The incidence of PC rent in Ultra soft cataracts varies from 0.5 to 15 % according to the underlying pathology and its association with the posterior capsule. Undoubtedly, posterior polar cataract continue to remain a leading cause of posterior capsular rents in up to 15 to 20% cases despite all the precautions and modifications in the technique. Inherent and very dense adhesions and rather the conversion of the posterior pole of the capsule into a plaque can lead to a rent in good number of cases. Dense posterior rosette pattern traumatic cataract or congenial cataracts with posterior plaque follow posterior polar cataract in terms of a higher incidence of PCR in up to 8 to 10% cases. However, remaining types of soft cataracts like Posterior Subcapsular, Grade one to two Sclerosis and Traumatic or Congenial cataracts without any association with the posterior capsule are likely to have less than 1% of chances for intraoperative complications.

Advanced application of fluidics and newer hydro based phaco techniques have shown a significant decline in the incidence of PC rent in soft cataracts.

How to Prevent/Minimise the Risk of Posterior Capsule Rupture

Meticulous and cautious dealing of the posterior plaque, dense posterior subcapsular cataract during phacoemulsification may decrease intraoperative and postoperative complications and are likely to reveal substantially improved postoperative visual acuity.

Following tips may be highly beneficial while managing any kind of soft cataract with densely adhered posterior subcapsular sheets:

(i) Slow and gradual hydrodissection: Initially confined upto the periphery of the posterior capsule and away from the thickened and adhered posterior cataract.

(ii) Gentle deep core hydrodelineation maintaining inside out pattern of fluid waves; thereby leaving superficial and most posterior layers free from hydrodelineation.

(iii) Least ultrasound energy on the zero degree tip.

(iv) No sculpting, rather relying upon Phacoaspiration, flip and chip, Cartwheel movements, hybrid or onion peeling techniques of nucleus management. Chopping may be possible in limited and selected type of soft cataracts.

(v) Moderate aspiration /irrigation settings

POSTOPERATIVE COMPLICATIONS

(i) Mild to moderate uveitis 4–6%

(ii) Secondary glaucoma 4–5%

(iii) Macular oedema 12–16%

(iv) PCO: 30 to 40% after interval of two years

(v) Residual posterior capsule plaque postoperatively, which required neodymium: YAG laser capsulotomy: 12 to 15%.

RESULTS

Overall, visual outcome following phacoemulsification surgery in cases of very soft cataract is encouraging and gratifying. More than 95% patients are likely to regain visual acuity of 20/40 or more. Pre-existing conditions like nebular corneal opacities, chronic anterior uveitis, or retinal involvements such as diabetic retinopathy, ARMD or any surgical complications are major factors known to influence outcome.

CONCLUSION

Surgical management of very soft cataracts demands much more attention than handling hard cataracts of any grade. Meticulous attention towards phaco energy modulation and utmost care against inadvertent injury to the posterior capsule due to unprecedented softness of the nucleus is the key to success.

BIBLIOGRAPHY

1. Judy Y.F Ku, MBChBa, Christina N Grupcheva, Keratoglobus and posterior subcapsular cataract: Surgical considerations and in vivo microstructural analysis Arch Ophthalmol May 2003.

2. R. C. Drews. Posterior subcapsular cataracts. Arch Ophthalmol, Aug 1979; 97: 1543.

3. Incidence of Age-Related Cataract: The Beaver Dam Eye Study. Arch Ophthalmol, Feb 1998; 116: 219–225.

4. Vitamin Supplement Use and Incident Cataracts in a Population-Based Study Arch Ophthalmol, Nov 2000; 118: 1556–1563.

5. Bickol N. Mukesh; Anhchuong Le; Peter N. Development of Cataract and Associated Risk Factors: The Visual Impairment Project Arch Ophthalmol, Jan 2006; 124: 79–85.

6. Sudha Cugati; Robert G. Cumming; Wayne Smith; Visual Impairment, Age-Related Macular Degeneration, Cataract, and Long-term Mortality: The Blue Mountains Eye Study.Arch Ophthalmol, Jul 2007; 125: 917–924.

7. Jie J. Wang; Paul Mitchell; Judy M. Simpson;.Visual Impairment, Age-Related Cataract, and Mortality. Arch Ophthalmol, Aug 2001; 119: 1186–1190.

8. M L Lopez, V Freidlin, M B Datiles. Longitudinal study of posterior subcapsular opacities using the National Eye Institute computer planimetry system., 3rdBritish Journal of Ophthalmology 1995;79:535–540.

9. Cathy A McCarty, Jill E Keeffe, Hugh R Taylor. The need for cataract surgery: projections based on lens opacity, visual acuity, and personal concern. Br J Ophthalmol 1999; 83: 62–65 (January).

10. N. A. Frost, J. M. Sparrow, and L. Moore. Associations of Human Crystalline Lens Retrodots and Waterclefts with Visual Impairment: An Observational Study. Invest. Ophthalmol. Vis. Sci., July 1, 2002; 43(7): 2105–2109.

11. J. Eshaghian; B. W. Streeten.Human posterior subcapsular cataract. An ultrastructural study of the posteriorly migrating cells.Arch Ophthalmol, Jan 1980; 98: 134–143.

12. V. Greiner; L. T. Chylack Jr.Posterior subcapsular cataracts: histopathologic study of steroid-associated cataracts. Arch Ophthalmol, Jan 1979; 97: 135–144.

13. T. W. Bochow; S. K. West; A. Azar; B. Munoz; A. Sommer; H.R. Taylor Ultraviolet light exposure and risk of posterior subcapsular cataracts Arch Ophthalmol, Mar 1989; 107: 369–372.

14. Anselm Hennis; Suh-Yuh Wu; Barbara Nemesure; M. Cristina Leske Risk Factors for Incident Cortical and Posterior Subcapsular Lens Opacities in the Barbados Eye Studies. Arch Ophthalmol, Apr 2004; 122: 525–530.

15. Cécile Delcourt; Isabelle Carrière; Alice Ponton-Sanchez; Annie Lacroux; Marie-José Covacho; Laure Papoz; and the POLA Study Group.Light Exposure and the Risk of Cortical, Nuclear, and Posterior Subcapsular Cataracts: The Pathologies Oculaires Liées à l'Age (POLA) Study Arch Ophthalmol, Mar 2000; 118: 385–392.

31

Phacoemulsification Surgery in a Miotic Pupil

Col JKS Parihar sm, vsm, and Col Neelam Puthran

INTRODUCTION

Good mydriasis is an important prerequisite to achieve smooth and good outcome following the phacoemulsification procedure. A pupillary dilatation of 7 mm or more is considered as ideal for phacoemulsification surgery. Till a few years ago, a small pupil used to be a relative contraindication for the phaco procedure. However, with increasing use of this technique, there is a desire to perform phacoemulsification surgery in each and every possible situation. Phacoemulsification surgery in miotic pupils (less than 4 mm in size) is gaining acceptance; the miotic pupil is invariably associated with several other structural and functional anomalies which may have the tendency to adversely influence ultimate surgical outcome. Poor mydriasis can pose difficulties in intraoperative management of the nucleus. This results in inadequate visualisation; leading to a sequence of events which can produce posterior capsular rupture, vitreous disturbance and nucleus drop. Capsulorrhexis can be small in diameter leading to difficulties in implantation and positioning of lens. Capsulorrhexis can be small subsequently lead to phimosis of the anterior capsule and the capsular contraction syndrome.

With appropriate precautions, planning and correct technique, the surgery can be safely performed in a miotic pupil. However, the surgical technique warrants meticulous planning and modifications in surgical technique, machine settings and fluidics. It should not be performed by residents in their training period as the margin for error in cases of miotic pupils is very small. Supplementary adjuvants in the form of pharmacological modulations or use of mechanical retractors are considerably beneficial. The choice of correct IOL to be implanted and postoperative care are equally important issues to discuss. The objectives include good pupillary function without producing unaesthetic scars, photophobia or diplopia.

In the days of intracapsular cataract surgery, large sector were performed. With better visual rehabilitation provided by intraocular lens, these techniques are not suitable as they give rise to glare and uniocular diplopia.

In this chapter we attempt to cover various aspects related with phaco in a miotic pupil.

CAUSES OF MIOTIC PUPIL (LESS THAN 4 MM IN SIZE)

Small pupil is one with less than 4 mm diameter. As per Gimbel, its incidence during phacoemulsification is about 1.5% of cases. It is necessary to dilate the pupil prior to phacoemulsification.

Small Pupil may be Functional (Hypo Reactive)

(i) Hyperopic patients and those having shallow anterior chambers.

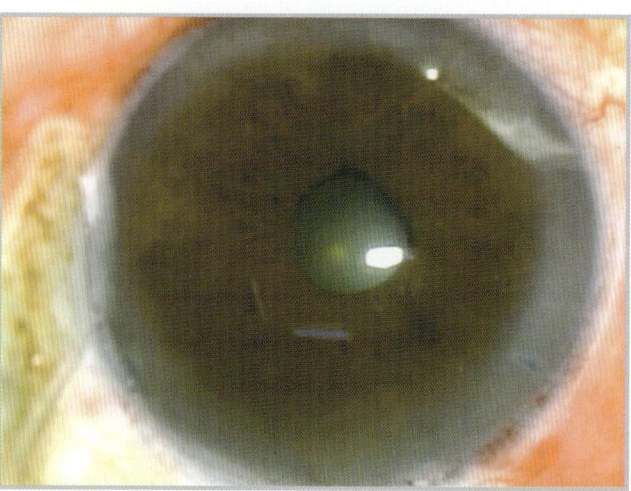

Fig. 31.1: Miotic pupil

(ii) Patients using anti-glaucoma medication (particularly Pilocarpine or Cholinesterases) for long periods.

(iii) Pseudo exfoliation syndrome.

(iv) Paediatric cases due to poorly developed dilator pupillae muscle.

(v) Iris atrophy in old age.

Fixed Pupil Mainly due to Posterior Synaechiae Following

(i) Uveitis   (ii) Trauma
(iii) Neurological   (iv) Iatrogenic
(v) Old age.

Intraoperative Floppy Iris Syndrome (IFIS)

This forms a separate entity as at the onset, the pupil is well dilated. Problems start after hydroprocedures with billowing and repeated prolapse of iris even through a well constructed incision and side port. Repeated manipulations and damage to iris with phacoprobe eventually leads to pupillary constriction. This condition has been noted to occur in male patients who are on alpha adrenergic blockers like terazosin (Hytrin), prazosin, alfuzosin or doxazosin for benign prostatic hypertrophy. These patients can be managed with preoperative instillation of atropine, intraoperative use of intracameral adrenaline and use of iris hooks, if pupil constricts.

PREOPERATIVE EVALUATION

History of uveitis and therapy for urinary problems is a must. Examination of the eye under the slit lamp is critical in detecting and evaluating these cases.

Irido-corneal or irido-lenticular synechiae, atrophy of the iris stroma (as detected by loss of iris pattern), ectropion of the pupillary edge and paralysis of the iris muscle are the conditions that influence mydriasis. Extent of mydriasis should be evaluated following instillation of mydriatic eye drops (10% phenylephrine and 1% tropicamide). These should be instilled twice at equal intervals, 30 minutes prior to the evaluation.

The mydriasis achieved then is classified as:

(i) Excellent   (ii) Good
(iii) Sufficient   (iv) Poor.

The pupillary diameter can also be recorded.

HOW TO MANAGE MIOTIC PUPIL

The following techniques can be used individually or in a combination for phacoemulsification in a patient with small pupils.

(i) Pharmacological treatment
(ii) Mydriasis using viscoelastic agent
(iii) Synechiolysis

(iv) Pupillary stretching
(v) Pupillary dilators
(vi) Iris surgery.

Pharmacological Treatment (Pharmacological Modulation of Miotic Pupil)

Pharmacological treatment can be done using eye drops. They are all instilled prior to surgery.

(i) **Pre-operative medications:** It is mandatory to instill drugs from both sympathomimetic and sympatholytic groups as they have synergistic effects. 10% phenylephrine and 1% tropicamide is the most commonly used combination. 1% cyclopentolate is also effective in causing quick and sustained mydriasis. Topical non steroidal anti-inflammatory agents like 0.03% flurbiprofen can be used pre-operatively to prevent intraoperative constriction following handling of iris and prostaglandin release. 2% Homatropine is not a good choice as its onset of action is longer and the extent of mydriasis is less.

(ii) **Intra-operative medications:** To increase mydriasis one can use preservative free adrenaline 1:1000 diluted in 10ml of BSS. This is injected into the anterior chamber at the commencement of the operation through the site of initial entry.

Visco-mydriasis

In this method, a viscoelastic substance (VES) is used to increase mydriasis. It can be used as an ideal follow up to the pharmacological therapy. The viscoelastic substance should have a very high molecular weight and must be transparent. A cohesive type of viscoelastic is preferred.

When the VES is injected into the eye, it produces good mechanical mydriasis. It also maintains the chamber depth during capsulorrhexis. It gives the surgeon control over iris tissue if it is atonic or tends to prolapse into the surgical wound and can tamponade any bleeding from the iris blood vessels.

Synechiolysis

If the pupil is fixed by posterior synechiae, synechiolysis is required to achieve uniform mydriasis. It should not be performed if there is any evidence of zonular compromise. The posterior synechiae are largely restricted to the pupillary edge and generally do not extend towards the iris root. These must be carefully identified during pre-operative evaluation and broken using a blunt spatula, avoiding excessive traction on the root of iris.

Pupillary Stretching

Luther Frye had introduced this technique. First the anterior chamber is filled with a VES, two iris hooks/ Y Pushers/

Iris spatule are introduced from the opposite sides, engaging the pupillary border. The hooks exert a centrifugal pressure causing controlled stretching of the pupillary edge to produce mydriasis. They stretch the pupil without damaging or tearing it. They are introduced through the side port and main incision. A small quantity of VES can escape from the anterior chamber during the stretching maneuvers; it must be replaced immediately to keep the anterior chamber deep.

One handed dilators are also available and they are safer and achieve good mydriasis. Bleeding is also limited and the pupil has good postoperative function.

Pupillary Dilators

Lack of iris tone may not produce sufficient mydriasis even after stretching. Use of dilating iris hooks or iris rings is indicated if stretching fails to dilate the pupil adequately.

Types of Iris Hooks

(i) **De Juan hooks:** De Juan hooks consist of segments in monofilament nylon thread and are curved at one end. A small silicone stopper is fixed on the segment to establish the desired length. They are inserted through one or more limbal paracentesis and hooked to the pupil edge. With centrifugal retraction, the silicone stopper is blocked on the limbus at the required distance. Normally four hooks are placed to produce a square shaped pupil.

(ii) **Mackool hooks:** Mackool hooks are made of titanium and are blocked at a preset distance.

(iii) **Siepser's hydrogel ring:** Siepser's hydrogel ring is oval in shape when dehydrated and is inserted through a 3 mm opening; when hydrated it expands. It is positioned over the pupillary collarette using a manipulator hook, allowing its flanges to capture the iris border thereby dilating the pupil. The ring is difficult to remove at the end of the surgical procedure.

(iv) **C-shaped PMMA dilators:** Here the ring is incomplete from where the phaco tip operates, to prevent the ring from being engaged by the tip. It produces a stable and uniform mydriasis.

(v) **Perfect Pupil (TM):** Perfect Pupil (TM): This device has been recently developed by John Milverton of Australia and is made of sterile, disposable polyurethane ring with an internal diameter of 7.0 mm. It can be inserted through a 3.2 mm clear corneal incision. The ring is open for 45 degrees to allow for the passage of instruments during the surgical procedure. After the use of this device, the pupil assumes its normal shape.

(vi) **Iris hooks:** Iris hooks are the most commonly used devices for pupillary dilatation. These are made of Prolene and have a silicon stopper. The tip of the hook is curved and the overall lengths approximately 10–12 mm. They are available in sets of four.

Technique of Phaco with Iris Retractors

Phacoemulsification surgery can be performed in a miotic pupil after stretching the pupil with the help of iris hooks. Most surgeons prefer to perform phaco after removing the iris hooks once the pupil has been stretched mechanically. The removal of iris hooks facilitates adequate depth of anterior chamber as well as providing a natural position of the iris diaphragm during the surgery. Surgical maneuvers remain very smooth and comfortable. However, removal of iris hooks prior to the commencement of phacoemulsification may revert the pupillary dilatation due to inadvertent touch of iris particularly in the presence of a very small and rigid pupil, like in certain cases of post uveitic cataract or in cases of advanced pseudoexfoliation syndrome. Author recommends judicious application and technique of iris hooks in these cases depending upon the type of pupil as well as on the basis of surgical technique of nucleotomy adopted by the surgeon himself.

The technique of phacoemulsification needs to be modified when operating in eyes with pupillary dilating devices in place. The aspiration flow rate and vacuum levels have to be reduced to prevent the phaco tip from catching the iris. The iris gets lifted up towards the cornea, thereby reducing the space in anterior chamber. Iris damage can occur while inserting and removing the probe, hence the number of times the phaco probe has to be removed from the eye has to be minimised. The chamber depth should be kept constant. Using continuous irrigation mode or an AC maintainer will help in achieving this. When performing the trenching techniques, the length of the trench should be kept short. One should aim to deepen the trench by keeping the superficial anterior nuclear plate intact. This reduces the chances of the iris being sucked into the phaco probe. This maneuver requires some skill and experience as the tip of phaco probe is not visible. The residual anterior nuclear plate can be removed last. Vertical chopping is the technique of choice in eyes with small pupils. The probe is embedded into the main central bulk of the nucleus and a chopper with a pointed tip is embedded close to the phaco probe. This is followed by a movement of lateral separation, thereby dividing the nucleus. Vertical chop technique has many advantages. There is minimal to and fro movement of the phaco probe, which minimises the risk of iris from being aspirated into the probe tip. There are minimal fluctuations in anterior chamber depth which helps in maintaining a stable iris diaphragm and prevents further constriction of the pupil.

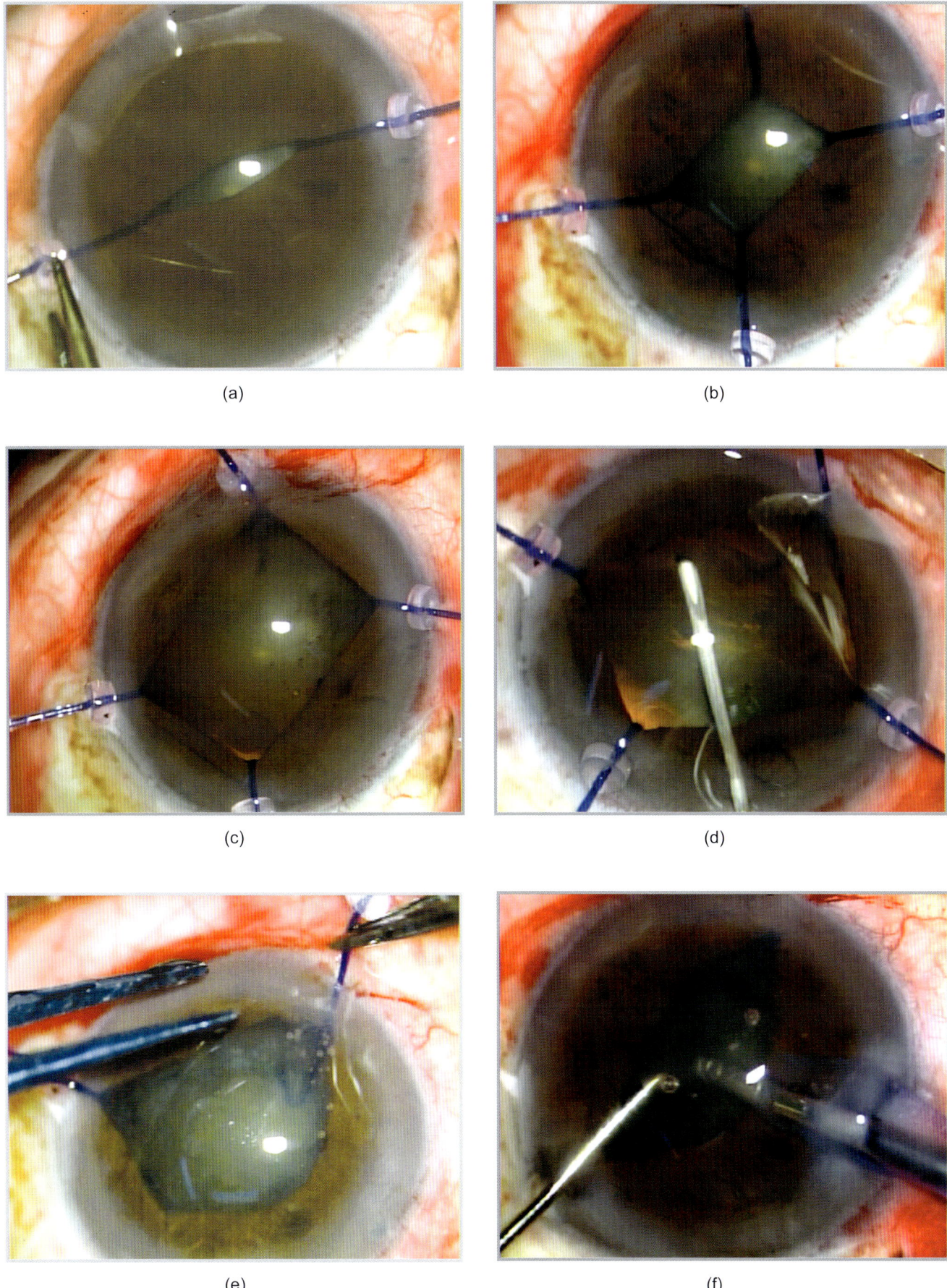

(a)

(b)

(c)

(d)

(e)

(f)

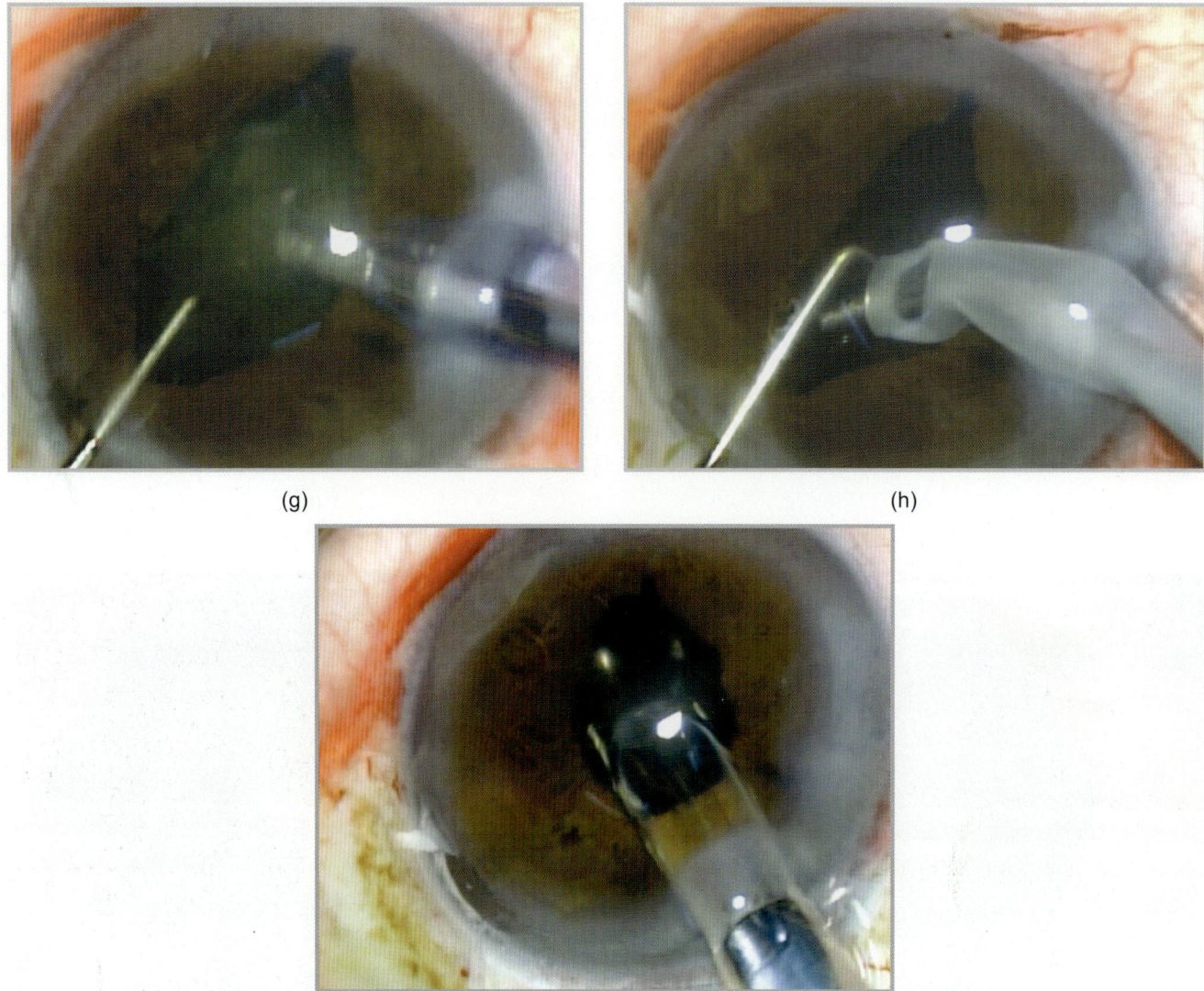

(g)

(h)

(i)

Fig. 31.2: (a) Miotic Pupil: Insertion of Iris hooks, (b) All four iris hooks are placed, (c) Miotic pupil is being stretched with the help of four iris hooks, (d) Capsulorrhexis under the presence of four iris hooks, (e) Iris hooks are being removed prior to the commencement of phacoemulsification, (f) Nucleotomy through mechanically stretched pupil, (g) Fragment removal, (h) Coaxial Irrigation/Aspiration, (i) Insertion of Acrylic Foldable IOL implantation

Intraoperative Complications/Constraints of Iris Hook Procedures

   (i) Additional incisions are required for insertion of four iris hooks.

  (ii) The hooks occupy space and in an eye with a narrow angle, this space in anterior chamber is at premium.

 (iii) Iris tear and bleeding from iris tissue.

 (iv) Anterior capsular tear. In cases where anterior capsule is fragile, tears can occur even with touch of a soft tipped hook.

Iris Surgery

It may be performed either in association or instead of the procedures described above. These methods can be useful in cases of iris atrophy but can cause bleeding, postoperative inflammation, iris traction and sometimes the need to leave iris sutures *in situ* permanently.

Sphincterotomy and Sphincterectomy

In sphincterotomy, six to eight radial partial cuts are made at the pupillary margin to disable the sphincter pupillae muscle: thereby aiding dilatation. This technique is useful in a senile miotic pupil, postinflammatory miosis and miosis following prolonged use of miotics. Sphincterectomy involves removal of a partial section of the iris tissue with sphincter pupillae muscle. The pupil is deformed in shape after this technique.

Removal of the Pupillary Membrane

This technique was first described by Oscher. It involves removal of membrane at the pupillary edge: a thin

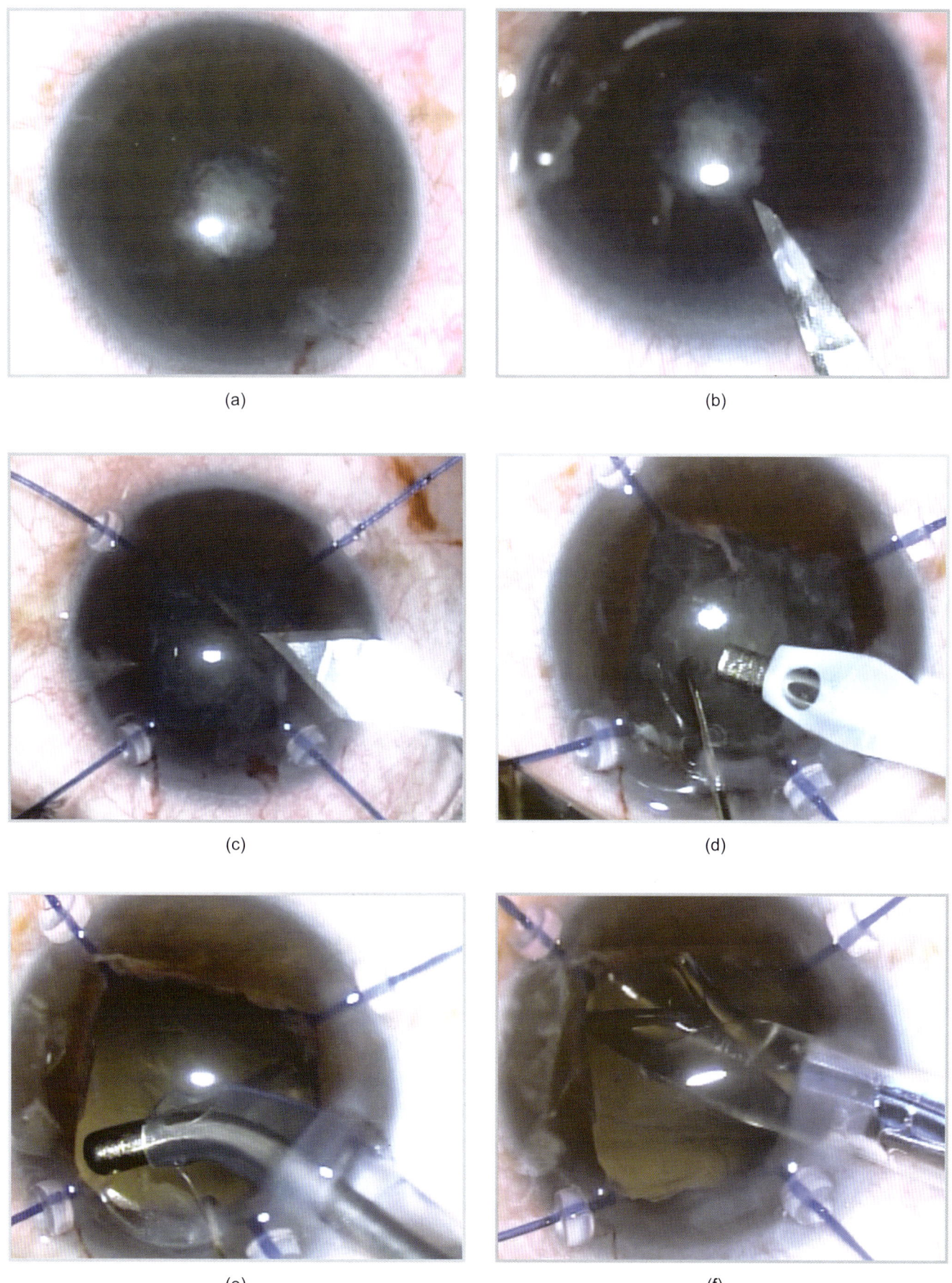

(a)

(b)

(c)

(d)

(e)

(f)

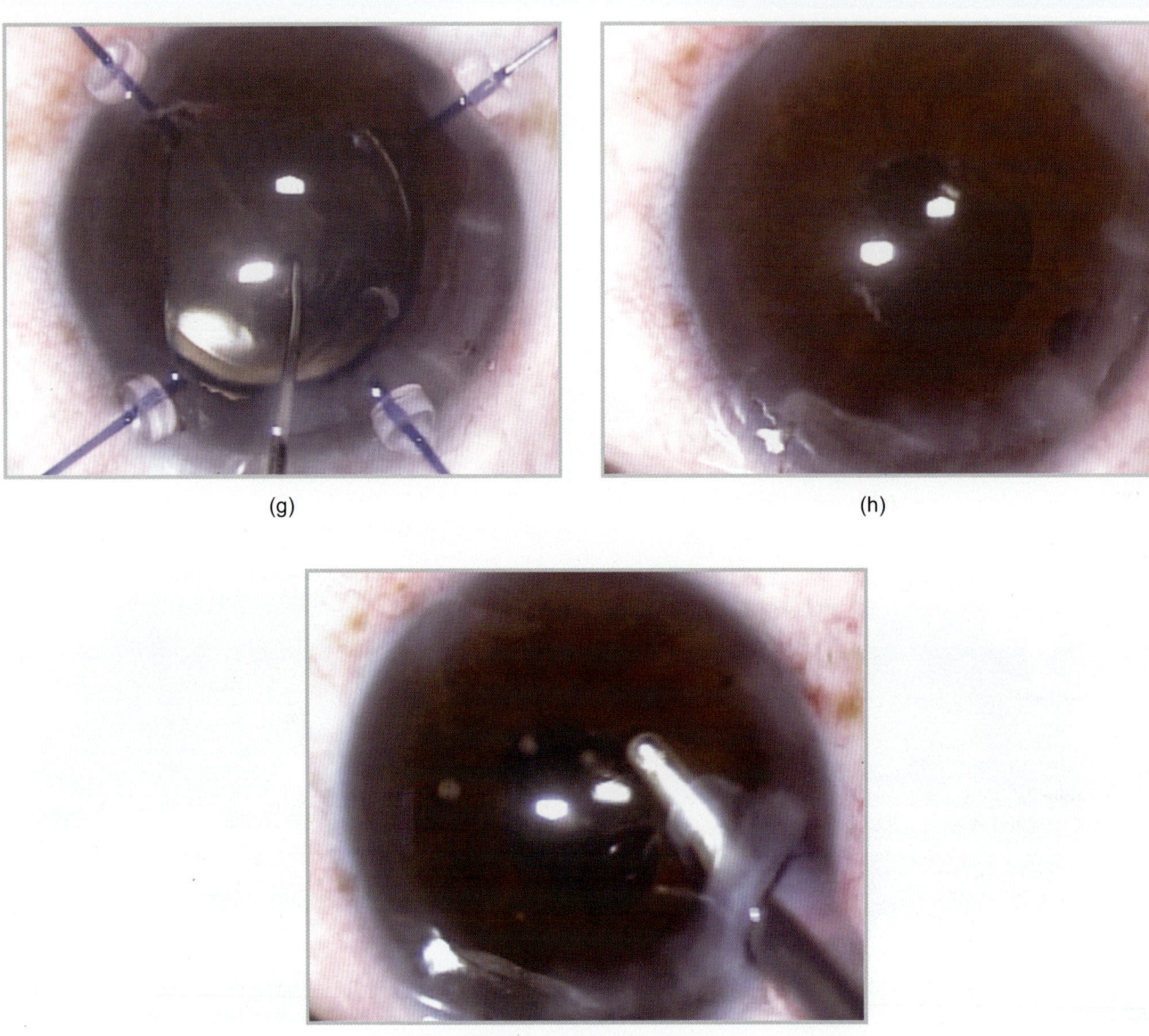

Fig. 31.3: (a) Post uveitic miotic pupil, (b) Miotic Pupil: Incision to introduce iris hooks, (c) 3.2 MM keratome clear corneal incision under the presence of four iris hooks, (d) Nucleotomy by direct chopping through mechanically stretched pupil, (e) Coaxial Irrigation/Aspiration under the presence of iris hooks *in situ*, (f) Insertion of Acrylic foldable IOL implantation, (g) Acrylic foldable IOL implant is being dialled, (h) Pilocarpine modulated pupil after insertion of IOL implants, (i) Post IOL implant Insertion wash

transparent membrane covering the pupillary margin can be dissected free from the iris using fine microtipped forceps under viscoelastic cover.

Iridotomy

Iridotomy may be the only option to expand the pupil when the iris is atrophic and sclerotic. The iridotomy may be proximal or distal to the surgical incision. When performed in a proximal position, a radial cut extends to the pupil edge starting from a basal surgical iridectomy made initially. When iridotomy is distal to the surgical incision, it is simply performed by cutting the iris radially from the pupillary edge towards the iris root. The surgeon must

ensure that the edge of cut iris is never engaged by the phaco tip. At the end of the surgery rearrangement of the iris anatomy is done by performing iridoplasty which requires suturing the ends of iris with 10/0 nylon sutures. Broad sector iridotomy can be performed if all fails.

Iris sutures

Placement of iris sutures to achieve mydriasis is rare. Suture is passed from the anterior to the posterior chamber: thereby transfixing the pupil which is pulled radially towards the periphery. The anterior capsule can be damaged while passing the suture and the suture can damage the iris tissue.

Tips for Phacoemulsification in a Small Pupil

(i) Thorough pre-operative clinical examination of the patient's eyes, especially studying the iris morphology and pupillary margin. These surgeries should not be performed by residents and those learning phaco.

(ii) Preoperatively, evaluate the maximum possible mydriasis.

(iii) Use pharmacological therapy to produce maximum mydriasis

(iv) Use of intracameral adrenaline diluted to 1 in 10.

(v) Use of abundant and appropriate VES.

(vi) Use a combination of surgical techniques to get optimal mydriasis without permanently compromising the pupil and iris function.

(vii) Always add 1ml of 1:1000 adrenaline to a 500 ml irrigation bottle.

(viii) Use direct vertical chop technique and keep aspiration flow rate and vacuum levels low. Keep the phacoprobe in the centre where there is the least chance of iris trauma and posterior capsular damage.

(ix) Always maintain a deep anterior chamber to prevent any further miosis.

(x) In presence of a small pupil, a large 6.0 mm IOL should be implanted preferably into the capsular bag. Heparin coated IOL's may also be used.

(xi) In the postoperative period expect more than routine inflammation in such patients and give appropriate drugs to control it.

CONCLUSION

Operating upon a cataract in the presence of a small pupil is every surgeon's nightmare. It requires an experienced surgeon, meticulous planning, good surgical technique and use of combinations of drugs and devices to achieve the desired surgical outcome.

BIBLIOGRAPHY

1. Kershner, RM. Management of the Small Pupil in Clear Corneal Cataract Surgery: J Cataract Refract Surg, 2002; 28.

2. Jampol LM, Jain S, Pudzisz, et al. Nonsteroidal anti-inflammatory drugs and cataract surgery: Arch Ophthalmol. 1994; 112:891–894.

3. Allaire C, Lablache Combier M, Trinquand C, et al. Comparative efficacy of 0.1% indomethacin eyedrops, 0.03% flurbiprofen eyedrops and placebo for maintaining perioperative mydriasis: J Fr Ophtalmol. 1994; 17:103–109.

4. Gaynes BI, Deutsch TA. Cost-effectiveness of topical 0.03% flurbiprofen in outpatient cataract surgery as measured by surgical time and vitreous loss: Am J Health Syst Pharm. 1998; 55(suppl 4):S23–S24.

5. Roberts CW. Comparison of diclofenac sodium and flurbiprofen for inhibition of surgically induced miosis. J Cataract Refract Surg. 1996; 22(suppl 1):780–787.

6. Solomon, KD, Turkalj JW, Whiteside SB, et al. Topical 0.5% ketorolac v/s 0.03% flurbiprofen for inhibition of miosis during cataract surgery. Arch Ophthalmol. 1997; 115:1119–1122.

7. Srinivasan R, Madhavaranga. Topical ketorolac tromethamine 0.5% versus diclofenac sodium 0.1% to inhibit miosis during cataract surgery. J Cataract Refract Surg. 2002; 28:517–520.

8. Flach AJ. Topical nonsteroidal drugs in ophthalmology. Int Ophthalmol Clin. 2002; 42:1–11.

9. Gimbel H, Van Westenbrugge J, Cheetham JK, et al. Intraocular availability and papillary effect of flurbiprofen and indomethacin during cataract surgery. J Cataract Refract Surg. 1996; 22:474–479.

10. Ozturk F, Kurt E, Inan UU, et al. The efficacy of 2.5% phenylephrine and flurbiprofen combined in inducing and maintaining papillary dilatation during cataract surgery. Eur J Ophthalmol. 2000; 10:144–148.

11. Osher R. The use of tpa in the management of small pupil phacoemulsification. Video J Cataract Refract Surg. 1995; 11:1.

12. Bartlett JD, Miller KM.Phacoemulsification techniques for patients with small pupils. Comp Ophthalmology Update. 2003; 4: 171–176.

13. Kershner RM. Sutureless one-handed intercapsular phacoemulsification–the keyhole technique. J Cataract Refract Surg 1991 ; 17(Supp):719–725.

14. Smith GT, Liu CSC. Flexible iris hooks for phacoemulsification in patients with iridoschisis. J Cataract Refract Surg 2000; 26:1277–1280.

15. Graether JM. Graether pupil expander for managing the small pupil during surgery. J Cataract Refract Surg 1996; 22: 530–535.

16. Chang DF, Campbell JR. Intraoperative floppy iris syndrome associated with tamsulosin. J Cataract Refract Surg 2005; 31:664–73.

17. Settas G, Fitt AW. Intraoperative floppy iris syndrome in a patient taking alfuzosin for benign prostatic hypertrophy. Eye 2006; 20:1431–2.

18. Pringle E, Packard R. Antipsychotic agent as an etiologic agent of IFIS. J Cataract Refract Surg 2005; 31:2240–1.

19. Chadha V, Borooah S, Tey A, Styles C Singh J. Floppy iris behaviour during cataract surgery: Associations and variations. Br J Ophthalmol 2007; 91:40–2.

20. Oshika T, Ohashi Y, Inamura M, Ohki K, Okamoto S, Koyama T, et al. Incidence of intraoperative floppy iris syndrome in patients on either systemic or topical alpha (1)-adrenoceptor antagonist. Am J Ophthalmol 2007; 143:150–1.

21. Bendel RE, Philips MB. Preoperative use of atropine to prevent intraoperative floppy-iris syndrome in patients taking tamsulosin. J Cataract Refract Surg 2005; 32:1603–5.

22. Miller KM, Keener Jr, GT. Stretch pupilloplasty for small pupil phacoemulsification. Am J Ophthalmol. 1994; 117: 107–108.

23. Brown DC. The phaco flip technique. Cataract & Refractive Surgery Today. 2001;2:18–20.

24. Dinsmore JC. Modified stretch technique for small pupil phacoemulsification with topical anesthesia. J Cataract Refract Surg. 1996; 22:27–30.

25. Fine IH. Pupilloplasty for small pupil phacoemulsification. J Cataract Refract Surg. 1994; 20:192–196.

26. Pham DT, Volkmer C, Leder K, et al. Partial Sphincterectomy in cataract surgery. Clinical and patho-histologic results. Ophthalmologe. 1998; 95:635–638.

27. Masket S. Preplaced inferior iris suture method for small pupil phacoemulsification. J Cataract Refract Surg. 1992; 18:518–522.

28. Masket S. Avoiding complications associated with iris retractor use in small pupil cataract surgery. J Cataract Refract Surg. 1995; 22:168–171.

29. Yuguchi T, Oshika T, Sawaguchi S, et al. Pupillary functions after cataract surgery using flexible iris retractor in patients with small pupil. Jpn J Ophthalmol. 1999; 43: 20–24.

30. Birchall W, Spencer AF. Misalignment of flexible iris hook retractors for small pupil cataract surgery: effects on pupil circumference. J Cataract Refract Surg. 2001; 27: 20–24.

31. Oetting TA, Omphroy LC. Modified technique using flexible iris retractors in clear corneal surgery. J Cataract Refract Surg. 2002; 28:596–598.

32. Akman A, Yilmaz G, Oto S, Akova Y. Comparison of various pupil dilatation methods for phacoemulsification in eyes with a small pupil secondary to psueudoexfolication. Ophthalmology 2004; 111:1693–1698.

33. Toshiaki Kubota, Ichiro Toguri, Naoko Onizuka, Toshie Matsuura. Phacoemulsification and Intraocular Lens Implantation for Angle Closure Glaucoma after the Relief of Pupillary Block, Ophthalmologica 2003; 217:325–328.

32

Phaco in Posterior Polar Cataract

Dr (Mrs) P Sadhotra, Col JKS Parihar SM, VSM and Lt Col Sandeep Gupta

A posterior polar cataract is a dense white opacity that is situated in the central posterior capsule. It consists of characteristic concentric rings around the central opacity (bull's eye). Posterior polar cataract (PPC) is a special situation that is more prone to intraoperative posterior capsular dehiscence and hence, tests the skills and experience of a phaco surgeon. If the diagnosis of PPC is missed or proper guidelines are not followed, the intraoperative course of surgery can be complicated by the occurrence of posterior capsular (PC) rent, vitreous disturbance, and nucleus dislocation.

MORPHOLOGY

Posterior polar cataracts are associated with remnants of the hyaloid system or the tunica vasculosa lentis. These cataracts may also occur without any relation to hyaloid remnants and appear as circular or rosette-shaped opacities; they are hereditary and usually transmitted as a dominant trait. The gene for this has been mapped to chromosome 16q22. PPCs are considered to arise before birth or in early infancy. They are generally bilateral without any sexual predilection. Autosomal dominance is the most common inheritance pattern, though sporadic and autosomal recessive cases have also been reported. The exact pathogenesis of the PPC is unclear, but is speculated to be due to the persistence of the hyaloid artery or invasion of the lens by mesoblastic tissue. PPCs are dense white, well-circumscribed plaques having concentric rings (onion-whorl pattern) with or without imprint opacity anteriorly); occupying the axial posterior cortical and the subcapsular regions. These cataracts have thicknesses unlike posterior subcapsular cataracts, which are thin occupying only the posterior subcapsular region. Duke-Elder classified PPC into two types; stationary and progressive. The stationary type as described above is more common and compatible with good visual acuity. The posterior polar opacity may sometimes get camouflaged by advancing nuclear sclerosis. The progressive type (less common) manifests earlier due to centrifugal extension of the opacity along the posterior capsule. The progression seems most common in young adults who seek early surgical relief due to their incapacitating visual symptoms.

CLASSIFICATION

This classification is important for a preoperative predication of complications and aids in forming a prognosis.

TYPE 1: Opacity confined to structures adjacent to the posterior subcapsular cataract.

TYPE 2: Opacity with ringed appearance like an onion.

TYPE 3: Opacity with dense white spots at the edge often associated with thin or absent posterior capsule.

TYPE 4: Combination of all the above three types with nuclear sclerosis.

Intraoperative constraints and risk of PC rent, proportionately increase with type 3 and 4, respectively.

CLINICAL FEATURES

(i) Patient remains symptomatic despite good corrected visual acuity. Such symptoms are more prominent with a dense opacity adjacent to the nodal point as compared to a central opacity involving the posterior capsule.

(ii) Better Mesopic vision than in bright illumination.

(iii) Significant glare.

DIFFERENTIAL DIAGNOSIS

(i) Posterior subcapsular cataract

(ii) Mittendorf dot

(iii) Injury to the posterior capsule.

How to differentiate from Posterior Subcapsular Cataract

Surgical management of posterior polar cataracts is a very challenging task as compared to the posterior subcapsular cataract. A posterior polar cataract is the first diagnosis of exclusion in case of any evidence of posterior cataract.

Anatomical Differences

See Table 32.1.

SURGICAL MANAGEMENT OF POSTERIOR POLAR CATARACT

Preoperative Evaluation

In addition to detailed preoperative examination, a thorough counselling should be conducted to apprise the

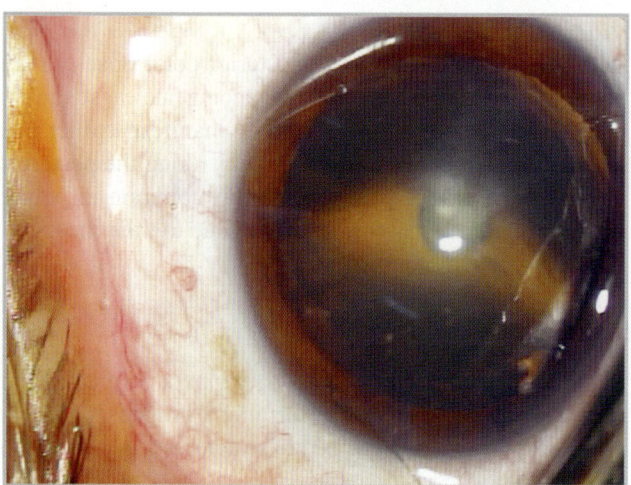

Fig. 32.1: Posterior polar cataract

patient about significant risk involved with higher incidence of intraoperative complications in posterior polar cataract surgery which may include the higher chances of intraoperative nucleus drop due to inadvertent posterior capsular rent and possible posterior segment intervention to deal with such situation. Patient should also be apprised about delayed visual recovery in certain cases. In addition, the surgeon should discuss Nd: YAG capsulotomy for residual plaque and emphasise the possibility of preexisting amblyopia, especially in cases of unilateral posterior polar cataract.

There is no sure way of knowing preoperatively whether a preexisting PC rent is there or not. Daljit Singh has described the presence of dense white spots without rings, encircling the PPC in some cases (Daljit Singh sign). Osher et al mentioned oil droplet like particles behind the plane of PPC with the same prognostic value. Okihiro Nishi denies there are any special signs or biomicroscopy findings for predicting intraoperative capsular stability. However, a PC rent in previously operated eye and a classic bull's eye appearance of a PPC in the fellow eye can be diagnostic. Since the preoperative clues for predicting the occurrences of intraoperative PC rent are not very reliable it is the authors' strategy to approach a PPC under the assumption that the PC is already open. Hence it is mandatory to discuss this complication with the patient and take an informed consent. A meticulous planning of the surgical strategy is desired.

Anaesthesia

The choice of anaesthesia technique or applications of general anaesthesia depends upon the merits and age of

Table 32.1: Anatomical differences		
	Posterior polar cataract	**Posterior subcapsular cataract**
Age	Younger age group	Not associated with age
Origin	Invariably developmental anomaly	No relation
Appearance	Bull's eye/Plaque/Mass	Uniform or vacuolar
Shape	Circular	Plate like
Rings	Concentric rings	No rings
Colour	Whitish brown	Golden yellow
Site	Adherent to PC	Not adherent to PC
Size	2.5–4 mm	May be up to equator
Thickness	Thicker, involves more structures than posterior capsule	Thinner, confined to only the posterior subcapsular region
Pre-existing PC tear	May be a presenting feature	Not seen
Associated nuclear/cortical opacity	Not a routine feature except posterior cortex may be affected	Usually not seen
Systemic disease	No	Usually associated with systemic or ocular diseases

the patients as well as on surgeon's preference. Peribulbar anaesthesia with oculopressure to soften the globe diminishes intraoperative posterior pressure. With increasing experience, one may use topical anaesthesia in a selective manner. We have switched over to topical anaesthesia about three years ago.

SURGICAL TECHNIQUE

We prefer a closed chamber technique. The contours of the cornea and the globe should be maintained throughout the procedure.

Capsulorrhexis

Ideally, the capsulorrhexis should not be larger than 5 mm. Although a size of 4 mm or less could be detrimental if the surgeon must prolapse the nucleus into the anterior chamber, a larger opening may not leave adequate support for a sulcus-fixated IOL if the posterior capsule is compromised.

As such, PPC is generally seen in younger patients where size of nucleus is invariably small. While keeping in mind the peculiarity of capsular elasticity and excessive tendency for extension of rhexis in such cases it is recommended to attempt a smaller rhexis as compared to the desired one so as to achieve optimal rhexis ultimately. Authors recommend the use of rhexis forceps over needle to complete the rhexis, since forceps provides better control over linear movements particularly in younger patients or in cases of thin and fragile capsule.

Hydroprocedures

The judicious application of hydroprocedures is one of the most important and crucial single aspect of smooth and uneventful outcome following surgery in cases of posterior polar cataracts.

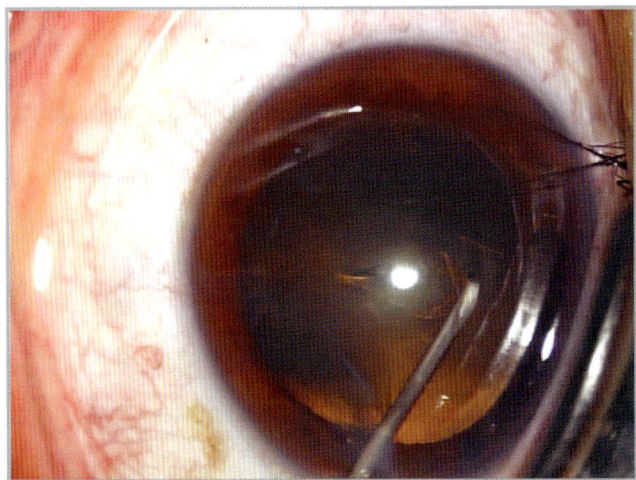

Fig. 32.2: Capsulorrhexis in posterior polar cataract

Cortical cleaving hydrodissection can lead to hydraulic rupture and should be avoided, i.e. "Hydrodissection free Phacoemulsification" is recommended. Instead it is logical to perform hydrodelineation to create a mechanical cushion of epinucleus. Fine et. al. performed hydrodissection in multiple quadrants and gently injected tiny amounts of fluid in such a manner that the fluid wave could not extend across the posterior capsule.

Vasavada et al have described inside out delineation for post polar cataracts, in which they sculpt a central trench using the slow-motion technique with care not to mechanically rock the lens. Injecting a dispersive viscoelastic through the side port incision before retracting the probe prevents the forward movement of the iris-lens diaphragm. They introduce a specially designed, right-angled cannula mounted on a 2-ml syringe filled with fluid through the main incision and place the tip adjacent to the right wall of the trench at an appropriate depth, depending on the density of the cataract. The tip then penetrates the central lenticular substance, and injects fluid through the right wall of the trench.

The fluid traversing inside out produces delineation (A golden ring within the lens indicates successful delineation). If the delineation is incomplete, the surgeon may inject fluid in the left wall of the trench with another right-angled cannula. The trench allows the surgeon to reach the central core of the nucleus. When fluid reaches a desired depth, it will create an epinuclear bowl that will act as a mechanical cushion to protect the posterior capsule during subsequent maneuvers. With conventional hydro-delineation, the cannula penetrates the lenticular substance and thus causes the fluid to traverse from the outside inward. It is sometimes difficult to introduce the cannula within a firm nucleus, and the effort can rock and stress the capsular bag and zonules. The surgeon may also inadvertently inject fluid into the subcapsular plane and thereby conduct unwarranted hydrodissection. Inside-out delineation is easy to perform, provides excellent surgical control, reduces stress to the zonules, and precisely demarcates the central core of nucleus.

Arup Chakraborty et al, instead, performed hydrofree-dissection. Hydrofreedissection involves sweeping under the anterior capsular surface with a cyclodialysis spatula along all the meridians. This is achieved by working the spatula through two side port incisions. The spatula tip is carefully advanced till the capsular fornix is reached and then the sweeping manoeuvre is initiated. This eliminates risk of PC rent with a fluid wave.

The Author's (Col JKSP) Preferences

Hydrodissection

Undoubtedly hydrodissection carries the higher risk of capsular rupture, in cases of posterior polar cataract due to obvious hurdles to the fluid wave at the site of plaque.

Hence, hydrodissection free phacoemulsification or selective hydrodissection is the best choice in such cases.

We prefer to inject a very small quantity of BSS fluid in all the four quadrants in such a manner so as to achieve partial cleavage between capsular bag and cortical matter without involving the posterior polar cataract. This is further augmented by the infiltration of sodium hylarunate at the same plane.

Hydrodelineation

The next step is deep hydrodelineation at the plane of mid-nucleus so as to achieve cleavage or the golden ring appearance around the core nucleus.

The visco separation is equally beneficial at this stage. One should avoid repeated and sequential hydrodelineation so as to ensure safety against posterior capsule dehiscence.

The Nucleus Rotation

The nucleus rotation must be avoided in these cases so as to prevent any capsular dehiscence or nucleus drop.

Nucleus Management

All of our techniques are geared towards facilitating the removal of the nucleus while it is cushioned by the epinucleus. Bimanual cracking and division of the nucleus involve outward movements and can distort the capsular bag. We recommend direct or stop and chop or cart wheel flip and chip technique. Most of the nuclei in posterior polar cataracts are soft nuclei, hence moderate energy and aspiration settings are much more beneficial. Conventional sculpting may not be a viable option in soft cataracts with posterior plaques since it may involve a higher risk of posterior capsular rent or direct injury to the capsule due to ultrasonic energy in soft cataracts.

The authors prefer to use the zero degree tip in these cases to minimise mechanical injury in case of soft cataracts. For nuclear sclerosis greater than 2+, we use the technique of step by step chop *in situ* with 10% to 15% ultrasound, vacuum of 150 to 225 mmHg, an aspiration flow rate of 20 mL/min, and a bottle height of 70 to 90 cm.

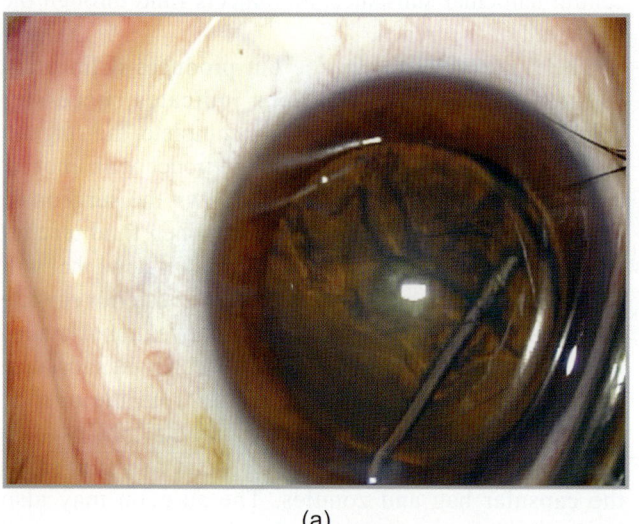

(a)

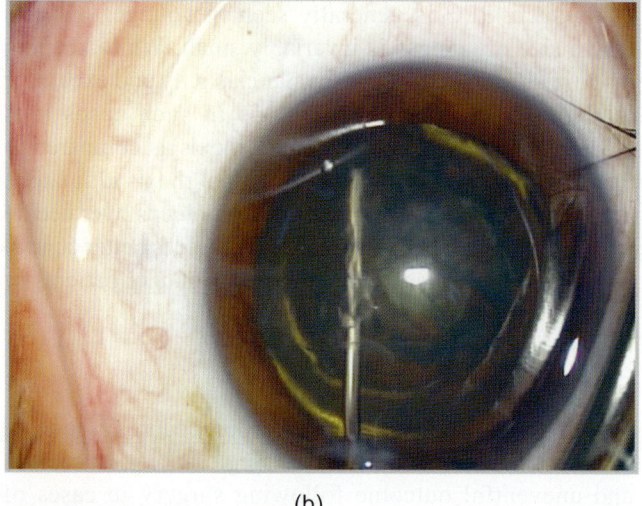

(b)

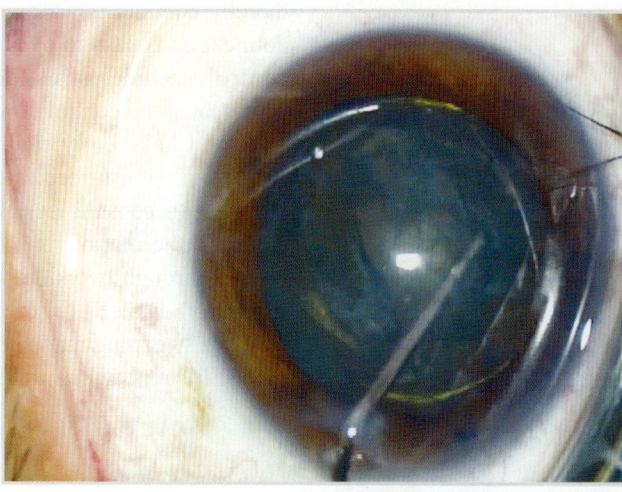

(c)

Fig. 32.3: (a) Hydrodissection in cases of posterior polar cataract, (b) Sequential hydrodelineation in posterior polar cataract, (c) Sequential hydrodelineation in posterior polar cataract

The resultant fragments are removed with a stop, chop technique. Our aim remains to remove central nucleus first followed by onion peeling separation and removal of the remaining nucleus and the epinucleus plate. For less dense nuclei, we aspirate the entire nucleus within the epinuclear shell. Thus, the slow-motion technique reduces turbulence in the anterior chamber.

Injecting viscoelastic prior to removing the instrument prevents the anterior chamber from collapsing and the posterior chamber from bulging forward. Posterior plaque along with adjacent cortical plate is left as such till the end of the procedure so as to maintain the integrity of posterior capsule at the maximum.

Depending upon the thickness and density of the plaque as well as its relations with the posterior capsule, plaque may require gentle dissection with the help of a fine needle and Synskey's hook.

We prefer to use the bimanual phacoaspiration – irrigation method to handle very soft nucleus without applying any ultrasonic energy.

Osher et al have also described the technique of slow motion phacoemulsification.

Lee and Lee described their use of the lambda technique to sculpt the nucleus, after which they cracked along both arms and removed the central piece. Vasavada and Singh described the use of step by step chop *in situ* and lateral separation to minimise stress on the capsule-zonule complex.

Arup Chakraborty et al employed a technique, which was not dependent on nucleus rotation. Majority of the cases of PPC had a soft nucleus. This was progressively debulked employing low phaco parametres like maximum ultrasound power of 40% to 70%, flow rate of 15 ml/min, a vacuum of 5–50 mmHG (depending upon the stage of the nucleus

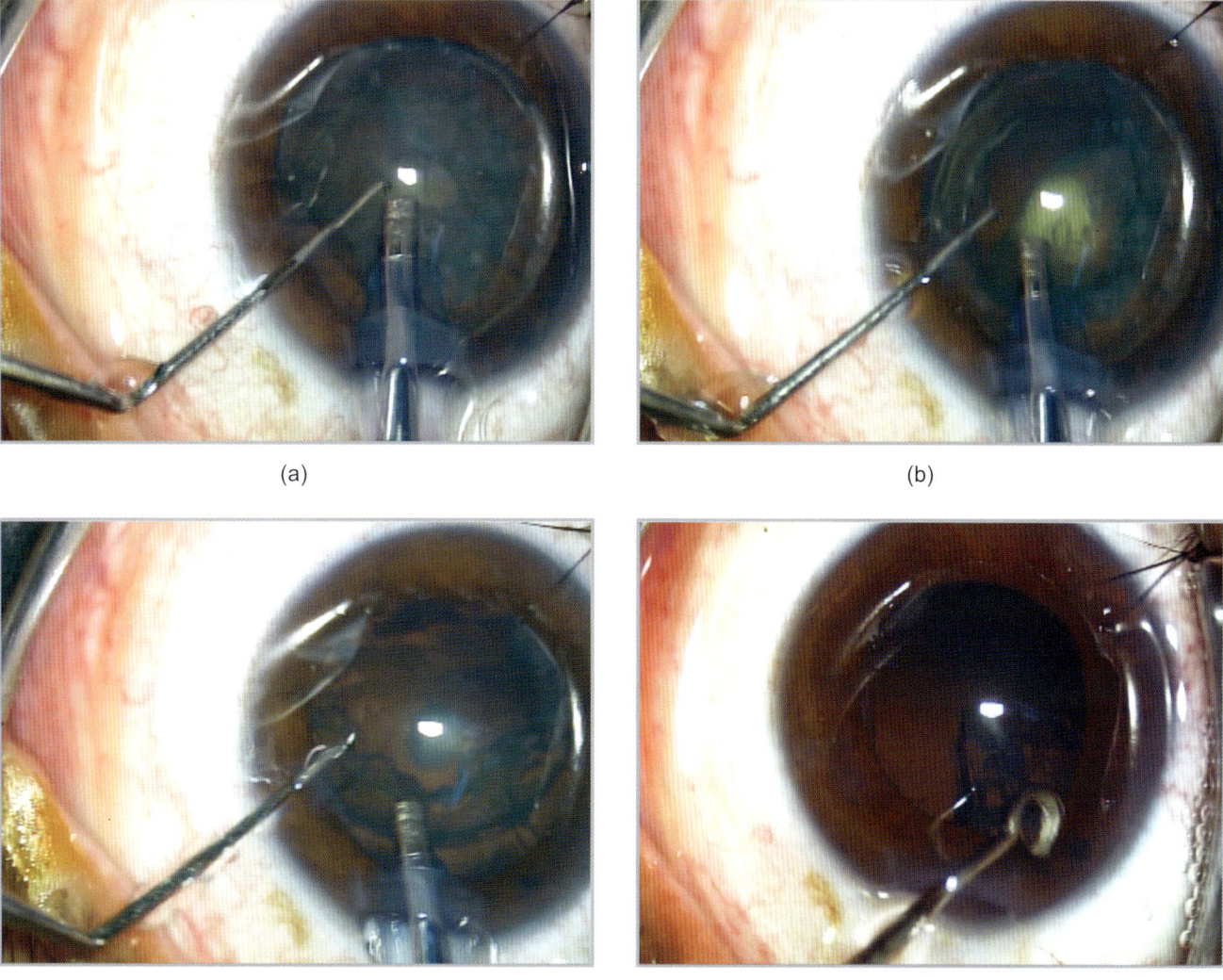

(a)   (b)

(c)   (d)

Fig. 32.4: (a) Nucleus management in posterior polar cataract (Removal of central core nucleus), (b) Nucleus management in posterior polar cataract: onion peeling separation and removal of the remaining nucleus, (c) Posterior plate management in posterior polar cataract: onion peeling separation and removal of the remaining posterior plate, (d) Posterior plaque management in posterior polar cataract

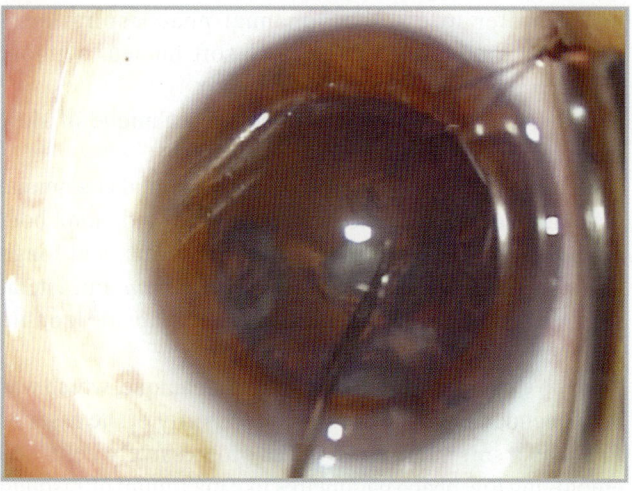

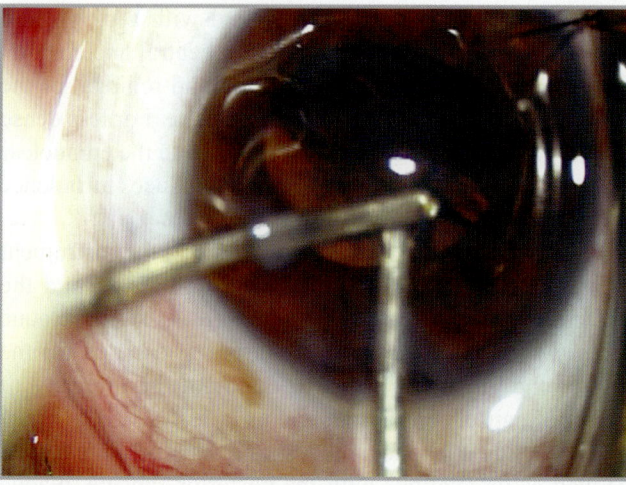

(e)   (f)

Fig. 32.4: (e) Posterior plaque management in posterior polar cataract: Dissection of posterior plaque, (f) Bimanual Irrigation and aspiration in posterior polar cataract

removal) and infusion bottle at 40 cm. Initially, most of the central and interior portions of the nucleus were debulked, thereby more space in the capsular bag was created. Subsequently, rest of the superior portions of the nucleus along with the epinucleus was displaced into the space created in the capsular bag inferiorly and emulsified. This was achieved by incremental injections of viscoelastic materials (VE) at the superior capsular fornix (limited viscodissection) till the superior portion of the nucleus and the epinucleus were displaced just up to the upper CCC margin from where it was flipped into the anterior chamber with a cyclodialysis spatula working through the side port. The residual cortex was removed by bimanual irrigation/ aspiration (I/A) working from periphery to centre. The central PC was never polished or vacuumed.

IOL Implantation

An atraumatic technique with minimal stress on the PC is employed for IOL insertion into the capsular bag. Single piece hydrophobic acrylic IOL implant remains the first preference. However if a PC tear is noticed, every effort is made to prevent extension of the tear and minimise vitreous loss. The basic principle followed is not to allow the anterior chamber to collapse by maintaining a closed system. This is achieved by injecting viscoelastics materials before withdrawing the phaco tip or the I/A probe from the anterior chamber. Cortex is removed by a dry technique using a cannula on a syringe. If vitreous presents in the anterior chamber at any stage, a thorough automated anterior vitrectomy (preferably bimanual) is performed. The possibility of posterior CCC is considered in the event of a small and central PC rent. All PMMA IOL implantation in the ciliary sulcus remained our choice till three years ago, when we switched over to the acrylic IOL implantation over CTR in cases of capsular dehiscence. However in certain very large and uncontrolled dehiscences, one may have to consider the IOL implantation into the ciliary

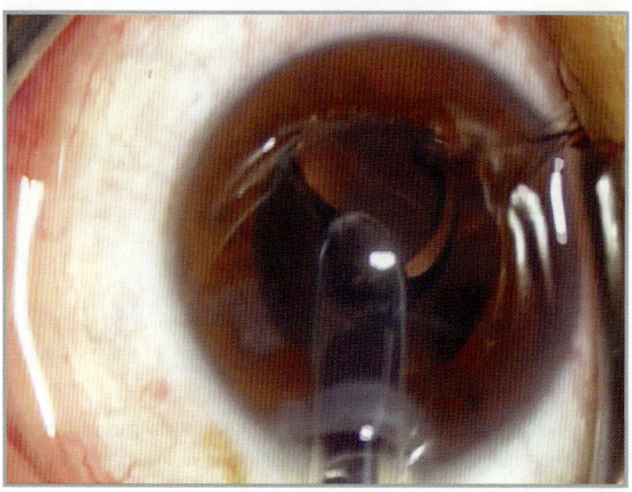

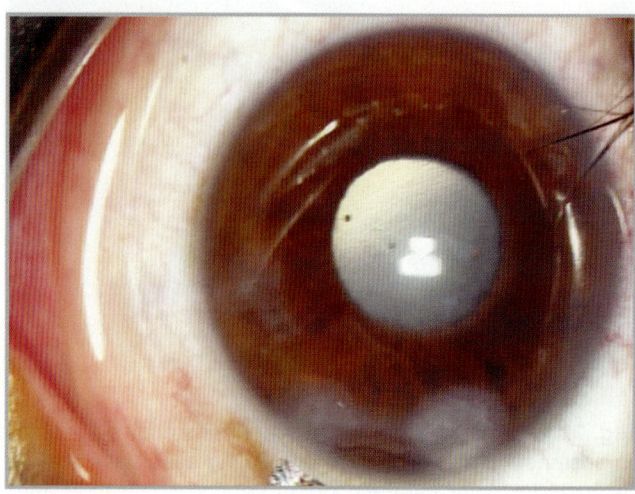

Fig. 32.5: Single piece hydrophobic acrylic IOL implantation   **Fig. 32.6:** Stromal hydration

sulcus. Viscoelastics material is removed very cautiously taking care to maintain the intraocular pressure and the anterior chamber depth throughout the procedure.

The status of the posterior capsule (PC) actually dictates the action of the surgeon. If the PC is absent or torn but with no vitreous loss, a dispersive viscoelastic is injected over the defect to tamponade and push the vitreous face backwards. A dispersive rather than a cohesive viscoelastic is preferable as it is more adapted to maintaining a space and stabilising the anterior vitreous face. If there is PCR with vitreous loss, a two port anterior vitrectomy is performed. Intraocular lens implantation in these cases would depend on the extent of the PCR and the integrity of the remaining PC.

Intraoperative Complications/Observations
   (i) Inherent preexisting posterior capsular dehiscence 3–4%
   (ii) PC rent: 12–20%
   (iii) Posterior dislocation of nucleus: Nil in our experience (5 to 20% in various series).

Postoperative Complications
   (i) Mild to moderate uveitis 5–11%
   (ii) Secondary glaucoma 8–10%
   (iii) Macular oedema 10–15%
   (iv) PCO: 30 to 40% after an interval of two years
   (v) Residual posterior capsule plaque postoperatively, which required Neodymium:YAG laser capsulotomy: 12 to 15%.

Incidence of PCR in PPC
As per our experience the incidence of intraoperative PC rent in PPC is around 12% encountered during last five years as compared to 24% observed by us during 1996 to 2001. In the studies reported by Osher et al (1990) and Vasavada et al (1997), the incidence of intraoperative rupture of the PC has been 26% and 36%, respectively. The lower incidence in current series is probably attributed to improvements in technology, availability of better and newer equipments, innovations in surgical techniques as well as overall enhancement in surgical experience and exposures. The incidence of PC rupture in other types of cataracts is only 1.1%.

Predisposing Factors for Higher Incidence of PCR in PPC
Various hypotheses have been put forward to explain this higher incidence of rupture. The cataract may be tightly adhered to the underlying posterior capsule, which may fail to separate during PE resulting in a tear. The posterior capsule beneath the PPC could also be abnormally thin and fragile and give way with the slightest manipulations. It is also possible that the central posterior capsule fails to develop and is simply absent (congenital posterior dehiscence). In our opinion, surgery should be delayed as long as possible and undertaken only if the patient finds it

difficult to perform routine activities. The highest incidence of capsular rupture occurred during removal of the posterior polar opacity or during cleaning of the posterior capsule after the opacity had been removed.

We believe that excessive adherence of the opacity to the posterior capsule and unusual thinness of the capsule predisposed these eyes to posterior capsular rupture.

Type 3 and 4 PPC are associated with increased chances of PC rupture and associated complications.

How to Prevent/Minimise Risk of Posterior Capsule Rupture

Dealing with the posterior plaque during phacoemulsification carefully may decrease intraoperative and postoperative complications and remarkably improve postoperative visual acuity.

Following tips may be very beneficial while managing posterior polar cataracts:
   (i) No hydrodissection or very selective hydrodissection.
   (ii) Gentle deep core hydrodelineation leaving superficial and most posterior layers free from hydrodelineation.
   (iii) Least US energy on zero degree tip.
   (iv) No sculpting rather relying upon Chopping or Cart wheel movements/onion peeling techniques of nucleus management.
   (v) Moderate aspiration /irrigation settings.

Results

Overall visual outcome following phacoemulsification surgery in cases of posterior polar cataract is encouraging and gratifying. More than 85% patients are likely to regain visual acuity of 20/40 or more. However, the remaining cases may have compromised and poor visual outcome due to preexisting conditions like amblyopia or retinal involvements like macular degeneration and retinitis pigmentosa.

CONCLUSION

Surgical management of posterior polar cataracts poses a special challenge to the cataract surgeon. It is important that the surgeon and the patient understand the technical difficulties associated and are aware of potential complications. It may be prudent to address these cases at the end of an operating list or to shorten the list in anticipation of prolonged surgical time. The surgeon should use a technique that he or she is most familiar and comfortable with. With emphasis on gentleness, together with patience and a well-practiced technique, the incidence of PCR can be minimised in phacoemulsification for posterior polar cataracts.

BIBLIOGRAPHY

1. Luntz MH. Clinical types of cataracts. Duane's Ophthalmology 1996; CD ROM.
2. Siatri H, Moghimi S: Posterior polar cataract: minimising risk of posterior capsule rupture. Eye. 2006 Jul; 20(7):814–6.
3. Fine IH, Packer M, Hoffman RS. Management of posterior polar cataract. J Cataract Refract Surg. 2003; 29:16–19.
4. Haripriya A, Arvind S, Vadi K, Natchiar G: Bimanual microphaco for posterior polar cataracts. J Cataract Refract Surg. 2006 Jun; 32(6):914–7.
5. Gavris M, Popa D Carcus C, Gusho E,Clocotan D, Horvath K. Ardelean A, Sangeorzan D: Phacoemulsification in posterior polar cataract Oftalmologia. 2004;48(4):36–40. Romanian.
6. Lee MW, Lee YC. Phacoemulsification of posterior polar cataracts—a surgical challenge. Br J Ophthalmol. 2003, 87:1426–1427.
7. Liu Y,Liu Y, Wu M, Zhang X: Phacoemulsification in eyes with posterior polar cataract and foldable intraocular lens implantation Yan Ke Xue Bao. 2003 Jun; 19(2):92–4. Chinese.
8. Hayashi K, Hayashi H, Nakao F, Hayashi F : Outcomes of surgery for posterior polar cataract. J Cataract Refract Surg. 2003 Jan; 29(1):45–9.
9. Vasavada A, Singh R. Phacoemulsification in eyes with posterior polar cataract. J Cataract Refract Surg. 1999 Feb; 25(2):238–45.
10. Vasavada A, Singh R. Step-by-step chop in-situ and separation of very dense cataracts. J Cataract Refract Surg 1998; 24:156–9.
11. Vasavada AR, Raj SM. Inside-out delineation. J Cataract Refract Surg. 2004; 30:1167–1169.
12. Osher RH, Yu BC, Koch DD. Posterior polar cataracts: A predisposition to intraoperative posterior capsular rupture. J Cataract Refract Surg. 1990 Mar; 16(2):157–62.
13. Osher RH. Slow motion phacoemulsification approach. J Cataract Refract Surg. 1993; 19:667.
14. Allen D, Wood C. Minimising risk to the capsule during surgery for posterior polar cataract. J Cataract Refract Surg. 2002; 28:742–744.
15. Budde WM, Jonas JB. Complications after rupture of the lens capsule with vitreous body prolapse during routine cataract operations Klin Monatsbl Augenheilkd. 1999 Oct; 215(4): 237–40. German.

33

Phaco in Myopic Eye

Col JKS Parihar SM, VSM

INTRODUCTION

Cataract surgery in the presence of high myopia remains a big challenge mainly due to the peculiarities of structural and refractive anomalies as well as the compounded risk of intra and postoperative complications. Despite the fact that modern technique of phacoemulsification cataract surgery has improved the operative safety and minimised the risk of complications substantially in all kinds of complex and complicated cataract, the high myopia still poses certain inherent problems.

In this chapter, we have analysed the overall view on the phacoemulsification surgery in the presence of myopia of more than 7 dioptres along with peculiarities of configuration of eye including the anterior chamber, lens and fundus traits like retinal thinning, staphyloma and axial elongation as well as intraoperative complications, their prevention and management strategies and ultimate postoperative refractive status are analysed.

STRUCTURAL VARIATIONS IN HIGHLY MYOPIC (MORE THAN 7 DIOPTERS) EYE FROM NORMAL EYE AND ITS CORRELATION WITH THE APPLIED ANATOMY OF LENS

The entire eye ball is large and prominent; the anterior chamber is deep, and the pupil usually large and somewhat sluggish.

Ophthalmoscopically, the main changes observed are the generalised atrophy of the retina and the choroid, the myopic crescent at the disc, the disturbances at the macula, the occurrence of a posterior staphyloma, and cystoid degeneration at the ora serrata,

At the macula an atrophic patch is common, and this is accompanied by the abolition of central vision. A similarly disastrous result is produced by the appearance of a dark pigmented area in this region (Forster-Fuchs fleck).

Complications in the form of tears and haemorrhages in the retina may occur spontaneously and may be accompanied by retinal detachment.

Most of the cases of myopia are axial. Axial length is shown to have an emmetropising effect on lens thickness, being more optically powerful (thicker) in hyperopic eyes. These values are useful in determining average sound velocities for use with ultrasound A-scan instruments for measuring the axial length of the eye. Patients with axial myopia are more likely to develop cataracts at an earlier age than those with shorter axial lengths.

Various studies have shown a strong association between nuclear and posterior subcapsular cataracts and myopia. A nuclear cataract is a frequent occurrence in high myopia. Posterior subcapsular cataract is also associated with deeper anterior chamber, thinner lens, and longer vitreous chamber, with vitreous chamber depth explaining most of the association between posterior subcapsular cataract and myopia.

CONSTRAINTS OF PHACOEMULSIFICATION SURGERY IN CASES OF HIGH MYOPIA

High myopia has several constraints in performing phacoemulsification surgery based on structural and functional variants. A larger anterior segment and wider pupil dilatation may induce significant problems right from the construction of incision, larger rhexis size, which will not cover intraocular lens edges. Inconsistent and abnormal depth of the anterior chamber are significant problems. The presence of elongated and lax zonules of the lens accompanied with degenerated vitreous may result in subluxation or dislocation of the lens and so this may contribute to the operative hazards of cataract surgery.

Intraoperative constrains compounded with sclerotic and posterior subcapsular cataract tend to have a higher incidence of posterior capsule opacification.

PREOPERATIVE EVALUATION INCLUDING FOR GLAUCOMA IN THE PRESENCE OF MYOPIA

Measurement of the axial length is of importance since an increase in the axial length or myopia of the eye is associated with a lower mean age at the time of surgery and higher grade of nuclear cataract.

A careful look for posterior lenticonus is suggested in cases in which there is a discrepancy between the biometry and refraction and no significant nuclear sclerosis to account for the high myopia. Surgeons should be aware of dehiscence or thinning of the posterior capsule while doing cataract extraction in these patients.

Active searching and prophylactic laser treatments for retinal tears developed before and after cataract extraction in patients with high myopia are recommended. This may lower the incidence of postoperative retinal detachment.

Amblyopia, maculopathy and other pathologies should be ruled out. History must accurately correlate the accuracy of symptoms with the clinical findings. Esophoria may occur in very high myopia without subjective trouble. Binocular motility should be examined in advance and patients warned in dubious cases that there would be a period of adaptation to the new condition.

High myopia is associated with-the-rule or oblique astigmatism. Its reduction requires tailored incisional approach, to avoid its postoperative increase and torque.

Various reports have documented the higher incidence of open angle glaucoma in cases of high myopia. However, enhanced scleral elasticity and decreased rigidity due to elongated eyeball and vitreous degeneration poses great challenge in early detection of glaucoma in such cases. Hence, meticulous attention is very much essential to rule out the presence of glaucoma despite so called normal intraocular pressure.

CALCULATION OF IOL POWER INCLUDING POST SURGICAL TARGET REFRACTION

Target Refraction in Myopic Eye after IOL Implantation

The presumed postoperative refractive status remains a challenging and the most difficult task in following modern cataract surgery in the present scenario. The changing pattern of professional and social activities based on the very high and excellent visual functions demands precision of a very high order following cataract surgery.

The ultimate postcataract surgery refractive status is based on several factors. The myopes with good retinal functions and reported to have good visual acuity prior to the cataract formation may remain comfortable with a refractive status of residual –0.5 to –1.0 D myopia, postoperatively.

However, in the presence of impaired visual functions, due to preexisting retinochoroidal abnormalities or unprecedent and compound myopic astigmatism, the patient may not be comfortable with emmetropia. The myopes with such functional and structural status are much more comfortable and tuned with a substandard distance visual acuity and to a good near vision. Hence, an emmetropic postoperative refraction with an added need of correction for near visual acuity may not be acceptable to this group of patient.

Considering various aspects, the postoperative refractive status should be customised as per the need of each and every patient. A younger patient or a very skilled professional will require the precise and accurate visual acuity in all the dimensions of visual need. Whereas, an elderly and high myopic will be more happy with excellent near and intermediate visual acuity. The postsurgical residual myopia of around –2.0 D is an excellent option as target refraction to achieve in cases of elderly myopic individuals. This will facilitate good near and intermediate functions and very good comfort with corrected visual acuity for distance. However, younger age group should be subjected to near emmetropic correction as per the demand of their professional and social activities.

Methods of Biometry and Challenges of High Myopia

IOL power measurement and biometry is often not accurate in eyes with high myopia or high hyperopia, particularly evaluated by conventional A-ultrasound method for the measurement of the axial length. Partial coherence interferometry biometry, a non-invasive method, has been found to be much more precise and accurate for measuring the axial length, thereby it is substantial in improving in the postoperative refraction.

Postcorneal refractive surgery cornea poses a greater challenge while evaluating the IOL power measurement which turns to be inaccurate and gives unpredictable refractive outcome with conventional methods of biometry.

In eyes with axial lengths longer than or equal to 27.0 mm, current third- and fourth-generation lens calculation formula's have a tendency to over minus patients between –1.0 and –4.0 D. The formula's appear to perform better for the plus-power IOL implantation than for the minus-power IOL implantation. Unevenness of the posterior pole caused by a staphyloma decreases the accuracy of axial length measurements. The longest values may not correspond to the visual axis, with postoperative hypermetropia, and reproducibility of the measurement being low. Hence, careful attention should be directed to locate macula relative to staphyloma on fundus examination. The undue myopic shift in the IOL power calculation can be minimised by occluding the other eye.

As compared to conventional IOL calculation formula, SRK-T formula provides better predictability in cases of large eyeball with axial length of more than 26.0 mm. One can also employ formulae like Holladay 1 and 2 and Hoffer Q in high myopic cases.

The precise position and depth of posterior pole staphylomas may be ascertained by the B Scan so as to achieve higher predictability and accuracy in the presumed IOL power in the presence of high myopia.

After corneal refractive surgery, various techniques to determine the current corneal power should be compared and the value around which results tend to cluster should be relied on to avoid hyperopia after cataract surgery with lens implantation. In those cases where keratometry and refraction before PRK/LASIK are available, the gold standard used is to subtract the change of the SEQ at the corneal plane from the preoperative central keratometric power, although in the present case report, the subtraction of 24 % of the SEQ change at the spectacle plane from the measured corneal power value seemed to produce the best result. Pure subtraction of the SEQ change at the spectacle plane from the corneal power value before refractive surgery has to be avoided in eyes with excessive myopia. The most reliable corrected power value should be inserted in more than one modern third-generation formula (such as Haigis, Hoffer Q, Holladay 2, SRK/T) and the highest power IOL should be implanted. In all instances, the cataract surgeon has to make sure that the corrected K-reading is not wrongly re-converted within the IOL power calculation formula used.

Clear lens extraction with negative-power IOL implantation using the SRK/T formula had good effective-ness, acceptable predictability, and a low morbidity in eyes with extreme myopia over a short follow-up. A longer follow-up with more cases is needed to assess the safety of the procedure.

Surgeons should be aware of the tendency for negative-powered lenses to overcorrect and lead to a hyperopic outcome when using the SRK/T biometry formula in highly myopic eyes. A weaker-powered negative IOL is recom-mended to aim for a more myopic postoperative outcome by about 1.00 to 2.00 D.

SURGICAL TECHNIQUE

Anaesthesia: Topical *vs* Peribulbar

Infiltrative anaesthesia carries a greater risk of eyeball perforation due to longer axial length and posterior staphyloma. The surgeon should pay maximum attention when peribulbar or retrobulbar infiltrations are performed in these patients. The axial length of the eye should be known, the patient should be asked to keep the eyes wide open during the block procedures, and the surgeon should not compress the eye ball to avoid rotating the posterior pole towards the expected needle passage. Perforation of the sclera provokes acute pain, which is exacerbated by the injection of local anaesthetic inside the eye. It should be suspected when there is marked hypotony, flattening of the anterior chamber, alteration of the reflex of the fundus, and vitreous haemorrhage. A common and serious result of the perforation is detachment of the retina.

The incidence of retrobulbar haemorrhage varies between 1 to 3%. The use of fine needles provokes smaller lesions to the vessels and bleeding that is easier to control.

Ptosis and diplopia are common during the first 48 hours after cataract surgery when performed on local blocks. The persistence of functional alterations of the extraocular muscles suggest a myotoxic effect of the anaesthetic or damage to the motor nerve. The most common cause of prolonged functional defects in the extraocular muscles is the intramuscular injection.

With the above in view, peribulbar technique should be preferred over retrobulbar. Topical anaesthesia appears more than appropriate.

Role of CTR

In high myopes, zonules are weak and sometimes the zonules are so weak that a vitreous strand from the base may gain entry into the anterior chamber, simulating a posterior capsule rupture. In such cases a capsular tension ring may help to stabilise the bag.

Incisions

In cases of preoperative astigmatism, the incision should be created in the steepest meridian. The incision causes flattening of the meridian it had cut along with steepening of the opposite meridian. As a result, the superior incision that causes against-the-rule astigmatism can be useful for correcting with-the-rule astigmatism.

The high myopic eye is invariably found to have abnormally deep anterior chamber which may pose intra operative constraints during the phacomanoeuvre. Hence, an ideal phaco tunnel should not be too long so as to avoid any undue pressure on the cornea while performing instrumentation.

The size of the incision depends on the size of the lens to be implanted. The incision should be large enough to consent the easy implantation of the lens without causing any trauma to the edges of the incision itself.

This is especially important in the case of myopia as the implanted lens may be large due to the large dimensions of the capsular bag.

Rhexis

There is a temptation not to deepen the anterior chamber too much because it makes the capsulorrhexis more difficult; it is safer to have the capsule flattened with viscoelastic.

Myopic pupil, by and large, dilates well. A judicious approach is very much essential to ensure the appropriate

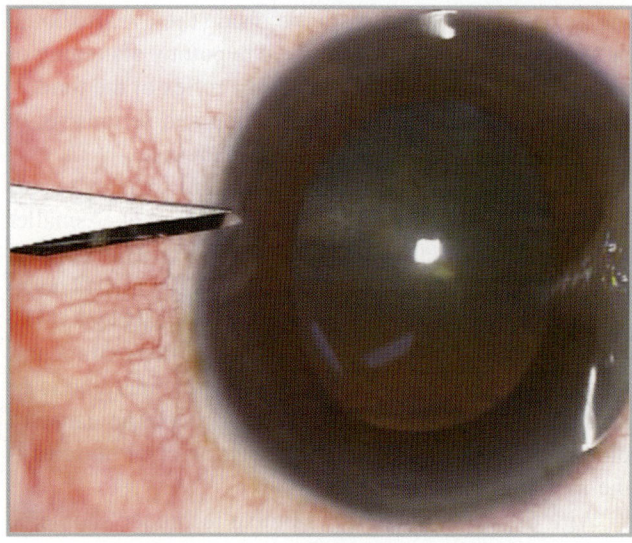 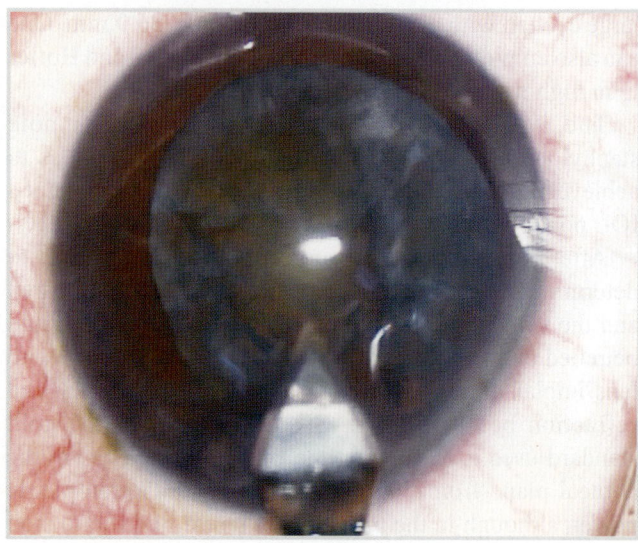
(a)   (b)

Fig. 33.1: (a) Side port incision, (b) Main incision (extended upto 2.8 mm after completion of hydroprocedures)

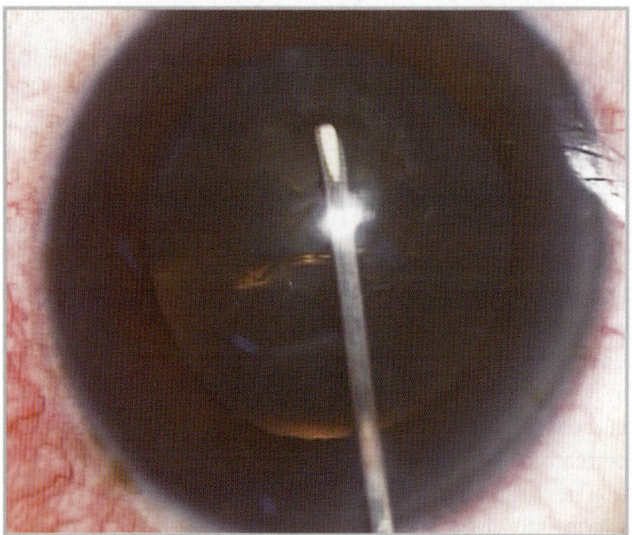

Fig. 33.2 : Rhexis

size of the rhexis which should not be too large so as to allow adequate approximation and cover of edges of optics of the IOL implant particularly in the presence of greater diameter of the anterior chamber.

Another important factor is unexpected elasticity of capsule with a tendency to extend and tear towards the periphery, specially in the presence of a large rhexis in a widely dilated pupil. This may lead to zonular disinsertion. The tear may then have a tendency to follow the radial course of the zonules rather than the desired circumferential course. Hence, the rhexis of 5 to 5.5 mm remains an ideal choice.

A widely dilated pupil, commonly seen in high myopes, favours the occurrence of peripheral extension of the capsulorrhexis because the zonular insertions may be encountered. The tear may then have a tendency to follow the radial course of the zonules rather than the desired

circumferential course. Hence, rhexis should be done with utmost care in these patients.

Hydroprocedures

Hydrodissection and hydrodelineation should be done taking care to decompress the capsule by depressing the central portion of the lens with the cannula so that fluid is forced around the lens equator from behind.

These manoeuvres should be done with utmost gentleness to prevent any undue force on the zonules, which may already be weak in such cases.

Techniques of Nucleotomy (Chopping *verses* Sculpting)

Sculpting being a basic technique has several safety features over chopping, particularly in the hands of a beginner or less

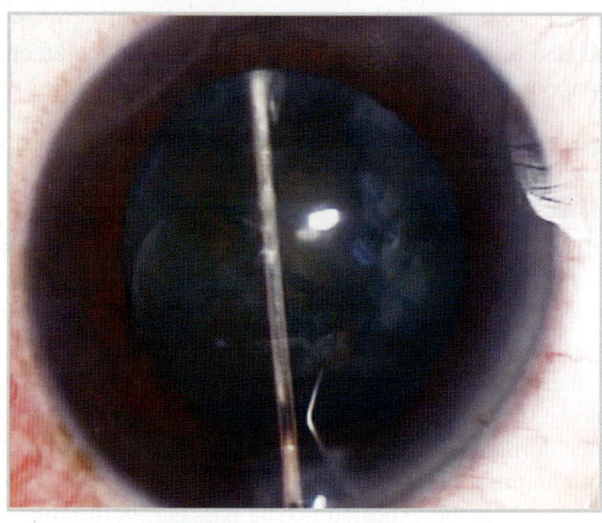

Fig. 33.3: Hydroprocedures

experienced surgeon, specially in the presence of uncomplicated cataracts. However, high myopia associated with the presence of deep anterior chamber, weak and stretched zonules and degenerated vitreous makes sculpting vulnerable to the enhanced risk of intraoperative complications. Such threat may be minimised by meticulous attention and the application of precise position of phaco tip during sculpting. The parallel movement in relation to the concave slope of the posterior aspect of the nucleus and posterior capsule is very much essential for ideal sculpting. A constant position of the residual nuclear material ahead of the phaco tip at the end of each sculpting manoeuvre is very crucial to maintain safety. It is equally important to ensure that the nucleus should not be engaged too deep, specially in the inferior pole so as to avoid disinsertion of superior zonules.

Author's Preference

In our view, chopping is a fairly safe technique particularly while dealing with situations like high myopia, vitreous degeneration, subluxated lens or zonular weakness. A good rhexis of 5.5 to 6.0 mm size, sequential hydroprocedures and adequate prechopping clearing of cortical material (except under surface of nucleus) enhances safety of chopping over sculpting.

The US energy demands is much less with chopping as compared to sculpting. The traction on zonules due to repeated linear movements of tip is much more during sculpting whereas mechanical force on zonules and the posterior capsule is greatly reduced while performing chopping due to freely floating nucleus over the posterior cortical plate under the presence of viscocushions.

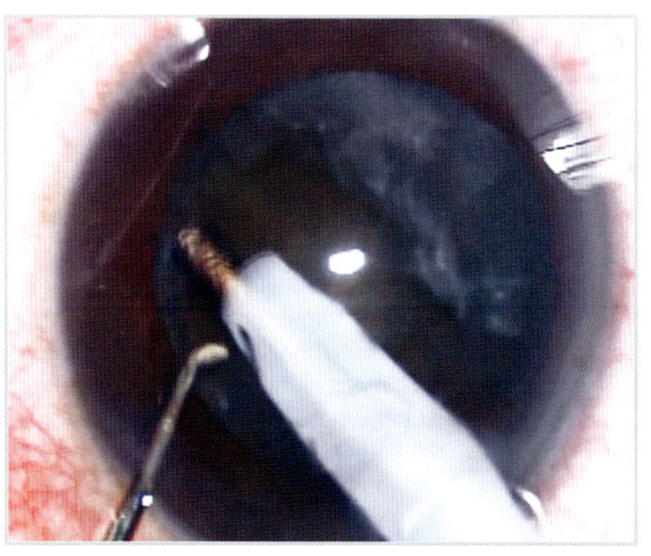

(a)

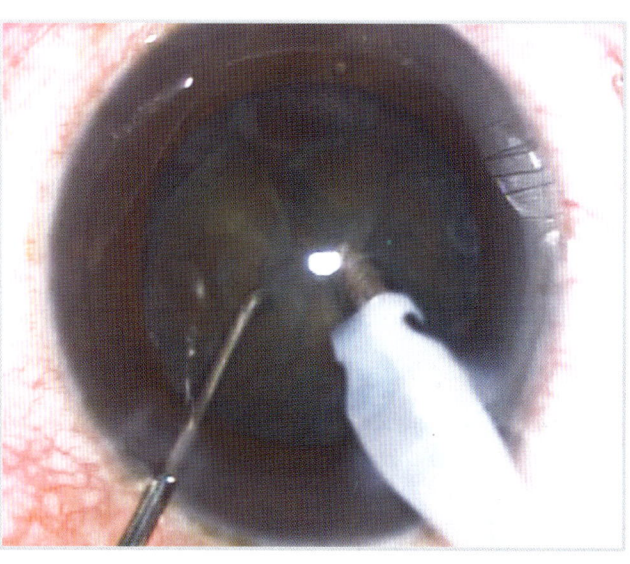

(b)

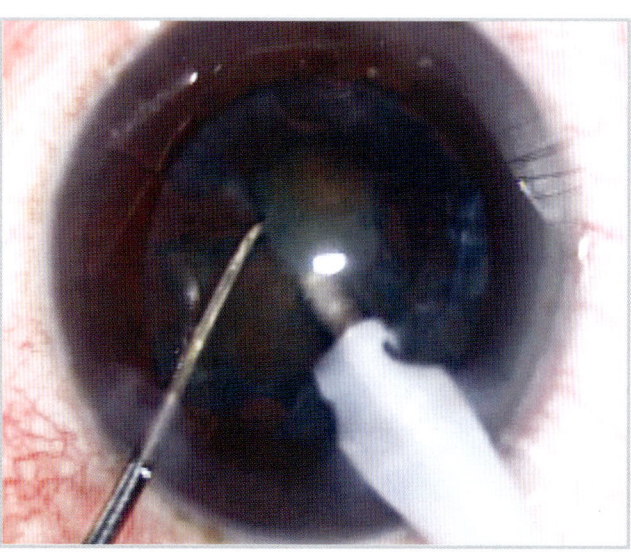

(c)

Fig. 33.4: (a) Nucleotomy in high myopia: Prechopping cortical clearing, (b) Nucleotomy in highmyopia: Direct central chopping, (c) Nucleotomy in high myopia: Fragment removal

The surgeon may even perform chopping at the iris plane in cases of high myopia, since such eyes have deep anterior chamber; thereby minimising the threat to endothelial cells as well as to zonules and posterior capsule.

Machine Settings

The present concept of moderate settings of US energy, flow rate and vacuum which is based on advanced applications of fluid dynamics and Hydroprocedures, has revolutionised the nucleotomy techniques. Such settings are of immense benefit in case of complicated cataracts or complex situations like high myopia and zonular weakness. Advance phaco chop technique has least stress on zonules and the posterior capsule as well. However, certain modifications are required while dealing with cataract in the presence of high myopia.

Bottle Height

The average bottle height of about 50–60 cm above the patient head level is sufficient enough to handle cataract in the high myopic eye by minimising the impending risk of deep anterior chamber as well as of downward push on the lens diaphragm thereby resulting in enhanced safety. The progressive sequences of vertical and steeper positions of the phaco tip and corneal burns are also less with lower bottle height and moderate settings.

Suggested Settings

(i) Peristaltic pumps
Initial prechop cortical clearing:
(a) Flow rate 14–20 cubic ml/mt.
(b) Aspiration 125–175 mmHg.
Direct groove and central chopping/fragment removal:
(a) Flow rate 20–24 cubic ml/mt.

(b) Aspiration 175–225 mmHg.
(c) US energy: 10 to 30 % (Based on nucleus grading).

(ii) Ventury pumps
Initial prechop cortical clearing
Aspiration 60/–75 mmHg.
Direct groove and central chopping/fragment removal
(a) Aspiration 100–125 mmHg.
(b) US energy: 10 to 25% (Based on nucleus grading).

Irrigation and Aspiration

Sequential hydroprocedure softens the cortical matter as well as enhances the procedure of prechopping, cortical clearing and further, opening of capsular fornices.

Prechopping cortical clearing all over the nucleus except beneath it reduces the bulk of cortical matter for final removal by irrigation and aspiration.

Hence I/A can be accomplished by moderate settings of 225 to 250 mmHg that too without compromising the safety of zonules and capsular bag.

Choice of IOL

In extreme myopia, the dimensions of the IOL should be increased to adjust to a larger bag. A total diameter of 12.3 or even 12.5 mm may be inadequate to achieve a broad equatorial arc of contact. Larger pupil size and the need for repeated fundus examinations warrant optic sizes of 6 mm or even 6.5 mm. In our view, high refractive indexed single piece hydrophobic acrylic IOL having square edge is a better choice over other IOL implants, especially over PMMA lenses, since high myopia is linked with higher incidence of PCO.

The presence of an acrylic IOL of low-power, zero-power, or minus-power with a sharp optic edge reduces

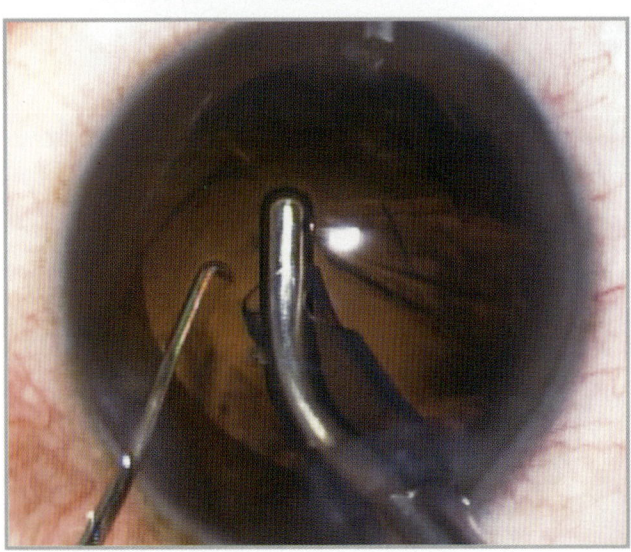

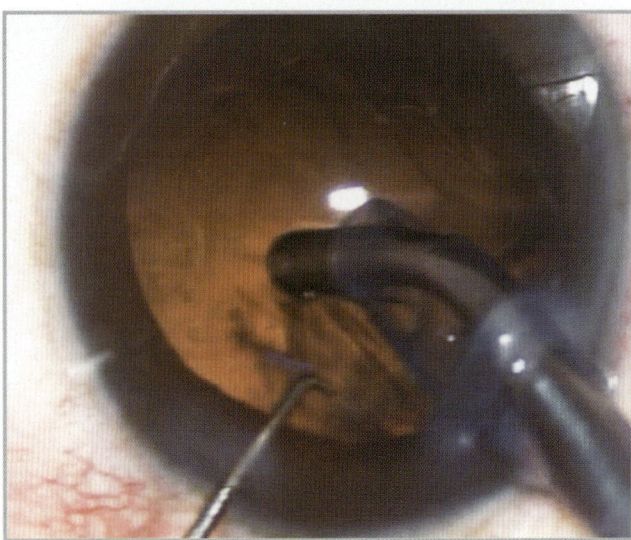

(a) (b)

Fig. 33.5: (a) Irrigation and aspiration in high myopia, (b) Irrigation and aspiration in high myopia: Removal of subincisional cortex

the incidence and severity of PCO as compared to the lens extraction alone in cases of high myopia.

COMPLICATIONS AND HOW TO PREVENT/ MINIMISE AND LINE OF MANAGEMENT

Intraoperative

Cataract surgery in the presence of high myopia poses several intraoperative risks and frequent occurrence of complications like zonular disinsertion, posterior capsular rent, dropped nucleus or fragment as well as possible dislocation of IOL implant. Undoubtedly, the incidence of above mentioned complications have declined to a great extent in the recent past.

The sole genesis of intraoperative risks are based on the presence of a frequently soft lens and thinner capsule and looser zonules. The sculpting procedure in a soft lens may excavate too deep. In addition to it, the disproportionate energy settings and undue mechanical force while attempting sculpting may aggravate zonular disinsertion in the condition of pre-existing zonular weakness. Lax zonules are preoperatively indicated by a deeper anterior chamber and slight lens subluxation. Lowering the infusion bottle height and flow is a better option to minimise the risk of retropulsion of the lens plane. Meticulous and relatively sloppy movement of the phaco tip parallel to the nuclear plane may decline the risk of impending damage to the zonules. However, in our view the cart wheel technique (modified by author) is very effective for soft cataract whereas direct groove and chopping remains the most effective and safe method in cases of all kinds of cataracts except soft cataract.

There are a number of surgical approaches available for the removal of subluxated lenses. Inatani et al have observed that lens extraction is effective in controlling intraocular pressure in eyes with secondary glaucoma associated with lens subluxation.

Earlier techniques like intra and extracapsular cataract extraction were associated with higher risks. However, the modern technique of phacoemulsification with the application of CTR or the use of iris hooks to provide support to the capsular bag has greatly enhanced the intraoperative safety as well as ease while handling subluxated cataract.

In addition to the above, the endocapsular lensectomy with vitrector, fragmatome removal via the pars plana may be a viable option in selected cases.

Postoperative Complications

(a) Immediate

The risk of complications in immediate postoperative period following phacoemulsification surgery in cases of high myopia remains same as seen in other cases. However, a close look is essentially required to keep a watch on the possibility of subluxation of IOL, secondary glaucoma and macular oedema in these cases despite the fact that we did not encounter any such occurrence in our practice so far.

(b) Intermediate and Late Complications

(i) Transient aesthenopia and diplopia

The high myopes may suffer from diplopia and transient aesthenopia following bilateral cataract surgery, mainly due to a sudden decline in the pre-existing high myopic status

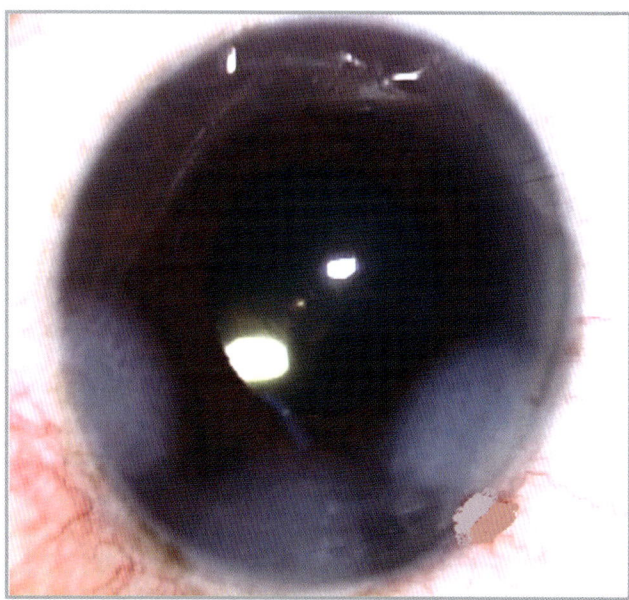

(a)   (b)

Fig. 33.6: (a) IOL Implantation in High Myopia: High refractive indexed single piece hydrophobic acrylic IOL, (b) IOL Implant is *in situ*

as well as precipitation or aggravation in the pre-existing or undetected esophoria. Such complaints invariably respond to appropriate use of prism and, by and large, do not warrant for any surgical intervention.

(ii) Dislocation of intraocular lens (IOL)

Dislocation of an intraocular lens (IOL) with the capsular bag is a late complication of cataract surgery, reported with increasing frequency in recent years. Pseudoexfoliation, uveitis, myopia, and other diseases associated with progressive zonular weakening and capsular contraction are the predisposing conditions. Capsular tension rings probably help but do not prevent this complication. Management includes IOL exchange, replacement with an anterior or a sutured posterior chamber IOL, or suturing the IOL through the bag to the iris or the sclera.

(iii) Rhegmatogenous retinal detachment

High myopes are vulnerable to have the occurrence of rhegmatogenous retinal detachment throughout life. This risk further increases following any ocular surgery or trauma. The various studies have reported the incidence of 4 to 5% following uncomplicated phacosurgery in this group. The myopes from the younger age group are more prone to retinal detachment due to the impending intraoperative risk of incomplete vitreous detachment. High myopes are found to have the known observation of retinal detachment following YAG laser capsulotomy.

Hence, a detailed preoperative and periodic post-operative fundus examination on a regular basis is strongly recommended. Early detection and treatment of peripheral retinal degenerations and holes has definitive role to reduce the incidence of retinal detachment.

(iv) Cystoid macular oedema

There is a rise in the incidence of postoperative cystoid macular oedema due to an increase in the incidence of vitreous loss during surgery or due to a postoperative disruption of the anterior hyaloid membrane. About 1 to 3 months after surgery, there may be a postoperative decrease of visual acuity. Ophthalmoscopy reveals loss of foveal reflex and a yellowish reflex or spot that appears to lie deep behind the retina. The cystoid spaces are best seen using the red-free light, which renders their inner walls visible.

(v) Choroidal neovascularisation (CNV) in patients with high myopia (>8 dioptres) who underwent cataract surgery

Various authors have studied the incidence and characteristics of choroidal neovascularisation (CNV) in cases of high myopia (>8 dioptres) following phaco-emulsification and intraocular lens implantation surgery. It has been observed that high myopia is linked with higher incidence of *CNV following cataract surgery which may vary upto 10 to 12%.* The eyes having pre-existing evidence of CNV preoperatively in the fellow eye were found to have high incidence of CNV (35 to 40%) following

cataract surgery as compared to 7 to 9% in cases of no evidence of CNV in the fellow eye.

(vi) PCO

High myopia has been found to have higher incidence of PCO following cataract surgery in earlier reports. These were linked with conventional ECCE and initial experiences with phacoemulsification surgery. Such an incidence has been reported from 20 to 30 % after 3 years of surgery. However, there has been significant decline in this incidence in recent past which is mainly based on the invention of newer hydrophobic square edge IOLs, CTR and viscoelastics, advanced techniques of phaco, based on judicious application of fluidics as well as availability of modern phacomachines and microscopes.

In our series, the incidence of PCO has declined upto 10 to 12% after 3 years of follow up which is at par with other uncomplicated cases.

(vii) Clear lens extraction by phacoemulsification and IOL implantation in a highly myopic eye.

Certain cases of high myopia particularly those who are having refractive and structural contraindications for keratorefractive procedures may be benefited by clear lens extraction by phacoemulsification and IOL implantation.

Various studies have documented wide acceptability and gratifying outcome. Authors have experienced gratifying results following clear lens extraction in a large series. We did not notice any significant complication following clear lens extraction. In our view, sub two mm MICS followed by IOL implantation through 2 mm incision appears to be a better option. However, IOL implantation remains more appropriate even of very small power or negative power in these cases so as to minimise the risk of subsequent PCO formation.

CONCLUSION

The structural and refractive peculiarities of the myopic eye particularly in high myopes pose significant challenges in phacoemulsification surgery.

Pre-existing zonular weakness or laxity, vitreous degeneration, retinal involvements both peripheral degeneration and maculopathy remain high risk factors for ultimate visual recovery. However, a detailed preoperative workup of the individual patient, including extensive retinal examination and a thorough assessment of the IOL power is of great significance. Meticulous attention towards fluidics, machine parametres and selection of appropriate techniques of nucleotomy are essential and key factors to minimise the risk of any complications. Needless to stress, the modern phacoemulsification technique has revo-lutionised the ultimate outcome of cataract surgery in highly complex situations as compared to the conventional extracapsular cataract surgery methods.

BIBLIOGRAPHY

1. H. Seward, R. Packard, and D. Allen. Management of cataract surgery in a high myope. Br J Ophthalmol. 2001 November; 85(11):1372–1378.

2. Tsai Ching-Yao; Chang Ting-Jia ; Kuo Li-Lin; Chou Pesus; Woung Lin-Chung. Visual outcomes and associated risk factors of cataract surgeries in highly myopic Taiwanese : Ophthalmologica 2007, vol. 221, (1) pp. 18–23.

3. Kohnen S, Brauweiler P. First results of cataract surgery and implantation of negative power intraocular lenses in highly myopic eyes. J Cataract Refract Surg. 1996 May; 22(4): 416–420.

4. Kora Y, Yaguchi S, Inatomi M, Ozawa T. Preferred postoperative refraction after cataract surgery for high myopia. J Cataract Refract Surg. 1995 Jan; 21(1):35–38.

5. Budak K, Friedman NJ, Koch DD. Limbal relaxing incisions with cataract surgery. J Cataract Refract Surg. 1998 Apr; 24(4):503–508.

6. Totan Y, Bayramlar H, Cekiç O, Aydin E, Erten A, Daðlioðlu MC. Bilateral cataract surgery in adult and pediatric patients in a single session. J Cataract Refract Surg. 2000 Jul; 26(7): 1008–1011.

7. Ramsay AL, Diaper CJ, Saba SN, Beirouty ZA, Fawzi HH. Simultaneous bilateral cataract extraction. J Cataract Refract Surg. 1999 Jun; 25(6):753–762.

8. Beatty S, Aggarwal RK, David DB, Guarro M, Jones H, Pearce JL. Simultaneous bilateral cataract extraction in the UK. Br J Ophthalmol. 1995 Dec; 79(12):1111–1114.

9. Galand A, van Cauwenberge F, Moosavi J. Posterior capsulorhexis in adult eyes with intact and clear capsules. J Cataract Refract Surg. 1996 May; 22(4):458–461.

10. Modarres M, Parvaresh MM, Hashemi M, Peyman GA. Inadvertent globe perforation during retrobulbar injection in high myopes. Int Ophthalmol. 1997; 21(4):179–185.

11. Osher RH, Yu BC, Koch DD. Posterior polar cataracts: A predisposition to intraoperative posterior capsular rupture. J Cataract Refract Surg. 1990 Mar; 16(2):157–162.

12. Alldredge CD, Elkins B, Alldredge OC Jr. Retinal detachment following phacoemulsification in highly myopic cataract patients. J Cataract Refract Surg. 1998 Jun; 24(6):777–780.

13. Jacobi FK, Hessemer V. Pseudophakic retinal detachment in high axial myopia. J Cataract Refract Surg. 1997 Sep; 23(7): 1095–1102.

14. Olsen G, Olson RJ. Update on a long-term, prospective study of capsulotomy and retinal detachment rates after cataract surgery. J Cataract Refract Surg. 2000 Jul; 26(7):1017–1021.

15. Kengo Hayashi, Kyoko Ohno-Matsui, Soh Futagami Seiji Ohno, Takashi Tokoro and Manabu Mochizuki : Choroidal Neovascularisation in Highly Myopic Eyes After Cataract Surgery :Jpn J Ophthalmol 2006; 50:345–348.

16. Nishi O, Nishi K, Sakanishi K. Inhibition of migrating lens epithelial cells at the capsular bend created by the rectangular optic edge of a posterior chamber intraocular lens. Ophthalmic Surg Lasers. 1998 Jul; 29(7):587–594.

17. Nishi O, Nishi K, Wickström K. Preventing lens epithelial cell migration using intraocular lenses with sharp rectangular edges. J Cataract Refract Surg. 2000 Oct; 26(10):1543–1549.

18. Peng Q, Visessook N, Apple DJ, Pandey SK, Werner L, Escobar-Gomez M, Schoderbek R, Solomon KD, Guindi A. Surgical prevention of posterior capsule opacification. Part 3: Intraocular lens optic barrier effect as a second line of defense. J Cataract Refract Surg. 2000 Feb; 26(2): 198–213.

19. Apple DJ, Peng Q, Visessook N, Werner L, Pandey SK, Escobar-Gomez M, Ram J, Auffarth GU. Eradication of posterior capsule opacification: documentation of a marked decrease in Nd:YAG laser posterior capsulotomy rates noted in an analysis of 5416 pseudophakic human eyes obtained postmortem. Ophthalmology. 2001 Mar; 108(3): 505–518.

20. Zaldivar R, Shultz MC, Davidorf JM, Holladay JT. Intraocular lens power calculations in patients with extreme myopia. J Cataract Refract Surg. 2000 May; 26(5):668–674.

21. Hoffer KJ. Clinical results using the Holladay 2 intraocular lens power formula. J Cataract Refract Surg. 2000 Aug; 26(8):1233–1237.

22. Vasavada AR, Chauhan H, Shah G. Incidence of posterior capsular plaque in cataract surgery. J Cataract Refract Surg. 1997 Jun; 23(5):798–802.

23. Apple DJ, Isaacs RT, Kent DG, Martinez LM, Kim S, Thomas SG, Basti S, Barker D, Peng Q. Silicone oil adhesion to intraocular lenses: an experimental study comparing various biomaterials. J Cataract Refract Surg. 1997 May; 23(4): 536–544.

24. Farbowitz MA, Zabriskie NA, Crandall AS, Olson RJ, Miller KM. Visual complaints associated with the AcrySof acrylic intraocular lens(1). J Cataract Refract Surg. 2000 Sep; 26(9): 1339–1345.

25. Davison JA. Positive and negative dysphotopsia in patients with acrylic intraocular lenses. J Cataract Refract Surg. 2000 Sep; 26(9):1346–1355.

34

Phaco in Severely Hyperopic Eye

Col JKS Parihar SM, VSM and Lt Col SK Mishra VSM

INTRODUCTION

The highly hyperopic eye is atypical in response to surgery because of its peculiar anatomy. Moreover, a significant percentage of hyperopic eyes develop narrowing of the angle of the anterior chamber (AC) later in life as the growth of the lens becomes disproportionate to the size of the remaining anterior segment. Also many of these eyes may have to be treated with prolonged miotic therapy, which causes rigid and miotic pupil, formation of pupillary membranes, and development of the cataract.

Cataract surgery in these severely hyperopic and/or microphthalmic eyes is difficult from both anatomical and functional points of view. Fortunately, cataract extraction by a closed chamber technique through a small incision in the first instance and under topical anesthesia in the second, has greatly improved the surgical outcome in these eyes and a series of maneuvers have been developed to further reduce complications.

At present, with advancement of machines and techniques, phacoemulsification can now be performed in severely hyperopic eyes with nearly the same safety as the average eye. This has given surgeons confidence to subject these eyes to cataract surgery and intraocular lens (IOL) implantation for solely refractive purposes.

Emmetropia following surgery in highly hyperopic eyes cannot be predicted and guaranteed due to difficulty of precise calculation of presumed power of the IOL. Eyes that are much longer or shorter than normal do not correlate well with the available statistical formulae, even with modifications. The theoretical formulae are not precise because they are based on estimations of optical and anatomical relations and/or on empirically derived constants, the imprecision of which is magnified in cases of extremes of axial lengths. Often, there is an under-correction, which is particularly discomforting when the operation is performed to correct the refractive error. Moreover, IOLs are normally difficult to procure in powers that exceed 34 dioptres. Intraocular lenses with greater power can be produced, but the optical characteristics of these lenses suffer due to high anterior curvature. As a result, more than one lens may be necessary for achieving emmetropia, using the technique polypseudophakia.

ANATOMICAL FEATURES IN A SEVERELY HYPEROPIC EYE THAT INFLUENCE CATARACT SURGERY

Knowledge of the surgical anatomy of hyperopic eyes is essential for discussing surgical techniques, complications and their prevention. Some features are common to all severely hyperopic or microphthalmic eyes, while others are observed in a smaller number. Generally speaking, hyperopic eyes fall into two categories:

(i) Those with a reduced anterior segment, and
(ii) Those with a normal anterior segment.

Hyperopic Eyes with a Reduced Anterior Segment

This is the most common cause of hypermetropia and is known as axial hypermetropia. About 1mm reduction of length can cause hypermetropia of 3 dioptres. These eyes do not have the same anterior chamber morphology as seen in cases of hyperopia with a normal anterior segment and depth. Reduced axial length can be an unexpected outcome of biometry.

Because of the dramatic presentation of acute glaucoma, we often consider hyperopic eyes as having an anterior segment that is proportional to the axial length with reduced size. Nevertheless, this is only true for a proportion of eyes. These eyes have reduced axial lengths, often less than 21 mm, the size of the crystalline lens is more or less normal and tends to push the iris forwards. This reduces the depth of the anterior chamber. The diameter of the cornea is relatively less but its thickness is nearly normal and this results in increased corneal rigidity. The iris is frequently dark and thick, the chamber angle is narrow (0–2 according to Shaffer). The posterior segment is typical of hyperopic eyes with an increase in scleral and choroidal thickness. These eyes may develop acute angle closure even in younger patients, those below 40. Often these eyes undergo a cataract surgery after a long history of narrow-angle glaucoma, Laser iridotomy, and probably a miotic pupil that does not dilate because of a prolonged miotic therapy. Prolonged use of miotics also exacerbates cataractous change and sometimes surgery may have been postponed for years because of the high risk of surgical complications. For example, due to shallow chamber Descemet's membrane can be easily damaged in the area close to the point of entry and the endothelial cell count is often reduced given the reduced space available in the anterior chamber and the typical considerable thickness of the cataractous lens.

Hyperopic Eyes with a Normal Anterior Segment

There are severely hyperopic or microphthalmic eyes with a normal-sized anterior segment which is not in proportion to the axial length. In these eyes, the size of the cornea is normal, the depth of the anterior chamber would appear to be normal, the chamber angle is wide and there is no risk of angle closure. In such cases, severe hyperopia is primarily a refractive disturbance due to a flatter curvature of cornea, lens, or both. About 1 mm increase in radius of curvature results in 6 dioptres of hypermetropia.

Prevalence of the Two Types

The two types of hyperopic eyes have a geographical distribution that is dependent on the characteristics of the local population. Closed angle glaucoma, with or without severe hyperopia, is more frequent among Eskimos. It has been seen that the prevalence of hyperopic eyes with a normal anterior segment is greater in extreme hyperopia (in excess of 10 dioptres) as compared to moderate hyperopia (between 3 and 6 dioptres). In a study of 93 hyperopic eyes, Holladay reported that 83% of eyes had a normal anterior segment, while the remaining 17% revealed a reduced anterior segment. The incidence of hyperopia in a reduced anterior segment has been found to vary between two and four percent. Contrary to this, myopic eyes are rarely associated with reduced anterior segment.

APPLIED ASPECTS OF CALCULATION OF THE IOL IMPLANT POWER

Keratometric Measurements

Keratometry can be measured using a routine keratometre or by using corneal topography. There are no specific problems in keratometry of severely hyperopic eyes and the imprecision observed are comparable to those for routine eyes.

Ultrasonic Biometry

Ultrasound biometry in the hyperopic eye on one hand is an apparently simple procedure, yet delicate on the other. Measurement of the axial length can be obtained easily using focalised probes, as the proximity to the posterior wall of the bulb permits return echo of considerable intensity. Sometimes, the intensity of this echo makes it necessary to reduce the gain. Use of immersion biometry avoids corneal flattening which can alter the calculation of the proper power of the IOL. Immersion technique permits a precise measurement of axial length that is comparable with measurements recorded by optical coherence biometry (OCB).

The depth of the anterior chamber and the thickness of the lens should be measured carefully, because the postoperative position of the IOL, and therefore the effective power in the pseudophakia will depend upon these anatomical structures.

Biometric measurement, and not the impression at the slit lamp, determines whether the anterior segment of the hyperopic eye is normal or shorter than normal.

Methods for Power Calculation

The statistical formulae for the calculation of the power of IOLs are highly unsatisfactory in severely hyperopic eyes because they tend to underestimate the ametropia. Moreover, they cannot consider the anatomical and biometrical differences between eyes with equal keratometric values and equal axial length, which in extreme hyperopia gives rise to two very different populations of eyes.

Recently optical formulae have been studied to provide better results in ametropic eyes, with attempts to reduce the approximations necessary with the statistical formula's or the more dated optical formula's. The basic concept is to identify the variables that can influence the result, including corneal diameter, keratometric values, ACD, thickness of the lens, and axial length. Holladay developed a formula (Holladay II), which appears to be particularly suited for severely hyperopic eyes.

Choice of the Implant

In highly hyperopic eyes, choice of implant must consider special conditions. Rigid polymethyl-methacrylate (PMMA) lenses should be reserved for exceptional cases, even though they are the only lens type available in powers greater than 30 D. Moreover, some foldable lenses are available with diameter of 5.5 mm, possibly too small for normal eyes but a valuable aid in microphthalmic eyes with a reduced anterior segment and pupil miosis. In eyes with a reduced anterior segment, a lens of total diameter of 12 mm is also suitable for implantation in the sulcus, in the event of rupture of the posterior capsule. Author prefers to use single piece hydrophobic IOL implants as a first choice essentially on the virtue of excellent IOL material, design as well as ease of the insertion technique.

PHACOEMULSIFICATION IN HIGHLY HYPEROPIC EYES

Before undertaking cataract surgery in severe hyperopia, one must consider the greater possibility of intra and postoperative complications if the anterior segment is reduced in size; furthermore, there will be considerable problems of postoperative refraction if the anterior segment is of abnormal dimensions.

Eyes with a Reduced Anterior Segment

Surgical difficulty in eyes with a reduced anterior segment is akin to the problem faced with narrow angle glaucoma. Extraction of the lens should preclude any possibility of an attack of acute glaucoma even years after surgery.

Increased Intraocular Pressure

Entering an eye with increased intraocular pressure (IOP) may jeopardize the safety of the entire operation. The sudden drop in pressure to atmospheric value, typically observed in extracapsular surgery, provokes dilation of the choroidal vascular bed which can lead to the rupture of choroidal vessels with suprachoroidal hemorrhage. Rarely, there can be an expulsive hemorrhage. Extracapsular extraction must be abandoned in these eyes. The eyes must be prepared for surgery by lowering the IOP to normal levels.

If the surgeon needs to operate under conditions of raised pressure, we recommend anesthesia that will cause a reduction in arterial pressure preferably general anesthesia with controlled hypotension. It is always recommended to give ocular hypotensive drugs like acetazolamide about 1–2 hrs before surgery if not contraindicated. Moreover, an eye under tension should be decompressed gradually to give the choroidal vessels time to adapt to the new lower pressure.

Low Endothelial Cell Count

The endothelial cell count may be very low in severely hyperopic eyes and the surgery has to be particularly delicate. An adhesive viscoelastic substance (viscoat) should be used liberally during phacoemulsification to maintain space and for providing protection to the corneal endothelium and also to prevent descemets stripping.

Reduced Depth of the Anterior Chamber

In a setting where closed angle glaucoma is also present, the AC may be less than 2 mm deep, obliging the surgeon to use a more corneal approach for the incision. The tunnel should be slightly shorter than normal so that the internal incision will not be excessively central. The objective is to avoid the prolapse or even minor damage of the iris, hence facilitating the maneuvers in a reduced space. The anterior chamber can then be deepened with a viscoelastic substance (VES) with high zero shear viscosity, such as Healon GV or Healon 5. The shorter and more central corneal tunnel may have to be sutured at the end of the surgery.

Miosis

Reduced pupil diameter is seen commonly in highly hyperopic eyes, particularly those on prolonged miotic therapy. Fibrosis of the pupillary margin is often associated with the formation of a pale or pigmented ring. Sometimes, a true pupillary membrane develops. Its consistency is similar to the anterior capsule but it is easily distinguished.

Miosis should not be resolved with strong sympathomimetics as these risk provoking an increase in arterial pressure that can dilate the choroidal vascular bed with an increase of vitreous pressure. It is safer to use a VES with high viscosity at zero shear-Healon GV or Healon 5 that deepens the anterior chamber, maintains pressure tension on the pupil margin and can be removed. The pupil should be dilated mechanically only if absolutely necessary. Capsulorrhexis is easily achieved if there is no posterior pressure.

If other measures fail, the surgeon can perform multiple sphincterotomies which involve no more that 1 mm of the iris. Following cataract surgery, many pupils dilated in this way return almost completely to their preoperative dimensions.

Posterior Pressure

Excessive vitreous pressure during cataract surgery is common in glaucomatous eyes, particularly those having narrow angle glaucoma. Posterior pressure begins shortly after the start of the operation and may be particularly evident towards the final phase of irrigation and aspiration. One of the main advantages of phacoemulsification is that it is a closed chamber surgery that can be interrupted at any stage and resumed after the pressure is controlled. Local infiltration anesthesia is risky for these eyes, while topical surface or general anesthesias create less orbital pressure. Sub-Tenon's anesthesia may be suitable but it may provoke uncomfortable subconjunctival hemorrhages.

Zonular Weakness

Zonular weakness, though otherwise rare in these eyes, may be a serious complication if induced during phaco-emulsification. Relaxation of the zonules is countered by the implantation of a ring for capsular tension (CTR), not a difficult manoeuvre in conditions of good visibility. Application of a CTR may be impossible under conditions of miosis.

The combination of miosis and relaxed zonules is a situation that may seriously compromise the outcome of surgery.

Hardness of the Cataract

If the consistency of the lens is not too firm, it causes few problems even under conditions of a small pupil. A very hard nucleus may make phacoemulsification very difficult through a small pupillary aperture. We prefer to perform sequential central chop including secondary central chopping of the core nucleus preceded by debulking of it. Moderately high vacuum and low power settings are ideal for this technique so as to ascertain due care to avoid burns at the site of sclerocorneal incision.

Surgical Complications in Hyperopic Eyes with Shallow Anterior Segment

Complications during or after phacoemulsification in highly hyperopic eyes with a shallow anterior chamber are frequently the same as those observed with more routine cataract surgery, though they appear with greater frequency. Some complications appear almost exclusively in eyes affected by angle closure glaucoma.

(i) *Floppy iris:* This is the most frequent complication. Due to increase in intraocular pressure, there is repeated prolapse of the iris making it floppy. Floppy iris tends to make phacoemulsification difficult increasing the risk of posterior capsule rupture.

(ii) *Rupture or disinsertion of the posterior capsule:* Rupture of the posterior capsule usually occurs through reduced visibility caused by pupillary miosis in eyes where the lens is hard and the capsule is fragile. This problem has to be managed by complete cleaning of the vitreous from the anterior segment and implantation of an IOL in the iridociliary sulcus. An endocapsular implantation of a foldable lens should be avoided since the field of view is significantly reduced and an accompanying zonular dialysis may have been missed.

(iii) *Transient postoperative increase in intraocular pressure:* In the majority of cases, raised IOP is due to the remaining viscoelastic that is left behind especially healon in the anterior segment at the end of surgery. Though, it has been demonstrated that a transitory increase in IOP does not cause further damage to the visual field, any degree of pressure increase can be corrected by giving oral acetazolamide or IV mannitol. If still very high, one can attempt paracentesis with a 30 G needle repeating the manoeuvre if necessary

(iv) **Ciliary block or malignant glaucoma:** Ciliary block or malignant glaucoma is a rare complication that may occur after any anterior and posterior segment surgery. It involves misdirection of aqueous into the vitreous instead of the posterior chamber. A large increase in pressure may follow with a reduction of the anterior chamber depth and secondary angle closure. Though a rare occurrence, this may occur in pseudophakic eyes. The biometric characteristics of eyes with malignant glaucoma are similar to severely hyperopic eyes. Medical treatment consists of cycloplegics and mydriatic eyedrops, while the surgical solution consists of a capsulotomy with Nd:YAG laser through an iridectomy if present, or a posterior vitrectomy performed in the more refractory cases.

Surgical Complications in Hyperopic Eyes with Normal Anterior Segment

When the anterior segment is normal, there are fewer surgical problems and they are similar to complications associated with routine cataract surgery; hence surgical strategies are essentially the same as in cases of any standard situation.

(i) *Zonular dehiscence:* Dehiscence of the zonules can be identified by a marked increase in depth of the anterior chamber during phacoemulsification. One must avoid further loss of zonules. It is advisable to lower the infusion bottle and vacuum level, and aspiration flow rate to avoid chamber fluctuations. These steps may lead to heating of the incision, particularly if the cataract is hard. Fortunately, many of these eyes are operated early, before the lens nucleus becomes hard and rigid. In case dehiscence is more than 3 O'clock hours, the endocapsular ring should be used before implanting the IOL.

(ii) *Rupture of disinsertion of the posterior capsule:* Rupture of the posterior capsule may occur because it is particularly thin in these microphthalmic eyes. In these eyes, zonular weakness becomes risk for both posterior capsules, in the event of a sudden shallowing of the previously deep anterior chamber, and for the integrity of the capsular attachments, with the possibility of partial or total zonular dialysis.

(iii) *Suprachoroidal effusion:* One feature of microphthalmic eyes, particularly those with an axial length of less than 20 mm have a tendency for suprachoroidal effusion when the pressure in the anterior chamber is reduced to atmospheric level. For this reason, extracapsular cataract extraction (ECCE) is considered risky, whereas with small incision phacoemulsification, this risk is greatly reduced. A recent study indicated a marked reduction of the prevalence of the uveal effusion during cataract surgery since phacoemulsification was introduced. However, if it appears, the operation must be interrupted and postponed until ophthalmoscopic examination of the posterior segment appears normal.

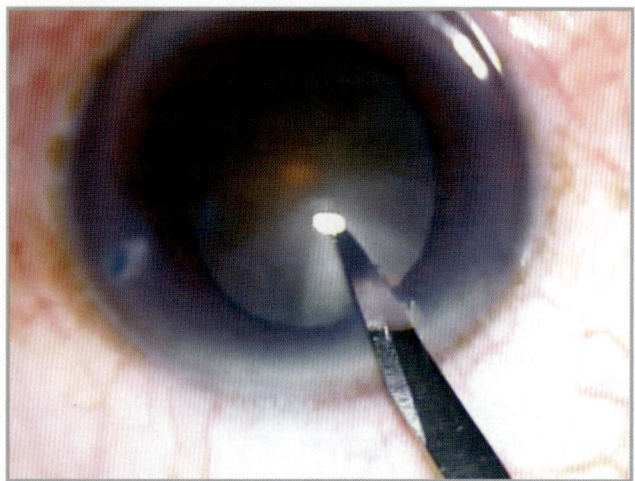

Fig. 34.1: Primary incision in a post YAG iridotomy hyperopic eye with shallow anterior chamber, poorly dilating pupil and hard brown cataract

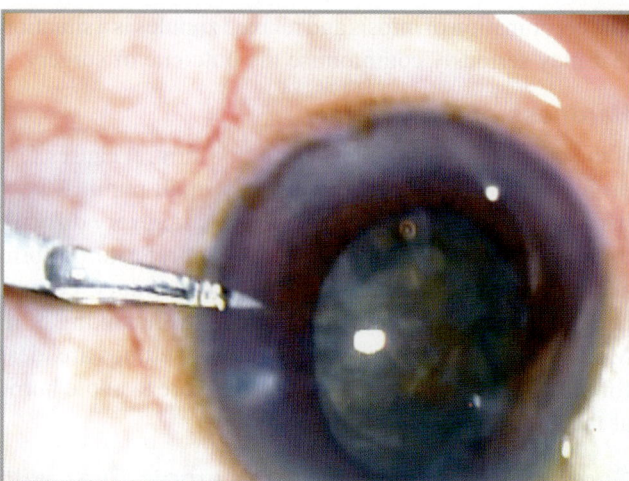

Fig. 34.2: Side port incision away from the site of YAG iridotomy in a hyperopic eye with shallow anterior chamber, poorly dilating pupil and hard brown cataract

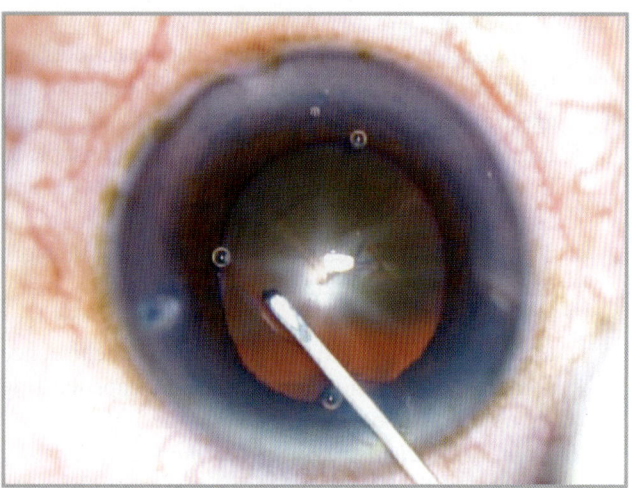

Fig. 34.3: Rhexis in a post YAG iridotomy hyperopic eye with shallow anterior chamber, poorly dilating pupil and hard brown cataract

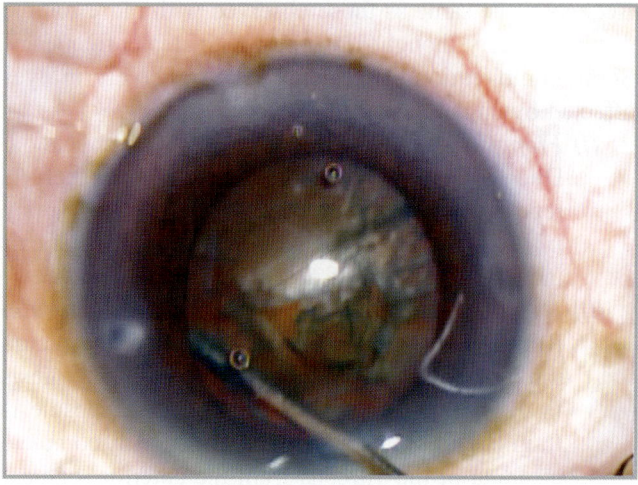

Fig. 34.4: Hydroprocedures in a post YAG iridotomy hyperopic eye with shallow anterior chamber

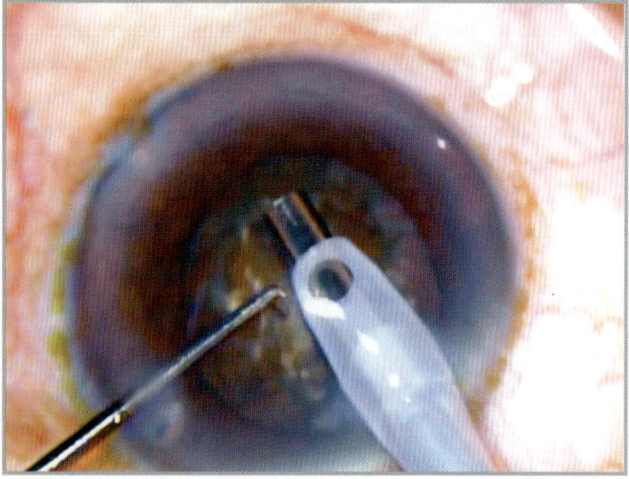

Fig. 34.5: Clearing of superficial cortex prior to the chopping in a post YAG iridotomy hyperopic eye with shallow anterior chamber

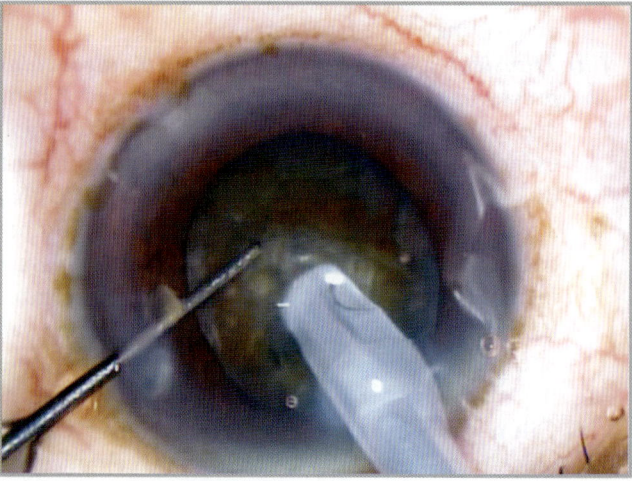

Fig. 34.6: Central chopping in a post YAG iridotomy hyperopic eye with shallow anterior chamber: Phaco tip is being embedded into the nucleus

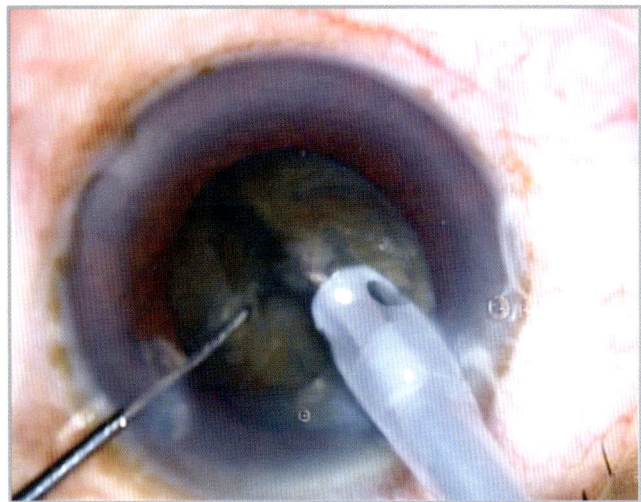

Fig. 34.7: Primary nucleotomy in a post YAG iridotomy hyperopic eye with shallow anterior chamber

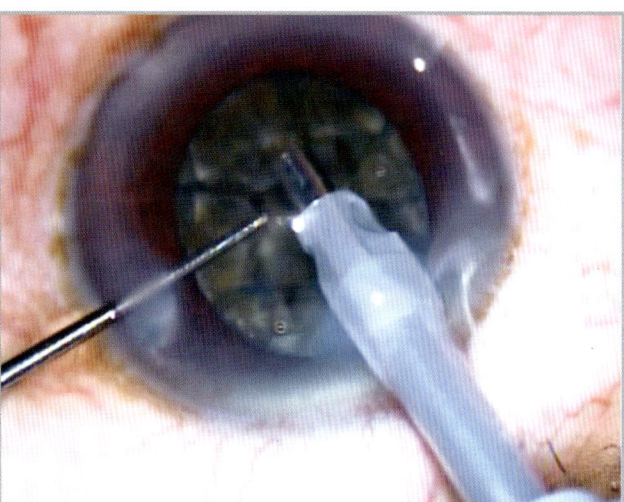

Fig. 34.8: Secondary nucleotomy in a post YAG iridotomy hyperopic eye with shallow anterior chamber

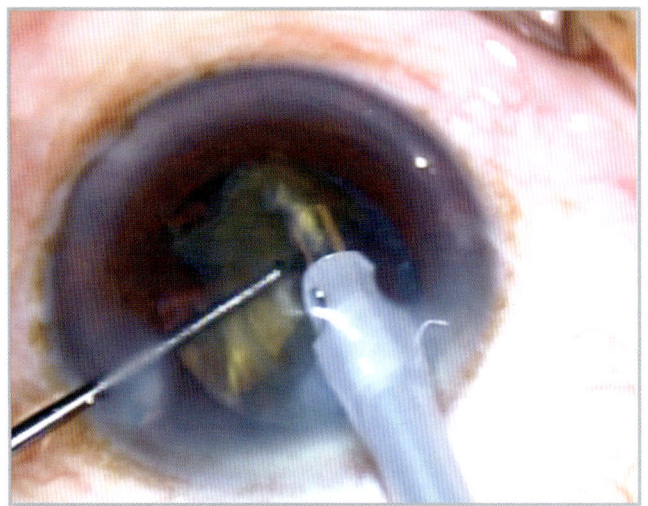

Fig. 34.9: Fragment removal in a post YAG iridotomy hyperopic eye with shallow anterior chamber

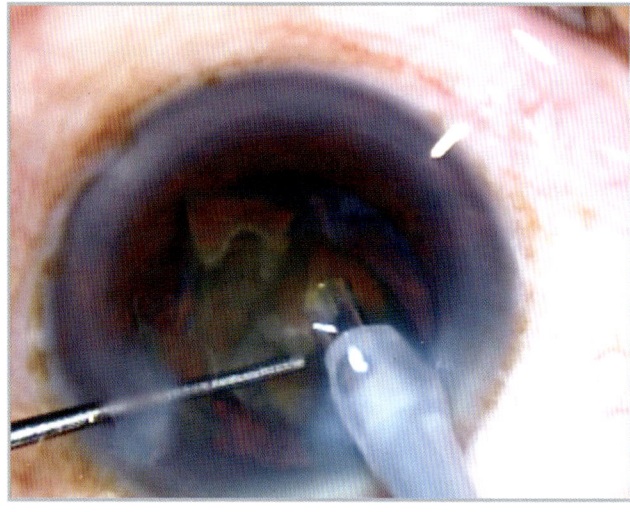

Fig. 34.10: Removal of thick posterior plate in a post YAG iridotomy hyperopic eye with shallow anterior chamber

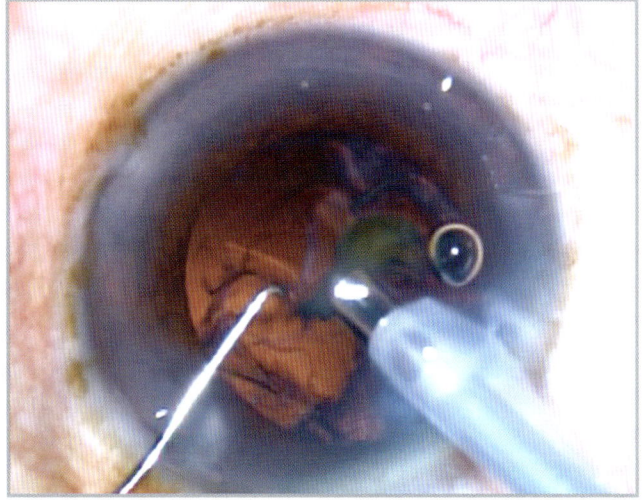

Fig. 34.11: Removal of tiny last fragment in a post YAG iridotomy hyperopic eye with shallow anterior chamber

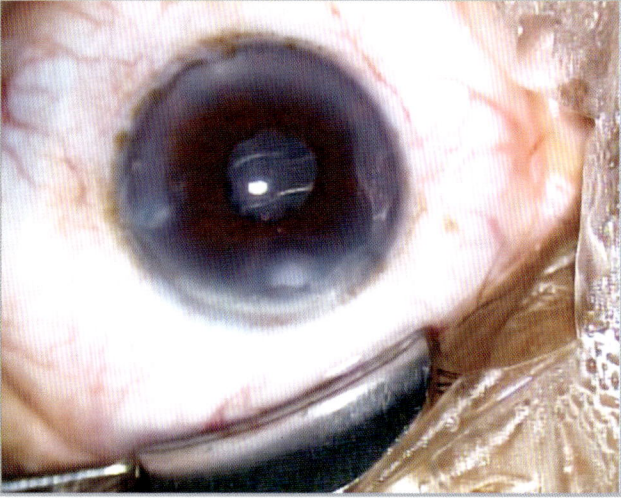

Fig. 34.12: PC IOL is well placed in a post YAG iridotomy hyperopic eye with shallow anterior chamber

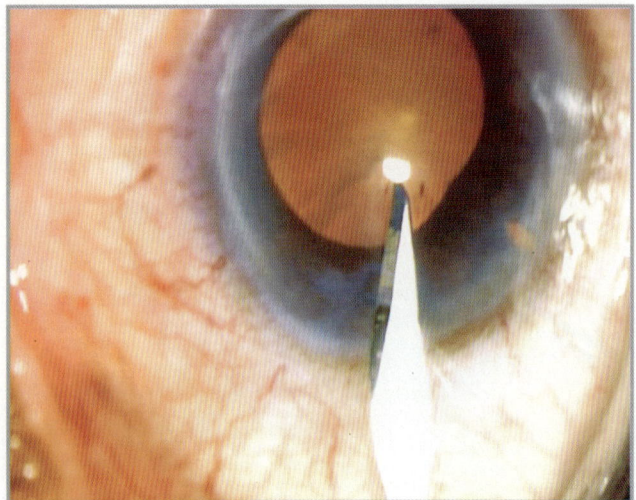

Fig. 34.13: Primary side port incision in a post YAG iridotomy hyperopic eye with normal anterior chamber depth

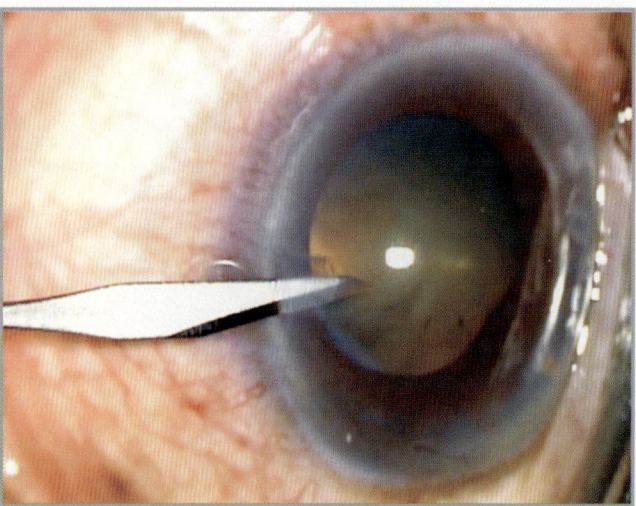

Fig. 34.14: Primary incision in a post YAG iridotomy hyperopic eye with normal anterior chamber depth

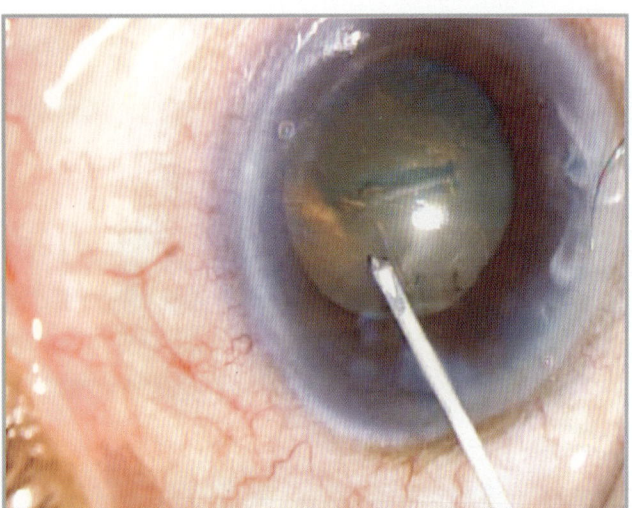

Fig. 34.15: Rhexis in a post YAG iridotomy hyperopic eye with normal anterior chamber depth

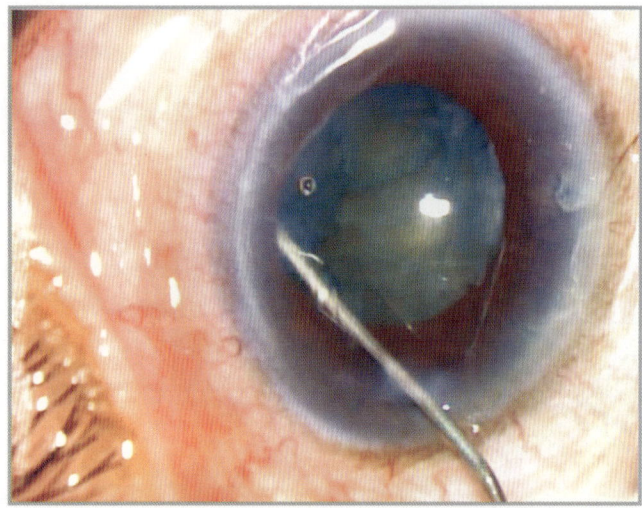

Fig. 34.16: Hydroprocedures in a post YAG iridotomy hyperopic eye with normal anterior chamber depth

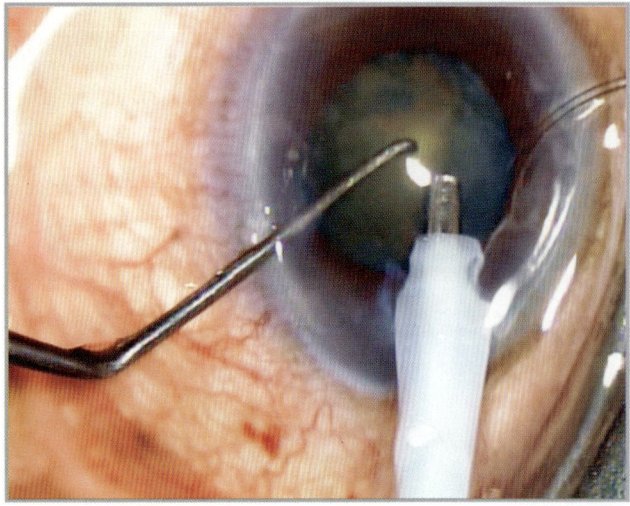

Fig. 34.17: Commencement of central chopping in a post YAG iridotomy hyperopic eye with normal anterior chamber depth

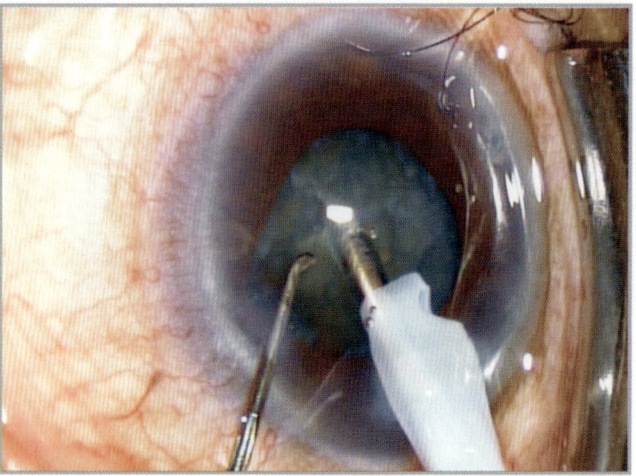

Fig. 34.18: Central chopping in a post YAG iridotomy hyperopic eye with normal Anterior chamber depth: Phaco tip is being embedded into the nucleus

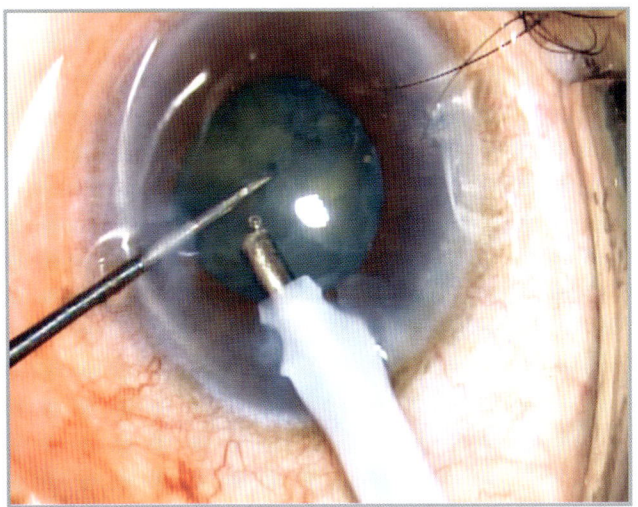

Fig. 34.19: Primary nucleotomy in a post YAG iridotomy hyperopic eye with normal anterior chamber depth

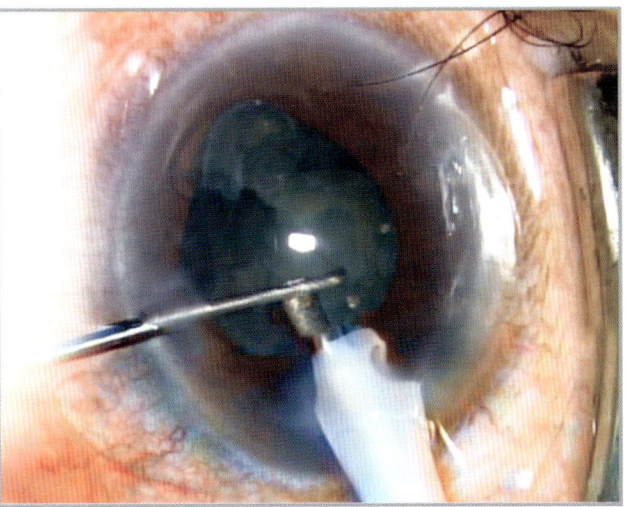

Fig. 34.20: Nucleus rotation for secondary nucleotomy in a post YAG iridotomy hyperopic eye with normal anterior chamber depth

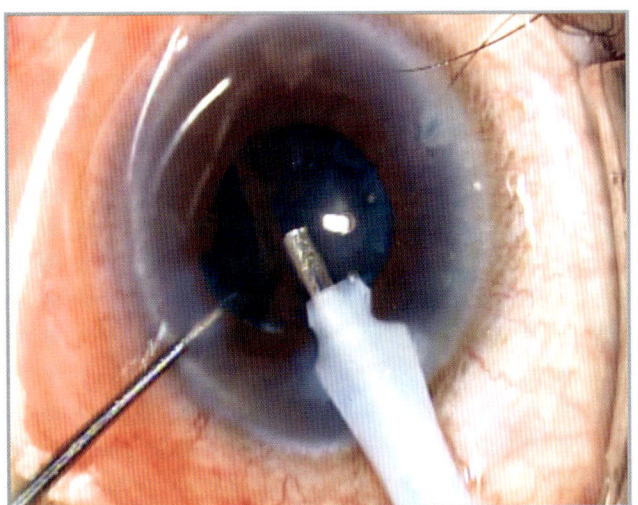

Fig. 34.21: Secondary nucleotomy in a post YAG iridotomy hyperopic eye with normal anterior chamber depth

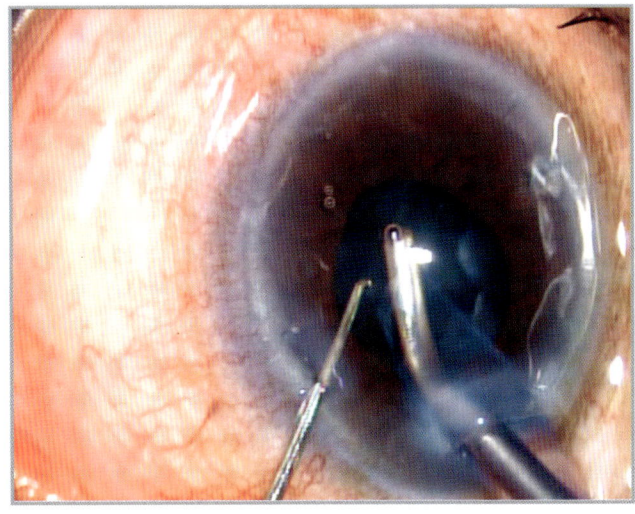

Fig. 34.22: I/A in a post YAG iridotomy hyperopic eye with normal anterior chamber depth

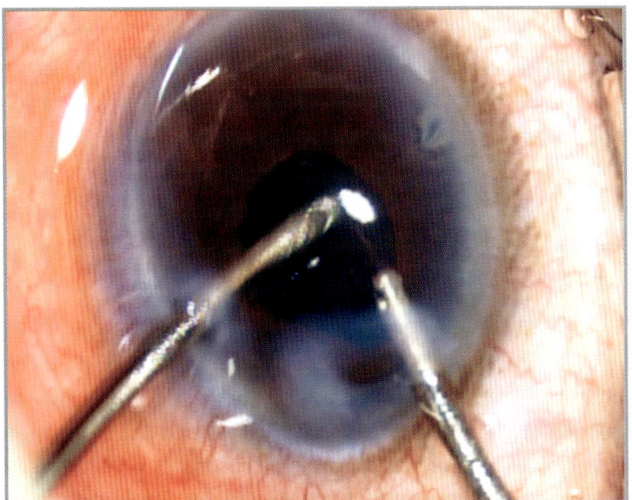

Fig. 34.23: Removal of sub iridotomy sticky cortex in a post YAG iridotomy hyperopic eye with normal anterior chamber depth

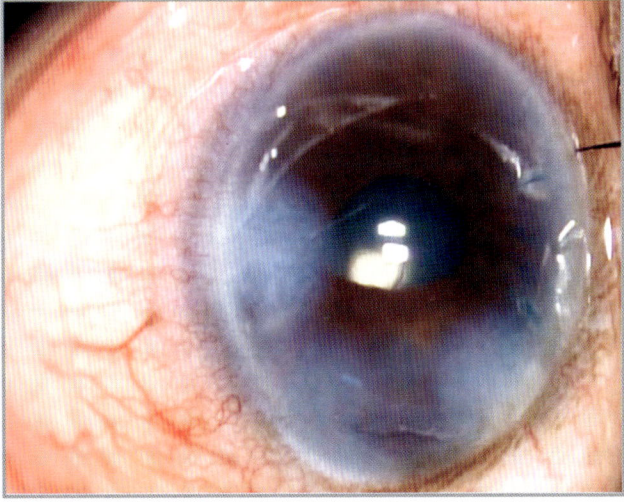

Fig. 34.24: C IOL is well placed in a post YAG iridotomy hyperopic eye with normal anterior chamber depth

(iv) Scleral fixation of the implant: The tendency for the microphthalmic eye to bleed may also be apparent during attempted scleral fixation of a lens implant following rupture of the posterior capsule. This manoeuvre risks hemorrhage in normal eyes also and the risk increases considerably in very short eyes. In the event that a large capsular rupture prevents fixation of the IOL in the iridociliary sulcus, the surgeon has very few truly valid options for these eyes. There is the choice of immediate or later scleral fixation, or iris fixation. The dimensions of the microphthalmic eye are rarely sufficient for an anterior chamber implant.

CLEAR LENSECTOMY FOR REFRACTIVE PURPOSES

Patients affected by severe hyperopia have problems in everyday life as they have poor uncorrected near and distance vision and always require optical correction. This problem is accentuated as the patient ages, because presbyopia obliges the addition of positive lens power to lenses that are already of high power. Moreover, these patients tolerate contact lenses less than their myopic counterparts. In practice, they often cannot manage insertion of contact lenses without using spectacles. The problems are augmented by the aesthetic and functional limitations of the thick spectacles. These lenses are often very heavy, with numerous residual aberrations, and are expensive. Severely hyperopic patients often use corrective lenses that are designed to correct aphakia.

These problems have lead some surgeons to consider the extraction of the clear lens and implantation of a refractive IOL in these hyperopic patients. The basic idea behind this surgery is that the severely hyperopic eye requires refractive surgery more than the severely myopic eye, but has fewer surgical options available. It is unlikely that corneal surgery can correct more than 4 to 5 D even when the best laser and Lasik techniques are used; phakic IOLs are currently being studied and are not suitable for eyes with a reduced anterior segment. Clinically, the hyperopic eye is less likely to be subjected to retinal detachment compared to the myopic eye because of the different anatomical conditions and may also benefit from lensectomy in the event of predisposition to closed angle glaucoma. As a result in recent, years, lensectomy has been used as a preventive measure and/or treatment of closed angle glaucoma in very short eyes.

Clinical Experience

Osher, at the European Society of Cataract and Refractive Surgeons (ESCRS) Congress in Innsbruck in 1993, first reported the clinical experience of lensectomy for refractive purposes in severely hyperopic eyes. He reported on four eyes operated with phacoemulsification, where the satisfaction of the patients was the counterpoint of the surgeon's dissatisfaction in terms of the refractive results. An error of +4 D was observed in one pseudophakic eye. This first report highlighted what were destined to be the most serious problem of this type of surgery; i.e. difficulty in calculating the correct power for the implant. According to Siganos, intraoperative endothelial cell loss may be greater than usual. However, the postoperative course of these eyes remains uneventful. The immediate postoperative period may witness malignant glaucoma in 2 to 5% cases. The incidence of secondary cataract is similar to that following cataract surgery in average eyes of the same age group.

The difficult problem linked to the extraction of the clear lens with implantation of an IOL as a form of refractive surgery in eyes with extreme hyperopia, is precise calculation for the power of the implant. Kolahdouz underlines that in an eye measuring 17.71 mm, the Sanders-Retzlaff-Kraff (SRK) II formula suggested a power of 37.5 D, and the Holladay 2 a power of 46 D with equal desired postoperative refraction. In agreement with Fenzl, the author concluded that the Holladay 2 formula was the most accurate, with refractive errors limited to between –1 D and +1.23 D in a further series of 10 operated eyes with axial lengths of between 16.11 mm and 22.23 mm.

POLYPSEUDOPHAKIA

Many highly hyperopic eyes subjected to cataract surgery require implantation of an IOL in excess of 30 D. Some necessitate a lens in excess of 34 D which is the maximum power available in serially produced lenses. The reasons for such high power requirements are the reduced axial length, and the posterior position of the optic disc with respect to the corneal apex. While hyperopic eyes, with a reduced anterior segment generally require lens power near 30 D, those with a normal anterior segment frequently require powers superior to 40 D, and sometimes as strong as 50 D.

Phakic IOL

Refractive predictability appears better for hyperopia than for myopia using the STAAR collamer foldable posterior chamber phakic intraocular lens. In hyperopic eyes, development of pupillary block may occur.

A high diopteric power can theoretically be obtained with custom-made IOLs, but the thickness of the lens creates optical aberration. Moreover, implantation of custom-built lenses is not practical due to the long time required for production. For these reasons, it was theorised that the problem could be resolved by implanting two IOLs selected from the power range normally used in surgery.

Among the first surgeons to suggest the possibility was Gayton in 1993. Shugar in 1996 reported on one of the first groups consisting of 6 operated eyes. While Gayton used two PMMA lenses, Shugar used two acrylic foldable lenses. Since then, polypseudophakia has spread as a routine technique for achieving emmetropia in severely hyperopic eyes and as a corrective means for pseudophakic refractive errors. The refractive results have proved to be good, with an acceptable complication profile.

Clinical Polypseudophakia

When two lenses are implanted, the lenses come into contact at the apex, the optical system obtained is considered as a single lens, according to the suggestions of physical optics as applied to thick lenses and to lens systems. The resulting power is the sum of the two powers. It has not yet been clarified whether there is benefit to splitting the diopteric power equally, or implanting lenses of different powers. Initial observations regarding a different depth of focus in pseudophakia as a result of the two methods have not been confirmed clinically. The issue is of interest when the two lenses are of different powers, in that, the anterior or posterior displacement of the stronger lens could reduce the precision of the postoperative refraction. Current opinion tends toward the backward displacement of the posterior lens. Therefore, it may be useful to split the total power equally between the two IOLs.

The contact area between the two lenses can be considered to be a spot where two convex PMMA surfaces come into contact. Recent studies clarified that with foldable lenses, there is a circular contact zone, with an extension depending on the type of IOL and the diopteric power. This contact zone may be responsible for modest visual reduction and for some of the multimodal phenomena that are sometimes observed in polypseudophakia.

However, there are also complications of polypseudophakia. A white precipitate may persist between the two lenses, this can reduce postoperative visual acuity. This material has been interpreted as residual viscoelastic. Also, postoperatively, Elsching's pearls may proliferate between the two lenses, reducing vision and increasing hyperopia. None of these problems has been reported following implants with PMMA. Elimination of the residual material and Elsching's pearls from the space between the two lenses is extremely difficult at surgery and may require explantation and lens exchange. For this reason, implantation of two acrylic lenses into the capsular sac is no longer recommended.

Calculation of Implant Power

The simplest method for calculating the power of the implants is to consider the total power to be implanted and to divide by two. According to Perrone, this leads to errors due to the posterior displacement of the first lens. The author proposes a correction of power, increasing it by 10% for every mm of the presumed posterior displacement.

Many severely hyperopic eyes have a postoperative hyperopic refractive error. These eyes can be aided with polypseudophakia, placing a secondary implant in the capsular bag or more often in the ciliary sulcus. In order to calculate the secondary implants in eyes with incorrect pseudophakia, this simple formula proposed by Gills can be used with or without the correction of Perrone, or by using the more complex Holladay 2 formula. This formula supplied results that were more precise.

Axial length < 21 mm   IOL power(d) = (Refraction x 1.5) + 1
Axial length 22–26 mm IOL power(d) = (Refraction x 1.4) + 1
Axial length > 27 mm   IOL power(d) = (Refraction x 1.3) + 1

The technique of the multiple implants has also been used with intraocular multifocal lenses and even in children (G Ravalico: Personal communication, 1999). The multifocal surface of the lens was positioned as the more posterior lens (diffractive optic) or as the more anterior lens (refractive optic). Despite being interesting, these applications must be considered experimental until long-term follow-up has clarified the results.

Polypseudophakia provides very good refractive outcome. More than 40% eyes attain emmetropia or refractive error of less than 0.5 dioptre, whereas more than 70% eyes fall within 1 dioptre of residual refractive error.

Better understanding of the exact position of the IOL in the postoperative period should lead to significant improvements in the estimated refractive outcome.

CONCLUSION

Cataract surgery for the severely hyperopic patient is now safer with phacoemulsification. These eyes should be operated precociously, in order to avoid the possibility of narrow-angle glaucoma in eyes with a reduced anterior segment, and to improve the vision of eyes with a normal-sized anterior segment.

The difficulties associated with the anatomical conditions of these eyes are combined with the problems linked to the calculation of the power and the availability of the lens implant. These problems are being resolved through renewed calculation formula's, and through the increasingly popular technique of polypseudophakia. Multiple implants, particularly if they can be associated with multimodal lenses, will offer a valid option for those eyes not affected with cataract, where lensectomy and implantation of an IOL or phakic IOL are performed for refractive purpose.

BIBLIOGRAPHY

1. Holladay JR: Achieving hemitropic in extremely short eyes. Presented at the 1996 Annual Meeting of the American Academy of Ophthalmology, Chicago, 1996.
2. Gills JP, Cherchio M: Phacoemulsification in high hyperopic cataract patients. In: Lu LW, Fine IH (Eds): Phacoemulsi-fication in Difficult and Challenging cases. New York: Thieme 1999, 21–31.
3. Brannnan SO, Kyle G: Bilateral micro cornea and unilateral microphthalmic resulting in incorrect intraocular lens selection. J Cataract Refract Surg 1999, 25:1016–18.
4. Greve EL: Primary angle–closure glaucoma–extracapsular cataract extraction or filtering procedure? Int Ophthalmol 1988, 12:157–62.
5. Gunning FP, Greve EL: Uncontrolled primary angle closure glaucoma–results of early intercapsular cataract extraction and posterior chamber lens implantation. Int Ophthalmol 1991, 15:237–47.
6. Gunning FP, Greve EL: Lens extraction for uncontrolled angle–closure glaucoma- long-term follow up. J Cataract Refract Surg 1998, 24:1347–56.
7. Krupin T, Feitl ME, Bishhop KI: Postoperative intraocular pressure rise in open-angle glaucoma patients after cataract or combined cataract-filtration surgery. Ophthalmology 1989, 96: 579–84.
8. Gills JP, Fenzl RE. Cherchio M: refractive and visual outcome of hyperopic cataract cases operated on before and after implementation of the Holladay II formula. Ophthalmo-logy1998,105: 1759–64.
9. Signanos DS, Signanos CS, Pallikaris IG: Clear lens extraction and intraocular lens implantation in normally sighted hyperopic eyes. Refract corneal surg. 1994, 10: 117–24.
10. Lyle WA, Jin GJC: Clear lens extraction for the correction of high refractive error. J Cataract refract surg. 1994, 20: 273–76.
11. Osher RH: clear lens extraction (letter). J Cataract Refract surg. 1994, 20:673–74 .
12. Signanos DS, Pallikaris IG, Signanos CS: Clear lensectomy and intraocular lens in normally sighted highly hyperopic eyes-three-year follow up . Eur J Implant Refract Surg 1995, 7:128–33.
13. Lyle WA, Jin GJC: Clear Jens extraction to correct hyperopia. J Cataract Refract surg. 1997, 23:1051–56.
14. Kolahdouz-Isfahani AH, Rostamian K, Wallace D et al: Clear lens extraction with intraocular lens implantation for hyperopia. Refract corneal surg. 1999, 15:316–23.
15. Vicary D, Sun XY, Montgomery P: Refractive lensectomy to correct ametropia . J Cataract Refract surg. 25:943–48,1999.
16. Accou M, Hennekes R: Implantation of posterior chamber lenses of more than 30 dptr. Bull soc Belge Ophthalmol 1996, 261:121–24.
17. Gayton JL, sanders VN: Implanting two posterior chamber intraocular lenses in a case of microphthalmos. J cataract Refract surg. 1993, 19:776–77.
18. Shugar JK, Lewis C, Lee A: Implantation of multiple foldable acrylic posterior chamber lenses in the capsular bag for high hyperopia. J cataract Refract surg. 1996, 22:1368–72.
19. Holladay IT: Gills JP, Leidlein J et al: Achieving hemitropic in extremely short eyes with two piggyback posterior chamber intraocular lenses. Ophthalmology 1996, 103:118–23.
20. Holladay JT: Standardising constants for ultrasonic biometry, keratometry and intraocular lens power calculations. J cataract Refract surg. 1997, 23:1356–70.
21. Perrone DM: Modified intraocular lens power formula in polypseudophakia. J cataract Refract surg. 1996, 22:1392–93.
22. Findl O, Menapace R, Rainer G et al: Contact zone of piggyback acrylic intraocular lenses. J cataract Refract surg 1999, 25:860–62.
23. Shugar JK, Schwartz T: Interpseudophakos Elsching. Pearls associated with late hyperopic shift—a complication of pigggyback posterior chamber intraocular lenses. J cataract Refract surg. 1999, 25:863–67.
24. Holladay JT: Preoperative refraction vs. axial length for intraocular lens calculations. Phaco and Foldables 1997. 10(1):1–7.
25. Pesando PM, Ghiringhello MP, Tagliavacche P: Posterior chamber collamer phakic intraocular lens for myopia and hyperopia. J Refract Surg. 1999 Jul–Aug; 15(4):415–23.

35

Phaco in
Pseudoexfoliation Syndrome

Col JKS Parihar SM, VSM and Lt Col Santosh Kumar

INTRODUCTION

Exfoliation syndrome is a relatively common condition affecting the anterior segment of the eye. It was first described by Lindberg in 1917 and Vagt in 1930, correlated its incidence to a specific form of secondary glaucoma. In 1954, Dvorak Theobald reported that this fibrillar exfoliative material involving the anterior segment was of unknown origin and he introduced the term pseudo-exfoliation to distinguish the condition from true lens exfoliation. True exfoliation is a rare entity in which the lens capsule is split into two layers with an evanescent sheet attached to the anterior lens capsule floating in the aqueous.

Pseudoexfoliation syndrome now is well recognised as a generalised systemic disorder involving abnormal production or turnover of extracellular matrix material throughout the systemic vasculature.

For ophthalmologists, it represents a spectrum of intraocular and extraocular manifestations caused by changes resulting from the deposition of pseudoexfoliation material in tissues of the eye. Phacoemulsification cataract surgery in the presence of pseudoexfoliation offers rather exceptional surgical challenges. It is imperative that all cataract surgeons be aware of the potential risks and complications of cataract surgery and IOL implantation in such cases.

Previously there were many reports in literature of an increased incidence of capsular rupture and tears, zonular dehiscence with manual extracapsular cataract extraction in patients with pseudoexfoliation syndrome.

Phacoemulsification cataract surgery has now emerged as a safe and effective management option in patients with cataract in pseudoexfoliation syndrome. Several recent studies have recommended that phacoemulsification with IOL implantation can be performed routinely in their patients if special care is exercised in preoperative evaluation as well as postoperatively.

INCIDENCE

(i) Exfoliation syndrome is found worldwide and occurs perhaps with varying frequency in all geographic regions of the world.

(ii) Its incidence increases with age and this has been documented by almost every researcher.

(iii) In most cases, it develops in the late seventh and early eighth decades of life.
Aramides et al reported that as much as 42.85% of the patients above 80 yrs. may be affected.

(iv) Various studies show that between 2% and 35% of patients and of 70 yrs. have the syndrome. Surprisingly, it is readily seen in patients who are more than 50 yrs of age.

(v) It is not more common in one sex.

(vi) It is probably inherited, possibly autosomal dominant with incomplete per entrance and varying expressivity.

(vii) The severity of damage to ocular structures including rigid pupil and zonules caused by pseudoexfoliative material is linked with ethnic variations which is more significant in the dark and markedly pigmented iris population.

PREVALENCE

(i) The overall prevalence of PSE varies from 0.4 to 9% in different ethnic groups (Chinese 0.4%, Japanese and south Indian 3.4%, and 7 to 9% among black South Africans) and by racial origins.

(ii) The prevalence of glaucoma in cases of pseudoexfoliation has been observed upto 13%.

(iii) The prevalence of pseudoexfoliation among all glaucoma cases are varying upto 15%.

(iv) The prevalence of pseudoexfoliation syndrome increased with increasing age from 3 to 3.5% in the age group of 40 years or above to 5 to 7% in the advanced age group of more than 60 years of age.

(v) The prevalence of pseudoexfoliation syndrome is associated with increased prevalence and severity among outdoor occupations.

SURGICAL ANATOMY AND HISTOPATHOLOGY

Exfoliation syndrome is a puzzling disease of the anterior segment of the eye. Since Lindberg first described the syndrome in 1917, the origin of the exfoliative material has been a matter of considerable controversy.

Currently, there is a consensus that the exfoliative material is synthesised by various cell types at multiple sites. In the anterior segment of the eye, the pseudo-exfoliation material appears to originate from various cell types lining the anterior and posterior chambers, including iris pigment epithelium, ciliary non-pigmented epithelium, pre-equatorial lens epithelium and corneal endothelium. Vogt and Bert Elson and co-authors believe that the material is lens derived.

In addition to multifocal, subsequent desquamation and aqueous dispersal accuses, which is responsible for deposits of non cellular structures such as the anterior hyaloids or zonular fibers, anterior vitreous phase, particularly in aphakic or psuedophakic and even on IOL implants. The syndrome adversely affects almost all intraocular tissue, from the corneal endothelium to the optic nerve.

There is format run and deposition of small flakes of whitish to light gray fibrillogranular material on various intraocular structures. Tissues affected are anterior lens capsule, iris, anterior chambers angle, zonules, ciliary body, anterior vitreous face and conjunctiva.

Ultrastructural studies show that the material has the appearance of a fibrillar protein and it could be a mucopalysaccharide, a basement membrane, or an amyloid group protein.

Accumulation of exfoliative material gradually coats the zonules with coarse marked changes of the normal architecture of the basement membrane of nonpigmented cells of ciliary processes where the zonules are anchored onto the pseudoexfoliation clumps between the zonules bundles. There is stretching, mechanical and internal breaking of the zonules at this ciliary body attachment. The presence of degenerative changes in the zonules fibers of patients with PES, especially near the ciliary processes as well as the lens, and the stretching capability observed in experimental studies are related to the higher incidence of phacodonesis in patients with pseudoexfoliation syndrome mentioned by various authors.

Also an iris is degenerated with defects in the pigmented pupillary margin and the iris vessels are pathological.

Mechanism of Glaucoma in Pseudoexfoliation Syndrome

The presence of pseudoexfoliative fibrillar material on the various structures of the anterior chamber and the angle of anterior chamber are responsible for manifestations of different types of glaucoma including open angle, angle closure or ciliary block glaucoma.

(i) *Pseudoexfoliation syndrome and open angle glaucoma:* The higher incidence of open-angle glaucoma has been associated with the pseudo-exfoliation syndrome. The diagnosis of open angle glaucoma is frequently made more in eyes with pseudoexfoliation. Exfoliative glaucoma accounted for approximately one fourth of open-angle glaucoma cases (OAG).

The presence of pseudoexfoliative fibrillar deposits into the Schwalbe's line and trabecular meshwork are essentially attributed to the origin of pseudoexfoliation induced open angle glaucoma.

(ii) *Pseudoexfoliation syndrome and angle closure glaucoma:* The progressive effect of pseudoexfoli-ation material production on zonular fibers may first be recognised clinically by phacodonesis which may lead to spontaneous subluxation or dislocation of the lens posteriorly into the vitreous or anteriorly precipitating angle closure or even ciliary block glaucoma.

The iridocorneal angle pigmentation has direct link with the angle closure and the status of IOP.

CLINICAL FEATURES

The syndrome occurs more often bilaterally, though appearing in one eye earlier than the other.

The syndrome is characterised by gray or white flakes on the anterior lens capsule having a classic deposition pattern involving the central and the peripheral lens.

The fine dust-like particles of fibrillar material initially visible across the surface of the lens is seen. However, pupillary movements in the form of regular constriction and dilatation redistribute the exfoliative material in classical, central and peripheral pattern of deposits on the lens surface while relatively maintaining the clear mid-peripheral zone.

The other features include deposits over pupillary margins of iris with an atrophic, almost transparent incomplete iris ring with a whitish border at the pupil area with increased melanin dispersion and trabecular meshwork pigmentation.

There is a presence of gray or white flakes on the anterior lens capsule, iris with increased melanin dispersion and trabecular meshwork pigmentation. A rigid pupil that does not easily respond to mydriatics and dilates submaximally. This poor mydriasis is related to iris infiltration and fibrosis from pseudoexfoliation.

In addition to multifocal production, subsequent desquamation and acquired dispersal occurs, which is responsible for deposits also on non cellular structures such as the anterior hyaloids, zonular fibers and even on artificial lenses.

The pseudoexfoliative fibrillar deposits seen on the endothelial surface of the cornea may simulate keratic precipitates and should be evaluated carefully.

Gonioscopy Evaluation

Gonioscopic evaluation is essential in all cases with coexisting glaucoma and cataract. The Gonioscopic examination may highlight the presence of pigments, Sampaolesi line, along the posterior terminus of Descemet's membrane (Schwalbe's line).

Selection of Surgical Technique: Phacoemulsification *vs* Conventional ECCE

Cataract extraction in a setting of pseudoexfoliation syndrome presents a spectrum of challenges ranging from miotic and poorly dilated pupils to zonular instability and relatively hard cataract. Such structural peculiarities in the pseudoexfoliation syndrome increases the occurrence of intraoperative and postoperative complications of cataract surgery.

The majority of the studies done primarily showed a relatively high incidence of capsular rupture, zonular breaks, intraoperative lens dislocation and vitreous loss particularly in patients undergoing ECCE.

In certain situations, serious complications like a nucleus drop may be encountered mainly in cases of hard cataract with miotic pupils and zonular dialysis of more than 30%.

At one time, even doing ECCE and poor pupillary dilatation was a relative contraindication in cases of pseudoexfoliation syndrome.

Advancements in phacotechnology, surgical techniques, capsular support devices and better understanding of the disease process have resulted in phacosurgery being performed with even fever complications.

Special care must be exercised while performing cataract surgery in patients with pseudo-exfoliation syndrome where it presents varied surgical challenges.

The results of phacoemulsification surgery are much more superior and gratifying over manual ECCE in eyes with pseudoexfoliation.

In our view, phacoemulsification surgery with or without glaucoma surgery is undoubtedly a preferred technique over conventional ECCE.

Preoperative Clinical Evaluation of Cataract in Pseudoexfoliation Syndrome

Types of Cataract

Slit lamp assessment in most cataracts revealed a combination of nuclear and posterior subcapsular cataracts. The pattern of lenticular changes has been found to have a wide spectrum of diversity in these cases. Posterior subcapsular cataract is the most common feature which is followed by the nuclear sclerosis type as reported by several workers.

However, in Indian scenario hard cataract is commonly seen which probably is a sequel of delayed changes in sclerotic type of cataract.

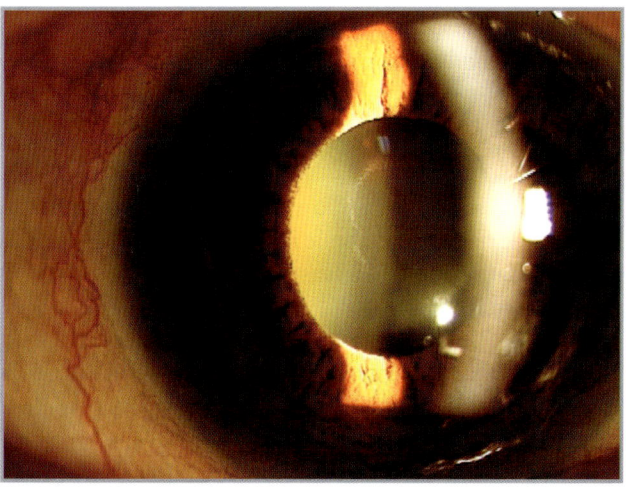

(a)

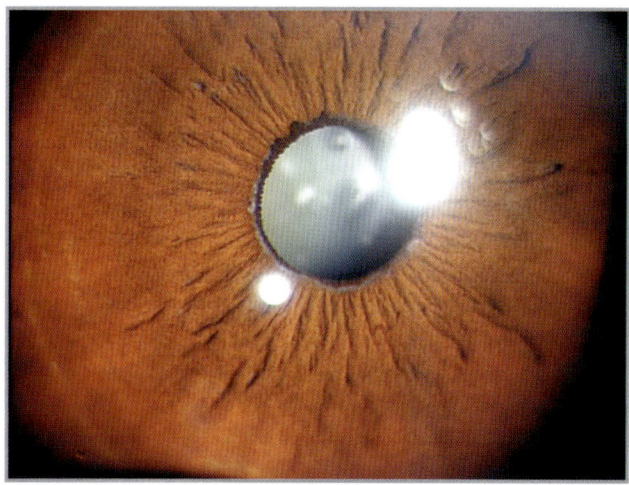

(b)

Fig. 35.1: (a) Pseudoexfoliation syndrome: Presence of gray or white flakes on the iris as well as in a circular ring manner on the anterior lens capsule, (b) Pseudoexfoliation syndrome: Presence of gray or white flakes on the iris

Iridophacodonesis

Pseudoexfoliation syndrome is the most common cause of lens instability. Iridophacodonesis is one of the factors that is related to a high frequency of capsular rupture, zonular disinsertion and consequent vitreous loss.

Careful preoperative examination is required to exclude patients with phacodonesis which an average examinee may not be able to note especially in cases of mild involvement since poor dilation is associated with pseudoexfoliation.

Iridophacodonesis is not seen until there is a certain degree of zonular weakness. When the zonular changes are advanced, iridophacodonesis becomes apparent and may even lead to spontaneous subluxation of the lens. Iridophacodonesis is significantly higher in light coloured iris than in dark coloured iris. Hence, iridophacodonesis is also seen more with light coloured iris and less in Indian eyes which is a composite effect of less significant damage to the zonular apparatus in the pseudoexfoliation syndrome in Indian eyes.

Evaluation of Pupil/Exfoliative Material

In advanced and mature cataracts, pseudoexfoliative material may be difficult to recognise. Preoperatively, one should vigorously attempt to dilate the pupil maximally; otherwise peripheral exfoliation may go unnoticed which occurs exclusively in cases of zonular weakness or disinsertion.

Rigid and smaller pupils are determined to be significant risk factors for vitreous loss and zonular dialysis.

Surgeons should consider various clinical measures to assess pupil size and consistency preoperatively, in a patient with pseudoexfoliation and with moderate dilatation so as to achieve best possible surgical outcome.

When to Intervene?

The considering complexity of the pseudoexfoliation syndrome and the risk involved which is directly proportional to the advanced stages of cataract and glaucoma, surgery should be planned more cautiously and cataract should be intervened at an early stage than in senile cataract. The following factors deserve special consideration while planning surgical intervention in these cases.

(i) The occurrence of spontaneous and intraocular lens dislocation in PES has been attributed to the weakness of the loose zonules.

This zonular weakness is greater in patients with mature and hypermature cataracts, poorly dilating pupils, glaucoma and uniform trabecular mesh-work pigmentation.

(ii) Corneal endothelium of eyes with PES manifested consistent morphologic changes when compared with age-matched controls and this was an early and essential sign of the syndrome. Thus, another risk factor of a frigate corneal endothelium is added to cases which require cataract surgery with IOL implantation. The precise and careful technologies with use of high viscous-cohesive ophthalmic surgical devices are essentially required when operating on eyes with PES.

Role of Antiglaucoma Medication Prior to the Surgical Intervention

Needless to emphasize the significance of good and adequate control of glaucoma which is always beneficial and should be achieved upto the optimal level. However, while considering the medical regimen, the role of each and every antiglaucoma medication, their inter-drug compatibility as well as any impending intra and postoperative adverse influence of any specific drug is of immense significance. While planning preoperative medical regimen, the drug combination should be based on their mechanisms of action based on different pathways like actions on trabecular meshwork, aqueous formation, angle structures or on supra choroidal pathway.

The drugs acting on prostaglandin inhibitory system deserve special consideration since these drugs are invariably associated with higher incidence of intra as well as postoperative complications like intraoperative bleeding, sphincteric atony, flappy iris as well as higher incidence of postoperative uveitis, CME as well as choroidal effusion. In our view, such drugs should be discontinued atleast six weeks prior to the surgery; while IOP is maintained with the help of substitute regimen.

Concurrent Phacoemulsification and Trabeculectomy or Phacoemulsification Surgery Alone

The knowledge of the IOP reducing effect of cataract surgery in normal eyes is useful for planning cataract management, especially in eyes with exfoliation and in those with combined cataract and glaucoma.

When to Perform Phacoemulsification Surgery Alone?

(i) Patients with PES, a visually significant cataract, and no advanced optic nerve damage, phacoemulsification alone is a reasonable option for initial IOP management.

(ii) For the patients who are well controlled with medications (two or less) do not need filtration surgery. At the time of cataract surgery, a clear corneal incision is performed from the temporal periphery. This phacoemulsification through the avascular corneal tissue does not jeopardize filtration surgery subsequently in a superior location.

Concurrent Phacoemulsification and Glaucoma surgery: Trabeculectomy/Glaucoma Drainage Devices

Studies have reported varied strategies in managing glaucoma with pseudoexfoliation syndrome. Honjo et al have found the combination of trabeculectomy, phacoemulsification and IOL implantation to be effective in treatment of PES with coexisting cataract, where the preoperative IOP was simply concurrent with antiglaucoma medication.

The authors recommend concurrent phaco and modulated trabeculectomy procedure when the patient has poorly controlled glaucoma in the presence of coexisting cataract and pseudoexfoliation. We prefer two port trabeculectomy and phaco through a clear corneal incision over single site phacotrabeculectomy through a limbal conjunctival incision with a self sealing scleral tunnel since risk of intraoperative complications and overall control of IOP is much superior after two port /site glaucoma and cataract procedure.

A combined phacoemulsification and glaucoma drainage device may be suitable in certain cases where IOP is still uncontrolled, despite application of three or more medications or after laser iridotomy and still on medication.

We finally recommend that any of the other combined techniques can be used by which a surgeon is comfortable including with, or without the use of antimetabolites.

Surgical Technique of Phacoemulsification in the Presence of Pseudoexfoliation Syndrome

Phacoemulsification in cases of pseudoexfoliation syndrome has to be performed with extreme caution and prudence, so as not to damage the already compromised zonules. Excellent results can be achieved with improvements in phacoemulsification technology, careful manipulation intraoperatively and the use of various surgical adjuncts such as hooks and capsular tension rings.

The Choice of Phacomachine

Usage of one of the high end machines (Sovereign, Legacy, and Millennium) ensures a better intraoperative control without much surge which prevents damage to the already compromised zonules.

High cavitations tips (Kelman tip) are recommended as they obliterate nuclear material in advance of the tip without exerting forces on the lens as the lens rotates. Also the configuration of the Kelman tip allows for a phaco sweep procedure wherein after initial trenching, without rotating the lens, a lateral and rotational movement of the phaco probe grooves in a lateral direction.

Anaesthesia: Topical *vs* Peribulbar

Topical anaesthesia is not an ideal choice for phacosurgery in cases of pseudoexfoliation syndrome since rigid, miotic pupil with hard cataract poses challenges which may require additional procedures like application of iris stretching devices and CTR. Over and above, these cases carry higher risk of intraoperative complications like vitreous disturbances or nucleus drop. The management of such eventuality may not be feasible under topical. As such, concurrent phaco and glaucoma procedures should be considered under peribulbar anaesthesia.

Procedures such as digital or mechanical pressure after peribulbar injection should be avoided as application of undue pressure on the eyeball following infiltrative anaesthesia may aggravate the zonular disinsertion which is invariably associated with compromised zonules in cases of pseudoexfoliation.

HOW TO MANAGE A SMALL PUPIL

Inadequate mydriasis is a major intraoperative difficulty observed by almost every surgeon and herein, gentle manipulation and special care is exercised while performing surgery in patients with pseudoexfoliation. Use of pupil stretching maneuvers/devices can overcome the problems of insufficient mydriasis effectively. A small pupil can be dealt with by sector iridectomy, iris hooks, iris rings and pupillary stretching with or without the use of multiple half width sphincterotomies.

It is possible to perform phaco without applying pupillary stretching devices in selective cases even with pupillary sizes of 3.5 to 4 mm in diameter by the central chopping technique while performing all phacoemulsification maneuvers within a small central place of the lens. However, use of stretching devices is highly beneficial if the pupil size is less than 5 mm particularly in cases of handling hard cataract with zonular disinsertion or other complications.

Technique of Application of Iris Hooks/ Retractors

Disposable nylon iris hooks are placed on the pupillary margins prior to the capsulorrhexis so as to facilitate adequate exposure of the anterior surface of the lens.

The technique involves making four stab incisions using 25 or 27 gauge needles. Each opposite pair is at mutually perpendicular meridians and straddles the subsequent phacoemulsification and side port incisions. Structuring of the anterior capsular opening into a square like configuration prevents rotational movement of the bag, whereas the mutually perpendicular distribution of each pair of fixation points presents significant anteroposterior capsular bag movement. It appears that phacoemulsification may be performed safely even when the lens is unstable. The use of hooks to support the lens is simple and they may be useful in cases of anticipated zonular weakness such as PES.

Fine et al found the use of pupil dilators to be uniformly applicable in the presence of small pupils. Beehler pupil dilator can stretch the pupil to 6.0 to 7.0 mm while creating tiny sphincterotomies circumferentially around the papillary margins.

Modified iris retractors can be placed on the pupillary margin without making sphincterotomies following identical procedures. These retractors are equally effective. Lee et al have found the use of only micromole retractors without complementary CTR, to be adequate for phacoemulsification and IOL insertion in eyes with PES induced lens instability. They have recommended that the two methods of capsule stabilisation are complimentary and may be used simultaneously in cases with severe lens instability.

Author prefers to stretch the pupil with iris retractors and performs rhexis while keeping retractors *in situ*. However, retractors can be removed prior to the commencement of phacoprocedures. Despite removing the retractors, adequate pupillary dilatation can be maintained throughout the phacoprocedures without compromising structural configuration of the anterior chamber and the iris diaphragm, particularly in cases of shallow anterior chambers where phacoprocedures may be partly inconvenient in the presence of pupillary stretching devices.

At the end of the surgical procedure the pupil is mechanically reduced with a lens hook supplemented with an intraocular miotic. Though majority of these pupils maintain a good cosmetic appearance and an ability to react to light postoperatively, a few may require miotic drops for some time after surgery to avoid synaechiae to the capsulorrhexis margin.

If hooks or pupil dilators are not available, sectioning the inner most part of the sphincter at three places, about 120 degrees apart, can achieve an acceptable degree of mydriasis.

CAPSULAR TENSION RING IN CASES OF PSE

Inserting a ring into the capsular bag fornix (equator) to support the zonular apparatus was first described by Hara and co-authors.

This is a useful adjunctive therapy in addressing cataract with PES. When placed in the capsular bag (approx 10 mm diameter), the ring keeps the bag stretched and provides several advantages:

(a) Presents concentration of forces on individual zonules by distributing all forces applied to any point on the capsulorrhexis to the entire zonular apparatus.

(b) They keep the bag stretched and maintain the capsular concavity throughout the procedure, thereby assuring great safety during all intraocular manipulations.

(c) They provide sufficient counter traction to avoid excessive postoperative shrinkage of the anterior capsular opening as a result of fibrosis leading to IOL decentration, zonular elongation and occasional ocular hypotony.

CTR's are made of PMMA which has expanded ends that contain positioning holes. The ring comes in two sizes: 10 mm diameter (type 14) for routine cases and 12 mm diameter (type 14A) for high myopia.

A modified CTR developed by Cionni has a fixation hook for severe or progressive cases of zonular deficiency. The hook arises from the loop to run centrally, then covers anteriorly into a parallel plane where it runs peripherally to end up with an eyelet for manipulation and suture placement. This design allows for additional surface fixation to the eye wall without distorting the capsulorrhexis opening.

Depending on when the zonular defect presents, a CTR may be inserted at any stage of the cataract procedure. By re-establishing the capsules contour, the CTR prevents the capsules fornix from being aspirated.

Fine et al recommended placement of the ring in the bag immediately after the completion of capsulorrhexis. The ring is slipped into the incision and fed under the capsulorrhexis with a forceps while the second hand goldens it with a latest hook through the side port incision. Once the ring is in place, cortical cleaning hydrodissection is performed followed by hydrodelineation.

In a few situations when the zonular laxity is not significant, CTR can be implanted after emulsifying the nucleus. This stretches the equatorial circumference of the capsule's bag and, as the ring expands against the intact zonules, resulting in better centration of the capsular bag. The rigidity of the expanded ring provides counter traction and facilitates safer cortical aspiration and IOL insertion.

Even during the stage of insertion of the trailing haptic of IOL, if one feels that zonules are overstressed, the CTR is inserted with the IOL partially in place and the trailing haptic is then inserted.

Excessive anterior capsules contraction could distort the single CTR with the IOL in the bag. Menapace et al recommended implantation of two larger rings in high risk cases.

CTR is a very useful tool to manage zonular dehiscence and cases of PES and every phaco surgeon should be familiar with the techniques of insertion. Though the procedure has a learning curve, yet it can be mastered easily. Another limitation of the CTR is in the procedure of irrigation / aspiration during which an additional force is required to remove the cortex which is held pressed up against the capsules fornices. Despite above mentioned constraints, the implantation of CTR prior to nucleotomy reduces the risk of preoperative complications like zonulysis, PCR and nucleus dislocation as well as facilitates the implantation of foldable IOL implant and ultimate visual outcome.

CAPSULORRHEXIS

CCC is definitely a challenge in cataract surgery in PES due to the presence of weak zonules and also a poorly dilating pupil. One has to exercise special care and caution during capsulotomy as any amount of traction can unzip the already weakened zonules. Capsulorrhexis in the presence of pseudoexfoliation syndrome has a very high risk of extension of rhexis, zonular disinsertion and aggravation of phacodonesis.

The lack of zonular integrity tends to restrict and make it difficult to perforate the capsule to begin a CCC. The dye enhanced rhexis is more suitable and preferred in the presence of pseudoexfoliation. It is better to make an initial opening with a cystitome under the care and support of an iris hook or spatula so as to hold the lens in the position against zonular disinsertion. The subsequent manoeuvre may be completed with the help of rhexis forceps which is invariably more precise and controlled.

Neumann has described a technique of two handed capsulotomy using tangential forces in eyes with weakened zonules. After starting the capsulotomy, the capsular flap is stabilised with the forceps through the main incision while a second instrument such as a bifurcated spatula, is introduced through the side-port incision. Slight backward traction is placed on the flap with the forceps while the second instrument directly advances the turn edge in a tangential manner.

The size of capsulorrhexis is a contentious issue as we have proponents both for a larger as well as a smaller CCC. Fine et al recommended a CCC of 6.0 mm or larger in cases of PES and it leaves a lesser number of lens epithelial cells (LECs) postoperatively than a smaller capsulorrhexis. These LECs undergo metaplasia leading to capsulorrhexis shrinkage as the weakened zonules fail to contain the unopposed forces of capsular contraction.

In another view, a smaller CCC is being advocated as a means to maintain the capsulorrhexis margin safely within the pupillary area, under the direct visualisation of the surgeon.

In one view, a CCC of 5.5–6 mm would work well in the majority of cases of PES undergoing phaco-emulsification.

HYDRODISSECTION AND HYDRODELINEATION

A good hydrodissection as well as hydrodelineation is imperative for the success of phacoemulsification in PES. A good hydrodelineation produces an epinucleus shell as an added safeguard.

If an adequate cortical clearing hydrodissection is achieved and there is free movement of the lens relative to the capsular bag, minimal force will be transmitted to the capsule by endocapsular lens manipulation.

Surgical clearing hydrodissection requires extremely careful manicures, especially when decompressing the bag after having performed the posterior fluid wave. One must depress the posterior lip of the incision with the cannula which ensures easy egress of fluid/viscoelastics out of the eye; thereby avoiding unnecessary pressure build up. The fluid should be injected very gently at multiple locations. Partial cortical clearing hydrodissection is performed along with a gentle central lens decompression. This alleviates the chances of depressing the posterior lens with excessive forces that would lead to tearing of the zonules.

NUCLEUS MANAGEMENT (Authors preference)

The author prefers to perform endocapsular phacoemulsification by direct central chopping techniques. The central chopping has several advantages in case of a smaller rigid pupil, hard cataract and zonular weakness/disinsertion, as chopping exerts the least stress to the capsular bag and zonules as well as minimal chances of iris touch and chaffing encountered due to an inadvertent touch of the phaco tip. It is recommended that extreme care be taken while performing rotations of the nucleus so as to avoid zonular traction. A tangential rotation/movement of the nucleus is much more beneficial to avoid any eminent traction on zonules.

However, Howard fine et al recommended non-rotational cracking, as they consider this method as the least traumatic method of emulsifying the nucleus into quadrants that are easy to mobilise.

In both these techniques a good hydrodelineation with the epinuclear shell helps to stabilise the nucleus and presents transfer of mechanical and phacoemulsification forces to the capsule and zonules.

The author has strong reservations against down slope sculpting as nudging the nucleus in the subincisional area can stress the compromised zonules. A second instrument is passed through side port which will help stabilise the nucleus as well as lift it up slightly so as to push and feed it into the phaco tip.

CORTICAL IRRIGATION/ASPIRATION

The greatest peril to zonular integrity is the step of cortical aspiration where the zonules are subjected to maximum stress. Here lies the importance of cortical cleaning: hydrodissection ensures that majority of cortical matter is removed during flipping and evacuation of the epinuclear shell.

Alternatively, one can perform viscodissection on the leftover cortical matter from the capsular bag.

Moreover, the cortical clean up must be restricted until after IOL stabilises the capsular bag and the remaining cortex can then be aspirated in a more controlled fashion.

Fine et al have proposed tangential traction during mitigation aspiration of the cortical matter rather than stripping centrally, as this manoeuvre would maximise forces on a few cortical/copular connections at a time. Also these are areas of zonular dehiscence; one should strip tangentially towards the dehiscence as it may lead to unzipping of the zonular dehiscence.

CHOICE OF IOLs

There is a limited choice of IOLs that would provide a good surgical outcome on a long term basis in cases of PES undergoing IOL implantation. The IOL tilt was demonstrated to be greater in pseudoexfoliation eyes and this suggests that capsular shrinkage after extracapsular cataract surgery may be stronger in pseudoexfoliation eyes than in healthy eyes.

There is an increased risk of capsular contracture after silicone lens implantation as it carries a higher risk of PCO and capsular contracture in cases of pseudoexfoliation. In addition to lens material, the design of optics and angulation of haptics also plays a significant role in reducing postoperative inflammation, migration of lens epithelial cells and subsequent PCO formation.

It has been observed that heparin surface modified IOL implantation reduces chances of compromise of blood aqueous barrier after surgery and causes fewer cell deposits both on endothelium and the IOL surface. In addition to it, these IOL's have been found to have less foreign body reactions and limited postoperative inflammatory response as compared to PMMA IOL implants. In-the-bag implantation of multipiece acrylic IOL with PMMA haptics can be considered an alternative option over all PMMA rigid IOL.

However, the author prefers the use of hydrophobic single piece foldable lenses as the first choice. The biocompatibility of any IOL implant is inversely proportionate to the severity of pre and postoperative inflammation. The design as well as the water content and permeability of IOL material has a significant role in influencing the postoperative biocompatibility of the IOL. The less the biocompatibility of hydrophilic IOLs the more the water content as compared to the hydrophobic acrylic materials. The hydrophobic acrylic IOLs are most suitable in all conditions especially in the presence of any associated ocular involvements like pseudoexfoliation. The square or sharp edged design of optics of IOL enjoys superiority over other designs in terms of postoperative inflammation and subsequent pattern and incidence of PCO.

In cases of intraoperative complications or large zonular dialysis of more than 30%, a large size, all PMMA IOL having optic size of 6.0/6.5 mm with overall length of 13/13.5 mm should be implanted over CTR so as to avoid decentration of IOL. The PMMA haptics increases the haptic resistance which would counteract the forces of capsular contraction and resist any till decantation of the IOL.

In cases of significant PES, it may be admissible to meticulously polish the anterior capsule leaf overlapping the optic with the CTR already in place and then insert an acrylic single piece/ Multi piece or PMMA IOL in the bag to minimise capsular bag contraction.

COMPLICATIONS

It is generally accepted that the presence of exfoliative material increases the incidence of intraoperative complications such as zonular dehiscence, posterior capsules rupture, phacodonesis, vitreous loss and dropped nucleus or fragment. These complications have partly been attributed to dilating pupils, brittle capsules, weak zonules, and hardness of cataracts. Despite above mentioned several constraints, surgical experience remains a crucial factor in obtaining favourable outcomes in cases of PES undergoing phacoemulsification.

Compromised corneal endothelium is among many factors limiting success in patients with PES undergoing cataract surgery. The use of sodium hyaluranate is highly beneficial since it provides adequate coat to the endothelium as well as stabilises the anterior chamber for a better surgical outcome.

In addition the availability of better instrumentation, IOL implants and tremendous improvements in surgical expertise in the intra as well as postoperative turmoil has shown marked decline in their incidence, severity as well as significant and qualitative improvement in terms of final outcome.

As such most of the initial studies have involved manual ECCE as the method of cataract extraction and hence, these results cannot be extrapolated in phacoemulsification.

Intraoperative Complications

We have observed a relatively higher incidence of intraoperative complications upto 5 to 7% in cases of phacoemulsification surgery in the presence of pseudoexfoliation syndrome as compared to the 2 to 3% in cases of phacoemulsification surgery in uncomplicated cases.

The noted complications related with phacoemulsification surgery in the presence of pseudoexfoliation syndrome are enumerated as follows:

(i) *Intraoperative zonular disinsertion:* The incidence of zonular disinsertion during phacoemulsification surgery is much less (2 to 3%) as compared to 25 to 30% in case of conventional ECCE and in cases of pseudoexfoliation syndrome. The application of CTR and nucleotomy by direct central chopping has further minimised the risk of preoperative zonulysis.

(ii) Posterior capsular rupture: Pseudoexfoliation, undoubtedly carries a higher risk of a posterior capsular rent/rupture due to the thin and fragile capsule. The incidence of such complications varies from 4 to 6% in phacosurgery as compared to the 14 to 17% during ECCE. Meticulous intraoperative manoeuvre and application of CTR minimises the risk of a PC rent. The technique of visco expansion of the anterior chamber and induced mydriasis with viscoelastic and excessive bottle height during phacoemulsification should therefore be done with extreme caution as this may lead to inadvertent rupture of the posterior capsule and zonulysis.

(iii) Vitreous loss: Vitreous loss is linked with zonulysis and subsequent PC rupture.

(iv) Nucleus/fragment drop: Nucleus/fragment drop is not an unusual complication in the presence of pseudoexfoliation syndrome. The presence of rigid and miotic pupil in association with hard cataract and generalised structural variations are responsible for this severe complication. However, we have not encountered any nucleus or fragment drop so far in the presence of pseudoexfoliation syndrome. The judicious application of CTR, nucleotomy technique and machine dynamics as well as anticipation of impending complications or their earliest detection definitely minimise the risk of such dreaded occurrence.

(v) Miscellaneous complications: The presence of miotic and rigid pupil along with hard cataract are at risk of minor problems like iris chaffing. The use of pupillary stretching devices and careful emulsification and confining to the central most pupillary zone reduces the incidence of iris chaffing.

Early/Immediate Postoperative Complications

(i) Uveitis: Despite the fact that pseudoexfoliation syndrome carries the inherent higher risk of intraoperative complications as well as the altered blood–aqueous barrier, the incidence and severity of postoperative uveitis is remarkably low probably owing to the refined instrumentation, phaco-dynamics as well as surgical technique. The judicious use of topical steroids alongwith cycloplegics takes adequate care to control postoperative inflammation.

(ii) Secondary glaucoma: The presence of exfoliative material and subsequent compromised angle as well as viscooccluded angle may precipitate secondary glaucoma during immediate postoperative period. Intraoperative complications like vitreous loss, improper cortical clearing are other contributing factors for this eventuality. Hence, careful evaluation of possibility of postoperative glaucoma should be scrutinised as a routine. One should not hesitate to commence antiglaucoma medication in anticipation where intraoperative eventuality has taken place or in other suspected cases.

(iii) Choroidal effusion/detachment: Choroidal effusion/detachment is not an uncommon occurrence following concurrent cataract and glaucoma or isolated cataract surgery in cases of long standing and complicated glaucoma. As described earlier the incidence of choroidal effusion/detachment further increases, following prolonged use of newer antiglaucoma medications having action on prostaglandin inhibitory system. Sudden lowering in IOP in cases of prolonged and uncontrolled glaucoma cases is also attributed to the higher incidence, of upto 5 to 7% of this complication. The use of systemic and topical steroids as well as cycloplegics is sufficient enough to revert the situation within two to three weeks duration. We did not experience the essentiality of surgical intervention to manage choroidal deta-chment even in a single case so far.

Needless to stress again the fact that drugs acting on prostaglandin inhibitory system should be discontinued atleast six weeks prior to the surgery while IOP is maintained with the help of a substitute regimen so as to minimise the risk of intra and postoperative complications.

Delayed Complications

Pre-existing weakness of zonular apparatus and a rigid and small pupil which is further exaggerated due to reduced pupillary dilatation are added risk factors for delayed complications following phacoemulsification surgery in the presence of pseudoexfoliation syndrome. Noted problems are as follows:

(i) Spontaneous dislocation/Subluxation of IOL: Postoperative fibrosis with subsequent shrinkage of the capsule is increased in these eyes, and these centripetal forces will further loosen the zonular fibres. Late in-the-bag intraocular lens dislocation, is therefore, anticipated to become a growing problem in the future. However, author has not experienced late in-the-bag intraocular lens dislocation so far in any case of pseudoexfoliation syndrome.

(ii) Corneal endothelial dysfunction: The presence of exfoliative material on the posterior surface of cornea, hard cataract, miotic pupil, pre-existing glaucoma as well as associated intra- and postoperative complications are contributing factors towards a higher incidence of corneal endothelial dysfunction which may lead to the formation of bullous keratopathy. Intraoperative use of sodium hyaluronate, pupillary stretching devices and optimal utilisation of ultrasonic energy definitively reduces the risk of endothelial dysfunction. In addition to it, prevention of postoperative ocular inflammation and secondary glaucoma are equally important to minimise the risk of endothelial dysfunction.

(iii) *Higher incidence of CME:* Higher incidence of CME is a known fact following any intraocular surgery in cases of uncontrolled glaucoma, prolonged medications as well as in the presence of intraoperative eventuality like vitreous disturbance or posterior capsule rent. The dysfunctioning of the blood–aqueous barrier is one of the attributing factors for the higher incidence of CME of upto 12% in eyes with pseudoexfoliation syndrome. The management of CME remains essentially the same as described in other cases.

(iv) *PCO:* Pseudoexfoliation syndrome is invariably associated with higher incidence of PCO following cataract surgery as compared to the concurrent procedures in cases of POAG. The incidence of PCO ranges from 12 to 15% after three years in cases of acrylic single piece hydrophobic IOLs in the presence of PSE as compared to 9 to 12% in other cases of glaucoma. The incidence of PCO following acrylic hydrophobic and all PMMA IOL was ranging upto 15 to 20% and 15 to 25%, respectively.

The poorly dilating pupil, difficulty in performing meticulous cortical cleaning as well as higher incidence of intra and postoperative complications encountered with cases of pseudoexfoliation syndrome are linked with the subsequent higher incidence of PCO.

Postoperative Management

The postoperative management is essentially the same after cataract surgery as in the presence of pseudoexfoliation syndrome. However, the frequency and duration of topical steroids and cycloplegics along with other supportive medication may be titrated in accordance with the need. Systemic steroids are, by and large, not required.

CONCLUSION

Phacoemulsification in the presence of pseudoexfoliation of the lens presents unusual surgical challenges.

Improvements in phacoemulsification technology, gentle and careful manipulation intraoperatively, better surgical techniques, capsules support devices and better understanding of the disease process has eventually facilitated cataract surgery in these eyes almost without complications.

Although in experienced hands, phacoemulsification in PES has resulted in better outcomes, special care should still be exercised.

BIBLIOGRAPHY

1. Schlötzer-Schrehardt UM, Koca MR, Naumann GOH, Volkholz H. Pseudoexfoliation syndrome: ocular manifestation of a systemic disorder? Arch Ophthalmol. 1992; 110: 1752–1756.

2. Wollensak J, Becker HU, Seiler T. Pseudoexfoliation syndrome and glaucoma: does glaucoma capsulare exist? Ger J Ophthalmol. 1992; 1:32–34.

3. Arvind H, Raju P, Paul PG, Baskaran M, Ramesh SV, George RJ, McCarty C, Vijaya L. Pseudoexfoliation in South India 1: Br J Ophthalmol. 2003 Nov; 87(11):1321–3.

4. Thomas R, Nirmalan PK, Krishnaiah S, Pseudoexfoliation in southern India: the Andhra Pradesh Eye Disease Study. Invest Ophthalmol Vis Sci. 2005 Apr; 46(4):1170–6.

5. Krishnadas R, Nirmalan PK, Ramakrishnan R, Thulasiraj RD, Katz J, Tielsch JM, Friedman DS, Robin AL. Pseudo-exfoliation in a rural population of southern India: the Aravind Comprehensive Eye Survey. 1: Am J Ophthalmol. 2003 Jun; 135(6):830–7.

6. Rao RQ, Arain TM, Ahad MA. The prevalence of pseudo-exfoliation syndrome in Pakistan. Hospital based study. BMC Ophthalmol. 2006 Jun 22;6:27.

7. A L Young AL, Tang W W T, Lam D S C. The prevalence of pseudoexfoliation syndrome in Chinese people. British Journal of Ophthalmology 2004; 88:193–195.

8. Miyazaki M, Kubota T, Kubo M, Kiyohara Y, Iida M, Nose Y, Ishibashi T. The prevalence of pseudoexfoliation syndrome in a Japanese population: the Hisayama study. 1: J Glaucoma. 2005 Dec; 14(6):482–4.

9. Rotchford AP, Kirwan JF, Johnson GJ, Roux P. Exfoliation syndrome in black South Africans: Arch Ophthalmol. 2003 Jun; 121(6):863–70.

10. Naumann GOH, Schlötzer-Schrehardt U. Corneal endothelial involvement in pseudoexfoliation syndrome. Arch Ophthalmol. 1994; 112:297–298.

11. Eagle RC, Font RL, Fine BS. The basement membrane exfoliation syndrome. Arch Ophthalmol. 1979;97:510–515.

12. Guzek JP, Holm M, Cotter JB, et al. Risk factors for intraoperative complications in 1000 extracapsular cataract cases. Ophthalmology. 1987; 94:461–466.

13. Lumme P, Laatikainen L. Exfoliation syndrome and cataract extraction. Am J Ophthalmol. 1993; 116:51–55.

14. Brooks AMV, Gillies WE. The development of microneovascular changes in the iris in pseudoexfoliation of the lens capsule. Ophthalmology. 1987; 94:1090–1097.

15. Asano N, Schlötzer-Schrehardt U, Naumann GOH. A histopathologic study of iris changes in pseudoexfoliation syndrome. Am J Ophthalmol. 1995; 102:1279–1290.

16. Küchle M, Vinores SA, Mahlow J, Green WR. Blood-aqueous barrier in pseudoexfoliation syndrome: evaluation by immunohistochemical staining of endogeneous albumin. Graefes Arch Clin Exp Ophthalmol. 1996; 234:12–18.

17. Kraff MC, Sanders DR, Liebermann HL. Monitoring for continuing endothelial cell loss with cataract extraction and intraocular lens implantation. Ophthalmology. 1982; 89: 30–34.

18. Jampel HD, Friedman DS, Lubomski LH, et al: Effect of technique on intraocular pressure after combined cataract and glaucoma surgery: An evidence-based review. Ophthalmology 109: 2215–24; quiz 2225, 2231, 2002.

19. Friedman DS, Jampel HD, Lubomski LH, et al: Surgical strategies for coexisting glaucoma and cataract: an evidence-based update. Ophthalmology 109:1902–13, 2002.

20. Pereira FA, Cronemberger S: Ultrasound biomicroscopic study of anterior segment changes after phacoemulsification and foldable intraocular lens implantation. Ophthalmology 110:1799–806, 2003.

21. Abela-Formanek C, Amon M, Schauersberger J, Schild G, Kolodjaschna J, Barisani-Asenbauer T, Kruger A. Uveal and capsular biocompatibility of 2 foldable acrylic intraocular lenses in patients with uveitis or pseudoexfoliation syndrome: comparison to a control group. : J Cataract Refract Surg. 2002 Jul; 28(7):1160–72.

22. Hayashi K, Hayashi H, Nakao F, et al: Changes in anterior chamber angle width and depth after intraocular lens implantation in eyes with glaucoma. Ophthalmology 107: 698–703, 2000.

23. Shuba L, Nicolela MT, Rafuse PE. Correlation of capsular pseudoexfoliation material and iridocorneal angle pigment with the severity of pseudoexfoliation glaucoma. J Glaucoma. 2007 Jan; 16(1):94–7.

24. Gunning FP, Greve EL: Lens extraction for uncontrolled angle-closure glaucoma: long-term follow-up. J Cataract Refract Surg 24:1347–56, 1998.

25. Hayashi K, Hayashi H, Nakao F, et al: Effect of cataract surgery on intraocular pressure control in glaucoma patients. J Cataract Refract Surg 27:1779–86, 2001.

26. Jacobi PC, Dietlein TS, Lüke C, et al: Primary phacoemulsification and intraocular lens implantation for acute angle-closure glaucoma. Ophthalmology 109:1597–603, 2002.

27. Merkur A, Damji KF, Mintsioulis G, et al: Intraocular pressure decrease after phacoemulsification in patients with pseudoexfoliation syndrome. J Cataract Refract Surg 27:528–32, 2001.

28. Shingleton BJ, Heltzer J, O'Donoghue MW: Outcomes of phacoemulsification in patients with and without pseudo-exfoliation syndrome. J Cataract Refract Surg 29: 1080–6, 2003.

29. Katsimpris JM, Petropoulos IK, Apostolakis K, Feretis D.Comparing phacoemulsification and extracapsular cataract extraction in eyes with pseudoexfoliation syndrome, small pupil, and phacodonesis. Klin Monatsbl Augenheilkd. 2004 May; 221(5):328–33.

30. Stefan C, Nenciu A, Neaciu A, Ilie G, Dachin L. Phacoemulsification and pseudoexfoliative syndrome. Oftalmologia. 2004; 48(4):44–50.

31. Bayramlar H, Hepsen IF, Yilmaz H. Mature cataracts increase risk of capsular complications in manual small-incision cataract surgery of pseudoexfoliative eyes.: Can J Ophthalmol. 2007 Feb; 42(1):46–50.

32. Yi DH, Sullivan BR. Phacoemulsification with indocyanine green versus manual expression extracapsular cataract extraction for advanced cataract. J Cataract Refract Surg. 2002 Dec; 28(12):2165–9.

33. Bayraktar S, Altan T, Küçüksümer Y, Yilmaz OF: Capsular tension ring implantation after capsulorhexis in phaco-emulsification of cataracts associated with pseudoexfoliation syndrome. Intraoperative complications and early postoperative findings. 1: J Cataract Refract Surg. 2001; 27(10):1620–8.

36

Challenges of Phacoemulsification Surgery in Paediatric Cataract

Col Vijay Mathur and Col JKS Parihar SM, VSM

INTRODUCTION

Paediatric cataract blindness presents an enormous problem to developing countries in terms of human morbidity, economic loss, and social burden. Managing cataracts in children remains a challenge: treatment is often difficult, tedious and requires dedicated team effort. To assure the best long term outcome for cataract blind children, appropriate pediatric surgical techniques need to be defined and adopted by ophthalmic surgeons of developing countries. The high cost of operative equipment and the uneven world distribution of ophthalmologists, paediatricians, and anaesthetists create unique challenges.

CHALLENGES IN PAEDIATRIC CATARACT

Structural and Anatomical Differences as Compared to an Adult Eyeball

Paediatric eyeball is quite different from an adult eyeball. There are various structural and anatomical differences as compared to an adult eyeball:

(a) **Cornea and the sclera are more elastic:** This leads to a tendency of collapse of the eyeball when the eyeball is open during any surgical procedure.

(b) **Structural changes in the first two years of age:** In children less than 0–2 yrs. of age, the eyeball is still growing and changes in its length and corneal curvature occur. There is no formula yet to accurately calculate the IOL power in a growing eye. Approximate changes in IOL power calculation have to be made by the surgeon based on the child's age.

(c) **Angle structures are not yet fully developed:** The angle structures of the anterior chamber are not fully developed till one year of age. There is a higher risk of secondary glaucoma when cataract is operated upon early in life.

(d) **Lens capsule is thicker and more elastic:** Difficulty in doing capsulorrhexis.

(e) **Shallow anterior chamber, microcornea and microophthalmos** are encountered in cataracts due to congenital rubella syndrome.

(f) **Pattern of pupillary dilatation:** Poorly and slowly dilating pupil due to poorly developed dilator pupillae muscle.

(g) **Opacities in the visual axis after cataract removal:** Remnants of hyperplastic primary vitreous and tunica vasculosa lead to opacities in the visual axis after cataract removal.

(h) **Strong attachment of the vitreous body with lens:** This along with a tendency of scleral collapse creates a strong posterior push during surgery.

Due to these structural and anatomical anomalies, paediatric cataract becomes a different entity altogether as compared to adult cataract.

Age for Surgery

(a) Cataracts present at the time of birth, unilateral or bilateral, should be operated upon as early as possible to allow development of optic tracts and lateral geniculate body.

(b) Once binocular vision has become established, one can wait. In cataracts due to JRA, uveitis and trauma, medical therapy can be given till inflammation is under control. Surgery should be done before amblyopia sets in.

Biometry in Children

In the first 0–2 yrs of life, the eyeball grows in size to adult proportions. A newborn child is hypermetropic to the extent of +5.0 to +6.0 Diopters. As the eyeball grows, there is a myopic shift and the eye becomes emmetropic by 0–3 yrs of age.

There is no separate formula for IOL power calculation for children.

(a) **A child less than 1 years of age:** Many surgeons keep the child less than 1 yr of age aphakic and do secondary IOL implantation at a later date.[23] However, aphakia is a strong stimulus for amblyopia.

Many surgeons would like a child operated in the first year of life to be hypermetropic by +5.0 to +6.0 Diopters and balance of correction given by glasses. As the eyeball grows, there is a myopic shift towards emmetropia.

(b) **1 to 2 year old child:** In the second year of life, the child may be kept +3.5 D Hypermetropic.

(c) **Child older than 2 years of age:** After the third year of life, same correction as given by IOL formula's for adults can be given. IOL implantation does not alter the normal growth of the eyeball in any way.[12]

Surgical Procedures Advocated

Surgical procedures for paediatric cataract have undergone tremendous changes with availability of modern equipment and techniques.

Phacoaspiration

Phacoaspiration has become the procedure of choice. A small sealed wound maintains the anterior chamber depth, prevents collapse of the eyeball and prevents pupillary constriction. It also protects the posterior capsule and corneal endothelium.

(i) Incision

A clear corneal or a corneo-scleral incision may be made. Due to high content of elastin in paediatric cornea and sclera, the edges of the wound tend to gape.

Many surgeons would use Flieringa's rings in days of open chamber surgery in paediatric cataract. Due to this tendency of wound gape, surgeons still prefer to use a suture at the end of the surgery even in a water tight wound after Phacoaspiration.

(ii) Capsulorrhexis

Due to the thick and elastic nature of the capsule, this is one of the most difficult steps in surgery. It is mandatory to keep the anterior chamber formed deep throughout this step. Cohesive viscoelastics like hyaluronic acid and chondroitin sulphate may be used. The capsulorrhexis has a tendency to run into the periphery and the direction of pull must always be towards the centre after gripping the capsular flap with capsulorrhexis forceps as close to the torn margin as possible. The grip must be changed frequently and the anterior chamber must frequently be reformed with viscoelastics.

If you plan a small Rhexis (less than 3.5 mm), you will be able to get the adequate size. The flap should be raised relatively towards the centre. The length of horizontal/linear nick should not be more than 3 mm. Use sodium hyaluronate into the bag after giving nick if you prefer rhexis forceps. In total cataracts, dye enhancement is beneficial. Trypan blue can be safely used to stain the anterior capsule. Despite all precautions, the capsulorrhexis may still run into the periphery and the surgeon may have to give a fresh cut in the capsular margin with needle or vanas scissors and complete the rhexis from the other side.

(iii) Hydroprocedures

Hydrodissection is extremely important to separate the cortex from its capsular adhesions as a thorough cortical cleanup is essential for prevention of posterior capsular opacification. A flattened 23G cannula is inserted just under the anterior capsular margin and 0.3–0.5 ml of fluid is injected. This may be repeated in two or more quadrants.

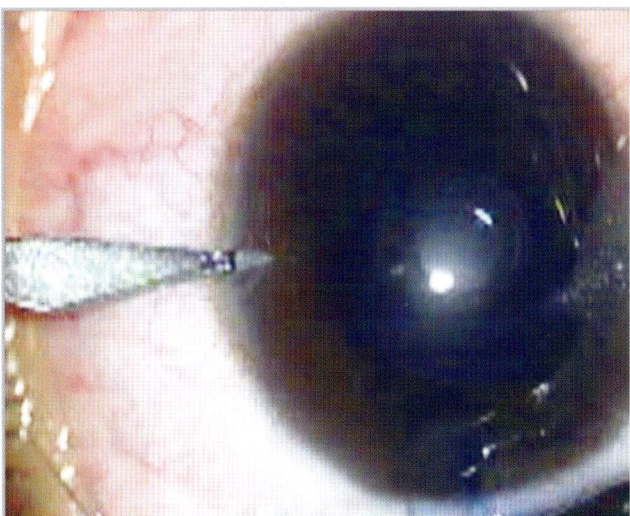

(a)

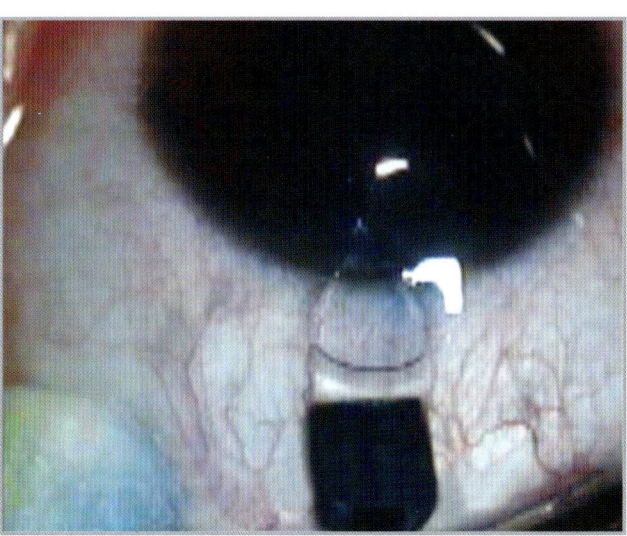

(b)

Fig. 36.1: (a) Side port incision, (b) Diamond knife incision (2.8 mm)

Hydrodelineation is generally not possible as there is no hard central nucleus.

Attempt to delineate the nucleus leads to prolapse of nucleus out of the capsular bag into the anterior chamber.

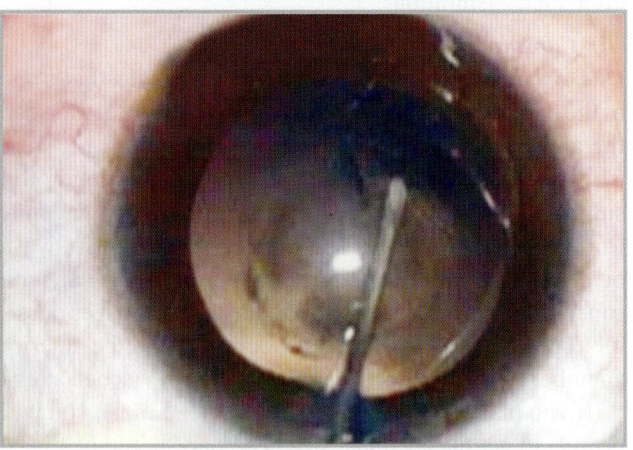

Fig. 36.2: Capsulorrhexis

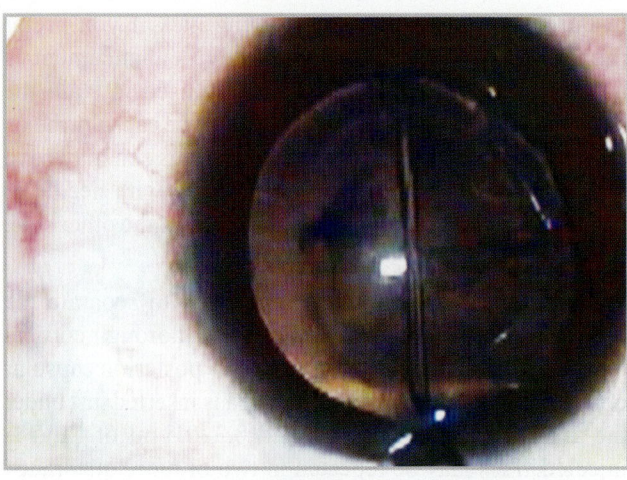

(a)

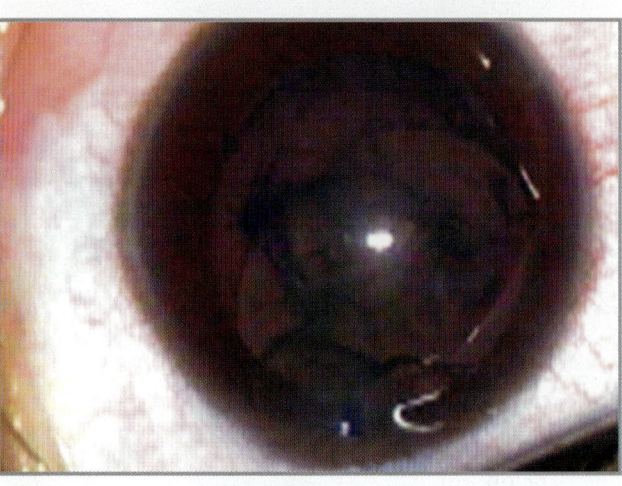

(b)

Fig. 36.3: (a) Hydroprocedures, (b) Hydroprocedures: Nucleus floated into the anterior chamber

In cases of posterior polar cataract, hydrodissection should be avoided.

(iv) Phacoaspiration

This is one of the easier steps of the procedure. Nucleus can be aspirated out in I/A mode with moderate vacuum. A Phacoprobe or an I/A probe maybe used for the purpose.

Cortical cleanup is difficult due to cortico-capsular adhesions, particularly in the sub-incisional area. In a micro-ophthalmic eye, it is difficult to manipulate the probe within the eyeball.

It is essential that all cortical matter be cleaned up or else remaining cells keep dividing to form Soemmering's ring which can lead to early PCO, incite uveitis and displace the IOL. A gentle and smooth manoeuvre of the capsule polisher over the posterior surface of anterior capsule and over the posterior capsule is recommended.

Viscoelastic cushion to remove adhered lens fibres and tiny plaque is very useful and beneficial to reduce the extent, severity and incidence of posterior capsular opacification particularly in case of paediatric cataract.

(v) Posterior Plaque Removal

Paediatric cataracts are very commonly associated with posterior plaques. Posterior plaques occurring as part of posterior polar cataracts are associated with the Mittendorf's dot (with persistent remnants of tunica vasculosa) or as a part of congenital Rubella syndrome. In cases of congenital rubella syndrome, the posterior plaque comprises of multiple dot like opacities. Removal of these plaques requires a lot of expertise and patience. One has to be very cautious while handling post plaque, else it may lead to PCR which may make further procedure very difficult even if you have planned PCCC subsequently. Planned PCCC controls vitreous disturbance whereas unplanned rents create total derangement of postcapsule and vitreous phase.

After forming the anterior chamber with viscoelastic, the plaque can be teased off the posterior capsule with the

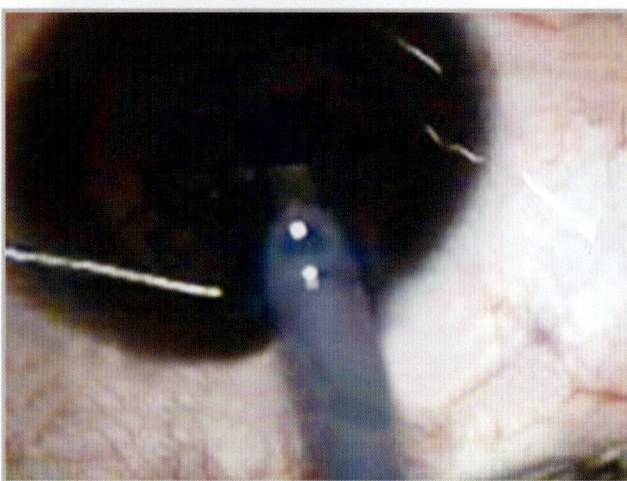

Fig. 36.4: Phacoaspiration: Zero power vacuum: 250 mmHg/ Peristaltic

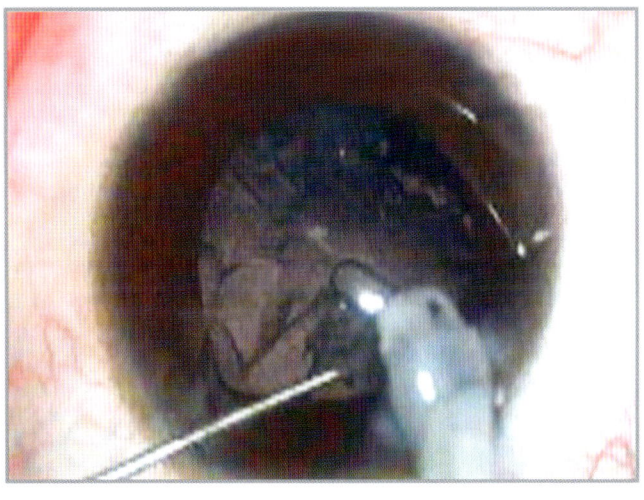
(a)

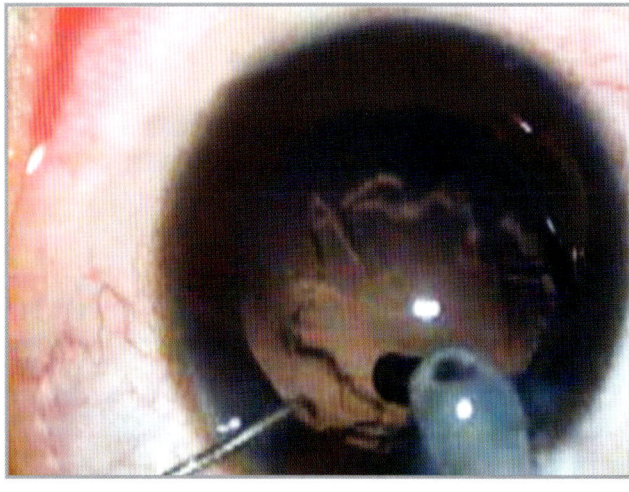
(b)

Fig. 36.5: (a) Removal of 12 O' clock cortex (co-Axial Method), (b) Hydroseparation and aspiration of posterior cortical plate

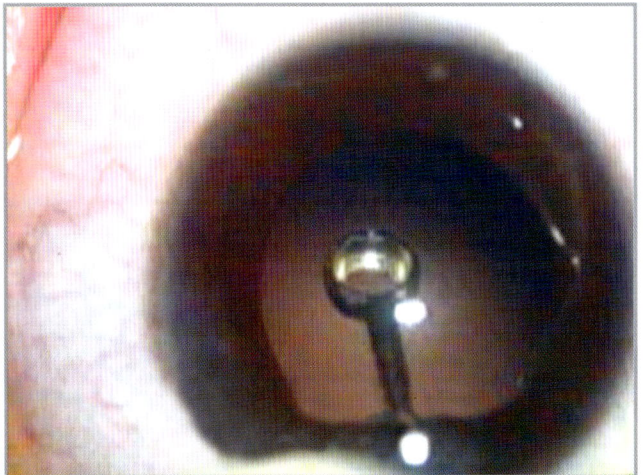

Fig. 36.6: Polishing of the anterior and posterior capsule

tip of an I/A probe. The vacuum and flow rate should be kept at the minimum. If this does not help, tip of a dialler is used to lift one end of the plaque; cohesive viscoelastic can now be injected under the plaque to dissect it off. In posterior plaques associated with persistent remnants of tunica vasculosa, PCCC with localised anterior vitrectomy has to be done.

Machine settings (peristaltic/ventury) for different types of paediatric cataract (hypermature/post subcap plaque/Dense post adhesions):

Phacoaspiration is very tricky in paediatric cataract compared to senile cataract. Machine settings are of moderate vacuum with a relatively high flow rate. It should be variable as per steps of surgery. One has to be very cautious while handling post plaque, else it may lead to PCR which may make further procedure very difficult even if you have planned PCCC subsequently. Planned PCCC controls vitreous disturbance whereas an unplanned rent creates total derangement of the post capsule and vitreous phase.

Suggested machine settings for paediatric cataract surgery are as follows:

Procedure	Peristaltic pump machines	Venturi pump machines
Nucleus aspiration	150–200 mmHg	50–80 mmHg
Cortex aspiration	200–250 mmHg	150–200 mmHg
Posterior capsule polishing	30–50 mmHg	Minimum (10 mmHg)

Phacoaspiration with Posterior Continuous Capsulorrhexis (PCCC)

After aspirating the cataractous lens, PCCC is performed in children who are in the pre-school age group. This alone can prevent posterior capsular opacification (PCO) in a large majority of cases. PCIOL with or without IOL capture can be placed. PCCC is performed under viscoelastic. An opening smaller than that of anterior capsulorrhexis is generally performed with the help of capsulorrhexis forceps. A cystitome does not help. It is not helpful as the posterior surface of posterior capsule is slippery due to vitreous. In cases of posterior capsular plaque, the plaque can be teased off with a sharp instrument. If the posterior capsule is thick and calcified, vitrectomy cutter can be used with low aspiration and high cutting rate to create an opening in the posterior capsule.

Phacoaspiration with Posterior Continuous Capsulorrhexis and Anterior Vitrectomy

Vitrectomy can be done if there is disturbance of vitreous or if there is opacification of anterior vitreous. High cutting rate with low aspiration is used to clear vitreous prolapsing into the anterior chamber. It is not essential to do vitrectomy in anterior vitreous cavity – this only leads to hypotony and makes further surgical steps difficult.

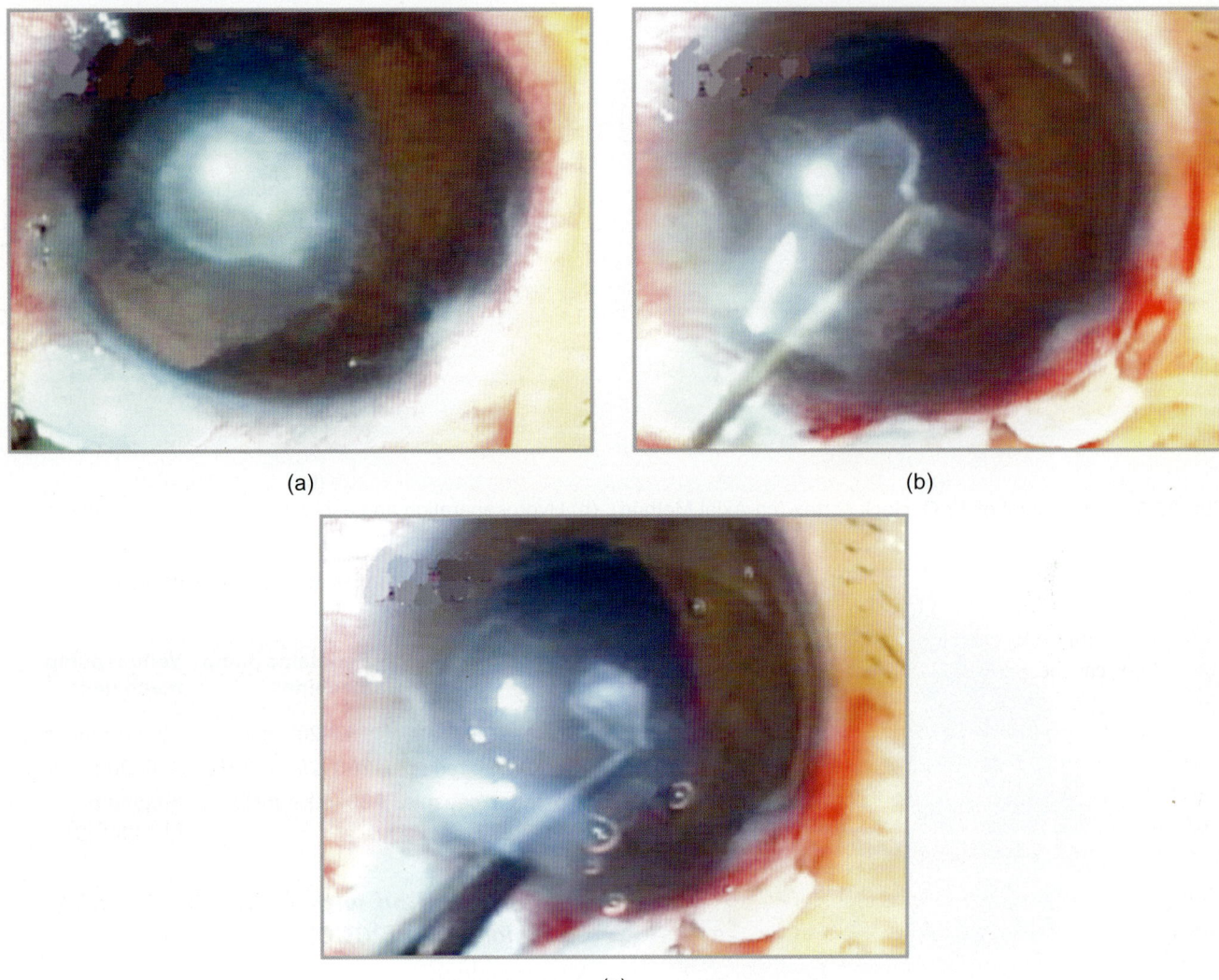

(a)   (b)

(c)

Fig. 36.7: (a) Posterior plaque, (b) Posterior plaque dissection with the help of a 26 gauze needle, (c) Posterior plaque dissection is being completed with the help of utrata capsulorrhexis forceps

Pars Plana Lensectomy and Vitrectomy

This technique ensures a clear visual axis but it is a more elaborate procedure. In addition to posterior segment complications like choroidal detachment, vitreous hemorrhage and retinal detachment, there is a risk of particles of lens matter dropping into the vitreous cavity and inciting severe postoperative vitritis. To implant an IOL over the capsular frill, a large Limbal incision is required which is associated with its own problems. It also takes cataract surgery out from the realm of anterior segment surgeons from the posterior segment surgeons who are few and far.

Posterior Chamber IOL Implantation

Except for very young children, PCIOL implantation is the preferred method of visual rehabilitation. For many years, PMMA lenses were being implanted and they have proven their worth in Paediatric cataract surgery. Heparin or Flourine surface modified IOL's have been used for years. They act by reducing cellular adhesion and protein deposit on IOL surface; thereby reducing incidence of IOL Opacification, formation of cyclitic membrane and PCO. Using PMMA or Foldable Acrylic IOL's with square edge design also help in preventing ingrowth of lens epithelial cells.

Recently, encouraging reports have started appearing in literature about foldable hydrophilic lenses. The lens material has been tested and found to incite minimal inflammation and prevent PCO. They have an added advantage of requiring smaller incisions for implanting which leads to lesser postoperative astigmatism and earlier rehabilitation[6]. However, in the presence of PCCC, their long term stability is to be seen.

Foldable IOL implanted in the bag have better visual outcome as compared to PMMA lenses.

This has become the procedure of choice. A small sealed wound maintains the anterior chamber depth, prevents collapse of the eyeball and prevents pupillary constriction. It also protects the posterior capsule and corneal endothelium. The nucleus is usually soft and can be aspirated without any phaco power. Ensuring intact Continuous Curvilinear Capsulorrhexis (CCC) and good Hydrodissection is a must. Meticulous cleanup of cortical matter is essential. Residual cortical matter can incite severe postoperative uveitis. Phacoaspiration with PCIOL implantation is the modality of choice in older children. Foldable IOL's implanted in the bag have a better visual outcome as compared to PMMA lenses.

Conventional Lens Aspiration

This procedure can be done, but difficulties can arise with shallow anterior chambers, high degree of postoperative astigmatism and suture related problems. Small Incision cataract can be safely done in children with the help of an Anterior chamber maintainer (ACM). Since the nucleus is small in size, it can be safely aspirated out through a small self sealing incision. If the incision is small and rhexis is intact, a foldable IOL can be placed in the bag. PCCC and vitrectomy can be done if required. This method can be safely done where automated I/A machine is not available as it is free from suture related problems. With an ACM in place the anterior chamber is always deep and formed thereby preventing collapse of the eyeball.

Examination under Anaesthesia (EUA)

Many children present to the ophthalmologist with Leucocoria. Often these children are agitated and uncooperative. Cataract maybe the commonest cause but other sinister conditions like retinoblastoma, primary hyperplastic persistent vitreous, toxocariasis, long standing retinal detachment, iridocyclitis and retinopathy of prematurity need to be ruled out.

Often EUA is the only opportunity to carry out a detailed examination of the eye in an uncooperative child. This

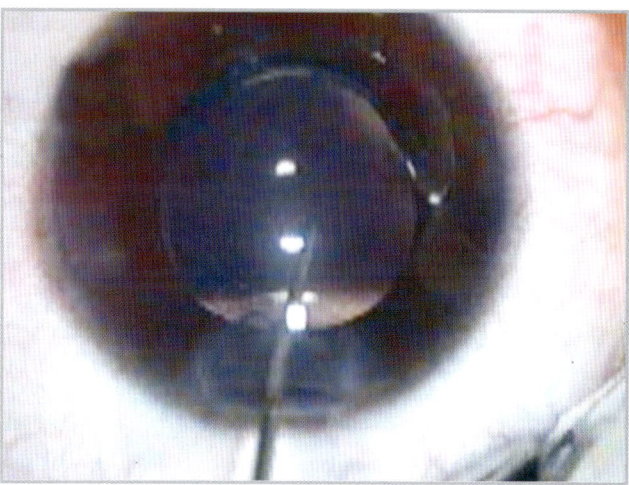

Fig. 36.9: Well placed IOL in the bag

examination maybe followed by cataract surgery. Both eyes must be examined. One should take this opportunity to carry out following examinations:

(a) **Detailed anterior segment examination** by operating microscope or a hand held slit lamp if available.

(b) **Axial length measurement using contact 'A' scan:** Contact with the child's eye should be very gentle, as even the slightest pressure can indent the cornea, causing a change in the axial length of the eye.

(c) Measurement of the corneal diameter.

(d) Intraocular pressure using Perkin's or Schiotz's tonometre.

(e) **Keratometry using a portable hand held Keratometre.** This along with axial length can be used for IOL power calculation.

(f) **Intraoperative biometry/refraction:** Is very useful as it may provide opportunity to adjust postop refraction to avoid subsequent amblyopia.

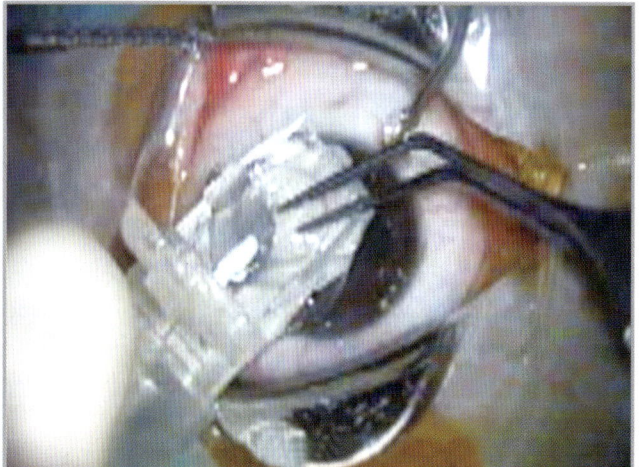

Fig. 36.8: Square edge acrylic foldable IOL implant

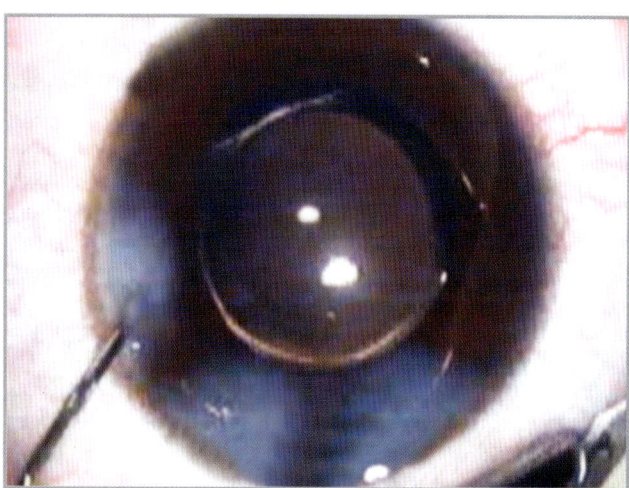

Fig. 36.10: Stromal hydration

(g) **Funduscopic examination using indirect or direct ophthalmoscope:** In cases of the congenital rubella syndrome the retina may have 'salt and pepper' appearance. In premature children, the retina is still immature, vascular arcade on the temporal side may not be extending up till the retinal periphery and the retina gives a grayish appearance. Coloboma of the optic disc and retina maybe associated with congenital cataracts. In others, persistent hyperplastic primary vitreous (PHPV) maybe seen. Optic disc should be evaluated for changes suggestive of glaucoma. Stereoscopic view with an indirect ophthalmoscope is invaluable.

The role of EUA is critical as it decides the further management and the prognosis.

Constraints and Peculiarities of Phacoemulsification

(a) **Structural variations in Tenons capsule:** Tenons capsule is thick, vascular and strongly adherent to conjunctiva. Cutting the tenons capsule may lead to granuloma formation.

(b) **Ill defined angle of anterior chamber:** Angle being immature, surgical limbus is not clearly defined. Attempted entry at limbus may be posterior than expected leading to problems like iris prolapse, iridodialysis, wound leak and shallow anterior chamber and difficulty in manipulation of the phaco probe. It is better to go for a clear corneal incision.

(c) **Difficulty in performing continuous curvilinear capsulorrhexis (CCC):** is a major hurdle. Owing to thick and elastic anterior capsule, the rhexis tends to run out to the periphery. Keeping the anterior chamber always deep and formed with viscoelastics like hyaluronidase, helps. One should aim to make a smaller rhexis (to begin with, 3.0 mm opening should be the aim) as the rhexis has a tendency to enlarge. Capsulorrhexis forceps are helpful in doing CCC. Cuts with vannas scissors in rhexis margins may be necessary and the CCC can be completed from the opposite direction whenever it extends irretrievably towards the periphery.

(d) **Constraints in attempting hydroprocedures:** Due to the soft nucleus, hydrodelineation is not possible. Thorough hydrodissection should be done. This alone is sufficient to loosen the lens cortex and the nucleus which can be aspirated in the I/A mode.

(e) **Posterior capsular rhexis:** Posterior capsule at times is opacified and requires PCCC to be done. Most surgeons would do PCCC in younger children (pre-school age group). PCCC opening has to be smaller than anterior CCC opening. It is imperative to use capsulorrhexis forceps as posterior surface has vitreous adhering to it and needle alone is not sufficient.

(f) **Role of anterior vitrectomy:** If there is vitreous disturbance or opacification, anterior vitrectomy has to be done. Most surgeons would do PCCC with anterior vitrectomy routinely in all children below 2 yrs of age.

(g) **Postsurgical visual rehabilitation:** In all children, visual rehabilitation is necessary in postoperative period to prevent amblyopia.

(h) **Difficulties encountered during general Anaesthesia:** All children are required to be operated under general anaesthesia. Attempt should be made to rule out any underlying co-morbid systemic disorder.

(i) **Traumatic cataracts:** Traumatic cataracts form an important group of childhood cataracts. Trauma can be associated with other derangements in the anterior and the posterior segments. 'Pentagon approach' maybe necessary in dealing with these cases.

Postoperative Peculiarities of Cataract Surgery in Children

Postoperative follow-up in a child presents with problems like difficulty in examination of the operated eye. Child may become very uncooperative and even refuses to yield to examination with torch light. A child who is able to open his eye and is looking around without too much of blepharospasm or lacrimation is a heartening sight for the surgeon. In this regard phaco surgery scores over conventional lens aspiration as there is no suture induced irritation, making it more comfortable for the child.

(a) **Postoperative uveitis:** Postoperative uveitis can be very severe and plastic in nature. Moderate to severe uveitis or severe fibrinoid reaction is a major postoperative threat to a good outcome in the paediatric age group. Children with JRA associated cataracts, rubella syndrome associated cataract and traumatic cataracts are more at risk and a preoperative course of systemic steroids may be justified in these cases. Cataracts due to other causes may develop uveitis in postoperative period because of remnant cortical matter or excessive intraoperative manipulation. This needs to be energetically treated with strong topical cycloplegics and steroids. Systemic steroids should be used provided they are not contraindicated. Many techniques, like using intracameral heparin infusion and recombinant tissue plasminogen activator (r-tpa) have been used to reduce postoperative inflammation in high risk cases. Use of heparin/flourine surface modified IOL's has been suggested in high risk cases. In-the-bag IOL implantation reduces the risk of postoperative uveitis.

(b) **Glaucoma**: Glaucoma is one of the major complications occurring in children who have been operated very early (before 3 mths of age). In addition, paediatric cataract may be associated with other congenital anomalies like microcornea and pre-existing angle anomalies which may also adversely affect the status of IOP or postoperative pupillary block may be responsible factors.

Intraoperative tissue handling and even surgical trauma despite uneventful surgery may trigger off chronic postoperative inflammation or secondary uveitis. Over and above, the most burning issue is that surgical procedure at a very young age itself is a predisposing factor for the manifestation of glaucoma in the paediatric age group, particularly in the first year of life. Older children are also at lifelong risk of developing glaucoma and require lifelong follow-up. Postoperative Glaucoma is compounded by the problem that it is very difficult to measure IOP in children, particularly in the postoperative period. They do not cooperate for applanation tonometry, and indentation tonometry is inaccurate due to altered scleral rigidity. Clinically, one has to rely on signs like corneal oedema, photophobia, circumcorneal ciliary congestion and digital tonometry. For more accurate assessment EUA has to be resorted to. ACIOL is generally contraindicated in children due to damage to the angle structures and tendency to cause UGH syndrome.

It is worth considering that glaucoma can manifest at any time following cataract surgery in the paediatric age group irrespective of the aetiology, though it is more common in the case of congenital cataract. Hence, consent and close follow-up in these cases is prudential.

(c) **Retinal complications:** Risk of retinal detachment after cataract surgery is relatively more in case of the paediatric age group.

(d) **Posterior capsular opacification:** Posterior capsular opacification occurs universally in all children. This is very thick and membranous and does not respond to YAG laser. Thus, many surgeons are in favour of primary posterior capsulotomy with anterior vitrectomy in all cases. Thorough cortical cleanup and polishing of the posterior capsule helps in delaying PCO. Others are in favour of PCCC with optic capture without vitrectomy. Using PMMA or Foldable Acrylic IOL's with square edge design also helps in preventing ingrowth of lens epithelial cells.

(e) **Aggressive treatment for amblyopia:** Severe Amblyopia is known as one of the most crucial factors in case of ultimate functional outcome. Preoperative status of the eye as well as postoperative factors influencing visual axis and refraction are the major factors to trigger off severe visual deprivation and amblyopia. Aggressive treatment for amblyopia should be started at the earliest, particularly in unilateral cataracts.

(f) **Opacification of the IOL:** Opacification of the IOL can occur even in absence of severe inflammation and PCO. This can lead to diminution of vision months or years following successful cataract surgery. The only treatment is to explant the opacified IOL and replace it with another lens.

Effect of IOL Surgery on the Pattern of Growth of Eyeball and Refraction in Paediatric Age Group

The presence of IOL implant and grossly affected accommodation due to absence of human crystalline lens are great challenges to the normal stimulus for the growth of the eyeball. Hence, unpredicted changes in the axial length and refractive status demands special attention during long term follow-up so as to avoid amblyopia. Age of the child at the time of surgery, time lapse between disease and surgery, status of refraction and optical media clarity also influence growth of the eyeball. The impact of genetic factors also cannot be undermined in this process.

Anisometropia and variation in the axial length from the contralateral eye, are other important factors responsible to influence the axial growth.

In our experience, axial growth of the eye is slightly less in pace in a psuedophakic eye as compared to the normal eye. The growth pattern is more affected in case of aphakic, anterior chamber IOL implants and sulcus or scleral fixated IOL implants as compared to in-the-bag foldable IOL implant.

CONCLUSION

Paediatric cataract surgery has become safer and predictable due to recent advances in cataract surgery, improvisation of lOLs and better understanding of its pathophysiology.

However, many controversies still exist and there are divergent views on issues like IOL implantation in very young children, IOL materials, and biometry. Despite these controversies, IOL implantation is gradually occupying the rider seat and is going to be accepted as an established and standard treatment regimen irrespective of age constraints in the near future.

REFERENCES AND BIBLIOGRAPHY

1. Wilson ME, Pandey SK, Thakur: Paediatric cataract blindness in the developing world: surgical techniques and intraocular lenses in the new millennium". Br J Ophthalmol. 2003 Jan; 87(1):14–9.

2. Foster A, Gilbert C, Rahi J. Epidemiology of cataract in childhood: a global perspective. J Cataract Refract Surg 1997; 23:601–604.

3. "Koc F, Kargi S, Biglan AW, Chu CT, Davis JS. The aetiology in paediatric Aphakic glaucoma". Eye. 2005 Nov 11; [Epub ahead of print].

4. Cetin E, Yaman A, Berk A. Etiology of childhood blindness in Izmir, Turkey. Eur J Ophthalmol 2004; 14:531–537.

5. Parihar JKS, Dash RG, Vats DP, Verma SC, Sahoo PK, Rodrigues FE. "Management of anterior segment penetrating injuries with traumatic cataract by Pentagon approach in paediatric age group: constraints and outcome". Indian J Ophthalmol. 2000 Sep; 48(3):227–30.

6. Zetterstrom C, Lundvall A, Kugelberg M. Cataracts in children. J Cataract Refract Surg 2005; 31:824–840.

7. "Comparison of epilenticular IOL implantation vs technique of anterior and primary posterior capsulorrhexis with anterior vitrectomy in paediatric cataract surgery". Eye. 2006 Jun 9; [Epub ahead of print].

8. Raghu H, Subhan S, Jose RJ, et al. Herpes simplex virus - 1 - Associated congenital cataract. Am J Ophthalmol 2004; 138:313–314.

9. "Intracameral tissue plasminogen activator to prevent severe fibrinous effusion after congenital cataract surgery". Br J Ophthalmol. 2005 Nov; 89(11):1458–61. Comment in: Br J Ophthalmol. 2005 Nov; 89(11):1390–1.

10. Pandey SK, Werner L, Escobar-Gomez M, et al. Dye enhanced cataract surgery. Part 1: anterior capsule staining for capsulorrhexis in advanced/white cataracts. J Cataract Refract Surg 2000; 26:1052–1059.

11. Bradfield YS, Plager DA, Neely DE, et al. Astigmatism after small incision clear corneal cataract extraction and intraocular lens implantation in children. J Cataract Refract Surg 2004; 30:1948–1952.

12. Mandal AK, Netland PA. "Glaucoma in aphakia and pseudophakia after congenital cataract surgery". Indian J Ophthalmol. 2004 Sep; 52(3):185–98.

13. Wilson ME. Anterior capsule management for pediatric intraocular lens implantation. J Pediatr Ophthalmol Strabismus 1999; 36:314–319.

14. Rowe NA, Biswas S, Lloyd IC "Primary IOL implantation in children: a risk analysis of foldable acrylic v PMMA lenses" Br J Ophthalmol. 2004 Apr; 88(4):481–5.

15. "Lundvall A, Kugelberg U. Outcome after treatment of congenital bilateral cataract". Acta Ophthalmol Scand. 2002 Dec; 80(6):593–7. Comment in: Acta Ophthalmol Scand. 2002 Dec; 80(6):569.

16. Tromans C, Haigh PM, Biswas S, Lloyd IC "Accuracy of intraocular lens power calculation in paediatric cataract surgery" Br J Ophthalmol. 2001 Aug; 85(8):939–41.

17. Dada T, Dada VK, Sharma N, Vajpayee RB."Primary posterior Capsulorrhexis with optic capture and Intracameral heparin in paediatric cataract surgery". Clin Experiment Ophthalmol. 2000 Oct; 28(5):361–3.

18. Mehta JS, Adams GG "Recombinant tissue plasminogen activator following paediatric cataract surgery". Br J Ophthalmol. 2000 Sep; 84(9):983–6.

19. Quo S, Wagner RS, Caputo A. Management of the anterior and posterior lens capsules and vitreous in pediatric cataract surgery. J Pediatr Ophthalmol Strabismus 2004; 41:330–337.

20. Flitcroft DI, Knight-Nanan D, Bowell R, Lanigan B, O'Keefe M. "Intraocular lenses in children: changes in axial length, corneal curvature, and refraction". Br J Ophthalmol. 1999 Mar; 83(3):265–9.

21. Vasavada AR, Trivedi RH, Nath VC. Visual axis opacification after Acrysof intraocular lens implantation in children. J Cataract Refract Surg 2004; 30: 1073–1081.

22. Lee HK, Kim CY, Kwon OW, et al. Removal of dense posterior capsule opacification after congenital cataract extraction using the transconjunctival sutureless vitrectomy system. J Cataract Refract Surg 2004; 30:1626–1628.

23. Lesueur LC, Arne JL, Chapotot EC, Thouvenin D, Malecaze F. "Visual outcome after paediatric cataract surgery: is age a major factor?" Br J Ophthalmol. 1998 Sep; 82(9):1022–5.

24. Churchill AJ, Noble BA, Etchells DE, George NJ "Factors affecting visual outcome in children following uniocular traumatic cataract" Eye. 1995; 9 (Pt 3):285–91.

25. Mullner-Eidenbock A, Amon M, Moser E, Kruger A, Abela C, Schlemmer Y, Zidek T. "Morphological and functional results of AcrySof intraocular lens implantation in children: prospective randomised study of age-related surgical management". J Cataract Refract Surg. 2003 Feb; 29(2): 285–93.

26. Jensen AA, Basti S, Greenwald MJ, Mets MB "When may the posterior capsule be preserved in pediatric intraocular lens surgery?". Ophthalmology. 2002 Feb; 109(2):324–7; discussion 328.

27. Koch DD, Kohnen T. "A retrospective comparison of techniques to prevent secondary cataract formation following posterior chamber intraocular lens implantation in infants and children" Trans Am Ophthalmol Soc. 1997; 95:351–60; discussion 361–5.

28. Koch DD, Kohnen T "Retrospective comparison of techniques to prevent secondary cataract formation after posterior chamber intraocular lens implantation in infants and children". J Cataract Refract Surg. 1997; 23 Suppl 1:657–63. Erratum in J Cataract Refract Surg 1997 Sep; 23(7):974.

29. Raina UK, Gupta V, Arora R, Mehta DK. "Posterior continuous curvilinear capsulorrhexis with and without optic capture of the posterior chamber intraocular lens in the absence of vitrectomy". J Pediatr Ophthalmol Strabismus. 2002 Sep-Oct;39(5):278–87. Comment in J Pediatr Ophthalmol Strabismus. 2003 May-Jun; 40(3):130–1; author reply 131.

30. Ram J, Brar GS, Kaushik S, Gupta A, Gupta A. "Role of posterior capsulotomy with vitrectomy and intraocular lens design and material in reducing posterior capsule opacification after pediatric cataract surgery". J Cataract Refract Surg. 2003 Aug; 29(8):1579–84.

31. Ahmadieh H, Javadi MA "Intraocular lens implantation in children." Curr Opin Ophthalmol. 2001 Feb; 12(1):30–34.

32. BenEzra D, Cohen E, Rose L "Traumatic cataract in children: correction of aphakia by contact lens or intraocular lens". Am J Ophthalmol. 1997 Jun; 123(6):773–82.

33. Plager DA, Yang S, Neely D, Sprunger D, Sondhi N. "Complications in the first year following cataract surgery with and without IOL in infants and older children". J AAPOS. 2002 Feb; 6(1):9–14.

34. Pavlovic S. "Cataract surgery in children" Med Pregl. 2000 May–Jun;53(5–6):257–61. [Article in Croatian]

35. BenEzra D, Cohen E "Cataract surgery in children with chronic Uveitis".Ophthalmology. 2000 Jul; 107(7):1255–60.

36. Zetterstrom C, Lundvall A, Kugelberg M "Cataracts in children". J Cataract Refract Surg. 2005 Apr; 31(4):824–40.

37. Stagner DR Jr, Weakley DR Jr, Hunter JS. Long term rates of PCO following small incision foldable acrylic intraocular lens implantation in children. J Pediatr Ophthalmol Stabismus 2002; 39:73–76.

37

Phacoemulsification Surgery in Traumatic Cataract with Subluxated Lens

Col JKS Parihar SM, VSM and Col Vijay Mathur

INTRODUCTION

Phacoemulsification surgery in cases of subluxated lens with zonulysis is a real challenging task. This particular situation may create significant complications unless and until great care and patience is observed while handling these cases. Other than subluxation and zonulysis, Vitreous herniation into anterior chamber, distortion of angle structures leading to secondary glaucoma and sphincter injuries may be added problems.

DYNAMICS OF STRUCTURAL DERANGEMENTS IN SUBLUXATED LENS

Derangements in Anterior Segment/Zonular Dehiscence

Zonular dehiscence, weakness, or zonulopathy is a very significant and crucial trauma-related derangement which is responsible for subluxation of lens along with adverse impact on vitreous base as well. The associated angle recession further enhances the complexity and magnum of anterior segment trauma-related problems.

The impact of zonular dialysis is directly proportionate to the extent of dehiscence and the underlying pathology which differentiates and quantifies the overall impact of zonulysis. For instance, segmental zonular dehiscence in cases of traumatic cataract will have different impact as compared to the same amount of zonulysis in cases of pseudoexfoliation which have generalised zonular pathology in addition to the selective dehiscence.

Classification of Zonular Dialysis (Parihar's Modified Classification)

The zonular dialysis can be graded as per the extent of dialysis in terms of clock hours and the severity of zonular instability. The author has modified the classification of zonular dehiscence, which is as follows:

Parihar's Modified Classification of Zonular Dehiscence

GRADE ONE:

I "A": Zonular dehiscence of less than one clock hour and without any capsular rent or vitreous derangement.

I "B": I "A" along with capsular rent or vitreous derangement.

GRADE TWO:

II "A": Zonular dehiscence of more than one clock hour but less than one quadrant but without any capsular rent or vitreous derangement.

II "B": II "A" along with capsular rent or vitreous derangement.

GRADE THREE:

III "A": Zonular dehiscence of more than one quadrant but less than two quadrants without any capsular rent or vitreous derangement.

III "B": III "A" along with capsular rent or vitreous derangement.

GRADE FOUR: Zonular dehiscence of more than two quadrants but less than three quadrants (invariably associated with capsular rent or vitreous derangement or both).

GRADE FIVE: Zonular dehiscence of more than three quadrants but less than four quadrants.

GRADE SIX: Complete zonular dialysis.

Derangements in Posterior Segment

Zonular dialysis in subluxated cataract is invariably associated with involvement of vitreous and retina particularly in cases of trauma since ocular trauma is bound to have some kind of impact on the vitreous and retina ranging from minimal to severe changes. Vitreous haemorrhage may lead to PVD or vitreous derangement. Macular oedema or peripheral retinal degeneration or both changes may be seen. Delayed changes like macular scarring, choroidal or retinal detachment may also be seen. Posterior segment change in the form of vitreous degeneration is invariably associated with other case of subluxation of lens including the cases of pseudo-exfoliation, myopia, and congenital anomalies. Retinal degeneration may also be seen in these cases. The higher incidence of CME following phacoemulsification surgery in complicated and trauma cases is a known entity hence; a thorough and detailed posterior segment evaluation is an essential prerequisite in all cases of anterior segment trauma and in other conditions where application of CTR is a mandatory requirement.

APPLICATION OF CTR IN SUBLUXATED LENS/PCR/ZONULOLYSIS

The capsular tension ring (CTR) is a very simple yet effective and beneficial device, which may be inserted into the capsular bag to enhance stability and centration of the subluxated lens or deranged capsular bag. CTR is a compressible circular ring which is made up of polymethyl methacrylate (PMMA). The ring possesses an eyelet at either end. The specific 'ski tip' configuration of the end terminals minimises the risk of entrapment of the capsular bag equator while inserting CTR. The CTR is available in various sizes and configurations. The uncompressed diameter varies between 12.3 mm (compresses to 10.0 mm), 13.0 mm (compresses to 11.0 mm), and 14.5 mm (compresses to 12.0 mm), whereas it is 0.18 mm thick. The CTR may be inserted manually with the help of forceps or with injectors. The injector system is preferred due to its inherent advantage of being less traumatic.

History of CTR

The first endocapsular device was designed and introduced by Hara, Nagamoto, and Bissa Miyajima in 1991. UFC Legler and BM Witschel further modified CTR which was made up of PMMA and comprised an oval-shaped open ring structure with eyelets at both the free ends. This work was presented for the first time in May 1993 at the American Society of Cataract and Refractive Surgery [ASCRS] Symposium on Cataract, IOL, and Refractive Surgery held at Seattle. However, CTR has been gaining wide acceptance and popularity in recent past as a very effective and useful surgical appliance in cases of zonular dialysis, PCR and several other conditions where derangement of capsules, zonules or vitreous is existing or anticipated.

Prior to the advent of the M-CTR, the management of subluxated cataract of grade four and above was a Herculean task as the conventional CTR may not be able to provide desired stability to the capsular bag in such situations. A sutured CTR through the capsular bag with or without a peripheral capsulorhexis was an alternative option to manage extensive zonular dehiscence until Cionni designed and introduced an open-ring design M-CTR (Morcher GmbH) in 1998. M-CTR possesses an excellent feature to reposition the subluxated lens in cases of marked zonular dialysis by making it possible to anchor the capsule bag to the eye wall.

Further modification in CTR was made by Ahmed in 2002 by adding a partial PMMA ring segment at 120° with a radius of 5 mm and anteriorly positioned fixation eyelet has facilitated the application of CTR even with the eventuality of excessive zonular dehiscence.

The Mechanics of the CTR

CTR provides stability to the capsular bag by following mechanics:

(i) Redistributes tension from existing zonules and augments effectively the areas of weak zonules by buttress, thereby stabilising the entire zonular apparatus.

(ii) Stretching the capsular bag thereby expanding equator of the capsular bag which ultimately maintains the circular contour of the bag and tautens the posterior capsule during surgery, thus enhances zonular support.

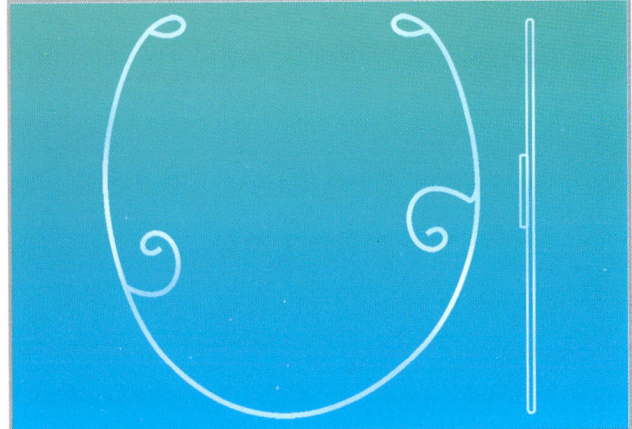

Fig. 37.1: Cionni M-CTR for suture scleral fixation

(iii) Reposition a subluxed capsular bag.

(iv) Provides intraoperative support during phaco-emulsification as well as to IOL implant for long-term IOL stabilisation.

Indications of Application of CTR (Capsular Tension Ring)

The CTR may be used in any of the conditions where the integrity of capsular bag and zonules are debatable. CTR may be applied in following conditions:

(a) Primary Indications

(i) Traumatic subluxation of lens.

(ii) Traumatic localised weakness/zonular dialysis.

(iii) Developmental/congenital anomalies of lens and zonules like Marfan's syndrome resulting in sub-luxation of the lens.

(b) Relative Indications

(i) Posterior capsular rent.

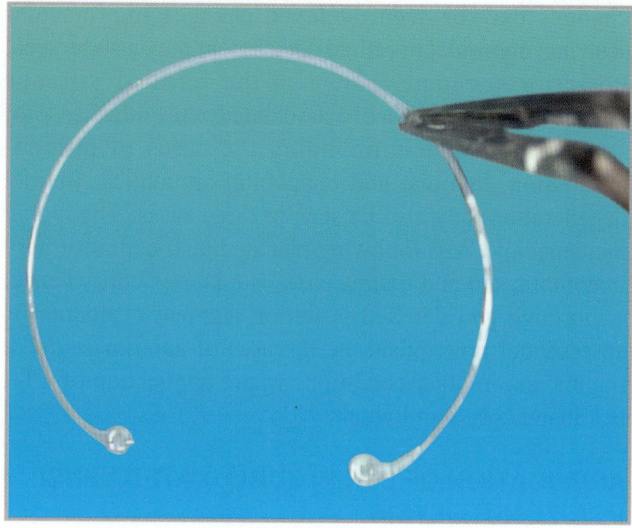

Fig. 37.2: CTR (capsular tension ring)

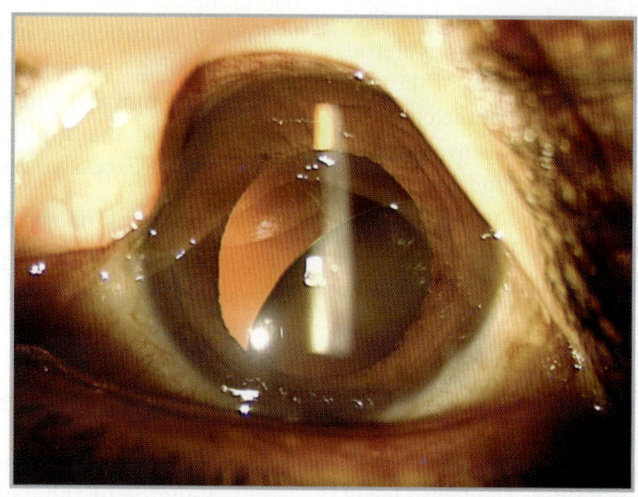

(a)

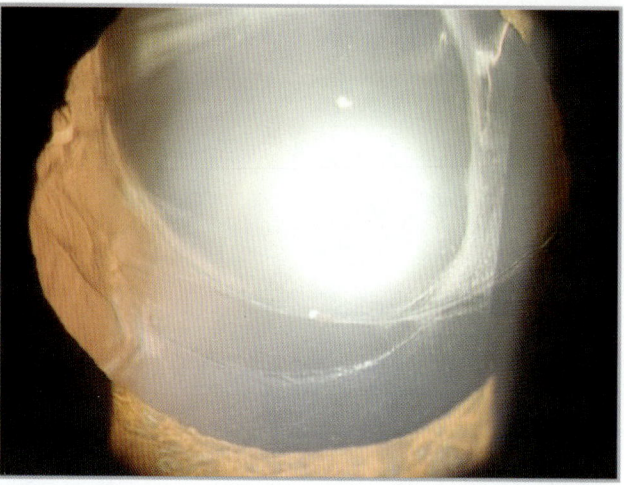

(b)

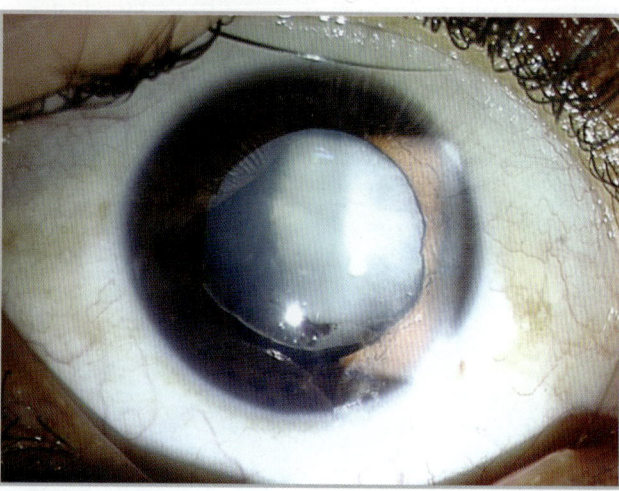

(c)

Fig. 37.3: Traumatic subluxation of lens

(ii) Intraoperative complications leading to zonular damage.

(iii) Axial myopia greater than 26 mm. Relative instability of the capsular bag.

(iv) Pseudoexfoliation syndrome.

(v) Phacoemulsification surgery in postvitrectomy cases.

(vi) Hypermature cataract.

(vii) Postradial keratotomy and glaucoma surgery cases. Both of these procedures may lead to shallow or flat anterior chambers, through perforation or excessive filtration, and thereby place stress on the zonular apparatus.

Merits of Application of CTR (Capsular Tension Ring)

(i) Minimises intraoperative risk. CTR alters the axis of traction /stretching force on capsular bag and zonules thereby providing redistribution of applied force on to the entire circumference of the capsule.

(ii) Stretches the posterior capsule in cases of PCR, zonulysis.

(iii) Reposition the subluxated lens into position by stretching force.

(iv) Facilitates various steps of phacoemulsification at ease due to the relatively stable position of the subluxated lens.

(v) The CTR minimises and restricts undesirable and annoying movement of the lens and zonules, thus reducing the risk of a capsular tear.

(vi) Facilitates and provides adequate support to the all PMMA large size IOL implant in case of zonulysis and posterior capsular rent of more than 4–5 mm in size. In-the-bag flexible or phaco profile PMMA IOL may also be possible with the support of CTR in cases of small PC rent of less than 3 mm of size.

(vii) CTR decreases prevalence of capsular contraction and posterior capsule opacification (PCO).

(viii) Prevents postoperative shrivelling of capsule, hence facilitates Nd:YAG capsulotomy.

(ix) Improves postoperative IOL centration and minimises the risk of IOL tilt.

Constraints/Complications Encountered with Application of CTR (Capsular Tension Ring)

(i) Dislocation of CTR into vitreous. This may lead to pars plana vitrectomy and removal of CTR.

(ii) Extension of zonulysis/PC tear particularly at the time of insertion of CTR.

(iii) Capsular phimosis (more common with silicon IOL implantation, particularly in cases of pseudo-exfoliation syndrome).

Selection of Types of CTR

(i) Less than 3 clock hours zonulysis – no eye CTR.

(ii) 3 to 6 clock hours zonulysis – one eye CTR.

(iii) More than 6 o'clock hours zonulysis – two eye CTR.

Surgical Technique Insertion of CTR in Subluxated Lens/PCR/Zonulolysis

It has been described in detail in subsequent para as part of surgical technique of phacoemulsification in these cases.

Phacoemulsification Surgery in Subluxated Lens

(a) **Anaesthesia technique:** The choice of anaesthesia depends upon the merits, age of the patient and, of course, on the surgeon's own preference. Author prefers to apply general anaesthesia in cases of paediatric and peribulbar in remaining cases. One should attempt to maintain adequate hypotony and akinesia in such cases.

(b) **Incisions:** The author prefers to construct clear corneal incision over scleral, since scleral incision may make further maneuvering more difficult. The main incision should be made at 90–120° in relation to the subluxation to avoid any further stretching the preexisting dehiscent posterior capsule.

(c) **Choice of viscoelastic material:** Dispersive visco-elastic material is the preferred choice. Viscoelastics should be injected into the anterior chamber through the second (side port) incision in such a manner, particularly while injecting in the subluxated quadrant, so as to minimise the risk of damaging the hyaloid and thus subsequent vitreous derangements.

(d) **Capsulorrhexis**

(i) **Constraints:** Zonulysis makes CCC difficult since there is no counter pressure while pulling reverted anterior capsular flap; rather there is a backward push and lens moves towards direction of needle movement. This may result in extension of zonulysis or vitreous disturbances.

(ii) **Technique:** Trypan blue dye enhanced rhexis is recommended in case of intumescent cataract.

(a) Gentle and guarded movements of the cystitome under sodium hyaluronate 1.4% cushion.

(b) Subluxated lens may be given support of dialler or Synskey's hook.

(c) Rhexis should be completed in sequences and without any downward pressure on the lens. A smaller rhexis mostly in the quadrant of the subluxation is beneficial for subsequent implantation of the CTR. However, the rhexis can be enlarged after the IOL implantation.

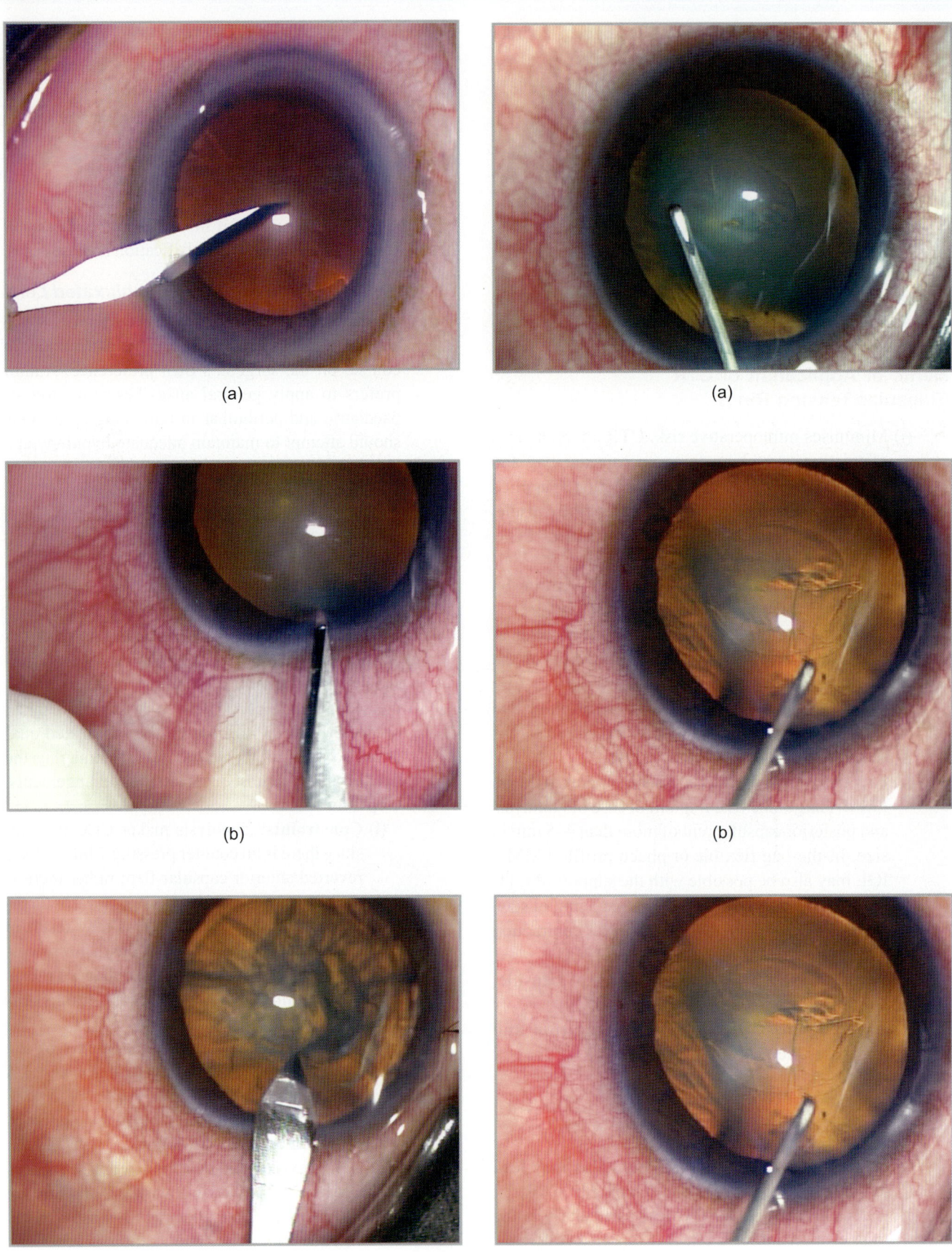

Fig. 37.4: (a) Side port incision, (b) Initial entry for the subsequent main incision, (c) Main incision

Fig. 37.5: (a), (b) and (c) Capsulorrhexis in subluxated lens with zonulysis

Application of CTR in Subluxated Lens/PCR/Zonulolysis

Selection of Capsular Tension Ring Size

The selection of CTR size is directly proportionate to the dimensions of the capsular bag. Ideal CTR should have an overlap of the end terminals so as to facilitate adequate circumferential support. Larger corneal diameter and axial length are invariably associated with a large capsular bag. However, a large size CTR (except in high hypermetropic or paediatric eye) enjoys preference by most of the surgeons including the authors' preference.

Ideal Intraoperative Time to Insert CTR

CTR offers better nuclear stability for phacoemulsification and subsequent cortical removal. The author recommends

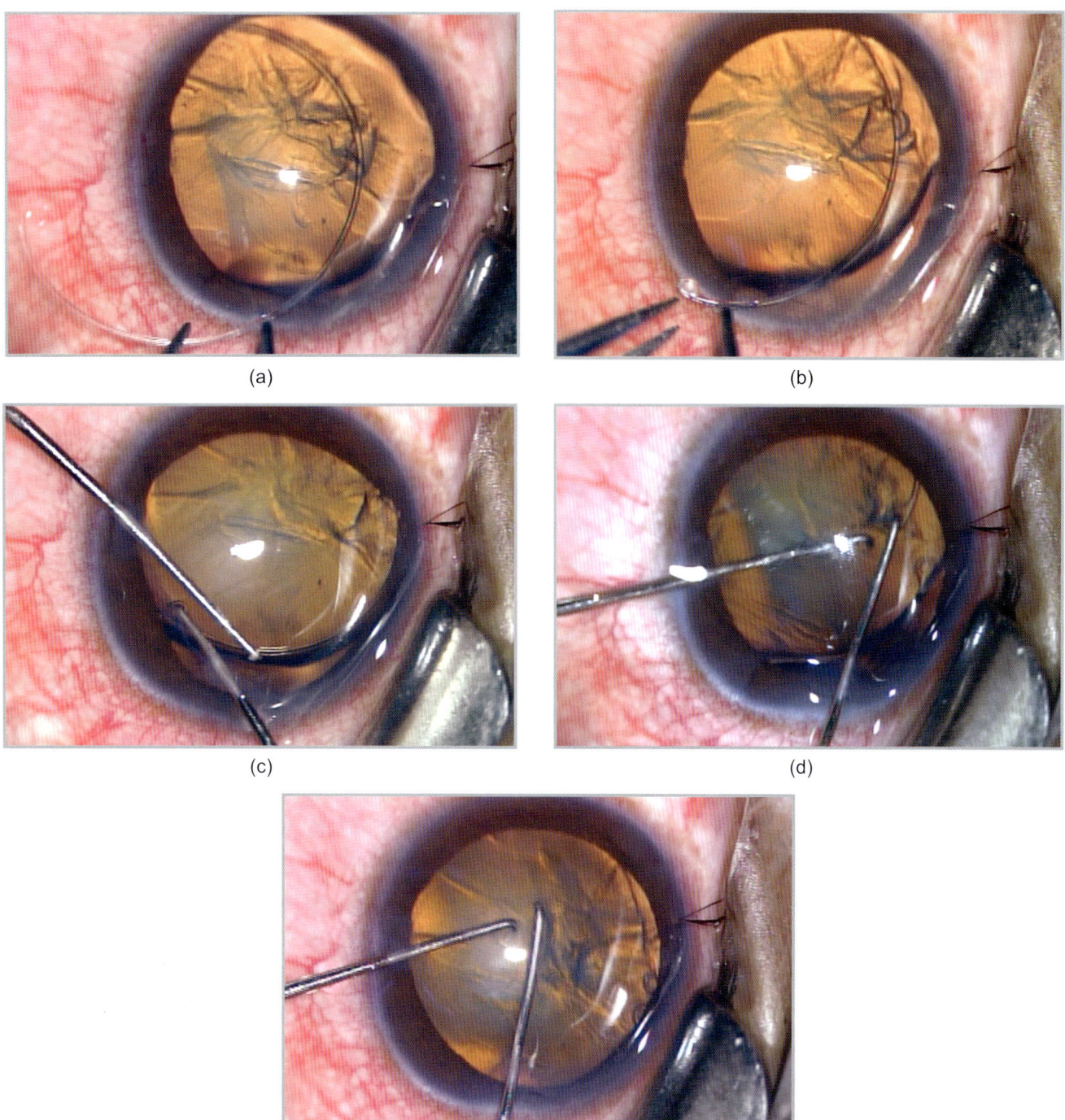

(a)

(b)

(c)

(d)

(e)

Fig. 37.6: (a) CTR is being pushed into the capsular bag in subluxated lens with zonulysis, (b) and (c) CTR is being pushed into the capsular bag in subluxated lens with zonulysis (9 to 2 O'clock), (d) CTR is being pushed into the capsular bag in subluxated lens with zonulysis with the support of two synskey's hook, (e) CTR is well placed in the capsular bag

CTR insertion just after completion of capsulorrhexis and prior to the commencement of hydroprocedure. However, CTR may pose certain constraints while handling dense lens which carries greater risk of iatrogenic zonular deinsertion. Presence of CTR and subluxated lens demands meticulous care while performing nucleotomy and subsequent cortical removal. The removal of peripheral cortex may be difficult due to entrapment of cortex by CTR. Despite such technical complexities, prenucleotomy insertion of CTR minimises incidence of intraoperative complications which resulted owing to inadvertent zonular dialysis.

Technique

(i) Intraoperative insertion of the CTR is through the main/side port incision depending upon the site of zonulysis. The direction of movements should not extend the zonulysis.

(ii) Insertion should be very slow and with the support of a dialler and McPherson's forceps.

(iii) All efforts ought to be made to put both open loops together and overlapping to each other and away from the site of zonulysis so as to facilitate starching of the capsular bag.

PHACOEMULSIFICATION PROCEDURE

Hydroprocedures

(i) Great care is to be observed while performing hydroprocedures. A very delicate and gentle hydroprocedure is of the greatest significance in subluxated cataract.

Hydrodissection should be done by using minimal fluid. The direction of cannula should remain forward and upward towards the anterior capsule.

(ii) Visco hydrodelineation with sodium hyaluronate 1.4% into perinuclear/cortical contents facilitates

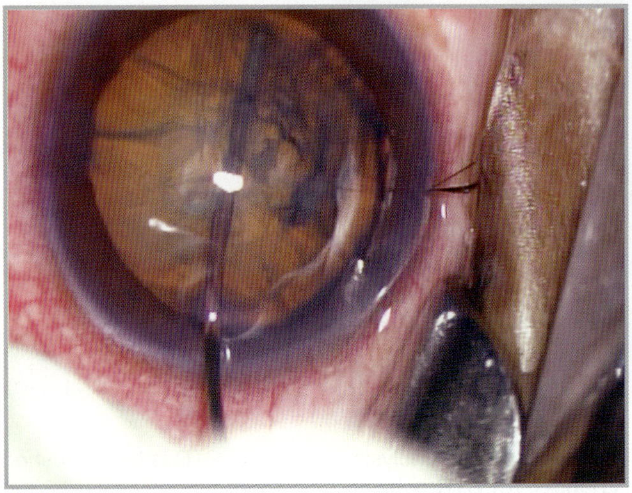

Fig. 37.7: Hydroprocedures in subluxated lens with zonulysis

hydrodelineation. Visco injection stretches CTR towards fornices of the capsular bag and pushes the lens in position, hence facilitates rhexis maneuver.

(iii) Position of the lens should be allowed to remain in horizontal and pupillary plane with the help of continuous support and backward movements of dialler.

Nucleus Rotation/Dialling of Lens Nucleus

Should be avoided or should be very gentle and slow. One should restrict rotation of the nucleus to the least and minimum. However, the author prefers to avoid nucleus rotation.

PHACOEMULSIFICATION SURGERY IN SUBLUXATED LENS: CONSTRAINTS

Nucleotomy

Nucleus management in subluxated lens is a real challenging task. This particular step may create significant complications unless and until great care and patience is being observed. The presence of subluxation of lens, zonulysis and dynamic movements of the lens during procedure thereby resulting in sustained and continuous pressure and traction on zonules and capsular bag remains the key issue. Undoubtedly, CTR will be an effective tool in above-mentioned situations, yet CTR does not make phacoemulsification absolutely safe. Hence, a surgeon remains on his toes during entire procedure.

Aim

To avoid (i) Extension of zonulysis, (ii) Vitreous prolapse, and (iii) Nucleus drop

Achieve

Successful completion of the phacoprocedure despite all odds.

Technique

Direct chop technique is preferred over sculpting.

(i) **Sculpting** should be avoided as it may lead to aggravation of zonulysis.

• Be alert of vitreous disturbance and nucleus drop.

(ii) **Chopping**

Advantages: No pressure on the posterior capsule. However, the nucleus should be attempted to be pulled out of the bag while keeping the direction of force perpendicular to the subluxation so as to avoid further zonulysis.

Machine settings should be of moderate power and low vacuum to avoid a pull; but it may make procedure slow (US 20–30%/ vacuum 70–100 mm, flow rate 24 to 28 mm/mt). Hence chopping carries some risks but is definitely superior to sculpting.

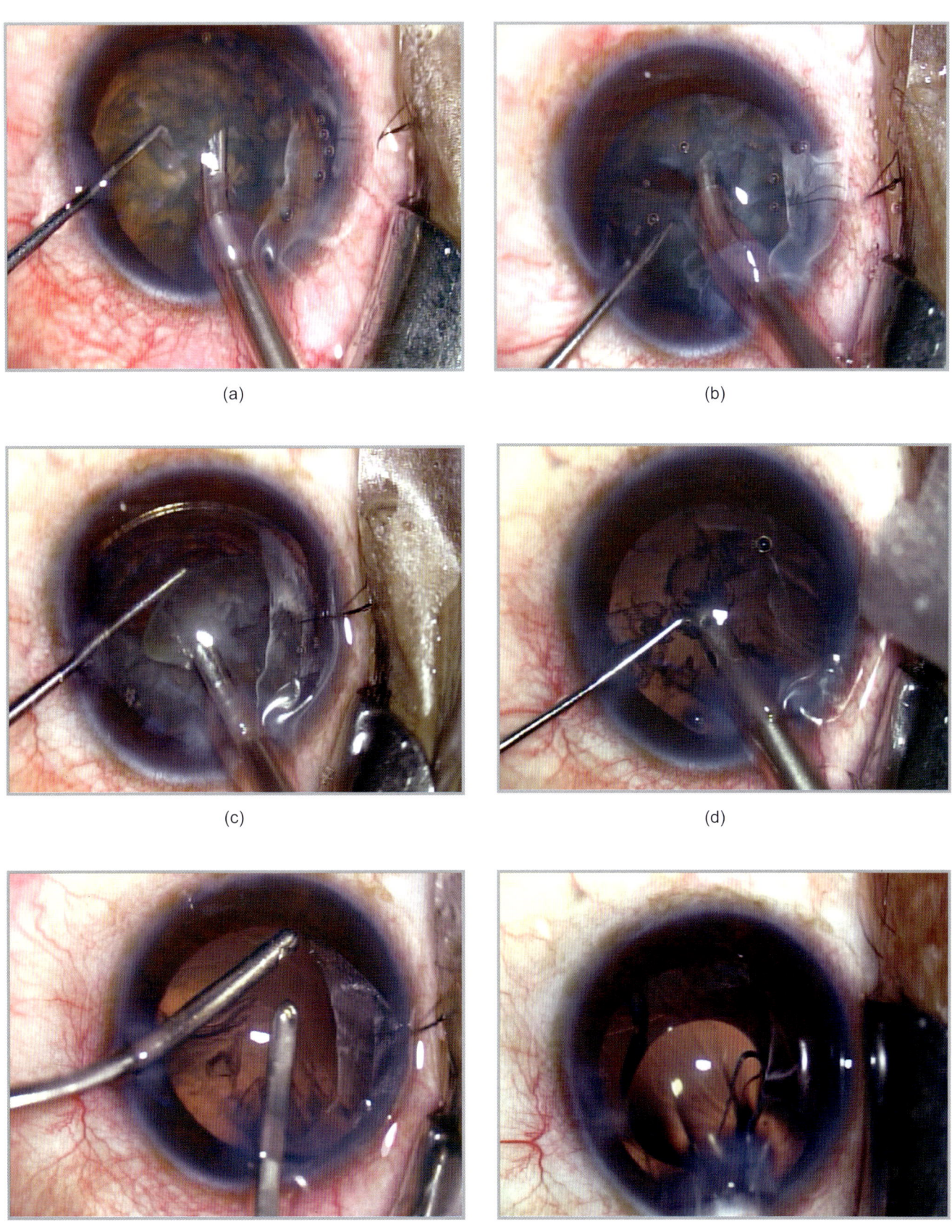

Fig. 37.8: (a), (b) Phacoemulsification by direct chop technique, (c) Fragment removal under the presence of the CTR ring, (d) Irrigation and aspiration with the help of automated coaxial I /A cannula, (e) Irrigation and aspiration with the help of automated bimanual I/A cannula, (f) Single piece hydrophobic foldable IOL is being placed over the CTR

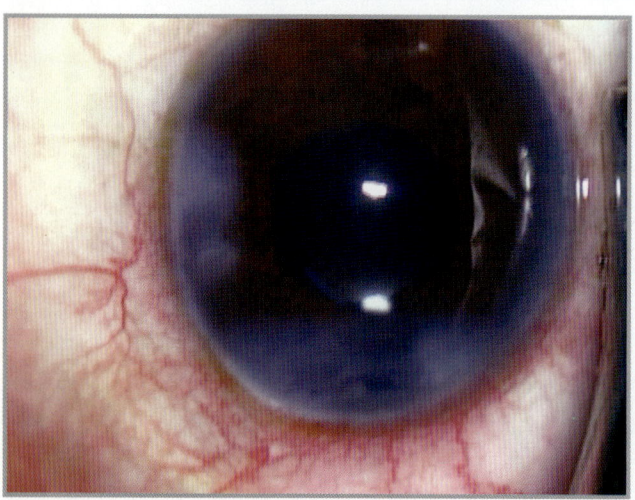

Fig. 37.8: (g) Single piece hydrophobic foldable IOL is placed over CTR

(iii) **Ice-cream scooping:** An ideal technique for subluxated and soft cataract. The combination of scooping and subsequent chopping is also a good option.

Frequent injection of sodium hyaluronate into the capsular bag to produce visco cushion effect has definitely proved to be effective to minimise a risk of complications.

Irrigation and Aspiration Technique

Carries maximum threat of dreaded complications which very much resembles something like risk of accidents while driving down the slope of a hill after a sustained but tiring and stretched efforts of driving uphill.

Technique

(a) Do not act like a rabbit or a deer but like a snail or a tortoise as slow and steady wins the race. The best phaco technique in subluxated cataract is a slow motion phaco.

(b) It is better to choose low aspiration flow rate and vacuum on low infusion bottle height (flow rate 30 ml/mt, vacuum 60 to 90 mmHG) rather than high rising vacuum in conventional I/A. Simcoe cannula may also be used in these cases.

(c) Continuous irrigation into the capsular bag enhances cortical matter hydration; hence facilitates aspiration. The procedure adopted should be very slow, gentle and the approach meticulous. Time is not the decisive factor as the ultimate results are more important.

(d) Last but not the least, do not hesitate to liberally use sodium hylarunate. This will not only allow adequate resistance against traction on zonules and the capsular bag during aspiration but will also keep the CTR at its place and keep fornices of the bag widely open.

IOL Implantation in Subluxated Lens with Zonulysis

It is possible to perform phacoemulsification surgery with IOL implantation successfully in cases of significant subluxation of lens with zonulysis. The preference of IOL is based on the extent of zonulysis and subluxation. In our experience, foldable IOL implantation is possible in up to 30–35% of zonulysis or 2–3 mm of PC rent. It is possible to place all PMMA large size IOL over the anterior capsular rim supported by the CTR up to 40–50 % zonulysis or 4–5 mm PC rent.

The surgeon must ensure the least traction and pressure on capsular bag while inserting an IOL implant. Great precaution is the order of the day while placing foldable IOL into the bag. The IOL haptics tend to follow unexpected and unprecedented courses of defolding during implantation through injector. This may lead to damage to the capsular bag, extension of zonulysis or in case of a small rent, may traverse into the vitreous cavity through a PC rent. Hence, all our efforts should be made to prevent extension of subluxation or zonulysis at the time of IOL implantation.

In the remaining cases where conventional PC IOL implantation is technically not a viable option, scleral fixated IOL should be considered over AC IOL implantation. We do not recommend AC IOL in any situation in subluxated lens due to the high risk of intraoperative constraints as well as obvious and very significant incidence of postoperative complications.

Postoperative Complications

In addition to the known incidence and pattern of pre and postoperative complications, encountered with phacoemulsification surgery, following complications have been found to have higher incidence:

(i) Damage to the anterior capsular rim and of iris.
(ii) Dislocation of subluxated lens, CTR or IOL implant.
(iii) Corneal oedema.
(iv) CME

CONCLUSION

Phacoemulsification in subluxated lens presented more problems and complications than usual. However, it seems to be safer than manual extracapsular surgery because it minimises the risk of intraoperative eye hypotony or collapse. Over the past decade, there have been dramatic advances in the management of zonular weakness. The application of CTR makes it possible to successfully perform phacoemulsification surgery with IOL implantation.

The preference of IOL is based on the extent of zonulysis and subluxation. In our experience, foldable IOL implan-tation is possible in up to 30–35% of zonulysis or 2–3 mm of PC rent. It is possible to place all PMMA large size IOL over the anterior capsular rim supported by the CTR upto 40–50% zonulysis or 4–5 mm PC rent. Scleral fixated IOL should be the choice in all the cases where any kind of PC IOL is not possible. AC IOL is not preferred by us in any situation in subluxated lens due to intraoperative constraints and significant postoperative complications.

BIBLIOGRAPHY

1. Leger U. MD, B.M. Witschel, MD, S.J. Lim, MD, et al. The Capsular Ring: A New Device for Complicated Cataract Surgery, film presented at the 3rd American–International Congress on Cataract, IOL and Refractive Surgery, Seattle, Washington, USA, May 1993.
2. Menapace R, Findl O, Georgopoulos M, et al. The capsular tension ring: designs, applications, and techniques. J Cataract Refract Surg 2000; 26: 898–912.
3. Osher RH. History and experience with capsular tension rings. In: Cataract and Refractive Surgery Today. January 2005. pp. 1–5. This paper provides a review on the history and uses of CTRs.
4. Hara T, Hara T, Yamada Y. 'Equator ring' for maintenance of the complete!) circular contour of the capsular bag equator after cataract removal. Ophthalmic Surg 1991; 22:358–359.
5. Nagamoto T, Bissen-Miyajima H. A ring to support the capsular bag after continuous curvilinear capsulorhexis. J Cataract Refract Surg 1994; 20:417–420.
6. Gimbel HV, Sun R. Clinical applications of capsular tension rings in cataract surgery. Ophthalmic Surg Lasers. 2002; 33: 44–53.
7. Gimbel HV, Sun R, Heston JP. Management of zonular dialysis in phacoemulsification and IOL implantation using the capsular tension ring. Ophthalmic Surg Lasers 1997; 28: 273–281.
8. Sun R, Gimbel HV. In vitro evaluation of the efficacy of the capsular tension ring for managing zonular dialysis in cataract surgery. Ophthalmic Surg Lasers 1998; 29:502–505.
9. Jacob S, Agarwal A, Agarwal A, et al. Efficacy of a capsular tension ring for phacoemulsification in eyes with zonular dialysis. J Cataract Refract Surg 2003; 29:315–321.
10. Hasanee K, Ahmed UK, Kranemann C, Crandall AS. Capsular tension segment: clinical results and complications. American Academy of Ophthalmology Meeting, New Orleans, Louisiana; October 2004. Paper Session.
11. Ahmed UK, Crandall AS, Kranemann C, Goldsmith J. Clinical Results of the Cionni Modified Capsular Tension Ring for Sever Zonular Weakness. American Academy of Ophthal-mology Meeting, New Orleans, Louisiana; October 2004. Paper Session.
12. Ahmed UK, Cionni RJ, Kranemann C, Crandall AS. Optimal timing of capsular tension ring implantation: A Miyake-Apple video analysis. J Cataract Refract Surg 2005; 31:1809–1813.
13. Ahmed IK, Butler M. Capsular Tension Devices for the Glaucoma Surgeon. In: Glaucoma Today. Nov-Dec 2004. pp. 1–4.
14. Ahmed IK, Chen SH, Kranemann C, Wong DT. Surgical repositioning of dislocated capsular tension rings. Ophthalmology 2005; 11 2:1725–1 733.
15. Ahmed IK, Crandall AS. Ab-externo scleral fixation of the Cionni modified capsular tension ring. J Cataract Refract Surg 2001; 27:977–981.
16. Kohnen T, Baumeister M, Buhren J. Scheimpflug imaging of bilateral foldable in the bag intraocular lens implantation assisted by a scleral-sutured capsular tension ring in Marfan's syndrome. J Cataract Refract Surg 2003; 29: 598–602.
17. Lam DS, Young AL, Leung AT, et al. Scleral fixation of a capsular tension ring for severe ectopia lentis. J Cataract Refract Surg 2000; 26:609–12.
18. Cionni RJ, Osher RH, Marques DM, et al. Modified capsular tension ring for patients with congenital loss of zonular support. J Cataract Refract Surg 2003:29 ;1668 –73.
19. Cionni RJ, Osher RH. Management of profound zonular dialysis we with a new endocapsular ring designed for scleral fixation. J Cataract Refract Surg 1998; 24:1299–1306.
20. Moreno-Montanes J, Rodriguez-Conde R. Capsular tension ring in eyes with pseudoexfoliation. J Cataract Refract Surg 2002; 28:2241–2242.
21. Moreno-Montanes J, Sainz C, Maldonado MJ. Intraoperative and postoperative complications of Cionni endocapsular ring implantation. J Cataract Refract Surg 2003; 29:492–497.
22. Moreno-Montanes J, Sanchez-Tocino H, Rodriguez-Conde R. Complete anterior capsule contraction after phacoemulsi-fication with acrylic intraocular lens and endocapsular ring implantation. J Cataract Refract Surg. 2002; 28:717–719.
23. Deliseo D, Longanesi L, Grisanti F, Negrini V. Prevention of posterior capsule opacification using capsular tension ring for zonular defects in cataract surgery. Eur J Ophthalmol 2003; 13(2):1 51–154.
24. Bayraktar S, Alton T, Kucuksumer Y, Yilmaz OF. Capsular tension ring implantation after capsulorhexis in phacoemulsi-fication of cataracts associated with pseudoexfoliation syndrome. Intraoperative complications and early postopera-tive findings. J Cataract Refract Surg 2001; 27:1620–1628.
25. Hayashi K, Hayashi H, Matsuo K, et al. Anterior capsular contraction and intraocular lens dislocation after implant surgery in eyes with retinitis pigmentosa. Ophthalmology 1998; 105:1239–43.
26. Mizuno H, Yamada J, Nishiura M, er al. Capsular tension ring used in a patient with congenital coloboma of the lens. J Cataract Refract Surg 2004; 30:503 –06.
27. Bopp S, Lucke K. Chronic cystoid macular edema in an eye with a capsule defect and posteriorly dislocated capsular tension ring. J Cataract Refract Surg 2003; 29:603–608.
28. Bhattacharjee H, Bhattacharjee K, Das A, et al. Management of a posteriorly dislocated endocapsular tension ring and a foldable acrylic intraocular lens. J Cataract Refract Surg 2004; 30:243–246.
29. Lang Y, Fineberg E, Garzozi HJ. Vitrectomy to remove a posteriorly dislocated endocapsular tension ring. J Cataract Refract Surg 2001; 27:474–476.
30. Vass C, Menapace R, Schetterer K, et al. Prediction of pseudophakic capsular bag diametre based on biometric variables. J Cataract Refract Surg 1999; 25:1376–1381.

31. Waheed K, Eleftheriadis H, Liu C. Anterior capsular phimosis in eyes with a capsular tension ring. J Cataract Refract Surg 2001; 27:1688–1690.

32. Crandall A. Capsular tension rings and pseudoexfoliation. In: Cataract and refractive surgery today. Jan 2004;46–7.

33. Tehrani A, Dick HB, Krummenauer F, et al. Capsule measuring ring to predict capsular bag diametre and follow its course after foldable intraocular lens implantations. J Cataract Refract Surg 2003; 29:2127–2134.

34. Jehan FS, Mamalis N, Crandall AS. Spontaneous late dislocation of intraocular lens within the capsular bag in pseudoexfoliation patients. Ophthalmology 2001; 108: 1727–1731.

35. Faschinger CW, Eckhardt M. Complete capsulorhexis opening occlusion despite capsular tension ring implantation. J Cataract Refract Surg 1999; 25:1013–1015.

36. Werner L, Pandey SK, Escobar-Gomez M, et al. Anterior capsule opacification: a histopathological study comparing different IOL styles. Ophthalmology 2000; 107:463–471.

37. Too CK, Shin JA, Kim JH. Capsular opening contracture after continuous curvilinear capsulorhexis and intraocular lens implantation, J Cataract Refract Surg 1996; 22: 585–590.

38. Nishi 0, Nishi K, Menapace R. Capsule-bending ring for the prevention of capsular opacification: a preliminary report. Ophthalmic Surg Lasers 1998; 29:749–753.

39. Ma PE, Kaur H, Petrovic V, nay u., vision ring from the vitreous. Ophthalmology.

40. Dick HB. Closed foldable capsular rings. J Cataract Refract Surg 2005; 31: 467–471.

41. Dick HB, Schwenn O, Pfeiffer N. Implantation of the modified capsular bending ring in pediatric cataract surgery using a viscoadaptive viscoelastic agent. J Cataract Refract Surg 1999; 25:1432–1436.

42. Praveen MR, et al: Phacoemulsification in subluxated cataract. Indian J Ophthalmol 2003 Sep; 51(3): 282

43. Saco S, Menapace R, Findl O, et al. Long-term efficacy of adding a sharp posterior optic edge to a three-piece silicone intraocular lens on capsule opacification: five-year results of a randomised study. Am J Ophthalmol 2005; 139:696–703.

44. Santoro S, et al: Subluxated lens: Phacoemulsification with Iris hooks. J cataract refract surgery 2003 Dec; 29(12): 2269–73.

45. Dux, et al, Phacofragmentation of dislocated lens in vitreous cavity. Zhonghua Yan Ke Za Zhi. 2001 Nov; 37(6): 428–30.

46. Lee DH, Shin SC, Joo CK. Effect of a capsular tension ring on intraocular lens decentration and tilting after cataract surgery. J Cataract Refract Surg 2002; 28:843–846.

38

Phaco in
Posterior Subcapsular Cataract

Col JKS Parihar SM, VSM **and Lt Col Anirudh Singh**

INTRODUCTION

Posterior subcapsular cataracts (PSC) account for only 10% of all cataracts. These are uniform and vacuolar plate like cataracts confined to the posterior subcapsular region only. The importance of these cataracts lies in the fact that they are most often associated with systemic or ocular diseases. Important risk factors in posterior subcapsular cataract development include exposure to excessive X-ray or gamma radiation, diabetes and steroid induced mechanisms that initiate cellular or molecular dysfunction are as yet poorly understood.

MORPHOLOGY

Posterior subcapsular opacities appear as sheets of vacuoles, water clefts, coronary flakes, focal dots, retro dots or fibre folds. Each lens feature is graded from 0.1 (minimal or absent) to 5.9 (severe) in 0.1 steps. Association of posterior polar cataract has been seen in around 10–15% of the cases of posterior subcapsular cataract.

CLASSIFICATION

Lens opacities classification system (LOCS III) 1993 is used for grading the cataract. It grades the lens opacity in steps of 0.1 degree from 0.1 to 5.9. However, another simplified and more practical method is to grade the posterior subcapsular cataract from P1 to P5 depending on the increasing area of posterior subcapsular opacity which the authors also follow in the authors' centre. It is important for preoperative prediction of complications and has prognostic value. Intraoperative constraints and risk of PC rent proportionately increase with type P4 and P5, respectively.

CLINICAL FEATURES

(i) Patient remains symptomatic, despite good corrected visual acuity. Symptoms are proportionate to the grade of PSC.

(ii) Better mesopic vision than in bright illumination.
(iii) Significant glare particularly noticed while driving in the night.

DIFFERENTIAL DIAGNOSIS

 (i) Posterior polar cataract
(ii) Mittendorf dot
(iii) Injury to the posterior capsule.

HOW TO DIFFERENTIATE IT FROM POSTERIOR POLAR CATARACT

See Table 38.1.

SURGICAL MANAGEMENT OF POSTERIOR SUBCAPSULAR CATARACT

Preoperative Evaluation

In addition to a detailed preoperative examination, a thorough counselling should be conducted to apprise the

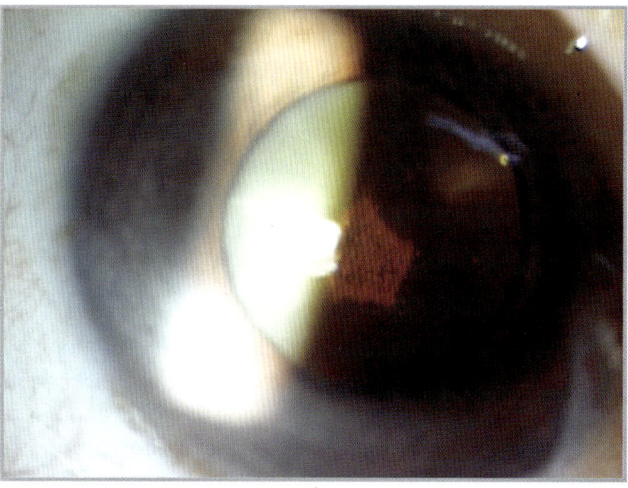

Fig. 38.1: Posterior subcapsular cataract

Table 38.1: Anatomical differences

S.No.		Posterior Polar Cataract	Posterior Subcapsular Cataract
1.	Age	Younger age group	Not associated with age
2.	Origin	Invariably a developmental anomaly	No relation
3.	Appearance	Bull's eye/plaque/mass	Uniform or vacuolar
4.	Shape	Circular	Plate-like
5.	Rings	Concentric rings	No rings
6.	Colour	Whitish brown	Golden yellow
7.	Site	Adherent to PC	Not adherent to PC
8.	Size	2.5–4 mm	Maybe up to the equator
9.	Thickness	Thicker, involves more structures than the posterior capsule	Thinner, confined to posterior subcapsular region only
10.	Preexisting PC tear	May be a presenting feature	Not seen
11.	Associated nuclear/ cortical opacity	Not a routine feature except that the posterior cortex may be affected	Usually not seen
12.	Systemic disease	No	Usually associated with systemic or ocular diseases

patient of about 10–15% association of posterior polar cataracts with the PSC and its consequent greater risk with higher incidence of intraoperative complications which may include higher chances of intraoperative nucleus drop due to inadvertent posterior capsular rent and possible posterior segment intervention to deal with such situation. Patient should also be apprised of delayed visual recovery in certain cases.

In addition, the surgeon should discuss Nd:YAG capsulotomy for residual plaque and emphasize the other effects of aetiological cause like diabetes, steroid induced or traumatic, if any.

Anaesthesia

The choice of anaesthesia technique or applications of general anaesthesia depends upon the merits and age of the patients as well as on the surgeon's own preference. Peribulbar anaesthesia with oculopressure to soften the globe diminishes intraoperative posterior pressure. With increasing experience, one may use topical anaesthesia in a selective manner. We did not notice any difficulty or constraint while handling posterior subcapsular cataract under topical anaesthesia at several occasions. In our view, it is a matter of surgical precision and personal comfort rather than essentiality of peribulbar over topical anaesthesia.

Surgical Technique

We prefer a closed chamber technique. The contours of the cornea and the globe should be maintained throughout the procedure. Any kind of incision is good enough to perform surgery in these cases. The author prefers to proceed with clear corneal temporal incision for its precision, safety and quicker application.

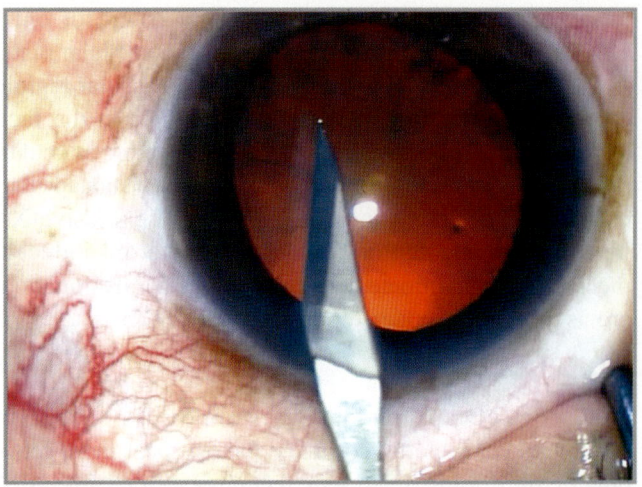

Fig. 38.2: Post subcapsular cataract: Incision

Capsulorrhexis

Ideally, the capsulorrhexis should not be larger than 5 to 5.5 mm in size. Although, a size of 4 mm or less could be detrimental if the surgeon must prolapse the nucleus into the anterior chamber, a larger opening may not leave adequate support for a sulcus-fixated IOL, if the posterior capsule is compromised.

The use of needle or rhexis forceps is exclusively the surgeon's preference. In our view, the rhexis forceps enjoys superiority over needle in certain situations like thin and fragile capsule especially in younger patients where forceps provides better control over linear movements by needle.

Hydroprocedures

(a) **Hydrodissection:** The judicious application of hydroprocedures is one of the most important and crucial single aspects of smooth and uneventful outcome following surgery in cases of posterior

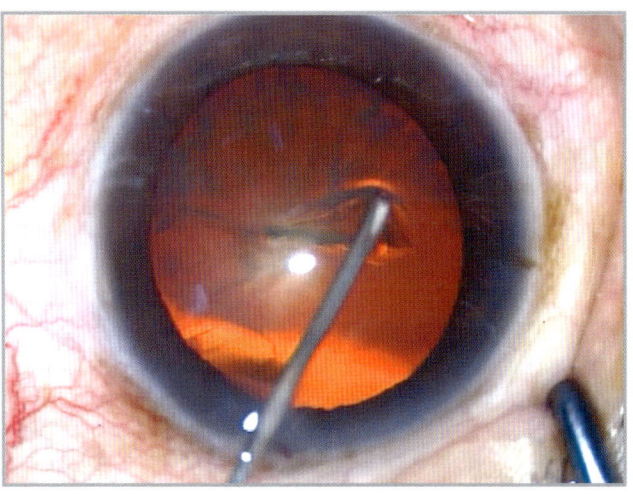

Fig. 38.3: Post subcapsular cataract: Rhexis

polar cataracts. Slow cortical cleaving hydro-dissection with only 0.5–1 ml of fluid is used in two quadrants to separate the capsule from the cortex. Rapid injection of fluid should be avoided as it can lead to hydraulic rupture.

The fluid traversing the subcapsular plane produces delineation (a golden ring within the lens indicates successful delineation). When fluid reaches a desired depth, it will create an epinuclear bowl that will act as a mechanical cushion to protect the posterior capsule during subsequent manoeuvres. Arup Chakrabati et al instead, performed hydrofree-dissection. Hydrofreedissection involved sweeping under the anterior capsular surface with a cyclo-dialysis spatula along all the meridians. This is achieved by working the spatula through two side port incisions. The spatula tip is carefully advanced till the capsular fornix is reached and then the sweeping manoeuvre is initiated. This eliminates the risk of PC rent with a fluid wave.

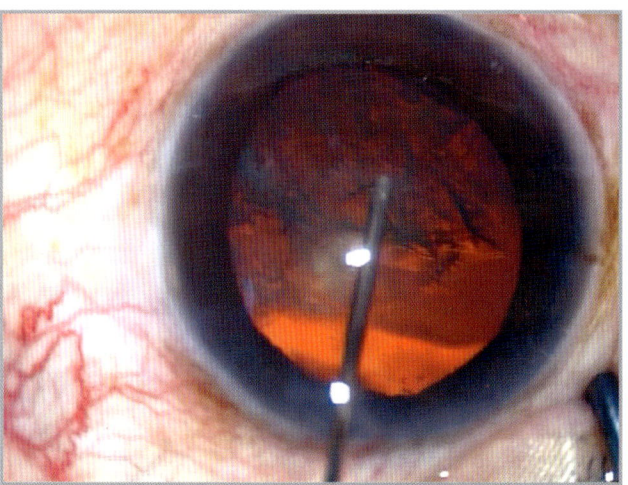

Fig. 38.4: Hydrodissection in cases of posterior subcapsular cataract

We prefer to inject a very small quantity of BSS fluid in at least two quadrants in such a manner so as to achieve cleavage between the capsular bag and the cortical matter. This is further augmented by the infiltration of sodium hyaluronate at the same plane.

(b) **Hydrodelineation:** The next step is deep hydro-delineation at the plane of mid nucleus so as to achieve cleavage or golden ring appearance around the core nucleus. The visco separation is equally beneficial at this stage. One should avoid repeated and sequential hydrodelineation so as to ensure safety against posterior capsule dehiscence.

Nucleus Management

All of our techniques are geared towards facilitating the removal of the nucleus while it is cushioned by the epinucleus. Bimanual cracking and division of the nucleus involve outward movements and can distort the capsular bag. We recommend direct or stop and chop or cart wheel flip and chip technique depending upon the grading of the nucleus. The majority of nuclei in posterior subcapsular cataracts are soft nuclei, hence moderate energy and aspiration settings are much more beneficial. Conventional sculpting may not be a viable option in soft cataracts with posterior plaques, since it may involve a higher risk of posterior capsular rent or direct injury to the capsule due to ultrasonic energy in soft cataracts.

We prefer to use a zero degree tip in these cases to minimise mechanical injury in case of soft cataracts. For nuclear sclerosis greater than 2+, we use the technique of sequential chopping *in situ* with 10% to 15% ultrasound, vacuum of 150 to 225 mmHg, an aspiration flow rate of 20 mL/min, and a bottle height of 70 to 90 cm. The resultant fragments are removed with a stop, chop technique. Our aim remains to first remove the central nucleus followed by an onion peeling separation and removal of the remaining nucleus and the epinucleus plate. For less dense nuclei, we aspirate the entire nucleus within the epinuclear shell. Thus, the slow-motion technique reduces turbulence in the anterior chamber.

Management of Epinuclear Shell

Posterior subcapsular plate with adjacent cortical plate is left as such till the end of the procedure so as to maintain the integrity of posterior capsule at the maximum.

In case of associated posterior plaque, depending upon the thickness and density of plaque as well as its relations with posterior capsule, plaque may require gentle dissection with the help of fine needle and Synskey's hook.

We preferred to use bimanual phacoaspiration–irrigation method to handle very soft nucleus without applying any ultrasonic energy.

Osher et al have also described the technique of slow motion phacoemulsification. Lee and Lee described their

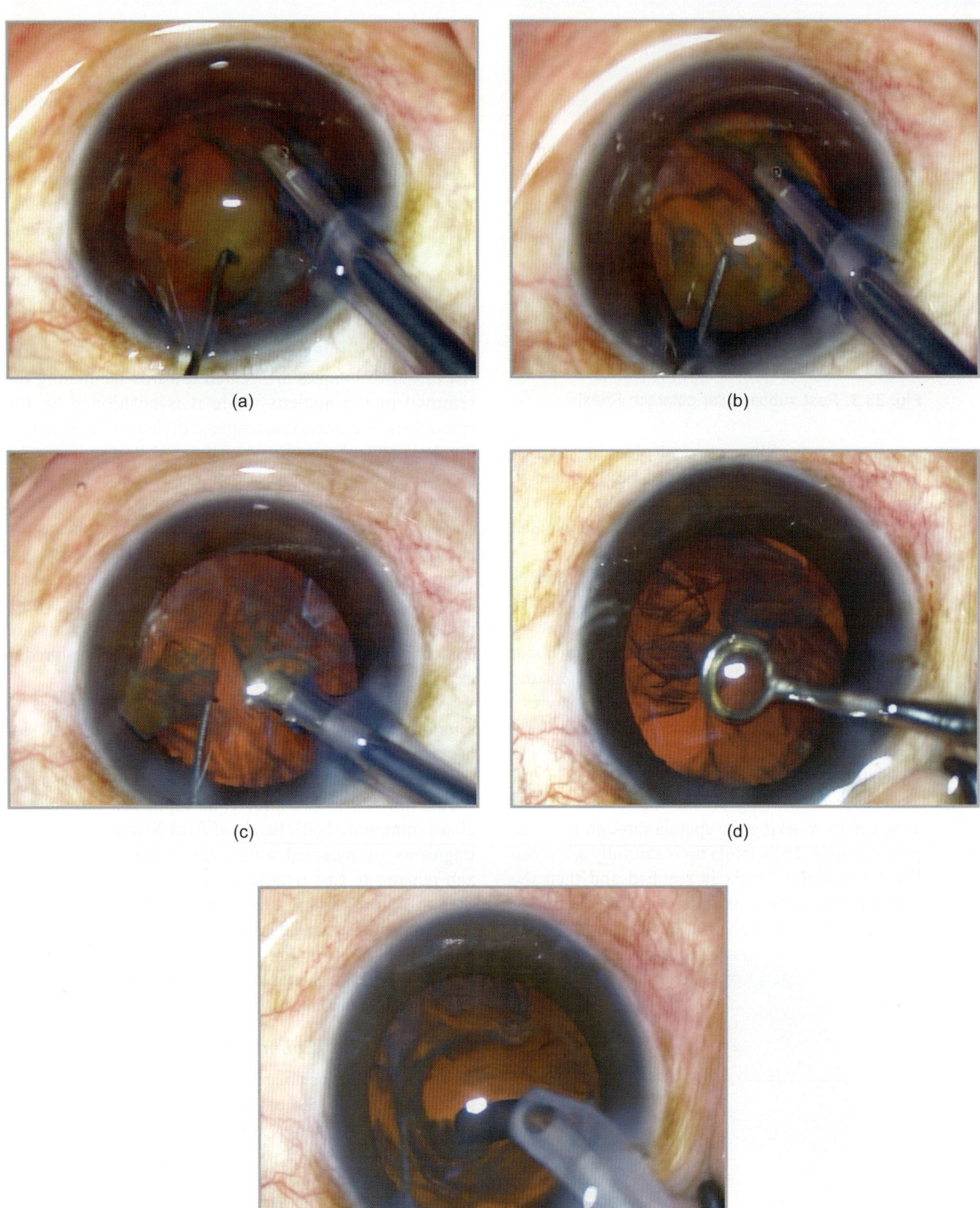

Fig. 38.5: (a) Post subcapsular cataract: Cortical clearing, (b) Post subcapsular cataract: Direct Chopping, (c) Nucleus management in posterior subcapsular cataract (removal of central core nucleus), (d) Posterior plate management in posterior subcapsular cataract: onion peeling separation and removal of the remaining posterior plate, (e) Post subcapsular cataract: IA aspiration

use of the lambda technique to sculpt the nucleus, after which they cracked along both arms and removed the central piece. Vasavada and Singh described the use of a step by step chop *in situ* and lateral separation to minimise stress on the capsule-zonule complex.

Arup Chakraborty et al employed a technique, which was not dependent on nucleus rotation. Majority of the cases of PSC had a soft nucleus. This was progressively debulked employing low phaco parametres like maximum ultrasound power of 40% to 70%, flow rate of 15 ml/min, a vacuum of 5–50 mmHg (depending upon the stage of the nucleus removal) and infusion bottle at 40 cm. Initially, most of the central and interior portions of the nucleus were debulked, thereby more space in the capsular bag was created. Subsequently, the rest of the superior portions of the nucleus along with the epinucleus was displaced into the space created in the capsular bag inferiorly and emulsified. This was achieved by incremental injection of viscoelastic materials (VE) at the superior capsular fornix (limited viscodissection) till the superior portion of the nucleus and the epinucleus were displaced just up to the upper CCC margin from where it was flipped into the anterior chamber with a cyclodialysis spatula working through the side port. The residual cortex was removed by bimanual irrigation/aspiration (I/A) working from periphery to the centre. The central PC was never polished or vacuumed.

IOL Implantation

An atraumatic technique with minimal stress on the PC is employed for IOL insertion into the capsular bag. Single piece hydrophobic acrylic IOL implant remains our first preference. However, if a PC tear is noticed, every effort is made to prevent extension of the tear and minimise vitreous loss. The basic principle followed is not to allow the anterior chamber to collapse by maintaining a closed system. This is achieved by injecting viscoelastic

materials before withdrawing the phaco tip or the I/A probe from the anterior chamber. Cortex is removed by a dry technique using a cannula on a syringe. If vitreous presents in the anterior chamber at any stage, a thorough automated anterior vitrectomy (preferably bimanual) is performed.

The possibility of posterior CCC is considered in the event of a small and central PC rent. All PMMA IOL implantation in the ciliary sulcus remained our choice till three years ago until we had switched over to the acrylic IOL implantation over CTR in cases of capsular dehiscence. However, in certain very large and uncontrolled dehiscences, one may have to consider the IOL implantation into the ciliary sulcus. Viscoelastic material is removed very cautiously taking care to maintain the intraocular pressure and the anterior chamber depth throughout the procedure.

The status of the posterior capsule (PC) actually dictates the action of the surgeon. If the PC is absent or torn but with no vitreous loss, a dispersive viscoelastic is injected over the defect to tamponade and push the vitreous face backwards. A dispersive rather than a cohesive viscoelastic is preferable as it is more adapted to maintaining a space and stabilising the anterior vitreous face. If there is PCR with vitreous loss, a two port anterior vitrectomy is performed. Intraocular lens implantation in these cases would depend on the extent of the PCR and the integrity of the remaining PC.

Intraoperative Complications/Observations

Incidence of PCR in PSC

The incidence of PC rent in PSC has been reported in around 5–9% in different studies as compared to 1.1% reported in other types of cataract. We have seen gradual decline in the incidence of PC rent in PSC from the initial 5 to 6% to less than 2% observed during the last five years. The changing pattern of application of fluidics as well as

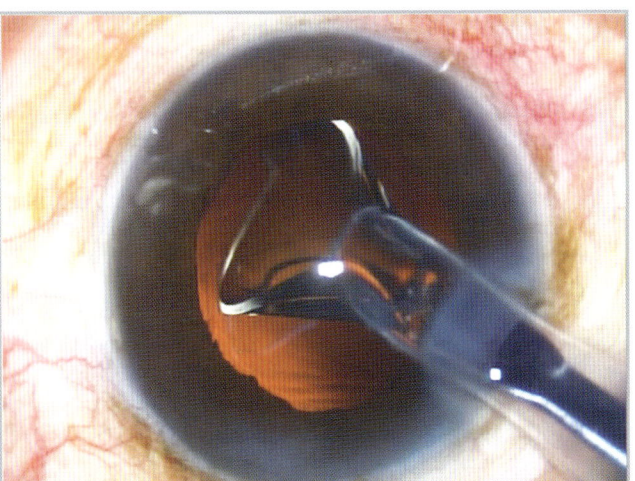

(a)

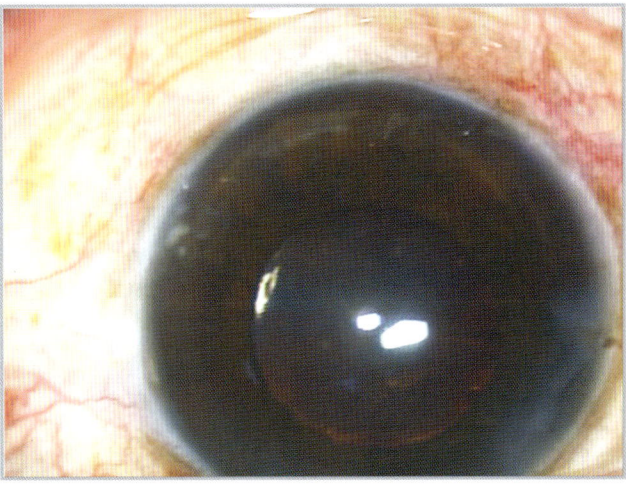

(b)

Fig. 38.6: (a) Single piece hydrophobic acrylic IOL implantation, (b) Post subcapsular cataract: IOL *in situ*

rapid advancement in surgical technique and availability of refined, advanced and better phacomachines are key factors to achieve this breakthrough.

How to Prevent/Minimise Risk of Posterior Capsule Rupture

Dealing carefully with the posterior plaque during phacoemulsification may decrease intraoperative and postoperative complications and remarkably improve postoperative visual acuity.

Following tips may be very beneficial while managing posterior subcapsular cataracts:

(i) Slow and gradual hydrodissection.
(ii) Gentle deep core hydrodelineation leaving superficial and most posterior layers free from hydrodelineation.
(iii) Least US energy on a zero degree tip.
(iv) No sculpting rather relying upon chopping or cart wheel movements/onion peeling techniques of nucleus management.
(v) Moderate aspiration/irrigation settings

Postoperative Complications

(i) Mild to moderate uveitis 3–5%
(ii) Secondary glaucoma 3–5%
(iii) Macular oedema 10–15%
(iv) PCO: 30 to 40% after an interval of two years
(v) Residual posterior capsule plaque postoperatively, which required neodymium: YAG laser capsulotomy: 12 to 15%.

Results

Overall visual outcome following phacoemulsification surgery in cases of posterior subcapsular cataract is encouraging and gratifying. More than 97% of patients are likely to regain visual acuity of 20/40 or more. However, the remaining cases may have compromised and poor visual outcome due to preexisting conditions like chronic anterior uveitis or retinal involvements like diabetic retinopathy or surgical complications.

CONCLUSION

Surgical management of posterior subcapsular cataracts is rather simple if the basic rules of phacoemulsification are followed. It is important that the surgeon and the patient understand the minor technical difficulties associated and are aware of potential complications.

BIBLIOGRAPHY

1. Judy Y.F Ku, MBChBa, Christina N Grupcheva, Keratoglobus and posterior subcapsular cataract: Surgical considerations and in vivo microstructural analysis Arch Ophthalmol May 2003.
2. R.C. Drews. Posterior subcapsular cataracts. Arch Ophthalmol, Aug 1979; 97: 1543.
3. Incidence of Age-Related Cataract: The Beaver Dam Eye Study. Arch Ophthalmol, Feb 1998; 116: 219–225
4. Vitamin Supplement Use and Incident Cataracts in a Population-Based Study Arch Ophthalmol, Nov 2000; 118: 1556–1563.
5. Bickol N. Mukesh; Anhchuong Le; Peter N. Development of Cataract and Associated Risk Factors: The Visual Impairment Project Arch Ophthalmol, Jan 2006; 124: 79–85.
6. Sudha Cugati; Robert G. Cumming; Wayne Smith; Visual Impairment, Age-Related Macular Degeneration, Cataract, and Long-term Mortality: The Blue Mountains Eye Study. Arch Ophthalmol, Jul 2007; 125: 917–924.
7. Jie J. Wang; Paul Mitchell; Judy M. Simpson;.Visual Impairment, Age-Related Cataract, and Mortality. Arch Ophthalmol, Aug 2001; 119: 1186–1190.
8. M L Lopez, V Freidlin, M B Datiles. Longitudinal study of posterior subcapsular opacities using the National Eye Institute computer planimetry system., 3rd British Journal of Ophthalmology 1995;79:535–540.
9. Cathy A McCarty, Jill E Keeffe, Hugh R Taylor. The need for cataract surgery: projections based on lens opacity, visual acuity, and personal concern. Br J Ophthalmol 1999; 83:62–65 (January).
10. N.A. Frost, J.M. Sparrow, and L. Moore. Associations of Human Crystalline Lens Retrodots and Waterclefts with Visual Impairment: An Observational Study. Invest. Ophthalmol. Vis. Sci., July 1, 2002; 43(7): 2105–2109.
11. J. Eshaghian; B. W. Streeten.Human posterior subcapsular cataract. An ultrastructural study of the posteriorly migrating cells. Arch Ophthalmol, Jan 1980; 98: 134–143.
12. V. Greiner; L. T. Chylack Jr.Posterior subcapsular cataracts: histopathologic study of steroid-associated cataracts.Arch Ophthalmol, Jan 1979; 97: 135–144.
13. T.W. Bochow; S.K. West; A. Azar; B. Munoz; A. Sommer; H.R. Taylor Ultraviolet light exposure and risk of posterior subcapsular cataracts Arch Ophthalmol, Mar 1989; 107: 369–372.
14. Anselm Hennis; Suh-Yuh Wu; Barbara Nemesure; M. Cristina Leske Risk Factors for Incident Cortical and Posterior Subcapsular Lens Opacities in the Barbados Eye Studies. Arch Ophthalmol, Apr 2004; 122: 525–530.
15. Cécile Delcourt; Isabelle Carrière; Alice Ponton-Sanchez; Annie Lacroux; Marie-José Covacho; Laure Papoz; and the POLA Study Group. Light Exposure and the Risk of Cortical, Nuclear, and Posterior Subcapsular Cataracts: The Pathologies Oculaires Liées à l'Age (POLA) Study Arch Ophthalmol, Mar 2000; 118: 385–392.

39

Phaco in Postuveitis Cataract

Col JKS Parihar SM, VSM and Lt Col SK Mishra VSM

INTRODUCTION

Cataract development is a very common occurrence in any form of anterior and intermediate uveitis, because of: (i) the recurrence and chronic inflammation, and (ii) the long term use of corticosteroid therapy. The reported incidence of cataract in uveitic patients varies between series but it approaches almost 50 percent in juvenile rheumatoid arthritis and other forms of posterior uveitis, and up to 75 percent in chronic anterior uveitis.

The indications for proceeding with cataract surgery are challenged in eyes with uveitis because the complications of this surgery are higher in these patients than in no uveitic patients. Uncontrolled inflammation, hypotony, phthisis bulbi, among others are important challenges to the postoperative period in uveitic patients. One has to weigh the benefits of surgery in such patients vis-à-vis the complications following the surgery, especially if the visual loss is not significant due to cataract.

FACTORS INFLUENCING SURGICAL APPROACH IN POSTUVEITIC CATARACT

There are some facts concerning these cataracts that make the therapeutical or surgical approach different from those associated with senior population:

(i) Cataracts associated with uveitis develop at an early age, affecting children and young adults.

(ii) A higher incidence of posterior subcapsular cataracts leads to glare disability and near vision difficulties.

(iii) Preoperative antiinflammatory regimens must be carefully planned for each individual patient which differs from the routine surgical protocol.

(iv) Postoperative follow-up should ensure control of inflammation and monitor the higher incidence of complications including posterior capsule opacification, glaucoma, iritis recurrences, macular oedema.

The improvement in surgical techniques and pre and postoperative control of inflammation, thanks to new and safer small incision surgeries and the usage of corticosteroids pre and postoperatively, has led to better results of surgery in patients with uveitis. This has increased the tendency to operate these eyes as early as possible to prevent more important complications.

Surgery should be performed when the inflammation of the eyes is quiet. However, in some patients it is impossible to clear every cell from the anterior chamber or vitreous. Furthermore, in patients with dense cataracts and primarily vitreoretinal inflammation, it is impossible to assess the activity of the disease behind the cataract.

PREOPERATIVE EVALUATION

Detailed Evaluation of Associated Systemic Involvements

It is worth considering to have a complete and detailed work up of coexisting systemic diseases since postuveitic cataract remains one of the manifestations of complex ocular systemic involvements. A consultation from rheumatologist, haematologist, pulmonologist or endocrinologist may be of immense benefit to the patient and the surgeon as well.

Clinical Examination

Symptoms

Complaints in those patients associated with the development of cataract will be in function of the age, type of uveitis and mostly the type of cataract. Decrease in vision is the most important symptom of the development of cataract in patients with uveitis. Glare, and sometimes halo, can be referred to by the patient as the first complaint.

Glare can be associated with posterior subcapsular cataract, anterior or intermediate uveitis or glaucoma that must be ruled out in such patients.

Slit Lamp Examination

Salient features: Chronic anterior uveitis

(i) **Conjunctiva:** The conjunctiva classically shows perilimbal injection (known as ciliary flush).

(ii) **Keratic precipitates:** The cornea may have keratic precipitates, which are clusters of WBCs collected on the endothelium. The types of keratic precipitates can provide a clue to the classification of anterior uveitis. Mutton-fat keratic precipitates are characteristic of granulomatous uveitis. Diffuse stellate keratic precipitates are classically seen in Fuchs heterochromic iridocyclitis. Interstitial keratitis is commonly seen in patients with syphilis and herpetic disease.

If enough white cells deposit on the bottom of the chamber, a hypopyon results. This finding is suggestive of HLA-B27 disease, Behçet disease, or endophthalmitis.

(iii) **Iris:** The iris can provide additional information about the possible aetiology or chronicity of the disease. Long-standing inflammation can cause posterior synechiae. Inflammatory nodules on the iris suggest granulomatous uveitis.

Heterochromia is the classic finding in Fuchs heterochromic iridocyclitis. Atrophy of the iris may point to *Herpes zoster* as the infection responsible for the inflammation.

(iv) **Pupil:** The pupil remains the most significant intra-operative constraint. The presence of posterior synechiae, rigid and irregular pupillary sphincter,

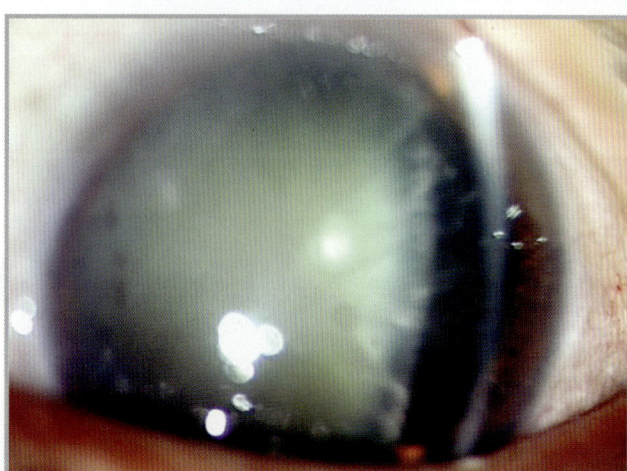

Fig. 39.1: Postuveitic cataract: Evidence of extensive iris atrophy with distortion of pupillary sphincter and presence of posterior synechiae. Diffuse perilimbal injection (known as ciliary flush) suggestive of chronic uveitis with secondary glaucoma is also visible

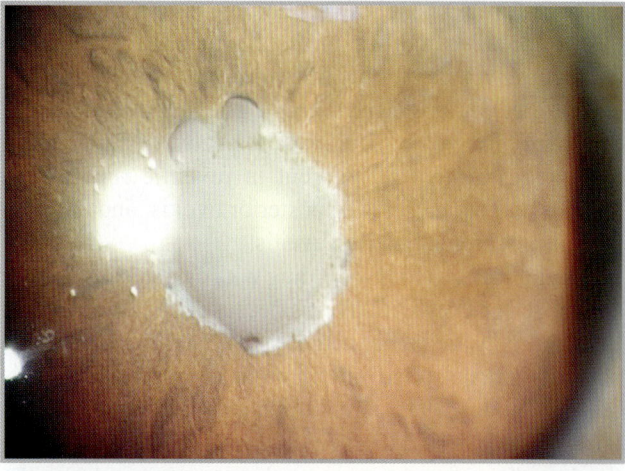

Fig. 39.2: Postuveitic cataract with nondilating miotic pupil

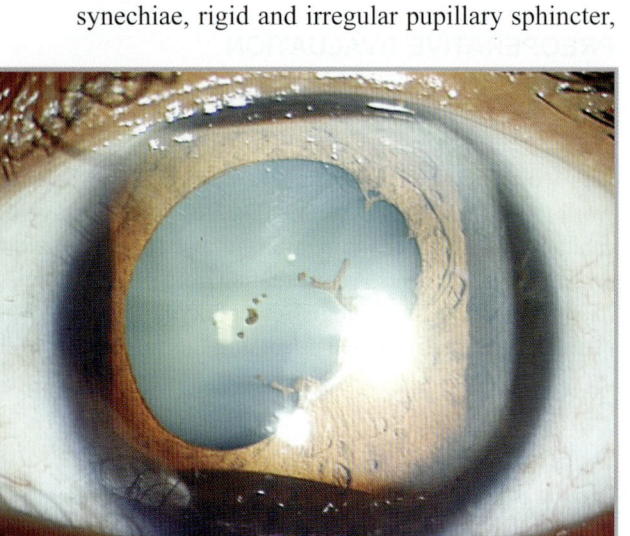

(a)

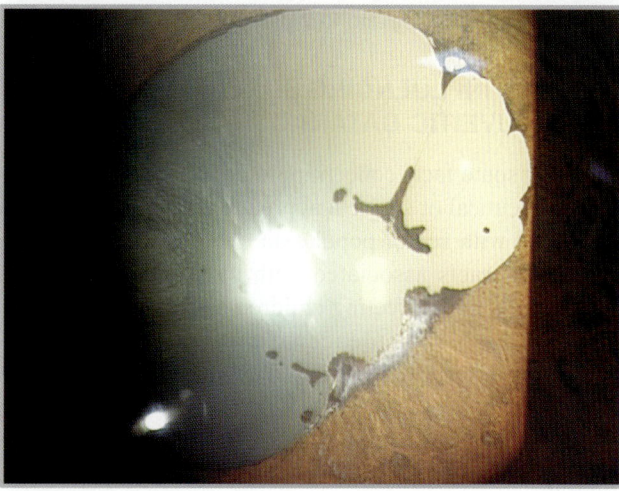

(b)

Fig. 39.3: (a) Postuveitic cataract (posterior subcapsular) showing multiple posterior synechiae with fibrous deposits on the pupillary margins, (b) Postuveitic cataract (posterior subcapsular) showing multiple posterior synaechiae with fibrous deposits on the pupillary margins (under retro illumination)

fibrous deposits around the pupillary deposits leading to poorly dilating or miotic pupil deserve special attention.

(v) **Lens:** The lens may show signs of cataractous change, which may suggest repeated bouts of iritis, or inflammatory precipitates may be present on the anterior lens capsule.

(vi) **Vitreous:** The anterior vitreous may have some cells that have "spilled over" from the anterior chamber. Some HLA-B27 diseases have varying amounts of vitritis and posterior pole involvement.

(vii) **Papillitis or disc oedema:** Papillitis or disc oedema may be seen in VKH disease, sarcoidosis, TB, Lyme disease, multiple sclerosis, toxoplasmosis, and toxocariasis.

(viii) **Intraocular pressure (IOP):** IOP is often low in acute cases of anterior uveitis (with the exception of herpetic uveitis) but may be elevated in chronic cases.

Intermediate Uveitis

Intermediate uveitis is an anatomical term suggested by the SUN Working Group. Intermediate uveitis is defined as intraocular inflammation that predominantly involves the peripheral retina, pars plana, and vitreous. Other terms used in literature include chronic cyclitis, peripheral uveitis, and pars planitis. The term pars planitis is reserved to describe a subgroup of patients with idiopathic intermediate uveitis with snow banking and/or snowball formation.

Intermediate uveitis accounts for approximately 8–15% of patients with uveitis in tertiary referral centres in the United States. Because characterisation of this disease (and terminology associated with it) has been ambiguous, the conclusions of some older epidemiologic studies have been called into question. However, the report by Rodriguez et al used IUSG criteria and reported incidence of 13%. We have found that intermediate uveitis share around 17% of all the cases of postuveitic cataract.

Symptoms

Patients typically present with painless blurred vision and floaters. Photophobia and redness are unusual.

Signs

(i) Ocular findings include mild-to-moderate anterior segment inflammation, although anterior cellular activity may be more pronounced in children and in patients with multiple sclerosis.

(ii) Presence of anterior vitreous cells is the *sin qua non* of this disorder and, occasionally, the vitritis is severe enough to cause profound loss of vision. White clumps of inflammatory cells (called snowballs) tend to accumulate at the vitreous base where perivascular exudation and neovascularisation may be present.

(iii) The presence of a whitish yellow exudative material on the peripheral retina and the pars plana (called snowbanking) is commonly seen. The presence of this material facilitates diagnosis but is not required to establish a diagnosis of intermediate uveitis. This finding is more consistent in patients with idiopathic intermediate uveitis and in children.

Since intermediate uveitis has been described in association with several systemic disorders, the initial diagnostic evaluation should exclude masquerade syndromes and infectious diseases in which immunosuppression may be ineffective or contraindicated.

The diagnostic approach to intermediate uveitis should focus on the history and clinical examination. Approximately, two-thirds of patients have idiopathic intermediate uveitis (pars planitis) followed by sarcoidosis in 20 to 25%, multiple sclerosis in 7 to 10% of patients.

WHEN TO INTERVENE: SURGICAL INDICATIONS

Cataract surgery may be considered in postuveitic cataract in the following situations:

1. Visually significant cataract if prospects for substantial improvement in visual acuity are good.
2. Cataract that impairs fundus assessment in a patient with suspected fundus pathology.

Visually Significant Cataract

Cataract is not a reversible disease, so if the cataract is causing marked decrease in vision, it will further decrease over subsequent years. Techniques to estimate postoperative visual acuity can be performed in patients where standard acuity scales are not sufficient and the health of the macula is unclear. Potential acuity metre (PAM) and laser interferometry are the most reliable techniques in these patients. OCT can be performed in patients suspected to have macular oedema, provided the cataract is not very dense.

Glare

Sometimes, a 20/20 visual acuity is present in a patient with uveitis but still the patient complains of blurred vision. Explanation of the potential risks and benefits must be carefully done including the fact that cataract is not reversible and that those symptoms will augment with time.

Improvement of Posterior Pole Visualisation

Those situations associated with visualisation of the posterior pole either to assess the evolution of a given disease (posterior uveitis, vasculitis, macular oedema) or the response to a treatment (systemic steroids or immunosuppressant) can be affected by the presence of a dense cataract or even a wide posterior subcapsular cataract.

PREOPERATIVE CONSIDERATIONS TOWARDS CASES OF POSTUVEITIC CATARACT

Line of preoperative management depends upon the severity and nature of postuveitic glaucoma. Hence, protocol may be grouped separately for complicated and uncomplicated nature of postuveitic cataract [based on the guidelines of the intraocular inflammation society (IOIS)].

Complicated Cases of Uveitic Cataract

Cases of postuveitic cataract that are essentially on systemic or periocular medication to control the uveitis as well as to maintain a quiescent state. In addition to it extensive derangement of the anatomical configuration of anterior segment as well as physiological functions like status of IOP is in question.

Uncomplicated Cases of Uveitic Cataract

Remaining cases of postuveitic cataract with excellent control of uveitis as well as a near normal anterior segment with adequate pupillary dilatation and minimal distortion of the pupillary sphincter. In addition to it, the absence of systemic steroid therapy to control uveitis in previous three months is also considered as a positive factor.

Preoperative Management of Uveitis

Control of Inflammation Prior to Cataract Surgery

The control of inflammation prior to cataract surgery in patients with a history of uveitis is very crucial and essential. There should not be any evidence of active uveitis as well as the eye should remain free of active inflammation at least for the last three months. These cases may require preoperative topical antiinflammatory drugs during this period to achieve optimum environment for surgery.

The single most important sign of inflammation is the presence or absence of inflammatory cells in the anterior-chamber. Chronic uveitis simply denotes vascular incompetence of the iris and ciliary body, a consequence of vascular damage from recurrent uveitis. Therefore, flare should not generally be used as a guidepost for inflammatory quiescence.

The presence of inflammatory cells in the vitreous may be extremely difficult to discern through an advanced cataract. The presence of vitreous cells does not necessarily signify active disease because inflammatory cells clear more slowly than in the anterior chamber. Vitreous inflammation does not appear to be significantly associated with the presence of cataract development in patients with Vogt-Koyanagi-Harada (VKH) syndrome.

Preoperative Regimen

It is recommended to commence standard preoperative regimen at least a week before the surgical intervention. Frequent instillation (three to four times in a day) of topical steroids should be instituted in each and every case of postuveitic cataract. In addition to it, systemic steroids should be given to all the cases defined as complicated uveitic cases.

All other medications for coexisting systemic disease should continue.

Surgical Technique: Conventional ECCE / Phacoemulsification/Concurrent Procedures

Problems in the Phacoemulsification Surgery in Postuveitic Cataract

Cataract surgery is sometimes complicated by the presence of:

(i) Iris atrophy, sclerosis of the pupillary sphincter,
(ii) Cyclitic membrane
(iii) Posterior synechiae
(iv) Anterior capsular sclerosis
(v) Possible haemorrhage from the iris and angle neovascularisation; as a result a precise and delicate surgery is mandatory.

Phacoemulsification allows a small wound, causes minimal trauma and may, therefore, minimise postoperative inflammation. Young patients and patients on high doses of corticosteroids are at an advantage with this technique. General anaesthesia is not necessary (though many patients are young and their treatment with general anaesthesia is compulsory), and regional anaesthesia by retrobulbar or peribulbar block are preferred. Topical anaesthesia is not contraindicated but we do not use it in these cases.

Clear corneal or scleral tunnel incision can be performed. Clear corneal incision has some advantages over scleral tunnels such as the absence of postoperative hyphaema, filtering blebs and need for cautery among others. This is our favoured approach for if foldable lens is implanted, and if the implantation of a rigid polymethyl-methacrylate (PMMA) lens is planned, a limbal approach with a short scleral tunnel is performed. In most of our cases we were able to implant a foldable lens. Viscoelastic substances are routinely used to release adhesions and aid mydriasis. Combinations of hyaluronic acid and chondroitin sulphate (Viscoat R) are preferred, and high viscosity viscoelastics can be sued (Healon GVR, Amvisc plus R). Many patients with uveitis have sclerosis of the dilator muscle of the pupil or intense posterior synechiae, and under viscoelastic aid synechiolysis is performed with an iris spatula. If further mydriasis is desired, four iris hooks in each quadrant may be used to stretch the pupil. If there is a cyclitic membrane over the iris margin, a utrata forceps may be used to peel the membrane from the pupillary margins, thus facilitating adequate pupillary dilatation. Continuous circular capsulotomy (capsulorrhexis) is always performed, even in intumescent cataracts, and if this is not possible a can-opener capsulotomy is opted for, but phacoemulsification is performed with caution.

The phacoemulsification procedure is accomplished by the most suitable technique for each case, with chop techniques if hardness of the nucleus is high. In general the nucleus is soft in young patients and phacoemulsification can be performed without any complications. Intensive cortical cleaning is mandatory to eliminate one of the sources of postoperative inflammatory reaction and the posterior surface of the anterior capsule must be aspirated with a low vacuum to eliminate proliferative cells and to remove one of the sources of posterior and possibly anterior capsule opacification. Bimanual techniques give excellent results in anterior cortical cleaning. Where there is extensive membrane formation in the vitreous, especially in the anterior part, vitrectomy after posterior central capsulorrhexis must be considered. If the vitreous cavity shows extensive fibrosis and exudates formation, trans-scleral pars plana vitrectomy may be indicated.

Type of Intraocular Lenses in Postuveitic Cataract

In the past, most surgeons regarded the existence of chronic uveitis as a relative contraindication to IOL implantation. For these reasons, sulcus or anterior chamber implantation has always been contraindicated and capsular bag placement has been controversial. Now, several studies have suggested that inserting a posterior chamber lens into the capsular bag is always recommended whenever possible, provided the inflammation has been controlled well.

The heparin surface-modified IOL is created by inducing electrostatic absorption of heparin onto the surface of a PMMA IOL. Heparin-coated IOLs are recommended for patients with uveitis as they decrease the number and severity of deposits on the surface of the IOL.

Several controlled studies comparing flexible IOL implantation through a 3.2 mm incision and conventional PMMA IOL implantation through 5.5 mm or larger incisions have been reported. Postoperative inflammation is significantly less with smaller incisions.

Polymethyl methacrylate (PMMA) has been the most commonly used IOL material in recent past. It has proved to be inert and stable and many companies manufacture numerous designs. New technology applied to PMMA lenses has enabled the development of new generation of acrylic foldable lenses for small incision surgery. Acrylic hydrophobic foldable IOL implantation in patients with chronic uveitis has also given good results and we routinely use such IOLs.

Silicone lenses have displayed greater inflammatory reaction in nonuveitic patients when compared to other IOL materials (PMMA, heparin-modified, hydrogel). After phacoemulsification procedures a number of complications have been described such as intense inflammatory reactions in the anterior chamber, total closure of the capsulorrhexis and an increase in posterior capsule opacification when compared with PMMA implants. We do not recommend the use of this material in patients whose blood-aqueous barrier is compromised. Also, one must keep in mind the later need for vitreoretinal surgery in such cases where silicone oil implantation may be required. Nevertheless, few reports of the use of silicone IOLs in patients with uveitis have been published. A 13 mm silicone IOL with a 6 mm optic was implanted through a 3.2 mm incision in a woman with sarcoidosis uveitis, and this case revealed perioperative tolerance to this silicone implant and rapid visual rehabilitation as compared with the fellow eye which received a rigid PMMA lens.

The issues surrounding IOL placement in uveitic eyes after cataract extraction remains a key concern in the management of the uveitic patient. Many features unique to a uveitic eye must be considered:

    (i) Different types of uveitis and their diagnoses
    (ii) Preoperative inflammation and
    (iii) Treatment, postoperative inflammation and specific complication.

With newer techniques and modern posterior chamber lenses, IOLs are being implanted with fewer complications. These IOLs are well tolerated in selected patients, especially when the lens is placed in the capsular bag. Many questions remain unanswered regarding the uveitic eye in conjunction with IOL biocompatibility and inflammation. However, in our experience, implantation of newer generation IOL implants in postuveitic cataract has been found to be very effective and safe in the long term follow up.

MANAGEMENT OF COEXISTING POSTUVEITIC CATARACT WITH GLAUCOMA/ POSTERIOR SEGMENT INVOLVEMENT BY CONCURRENT CATARACT WITH GLAUCOMA/VITRECTOMY PROCEDURES

Postuveitic Glaucoma/Cataract and Glaucoma

Management of singular postuveitic glaucoma or coexisting with cataract remains a big challenge to handle, particularly in the relatively younger age group. The functional and anatomical results following conventional trabeculectomy remains debatable in the long term follow up due to inherent constraints of intraocular inflammation. The nature, duration and severity of the inflammation as well as the mechanism of underlying inflammation and associated systemic disease play a significant role to determine the prognosis and success of the management strategy.

Various mechanisms produce secondary glaucoma, and it is important to identify them to institute the appropriate therapy. Special considerations should be given to the management of acute or chronic intraocular inflammation and if it is certain that corticosteroids are not the cause of the elevated pressure, pharmacological intervention to control inflammation or uveitic glaucoma remains the most initial step in the treatment of uveitic glaucoma. However, results of medical management or of conventional surgical intervention remained debatable and, by and large, unsatisfactory.

Various procedures like laser iridotomy, surgical iridectomy, trabeculodialysis, trabeculectomy, ab interno laser sclerotomy, pharmacologically modulated trabeculectomy, drainage implantation and Cycloablation are among different modalities. However, pharmacologically modulated trabeculectomy and Glaucoma drainage device implantation are most preferred surgical procedures in this complex group of uveitic glaucoma.

Pharmacologically Modulated Trabeculectomy

The use of antimetabolites in association with trabeculectomy has been used for at least 10 years. Good surgical results have been reported for secondary glaucomas such as traumatic, aphakic, and postuveitic glaucomas with the use of mitomycin-C. Mitomycin-C has replaced the use of 5-fluorouracil in preventing excessive fibrosis after trabeculectomy. However, the application of these drugs do carry certain risks and problems despite adequate control of intraocular pressure. Increased risk of hypotony, bleb leaks, and late bleb-related endophthalmitis are well documented problems. 0.02 mg/ml concentration of mitomycin-C covered by the scleral flap for two minutes and thorough washing of the remnants before suturing is being recommended as the preferred technique.

Glaucoma Drainage Devices Implantation

This surgical strategy seems to be promising when facing a progressive secondary glaucoma with uveitis. We have used valved drainage device like the Ahmad Glaucoma valve (FP-7 and FP-8) in more than fifty cases of postuveitic coexisting cataract and glaucoma or postuveitic glaucoma alone with promising results. These drainage devices have been found to be very effective in controlling the IOP. The surface area of this plate allows for the elaboration of a fibrotic bleb from across which there is absorption of the accumulated aqueous.

These devices are commonly used for the intractable glaucoma patients with uveitis who have failed to improve with other medical procedures and if intercurrent or recurrent inflammation is believed to be the reason for a standard filter drainage procedure.

Cataract Removal and Vitrectomy

Combined phacoemulsification and pars plana vitrectomy technique has shown several advantages over two step

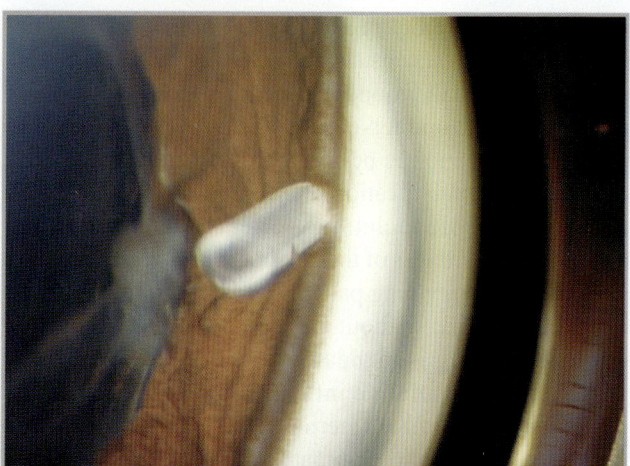

Fig. 39.4: Gonioscopic photograph revealing the presence of silicon tube of Ahmed Glaucoma drainage device in the angle in a case of postuveitic glaucoma and cataract

conventional ECCE or phacoemulsification surgery followed by vitrectomy.

A clear corneal self-sealing valve incision maintains excellent anterior chamber integrity and ocular configuration during concurrent vitrectomy following phacoemulsification cataract surgery. Postuveitic cataract may have certain peculiarities in relation to the configuration and hardness of the lens nucleus. However, an intact posterior capsule and subsequent in-the-bag IOL implantation takes precedence over lensectomy and vitrectomy.

However, if a limbal approach to the cataract and posterior pars plana vitrectomy is intended, the scleral incisions for the vitrectomy should be made first, fixed infusion method and upper sclerotomies should be occluded with scleral plugs. The advantage of this procedure lies in preserving part of the posterior capsule for the secondary implant of an IOL.

The authors prefer this approach whenever possible, first performing phacoemulsification of the crystalline lens followed by pars plana vitrectomy. A capsulotomy or posterior capsulorrhexis must be performed on completion of the vitrectomy due to the fast opacification occurring and because it allows decompartmentalisation of the eye, facilitating the access of antiinflammatory drugs in the postoperative stage. The authors recommend implanting IOL implant after completion of vitrectomy so as to enable good and final cortical wash following vitrectomy as well as surgical ease during vitrectomy. This procedure provides quick and early visual rehabilitation and good visual recovery.

Postoperative Treatment

A strategy for blocking postoperative inflammation, thereby avoiding potential ocular complications, is desirable. Topical steroids have become the standard care during the immediate postoperative period to reduce the morbidity associated with ocular inflammation so as to prevent structural damage to the eye, and to reduce the patient's discomfort. In addition to topical steroids, cycloplegics and antiglaucoma medication should also be instituted.

Prednisolone or dexamethasone, six to eight times daily beginning from day one after surgery up to one week then tapering the dosage over the following four to six weeks is usually recommended. Acetate or alcohol vehicles are the most adequate due to their superior ocular penetration.

Although, topical steroids are currently the most widely used antiinflammatory agents after cataract extraction, their potential side effects limit their clinical effectiveness in some settings. This is particularly true for steroids that have a predilection for elevating intraocular pressure (IOP). Thus, antiinflammatory agents that control postoperative inflammation with little effect on IOP would be a useful adjunct to the surgeon's therapeutic armamentarium.

Several recent studies have assessed the effectiveness of nonsteroidal anti inflammatory drug (NSAID) to treat ocular inflammation. Most NSAIDs used today act by inhibiting the enzyme cyclo oxygenase and thereby decreasing the formation of prostaglandins, which play a major role in ocular inflammation by producing and maintaining the rupture of the blood-aqueous barrier. Diclofenac drops were shown to reduce inflammation after argon laser trabeculoplasty, and after cataract surgery. The role of these drugs is then controversial in the postoperative control of inflammation even in uncomplicated senile cataracts. We cannot offer these drugs as an alternative to corticosteroids or even as an adjunct to treatment in uveitis patients with cataract.

A current strategy underlying the development of new steroidal compounds for ocular use is, therefore, to identify drugs that exhibit marked anti inflammatory activity while decreasing the propensity to raise IOP or induce other side effects.

Systemic steroids may also be required in certain cases of postuveitic cataract. When a previous uveitis is present, a severe postsurgical exacerbation of preexisting, inflammation should be expected. Depending upon the severity of the case one week prior to surgery, systemic corticosteroids in the form of oral prednisolone in dosage of 1 mg/kg body weight may be administered. At the time of surgery, a subconjunctival corticosteroid should be injected periocular far from any ocular wounds.

During the postoperative period, both topical and systemic corticosteroids may be tapered, based on the severity of ocular inflammation. In the most severe cases moderate to high doses of oral prednisone from 1 to 1.5 mg/kg/day, and intensive once per hour topical corticosteroid drops should be given prior to and tapered after surgery. In cases of steroid-induced glaucoma, the management may be much more difficult. In these cases temporary immuno-suppressive therapy may need to be substituted to control inflammation in the early postoperative period. These guidelines may be applied for all intraocular procedures in uveitis eyes.

Follow-up

Generally, a low inflammatory reaction is observed after IOL implantation in patients with chronic anterior uveitis, if preoperative and postoperative anti inflammatory measures are undertaken. Complications associated with these patients in the follow-up are as follows :

Posterior Capsule Opacification

Postuveitic cataract has been found to have a relatively higher incidence of posterior capsule opacification as high as 25 to 35%.

Membranes

The appearance of fibrous membranes mostly in pars planitis patients have been described. These membranes are dense enough to resist Nd: YAG laser rupture with high levels of energy. The tendency to reform is known and they are associated with displacements of the lens and retinal detachment.

Decreased Visual Acuity

The major causes of decreased visual acuity in these patients are cystoid macular oedema, epiretinal membrane, and glaucomatous optic nerve damage. Nevertheless, a proper visual acuity can be achieved in the majority of patients in the most important series of patients published. Visual acuities better than 20/40 can be achieved in 20 to 75 percent of patients.

Even low-grade chronic inflammation can result in permanent damage to the optic nerve, retina, anterior chamber angle and other structures that may preclude our efforts for a visual rehabilitation after cataract surgery. Early surgical intervention prior to the development of permanent structural damage from inflammation or corticosteroid therapy may be the option for the future. Better surgical approaches and the choice of the ideal lens for each patient is the goal for the present and the future in the surgical management of cataract in patients with uveitis.

CONCLUSION

Cataract in patients with uveitis is a frequent event that must be managed by surgical intervention. The surgical approach must always be individualised attending to the symptoms referred to by the patient, especially visual acuity, the aetiology of uveitis, the treatment necessary to maintain a quiescent state, and the expected difficulties of surgery. Preoperative and postoperative control of inflammation is mandatory and none of these patients should be enrolled in a standard surgical approach for senile cataracts.

BIBLIOGRAPHY

1. Kanski JJ, Shun Shin GA: Systemic uveitis syndromes in childhood-an analysis of 340 cases. Ophthalmology 91:1247–52, 1984.
2. Tabbara KF, Chavis PS: Cataract extraction in patients with chronic posterior uveitis. Int Ophthalmol Clin 35:121–31, 1995.
3. Ganesh SK, Babu K, Biswas J. Phacoemulsification with intraocular lens implantation in cases of pars planitis. J Cataract Refract Surg. 2004 Oct; 30(10):2072–6.
4. Tessler HH, Faber MD: Intraocular lens implantation versus no implantation in patients with chronic iridocyclitis and pars planitis. Ophthalmology 100:1026–29, 1993.
5. Kaufman AH, Foster CS: Cataract extraction in patients with pars planitis. Ophthalmology 100:1210–17, 1993.
6. Javadi MA, Jafarinasab MR, Araghi AA, Mohammadpour M, Yazdani S.Outcomes of phacoemulsification and in-the-bag intraocular lens implantation in Fuchs' heterochromic iridocyclitis. J Cataract Refract Surg. 2005 May; 31(5):997–1001.
7. O'Neill D, Murray PI, Patel BC, Hamilton AM.Extracapsular cataract surgery with and without intraocular lens implantation in Fuchs heterochromic cyclitis.Ophthalmology. 1995 Sep; 102(9):1362–8.
8. Ram J, Jain S, Pandav SS: Postoperative complications of intraocular lens implantation in patients with Fuchs' heterochromic cyclitis. J Cataract Refract Surg 21: 548–51, 1995.
9. Kaplan I IJ, Foster CS, Fong LP et al: Cataract surgery and intraocular lens implantation in patients with uveitis. Ophthalmology 96: 287–88, 1989.
10. Moorthy RS, Rajeev B, Smith RE et al: Incidence and management of cataract in Vogt-Koyangi-Harada syndrome. Am J Ophthalmol 118:197–204, 1994.
11. Tabbara KF, Chavis PS.Cataract extraction in Behçet's disease.Ocul Immunol Inflamm. 1997 Mar; 5(1):27–32.
12. Alio JL, Chipont E: Multicentrical IOIS study on surgery of cataract in the uveitic patient. First combined International symposium on Ocular Immunology and Inflammation. Amsterdam June 1998 (Personal communication).
13. Hooper PL, Rao N: Cataract extraction in uveitis patients. Surv Ophthalmol 35:120–45, 1990.
14. Alio JL, Ben Ezra D, Chipont E: Cataract in patients with uveitis. Symposium on Cataract IOL and Refractive Surgery, Seattle 1999 (Personal communication).
15. Alio JL, Chipont E: Inflammacion en Cirugia de la catarata. Inflamaciones Culares EDIKAMED (Ed): Barcelona 407–28, 1995.
16. Akova YA, Küçükerdönmez C, Gedik S.Clinical results of phacoemulsification in patients with uveitis. Ophthalmic Surg Lasers Imaging. 2006 May-Jun; 37(3):204–11.
17. Chaudhry NA, Cohen KA, Flynn HW Jr, Murray TG. Combined pars plana vitrectomy and lens management in complex vitreoretinal disease. Semin Ophthalmol. 2003 Sep; 18(3):132–41. Review.
18. Androudi S, Ahmed M, Fiore T, Brazitikos P, Foster CS. Combined pars plana vitrectomy and phacoemulsification to restore visual acuity in patients with chronic uveitis. J Cataract Refract Surg 2005;31:472–8.
19. Demetriades AM, Gottsch JD, Thomsen R, Azab A, Stark WJ, Campochiaro PA, et al . Combined phacoemulsification, intraocular lens implantation and vitrectomy for eyes with coexisting cataract and vitreoretinal pathology. Am J Ophthalmol 2003; 135:291–6.
20. Alio JL, Chipont E, Sayans JA: Flare-cell metre measurement of inflammation after uneventful cataract surgery with intraocular lens implantation. J Cataract Refract Surg 23:935–39, 1997.
21. Lowenstein A, Bracha R, Lazer I: Intraocular lens implantation in an eye with Behcet's uveitis. J Cataract Refract Surg 17:95–97, 1991.
22. Percival SPB, Pai V: Heparin-modified lenses for eyes at risk for breakdown of the blood-aqueous barrier during cataract surgery. J Cataract Refrc Surg 19:760–65, 1993.
23. Drews RC: Lens implantation lessons learned from the first million. Trans Ophthalmol Soc UK 102:505–09, 1982.
24. Alio JL, Sayans J, Chipont E: Laser flare-cell measurement of inflammation after uneventful extracapsular cataract extraction and intraocular lens implantation. J Cataract Refract Surg 22:775–79, 1996.
25. Martinez JJ, Artola A, Chipont E: Total anterior capsule closure after silicone intraocular lens implantation. J Cataract Refract Surg 22:269–71, 1996.
26. Palmer SS: Mitomycin as an adjunct chemotherapy with trabeculectomy. Ophthalmology 98:317–21, 1991.
27. Wolnetr B, Liebmann JM: Late bleb related endophthalmitis after trabeculectomy with adjunctive 5 Fluorouracil. Ophthalmology 98:1053–60, 1991.
28. Hill RA, Nguyen QH: Trabeculectomy and Molteno implantation for glaucomas associated with uveitis. Ophthalmology 93:903–08, 1993.
29. Koening SB, Han DP, Msfieler WF: Combined phacoemulsification and pars plana vitrectomy. Arch Ophthalmol 108:362–64, 1990.
30. MacKool RJ: Pars plana vitrectomy and posterior chamber intraocular lens implantation in diabetic patients. Ophthalmology 96:1679–80, 1989.
31. Jaanus SD: Anti-inflammatory drugs. In Bartlett JD, Jaanus SD (Eds): Clinical Ocular Pharmacology. Butterworth Publishers: Boston 163–97, 1989.
32. Herbort CP, Mermoud A: Anti-inflammatory effect of Diclofenac drops after argon laser trabeculoplasty. Arch Ophthalmol 111:481–83, 1993.
34. Othenin P, Borruat X: Association diclofenac-dexamethasone dans le traitement de inflammation postoperatorie. Klin Monatsbl Augenheilkd 200: 362–66, 1992.
35. Akova YA, Foster CS: Cataract surgery in patients with sarcoidosis-associated uveitis. Ophthalmology 101: 473–79, 1994.

40

Phacoemulsification in Vitrectomised Eyes

Col JKS Parihar, SM, VSM and Dr Sheshadri Mahajan

INTRODUCTION

Cataract formation and progression is a common event after pars plana vitrectomy (PPV). Up to 76% of patients undergoing PPV, experience cataract progression within 2 years. With the ever widening application of vitrectomy, one can expect an increase in the number of such cataracts referred to a general ophthalmologist. Phacoemulsification in such cases is a challenging task because of various anatomical changes within the eye such as a miotic pupil, posterior synechiae, deeper anterior chamber, unstable lens zonules, posterior capsular plaque, and positive pressure. These peculiarities present a higher incidence of complications than those performed in nonvitrectomised eyes.

Manual extracapsular extraction is difficult when performing an expression because of the absence of vitreous counter pressure. During expression, vitreous fluid may flow away through the corneoscleral wound leaving the nucleus in situ or even displacing it backward. The loss of intraocular fluid may lead to a posterior segment collapse. In cases of viscoexpression, the surgeon can get into the same situation. During phacoemulsification, these problems are not encountered because it provides better control of the fluid dynamics, so the risk of hypotony is minimised. Phacoemulsification is the best solution nowadays, and is increasingly used for cataract surgery on vitrectomised eyes, but the surgical procedure is always a great challenge even in skilled and experienced hands.

RISK FACTORS FOR THE DEVELOPMENT OF CATARACT IN VITRECTOMISED EYES

1. Preexisting cataractous changes
2. Secondary to the use of tamponading agents such as C3F8 or silicone oil
3. Progression of cataract in the long term follow up period.
4. Intraoperative lens touch
5. Diabetic patients

PREOPERATIVE EVALUATION

Preoperative evaluation should include slit lamp evaluation of lens, the detailed operative steps of vitreoretinal surgery, type of vitrectomy (core/ base excision), intraoperative areas of lens touch and vitreous substitute (saline/silicone oil). Isolated Traumatic Vitreous Haemorrhage, Vitreous Haemorrhage with Retained IOFB, Post Eales, Diabetic Retinopathy and Post RD surgery are common causes of Vitrectomy.

Investigations such as ultrasonography B scan in case of a dense cataract, UBM to note the status of the zonules in cases of silicone oil filled eyes with cataract and migration of the oil bubble in the anterior chamber are mandatory in addition to a thorough clinical work up.

CALCULATION OF INTRAOCULAR LENS POWER IN POST VITRECTOMY EYES

Calculation of Intraocular Lens Power in post vitrectomy eyes particularly in the presence of Silicon oil deserves special attention and require certain modifications in A-Scan settings and the calculation of presumed IOL power. The presence of Silicone oil attenuates sound velocity which gives a false impression of an elongated and a large eyeball. Hence IOL power calculation remains compromised in these situations. However, IOL power calculation is not difficult to measure in the absence of silicone oil in the vitrectomised eyes. Since pre-existing posterior segment pathology invariably influences functional results, an empirical estimate of the lens power may be sufficient.

In cases where concurrent or subsequent removal of silicone oil is planned, the axial length pertaining to the fellow eye is an ideal choice in calculating suitable presumed IOL power in the silicon filled eye.

However, if concurrent removal of silicon oil is not considered, certain modifications in calculation of power as described by Meldrum et al is worth considering. As per his method, refractive index of the silicon oil needs to be kept in mind.

SELECTION OF AN IOL IMPLANT

Undoubtedly, in-the-bag hydrophobic IOL implant remains the most preferred choice over any other acrylic or PMMA IOL implants. However, in cases of unfavourable situations like a posterior capsule rupture, the sulcus fixated IOL remains a good option.

While considering an IOL, silicone material based IOL implants are not preferred since such IOL implants are invariably prone to develop incompatibility between the IOL material and silicone oil. Over and above, the persistent touch and friction between the silicone based IOL implant and silicone oil are likely to trigger irreversible adherence of silicone oil droplets on the posterior surface of the IOL which may result in poor and distorted visual recovery.

SURGICAL TECHNIQUE

Phacoemulsification can be done as a sole procedure or combined with silicone oil removal.

Phacoemulsification Combined with Silicone Oil Removal

In combined cases, silicone oil is preferably removed first through pars plana sclerotomies made 3.5 mm from the limbus and an infusion cannula fixed in the inferotemporal quadrant. At the end of the oil removal, the upper quadrant sclerotomies are closed. We prefer to leave the infusion cannula in place till the completion of IOL implantation in the bag in such cases, as it gives us the advantage in case of inadvertent complications during phacoemulsification. Few surgeons prefer phacoemulsification prior to silicone oil removal and in our view management of intraoperative complications during phacoemulsification in such cases becomes tedious.

Poor fundus glow in silicone filled eyes is expected. Scleral tunnel incision gives an advantage of closed chamber dynamics but might not be feasible in cases with previous multiple PPV surgeries, wherein sclera is scarred and thinned at the sclerotomy sites. Clear corneal incision helps in easy manoeuvreing in such cases. However some surgeons avoid corneal tunnels in diabetic patients owing to concerns over an increased risk of delayed healing and epithelial complications. Intra operative abnormal deepening of the anterior chamber and wide pupillary dilatation is a universal phenomenon in vitrectomised eyes. Several explanations have been proposed for this phenomenon and range from the loss of vitreous scaffolding to the stretching of zonules by expansile gas and damage to the zonular apparatus during base excision vitrectomy. Capsulorrhexis should not be excessively large as an unstable anterior chamber increases the risk of extension of capsulorrhexis margin. Rarely, an inelastic anterior capsule in silicone oil filled eyes is a messy problem. Forceful hydrodissection can immediately terminate in lens dislocation. Zonular laxity particularly poses a constant threat at each stage of phacoemulsification. Decreasing the bottle height and changing the vacuum settings might not help with certainty. The so-called 'infusion deviation syndrome' can be observed in a few cases where initial deepening of the anterior chamber is followed by sudden and unpredictable shallowing. Paradoxically, increasing the bottle height so as to improve fluid inflow aggravates the problem. Minimising the bottle height and in-the-bag phaco seems to be the solution to the latter problem. Phacomachine with settings that prevent post occlusion surge is a safer bet in vitrectomised eyes. Liberal use of viscoelastics helps in maintaining the anterior chamber stability. Cortical aspiration needs to be done at a lower aspiration rate so as to avoid capturing flaccid posterior capsule. Posterior capsular plaque is the commonest encountered problem. Post surgery Yag-Capsulotomy is preferred unless a very thick plaque necessitates primary posterior capsulotomy after IOL implantation. Fundus examination with indirect ophthalmoscopy is a must before implanting an IOL. Silicone IOLs are best avoided, in view of chances of retinal surgery with oil infusion in future, whereas acrylic foldable IOLs are the preferred choice. Ensuring non leaking incisions at the end reduce the chances of postoperative hypotony.

Phacoemulsification as a Sole Procedure

Phacoemulsification surgery through a clear corneal incision and direct chop technique is preferred by the principal author in cases of moderate to hard cataract. Sculpting remains practically impossible in such situations, due to the unusual mobility and flaccidity of the capsular bag probably due to the absence of a tough vitreous cushion. Over and above, per operative zonular stress is a constraint with sculpting while handling this peculiar type of cataract. Flip and Chip technique should be given consideration in cases of a soft cataract.

Peroperative Constraints

The incidence of surgical problems and complications is invariably higher in post vitrectomy eyes compared to the standard cataract cases. Most common intraoperative observations and constraints faced by the authors are as under:

Rigid and Miotic Pupil (less than 3.5 mm)

In addition to the vitrectomised condition of eyes, pre-existing glaucoma and posterior segment involvement are also responsible for inadequate and ill sustained preoperative mydriasis. If, intracameral adrenaline and other conventional modes do not help, the anterior chamber infusion may result in adequate mydriasis in addition to a deep anterior chamber. However, the author prefers to go ahead with mechanical stretching devices.

Posterior Synechiae

The presence of posterior synechiae may lead to poor dilatation of the pupil. The use of mechanical pupillary stretching devices like iris hooks are a good option in these situations.

Fragile Texture of Anterior Capsule with Adhered Cortex

Fragile texture of the anterior capsule along with capsular adherence to the cortex entails a trypan Blue assisted Capsulorrhexis.

Abnormal Depth of AC Following Visco Administration

Abnormal depth of the AC following visco administration is a major constraint during the Phacoemulsification procedure mainly during capsulorrhexis.

Unprecedented and sudden changes in the anterior chamber depth and pupillary size during surgery are frequent occurrences. Irrigation and aspiration of sticky and cheesy cortex is also very difficult due to the same reasons.

Complications

(a) Intraoperative

   (i) Unprecedented and sudden changes in the anterior chamber depth and pupillary size during surgery.
  (ii) Significant difficulty while performing sculpting due to unusual mobility and flaccidity of the capsular bag probably due to the absence of tough vitreous cushion.
 (iii) Hyphaema.
 (iv) Pupillary sphincter injury or atony.
  (v) Posterior capsular tear.
 (vi) Nucleus drop.
(vii) Vitreous haemorrhage.

(b) Postoperative

(i) Immediate
  • Higher chances of corneal oedema in the immediate postoperative period could be due to a higher incidence of nuclear sclerosis in vitrectomised eyes which requires longer phaco time.
  • Postoperative uveitis (Mild to moderate)

  • Dispersion of uveal pigment in all types of IOL implants, however they are less in frequency and severity with hydrophobic IOL implantation.
  • Secondary glaucoma
  • Vitreous haemorrhage
  • Endophthalmitis
  • Macular oedema

(ii) Delayed
  • Corneal oedema (could be due to a higher incidence of nuclear sclerosis in vitrectomised eyes which requires a longer phaco time).
  • Macular oedema
  • Vitreous haemorrhage
  • Endophthalmitis
  • Retinal detachment
  • Posterior capsular opacity is the most common long term complication.
  • Peaking pupil
  • Ocular hypertension and Seidel phenomenon are relatively uncommon.

Visual Results

Moderate myopic shift of around one to two dioptres is expected despite meticulous IOL power calculation. In our experience, altered position of an IOL and capsular bag due to lack of vitreous support in post vitrectomy eyes may be responsible for this phenomenon. However, we designed our own modifications in biometry for subsequent IOL power calculations by readjusting this probable myopic shift to minimise induced myopia by predicting two dioptre of myopia in our remaining cases which has resulted in gratifying post phaco refractive status. However, overall compromised visual acuity of less than 6/12 is a known fact and probably considered as a good visual outcome. The extent of improvement may be limited by retinal co-morbidity, intraoperative constraints, and unexpected postoperative behaviour.

CONCLUSION

Cataract surgery after pars plana vitrectomy is a challenge for the anterior segment surgeon even with skilled hands and experience. Phacoemulsification in vitrectomised eyes has a higher incidence of intra and postoperative complications and constraints as compared to phacoemulsification in uncomplicated cataract. However, phaco with foldable IOL implantation is undoubtedly, preferred over conventional manual extra capsular surgery since closed chamber surgical technique imposes less risk of intra-op complications like choroidal haemorrhage due to sudden and profuse hypotony. The surgeon must be aware of the morphological and anatomical findings of these eyes. An alert phaco surgeon anticipating problems at each step would rarely need a backup vitreoretinal surgeon during phacoemulsification in postvitrectomised eyes.

Visual rehabilitation will generally be determined by the presence of underlying vitreo-retinal pathology. Considering the overall scenario, phacoemulsification is a safe and effective technique in eyes after pars plana vitrectomy that requires cataract surgery.

REFERENCES

1. Ahfat FG et al. Phacoemulsification and intraocular lens implantation following pars plana vitrectomy: a prospective study. Eye. 2003 Jan; 17 (1):16–20.
2. Miller KM et al. Phacoemulsification and lens implantation after pars plana vitrectomy. Ophthalmology.1998 Feb; 105 (2):287–94.
3. Chang MA, Parides MK, Chang S, Braunstein RE :Outcome of phacoemulsification after pars plana vitrectomy. Ophthalmology. 2002 May; 109 (5):948–54.
4. Murube J et al. Phacoemulsification in previously vitrectomised patients: an analysis of the surgical results in 100 eyes as well as the factors contributing to the cataract formation. Eur J Ophthalmol. 2006 Jan-Feb; 16 (1):52–9.
5. Villar Kuri J et al. Phacoemulsification cataract surgery in vitrectomised eyes. Arch Soc Esp Oftalmol. 2004 Nov; 79 (11):531–6.
6. Cekic O, Batman C. Phacoemulsification cataract surgery in vitrectomised eyes. J Cataract Refract Surg. 1999 Mar; 25 (3):305.
7. Yeoh R. Phacoemulsification in vitrectomised eyes. J Cataract Refract Surg. 1999 Aug; 25 (8):1038.
8. Diaz Lacalle V et al. Phacoemulsification cataract surgery in vitrectomised eyes. J Cataract Refract Surg. 1998 Jun; 24(6):806–9.
9. Leung ATS, Lam DSC, Rao SK: Phacoemulsification after vitrectomy (letter). J Cataract Refract Surg 1999,25: 1176.
10. McDermott, ML, Puklin, JE, Abrams GW et al: Phacoemulsification for cataract following pars plana vitrectomy. Ophthalmic Surgery and Lasers1997, 28: 558–647.
11. Grusha YO, Masket S, Miller KM: Phacoemulsification and lens implantation after pars plana vitrectomy. Ophthalmology 1998,105: 287–94.
12. Neuhann T: Overcoming the challenge of cataract surgery in vitrectomised eyes. 13th Symposium of the Greek Intraocular Implant and Refractive Surgery Society Athens, 1999.
13. Saunders DC, Brown AJ. Extracapsular cataract extraction after vitrectomy. J Cataract Refract Surg 1996; 22:218.221.
14. Smiddy WE, Stark WJ, Michales RG et al. Cataract extraction after vitrectomy. Ophthalmology 1998;94:483–7.
15. Sneed S, Parrish RK II, Mandelbaum S., et al: Technical problems of extracapsular cataract extraction after vitrectomy (letter). Arch Ophthalmol 1986,104: 1126–27.
16. Moisseiev J, Bartov E, Cahane M et al: Cataract extraction in eyes filled with silicone oil. Arch Ophthalmol 1992, 110: 1649–51.
17. Meldrum ML, Aaberg TM, Patel A et al: Cataract extraction after silicone oil repair of retinal detachments due to necrotising retinitis. Arch Ophthalmol 1996, 114: 885–92.
18. Shugar JK, de Juan E, Machemer R: Ultrasonic examination of the silicone filled eye: theoretic and practical considerations. Graefe's Arch clin Exp Ophthalmol 1986,224:361–67.
19. Jonas J, Budde WM, Songhomitra Panda-Jonas: Cataract surgery combined with transpupillary silicone oil removal through planned posterior capsulotomy. Ophthalmology 1996, 105: 1234–8.
20. Tanner V, Haider A, Rosen P: Phacoemulsification and combined management of Intraocular silicone oil. J Cataract Refract Surg 1998,24: 585–91.
21. Kusaka S, Kodama T, Ohashi Y: Condensation of silicone oil on the posterior surface of silicone intraocular lens during vitrectomised eyes. Am J Ophthalmol 1996,121: 574–75.
22. Apple DJ, Federmann JL, Krolicki TJ et al: Irreversible silicone oil adhesion to silicone intraocular lenses. A clinico-pathologic analysis. Ophthalmology 1996,103: 1555–61.
23. Ando F: Intraocular hypertension resulting from pupillary block by silicone oil. Am J Ophthalmol 1985,99: 87–88.
24. Hutton WL, Pesacka GA; Fuller DG. Cataract extraction in the diabetic eye after vitrectomy. Am J Ophthalmology 1987; 104:1–4.
25. Boyd Benjamín. Facoemulsificación. Highlights of Ophthalmology. 1995:65–99.
26. Batman C. Phacoemulsification cataract surgery in vitrectomised eyes, (Letter). J Cataract Refract Surg 1999;25(Mar):305.
27. Sha YO, MASKET S. Phaco and lens implantation after pars plana vitrectomy. Ophthalmology 1998; 105(Feb):287–293.
28. Pinter S, Sugar A. Phacoemulsification in eyes with past pars plana vitrectomy. J Cataract Refract Surg 1999;25(Apr):556–61.
29. Melberg NS, Thomas MA. Nuclear sclerotic cataract after vitrectomy in patients younger than 50 years of age. Ophthalmology 1995;102:1466–1471.
30. Tielsch JM, Legro MW, Cassard SD et al. Risk factors for retinal detachment after cataract surgery. Ophthalmology 1996; 103:1537–45.
31. Blakenship GW, Machermer R. Long term diabetic vitrectomy results. Report of 10–year follow-up. Ophthalmology 1985;92:503–6.
32. Novak MA, Rice TA, Michels RG, Auer C. The crystalline lens after vitrectomy for diabetic retinopathy. Ophthalmology 1984; 91:1480–4.
33. Margheiro RR, Cox MS Jr, Trese MT et al. Removal of epimacular membranes. Ophthalmology 1985;92:1075–83.
34. Koeenig SB, Han DP, Mieler WF et al. Combined phacoemulsification and pars plana vitrectomy. Arch Ophthalmol 1990;108: 362.4.

41

Phacoemulsification in Postkeratoplasty Cataract

Prof SK Angra FAMS, Col JKS Parihar SM, VSM, and Dr Vivek Angra

INTRODUCTION

Simultaneous cataract and corneal surgery is indicated in those cases in which coexisting disease reduces vision to unacceptable levels. It may also be indicated for those patients in whom subsequent cataract surgery is likely to result in corneal decompensation or in whom corneal surgery is likely to accelerate cataract formation. In general, simultaneous surgery is preferred as the patient is subjected to a single surgical exposure. However, this may not be indicated in all cases where isolated corneal opacity with clear lens is present, such cases may be subjected to keratoplasty alone. Another noted problem associated with combined cataract and corneal surgery is the calculation of presumptive intraocular lens power to be implanted in such cases as it may not be possible to calculate the corneal curvature of the eye to be operated upon due to the presence of corneal opacity, irregular curvature and altered length of the eyeball due to presence of a corneal scar. The final refractive status depends on the corneal curvature, power of the IOL and the axial length of the eye. For a simple cataract extraction, the major variable is the IOL power. However, following PK (penetrating keratoplasty), this remains highly uncertain owing to the high and irregular astigmatism following PK. Over and above, post PK cataract extraction may provide an opportunity to overcome annoying post PK astigmatism as well as to refashion refractive status of eye according to post PK astigmatism by adjustment in IOL power calculation during subsequent surgery. Logically, small incision phacoemulsification (phaco) with flexible IOL implantation should be a better choice in these cases, considering least adverse optical effect on corneal graft, as well as minimal surgically induced astigmatism, However, adverse impact on the graft status both pre and postoperatively in the form of intra-operative endothelial trauma, postoperative complications and graft behaviour have to be evaluated.

MERITS

The advantage of post PK phaco is the more precise and stable refractive status. This approach is considered more safe by some surgeons and allows adjustment of the IOL power to the power of the actual corneal graft. Other advantages include reduced chances of suprachoroidal effusion and expulsive haemorrhage as it is not an open sky surgery.

CONSTRAINTS AND DEMERITS

Cataract surgery in postkeratoplasty patients needs extra precautions, as the risk of graft failure is high. The disadvantages of post PK phaco include corneal graft decompensation, secondary glaucoma, uveitis, corneal oedema and repeat keratoplasty.

Special Considerations

Biometry

The average central spherical equivalent power of an 8.0 mm donor graft in an 8.0 mm recipient bed is generally stable from one month after penetrating keratoplasty until suture removal. It is also important to perform preoperative corneal topography. A two-stage procedure with cataract surgery performed 3 months after PK, as compared to the triple procedure, reduces postoperative ametropia at 12 months, if graft topography is taken into consideration at the time of cataract surgery. Keratometry is helpful for giving us the idea of the extent of the cylinder, but topography is important for quantifying and localising it. One can then treat the cylinder during the surgery, varying the site of incision and using limbal relaxing incisions. IOL power calculated should be so adjusted that it minimises keratoplasty induced astigmatism upto 1.5 to 2.5 D.

How to Reduce Astigmatism

Small incision: The smaller astigmatically neutral incisions enable us to deal more accurately during cataract surgery with preexisting astigmatism. Phaco incision is 3 mm wide, ECCE incision is 10–12 mm wide. Induced astigmatism is proportional to incision length. Phaco is obviously better.

Astigmatic keratotomy: These are additional incisions, usually paired, placed on the steep meridian of astigmatism. These cause flattening of the steep meridian. Relaxing incisions into the steep meridian of the cornea (arcuate keratotomy or limbal relaxing incisions) are useful for reducing up to 5 dioptres of preexisting astigmatism.

Toric IOLs: Another way of correcting preexisting astigmatism during cataract surgery is to use a new "toric" intraocular lens into which the astigmatism correction has already been incorporated. This lens has to be placed in the proper meridian. It is a nice but expensive and difficult to use idea because even a slight misalignment between the axis of the IOL and the axis of the astigmatism will cause an unpredictable refractive outcome.

Place incision on steep meridian: Any surgical incision made in the cornea weakens the cornea causing flattening. Flattening reduces the focusing power of cornea. The amount of flattening is proportional to the incision depth, length and closeness to the corneal apex. These parameters can all be manipulated by the surgeon. The surgeon will place the incision on the steepest meridian of cornea power (at 90 degree to the axis of the astigmatism on refraction).

For patients with even greater astigmatism, limbal relaxing incisions can be made several weeks before cataract surgery, followed by the insertion of a toric intraocular lens to treat the residual astigmatism. In addition, LASIK (laser in-situ keratomileusis) can be used to pretreat corneal astigmatism and can be combined with limbal relaxing incisions, toric intraocular lenses or a combination of all the three.

Role of Ocular Viscoelastic Devices (OVD)

During phacoemulsification, an OVD that satisfies the following requirements should be used:

(a) **Persistence in the anterior chamber and maintenance of an adequate chamber depth:** The dispersive OVDs are better. The cohesive substances, on the other hand, tend to escape in block, once the irrigation and the surgical maneuvers have caused an increase in the shear rate.

(b) **Protection of the intraocular surfaces:** In particular the endothelium, from the damage caused by the ultrasound emission, the nuclear fragments, the liquid flow, etc. The greater adhesive properties of OVDs, like viscoat play an important role from this point of view.

(c) **During aspiration of cortex**, the surgeon should use an OVD that will persist in the anterior chamber (to protect the endothelium) despite the high liquid flow.

(d) **During implantation of an IOL,** an OVD must maintain the spaces in the anterior chamber (and avoid traumatic contact of the IOL with the cornea and the iris). The ideal OVD should maintain good aperture of the capsular bag during all the implantation maneuvers.

(e) **The effects of the residual OVD** on the intraocular pressure during the early postoperative period, are well-known. As a result, it is essential that the surgeon performs an accurate and complete aspiration of the OVDs at the end of phaco to prevent graft failure due to early postoperative rise in IOP.

Surgical Technique

Visual acuity, refractive status and central corneal endothelial cell density should be taken into consideration before contemplating this procedure. Various studies have recommended that cataract surgery with IOL implantation can take place from 3 months after penetrating keratoplasty. Preoperatively, the patient should be started on topical prednisolone acetate 1% (6 times a day) and preferably systemic prednisolone (2 mg/kg).

Anaesthesia

Local anaesthesia using peribulbar anaesthesia technique, comprising lignocaine hydrochloride and bupivacaine injections should be used for adult patients, children should be taken up under general anaesthesia.

Incision

Extensive subconjunctival scarring, sometimes makes it very difficult to raise a conjunctival flap and the anatomy of the limbus is not well defined. The site of incision should be selected with a view to minimise any possible damage

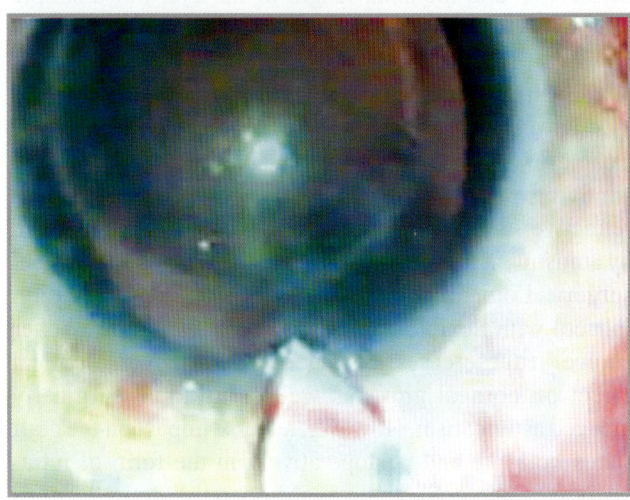

Fig. 41.1: Post PK phaco: Incision

to the limbal grafts. Most of the times it is difficult to raise a conjunctival flap due to extensive scarring in the subconjunctival tissues. A linear 3.2 mm posterior limbal incision is a very good option.

Extreme caution has to be exercised for construction of the wound because of difficult visualisation of the intracorneal dissection of the tunnel. A clear corneal entry is better in terms of visualisation but carries a risk of damage to the graft endothelium.

Rhexis

A small 4 mm sized, continuous curvilinear anterior capsulorrhexis (CCC) is made with the help of a cystitome, as a small rhexis protects the graft endothelium from damage.

Rhexis should be done, preferably after staining the anterior capsule with trypan blue under air cushion, to enhance visualisation of capsule.

Nucleotomy

The technique of nucleotomy, by and large, depends upon the surgeon's own preference as well as on the density of the nucleus. A surgeon should aim intercapsular phacoemulsification so as to avoid any undue insult to the corneal endothelium and prevent subsequent loss of endothelial cells. The author has preferential inclination towards the phaco chop technique, as less power is used in this maneuver. Thus, chances of endothelial damage and consequently graft failure are much less. However, a well practised sculpting can also provide excellent results.

Excellent rhexis and adequate hydroprocedures followed by moderate application of ultrasonic energy accompanied by low vacuum and moderate aspiration remain the most vital combination to achieve the best outcome in the presence of a graft.

Irrigation/Aspiration

Low aspiration flow rate and vacuum should be used as it reduces the turbulence within the anterior chamber during phacoemulsification and decreases endothelial cell loss. Phacoaspiration should be performed through a superotemporal posterior limbal incision with the corneal valve. The bottle height should be adjusted in such a way as that it prevents collapse of the anterior chamber during the surgery.

The viscoelastic should be completely aspirated out with the help of an I/A handpiece and the anterior chamber should be reformed with the help of BSS. Bimanual I/A is more suitable in the presence of graft, in terms of controlled aspiration and irrigation from all the quadrants that too without compromising the graft safety.

IOL Implantation

Single piece hydrophobic acrylic foldable intraocular lens is a safe choice of IOL in these cases. However, PMMA

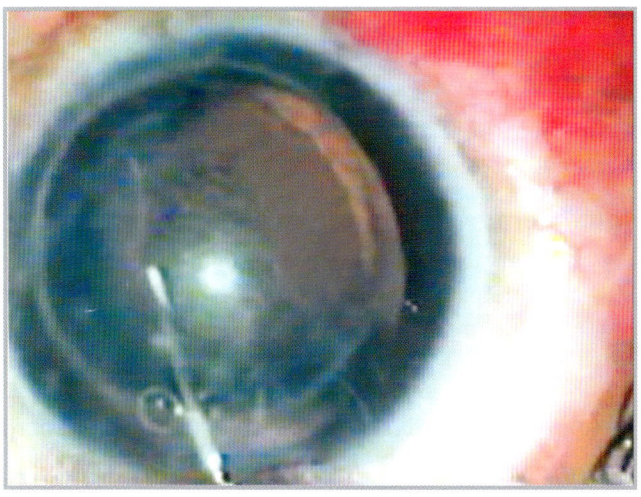

Fig. 41.2: Post PK phaco: Rhexis

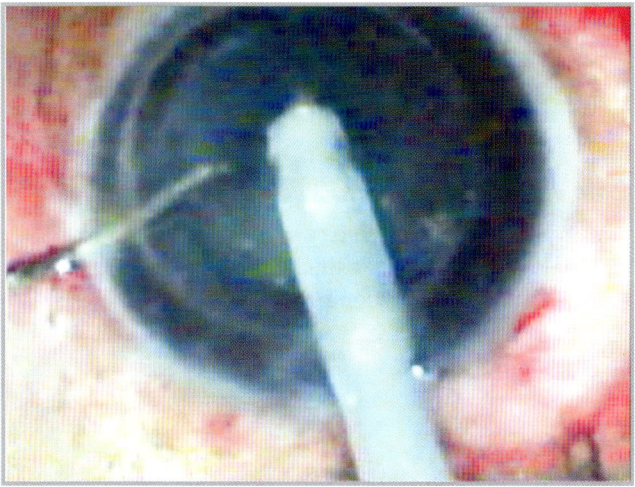

Fig. 41.3: Post PK phaco: Nucleotomy

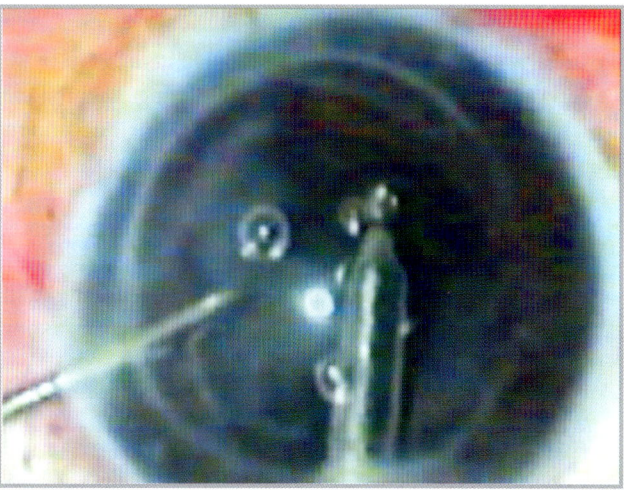

Fig. 41.4: Post PK phaco: Irrigation/aspiration

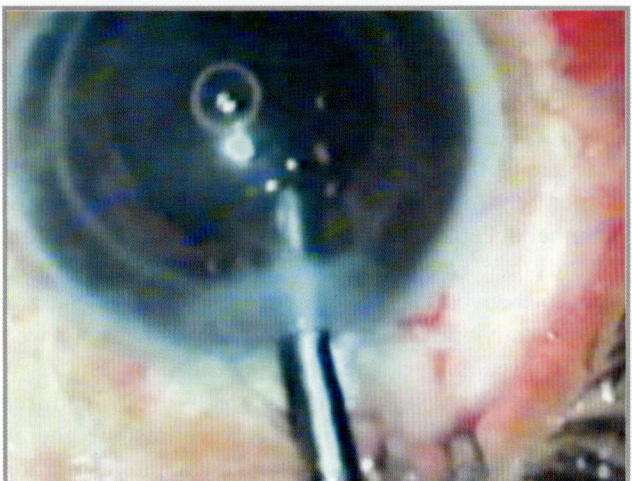

Fig. 41.5: Post PK phaco: IOL implantation

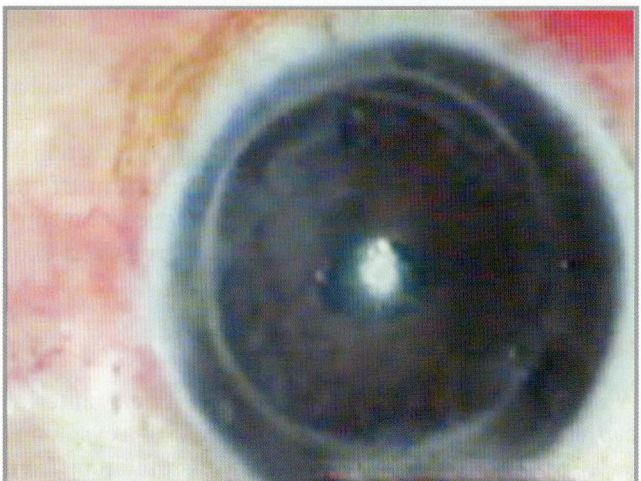

Fig. 41.6: Post PK phaco: IOL implantation is in situ

lenses can also be used in certain situations where posterior capsule is compromised. Cataract surgery with toric intraocular lenses allows the correction of a high degree of regular corneal astigmatism. By implanting a toric IOL, the overall astigmatism is reduced on an average to less than 1 D. The implantation of a foldable toric IOL (MS-6116-TU; Human optics) is a safe and predictable procedure to correct high preexisting corneal astigmatism (>2.0 D) in cataract surgery.

Postoperative Management

Postoperatively, all patients may be subjected to systemic as well as frequent topical instillation of steroids, cycloplegics and ocular hypotensives at least for a period of eight to twelve weeks. Topical steroids should be continued in a low dose for another period of one year as indicated in other post PK cases. In cases of steroid induced glaucoma, immunosuppressant can be added and steroids can be tapered off.

Postoperative Evaluation

Postoperatively patients should be evaluated for:
  (i) Corneal thickness /endothelial changes which can predict the impending corneal graft decompensation.
 (ii) Primary graft failure
(iii) Intraocular pressure: any increase should be treated promptly and aggressively
(iv) Macular oedema, if present, should be treated with nonsteroidal antiinflammatory drugs or a short course of oral steroids.

Follow-up

Postoperative followup should preferably be for a longer period to evaluate visual acuity, refraction, graft status including graft clarity, any evidence of uveitis, glaucoma, positioning of IOLs, posterior capsular thickening or any other complications or other significant observations, if any.

Astigmatism can be corrected by suture removal and relaxing the incision.

Complications

Complications of phacoemulsification following keratoplasty can be divided into:

Intraoperative

  (a) Injury to corneal endothelium which can occur while placing the graft on the recipient button or while implanting IOL
  (b) Posterior capsular rupture can occur due to decreased visibility
  (c) Zonular dialysis due to small rhexis and hard cataract

Immediate Postoperative

  (a) Uveitis
  (b) Secondary glaucoma
  (c) Mild striate
  (d) Primary graft failure/rejection
  (e) Macular oedema

Late Postoperative

  (a) Secondary glaucoma
  (b) Posterior capsular thickening
  (c) Late corneal decompensation
  (d) Macular oedema
  (e) High astigmatism

Visual Outcome

Visual results of cataract surgery following penetrating keratoplasty are definitely superior to those following concurrent cataract surgery and optical keratoplasty. Combining a repeat keratoplasty for a failed graft with the cataract surgery does not significantly affect the final outcome.

Though there is no significant difference in the optical clarity of post PK graft status following cataract surgery, the impending threat to graft endothelium due to obvious exposure of subsequent intraocular surgery remains unpredicted until extended follow-up is being observed .

Alternative Technique for Cataract Removal in Post PK Cases

Aqualase Cataract Removal

(i) As there is no ultrasonic energy, there is no heat generated due to friction and thus, no chance of thermal damage at the incision site. Fluid pulses are capsule-friendly and will not break or tear the posterior capsule. On the other hand, the capsule can still be broken by vacuum, so care must be taken as with any intraocular procedure.

(ii) Another advantage of Aqualase is the reduced amount of cortex remaining after nuclear removal.

Hence lesser chances of postoperative rise in IOP and subsequent graft failure.

However, in hard cataracts (more than grade 3 the efficiency of Aqualase is still in evolution.

CONCLUSION

In-the-bag phacoemulsification with IOL implantation is a safe and effective approach in cases of post PK cataract. The refractive outcome is statistically and significantly better after post PK phacoemulsification as compared to concurrent phaco and keratoplasty due to more accurate IOL power calculation with post PK keratometry readings and better centration of it as well as effective control of induced astigmatism and myopia. However, predictability of such refractive outcome is not as good as in the non-corneal grafted eye. Despite several constraints, intracapsular (in-the-bag) phacoemulsification with IOL implantation remains the most effective and preferred option in such cases if the postpenetrating keratoplasty eye needs to undergo cataract surgery.

BIBLIOGRAPHY

1. Akpek EK, Altan-Yaycioglu R, Karadayi K, Christen W, Stark WJ. Long-term outcomes of combined penetrating keratoplasty with iris-sutured intraocular lens implantation. Ophthalmology. 2003 May; 110(5):1017–22.

2. Amm M, Halberstadt M. Implantation of toric intraocular lenses for correction of high post-keratoplasty astigmatism. Ophthalmologe. 2002 Jun; 99(6):464–9.

3. Arora R, Narayanan R, Jain S, Raina UK, Mehta DK. Phacoemulsification after penetrating keratoplasty with auto-logous limbal transplant and amniotic membrane transplant in chemical burns. Indian J Ophthalmol 2005; 53: 121–3.

4. Arshinoff SA. Dispersive-cohesive viscoelastic soft shell technique. J Cataract Refract Surg 1999; 25:167–73.

5. Böhringer D, Reinhard T, Spelsberg H, Sundmacher R. Posterior chamber lens implantation after penetrating keratoplasty. Is this partly responsible for late transplantation failure? Ophthalmologe. 2004 Nov; 101(11):1093–7.

6. Brunett I, Rinne JR, Gemmil M, Arch Ophthalmol 1994: 112 (10):1311–19

7. Binder PS. Intraocular lens implantation after penetrating keratoplasty. Refractive corneal surgery 1989, 5(4):224–30.

8. Caporossi A, Traversi C, Simi C, Tosi GM. Closed-system and open-sky capsulorrhexis for combined cataract extraction and corneal transplantation. J Cataract Refract Surg. 2001; 27:990–993.

9. Chiou AG, Bovet J, de Courten C. Management of corneal ectasia and cataract following photorefractive keratectomy. J Cataract Refract Surg. 2006 Apr; 32(4):679–80.

10. Chang, Daniel H, Hardten, David R. Refractive surgery after corneal transplantation. Current Opinion in Ophthalmology. 16(4):251–255, August 2005.

11. Davis EA, Azar DT, Jakobs FM & Stark WJ: Refractive and keratometric results after the triple procedure. Experience with early and late suture removal. Ophthalmology (1998):105: 624–630.

12. Farjo AA, Rhee DJ, Soong HK, Meyer RF, Sugar A. Iris-sutured posterior chamber intraocular lens implantation during penetrating keratoplasty: Cornea. 2004 Jan; 23(1): 18–28.

13. Green M, Chow A, Apel A. Outcomes of combined penetrating keratoplasty and cataract extraction compared with penetrating keratoplasty alone. Clin Experiment Ophthalmol. 2007 May-Jun; 35(4):324–9.

14. Geggel HS. Intraocular lens implantation after penetrating keratoplasty. Ophthalmology 1994; 101:113–9.

15. Hughes WF. The treatment of cornea dystrophies by keratoplasty. Am J Ophthalmol 1960;50:1100–14.

16. Hayashi K, Hayashi H. Simultaneous versus sequential penetrating keratoplasty and cataract surgery. Cornea. 2006 Oct; 25(9):1020–5.

17. Hjortdal JO, EhlersN, Erdmann L : Topography of corneal grafts before and after penetrating keratoplasty. Acta Ophthalmol Scand 1997, 75: 645–648.

18. Jiang Y, Le Q, Yang J, Lu Y. Changes in corneal astigmatism and high order aberrations after clear corneal tunnel phaco-emulsification guided by corneal topography. 1: J Refract Surg. 2006 Nov; 22(9 Suppl):S1083–8.

19. Jonas JB, Rank RM, Budde WM. Visual outcome after allogenic penetrating keratoplasty. Graefes Arch Clin Exp Ophthalmol. 2002 Apr; 240(4):302–7.

20. Jonas JB, Rank RM, Budde WM, Sauder G. Factors influencing visual outcome after penetrating keratoplasty

combined with intraocular lens implantation: Eur J Ophthalmol. 2003 Mar; 13(2):134–8.

21. Kersey James P, O'Donnell, Annie; Illingworth, Christopher D: Cornea. 26(2):133–135, February 2007.

22. Karabatsas CH, Cook SD, Powell K and Sparrow JM (1998): Comparison of keratometry and videokeratography after penetrating keratoplasty. J Refract Surg 14: 420–426.

23. Liesegang T, Bourne W, Ilstrup DM. Short and long term endothelial cell loss associated with cataract extraction and intraocular lens implantation. Am J Ophthalmol 1984; 97: 32–9.

24. Lindquist TD. Open-sky phacoemulsification during corneal transplantation. Ophthalmic Surg 1994; 25:734–6.

25. Muraine MC, Collet A, Brasseur G.. Deep lamellar keratoplasty combined with cataract surgery. Arch Ophthalmol. 2002 Jun; 120(6):812–5.

26. Malbran ES, Malbran E, Buonasanti J, Androgen E. Closed-system phacoemulsification and posterior chamber implant combined with penetrating keratoplasty. Ophthalmic Surg 1993; 24:403–6.

27. Price FW Jr, Whitson WE, Marks RG. Progression of visual acuity after penetrating keratoplasty: Ophthalmology. 1991 Aug; 98(8):1177–85.

28. Polack FM . Keratoplasty and intraocular lenses; Cornea1985: 4(3) : 137 – 47

29. Powe NR, Schein OD, Gieser SC, Tielsch JM, Luthra R, Javitt J. Synthesis of the literature on visual acuity and complications following cataract extraction with intraocular lens implantation. Arch Ophthalmol 1994; 112:239–52.

30. Robin H, Hannouche D, Hoang-Xuan T. Triple procedure with phacoemulsification prior to grafting. J Fr Ophthalmol 1997; 20: 701–3.

31. Rao SK, Padmanabhan P. Combined pahcoemulsification and penetrating keratoplasty. Ophthalmic Surg Lasers 1999; 30:488–91.

32. Schein OD, Kenyon KR, Steinert RF, Verdier DD, Seabrook S: A randomised trial of intraocular lens fixation technique with penetrating keratoplasty: Ophthalmology 1993: 100 (10): 1437–43.

33. Shi WY, Zeng QY, Li SW, Xie LX. Cataract extraction and intraocular lens implantation after high-risk penetrating keratoplasty. Zhonghua Yan Ke Za Zhi. 2003 Nov; 39(11): 678–82.

34. Shimmura S, Ohashi Y, Shiroma H, Shimazaki J, Tsubota K. Corneal opacity and cataract: triple procedure versus secondary approach : Cornea. 2003 Apr; 22(3):234–8.

35. Tahzib NG, Cheng YY, Nuijts RM. Three-year follow-up analysis of Artisan toric lens implantation for correction of post-keratoplasty ametropia in phakic and pseudophakic eyes. Ophthalmology. 2006 Jun; 113(6):976–84. Epub 2006 Apr 27.

36. Vail A, Gore SM, Bradley BA, Easty DL, Rogers CA, Armitage WJ. Clinical and surgical factors influencing corneal graft survival, visual acuity, and astigmatism. Ophthalmology 1996; 103:41–49.

42

Phacoemulsification Surgery in Cases of Congenital Anomalies

Col JKS Parihar SM, VSM, Lt Col Anirudh Singh and Lt Col Sandeep Gupta

INTRODUCTION

Congenital anomalies are rare but visually significant group of disorders which were considered beyond hope not a long time back due to the presence of a multitude of ocular pathologies, amblyopia, media opacities, subluxated lenses and vitreoretinal pathologies. However, with advances in technology especially in the form of phacoemulsification and its advanced variants and adjuvants, it is possible to visually rehabilitate these patients at an early stage to give them a reasonable chance of social acceptability.

The procedure of phacoemulsification has to be modified in these patients according to the presence of various anatomical variations in the ocular structures in these patients. A reasonable degree of proficiency in the techniques of phacoemulsification is also needed to manage various complications in these cases. In the following paragraphs, there is a brief description of different accepted techniques in these cases and our experiences with them.

CLASSIFICATION

The various congenital anomalies which are associated with cataract and may require special consideration and precautions while performing phacoemulsification are:

- (i) Coloboma
- (ii) Aniridia
- (iii) Microphthalmos and nanophthalmos
- (iv) Subluxated lenses associated with congenital anomalies
  - Marfan's syndrome
  - Weil Marchesani syndrome
  - Ehler Danlos syndrome
  - Reiger's syndrome
  - Ectopia lentis et pupillae.

Iris Coloboma

Phacoemulsification of intumescent cataract, IOL implantation and reconstruction of congenital iris coloboma through one anterior chamber superior opening is the accepted mode of treatment in today's scenario. Cataract surgery in most cases is performed through a superior incision. No major modification in surgical technique is needed while doing phacoemulsification except of being aware of the possibility of zonular absence and lens subluxation in these cases.

Congenital iris coloboma repair using the modified McCannel suture technique via the same incision is difficult but is a technique, which provides good cosmetic and functional results. In certain situations, repair of coloboma may be done through a separate incision or may be left as such, in cases of well placed in-the-bag IOL where a smaller rhexis is covering the optic margins and providing good centration of it.

There is efficacy of surgical implantation of prosthetic iris devices in patients with iris deficiency such as traumatic iris defects, iris coloboma, and surgical or optical iridectomies. In these patients, implantation of a prosthetic iris device like tinted capsular tension ring with an integrated 60–90 degrees sector shield (Morcher L & G), and intraocular lens implant following cataract surgery appears to be safe and effective in reducing glare disability and improving visual outcomes. If more than 90 degrees of defect is present, more than one capsular tension rings with shields can be used.

Coloboma of Lens

Typically, there is lower zonules deficiency and zonular weakness in one or both eyes, leading to suspicion of congenital coloboma of the lens or the coloboma is obvious. Capsular tension ring implantation improves cataractous lens rotation and phacodonesis, enabling central IOL implantation in the capsular bag. Capsular tension ring implantation can facilitate cataract surgery in coloboma of the lens, even in long-term and continuous lens capsule deformity.

Phacoemulsification in Eyes with Cataract and Congenital Coloboma

Clinically significant cataract develops at a younger age in eyes with congenital coloboma than in eyes with typical age-related nuclear sclerotic cataract. The cataract may have a dense hard nucleus despite the younger age of the patient. Hence, phacotechnique may be rescheduled to meet the need of nucleotomy which is invariably not required in the case of cataract in the younger age group where phacoaspiration may suffice the purpose. The presence of coloboma and a rigid pupil are added constraints during nucleotomy and subsequent cortical removal. The coloboma defects may be associated with zonular weakening or deficiency. Spontaneous and delayed subluxation or dislocation of IOL is a known complication of cataract surgery even after uncomplicated intraoperative period. Hence, CTR application should be performed as a part of the standard protocol. However, the timing of CTR insertion may be chosen at any stage depending upon the intraoperative need or the surgeon's own preference since most coloboma iris are not associated with pre-existing subluxation of the lens. We recommend CTR insertion just prior to the IOL implantation as a standard protocol. Monocular diplopia from exposure of the intraocular lens (IOL) edge within the typically inferonasally located corectopia associated with the coloboma, a potential complication after cataract surgery in these eyes, can be managed by pupilloplasty as a primary or secondary procedure, if warranted.

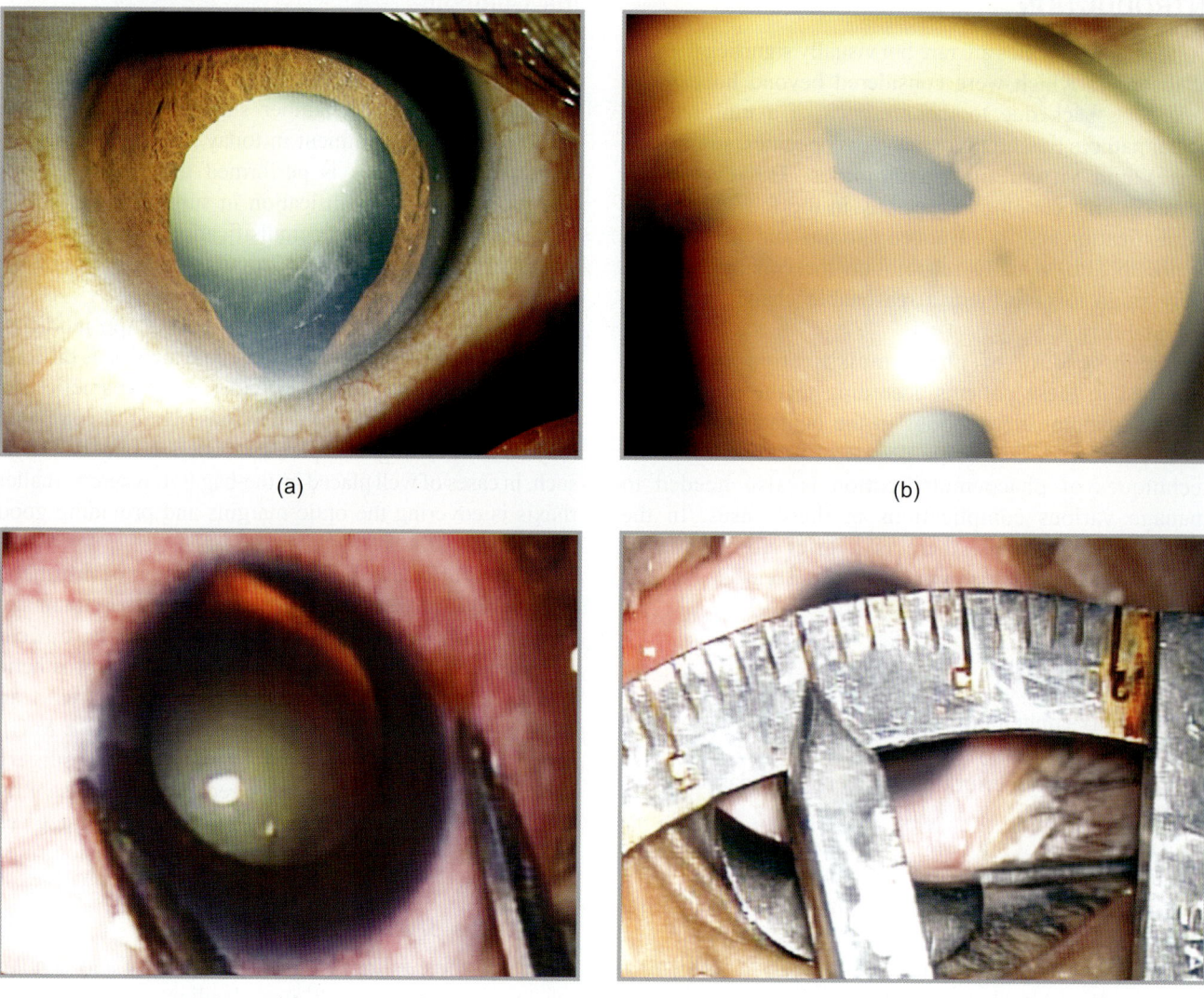

(a) (b)

(c) (d)

Fig. 42.1: (a) Typical inferonasal uveal coloboma with cataract, (b) Gonioscopic view, (c) Relative microcornea with typical inferonasal uveal coloboma and cataract, (d) Relative microcornea (less than 10 mm corneal diameter) with typical inferonasal uveal coloboma and cataract

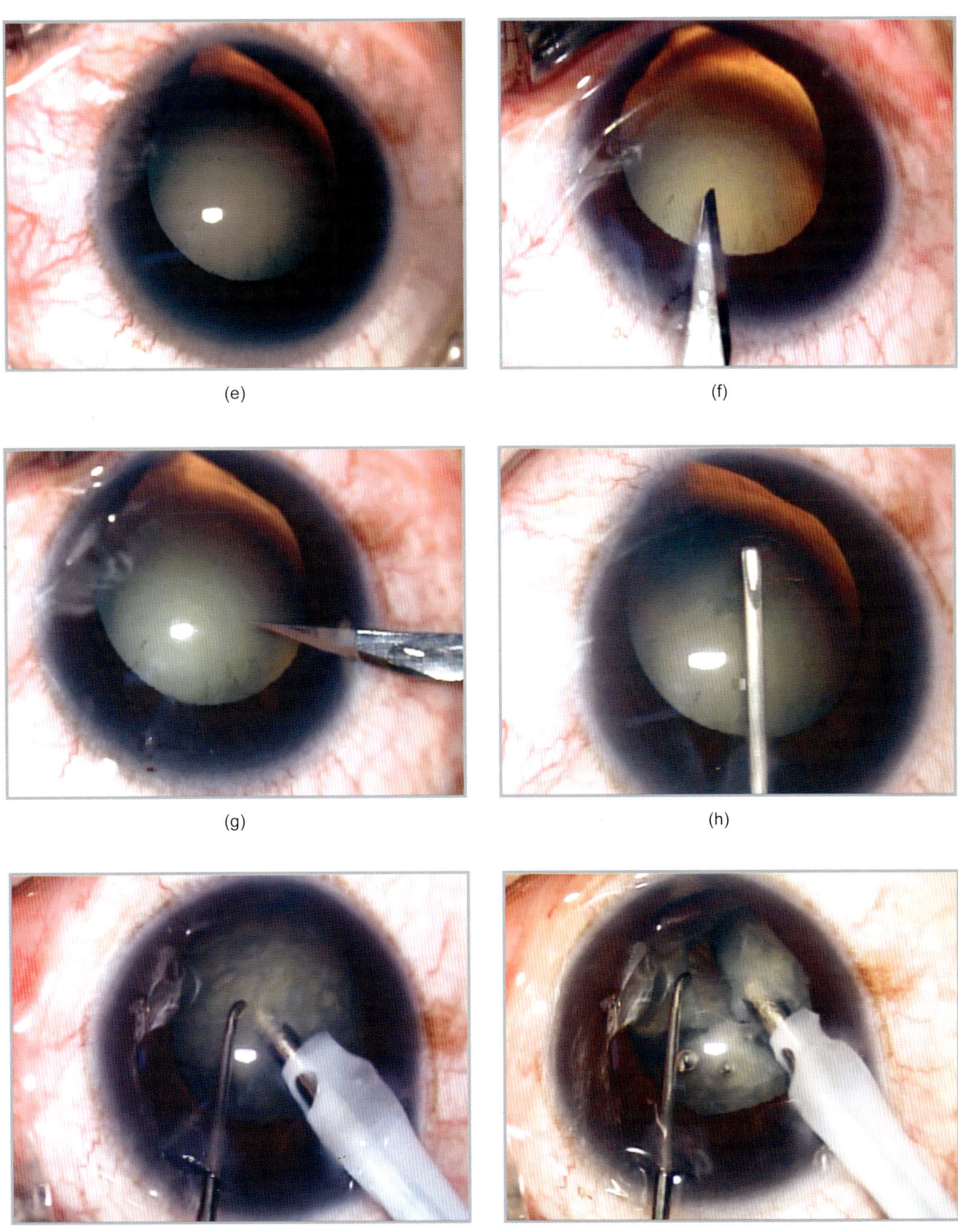

Fig. 42.1: (e) Typical inferonasal uveal coloboma with cataract: Good intraoperative mydriasis, (f) side port incision (right eye), (g) Initial 1 mm incision to be converted into 2.8 mm main incision (right eye), (h) Rhexis, (i) Nucleotomy by direct groove and central chopping, (j) Secondary central chopping

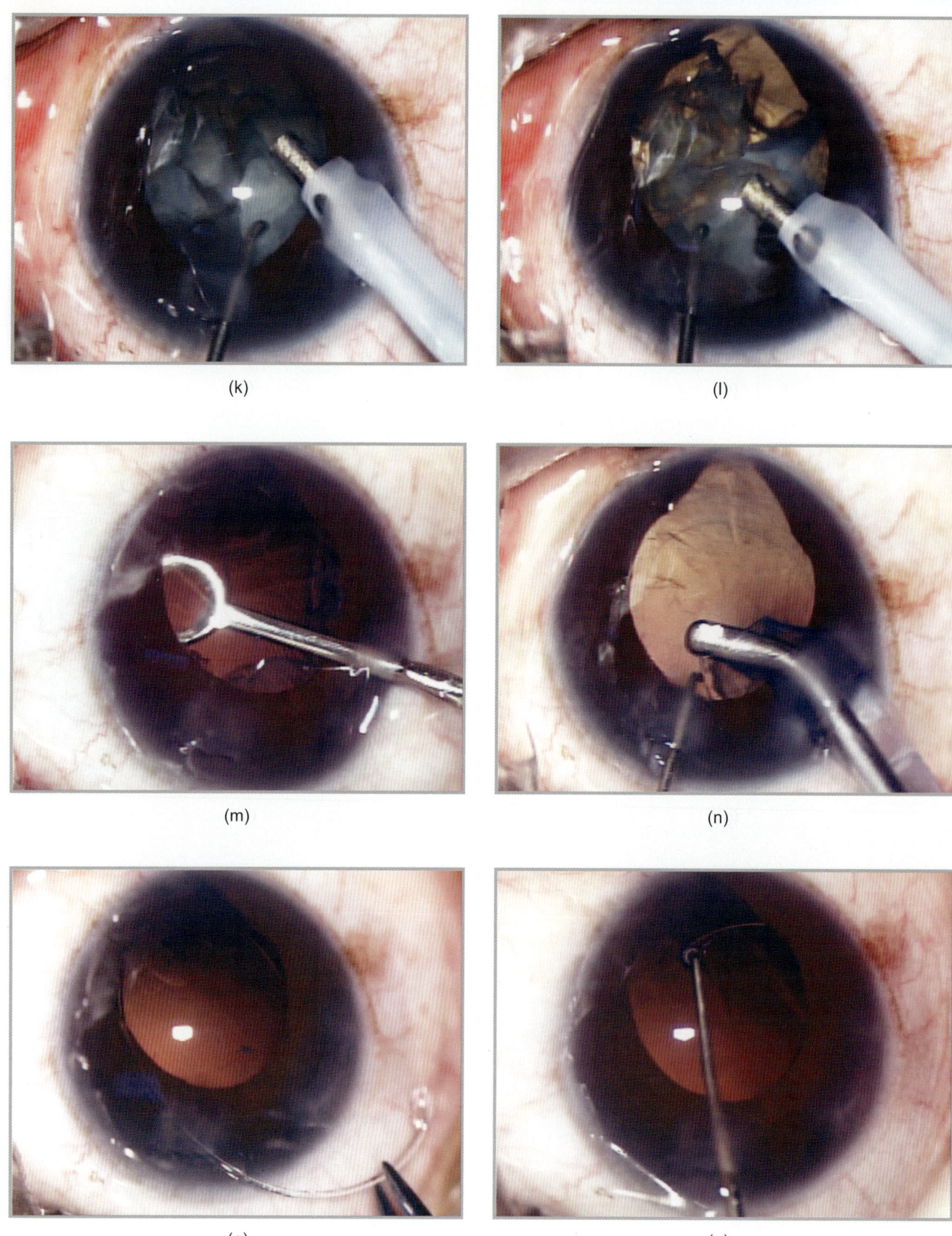

Fig. 42.1: (k) Tertiary and subsequent multiple nucleotomy by repeated central chopping, (l) Fragment removal, (m) Cortical separation from the capsular bag fornices, (n) Removal of subincisional cortex, (o) and (p) Insertion of CTR just prior to the implantation of IOL

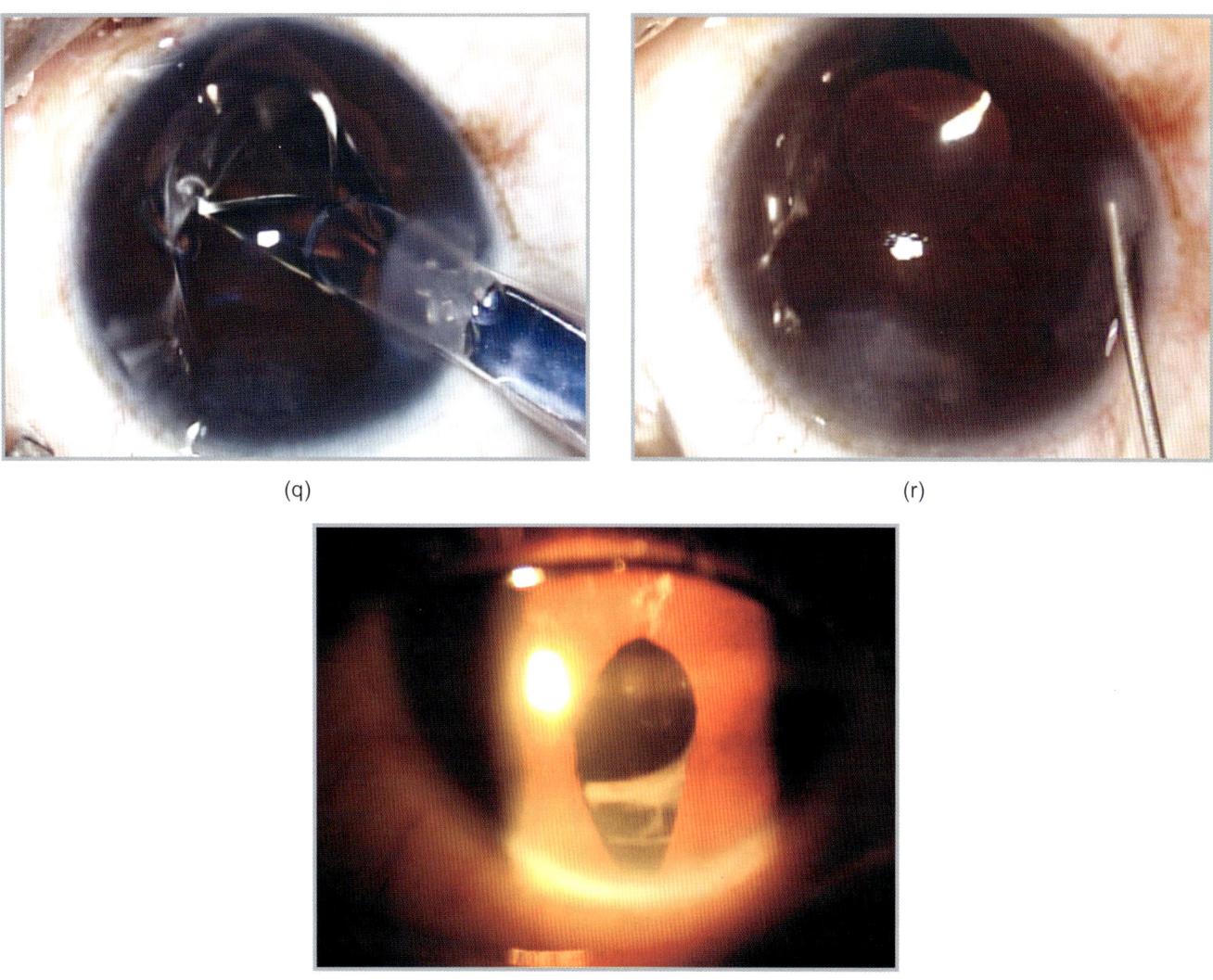

Fig. 42.1: (q) Insertion of acrylic single piece hydrophobic IOL implant, (r) IOL is well placed, stromal hydration is being performed, (s) Postoperative follow up: Three months postoperative photographs revealing anterior capsular rim is providing artificial pupil effect in the inferior quadrant

The improved vision in various studies indicates that phacoemulsification and IOL placement are safe and beneficial in patients with typical congenital coloboma and cataract. Cataract surgery was performed in our centre in six eyes of four patients with typical coloboma of the iris, choroid, and retina by phacoemulsification and the use of capsular tension ring. Contrary to previous reports of poor surgical results in these eyes, we saw no surgical or postoperative complications. Final visual acuity was excellent in four eyes. The other two had preexisting amblyopia that is the main cause of low postop visual acuity in most of the cases in most series. Most previous reports describe outmoded extracapsular techniques or contemporary intracapsular cataract extraction, all without an intraocular lens, hence the perceived poor results of surgery in these cases. Phacoemulsification surgery with minimal modification in technique and keeping in view the possibility of lens subluxation is very safe and accepted modality in these cases.

Phacoemulsification in Cases of Aniridia

Aniridia is an infrequent disease (1:65,000–95,000) caused by a bilateral alteration in the eye's development. It has no gender or racial preference. It is a well-documented genetic anomaly, which may appear sporadically or within families, exhibiting a dominant autosomal inheritance pattern with variable expression amongst the members of a family. The gene, which accounts for the disease (PAX6) is located in the short arm of chromosome 11 and finds broad expression in the development of various eye structures including the cornea, lens, angle, ciliary body and all retina layers. Therefore, aniridia is a global eye disorder in which only iridian hypoplasia (which gives its name to the disease) is the most evident clinical sign. The alterations in the anterior segment include keratopathy due to limbus dysfunction, dry eye, glaucoma, cataract, lens subluxation and a number of abnormalities in the angle. The posterior segment alterations include macular and optic nerve hypoplasia with a frequent association of strabismus and nystagmus which worsen the visual prognosis since an early age. In humans, PAX6 gene mutations were found not only in patients with aniridia, but also in some case of Peter's anomaly. Among the most important extraocular alterations, we find the development in sporadic cases of Wilms' tumor, frequently as a part of the WAGR syndrome (Wilms' tumor, aniridia, genitalurinary abnormalities and mental retard). The phenotype may vary considerably, even among members of the same family.

The visual defect appears in the first decade of life with visual acuity values ranging between 10 and 20% of normal due to foveal hypoplasia combined with the possible existence of congenital cataract, nystagmus and amblyopia. In contrast with the stability of retinal alteration, the progressive deterioration of the eyesight is mainly due to the development of glaucoma, cataract and keratopathy. One of the causes of progressive loss of vision and morbidity in aniridia patients is keratopathy derived from the dysfunction of limbal stem cells (LSCs). The progress in the understanding of the mechanisms involved in cellular renewal of the cornea, in recent years has allowed an adequate therapeutic approach of these patients in any phase of the disease. Supplying LSC by means of a limbus transplant. (Aniridia being a bilateral disease excludes a self-transplant, which are substituted by allografts with tissue from healthy relatives having high HLA compatibility, or from cadavers). In addition to keratopathy, these patients frequently exhibit other anterior segment alterations such as cataract, glaucoma or corneal opacity requiring on some occasions combined surgical procedures such as

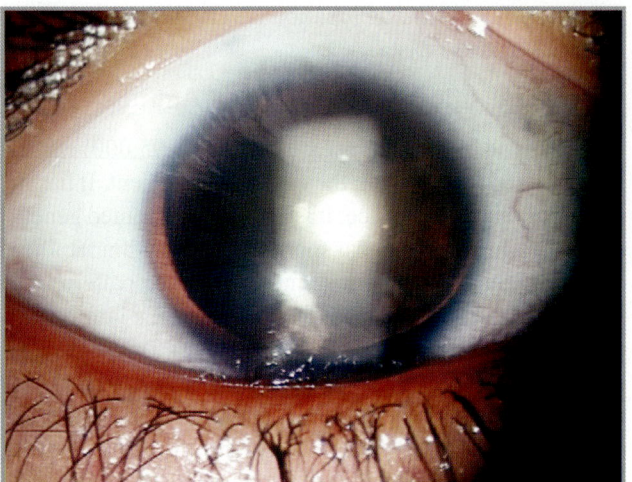

Fig. 42.2: Developmental cataract with glaucoma and aniridia: Ahmed glaucoma drainage device and IOL implant is visible

trabeculectomy, corneal transplant or phacoemulsification, with or without intraocular diaphragm implants.

Cataract surgery may be complicated by poor corneal clarity, keratopathy and zonular dehiscence. Phacoemulsification with minimal anterior chamber turbulence, minimal endothelial injury and in the bag placement of IOL with or without capsular tension ring is the desired modality of treatment.

Implantation of Iris Devices in Congenital and Traumatic Aniridias

Now we have a feasibility of an artificial iris implantation for traumatic or congenital aniridia. Patients can receive a black diaphragm intraocular lens (IOL) in capsular bag after phacoemulsification. Aniridia prosthesis, sulcus sutured, in front of a previous IOL can be implanted in these patients. A black diaphragm IOL, sulcus sutured, or iris diaphragm rings, in front of the previous IOL, and a sector iris prosthesis in front of an IOL in these eyes can be implanted. The glare disability was subjectively better in all cases. Several kinds of artificial iris implants are available. In all our patients with aniridia, iris artificial prostheses improved VA and diminished visual discomfort. Glaucoma is the most important complication after artificial iris implant. It is possible to implant the iris prosthesis in the capsular bag, but this requires a large capsulorrhexis and presents a surgical challenge.

Multisegmented coloboma rings (Rasch-Morcher type 50 C) are used with one or more of the same kind so that the interspaces of first rings are covered by the sector shields of the second forming a contiguous artificial iris.

Phacoemulsification Cataract Surgery in Relative Anterior Microphthalmos and Nanophthalmos

Relative anterior microphthalmos is defined as a condition with a horizontal corneal diameter (HCD) ≤ 11 mm, anterior chamber depth (ACD) ≤ 2.2 mm, and axial length (AL) >20 mm, with no other morphologic malformation. The prevalence of RAM is 6% in various studies. In suspicious eyes, examination is done preoperatively for HCD, ACD, and AL. Horizontal corneal diameter is measured with calipers. Anterior chamber depth and AL is measured with immersion shell with water. Associated ocular pathologic conditions are also recorded.

Major problem in these cases is calculation of accurate IOL power. The accuracy of IOL power calculated using the SRK, SRK II, S-SRK, SRK/T, Holladay, and Hoffer Q formula's has been evaluated in various studies in eyes with axial lengths less than 19.0 mm. Postoperative measurement of refraction showed a tendency toward hypermetropia compared with the refraction predicted by each formula. The best predicted refraction was calculated using the SRK/T formula. The tendency for hyperopic estimation was related to the axial length, particularly in eyes with a shorter axial length. However, there was no relationship between the refractive power of the cornea and the error in the predicted refraction by the SRK/T formula. Two eyes with an IOL power of 30.0 diopters (D) had severe hypermetropia in one study. Theoretical formula's were more accurate than the empirical ones in eyes with microphthalmos. The severe hypermetropia in the two eyes with a 30.0 D IOL indicates that such patients require a higher IOL power. However, the rest of phacoemulsification proceeds as routine keeping in mind the shallow anterior chamber and less space for maneuverability of the phacoemulsification probe and chances of endothelial damage.

Relative anterior microphthalmos is associated with the presence of a small pupil, corneal guttae, glaucoma, and pseudoexfoliation. Intraoperatively, RAM was associated with overall surgical difficulty because of less working space in AC, uveal trauma, descemet's detachment, and posterior capsule rupture. Postoperatively, RAM was associated with transient corneal edema of almost 75% on the first postoperative day. Relative anterior microphthalmos with its associations pose significant intraoperative difficulties. The occurrence of transient corneal edema was the most frequent postoperative complication in phacoemulsification.

With improvements in surgical skills, most patients of nanophthalmos have cataract extraction with posterior chamber intraocular lens (IOL) implantation, mainly by phacoemulsification and rarely by extracapsular cataract extraction, and in some eyes there is a need of lamellar scleral resections. Additional surgeries needed include glaucoma laser treatment cyclocryotherapy trabeculectomy with scleral resection trabeculectomy combined with phacoemulsification and neodymium: YAG laser capsulotomy. Common complications include severe iritis, broken IOL haptic with vitreous loss, posterior capsule opacity, choroidal hemorrhage, phthisis, and aqueous misdirection. Results indicate that echography should be used to assess retinal-choroidal-scleral thickness in eyes that are hyperopic and at risk of narrow-angle glaucoma. Thickening may confirm the diagnosis of nanophthalmos and allow careful preoperative assessment and appropriate operative procedures in these high-risk eyes. With advances in cataract, glaucoma, and uveal effusion treatments, surgical results in patients with nanophthalmos are improving.

Phacoemulsification in Subluxated Lenses in Patients with Marfan's Syndrome

The French paediatrician Antoine Marfan described the Marfan's syndrome in 1896 as an autosomal dominant connective tissue disorder with a high expressivity.

Its prevalence is approximately 4:10,000 and it affects different races and both sexes equally. The classic triad consists of subluxated lenses (ectopia lentis), skeletal deformities (tall stature, long limbs, kyphoscoliosis, pectus deformities and arachnodactyly) and cardiovascular abnormalities (degeneration of the heart valves and aortic dilatation, dissection and rupture).

The most common ocular feature found is ectopia lentis seen in almost 50–60% of patients due to marked zonular weakness. It is generally bilateral and superotemporal in direction. Other ocular features include: astigmatism, axial myopia, flat cornea, glaucoma (due to incomplete development of angle structures), and retinal detachment (due to myopia and aphakia). There is also presence of poor pupillary dilation, which may also be eccentric in location making the surgery even more difficult.

In patients with Marfan's syndrome and with ectopia lentis, the main surgical indications are:
(i) Low corrected vision
(ii) Subluxated lens with its margin over visual axis causing glare
(iii) Monocular diplopia
(iii) Cataract

Various surgical techniques have been described for the treatment of ectopia lentis, among these the following had been more popular: sectorial iridectomy, intra and extracapsular extraction of the lens, phacoemulsification, and limbal or pars plana lensectomy.

The procedures most commonly used today are phacoemulsification and limbal or pars plana lensectomy, with or without IOL implantation. In eyes with only focal zonular weakness or dialysis, use of an endocapsular capsular tension ring may permit placement of a PCIOL in the bag after phacoemulsification.

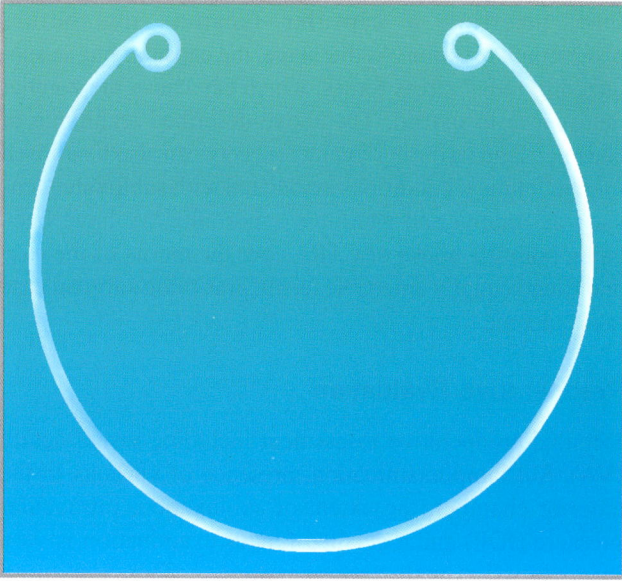

Fig. 42.3: Standard capsular tension ring

Phacoemulsification in Subluxated Cataract Associated with Congenital Anomalies

Surgical management of subluxated cataract presents a challenge to anterior segment surgeons. With recent advances in equipment and instrumentation, better surgical techniques and understanding of fluid dynamics, the surgeon is able to perform relatively safe cataract surgery in the presence of compromised zonules.

The management of subluxated lenses has remained a controversial issue for many years. Jarret retrospectively analysed the indications and techniques for surgical intervention in a series of 114 cases of subluxated or dislocated lenses. Both intracapsular and extracapsular cataract extraction (ECCE) had been documented for the management of subluxated lenses. Techniques used include discission, aspiration and cryoextraction. Recently, several authors have reported using pars plana lensectomy for subluxated lenses with good surgical outcome. In recent years, transscleral suture fixation of posterior chamber IOL has become an alternative to anterior chamber IOL implantation in eyes lacking capsular support. There are a number of surgical approaches available for the removal of subluxated lenses. Inatani et al. have observed that lens extraction is effective in controlling intraocular pressure in eyes with secondary glaucoma associated with lens subluxation. Anterior phacoemulsification with the use of a capsular tension ring to provide stability for phacoemulsification or the use of iris hooks to provide support to the capsular bag are both very useful in reaching a acceptable visual goal.

The use of iris hooks is a good option as most surgeons are familiar with and frequently use iris hooks; however, care needs to be taken as iris hooks can occasionally tear the margins of the capsulorrhexis. The iris hooks application is technically easier to stabilise the capsular bag rather than inserting a capsular tension ring before phacoemulsification. At this stage, the capsular bag is subjected to radial stress forces, which can cause the zonular dehiscence to extend. The above-described technique of capsular support during cataract surgery can also be utilised in other clinical conditions associated with subluxated lens such as trauma and Marfan's syndrome. We have been using both iris hooks or CTR as per the merits of the case and found equally amenable result, gratifying surgical ease and outcome.

Preoperative Evaluation

Detailed preoperative assessment including visual acuity (VA), Slit lamp examination, presence of vitreous in the anterior chamber, the extent of subluxation, intraocular pressure (IOP) and a detailed fundus examination is very important in each and every case. The Slit lamp examination should assess evaluation of the anterior chamber depth, the pupil for presence of traumatic mydriasis, the presence or absence of zonules, and the type and grade of cataract.

The Cataract is classified as Type-I nuclear sclerosis, Type-II anterior cortical. Type-III posterior cortical, and Type-IV posterior subcapsular cataract in these cases. The assessment of density of cataract is graded as G1–2 Soft, G3–4 Hard, and G5 Brunescent. The extent of subluxation should be documented in terms of quadrant involvement in clock hours. Slit lamp biomicroscopic examination with +90D. Keratometry, axial length, 'A' Scan biometry and ultrasound 'B' Scan is equally significant prior to the surgery.

Surgical Technique (Authors preference)

We followed the closed chamber technique, which is achieved only by phacoemulsification. Our surgical paradigms included a 3-plane valvular incision, injection of viscoelastic in the anterior chamber before removing any instrument from the eye, bimanual irrigation and aspiration and 2-port anterior chamber vitrectomy.

Temporal corneal tunnel was preferred for reasons of surgeon comfort and convenience.

Many surgeons locate the incision away from the area of the subluxation. We did not feel this was necessary. Capsulorrhexis is difficult and it is better to begin in the area where the zonules are whole and offer sufficient resistance. Capsulorrhexis can also be performed after the zone of zonular dehiscence and iridocrystalline diaphragm have been stabilised with iris hooks or CTR. We strictly adhered to the principle of initially performing smaller rhexis and later on enlarging it and care was taken to stay away from the site of subluxation. Greishabers flexible iris retractors were used. These were positioned parallel to the iris plane through small, short tract, peripheral paracentesis. The hooklets were placed around the edge of the anterior capsulorrhexis. The stop on the hook was adjusted to hold the rhexis edge to the scleral wall. In case of CTR, the ring is invariably introduced soon after making a small rhexis and prior to the commencement of hydroprocedures.

The application of such devices are of immense benefit by preventing fibrosis of the capsule and further decentration of IOL along with the capsular bag. Secondly, an initial small rhexis helped to restrict the turbulence in the bag and prevented vitreous aspiration during phacoemulsification. Iris retractors were used to temporarily support the dialysis for safer phacoemulsification and IOL placement. It also stabilised the bag.

Thorough but gentle multiquadrant hydrodissection helped us reduce the stress on the zonules during phacoemulsification. Secondly it helped in thorough cortical clean up and prevention of posterior capsule opacification.

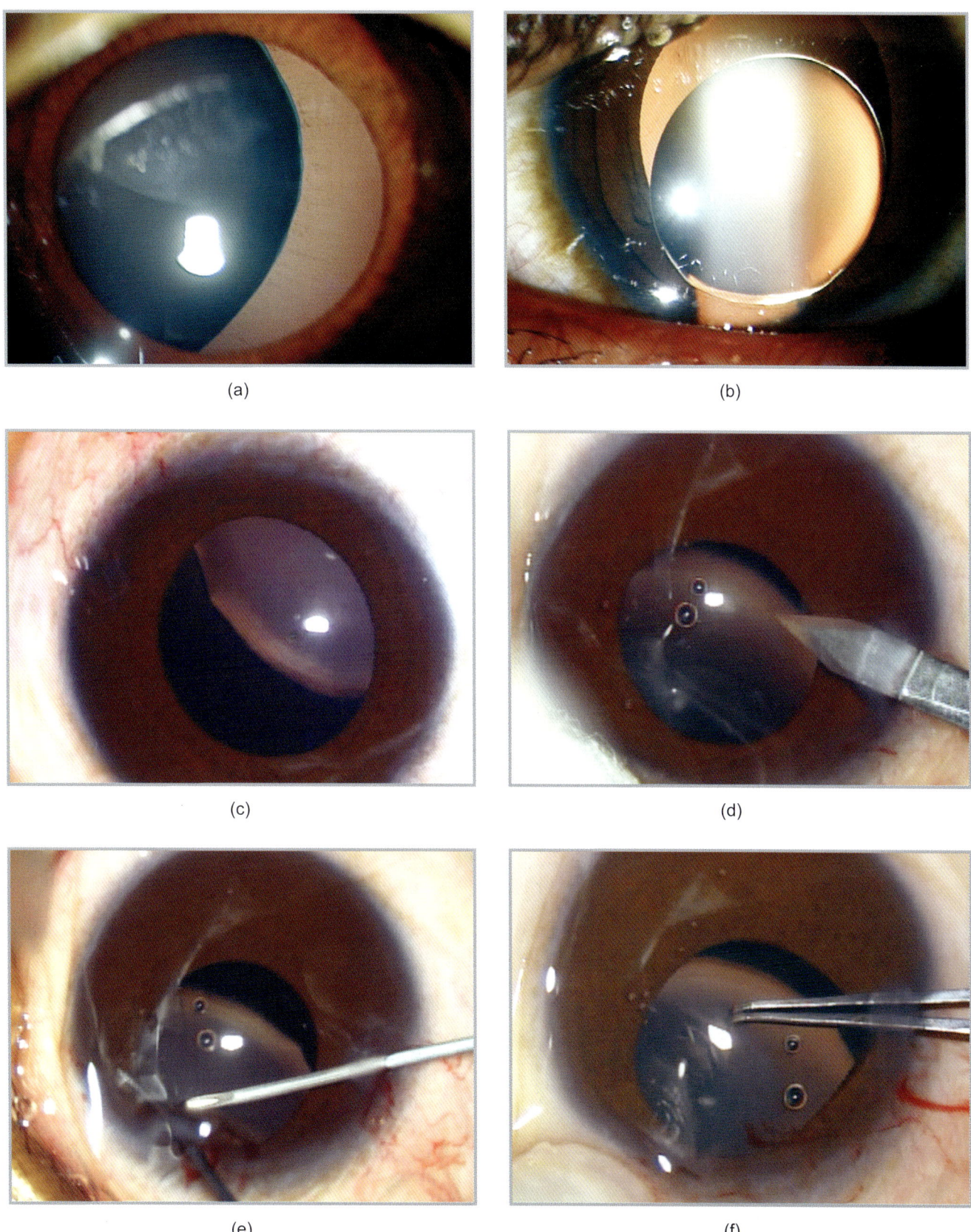

Fig. 42.4: (a) Marfan's syndrome (Subluxated cataract associated with other congenital anomalies), (b) Marfan's syndrome (anterior dislocation of lens associated with other congenital anomalies), (c) Marfan's syndrome: Subluxated lens with zonular defects is visible through intraoperative mydriasis, (d) A one mm incision for phacoaspiration, (e) Commencement of small rhexis with the help of a needle cystitome, (f) Completion of the small rhexis with the help of rhexis forceps

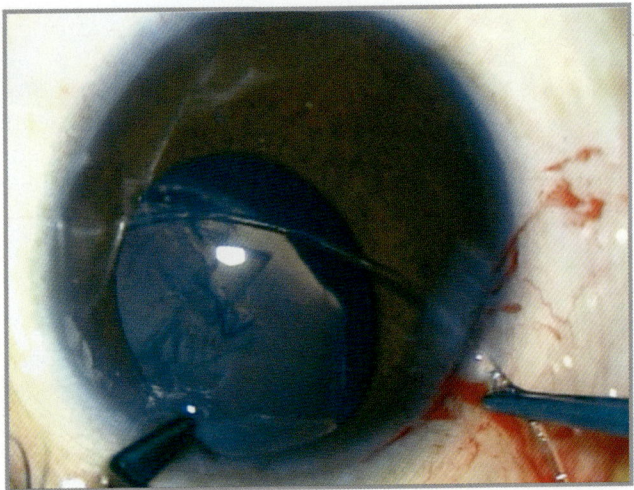

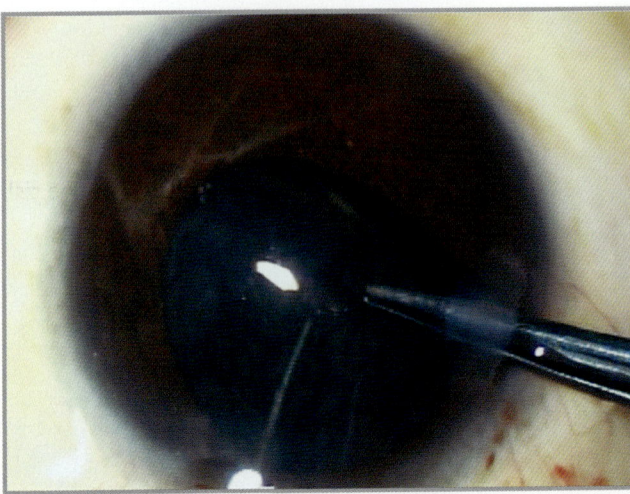

(g)   (h)

Fig. 42.4: (g) Insertion of CTR through small rhexis prior to the hydroprocedure, (h) Insertion of CTR is being pushed into the capsular bag

A cannula is inserted in the direction of the zone of disinsertion as the opposite direction would have led to enlargement of disinsertion. No deliberate hydro-delineation was performed.

Endocapsular phacoemulsification with our phaco technique allowed nucleus division with minimal stress on the capsular bag and produced multiple small nucleus fragments that were easy to consume in the central space. Being the soft nucleus in the younger age group, the conventional nucleotomy techniques like sculpting and chopping may neither be required nor feasible.

Bimanual phacoaspiration under low vacuum and power settings or direct bimanual phacoaspiration on the I/A mode may be good enough in most cases. Most of the time, the tip of the phaco probe is directed at the 6 O'clock position.

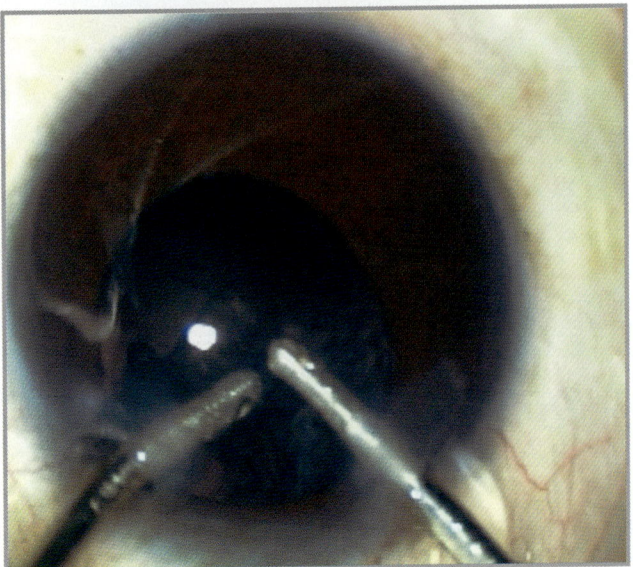

Fig. 42.4: (i) Removal of cataract by bimanual phacoaspiration technique

In case nucleotomy is planned by the sculpting method, the moderate parameters based on the grade of cataract, like 12 cc flow rate and 40 mmHg vacuum may be appropriate. In case of nucleotomy by chopping, step-by-step chop *in situ* and lateral separation followed by stop chop and cortical aspiration is performed. The step down principle was used for fragment removal (endless endeavor for endocapsular phacoemulsification).

The remaining cortex is removed by bimanual irrigation and aspiration with low aspiration flow rate, minimal bottle height and appropriate vacuum. In young patients with soft cataracts where chopping is not possible, we aspirated the nucleus with a phaco probe and removed the residual cortex by bimanual irrigation and aspiration.

It was mandatory to perform vitrectomy in the presence of vitreous before or during phacoemulsification. It is an established fact that contingent vitrectomy prevents any traction on the vitreous base and peripheral retina which may lead to retinal detachment and macular oedema. Bimanual I/A was performed to maintain a closed chamber. By using a low aspiration flow rate and low bottle height we maintained minimal turbulence within the anterior chamber and minimised the anterior chamber depth fluctuation.

The CTR was found to be useful in most of the cases in our series. The confirmation of the ring in the bag included dramatic expansion and stabilisation of the bag. Presence of CTR in the bag was visualised by retracting the iris. The presence of CTR in the bag had proved the enhanced safety and efficacy during phacoemulsification and IOL implantation, maintained the circular contour of the capsular bag and avoided collapse of the bag after the lens was removed from the capsule. Our main aim was to retain the natural bag support for placement of IOL. CTR can be applied at any stage of the surgery. We recommend insertion through small rhexis prior to the hydroprocedures particularly in cases of congenital anomalies where lens nucleus and cortex is invariably soft thus CTR insertion is quite possible prior to the hydroprocedures or removal of cortex. Over and above, the stretched bag facilitates subsequent phacoprocedures as well as minimises the risk of intraoperative complications.

We did not adapt any specific measurement for insertion of CTR except for axial length. Before inserting the CTR we injected viscoelastics just under the anterior capsulorrhexis to create a path for the CTR insertion. CTR of 10.0 mm/12.0 mm diameter was used to maintain the stability and stretch of the capsule during IOL implantation. In some cases, the ring was implanted by simple suture tie

forceps and in others with a shooter CTR was introduced through the main incision.

In eyes with total anterior dislocation of the lens, and in cases where we could not retain the bag during phacoemulsification, we performed scleral fixation. Scleral fixation was also attempted in cases where we could not retain the natural bag support during phacoemulsification and also in eyes where we could not achieve good centration even after implantation of CTR.

In summary, we could achieve in-the-bag implantation in most of the eyes due to application of the closed chamber technique, which allowed us to retain the natural bag support till the end of phacoemulsification. We could implant IOLs in all eyes. No major intraoperative

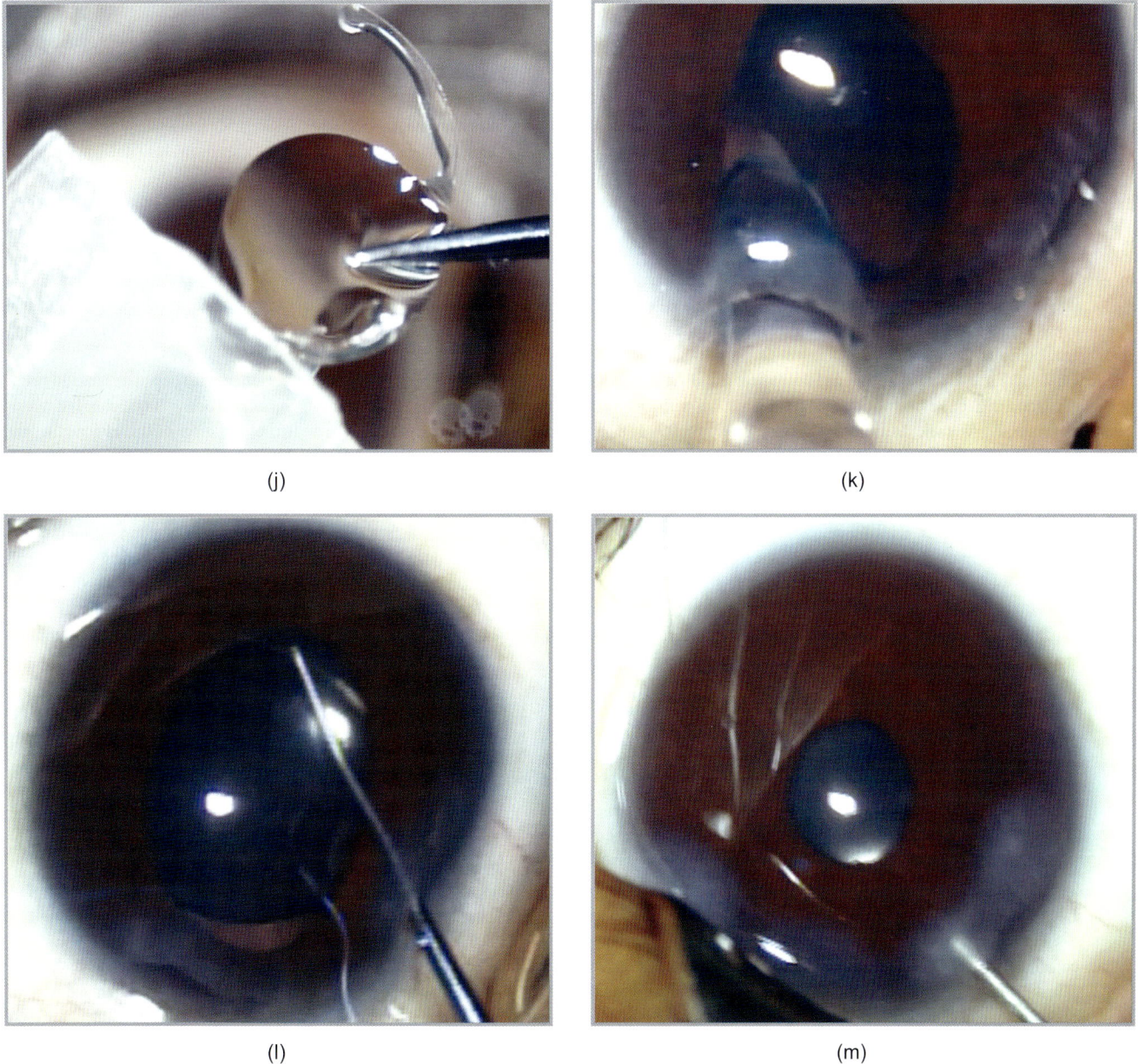

(j)

(k)

(l)

(m)

Fig. 42.4: (j) IOL implantation: Loading of IOL into cartridge, (k) Insertion of IOL into capsular bag, (l) IOL is being positioned over CTR in the capsular bag, (m) IOL is well positioned in the capsular bag and stromal hydration is being performed

complications were noted. The endocapsular ring in some eyes did not correct for centration of IOL. In these cases, Cionni Ring (Type 1L NONE MORCHER, MCTR) could be an alternative for better centration and stability of the bag and IOL.

CONCLUSION

The various congenital anomalies present with the multitude of ocular and systemic deformities have as such already exhausted all the hope by the time the patients reach us. However, our endeavor is to be cautious but optimistic in assessment and explanation of the prognosis.

A careful ocular and systemic examination is mandatory to find out the treatable causes of visual disturbance and to be aware the potential complications during surgery.

Phacoemulsification for cataract and subluxated lenses in these cases has offered a lot of hope, however the technique has to be modified for each patient, keeping in view the anatomical peculiarities in these cases.

The visual prognosis has to be guarded, as there might be presence of amblyopia and posterior segment pathologies associated.

Timely and proper intervention in many of these cases has led to socially acceptable positioning of many of these patients in recent past; hence a ray of hope is always there.

BIBLIOGRAPHY

1. Irit Bahar, Igor Kaiserman, David Rootman: Cionni endocapsular ring implantation in Marfan's Syndrome: Br. J. Ophthalmol., Nov 2007; 91:1477–1480.
2. Autosomal dominant Weill-Marchesani and Marfan syndromes are two sides of the same coin: Br. J. Ophthalmol., Jul 2003; 87: 846.
3. Thomas S Dietlein: Cionni capsular tension ring implantation in Marfan's syndrome: Br. J. Ophthalmol., Nov 2007; 91: 1419–1420.
4. Michael L. Nordlund MD, PhD, Alan Sugar MD and Sayoko E. Moroi Phacoemulsification and intraocular lens placement in eyes with cataract and congenital coloboma: visual acuity and complications.
5. Lu Lw, Fine I. H. Phacoemulsification in difficult and challenging cases: Phacoemulsification in subluxated Cataract. New York, Stuttgart: Thieme, 1999. pp 99–110.
6. Merriain JC, Zheng L. Iris hooks for phacoemulsification of the subluxated lens. J Cataract Refract Surg 1997; 23:1295–97.
7. Cionne RJ, Osher RH. Endocapsular ring approach to subluxated cataractous lens. J Cataract Refract Surg 1995; 21:245–49.
8. Buratto L, Osher RH, Masket S. Cataract surgery in complicated cases. Congenital subluxation of the crystalline lens and the surgical treatment. New York: Slack Incorporated. 2000. pp. 15–23.
9. Gimbel HV, Sun R, Heston JP. Management of zonular dialysis in phacoemulsification and IOL implantation using the capsular tension ring. Ophthalmic Surg Lasers 1997; 28:273–81.
10. Cionni RJ, Osher RH. Management of profound zonular dialysis or weakness with a new endocapsular ring designed for scleral fixation. J Cataract Refract Surg 1998; 24:1299–306.
11. Lam DSC, Young AL, Leung ATU, Rao SK, Fan DSP, Joan SK Ng. Scleral fixation of a capsular tension ring for severe ectopia lentis. J Cataract Refract Surg 2000; 26:609–12.
12. Gimbel HV, Sun R. Role of capsular tension rings in preventing capsule contraction. J Cataract Refract Surg 2000; 26:791–92.
13. Menapace R, Findl O, Georgapoules M, Rainer G, Vass C, Schmetterer K. The capsular ring: Design, applications and techniques. J Cataract Refract Surg 2000; 26:898–12.
14. Jensen AD, Cross HE. Surgical treatment of dislocated lenses in the Marfan syndrome and homocystinuria. Trans Am Acad Ophthalmol Otolaryngol 1972; 76:149–59.
15. Praveen MR, Vasavada Abhay R, Singh R: Phacoemulsification in subluxated cataract: Indian Journal of Ophthalmology. Apr 2003.
16. Gimbel HV, Sun R, Heston JP. Management of zonular dialysis in phacoemulsification and IOL implantation using the capsular tension ring. Ophthalmic Surg Lasers 1997; 28: 273–81.
17. Ahmed IK, Chen SH, Kranemann C, et al. Surgical repositioning of dislocated capsular tension rings. Ophthalmology 2005; 112:1725–33.
18. Osher RH. History and experience with capsular tension rings. Cataract and Refractive Surgery Today 2005; Jan:1–5.
19. Sun R, Gimbel HV. In vitro evaluation of the efficacy of the capsular tension ring for managing zonular dialysis in cataract surgery. Ophthalmic Surg Lasers 1998; 29:502–5.
20. Kohnen T, Baumeister M, Buhren J. Scheimpflug imaging of bilateral foldable in-the-bag intraocular lens implantation assisted by a scleral-sutured capsular tension ring in Marfan's syndrome. J Cataract Refract Surg 2003; 29:598–602.
21. Ahmed IIK, Crandall AS, Kranemann C, et al. Clinical results of the Cionni modified capsular tension ring for sever zonular weakness. Presented at the American Academy of Ophthalmology Meeting, New Orleans, October 25, 2004.
22. Moreno-Montanes J, Sainz C, Maldonado MJ. Intraoperative and postoperative complications of Cionni endocapsular ring implantation. J Cataract Refract Surg 2003; 29:492–7.
23. Ahmed IIK, Cionni RJ, Kranemann C, et al. Optimal timing of capsular tension ring implantation: a Miyake-Apple video analysis. J Cataract Refract Surg 2005; 31:1809–13.
24. Ahmed IK, Butler M. Capsular tension devices for the glaucoma surgeon. Glaucoma Today 2004; Nov-Dec:1–4.
25. Dick HB. Closed foldable capsular rings. J Cataract Refract Surg 2005; 31:467–71.
26. Cionni RJ, Osher RH. Management of profound zonular dialysis or weakness with a new endocapsular ring designed for scleral fixation. J Cataract Refract Surg 1998; 24:1299–306.
27. Ahmed II, Crandall AS. Ab-externo scleral fixation of the Cionni modified capsular tension ring. J Cataract Refract Surg 2001; 27:977–81.

28. Waheed K, Eleftheriadis H, Liu C. Anterior capsular phimosis in eyes with a capsular tension ring. J Cataract Refract Surg 2001; 27:1688–90.

29. Crandall A. Capsular tension rings and pseudoexfoliation. Cataract and Refractive Surgery Today 2004; Jan: 46–7.

30. Kurz S, Dick HB. Spring constants and capsular tension rings. J Cataract Refract Surg 2004; 30:1993–7.

31. Kurz S, Krummenauer F, Hacker P, et al. Capsular bag shrinkage after implantation of capsular bending or capsular tension ring. J Cataract Refract Surg 2005; 31:1915–20.

32. Moreno-Montanes J, Heras H, Fernandez-Hortelano A. Surgical treatment of a dislocated intraocular lens-capsular bag-capsular tension ring complex. J Cataract Refract Surg 2005; 31:270–3.

33. Bopp S, Lucke K. Removal of a capsular tension ring. Ophthalmology 2004; 111:196–7.

34. Ma PE, Kaur H, Petrovic V, et al. Technique for removal of a capsular tension ring from the vitreous. Ophthalmology 2003; 110:1142–4.

35. Dick HB, Schwenn O, Pfeiffer N. Implantation of the modified capsular bending ring in pediatric cataract surgery using a viscoadaptive viscoelastic agent. J Cataract Refract Surg 1999; 25:1432–6.

36. Kim JH, Kim H, Joo CK. The effect of capsular tension ring on posterior capsule opacity in cataract surgery. Korean J Ophthalmol 2005; 19:25–8.

37. Menapace R, Findl O, Georgopoulos M, et al. The capsular tension ring: designs, applications, and techniques. J Cataract Refract Surg 2000; 26:898–912.

43

Cataract with Concurrent Age-Related Macular Degeneration: Current Concepts

Col JKS Parihar SM,VSM **and Surg Cdr Tarun Choudhary**

INTRODUCTION

It is not uncommon to find patients with senile cataract with age-related maculopathy as both these afflictions occur in the elderly. Though not holding that position of importance in the developing countries, age-related macular degeneration (ARMD) is the leading cause of severe loss of vision in patients greater than 65 years of age in the developed world.

Due to the varying factors, in addition to better awareness and diagnostics—the incidence and prevalence of ARMD in India is on the rise. Dr AK Gupta et al, at the Dr RP Centre for Ophthalmic Sciences (AIIMS) found the prevalence of ARMD in rural North Indian population comparable to that recorded in the western settings.

ARMD has previously been known by other names as age-related maculopathy or senile macular degeneration, but the term ARMD is universally accepted. Though a detailed discussion on ARMD is beyond the scope of this chapter, a brief discussion of the disease is in order so as to better understand its interplay with senile cataract and cataract surgery.

ARMD

ARMD has been traditionally classified as dry ARMD or non-neovascular ARMD (NNV-ARMD) and wet ARMD or neovascular ARMD (NV-ARMD). The characteristics of NNV-ARMD include drusen with or without abnormalities of the RPE. The characteristic manifestation of NV-ARMD is the presence of Choroidal Neovascularisation (CNV). This occurs due to micro breaks in the Bruchs membrane allowing the microvascular tissue and fibroblasts to proliferate within the inner aspect of the Bruchs membrane.

The average age of onset of visual loss is about 65 years. After the age of 50 years, the incidence progressively increases till more than 35% people are affected by the age of 80 years.

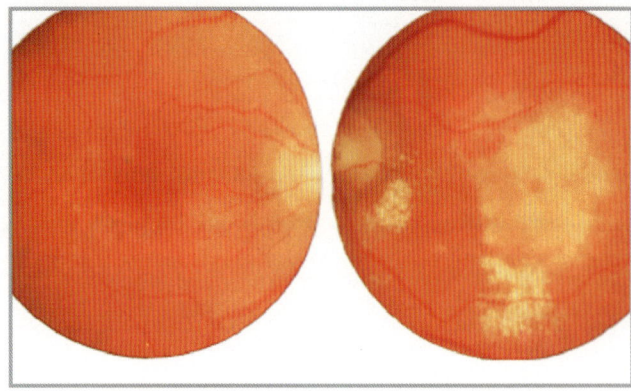

Fig. 43.1: NNV-ARMD(Rt) and NV-ARMD(Lt)

Treatment of NNV-ARMD

Counselling and Patient Education

The patient needs to be told the status of his ocular condition along with the natural course and variations of the disease. The patient also needs to be taught how to recognise symptoms of advanced ARMD like metamorphopsia, scotoma, etc.

Anti-oxidants

AREDS (Age-Related Eye Diseases Study) has demonstrated the advantage of anti-oxidants and zinc supplements in reducing the risk of progression of NNV-ARMD to advanced ARMD and in risk reduction for visual loss.

Avoiding UV Light

No study has proven a cause effect relation between UV light and ARMD. Still, use of sunglasses and shades in harsh sunny climates like ours has its advantages.

Laser Photocoagulation

Prophylactic laser photocoagulation of NNV-ARMD does not appear to offer any benefit in terms of retarding the progress to NV-ARMD as brought out in the Choroidal Neo-Vascularisation Prevention Trials (CNVPT).

Rheophoresis

Rheophoresis or differential membrane filtration of circulating macromolecules from blood to retard ARMD changes is in the experimental stage and is not recommended for NNV-ARMD.

Treatment of NV-ARMD

Laser Treatment

Laser treatment is used for classic CNV with well-defined borders or for lesions with classic and occult mixed components when the extent of the CNV has been accurately mapped. Laser is generally reserved for extra-foveal and distal juxta-foveal lesions. In proximal juxta-foveal lesions, where the fovea is likely to be damaged, other modalities are preferred.

Ocular Photodynamic Therapy (OPDT) or Photodynamic Therapy (PDT)

PDT is a two-step process which includes systemic administration of photo-sensitising drug followed by an application of a light of a particular wavelength to incite a localised photochemical reaction. This reaction generates reactive oxygen radicals which cause capillary endothelial cell damage and vessel thrombosis.

Nutritional Supplements

Anti-oxidants and zinc supplements have been shown to have a beneficial effect on NV-AMD by AREDS.

Trans-pupillary Thermotherapy (TTT)

Here, the lesion is cooked with sub-threshold laser irradiation with long exposure duration and large spot size. 810 nm diode laser is used and the energy penetrates the RPE and choroid minimising absorption by the neurosensory retina and also causing an induced tissue temperature rise of only 10° as compared to 42° with OPDT.

Pharmacological Inhibition of Angiogenesis

Current studies are focussing on pharmacological inhibition of angiogenesis using anti-vascular endothelial growth factor (anti-VEGF) chemicals. Clinical studies have shown significant beneficial effect of pegaptanib sodium (Macugen). Ranibizumab (Lucentis) and off label use of bevacizumab (Avastin) has shown similar benefit but long-term data is still not available. In its infancy, such treatment leaves unanswered questions like recurring cost, possible long-term effect on physiological functions of VEGF and the determination of end point of treatment.

Effect of Cataract on ARMD

It is not surprising to find the co-existence of cataract and ARMD in a patient as the age profile and many of the implicated risk factors for both the diseases, like UV light exposure, smoking and age are common. With rapidly ageing population and greater life expectancy, the number of patients with both cataract and ARMD will increase.

The question remains whether cataract has any effect on ARMD? The many confounding factors and the variable course of the disease have made the answer to this question elusive despite many large population-based and well modelled studies. A majority of the authorities believe that there is no correlation between the progression of cataract and ARMD in a patient.

Effect of Cataract Surgery on ARMD

Voluminous data exists on the effect of cataract surgery—whether ECCE or conventional phacoemulsification on ARMD. This matter has been the subject of many a study and the salient outcomes of validified studies are discussed below.

Although rigorous clinical trials are equivocal, there is a commonly held belief by the retina specialists that cataract surgery hastens the progress of NNV-ARMD to NV-ARMD. The Blue Mountain Eye Study and the Beaver Dam Eye Study both suggest that cataract surgery increases the chances of subsequent diagnosis of NV-ARMD. However, the methodology employed in these studies does not support a simple cause-effect relationship.

AREDS (Age-Related Eye Diseases Study) explored the possibility of association between cataract surgery and progression to NV-ARMD. The study concluded that there was no significant association between the two events, viz. cataract surgery and progression of NNV-ARMD to NV-ARMD. At 5 years after cataract surgery, the risk of progressing to NV-ARMD was about 10% higher than in the population that did not undergo cataract surgery.

Similar studies by AM Ambrecht et al have demonstrated the benefit in quality of life after cataract surgery in patients with ARMD over a follow-up period of five years.

Effect of ARMD on Cataract

The patients with ARMD have impaired macular function from the beginning of the disease but have decreased visual acuity only in the late stages of the disease, when the drusen resolve or the RPE detachment flattens, leaving an area of geographical atrophy affecting the fovea or when CNV arises. An early manifestation of decreased macular function is decreased contrast sensitivity. Since, this is also an effect caused by early cataract, the two pathologies augment each other's contrast sensitivity lowering effect, leaving the patient visually much more handicapped.

As ARMD occurs in the elderly, the vagaries of phacoemulsification in difficult situations as elucidated in other chapters of this book hold good. The higher risk of zonular weakness, low corneal endothelial cell count and liquefied vitreous are all factors which make the phacoemulsification surgery in the patient with ARMD more challenging.

APPROACH TO PHACOEMULSIFICATION IN A PATIENT WITH CONCURRENT CATARACT AND ARMD

Timing of Surgery

The first step in a patient with concurrent cataract and ARMD is to be aware that ARMD is present in the patient to some degree. Next, we need to find out whether the ARMD is NNV-ARMD or NV-ARMD. Towards this goal, an indirect ophthalmoscopy or a 78D fundus examination is invaluable as it can give a view of the fundus in an eye with a reasonably dense cataract. FFA and ICGA can also help in arriving at an answer to this question, media haze permitting. Aid of a B-scan can be taken in case of dense cataract which cannot be overcome by IDO.

In NNV-ARMD, the patient needs to be counselled to plan his surgery to the time when daily activities are hampered by his decreased visual acuity.

A new diagnosis of NV-ARMD on preoperative workup will result in the postponement of the patient's cataract surgery till the NV-ARMD has stabilised and vision has been optimised.

Preoperative Assessment

When the appearance of cataract is not commensurate with the degree of visual deterioration, additional testing is necessary.

The easiest tests, depending on the density of the cataract, are the amsler grid testing, pin-hole visual acuity and potential acuity meter. Diagnostic evaluation of the macula with the Optical Coherence Tomography (OCT) is a quick and noninvasive method of detecting the presence of macular pathology. NV-ARMD may show cystoid macular oedema, PED or subretinal fluid. In such cases, doing an FFA becomes a must to arrive at a decision about the extent of the visual loss due to NV-ARMD.

It is a good practice to examine the posterior segment of the other eye in detail, as more often than not, it gives an indication of what might be going on in the other eye. Though ARMD is asymmetrical, the two eyes generally progress in tandem.

Studies like AREDS provide us with useful prognostic indicators to identify the patients who are at a risk to progress from NNV-ARMD in one or both eyes to advanced ARMD in one eye over the next 5 to 10 years. An individual with a high risk of ARMD progression and vision loss would typically be an obese, hypertensive, myopic smoker with a family history of ARMD and with:

(i) Extensive Intermediate Drusen
(ii) At least one large Drusen
(iii) Non-central geographical atrophy
(iv) Advanced ARMD in the other eye

In addition, if OCT is available, the degrees of irregularities of the outer retinal contour also give a clue of the risk of progression from NNV-ARMD to NV-ARMD. A perfectly linear RPE-Bruchs membrane complex on OCT, generally confirms a low likelihood of progression from NNV-ARMD to NV-ARMD in the short term. On the other hand, an OCT with a saw-tooth like configuration of the RPE-Bruchs membrane contour indicates a poor prognosis for progression from NNV-ARMD to NV-ARMD. Such patients need supplementation with combined antioxidants and minerals to decrease the risk of disease progression and visual loss. In smokers, supplementation without betacarotene is preferred as betacarotene has been shown to increase the risk of lung cancer in smokers.

Patient Counselling

This is aimed at:

(i) Lifestyle modification of the patient to decrease the risk of progression of severe visual loss due to ARMD and its sequel.
(ii) Educating and informing the patient about both the disease process and their interactions as known to the medical world at present.

Giving the patient all the information and inputs he needs, the patient should be allowed to make an informed decision as to the timing of surgery. As the majority of available literature on the topic has concluded that there is no relationship between cataract surgery and acceleration of severity of vision loss due to ARMD, the surgeon needs to simply inform the patient that neovascular transformation is possible and what it means for the patient. The patient needs to be told in no uncertain terms that NV-ARMD is associated with continually decreasing visual acuity over several years and eventual disciform scar formation if not treated energetically. This will make him more compliant for the postoperative reviews.

Intraoperative Peculiarities

Phacoemulsification surgery in a patient with ARMD does not differ in any way from conventional phacoemulsification surgery in a patient with normal posterior pole. A few points worth noting are:

Blue Light Filtering IOL

As there is a growing body of evidence implicating blue light and UV light as a potential risk factor for progression of ARMD, it is advisable to implant any blue light filtering IOL when possible. Though evidence is inconclusive, these IOLs may play a role in preventing or decelerating the ARMD progression.

Telescopic IOL

A landmark study by Megumi Iizuka et al from the University of Toronto was based on the principle that the most desirable effect following cataract surgery in the presence of ARMD is to obtain an improvement in the distance resolution acuity, and the only optical solution to this is to use telescopic magnification. In this study, standard cataract surgery was performed, with the power of the IOL being derived from the reduced Gullstrand model of the eye in such a way that at the IOL plane, a negative lens was created. This together with the positive convex lens at the spectacle plane in the matching glasses formed a Galilean Telescope system with magnification of up to 33%. The authors reported considerable success with this technique. The critics of the study cited that in central retinal pathologies like ARMD, the patient depends on a large extent on his peripheral vision for his day-to-day activities. So, can a telescope-like device reduce the patient's field of vision considerably and cause him more discomfort than benefit?

To get over this problem, Dr Amar Agarwal et al from Dr Agarwal's Eye Hospital and Eye Research Centre, Chennai, India, did a pilot study to evaluate the visual and surgical outcome of an Intraocular Mirror Telescopic lens – the Lipschitz Macular Implant (LMI). Patients with vision less than 20/200 and in whom vision improved with x 2.5 external telescope were implanted with LMI after conventional phacoemulsification cataract surgery. The LMI is claimed to increase the central image on the retina while preserving the peripheral vision.

Postoperative Follow-up

It goes without saying that a meticulous and early postoperative retinal evaluation is a must in patients with ARMD who have undergone cataract surgery. The reason for this is that the limiting factor of the media opacities in the form of cataract interfering with the diagnosis and treatment of ARMD is removed. Also, patients may present with poor visual acuity few weeks following cataract surgery due to new NV-ARMD appearance that may be erroneously attributed to other causes. Thus, it is imperative to have a detailed postcataract surgery retinal evaluation, preferably by a retina specialist to reassess the existing ARMD lesions and lookout for any new lesions indicating progression from NNV-ARMD to NV-ARMD.

CONCLUSION

With early diagnosis and early treatment of NV-ARMD with anti-VEGF factors, excellent visual outcomes can be achieved. The patient should initially be told to assess his visual disabilities (inability to read, drive, indulge in favourite hobbies, etc). The ophthalmologist should then try and give the patient an idea of how much visual disability is due to ARMD and how much is due to cataract. Counselling and an interactive session with the patient goes a long way in meeting the patient's expectations making them in synch with reality. The patients with a high risk for progression and vision loss due to ARMD should be informed about this possibility and the importance of early and frequent exhaustive postoperative evaluations and follow-up in addition to being prescribed antioxidant and zinc formulations.

While the exact risk that cataract surgery confers upon the dry ARMD patient is debatable, the patient's expectations need to be carefully managed and progression to NV-ARMD constantly suspected in the early and immediate postoperative period.

REFERENCES

1. Cugati S, Cumming RG, Smith W, Burlutsky G, Mitchell P, Wang JJ. Visual impairment, age-related macular degeneration, cataract, and long-term mortality: the Blue Mountains Eye Study. Arch Ophthalmol. 2007 Jul; 125(7): 917–24.

2. Wang JJ, Klein R, Smith W, Klein BE, Tomany S, Mitchell P. Cataract surgery and the 5-year incidence of late-stage age-related maculopathy: pooled findings from the Beaver Dam and Blue Mountains eye studies. Ophthalmology. 2003 Oct; 110(10):1960–7.

3. Alió JL, Mulet EM, José M, Ruiz-Moreno, Sanchez MJ, Galal A. Intraocular telescopic lens evaluation in patients with age-related macular degeneration. J Cataract Refract Surg. 2004 Jun; 30(6):1177–89.

4. Velez G, Weiter JJ. Cataract extraction and age-related macular degeneration: associations, diagnosis and management. Semin Ophthalmol. 2002 Sep-Dec; 17(3-4):187–95

5. Armbrecht AM, Findlay C, Aspinall PA, Hill AR, Dhillon B. Cataract surgery in patients with age-related macular degeneration: one-year outcomes. J Cataract Refract Surg. 2003 Apr; 29(4):686–93.

6. Kaþkaloðlu M, Uretmen O, Yaðci A. Medium-term results of implantable miniaturised telescopes in eyes with age-related macular degeneration.J Cataract Refract Surg. 2001 Nov; 27(11):1751–5.

7. Armbrecht AM, Findlay C, Kaushal S, Aspinall P, Hill AR, Dhillon B.Is cataract surgery justified in patients with age related macular degeneration? A visual function and quality

of life assessment.Br J Ophthalmol. 2000 Dec; 84(12): 1343–8.

8. Is cataract surgery justified in patients with age related macular degeneration? A visual function and quality of life assessment.

9. BritishJournal of Ophthalmology2000. 84(12):1343–1348, Armbrecht, A M 1; Findlay, C 1; Kaushal, S 2; Aspinall, P 1; Hill, A R 2; Dhillon, B 1

10. Agarwal A, Lipshitz I, Jacob S, Lamba M, Tiwari R, Kumar DA, Agarwal A. Mirror telescopic intraocular lens for age-related macular degeneration: design and preliminary clinical results of the Lipshitz macular implant. J Cataract Refract Surg. 2008 Jan; 34(1):87–94.

11. Michael Casasnovas. No Association Between Cataracts and Macular Degeneration Seen in Large Study: Presented at ARVO. Archives Of Ophthalmology; 98:12, December 1980

12. Armbrecht AM, Findlay C, Kaushal S, Aspinall P, Hill AR, Dhillon B.Is cataract surgery justified in patients with age related macular degeneration? A visual function and quality of life assessment. Br J Ophthalmol. 2000 Dec; 84(12): 1343–8.

13. Megume Iizuka, John Gorfinkel, Mark Mandelcorn, Wai-Ching Lam, Robert Devenyi, Samuel N. Markowitz. Modified cataract surgery with telescopic magnification for patients with age related macular degeneration. Can j ophthalmol; 42:6, 2007

Cataract with Concurrent Retinitis Pigmentosa: Current Concepts

Col JKS Parihar SM,VSM and Surg Cdr Tarun Choudhary

INTRODUCTION

Retinitis pigmentosa (RP) was defined by the working conference of retinitis pigmentosa specialists in 1984 as a group of hereditary disorders that diffusely involve the photoreceptor and pigment epithelial function characterised by progressive visual field loss and abnormal Electro-Retino Gram (ERG). Though the word "Retinitis" implies an inflammatory or infectious pathology, there is no histopathological evidence of any inflammatory response in the photoreceptor layer or anywhere else in the retina. The present view is that RP has a genetic basis and classically involves the slow and progressive apoptosis of the photoreceptors.

There is no racial predilection and males are slightly more affected than females due to RP inheritance being X-linked in some cases. As of the present, more than 84 different genetic types of RP have been identified, with new ones being added with great frequency.

The patient generally becomes symptomatic in the third decade of life with the chief complaint being difficulty in dark adaptation in the initial stages and nyctalopia in the later stages. The typical signs of retinitis pigmentosa are retinal arteriolar attenuation, the coarse bone spicule, pigmentary changes, tessellated and tigroid appearance of the fundus, waxy pallor of the disc, macular atrophy/cellophane maculopathy/cystoid macular oedema.

Other ocular manifestations of RP include cataract, cystoid macular oedema (CME), open angle glaucoma, Posterior vitreous detachment, myopia, optic disc drusen and intermediate uveitis.

DIFFERENTIAL DIAGNOSIS

In a case of RP it is imperative to make a note of the acquired causes of retinal degeneration which can mimic RP. A few of such conditions are:

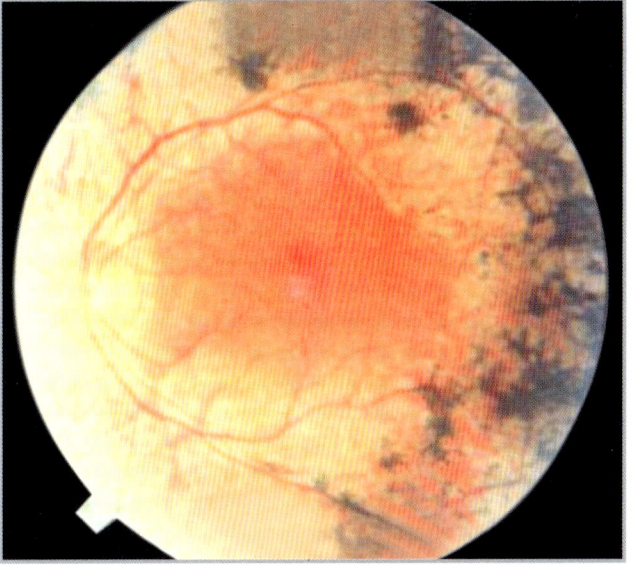
Fig. 44.1: Typical fundus in an RP patient

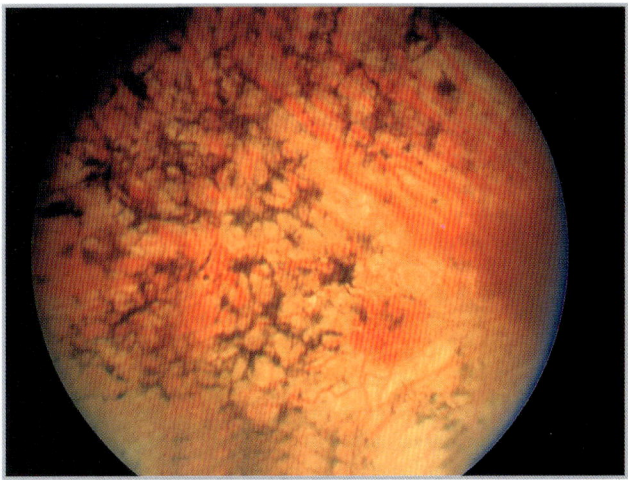
Fig. 44.2: Typical bone spicule pigmentation

- Previous ophthalmic artery occlusion
- Diffuse posterior uveitis
- Syphilis
- Paraneoplastic syndromes
- End stage chloroquine retinopathy treatment of RP

Treatment

Treatment of RP includes confirmation of the diagnosis, counselling, follow-up, low vision aids (LVA) treatment of cystoid macular oedema with tablet acetazolamide 250–500 mg OD for weeks to months, nutritional supplements in the form of vitamin A a palmitate (15,000 IU/day) and anti-oxidants and cataract surgery which is discussed in detail here.

CATARACT IN RP

Genesis

Cataract is one of the inherent manifestations of the disease process of RP, as also other tapetoretinal degenerations. Cataract was found in 46.4% of cases of RP in a study, out of which the overwhelmingly predominant form was the posterior subcapsular cataract (PSC) (94.3%).

There are two schools of thought regarding the aetiology of PSC in RP. One group believes that the cataract is a direct manifestation of gene expression. A second theory, which finds more favour, was proposed by Berliner in 1949. This stated that PSC are secondary to the primary retinal pathology. The progressive apoptosis of the photoreceptor cells releases a toxic substance to the crystalline lens. J Heckenlively stated that the primary metabolic abnormality occurs at the level of the photoreceptor-RPE complex. Photoreceptor outer segments are continually renewed and the terminal outer segment discs are removed by the RPE. Any metabolic disorder that imbalances the interaction of the photoreceptors with the RPE leads to the accumulation and deterioration of the outer segment membranes. Outer segment membranes contain a high amount of aecosahexinoic Acid which is very susceptible to peroxidation. Anterior migration of toxic radicals and lipid aldehydes formed by decosahexinoic acid peroxidation could cause vitreous changes and PSC, characteristic of RP.

Pathoanatomical Configuration

Pathoanatomical configuration of the PSC lens in RP patients by transmission electron microscopy and quantitative microradiography reveals:

- Extensive extracellular vacuolisation in the lens epithelium
- Focal degeneration in epithelial cells
- Mitochondrial swelling in epithelial cells
- Extensive swelling of hydrated lens fiber cells with a decrease in their dry mass content.

- Presence of elongated migrating nuclei containing cells on the posterior capsule
- Severe lens fiber disorganisation
- New, ill-formed basement membrane

APPROACH TO PHACOEMULSIFICATION IN A PATIENT WITH RP

Timing of Surgery

As the patient with RP develops cataractous lens opacities (mostly PSC) earlier than the normal population, cataract surgery is required earlier in these patients than in the normal population. There is no rationale for withholding cataract surgery in a patient of RP with optically significant cataract. As contrast sensitivity lowering is both a result of the retinal changes and PSC, it is better to remove the cataract to partially improve the contrast sensitivity.

Patient Counselling

In addition to the points mentioned earlier regarding patient education and counselling, it is essential to explain that cataract surgery will only partially improve the visual status.

Preoperative Assessment

Assessment of macular function in such patients can be done with the PAM or laser interferometers as generally the cataract density is not severe enough to prevent these tests. Also, studies have shown that conductive high frequency rhythmic ERG (40 Hz) and determination of electric sensitivity threshold for retina and the optic nerve axial bundle liability (ESL) are most accurate in the prediction of visual function. Out of the two, rhythmic ERG is much more sensitive to the macular area involvement and therefore, preferred.

Concurrent Glaucoma

Open angle type of glaucoma is known to coexist with RP in 3% cases and needs to be taken into consideration while planning a cataract surgery. As discussed in detail elsewhere, medical therapy to control IOT before surgery is a must. Thereafter, depending on the control, a combined filtering surgery with phacoemulsification and PCIOL or only phaco and PCIOL can be undertaken. Any prostaglandin inhibitors, which are finding more and more use as first line drugs in glaucoma management, must be discontinued at least four weeks prior to surgery. As the cataract of RP is not a uniformly dense cataract, a thorough fundus evaluation and if possible field analysis or macular function tests can be undertaken. Intraoperatively, a more thorough viscoelastic clean up after surgery is mandated in view of the already compromised trabecular meshwork drainage.

Coexisting Intermediate Uveitis

There is an established correlation between RP and intermediate uveitis with intermediate uveitis of RP than in the general population. A proper preoperative assessment including an indirect ophthalmoscopy and UBM if available is mandatory. Any evidence of intermediate uveitis should be treated with topical and oral steroids and NSAID. A posterior subtenons (4 mg) or intravitreal (0.4 mg) injection of triamcinolone acetonide may also be required. Intravitreal triamcinolone is used only as a last ditch method as it can raise the IOT in a significant number of patients. Whatever the treatment modality employed for the treatment of the coexisting uveitis, a close watch needs to be kept on the IOT as glaucoma also coexists with RP and may get aggravated due to the treatment offered for uveitis, especially in steroid responders. Also, the phaco-emulsification surgery needs to meticulous be much more atraumatic. Any retained cortical matter or leftover viscoelastic may reactivate a quiescent uveitis.

Concurrent Myopia

The eyes with RP generally have axial myopia and therefore, all discussions in the chapter on phacoemul-sification in cases of myopia of this volume hold good.

INTRAOPERATIVE AND POSTOPERATIVE PECULIARITIES

Anterior Capsular Contraction

The reported incidence of anterior capsular contraction after cataract surgery in patients with RP is significantly higher (9.6%) than in normal patients (1.4%). This in turn leads to a higher incidence of IOL decentration and tilt. Thus, the CCC made for phacoemulsification should be absolutely central and on the larger side (5.5 to 6 mm). Also, meticulous polishing of the under-surface of the remaining anterior capsular rim in the cap-vac mode of the machine is a good idea. This reduces anterior capsular contraction and phimosis as well as posterior capsular opacifications. Anterior capsular contraction can be treated with Nd:YAG anterior capsulotomy without any complications.

Posterior Capsular Opacifications (PCO)

The incidence of PCO in patients with RP undergoing surgery is also more (63% after 1 year) as compared to the normal population (26% after 1 year). This can be reduced by meticulous cortical cleanup, cap-vac capsular polishing and using square edge IOL in addition to ensuring that though large, the edge of the anterior capsular frill of the CCC overlies the IOL and does not touch the posterior capsule in any quadrant. Thus, more care needs to be given

to make a perfectly circular, central, correct sized CCC. In case it occurs, PCO can be treated with Nd:YAG posterior capsulotomy, making a smaller opening. In case the patient has RP related CMO, it is better to actively treat and wait for the improvement of this macular oedema by giving tablet acetazolamide 250 mg a day for at least 6 weeks prior to Nd:YAG capsulotomy.

Postoperative Macular Oedema

The incidence of postoperative CMO after cataract surgery in RP patients is 14% as compared to 4 to 6% in the normal population with various methods of cataract extraction. The macular oedema, if it occurs, needs to be treated conventionally along with oral carbonic anhydrase inhibitors. Rarely intravitreal triamcinolone acetate may be warranted.

Postoperative Refraction

As the patient of RP has lost his peripheral fields and generally, the fields are restricted to the central ten to fifteen degrees, it is better to leave the patient slightly myopic so as to create an inverse telescope effect and increase the field of vision to some extent. This is also desirable as preoperatively, most of the patients of RP are myopic.

Postoperative Care

Generally, the postoperative care after cataract surgery in a patient with RP does not vary from the normal. A special watch needs to be kept on the intraocular pressure and uveitis for any deviation from the normal. The points mentioned under the management of RP including counselling form an ongoing process and should continue unchanged irrespective of the cataract surgery.

CONCLUSION

Cataract is one of the inherent manifestations of the disease process of RP, as also other tapetoretinal degenerations. As a patient with RP develops cataractous lens opacities (mostly PSC) earlier than the normal population, cataract surgery is required earlier in these patients than in the normal population. There is no rationale for withholding cataract surgery in a patient of RP with optically significant cataract. Preoperative assessment to assess the macular functions and to rule out concurrent glaucoma, uveitis and myopia with its inherent retinal abnormalities play an important part in managing these patients. Postoperatively also, these patients require closer follow-up. The reported incidence of anterior capsular contraction after cataract surgery in patients with RP is significantly higher than in normal patients. This in turn leads to a higher incidence of

IOL decentration and tilt, which needs to be actively looked out for. The incidence of PCO in patients with RP undergoing surgery is also more (63% after 1 year) as compared to the normal population (26% after 1 year). This can be reduced by meticulous cortical cleanup, cap-vac capsular polishing and using square edged IOL. The incidence of postoperative CMO after cataract surgery in RP patients also high and needs treatment on conventional lines, if it occurs. Postoperatively, it is better to leave the patient slightly myopic so as to create an inverse-telescope effect and increase the field of vision. A special watch needs to be kept on the intraocular pressure and uveitis for any deviation from the normal. With adherence to the guidelines mentioned in this chapter, it is possible to have an un-eventful cataract surgery and postoperative period, resulting in a satisfied and happy patient.

REFERENCES

1. Eshaghian J, Rafferty NS, Goossens W. Ultrastructure of human cataract in retinitis pigmentosa. Arch Ophthalmol 1980 Dec; 98(12):2227–30

2. Bastek JV, Heckenlively JR, Straatsma BR.Cataract surgery in retinitis pigmentosa patients. Ophthalmology. 1982 Aug; 89(8):880–4

3. Fagerholm PP, Philipson BT. Cataract in retinitis pigmentosa. An analysis of cataract surgery results and pathological lens changes. Acta Ophthalmol (Copenh). 1985 Feb; 63(1): 50–8

4. Newsome DA, Stark WJ Jr, Maumenee IH. Cataract extraction and intraocular lens implantation in patients with retinitis pigmentosa or Usher's syndrome. Arch Ophthalmol. 1986 Jun; 104(6):852–4.

5. Hayashi K, Hayashi H, Matsuo K, Nakao F, Hayashi F. Anterior capsule contraction and intraocular lens dislocation after implant surgery in eyes with retinitis pigmentosa. Ophthalmology. 1998 Jul; 105(7):1239–43.

6. Jackson H, Garway-Heath D, Rosen P, Bird AC, Tuft SJ. Outcome of cataract surgery in patients with retinitis pigmentosa.Br J Ophthalmol. 2001 Aug; 85(8):936-8

7. Sudhir RR, Rao SK.Capsulorrhexis phimosis in retinitis pigmentosa despite capsular tension ring implantation. J Cataract Refract Surg. 2001 Oct; 27(10):1691–4

8. Armbrecht AM, Findlay C, Kaushal S, Aspinall P, Hill AR, Dhillon B.Is cataract surgery justified in patients with age related macular degeneration? A visual function and quality of life assessment.Br J Ophthalmol. 2000 Dec; 84(12):1343–8.

9. Megume Iizuka, John Gorfinkel, Mark Mandelcorn, Wai-Ching Lam, Robert Devenyi, Samuel N. Markowitz. Modified cataract surgery with telescopic magnification for patients with age related macular degeneration. Can J ophthalmol; 42:6, 2007

10. John D. Goosey, Wei Ming Tuon, and Charles A. Garcia. A Lipid Peroxidative Mechanism for Posterior Subcapsular Cataract Formation in the Rabbit: A Possible Model for Cataract Formation in Tapetoretinal Diseases. Investigative Ophthalmology & Visual Science; 25: May 1984

45

Phacoemulsification in Eyes with Previous Keratorefractive Surgery

Dr Rajesh Sinha MD, DNB, FRCS, Dr Ritika Sachdev MS and Dr Jeewan S. Titiyal MD

INTRODUCTION

Most patients who undergo refractive surgery are in their twenties or early thirties. With time, these patients come into an age when they require cataract surgery. However, these patients differ from other senile cataract patients. Guidelines have been formulated in order to perform the procedure and more importantly calculate accurately the power of the intraocular lens (IOL) to be implanted. Refractive surprises can be encountered if the surgeon acquires a casual approach towards these patients. Moreover, post-refractive surgery patients often present the same high expectations they had for their refractive procedures. The most demanding task in these patients is an accurate IOL power calculation apart from some other adjustments needed while performing the procedure.

WOUND CONSTRUCTION

The need for the modification in the wound construction is more in eyes that have undergone an incisional refractive surgery (Fig. 45.1).

The incision for phacoemulsification can either be clear corneal or scleral tunnel. Clear corneal tunnel incision can be considered in an eye with four or less radial incisions or in patients with previous photorefractive keratectomy (PRK) or laser in situ keratomileusis [LASIK] (Fig. 45.2).

In an eye with six or more radial incisions, a scleral tunnel incision should be made, particularly if incisions are traversing the limbus.

INTRAOPERATIVE VISUALISATION AND CORNEAL PROTECTION

Intraoperative visualisation may not be as good in an eye with radial incision as compared to any routine cataract patient with clear cornea. One should attempt to visualise the cataract through a central optical zone.

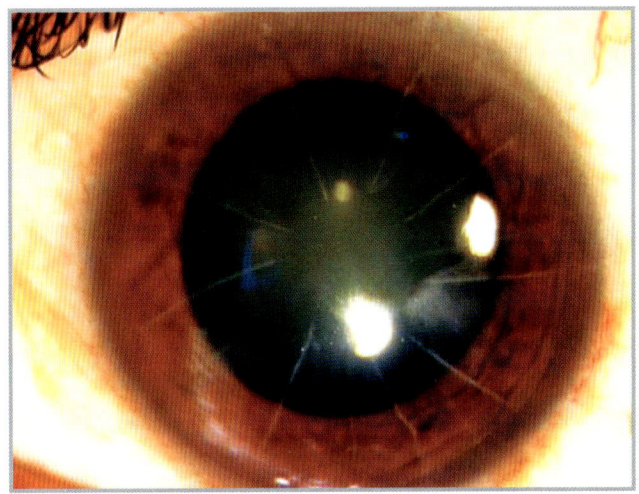

Fig. 45.1: Radial keratotomy

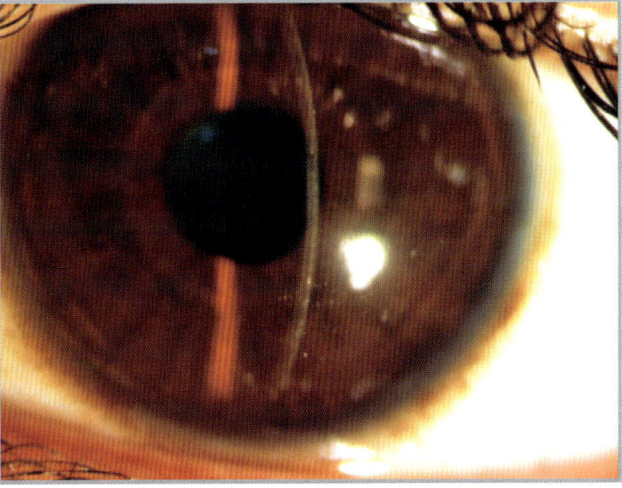

Fig. 45.2: Laser-in-situ keratomileusis

While removing the peripheral cortex, the eye can be rotated so that the visualisation of the periphery is through the central zone.

The endothelium should be coated with viscoelastic to minimise endothelial loss, which might have occurred previously due to keratorefractive surgery.

One should avoid excessive irrigation with low aspiration rates as it may lead to gaping of radial incisions.

CALCULATION OF IOL POWER: SOURCES OF ERROR

Corneal Power

The difficulty of IOL power calculation after refractive surgery lies in the ability to accurately calculate corneal power. The altered corneal shape can result in multiple ranges of corneal power throughout the central corneal surface. The average keratometric readings from the standard intraocular lens formulae are inaccurate for these patients.

Conventional manual keratometry measures point at a 3 mm zone, which can vary with steeper or flatter corneal shapes. Another factor introduced by corneal tissue removing surgeries, such as LASIK, has been the change in the standardised refractive index of the cornea due to a change in the power of the front surface of the cornea.

It is difficult to measure the true corneal power by keratometry, or corneal topography following refractive surgery. The reasons for this are as follows:

Keratorefractive surgery for myopia flattens the anterior corneal surface, but leaves the posterior corneal radius mostly unchanged. This disparity is greater with LASIK and somewhat less with RK. Because the central cornea has been flattened, keratometry may read a falsely large area. Manual and automated keratometers evaluate the radius of curvature designated by four points in orthogonal meridians separated about 3.2 mm apart with manual keratometers, or about 2.6 mm apart in automated keratometers. Rather than measuring several points within a central 2.5 to 3.5 mm area, the measurement may instead be at 5.0 to 6.0 mm. With the non-incisional forms of keratorefractive surgery, such as LASIK and PRK, the index of refraction of the cornea is probably changed. Automated keratometry and corneal topography analysis therefore might be using incorrect assumptions in measuring the corneal power.

Corneal optics in keratometers is assumed to be spherocylindrical. Normal corneas are nearly spherical, or prolate. The cornea can no longer be compared to a sphere centrally after refractive surgery. Post-refractive corneas, however, are oblate, i.e. a relatively flatter cornea in the centre and steeper in the periphery. Further, the back surface is no longer 1.2 mm steeper than the front surface as in a normal cornea.

For these reasons, keratometry and corneal topography will typically overestimate central corneal power following keratorefractive surgery for myopia. For low power myopic corrections by RK (less than –2.00 D), this effect is minimal. However for higher power myopic corrections, and especially those by LASIK, this overestimation can be quite significant. Failure to keep this important fact in mind will often result in an unexpected and unpleasant postoperative hyperopic surprise.

In a post-myopic refractive laser in-situ keratomileusis patient, the practitioner will be measuring the keratometry values from the steeper part of the cornea rather than the centrally flattened portion. The K is going to be estimated higher, thereby providing a falsely lower IOL power giving rise to a hyperopic surprise.

In post-hyperopic LASIK patients, the corneas are steeper in the centre and flatter in the periphery. The keratometry values are recorded from the flatter part of the cornea and are falsely estimated to be low. Therefore, IOL power will be overestimated giving rise to a myopic surprise. Potentially adding to the error is the fact that manual and automated keratometers do not take into account irregular astigmatism, which may occur after radial keratotomy, or central islands and decentrations with LASIK or photorefractive keratectomy.

Direct Change of Central Anterior Corneal Curvature

During excimer laser photorefractive keratectomy (PRK), selective removal of tissue across the anterior corneal surface results in a change of the anterior corneal curvature. Although the central anterior surface of the cornea may become flatter (to treat myopia) or steeper (to treat hyperopia), the posterior surface is presumed to remain stable. The same may be true for uncomplicated LASIK in which direct flattening or steepening of the central anterior corneal surface is achieved by focal keratectomies under a plano hinged flap.

Indirect Change of Central Anterior and Posterior Corneal Curvature

To correct myopia with radial keratotomy (RK), deep radially oriented incisions are applied in the midperiphery of the cornea to induce midperipheral bulging of the cornea, and flattening of the central cornea. Since no tissue is removed, it is assumed that the anterior and posterior surfaces of the cornea react in an analogous way.

Effective Lens Position

The effective lens position is the effective position of the IOL in relation to the anterior corneal vertex. The use of post-myopic correction corneal power (which is flatter) would underestimate the effective lens position (calculates a more forward lens position), and the IOL power.

HOW TO CALCULATE ACCURATE IOL POWER?

Measuring K

(a) Manual Keratometry
(b) Automated Keratometry
(c) Corneal topography
(d) Direct corneal power measurement

Manual Keratometry

Manual keratometry is the method that IOL power calculation formulae were originally based upon. Keratometry evaluates only four points separated 3 to 4 mm in two orthogonal meridians on the paracentral cornea, and the corneal optics are assumed to be spherocylindrical. Thus, asphericity or asymmetry of corneal shape cannot be measured with standard keratometry.

Manual keratometry probably represents the least accurate method since current instruments, such as the Zeiss, Javal-Schiotz, or Bausch & Lomb keratometers make too many assumptions that do not take into account irregular corneal astigmatism.

Automated Keratometry

Automated keratometers may be more accurate than manual keratometers in corneas after RK that have small clear zones (i.e., less than 3 mm) because they sample a smaller central area of the cornea (normally 2.6 mm). The smaller the clear zone and the greater the number of RK incisions, the greater the probability and magnitude of error. This error occurs because the samples at 2.6 mm are close to the paracentral transition zone (knee) after RK. After PRK or LASIK, automated keratometers accurately measure the front radius of the cornea, because the transition areas are far outside the 2.6 mm zone that is measured. However, derivation of keratometric diopters from the radius of curvature is still wrong.

Corneal Topography

Simulated Keratometry (Sim-K): The simulated keratometry value (Sim-K) is determined from the power of Placido mires 7, 8, and 9 of the videokeratoscope for 128 equally spaced meridians. Measuring more than 5000 points over the entire cornea and more than 1000 points within the central 3 mm, videokeratography provides greater accuracy in determining the power of corneas with irregular astigmatism as compared to keratometers. However, Sim-K value derivation may vary among different videokeratoscopes.

Average Central Power (ACP): A new parameter, average central power, is derived from the average of corneal powers inside the region demarcated by the entrance pupil of the TMS-1 videokeratoscope. Because the density of measured points with the videokeratoscope is highest in the central cornea and decreases toward the periphery, area-corrected power was used for compensation. This modified method is supposed to have major advantages over the classic Sim-K after RK with small clear zones, but not after PRK and LASIK.

Direct Corneal Power Measurement

Using the Orbscan scanning slit-beam videokeratoscope, a three-dimensional location of several thousand points of the corneal and anterior chamber surfaces can be determined. Two scanning slit lamps project 40 calibrated beams onto the eye, angled at 45° to the left and to the right of the video camera axis, covering the whole cornea from limbus to limbus and overlapping in the central 5 mm zone. This system has the potential to provide topographical height and power maps of the anterior and posterior corneal surfaces.

More recently the oculus pentacam, a rotating Scheimpflug camera, is being used to determine both the anterior and the posterior corneal curvatures.

Predicting the IOL Power

A combination of the clinical history and contact lens method is considered as one of the most accurate methods of determining the IOL power after refractive surgery.

However, newer modalities of IOL power calculation like the Borasio Edmondo Smith and Stevens (BESSt) formula, circumvent the limitation of these methods as they do not require any historical (preoperative) data.

(a) Clinical history method
(b) Contact lens method
(c) Double K method
(d) Nomogram based method (Feiz Mannis)
(e) Masket method
(f) Haigis-L formula
(g) BESSt formula
(h) Shammas-PL formula

Clinical History Method (CHM)

This method requires the following information:
- Pre-Refractive surgery refraction
- Pre-Refractive surgery K readings
- Post-Refractive surgery refraction (preferably current, but before significant cataract formation).

With the CHM, the number of diopters corrected by the refractive procedure is subtracted from the keratometric reading obtained before refractive surgery. The formula is

K = Preoperative Average K – Change in Manifest Refraction Prerefractive and Postrefractive Surgery at the corneal plane, i.e.

K = Pre-RS K+ (Pre-RS SE" Post-RS SE)

where K is the current keratometric reading, Pre-RS K is the prerefractive surgery keratometry, and Pre-RS SE and Post-RS SE are the prerefractive and postrefractive surgery spherical equivalents (SEs) at the corneal plane, respectively. An example of the calculation method has been illustrated in Table 45.1.

Contact Lens Method (Over-refraction)

After performing refraction, a plano hard contact lens with a known base curve is placed on the eye and an over-refraction is performed. If the refraction does not change with the lens, then the power of the cornea must be the same as the base curve of the contact lens. If there is a myopic shift, the power of the base curve is greater than that of the cornea by the amount of the shift. If there is a hyperopic shift, the power of the base curve of the contact lens is less than that of the cornea by the amount of the shift. Corneal power is calculated by the following formula:

K = Base Curve + (Difference in Refractive Error without Contact Lens and with Contact Lens)

K = C base + C power + R cl – R bare

Here, K is the true corneal power after refractive surgery, C base is the base curve of the contact lens in diopters, C power is the spherical refractive power of the contact lens in diopters, R cl is the spherical equivalent refractive error with the contact lens, and R bare is the spherical equivalent refractive error without the contact lens. An example of the method of calculation has been shown in Table 45.2.

To give accurate information, the refractive numbers (R cl and R bare) must retain their corresponding plus (hyperopic) and minus (myopic) signs, and be corrected for vertex distance.

However, this method works only if the visual acuity is better than 6/24.

Double K Method

This is a new method[7] for calculating postrefractive surgery IOL power, using modified SRK-T formula (Table 45.3). In this method, the SRK/T formula is programmed into a spreadsheet program (Microsoft® Excel 2000) using the corrected version of the formula. The programming is done so that effective lens position (ELP) calculation algorithms use Kpre and vergence formula algorithms use Kpost. The modified formula is shown in Table 45.3. Independent

---

Table 45.1: Calculation method

Mean preoperative K = 42.50 at 90° and

41.50 at 180° = 42 D

Preoperative refraction = –10 + 1 × 90°

Vertex = 14 mm

Postoperative refraction = –0.25 + 1 × 90°

Vertex = 14 mm

STEP 1.

Calculate the spheroequivalent refraction for refractions at the corneal plane (SEQC) from the spheroequivalent refractions at the spectacle plane (SEQS) at a given vertex, where

(a) SEQ = Sphere + 0.5 (Cylinder)

(b) $SEQ_C = \dfrac{1000}{\dfrac{1000}{SEQs} - \text{Vertex (mm)}}$

Calculation for preoperative spheroequivalent refraction at corneal plane

(a) $SEQ_R = -10.00 + 0.5 * (1.00) = \textbf{–9.50 D}$

(b) $SEQ_C = \dfrac{1000}{\dfrac{1000}{-9.50} - 14} = \textbf{–8.38 D}$

Calculation for postoperative spheroequivalent refraction at corneal plane

(a) $SEQ_R = -0.25 + 0.5 * (1.00) = +0.25\ D$

(b) $SEQ_C = \dfrac{1000}{\dfrac{1000}{-0.25} - 14} = \textbf{+0.25}$

STEP 2.

Calculate the change in refraction at the corneal plane.

Change in refraction =

Preoperative SEQC – Postoperative SEQC

Change in refraction = –8.38 – (+.025) = **–8.63 D**

STEP 3.

Determine calculated postoperative corneal refractive power.

Mean postoperative K = Mean preoperative K – Change in refraction at corneal plane

Mean postoperative K = 42.00 – 8.63 = **33.37 D**

Table 45.2: Contact lens method

Suppose, the current refraction = **+0.25 D**.

With a plano hard contact lens BC of 35 D placed on the cornea, the spherical refraction changes to –2 D. Because the patient had a myopic shift with the contact lens, the cornea must be weaker than the base curve of the contact by **2.25 D**.

Therefore, the cornea must be **32.75 D (35–2.25)**, which is slightly different than the value obtained by the calculation method.

SEQ refraction without hard contact lens = **+0.25 D**

Base curve of plano hard contact lens = **35.00 D**

SEQ refraction with hard contact lens = **–2.00 D**

Change in refraction = –2.00 – (+0.25) = **–2.25 D**

(myopic shift)

Mean corneal power = Base curve of plano HCL + Change in refraction

Mean corneal power = **35.00 + (–2.25)**

Mean corneal power = **32.75 D**

Table 45.3: Double-K SRK/T Formula

Equation 1: Preoperative corneal radius of curvature:

$$r_{pre} = 337.5/Kpre$$

Equation 2: Corrected axial length (LCOR):

If　L ≤ 24.2,　LCOR = L

If　L > 24.2,　LCOR = −3.446 + 1.716 × L − 0.0237 × L2

Equation 3: Computed corneal width (Cw):

Cw = −5.41 + 0.58412 × LCOR + 0.098 × Kpre

Equation 4: Corneal height (H):

H = r_{pre} − Sqrt [r_{pre}2 − (Cw2/4)]

Equation 5: Offset value:

Offset = ACD_{const} − 3.336

Equation 6: Estimated postoperative ELP (ACD):

ACD_{est} = H + Offset

Equation 7: Constants:

V = 12; n_a = 1.336; n_c = 1.333; n_cm1 = 0.333

Equation 8: Retinal thickness (RETHICK) and optical axial length (LOPT):

RETHICK = 0.65696 − 0.02029 × LLOPT

= L + RETHICK

Equation 9: Postoperative corneal radius of curvature:

$$r_{post} = 337.5/Kpost$$

Equation 10: Emmetropia IOL power (IOL_{emme}):

$$IOL_{emme} = \frac{[1000 \times n_a \times (n \times r_{post} - n_c m1 \times LOPT)]}{[(LOPT - ACD_{est}) \times (n_a \times r_{post} - n_c m1 \times ACD_{est})]}$$

Variables

L = axial length; K_{pre} = pre refractive surgery K-value; K_{post} = post refractive surgery K-value; ACD_{const} = IOL constant (can be computed from A-constant).

Table 45.4: Nomogram for Intraocular Lens Power Adjustment for Emmetropia after Myopic Excimer Ablation[9]

Change in Spherical Equivalent at the Spectacle Plane Induced by LASIK/Photorefractive Keratectomy (Diopters)	Increase in Intra-ocular Lens Power (Diopters)
1.00	0.36
1.50	0.66
2.00	0.96
2.50	1.26
3.00	1.55
3.50	1.85
4.00	2.15
4.50	2.45
5.00	2.74
5.50	3.04
6.00	3.34
6.50	3.64
7.00	3.93
7.50	4.23
8.00	4.53
8.50	4.83
9.00	5.12
9.50	5.42
10.00	5.72
10.50	6.02
11.00	6.31
11.50	6.61
12.00	6.91

variables are AL, Kpre, Kpost, and the A-constant of the IOL.

Equations 1 to 6 calculate the ELP. Therefore, Kpre is programmed to be used in equations 1 and 3. The Kpost value is used in equation 9, which converts the dioptric power value in millimeters or corneal radius of curvature, which goes into the vergence formula (equation 10). This calculates the emmetropic IOL power.

By calculating IOL power using this formula in postrefractive surgery patients, a hyperopic refractive error is noted in many patients.

Nomogram based Modification of IOL Power (Feiz-Mannis)

Feiz V et al have developed a nomogram (Table 45.4) that guided the theoretical adjustment of IOL power based solely on post-LASIK keratometry and the refractive change induced by LASIK without the need for pre-LASIK keratometry. To develop the nomogram, they used the following formula:

IOL power underestimation = −0.231 +

(0.595 × Change in SE)

The following assumptions were made:
1. IOL power after myopic LASIK would be higher than the IOL power before LASIK.
2. To achieve emmetropia after LASIK, the change in IOL power has to balance the refractive change induced by LASIK.
3. For every diopter (D) of change in IOL power, the refraction at the spectacle plane changes only by 0.67 D, as shown by Sanders and Kraff[10] in an analysis of 2500 eyes after cataract surgery. They found that after cataract extraction, by use of nomogram adjustment, 63.2% of eyes were within

0.5 D of the intended spherical equivalent, 84.2% were within 1.0 diopter of the intended spherical equivalent, and 100% were within 1.5 D of the intended spherical equivalent.

The Masket Method

This method uses a simple IOL power corrective adjustment regression formula.

The IOL power adjustment equation is as follows:

IOL power adjustment = LSE X (–0.326) + 0.101

(LSE= spherical equivalent of the laser treatment, adjusted for the vertex distance)

The Haigis-L Formula

This new algorithm precisely allows predictable outcomes in eyes after corneal refractive laser surgery solely for myopia on the basis of current measurements. Previous patient data are not required.

The Haigis-L formula is characterised by the following stages:

1. Use the correction curve to correct the current IOL Master the measurement of corneal radius and derive the effective equivalent corneal power.
2. Subtract 0.35 D from the obtained value to allow for the effective lens position prediction error.
3. Reconvert this value into an effective corneal radius on the basis of a keratometer index of 1.3315 and enter it into the regular Haigis formula (because this formula calls for a radius input and internally uses the 1.3315 conversion).

Hence, if $r$meas is the corneal radius (mm) measured with the IOL Master in an eye after laser surgery for myopia, the corrected radius $r$corr to be entered into the regular Haigis formula is calculated according to

$$r_{corr} = \frac{331.5}{-5.1625 \times r_{meas} + 82.2603 - 0.35}$$

The study of 187 eyes by Haigis documents the percentages of refraction predictions within ± 2.00, ± 1.00, and ± 0.50 D to be 98.4%, 84.0%, and 61.0%, respectively.

BESSt Formula

The BESSt formula, based on the Gaussian optics formula, was developed using data from 143 eyes that had keratorefractive surgery. This method does not require any historical data and thus may be applicable to those cases where lack of preoperative data precludes the use of other methods like the clinical history method.

Development of the BESSt formula:
- The accuracy of the Gaussian optics formula in estimating the corneal power in virgin corneas before refractive surgery was assessed, and the results were compared to the actual values measured with corneal topography. The Gaussian optics formula was then

modified on the basis of the results of regression analysis to take these differences into account. The modified version of the Gaussian optics formula was termed BESSt_vc (vc = virgin corneas) formula.
- The BESSt_vc formula was then refined on the basis of the results of the regression analysis until the closest possible fit with the K-values calculated with the history method was obtained. A correction factor was introduced to compensate for steep and flat corneas after laser refractive surgery. This final version of the formula was named the BESSt formula and, together with the history technique and the SRK/T and Hoffer Q formula (with or without the double-K adjustment), was implemented in a Microsoft Windows software program, the BESSt Corneal Power Calculator.

The formula takes the anterior and posterior corneal radii and pachymetry (Pentacam, Oculus) into account and does not require pre-keratorefractive surgery information. A software program has been developed (BESSt Corneal Power Calculator) based on this formula. (Table 45.5)

The early reports seem quite promising. Using the BESSt formula, 46% of eyes were within ± 0.50 D of the intended refraction and 100% were within ± 1.00 D. This study however, was carried out only on 13 eyes—7 with myopic laser correction and 6 with hyperopic correction.

Further studies are, however, warranted to establish the efficacy of this formula.

(h) The No-history Method: Shammas-PL formula

The no history method uses the Shammas-PL formula (Table 45.6), a post-LASIK modification of a previously described formula[14], in which the average corneal power, K, is replaced by the corrected mean corneal power, Kc, and where Kc = 1.14 Kpost – 6.8, with Kpost being the post-LASIK K-readings in diopters (D)[15]. No other modification was made to the original formula. The estimated postoperative anterior chamber depth (pACD) is expressed as the C-value in the formula. The conversion equation from the A-constant of a specific IOL to the C-value used in this formula reads as follows:

C = pACD = (0.5835 × A) – 64.40

The authors reported promising results with 93.3% of the eyes within ±1.00 D.

Methods to Bypass the Intraocular Lens Power Calculation

- Intraoperative Retinoscopy
- Hand held Autorefractometers

In this method, aphakic refractive correction can be used to calculate the IOL power for emmetropia. The measurements are obtained after the cataract has been removed, but prior to the lens implantation. The aphakic refraction

Table 45.5: Snapshot of the BESSt corneal power calculator

BESSt© Corneal Power Calculator ⊠

Patient

| Surname: | xxxxxxxxxxxxxxx | Name: | xxxxxxxxxxxxxx | Hospital Nc: | xxxxxxxxxxxxxx | Eye: | Right ▼ |

Required post-keratorefractive surgery data for BESSt Formula (Oculus PentacamTM)

CCT: 476   Ant r: 8.84   Post r: 6.51   AL: 25

Measuring units:

CCT: Central Corneal Thickness (microns)   Ant r: Anterior corneal radius of curvature (mn)
Post r: Posterior corneal radius of curvature (mm)   AL: Axial Length (mm)
Steep K: Steep corneal meridian (D)   Flat K: Flat corneal meridian (D)

Please select one of the following:

This cornea has undergone Kerato-Refractive Surgery ▼

OPTIONAL FIELDS (Post-refractive surgery Ks)

IOL Master Steep K: 41.12   IOL Master Flat K: 40.00

Desired post-phaco refraction and IOL A-constant

Target Refraction: -0.25

A-Constant IOL: 118.0 ▼

Clear All   Clear Results

OPTIONAL FIELDS: only needed to show the results of the Clinical History & double-K Method

Pre-keratorefractive surgery data

K1: 45.25   K2: 45.50   Sph: -7.25   Cyl: -0.66   BVD: 10

Post-keratorefractive surgery data

Sph: -0.37   Cyl: -0.25

Note: Note: The difference between Ant r (PentacamTM) and K average (IOL MasterTM) is >0.50 D.

Results

	Corneal Power:	IOL Power (bag): SRK®/T:	Hoffer Q:	IOL Power (bag): dk SRK/T	dk HofferQ
IOL Master®:	40.56	19.12	19.67		
BESSt® Formula:	37.97	21.79	23.06		
History cp	39.15	20.59	21.52	23.10	22.20
History sp	38.29	21.46	22.62	24.32	23.40

Cancel   Calculate

Table 45.6 : The Shammas-PL formula

Calculations of an emmetropic IOL:

$$IOLemm = \frac{1336}{L - 0.1(L - 23) - (C + 0.05)} - \frac{1}{\dfrac{1.0125}{Kc} - \dfrac{C + 0.05}{1336}}$$

where L = axial length in millimeters, C = pACD (estimated postoperative anterior chamber depth) in millimeters, the corrected K-readings Kc = 1.14 Kpost – 6.8, with Kpost being the post-LASIK K-readings in diopters.

For converting the A-constant of a specific IOL, to the Shammas pACD:

$$C = pACD = (0.5835 \times A) - 64.40$$

where A is the A-constant of the IOL being used. This conversion equation is different than the equation used to calculate other the pACD in other formula's.

Calculations for an ametropic IOL:

$$IOLam = \frac{1336}{L - 0.1(L - 23) - (C + 0.05)} - \frac{1}{\dfrac{1.0125}{Kc + R} - \dfrac{C + 0.05}{1336}}$$

where R is the desired refraction at the corneal plane.

can be performed by retinoscopy or using a portable autorefractor. The IOL power can then be calculated, taking the aphakic correction into account, with the aid of various formulae. The formula proposed by Mackool, for example, calculates the IOL power as follows:

$$P = 1.75 \times AR + (A - 118.84)$$

Where P = IOL power; AR = Aphakic correction; A = A constant of the intended IOL

Till date, none of the formula's is absolutely accurate for the calculation of the IOL power after previous keratorefractive surgery. However, each of these methods will assist the cataract surgeons to more accurately select the proper IOL power for patients who have had previous corneal surgery. The most difficult challenge for cataract surgeons is that much of the data necessary are often not present because of the long time interval between a patient's cataract surgery and the refractive surgical procedure. A working knowledge of these methods combined with trying to gather as much preoperative patient information as possible, will help surgeons overcome this problem, which will certainly grow in significance as the number of patients receiving refractive surgery increases worldwide. Newer formulae are however, constantly being developed and refined to circumvent the need for historical data.

The clinical history method and hard contact lens method, can be used for incisional surgery as well as excimer laser surgery. Care must be taken with the topographic method when analysing patients who have had previous PRK or LASIK due to a change in effective refractive corneal index of refraction.

Postoperative Results after RK

On the first postoperative day, there is some hyperopic shift, due to the transient corneal edema. Daily fluctuations cause a myopic shift during the day due to the regression of corneal edema after awakening in the morning.

Long-term Results after RK

Long-term results of cataract surgery after RK are very good. The long-term hyperopic shifts and against-the-rule astigmatism over time following cataract surgery should be the same as following RK. Glare and starburst patterns are usually minimal as these patients are adjusted to these unwanted optical images following the initial RK. If the patient's primary complaint before cataract surgery is glare and starbursts, it should be made clear to the patient that only the glare due to the cataract will be eliminated by surgery, and the symptoms that are due to the RK will remain unchanged.

Results after PRK/ LASIK

Hyperopic shift on the first day and daily fluctuations appear to be much less.

Practical Tips

1. Make sure that the patient has realistic expectations.
2. Discuss the desired target refraction. Aiming for –1.00D seems to be a good compromise.
3. Perform corneal topography analysis in all patients to assess the amount of irregular astigmatism and asphericity.
4. If keratometric power and refraction before refractive surgery are known, use the clinical history method, considering the change of spherical equivalent refraction at the corneal plane after RK, PRK, or LASIK. If those values are not known, you may want to use the respective calculations at the spectacle plane to be on the safe (i.e. myopic) side. Some experts in this field even recommend the use of spherical equivalent refraction change at the spectacle plane routinely and add another 1.00 to 2.00 D to the resulting IOL power, being sure to avoid any potential undercorrection. The clinical history method seems to be a reliable method after RK, PRK or LASIK.
5. If keratometric diopters but not refraction before refractive surgery is known, use the change in anterior surface keratometry readings after PRK or LASIK.
6. If preoperative keratometric diopters and refraction are not known and the visual acuity is 6/24 or better, try the hard contact lens method after RK or one may use the nomogram (Table 45.4).
7. If preoperative keratometric diopters and refraction are not known and visual acuity is less than 6/24 or plano hard contact lenses are not available, use average central power or the average keratometric diopters at multiple paracentral cursor points of videokeratography after RK, but use refined calculation of keratometric diopters from radius of anterior and posterior corneal surface after PRK or LASIK. A reasonable option in such a situation would be the use of nomogram (Table 45.4).
8. Use more than one modern third-generation formula (Hoffer Q, Holladay 2, SRK/T, Haigis). Do not use a regression formula (SRK I or SRK II) to calculate the IOL power and choose the highest value for your implant.
9. Newer formulae like the Haigis-L formula, the BESSt formula and the No-history method (Shammas-PL) are very useful in predicting the IOL power in patients with no prior data of their refractive procedure. The intial reports of these formulae seem to be quite promising.

The Haigis-L can be incorporated in the IOL Master software and the BESSt formula is available as a software known as the BESSt Corneal Power Calculator.

10. During the first days after cataract surgery following RK, patients may experience a significant hyperopic shift similar to the first postoperative days following their RK. This is due to corneal edema. These patients may also exhibit diurnal fluctuations of refraction during the early time period after cataract surgery. No lens exchange should be contemplated until the refraction has stabilised (1 week to 3 months).

11. Following PRK and LASIK, early hyperopic shift or diurnal fluctuations appear to be much less after cataract surgery. In most cases, stability of the cornea makes these cases no different than patients who have had no previous refractive corneal surgery.

To be on the safe side, it would be wise that refractive surgeons might consider giving their patients a wallet card indicating their preoperative keratometric reading, preoperative refraction, and postoperative refraction at some stable time point to allow for the application of the clinical history method.

At this time, no definite statement can be made concerning IOL power calculation in patients with intracorneal rings. However, reversing the refractive corneal effect by timely removal of the ring before assessment of keratometric diopters might be a valid option. This seems even more reasonable in the face of the multiple reports about complete reversibility of the refractive effect after ring removal.

The fool-proof methodology for calculation of accurate IOL power in an eye that has undergone prior refractive surgery has not yet been discovered. In the future, our ability to more accurately measure the corneal surfaces including the anterior and posterior curvature, as well as newer IOL technologies that allow for more surgeon customisation will help improve the outcome of this difficult surgical situation.

REFERENCES

1. Holladay JT, Prager TC, Ruiz RS, Lewis JW. Improving the predictability of intraocular lens calculations. Arch Ophthalmol 1986; 104: 539–541.

2. Holladay JT, Prager TC, Chandler TY, Musgrove KH, Lewis JW, Ruiz RS. A three part system for refining intraocular lens power calculations. J Cataract Refract Surg 1988; 13: 17–24.

3. Lowe RF, Clarke BA. Posterior Corneal Curvature. Br J Ophthalmol 1973; 57: 464–470.

4. Shammas HJ, Shammas MC, Garabet A, Kim JH, Shammas A, LaBree L. Correcting the corneal power measurements for intraocular lens power calculations after myopic laser in situ keratomileusis. Am J Ophthalmol. 2003 Sep; 136(3): 426–32.

5. Chen L, Mannis MJ, Salz JJ, Garcia-Ferrer FJ, Ge J. Analysis of intraocular lens power calculation in post-radial keratotomy eyes. J Cataract Refract Surg. 2003 Jan; 29(1): 65–70.

6. Gimbel HV, Sun R. Accuracy and predictability of intraocular lens power calculation after laser in situ keratomileusis. J Cataract Refract Surg. 2001 Apr; 27(4): 571–6.

7. Aramberri J. Intraocular lens power calculation after corneal refractive surgery: double-K method. J Cataract Refract Surg. 2003 Nov; 29(11): 2063–8.

8. J. A. Retzlaff, D.R. Sanders and M.C. Kraff, Development of the SRK/T intraocular lens implant power calculation formula. J Cataract Refract Surg 1990; 16: 333–340; correction, 528.

9. Feiz V, Moshirfar M, Mannis MJ, Reilly CD, Garcia-Ferrer F, Caspar JJ, Lim MC. Nomogram-Based Intraocular Lens Power Adjustment after Myopic Photorefractive Keratectomy and LASIK: A New Approach. Ophthalmology 2005; 112 (8): 1381–1387.

10. Sanders DR, Kraff MC. Improvement of intraocular lens power calculation using empirical data, J Am Intraocular Implant Soc 1980; 6: 263–267.

11. Masket S, Masket SE. Simple regression formula for intraocular lens power adjustment in eyes requiring cataract surgery after excimer laser photoablation. J. Cataract Refract Surg 2006; 32:430–434.

12. Haigis W. Intraocular lens calculation after refractive surgery for myopia: Haigas-L formula.. J. Cataract Refract Surg 2008; 34(10):1658–63.

13. Borasio E, Stevens J, Smith GT. Estimation of true corneal power after keratorefractive surgery in eyes requiring cataract surgery: BESSt formula. J. Cataract Refract Surg, 2006; 32(12): 2004–14.

14. Shammas HJ, Shammas MC, Garabet A, et al. Correcting the corneal power measurements for intraocular lens calculations after myopic laser in situ keratomileusis. Am J Ophthalmol. 2003; 136:426–432.

15. Shammas HJ, Shammas MC. No-history method of intraocular lens power calculation after myopic laser in situ keratomileusis.J. Cataract Refract Surg 2007; 33: 31–36.

16. Mackool RJ, Ko W, Mackool R,. Intraocular lens power calculation after laser in situ keratomileusis: Aphakic refraction technique. J. Cataract Refract Surg. 2006; 32: 435–437.

Phacoemulsification and Concurrent Procedures

▼ **Concurrent Phaco and Penetrating Keratoplasty**
Col JKS Parihar SM, VSM and Maj SK Dhar

▼ **Concurrent Phaco and Ahmed Glaucoma Valve Surgery**
Col JKS Parihar SM, VSM, Maj Jaya Kaushik

▼ **Phacotrabeculectomy: Different Techniques**
Dr Mahipal S Sachdev, Dr Tanuj Dada, Dr Anand Aggarwal and Col JKS Parihar SM, VSM

▼ **Post Phaco Psuedophakic Bullous Keratopathy: IOL Exchange and Scleral Fixated IOL Implantation**
Col JKS Parihar SM, VSM and Col Vijay Mathur

▼ **Concurrent Phacoemulsification and Pars Plana Vitrectomy**
Col VS Gurunadh, Brig Ajay Banarji, Col JKS Parihar SM, VSM and Wing Cdr HS Trehan

46

Concurrent Phaco and Penetrating Keratoplasty

Col JKS Parihar SM, VSM and Maj SK Dhar

INTRODUCTION

The patient presenting with both a cataract and corneal opacity requires special consideration. The surgeon has the option of removing the cataract without a corneal transplantation, performing a corneal transplantation as a primary procedure, or doing a combined cataract extraction and corneal transplantation.

The examination should start with an evaluation of the patient's cataract. This may be difficult in the presence of significant corneal opacity. Often, instilling 10% glycerin drops after topical anesthesia will dramatically clear the cornea as to permit an accurate view of the cataract. The pupil should be dilated for the best possible slit lamp view. The second eye should also be evaluated for the presence of a cataract. Often it will be at a similar level of development as the fellow eye. If the lens is not significantly cloudy, it may be wise to perform the penetrating keratoplasty alone. The success of corneal transplant is greater in the phakic eye. In addition, if the cataract surgery is performed at a later date, a more accurate determination of the intraocular lens power can be made. On the other hand, if the cataract is significant, a corneal transplant alone may accelerate its growth.

The evaluation of the cornea is more complex. The optical significance of surface irregularities may be difficult to assess by slit lamp examination. Such corneas often have irregular astigmatism that can be discovered by using computerised corneal topography. Irregular astigmatism can arise from epithelial or stromal causes. Some examples are Meesman's dystrophy, superficial punctate keratitis, and herpetic scars of the cornea. A hard contact lens can often help to identify the amount of visual loss caused by corneal surface irregularities.

Since the introduction of the triple procedure (simultaneous penetrating keratoplasty [PK], extracapsular cataract extraction [ECCE] and implantation of a posterior chamber intraocular lens [PCIOL]) in the mid-seventies, there is an ongoing discussion among corneal surgeons concerning the best approach for combined corneal disease and cataract. The age limits for this procedure are steadily being lowered, and with the advent of newer intraocular lens (IOL) technology including multifocal IOLs, the procedure may be a good choice for those in presbyopic age groups in near future. However, the present status of knowledge and experience, particularly limitations on accurate IOL power calculation and presumed postoperative refraction methods to induce least astigmatism does not advocate multifocal IOLs in PK and IOL surgery. The combined procedure reduces surgical and visual morbidity and is more effective than performing surgery in two or more stages. Early and recent clinical results have been extremely encouraging, as reported by multiple authors over the past twenty years.

Two microsurgical approaches feasible are: First ECCE + PCIOL prior to PK and Second ECCE + PCIOL after PK. For the refractive results after triple procedure some intraoperative details are crucial: Trephination of recipient and donor from the epithelial side without major oversize should preserve the preoperative corneal curvature. Graft and the PCIOL placed in the bag after continuous curvilinear capsulorrhexis should be centred along the optical axis. If possible, performing the capsulorrhexis under controlled intraocular pressure conditions prior to trephination may help to minimises the risk of capsular ruptures.

ECCE + PCIOL prior to PK requires a cornea that is still transparent enough to perform cataract surgery, and the risk of intraocular pressure rise after PK seems to be increased.

ECCE + PCIOL after PK has the potential of a simultaneous reduction of astigmatism during ECCE (appropriate location of the incision, simultaneous refractive keratotomies or implantation of a toric PCIOL). Disadvantages may include the loss of graft endothelial cells and the theoretically increased risk of immunological allograft reactions.

INDICATIONS FOR TRIPLE PROCEDURE

The triple procedure should be considered in following situations:

(i) Both corneal (moderate corneal opacity) and cataract diseases affected patients who require improvement in vision within their own reasonable lifestyles are excellent candidates for the procedure.

Several authors have examined the success of combined versus non simultaneous surgery and have found the results to be comparable. If the improvement in visual function can be achieved either by cataract and lens implant surgery or by corneal surgery separately; the simpler procedure should be the procedure of choice.

(ii) Coexisting cataract and corneal opacity—The assessment of the extent of corneal disease and lens opacity is based on the preoperative evaluation; however, occasionally the surgeon may not determine the severity of the cataract until the cloudy cornea has been removed partially in surgery and the lens can be inspected directly. If the cataract appears to be sufficiently dense to decrease the vision to 20/50 or worse postoperatively, the lens should be removed at the time of keratoplasty. The corneal specialist will have to make a judgement call based on clinical appearance, potential acuity measurements, specular microscopy, and pachymetry. In general, the endothelial dystrophy patient with less than 1000 mm^2 healthy endothelial cells, a corneal thickness greater than 0.62 mm, and a cataract should have a combined (triple) procedure.

CONTRAINDICATIONS FOR TRIPLE PROCEDURE

Contraindications for triple procedures are identical to those for noncombined keratoplasties. However triple procedure may not be an ideal option in under mentioned conditions:

(i) Uncontrolled ocular cicatricial pemphigoid or infiltrative keratitis with corneal melting.
(ii) Patients with proliferative diabetic retinopathy.
(iii) Uncontrolled glaucoma.
(iv) Uncontrolled recurrent episodes of moderately severe or severe uveitis are poor candidates for the triple procedure.
(v) History of severe herpetic stromal keratitis.
(vi) Active keratouveitis may have complicated

postoperative courses and will require pre- and postoperative oral antiviral prophylaxis and intensive follow-up.

Advantages

The major advantage of the triple procedure is the faster visual rehabilitation and less efforts for the most elderly patients

Disadvantages

Disadvantages may include the loss of graft endothelial cells and the theoretically increased risk of immunological allograft reactions. After triple procedure , major deviations from target refraction have been reported. However, individual multiple regression analysis may help to minimise this problem with appropriate methods of trephination. The postulated better refractive outcome and better uncorrected visual acuity after the sequential approach is opposed by a markedly delayed visual rehabilitation. For this reason, triple procedure including CE should be the method of choice for combined lens and corneal opacities where feasible. Often because of the rapidly progressive nuclear cataracts after PK, the simultaneous approach in elderly patients with Fuchs' dystrophy even with incipient lens opacities is a better option.

However, the prolonged operating time associated with the combined procedure is potentially associated with the devastating complication of expulsive choroidal haemorrhage. Although the complication can occur with corneal transplant or cataract surgery alone, it is more likely to occur in triple procedures. Most cases seem to occur in patients who move, cough, or squeeze the eyelids during the "open sky" portion of the operation (ECCE), and the importance of an adequate lid block cannot be overemphasised. The surgeon may be wise to stage the procedures or perform the cataract portion of the procedure in a more closed system (phacoemulsification) for patients who are at risk for expulsive choroidal hemorrhage (advanced age, glaucoma) or who are likely to be restless during surgery.

PHACOEMULSIFICATION vs ECCE IN TRIPLE PROCEDURE

The technique described allowed controlled capsulorrhexis, cataract removal and in-the-bag IOL implantation. With an open-sky technique, the posterior capsule and vitreous tend to move anteriorly. This makes cortex removal and intraocular lens implantation more difficult. The removal of the nucleus is often more difficult than during a closed system technique. Classic bimanual expression cannot be performed. The surgical technique described in this report can only be used in selected patients undergoing combined corneal transplant and cataract surgery. In this group of patients, however, the technique offers many intra- and postoperative advantages.

Advantages of Phacoemulsification over ECCE

(i) **Continuous curvilinear capsulorrhexis (CCC):** Continuous curvilinear capsulorrhexis (CCC) is performed in a closed system when corneal transparency is sufficient. With the open-sky method, the CCC is created while counter pressure is applied to the centre of the lens with a large spatula, reducing posterior pressure and thus, the risk of capsule tear.

(ii) **Less chances of uncompensated posterior pressure:** Less chances of uncompensated posterior pressure created when the cornea is open, include incomplete capsulorrhexis, incomplete aspiration-irrigation of the cortex, uncertain placing of the IOL, posterior capsule rupture, choroidal effusion, and even expulsive haemorrhage.

(iii) **Reduced risk of uveitis and secondary glaucoma:** Risk of intraocular pressure rise after PK and phaco seems to be less as compared to the ECCE and PK since in-the-bag implantation of IOL provides better configuration of anterior chamber in terms of more depth as compared to the sulcus fixated IOL, uniform surface of iris IOL diaphragm, practically no contact between the posterior surface of iris and IOL. Hence overall compound effect of such a configuration results in significant reduction in the chances of chronic uveitis, posterior synaechiae and subsequent secondary glaucoma.

(iv) **Less insult to graft endothelial cells:** The presence of in the bag IOL implant is much superior to the sulcus fixated IOL implant. The overall impact of in-the-bag IOL is seen as there is a reduced risk of uveitis, secondary glaucoma as well as better protection of endothelium and lesser chances of endothelitis.

Lower incidence of PCO: Phacoemulsification provides closed chamber manipulations while performing irrigation and aspiration procedures as compared to the ECCE and thereby provides a stable capsular bag with wide open fornices of the capsular bag. Such an intraoperative structural configuration facilitates adequate removal of cortical matter and thus reduces the risk of PCO formation. Over and above, the in-the-bag IOL position is substantially suitable to minimise the possibilities of proliferation of secondary fibres. Hence, concurrent phaco and PK has much superiority over ECCE in terms of reduced risk of PCO formation.

Disadvantages of Phacoemulsification over ECCE

Phacoemulsification with penetrating keratoplasty is difficult in cases of:

(i) Central corneal thinning and perforation
(ii) Peripheral corneal thinning
(iii) Corneal regrafting
(iv) Infectious keratitis
(v) In pediatric age group due to the need of posterior capsulotomy

ECCE is a safer option in all of these cases.

PROBLEMS RELATED TO CONCURRENT PHACOEMULSIFICATION AND PK

Biometry

After the decision has been made to proceed with the triple procedure, the lens-implant power calculation should be performed. Binder and Crawford and coworkers have evaluated the parameters that assist in proper lens-implant power selection and have developed linear-regression formula's based on their clinical experience. Retzlaff reported a linear-regression formula that has been used for cataract extraction with lens implantation. One author used this published regression formula, using the standard A-constant for the chosen IOL and inserted a prospective, postoperative keratometric value into the formula. After reviewing a series of 100 patients, the mean keratometric value was 44 dioptres in patients, atleast 1 year after operation and suture removal. The measurements were taken at least 1 month after suture removal. The formula is as follows:

$$\text{IOL power} = \text{A} - \text{constant (usually 116 dioptres)} - 2.5 \times \text{axial length} - 0.9 \times 43.5 \text{ dioptres}$$

Each corneal surgeon should individualise IOL power calculations by noting the average keratometry readings for a series of patients after keratoplasty. Several authors have reported that the choice of IOL power formula does not affect IOL power predictions in triple procedures, and the more important factor in postoperative refractive accuracy is the use of personalised constants within a given formula. Current technique for IOL power calculation uses theoretical formula's based on the axial length as recommended by Hoffer.

Axial Length (mm)	Formula	Percent Used
Table 46.1: Hoffer Technique for Intraocular Lens Power Calculation		
<22	Hoffer Q	8
22.0–24.5	Average of all three	72
24.5–26.0	Holladay	15
>26	Senders-Retzlaff-Kraff	5

The keratometry value selected is based on results of numerous triple procedures with the same trephine and suture techniques and yielded an average value close to 44.5 dioptres at 12 months postoperatively.

Combined surgery also poses a problem for proper lens power selection. It can be very difficult to get accurate keratometric readings on a pathologic cornea. The keratometric readings will often differ significantly from preoperative values. Unless the surgeon creates consistent keratometric values, he or she cannot accurately predict what the refractive outcome will be. The keratometric readings of the transplanted cornea are often less (flatter) than those of the host cornea. For this reason, we tend to choose a lens power 2 to 2.5 D greater than what the formula predicts. It is usually better to err in the myopic direction. Each surgeon must develop his or her own approach regarding lens power selection.

Inadequate Visualisation during Surgery

Pre-existing corneal opacity is bound to affect phacoprocedures adversely. The most significant constraints have been faced during rhexis and initial stage of irrigation/aspiration where corneal opacity and partly compromised red reflex pose significant difficulties. However, proper selection of cases and technique reduces the risk of such obstacles.

SURGICAL TECHNIQUE

Anaesthesia

The surgeon is ready to proceed once suitable corneal donor tissue has been obtained, the IOL power has been calculated as per methods described earlier. On the day of surgery, either a local or general anesthetic may be used. In our practice, most cases are done under local anaesthesia with minimal preoperative sedation. Equal parts of 0.75% bupivacaine and 4% lidocaine are mixed to give a solution that is 0.375% bupivacaine and 2% lidocaine. Hyaluronidase is also incorporated with the anesthetic to aid in tissue spread.

Methods to Improve Visualisation

Successful phacoemulsification may be difficult in cases of corneal haze because of poor or suboptimal visualisation of the lenticular morphology caused by the presence of corneal opacification/haze. Vital steps such as capsulorrhexis, nuclear emulsification, residual cortex removal, and foldable intraocular lens implantation are dependent upon the ability to visualise the capsular bag anatomy.

With poor visibility, errant capsular tearing is very common and difficult to control, thus jeopardising in-the-bag IOL implantation. The accepted recommendations to aid CCC in such cases are: dimming the operation room lights, increasing the operating microscope magnification and coaxial illumination, and using high density viscoelastics. The use of air, diathermy, endoilluminator, vitrector, scissors, and the two-stage CCC approach have also been suggested.

Removal of Epithelium

In addition to improving the results of corneal transplantation in selected cases, the removal of epithelium also enhances the visibility of the anterior capsule and lens which is of great help in performing phacoemulsification surgery under opaque or translucent cornea.

In cases in which no minimal peripheral epithelial oedema exists, removal of healthy peripheral recipient epithelium is unnecessary. In eyes with Fuchs's corneal dystrophy, several pathological changes may have occurred by the time of surgery including epithelial oedema, bullae, and striate keratopathy (resulting in significant corneal thickening), frank corneal decompensation, dense, nuclear cataract formation, and occasionally, tremendous epithelial hypertrophy (associated with superficial vascularisation). Some physicians prefer to remove oedematous corneal epithelium with or without fibrovascular pannus with a No. 64 Beaver blade. This approach decreases the chance of trephine slippage and irregular cutting of Bowman's membrane and the anterior lamellae of the cornea. In addition, this step ensures the sutures will be passed securely into corneal stroma, rather than into thickened fibrous tissue or epithelium. Occasionally, some cautery is required for prolific vessels, but bleeding normally ceases on its own.

Role of Trypan Blue Dye

Ophthalmic dyes such as 2% fluorescence sodium, 0.5% ICG and 0.1% trypan blue have been successfully used for performing CCC. Two main surgical techniques have been used for fluorescein sodium: (a) staining from above, under an air bubble, and (b) intracameral subcapsular injection.

Hydrodelineation associated with the formation of a golden ring, is sometimes difficult to notice. With the injection of a capsular dye solution, however, the surgeon can successfully visualise the demarcation between the nucleus and the epinucleus. In this situation, an incomplete hydrodissection/delineation can be easily identified and completed by injecting more stained fluid in that particular quadrant, if needed. After achieving complete hydrodissection and hydrodelineation it is easier to perform nuclear emulsification with less ultrasound power and time, decreasing the need for cortical cleanup and the risk of posterior capsule tears.

The staining of the nucleus (lens substance) helps in visualising the position of the phaco tip and its relation with the posterior capsule, thus enhancing the safety margin of the procedure.

Capsulorrhexis

In our view, capsulorrhexis is the most difficult step to perform under opaque cornea. The presence of opaque or translucent cornea poses significant hindrance to create a good central circular and curvilinear rhexis. One may prefer rhexis forceps over needle cystitome. However, the surgeon should go ahead with his own preference. It is very important to maintain the persistent contact with the leading edge of rhexis since it is extremely difficult to reorganise the continuity of rhexis movement under opaque cornea once it is lost. The author strongly recommends visualisation enhancing procedures/adjuvants like trypan blue staining of anterior capsule, retro illumination with the help of endoilluminator or partial excision of the anterior surface of cornea. The preference over different methods as described above are based on the merits of the case as well as on individual surgeon's experience and choice.

After excess viscoelastic and fluid is removed, a round capsulotomy is performed by capsulorrhexis. If there is any posterior vitreous pressure, the capsule edge often begins to tear radially. If this complication occurs, completion is best done with scissors. It is wise to avoid contact with the iris to prevent premature miosis before removal of the nucleus. The central piece of anterior capsule is removed, and any excess tags of peripheral AC can also be removed at this point. A nice, round opening approximately 6 mm in diameter is preferred.

Hydroprocedures

The author recommends slow and gradual hydroprocedure in the presence of opaque cornea, since poor visualisation may not allow early detection of signs of impending complications like extension of rhexis, zonulysis or posterior capsule rent. Hence, it is most important to maintain a very vigilant approach throughout the procedure

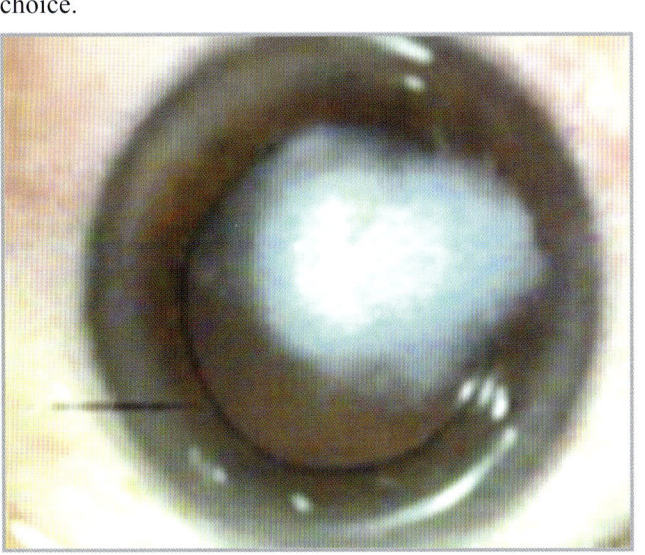

(a)

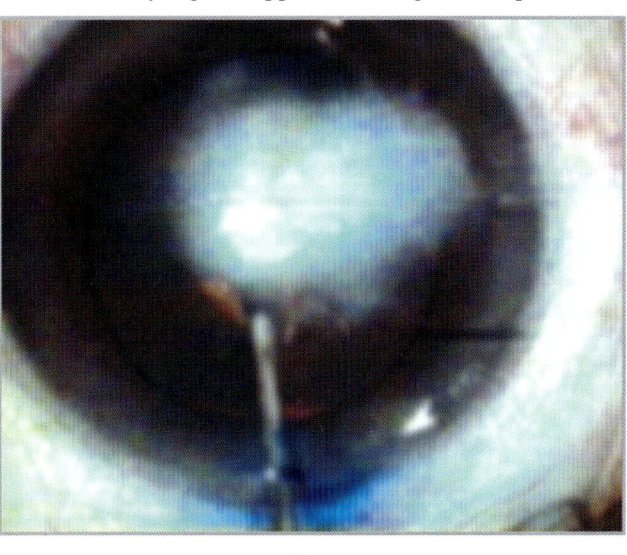

(b)

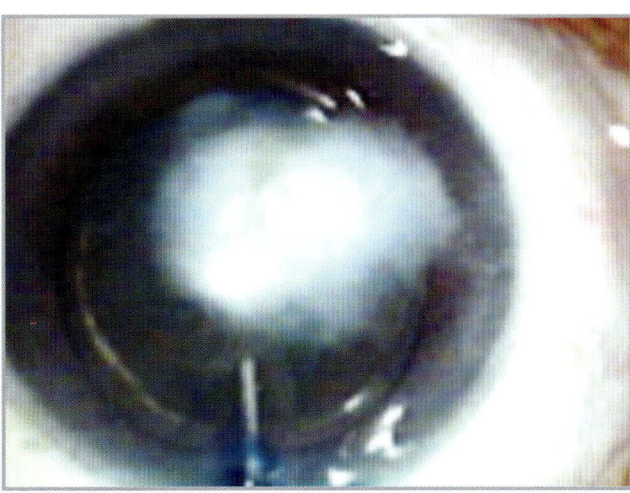

(c)

Fig. 46.1: (a) Coexisting cataract and corneal opacity, (b) Trypan blue enhanced rhexis, (c) Phaco in corneal opacity: Hydroprocedure

particularly while performing hydrodelineation which is linked with the possibility of hydroprocedure linked complications.

Nucleotomy in the Presence of Corneal Opacity

Nucleotomy may be performed by applying any technique of phaco fragmentation in the presence of corneal opacity. However, the author prefers to use chopping over divide and conquer technique since the latter technique demands several intraoperative manipulations like repeated nucleus rotation as well as sculpting movements. Chopping keeps nucleus away from posterior capsule throughout the procedure. Over and above, chopping applies relatively less energy as compared to sculpting which is very crucial in terms of its impact on peripheral corneal endothelium of a diseased cornea.

We recommend moderate settings of fluid dynamics so as to enhance safety during intraoperative manoeuvre in the presence of opaque cornea.

Irrigation and Aspiration

It is important to use relatively little fluid irrigation because excess fluid obscures the surgeon's view of the red reflex and creates multiple-mirrored images from the fluid surface, obscuring a good view of the cortex and posterior lens capsule.

Posterior Chamber Intraocular Lens Insertion

Viscoelastic is used to separate the anterior and posterior lens capsules to facilitate in-the-bag loop placement. Constant gentle downward pressure should be maintained on the IOL during insertion as the vitreous pressure tends to push the IOL back out of the bag. If necessary, the position of the lens can be inspected with a hook, and the lens implant rotated to achieve centration. A small peripheral iridotomy is optional, but it is not routinely done.

After the IOL is positioned, intracameral pilocarpine or acetylcholine chloride is used for miosis and to ensure the final placement of the lens behind the iris.

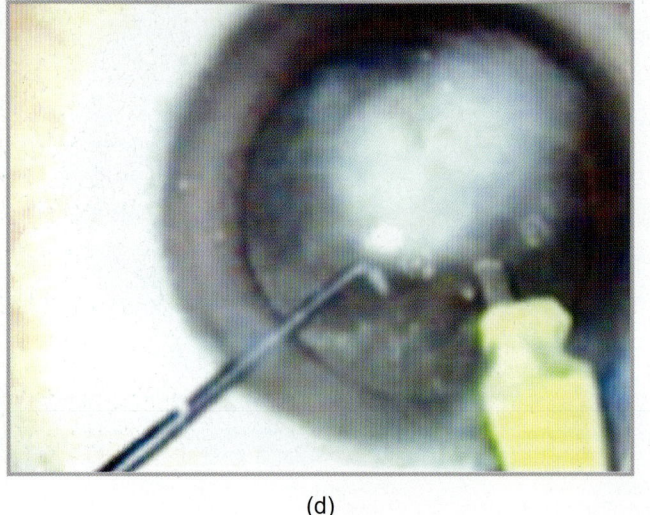

(d)

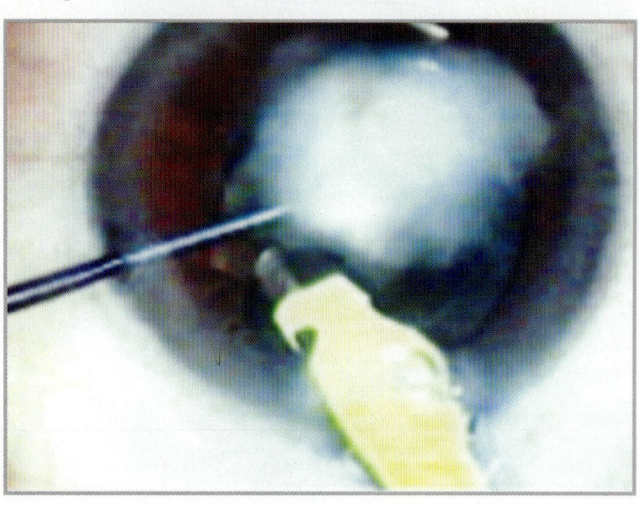

(e)

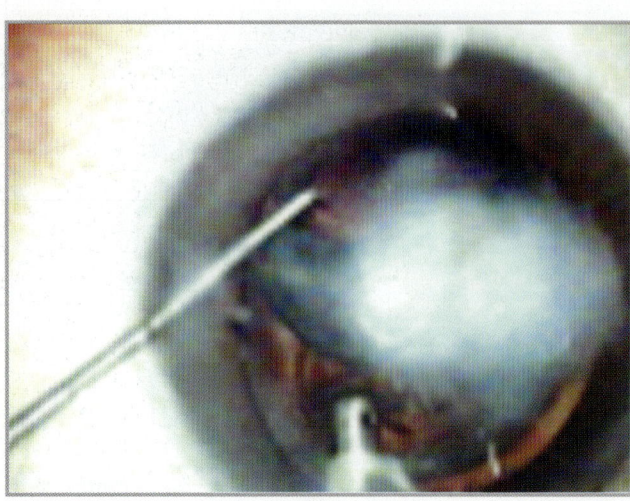

(f)

Fig. 46.1: (d) Phaco in corneal opacity: Direct chopping, (e) Phaco in corneal opacity: Fragment removal, (f) Phaco in corneal opacity: I/A

Residual viscoelastic material is left in situ so as to facilitate subsequent excision of opaque cornea and transplantation of donor cornea.

Donor Tissue Preparation

Donor tissue should be prepared before trephination of the patient's cornea to ensure that adequate donor tissue is available immediately upon entry into the anterior chamber. There are a variety of techniques for the trephination of donor tissue. Most surgeons cut the donor tissue endothelial side up with an Iowa, Troutman, or Hanna corneal trephine punch. The author has been using disposable trephines with ease and good results. The size of the trephine selected should be 0.25 mm greater than the opening to be made in the recipient cornea. The slight oversize of the button allows for some tissue compression effect of the sutures without significant flattening of the central graft curvature.

Recipient Cornea Trephination

Recipient cornea trephination is done in a usual manner. Needless to emphasise the significance of centration of cornea in terms of least induced astigmatism as well as ultimate graft survival. The most simple way of making centration is to mark the centre of the operating microscope light reflex on the recipient cornea.

The centre of the patient's cornea may be marked by measuring with 6 mm calipers from the periphery to the centre at all the four cardinal positions at 3, 6, 9 and 12 O'clock meridians. A 3 mm optical zone marker marked with gentian violet is centred over the four indentations in the cornea so as to ascertain the presumed position of the optical zone.

The position of subsequent interrupted or continuous suture placement may be marked with the help of an inked 12-incision radial keratotomy marker. The viscoelastic

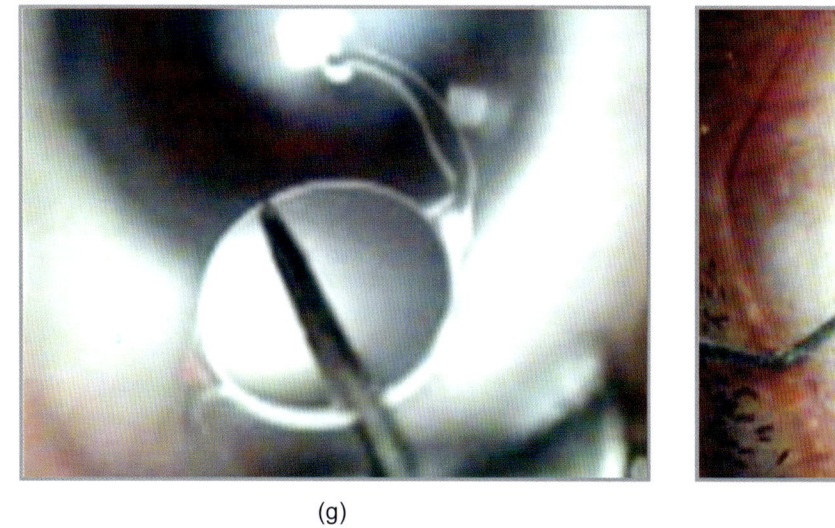

(g)

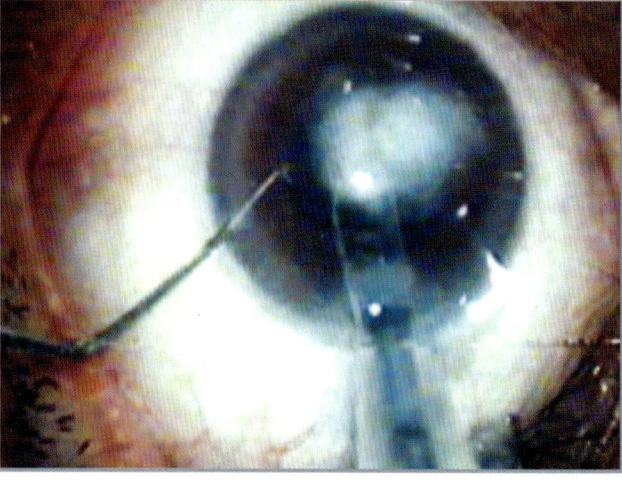

(h)

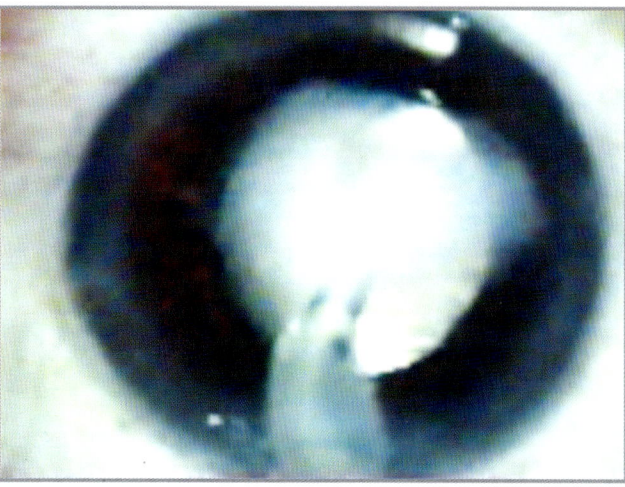

(i)

Fig. 46.1: (g) Phaco in corneal opacity: Hydrophobic acrylic IOL implantation, (h) IOL insertion under opaque cornea, (i) Phaco in corneal opacity: Post IOL implant wash

material is being injected into the anterior chamber prior to the excision of recipient cornea with the help of 26 gauze needle so as to protect the intraocular structures while manipulating the trephine.

Transplantation of Donor Graft

The donor cornea is removed from the polyteflon block with the help of corneal spatula or fine colibri forceps and placed over the recipient bed where it is secured with four cardinal sutures placed sequentially at the 12 O'clock, 6 O'clock, 3 O'clock, and 9 O'clock positions. The chamber is being reformed with viscoelastic material. The presence of visco material is highly beneficial to secure an adequate depth of the anterior chamber throughout the period of suturing.

The surgeon may choose a suture technique of his own preference like interrupted sutures alone, single or double continuous sutures or a combination of interrupted and continuous suture techniques.

Adjustment of Suture Tension

Intraoperative adjustment of suture tension to minimise postkeratoplasty astigmatism is vital to the success of corneal grafts.

Suture tension is adjusted twice during the operation; One, after the interrupted sutures and again, after the running suture is tied.

CHANCES OF GRAFT FAILURE IN CONCURRENT PHACO AND PK

(i) Concurrent phaco and penetrating keratoplasty show a similar risk of graft failure or allogenic graft rejection as with keratoplasty alone.

(ii) Postoperative complications (increased chances of raised IOP) and postoperative surgical interventions may increase the risk of graft failure in simultaneous phacoemulsification and PKP.

(iii) Intraocular lens implantation did not increase the risk for graft failure.

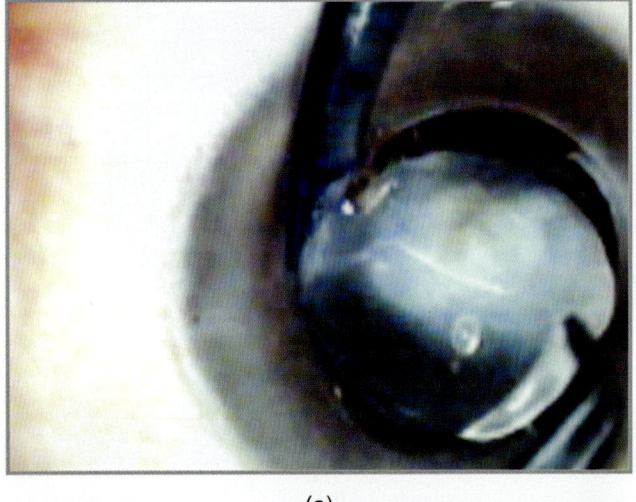

(a)

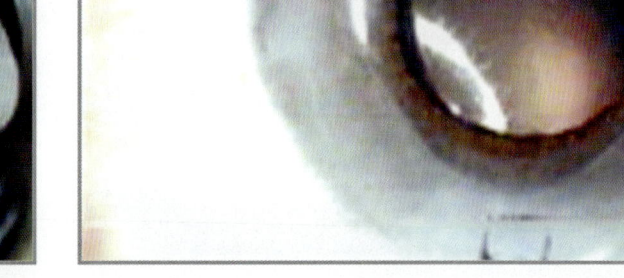

(b)

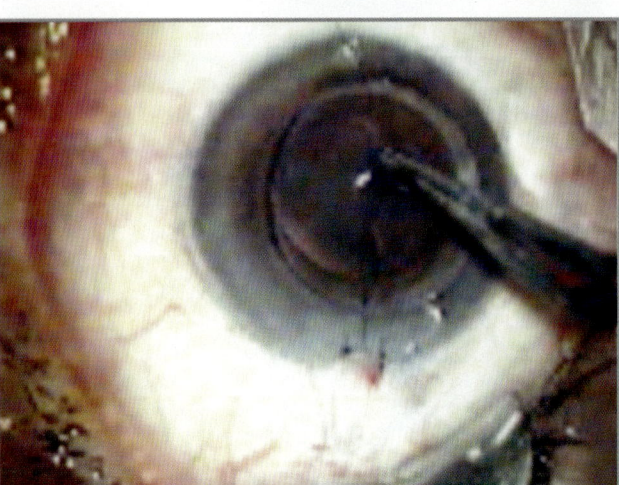

(c)

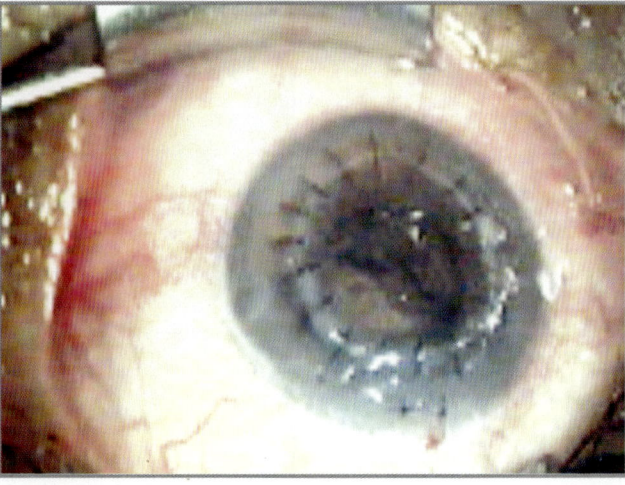

(d)

Fig. 46.2: (a) Post Phaco excision of opaque cornea, (b) Recipient bed prepared: In-the-bag IOL is visible, (c) Suturing of donor corneal graft following phaco and IOL implantation, (d) PK with phaco and IOL implantation

FACTORS INFLUENCING VISUAL OUTCOME AFTER CONCURRENT PHACO AND PK

The most important factors influencing visual outcome after concurrent phacoemulsification and penetrating keratoplasty are:

(a) Preoperative visual acuity, graft size, and the reason for keratoplasty.

(b) Other factors such as age, sex, diabetes mellitus, and preoperative refractive error do not substantially influence the postoperative visual outcome.

CONCLUSION

The concurrent PK and phacoemulsification with in-the-bag intraocular lens implantation being a closed system procedure, has definite superiority and several merits over the PK with ECCE which, has the potential risk of several constraints and complications. In view of the above, the author recommends phacoemulsification as the procedure of choice for cataract removal in cases of moderate grade corneal opacity.

BIBLIOGRAPHY

1. Malbran ES, Malbran E, Buonsanti J, Adrogue E. Closed-system phacoemulsification and posterior chamber implant combined with penetrating keratoplasty. Ophthalmic Surg. 1993 Jun; 24(6):403–6.

2. Groden LR. Continuous tear capsulotomy and phacoemulsification cataract extraction combined with penetrating keratoplasty. Refract Corneal Surg. 1990 Nov-Dec; 6(6): 458–9.

3. Nishida T. Basic science: cornea. In: Krachmer JH, Mannis MJ, Holland EJ, eds. Cornea, Volume I: Fundamentals of Cornea and External Disease. St Louis, Mo: Mosby–Year Book Co Inc; 1997:3–27.

4. Nardi M, Giudice V, Marabotti A, Alfieri E, Rizzo S. Temporary graft for closed-system cataract surgery during corneal triple procedures. J Cataract Refract Surg. 2001; 27:1172–1175.

5. Baca LS, Epstein RJ. Closed-chamber capsulorrhexis for cataract extraction combined with penetrating keratoplasty. J Cataract Refract Surg. 1998 May; 24(5):581–4.

6. Caporossi A, Traversi C, Simi C, Tosi GM. Closed-system and open-sky capsulorrhexis for combined cataract extraction and corneal transplantation. J Cataract Refract Surg. 2001; 27:990–993.

7. Bhartiya P, Sharma N, Ray M, Sinha R, Vajpayee R B. Trypan blue assisted phacoemulsification in corneal opacities; British Journal of Ophthalmology 2002; 86:857–859.

8. Nishimura Akira; Kobayashi Akira ; Segawa Yasunori ; Sugiyama Kazuhisa. Endoillumination-assisted cataract surgery in a patient with corneal opacity. J. cataract refractive surg 2003 (29)12, 2277–80

9. Marc C. Muraine, Amélie Collet, Gérard Brasseur, Deep Lamellar Keratoplasty Combined With Cataract Surgery: Arch Ophthalmol. 2002; 120:812–815.

10. Seitz B, Langenbucher A, Viestenz A, Dietrich T, Kuchle M, Naumann GO.Cataract and keratoplasty—simultaneous or sequential surgery? Klin Monatsbl Augenheilkd. 2003 May; 220(5):326–9. German.

11. Rao SK, Padmanabhan P. Combined phacoemulsification and penetrating keratoplasty. Ophthalmic Surg Lasers. 1999 Jun; 30(6):488–91.

12. Dangel ME, Kirkham SM, Phipps MJ. Posterior capsule opacification in extracapsular cataract extraction and the triple procedure: a comparative study. Ophthalmic Surg. 1994 Feb; 25(2):82–7.

13. Robin H, Hannouche D, Hoang-Xuan T. Triple procedure with phacoemulsification prior to grafting]J Fr Ophtalmol. 1997; 20(9):701–3.

14. Kocak-Altintas AG, Kocak-Midillioglu I, Dengisik F, Duman S. Implantation of scleral-sutured posterior chamber intraocular lenses during penetrating keratoplasty. J Refract Surg. 2000 Jul-Aug; 16(4):456–8.

15. Borderie V, Touzeau O, Laroche L. Value of implantation in the capsular bag during combined operation of penetrating keratoplasty and cataract surgery.J Fr Ophtalmol. 1997; 20(3):200–6. French.

16. Lois N, Kowal VO, Cohen EJ, Rapuano CJ, Gault JA, Raber IM, Laibson PR. Indications for penetrating keratoplasty and associated procedures, 1989–1995.Cornea. 1997 Nov; 16(6): 623–9.

17. Busin M, Arffa RC, McDonald MB, Kaufman HE. Combined penetrating keratoplasty, extracapsular cataract extraction, and posterior chamber intraocular lens implantation. Ophthalmic Surg. 1987 Apr; 18(4):272–5.

18. Kawamoto K, Morishige N, Chikama T, Nishida T. Modification of a soft contact lens for use during irrigation and aspiration in the penetrating keratoplasty triple procedure. Arch Ophthalmol. 2006 Apr; 124(4):550–1.

19. Kirkness CM, Cheong PY, Steele AD. Penetrating keratoplasty and cataract surgery: the advantages of an extracapsular technique combined with posterior chamber intraocular implantation. Eye. 1987; 1 (Pt 5):557–61.

20. Keates RH, Rothchild EJ, Bloom R. Endocapsular triple procedure—a new triple procedure technique. J Cataract Refract Surg. 1989; 15(3):332–5.

21. Shimmura S, Ohashi Y, Shiroma H, Shimazaki J, Tsubota K. Corneal opacity and cataract: triple procedure versus secondary approach.Cornea. 2003 Apr; 22(3):234–8.

22. Hunkeler JD, Hyde LL. The triple procedure; combined penetrating keratoplasty, cataract extraction and lens implantation. J Am Intraocul Implant Soc. 1979 Jul; 5(3):222–4.

23. Jonas JB, Rank RM, Budde WM, Sauder G. Factors influencing visual outcome after penetrating keratoplasty combined with intraocular lens implantation. Eur J Ophthalmol. 2003 Mar; 13(2):134–8.

24. Kuchle M, Handel A, Naumann GO. (Results of implantation of transsclerally sutured posterior chamber lenses in combination with penetrating keratoplasty) Ophthalmologe. 1998 Oct; 95(10):671–6.(German).

25. Borderie VM, Touzeau O, Bourcier T, Carvajal-Gonzalez S, Laroche L. The triple procedure: in the bag placement versus ciliary sulcus placement of the intraocular lens. Br J Ophthalmol. 1999; 83(4):458–62.

26. Asparov AA, Subbotina IN. Indications, terms and classification of reconstructive interventions based on penetrating keratoplasty with implantation of posterior chamber intraocular lens. Vestn Oftalmol. 2000 Nov-Dec; 116(6):3–7.(Russian).

27. Chiou AG, Bovet J, de Courten C. Management of corneal ectasia and cataract following photorefractive keratectomy. J Cataract Refract Surg. 2006; 32(4):679–80.

28. Bersudsky V, Rehany U, Rumelt S. Risk factors for failure of simultaneous penetrating keratoplasty and cataract extraction. J Cataract Refract Surg. 2004 Sep; 30(9):1940–7.

47

Concurrent Phaco and Ahmed Glaucoma Valve Surgery

Col JKS Parihar sm, vsm, Maj Jaya Kaushik

INTRODUCTION

Management of coexisting cataract and glaucoma, particularly in cases of refractory glaucoma associated with cataract is a highly complex situation in which conventional phacotrabeculectomy has been found to be disappointing particularly in cases of refractive glaucoma.

The term refractory glaucoma is being used for any kind of glaucoma which has not responded to medical or surgical treatment and needs subsequent surgical re-intervention.

The peculiarities involved with deranged anatomical configuration, physiology and dynamics of aqueous circulation in these cases are far different from the other glaucoma cases and were found to have a highly disappointing outcome. Such complexity further adds to limited and short term success despite repeated surgical intervention in the form of trabeculectomy or combined modulated trabeculectomy and trabeculectomy. Since the usual line of management of both medical and surgical procedures have invariably proved ineffective in this particular glaucoma group, the application of various glaucoma drainage devices have been tried in the recent past. However, such devices were not accepted in general due to complexity of procedure, constraints of follow up, as well as bioacceptance of valve material and design itself. The newer generation drainage devices have been found to have significant qualitative improvement in terms of design and materials as well. These changes have encouraged wider acceptance of such devices in refractory glaucomas. We have a vast experience in glaucoma drainage device application with several modifications and innovations in instrumentation and techniques including combined phaco and glaucoma drainage device applications and their subsequent long-term evaluation.

HISTORICAL BACKGROUND OF GLAUCOMA DRAINAGE DEVICES

Surgical procedures for glaucoma remained an uneven road until trabeculectomy was introduced for adult onset glaucoma. However, despite reasonably good results in moderate and uncomplicated glaucoma, the management of infantile and complicated glaucoma in both adult and paediatric cases remains a nightmare for most of the glaucoma surgeons. Over and above, management of concurrent glaucoma and cataract or corneal opacities remains the most frustrating outcome for patients as well as the surgeons. Poor response to filtering procedures had attracted invention of an ideal alternative device to control nonresponsive glaucoma which continues to remain a quest for all ophthalmic surgeons with great imagination and impending application of diverse resources such as suture materials like silk, catgut or metal, crystal and gelatin to cellulose and many more.

In 1906, Rollet and Moreau had placed horse hair through a corneal paracentesis in an attempt to drain a hypopyon externally. The same technique was later used to treat two patients with painful absolute glaucoma as an adjuvant to filtering surgery presuming to attain an alternative communicating medium. Sporadic attempts using implants to shunt aqueous to a variety of unconventional sites, including the vortex veins and the nasolacrimal duct, have since been reported. Since results were generally unfavourable or too poorly documented to evaluate, attention is now focused on devices shunting aqueous fluid to the subconjunctival space as with conventional GFS.

The first translimbal GDD, reported by Zorab in 1912, was silk thread used as a seton to aid drainage of anterior chamber fluid to the subconjunctival space. This was followed by similar use of gold, tantalum, and platinum thread/wire. Results were universally poor as these and other early translimbal setons did not address lack of flow control and hypotony associated with full thickness (unguarded) GFS, and added a foreign body chronic inflammatory stimulus. Simple translimbal tube devices were similarly unsuccessful, with high rates of early filtration failure.

The Molteno implant is considered the prototype device of this generation of filtration devices to control intraocular pressure. Other types of nonvalved devices developed after Molteno's design are such as the ones described by Krupin and Baerveldt, to mention some.

In 1969, Molteno introduced the concept that a large surface area was needed to disperse the aqueous beneath the conjunctiva. He inserted a short acrylic tube that was attached to a thin acrylic plate. The plate was sutured to the sclera close to the limbus. Most of the operations failed after the first 3–6 months because of plate exposure, tube erosion and scar formation.

In 1973, Molteno improved his device with the idea of draining the fluid away from the source to increase the success rate. He introduced the Molteno implant with a long silicone tube attached to a large end plate made up of polymethyl methacrylate placed in the subconjunctival space around 9–10 mm posterior to the limbus This device allows the aqueous humor to flow into the subconjunctival space and forms a filtration bleb in the site where the receptacle plate is located. (Molteno, 1976).

All the currently available GDDs are based on this concept by Molteno. The Molteno implant and similar implants offer no resistance to the outflow, resulting in hypotony, flat ACs, and choroidal effusions.

Since then, two major concepts have been introduced to modify the GDD. The first concept was that of a valve to offer resistance to the outflow, thereby reducing the incidence of postoperative hypotony. In 1976, Theodore Krupin developed a pressure-sensitive, unidirectional valve that provides resistance to the flow of aqueous and prevents early postoperative hypotony. This "slit valve" is designed to open at a pressure of 11 mmHg and to close at a pressure of 9 mmHg. In 1993, Mateen Ahmed introduced the Ahmed glaucoma valve (AGV), a pressure-sensitive, unidirectional valve that is designed to open when the intraocular pressure (IOP) is 8 mmHg (Ayyala, 1998; Huang, 1999; Topouzis, 1999).

The second major change has been the realisation that by increasing the surface area of the end plate, the surface area of drainage could be increased, resulting in lower IOPs (Freedman, 1992; Lloyd et al, 1994; Smith et al, 1992). In 1981, Molteno introduced the double plate implant with a surface area of 270 mm^2. In 1992, George Baerveldt introduced a nonvalved silicone tube attached to a large barium-impregnated silicone plate with a surface area of 250 mm^2, 350 mm^2, or 500 mm^2 (Mills, 1996; Smith, 1993; Lloyd, 1994; Siegner, 1995; Nguyen, 1998).

FDA-approved aqueous drainage/shunt implants are medically necessary for the treatment of members with refractory primary open-angle glaucoma when first-line drugs (e.g. timolol or latanoprost) and second-line drugs (e.g. brimonidine or dorzolamide) have failed to control intraocular pressure.

Translimbal drainage implants, or anterior GDDs, were implanted with the intention of preventing filtration failure by maintaining patency of a drainage fistula or sclerotomy. Anterior GDDs failed to improve filtration failure rates in comparison with conventional GFS, but it took almost half a century for investigators to begin to rationalise this lack of success.

In 1969, Molteno hypothesised that filtration failure was primarily attributable to subconjunctival fibrosis, with fistula closure occurring as a secondary event. This was later confirmed in histological studies of animal models of GFS. Realising that simple anterior GDDs would have little impact on this process, Molteno launched the concept of tube and plate GDDs, in which aqueous fluid is shunted to a plate device designed to maintain patency of a subconjunctival filtration reservoir in the face of continuing subconjunctival fibrosis. Although, confined to the use in complex cases by the advent of trabeculectomy and relatively successful conventional guarded GFS, these were the first GDDs to gain widespread acceptance and the Molteno tube remains the benchmark against which other tube devices are compared.

Tube and plate devices still dominate the contemporary GDD market. Prominent examples, in chronological order, are the Molteno, Krupin, Baerveldt, Ahmed, and OptiMed GDDs. Molteno moved the plate element of his early devices posteriorly away from the limbus to avoid problems with dellen formation and poor filtration associated with pre-existing anterior conjunctival scarring. Posterior placement beneath Tenon's capsule was also thought to improve protection from extrusion. 21 subsequent tube and plate GDDs share the essential design concept of posterior filtration via a tube in the anterior chamber to a plate element secured beneath Tenon's capsule, but differ in plate design and their provision for a flow control mechanism to protect from early postoperative hypotony.

Most GDDs have been developed in a virtual publication vacuum, with little available data to substantiate the manufacturers' claims for flow performance or biocompatibility. Clinical data are largely restricted to uncontrolled retrospective case series with variable follow up and differing definitions of surgical success. Evaluation is further complicated by the heterogeneity of inclusion criteria. Series included a variable proportion of complex cases, neovascular glaucoma in particular, with a predetermined high risk of filtration failure. Overall success rates, in terms of IOP control, appear similar between devices, with a reasonably high proportion of cases achieving a final IOP in the target range at 1 year after surgery. Half to two-thirds of these cases still require glaucoma medications, however, and target IOPs in the low teens ($\leq$ 16 mmHg) may be more realistic in terms of preventing disease progression than commonly adopted target levels ($\leq$ 21 or 22 mmHg), particularly where glaucomatous optic neuropathy is already advanced.

Evaluation is difficult, with few series including either long-term data or survival analysis. Despite certain reservations GDD offers definitive superiority and edge over conventional filtering surgeries particularly in case of non-responsive glaucoma.

AHMED GLAUCOMA DRAINAGE IMPLANT (VALVE)

Nonvalvular designs of initial GDD was the major constraint and inhibition towards wide acceptance of GDD as a useful measure to control nonresponsive glaucoma. Uncontrolled, excessive filtrations leading to significant and threatening complications were the genuine concerns. This has triggered the need for valved (restrictive) devices. Early nineties witnessed the modification and gradual transformation of free pass device (nonrestrictive) into valved (restrictive) device. Dr Mateen Ahmed, a US based medical engineer

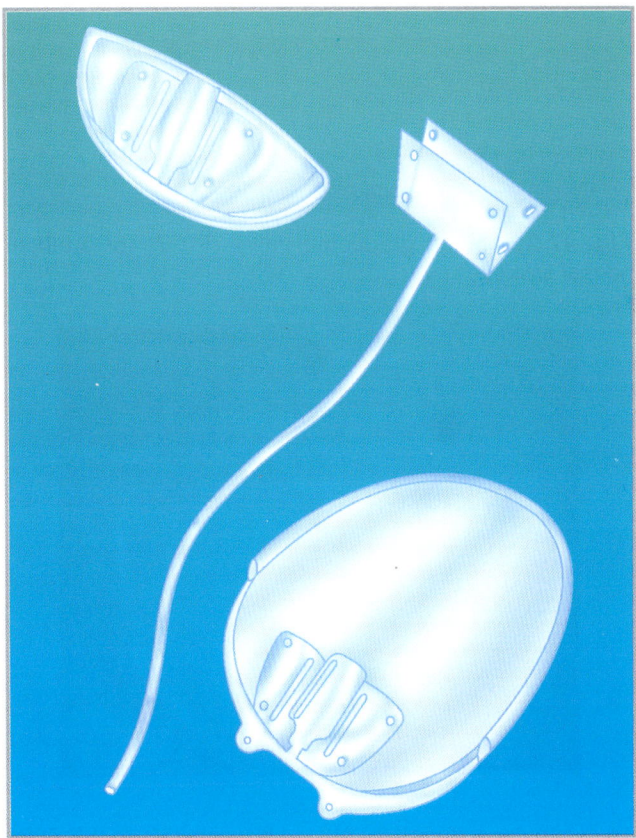

Fig. 47.1: Ahmed glaucoma valve: Components

from Central India, is amongst the pioneers to develop a unique restrictive valvular device, which consists of a receptacle plate and a connector tube of the plate with the anterior chamber. The receptacle plate possesses a bivalved valvular system that functions on Ventury flow principle. The first generation Ahmed valve basically had three components made up of different materials.

The receptacle plate was made of polypropylene whereas the communicating tube was made out of silicone of 0.635 mm of external diameter and an inner diameter of 0.317 mm. The third component was the silicone membrane acting as a unidirectional valvular device once attached to silicone tube so as to maintain aqueous communication from the anterior chamber.

However, polypropylene devices had witnessed significant fibrosis around valve plate resulting in gradual reduction in the functional capability of the valve in the due course of time. The present generation of Ahmed drainage device is essentially made of silicone including a receptacle plate that has shown excellent outcome. The research is still on to improve the valve functions, better control of aqueous flow, as well as biocompatibility to minimise fibrosis and other allogenic tissue reactions.

Principle and Components of AG Valve

AG Valve consists of Four Essential Components

   (i) The receptacle plate made of silicone/ polypropylene (13 × 16 mm) and having a surface area of 184 mm^2.

  (ii) The communicating tube made out of silicone (external diameter 0.635 mm and an inner diameter of 0.317 mm).

 (iii) The silicone membrane

 (iv) Cover shield

(i) The receptacle plate

The receptacle plate measures 13 × 16 mm and has a surface area of 184 mm^2. The plate is made of silicone/ polypropylene and has two lineal supports in the form of a bar, and four posts that are sealed through the tension cover and are responsible for the quality of the tension of the membrane and the valves. Besides, such plate has the tube on its edge in the proximal portion and, in each side of it, two small outbounds perforated in the centre that constitute the fixation element of the device to the sclera, since it is through there where the material with which the valve will be sutured to the sclera passes.

(ii) The communicating tube

The communicating tube is made up of silicone and have an external diameter of 0.635 mm and an inner diameter of 0.317 mm in all the models and sizes including smaller or paediatric valve. This silicone tube has direct attachment with the middle of inner silicone membrane through a perforation in it. The communicating tube provides direct access to the aqueous flow from the anterior chamber upto the inner silicone membrane, which in turn regulates the aqueous flow as per pressure equilibrium.

(iii) The silicone membrane

The silicone membrane possesses a unique feature of unidirectional pressure regulating system based on the surface tension on the membrane. Thus it achieves adequate pressure by virtue of a cover shield made of silicone or polypropylene. Hence, the membrane acts as a unidirectional bivalved valve.

(iv) Cover shield

The cover shield, as mentioned earlier, is an essential feature of pressure regulating unidirectional bivalved valve system. This cover or shield is made of silicone or polypropylene depending upon the type of valve.

This cover is responsible to attain a desired level of tension in the silicone membrane so as to have valve function. The cover provides support to the receptacle plate.

Mechanism of Pressure Regulating Action of the Glaucoma Drainage Device

The Ahmed glaucoma valve acts on the physics of "Ventury flow" system which is based on Bernoulli's equation.

All modern glaucoma drainage devices have the same basic design that consists of a silicone tube leading to a plate or a disc or an encircling element posteriorly beneath the conjunctiva or the Tenon's capsule. The plate or the discs placed posteriorly have a large surface area, which promotes formation of a filtering bleb posterior to the equator. Immediately following implantation of any such a device, there is a granulomatous reaction, which gradually resolves over a period of 04 to 05 months. The fibrous capsule matures over 06 months making the bleb thinner. Histologically, the bleb develops microcystic spaces, which serve as channels to shunt the aqueous into orbital tissues. The control of IOP depends upon the morphology of the filtering bleb. It is this fibrous capsule which offers resistance to aqueous outflow. Disruption of conjunctival bleb leads to hypotony.

SPECIFICATIONS OF AHMED GLAUCOMA DRAINAGE DEVICES

Glaucoma drainage devices are available in various designs basically to meet the needs of adult as well as of paediatric cases or of a smaller eyeball. Most common designs and their specifications are as follows:

1. **Anterior Chamber insertion of Ahmed Glaucoma Valve drainage tube:**
   (a) For adult eye: S2 & FP7
   (b) For paediatric or small globes: S3 & FP8 models

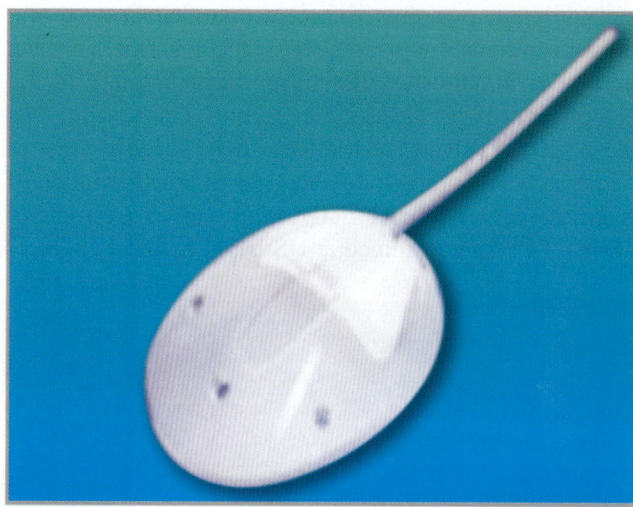

Fig. 47.2: Ahmed glaucoma valve (FP 7) for adult or normal size eye

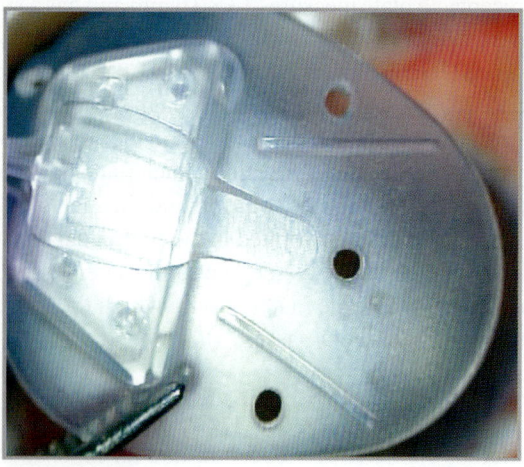

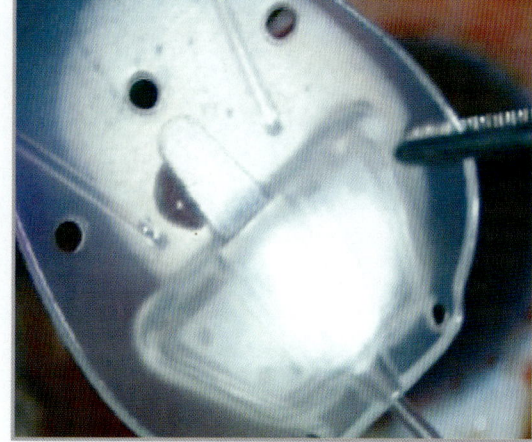

| (a) | (b) |

Fig. 47.3: (a) Ahmed glaucoma valve (FP 7) for adult or normal size eye (outer surface), (b) Ahmed glaucoma valve (FP 7) for adult or normal size eye (inner surface)

2. Posterior chamber insertion of Ahmed Glaucoma Valve drainage tube through pars plana

(a) PC 7 for adult eye

(b) PC 8 for paediatric or small globes

The configuration of pars plana clip valve is identical to that of FP 7 and 8 except that the valve tube possesses a clip which protects and secures its insertion through pars plana incision. However, a good vitrectomy is a prerequisite for the insertion of drainage tube into the posterior segment. AGV with pars plana clip is most suitable in certain situations where postoperative shallow anterior chamber is anticipated or poor corneal endothelial cell reserve may trigger corneal endothelial cell loss and decompensation. However good vitrectomy is a pre requisite for this procedure. PC7 is being used in adult eyes where as PC 8 is ideal for Paediatric or Small Globes.

Indications of AGV with Pars Plana Clip in Concurrent Procedures

(i) Angle closure glaucoma

(ii) Post PK glaucoma

(iii) Secondary glaucoma with aniridia

(iv) Traumatic cataract with angle recession glaucoma

(v) Neovascular glaucoma

S2 and S3 are older generation Ahmed Glaucoma Valves. In these models valve plate body and elastomer membrane of valve are made up of medical grade polypropylene and the drainage tube of valve is made up of Silicone. Whereas all components of newer generation FP 7, FP8, PC 7 and PC 8 models are made-up of silicone which provides better control of IOP.

Specifications of Adult Eye Ahmed Glaucoma Valve

Thickness	: 1.9 mm
Width	: 13.00 mm
Length	: 16.00 mm
Surface Area	: 184.00 mm
True Length	: 25.00 mm
Tube inner Diameter	: 0.305 mm
Tube Outer Diameter	: 0.635 mm

Specifications of Paediatric or Small Globes Ahmed Glaucoma Valve

Thickness	: 0.9 mm
Width	: 9.60 mm
Length	: 10.00 mm
Surface Area	: 96.00 mm
True Length	: 25.00 mm
Tube inner Diameter	: 0.305 mm
Tube Outer Diameter	: 0.635 mm

PATIENT SELECTION

Most of the cases of coexisting cataract and glaucoma may be considered suitable for combined phacoemulsification and glaucoma valve implantation. However, as a general guideline and on the basis of expected good functional outcome, preference may be drawn as per the undermentioned order:

(i) All cases of refractive glaucoma with coexisting cataract.

(ii) Cases which are nonresponsive to the glaucoma surgery in the form of progressive glaucomatous changes irrespective of IOP status.

(iii) Cataract with neovascular, uveitic glaucoma.

(iv) IOP of more than 21 mmHG despite filtering surgery and more than three drug regimen.

(v) All elderly cases of more than 60 years of age having mild to moderate cataract along with poor glaucoma control.

(vi) Elderly patients having uncontrolled IOP despite three drug regimen or laser iridotomy associated with or without significant cataract.

(vii) Moderate glaucoma with cataract having existing IOP of 21 mm or less but had initial uncontrolled IOP of more than 27 mmHg.

(viii) Glaucoma with coexisting cataract despite controlled IOP but had initial uncontrolled IOP of more than 30 mmHg.

(ix) All cases of congenital or juvenile glaucoma and cataract.

(x) Traumatic subluxated cataract with angle recession glaucoma.

Relative Contraindications

(i) Eyes with severe scleral and/or corneoscleral limbus thinning which may adversely influence proper fixation of the implant, or produces an unstable situation of the tube inside the anterior chamber due to poor resistance at the limbus.

(ii) Excessive conjunctival scarring or scleral thinning due to a previous surgery or trauma where dissection of conjunctival flap may not be suitable. However, such cases or cases of previous vitreoretinal surgery or multiple previous filtering procedures may be considered for glaucoma valve implant with scleral or pericardium graft along with amniotic membrane/conjunctival grafting. However, cases with existing retinal explants may be considered for valve implant.

(iii) Ciliary block glaucoma.

(iv) Cataract and glaucoma with intraocular silicone oil due to vitreoretinal surgery, as silicone IOL may travel into subconjunctival space through the tube. However, valve implant may be considered in the inferior-temporal quadrant in selected cases so as to allow the tube position far away from the silicone, which has a lower density than the aqueous humor.

PHACO AND AGV SURGICAL TECHNIQUES

The surgical technique of combined Ahmed glaucoma valve implantation and phacoemulsification cataract surgery needs to be modified and various steps have to be taken in different sequences as compared to the traditional isolated valve implant or phacoemulsification surgery so as to accord surgical ease and ultimately a better performance.

The initial steps just short of tube insertion into the anterior chamber through sclerotomy are performed prior to the commencement of cataract surgery. Cataract removal is performed in a usual manner of phacoemulsification by clear corneal incision and the direct chop technique except in case of a soft lens in paediatric cases where phacoaspiration by irrigation-aspiration (I/A), either co-axial or bimanual method is an ideal choice. The author prefers to implants a single piece hydrophobic acrylic foldable IOL implant in most cases. However, any other kind of IOL can be used.

Anaesthesia

The choice of anaesthesia between general and peribulbar anaesthesia is based on the age of the patient. General anaesthesia is essential in paediatric cases, whereas peribulbar anaesthesia is most suitable for adult cases. In our view, topical anaesthesia is not an ideal choice for drainage device implant or for combined glaucoma and cataract surgery due to obvious reasons of comparatively prolonged duration of surgery and relatively more manipulations over the conjunctiva and the sclera to place the valve over it.

The Quadrant Selection for Placement of Glaucoma Valve

The implant can be put in any quadrant of the eyeball which should be ascertained preoperatively. However, the most preferred quadrant remains superiortemporal quadrant due to the following reasons:

  (i) Placement of valve is smooth and easy.
 (ii) Relatively safer as superiortemporal quadrant has an adequate space between the valve and muscular structures, hence subsequent fibrosis around the valve plate is unlikely to affect ocular motility.

Valve can be implanted in other quadrants in the order of preference which are as following:

  (i) Inferior temporal
 (ii) Superior-nasal and
(iii) Inferior nasal.

Caution

The optic nerve is relatively closer to the limbus in the nasal quadrant due to the shorter distance in the nasal side between the ocular globe, and the optic nerve.

Hence while placing the implant in the nasal quadrants the valve should be fixed to the episclera at a maximal distance of 6 to 8 mm from the limbus so as to avoid any injury or proximity to the optic nerve. Needless to emphasise the significance of intraoperative evaluation of the conjunctiva, sclera, limbus and iris prior to the final consideration of the entrance site.

Insertion of Superior Rectus Suture

Contrary to the conventional clear corneal phaco surgery, combined procedure demands the superior rectus bridle suture as an essentiality.

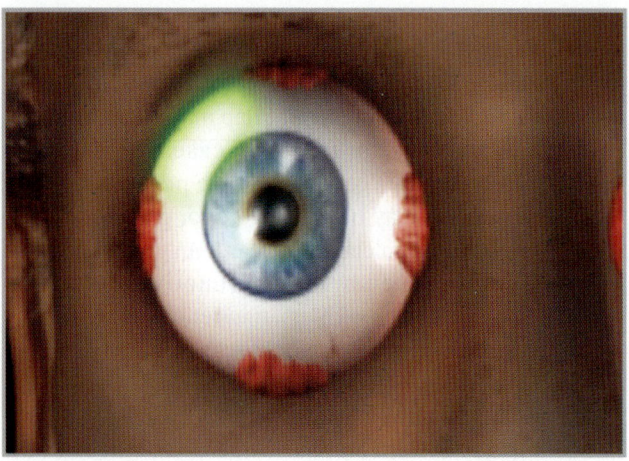

(a)

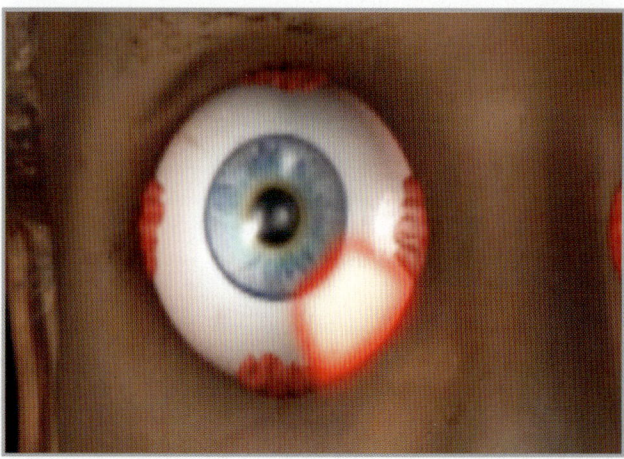

(b)

Fig. 47.4: (a) and (b) The quadrant selection for placement of glaucoma valve

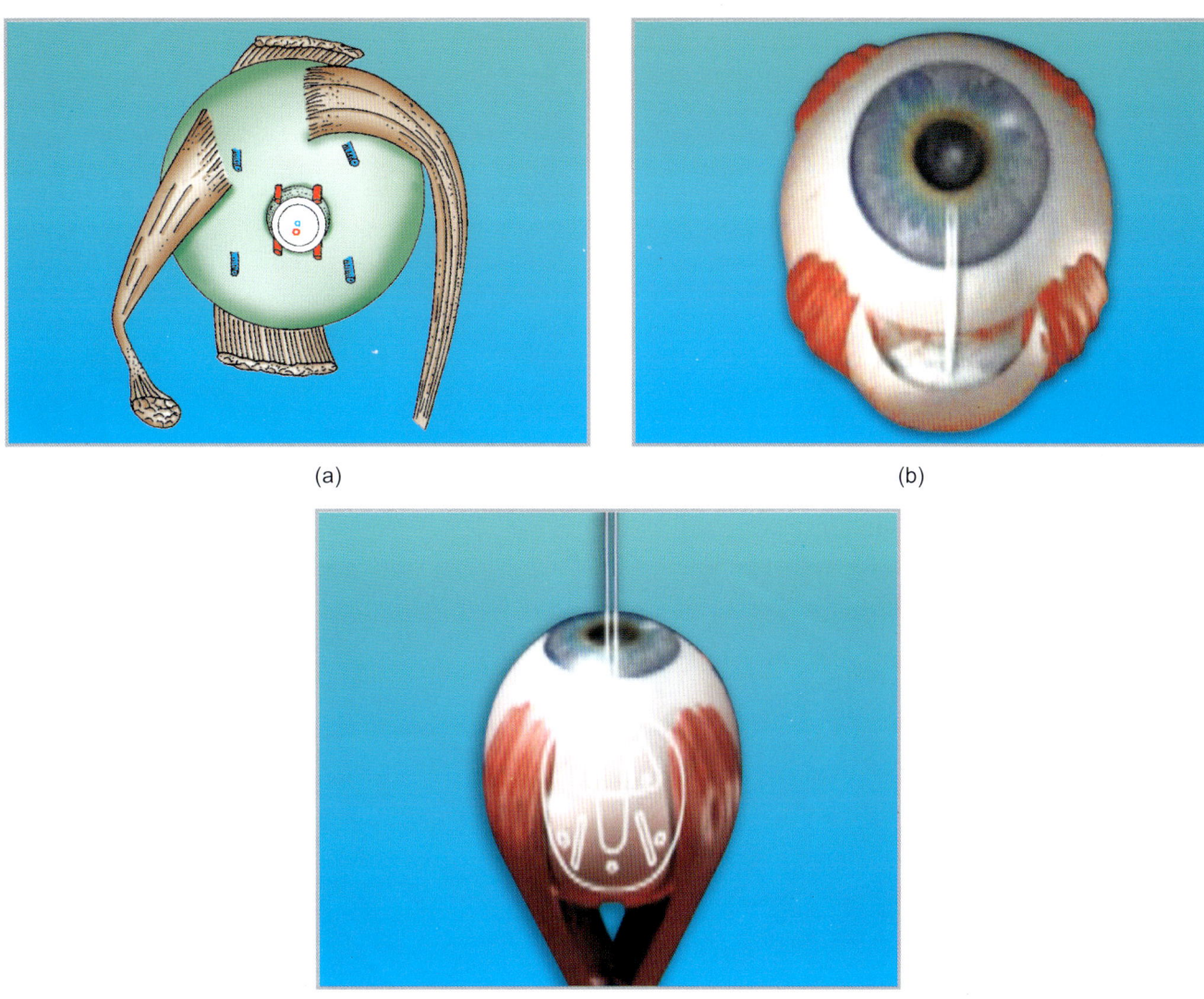

(a)　　　　　　　　　　　　　　　　　(b)

(c)

Fig. 47.5: (a) and (b) Valve implant in the superiortemporal quadrant and its relation with the postequator structures, (c) Valve implant in the superiortemporal quadrant and its relation with the optic nerve

Conjunctival Flap (Fig. 47.6)

Conjunctival dissection should include the quadrant where the valve is going to be placed. After the insertion of superior rectus suture, fornix based conjunctival flap is raised by 90 degree peritomy. Subconjunctival infiltration of a small quantity of 2% lignocaine hydrochloride into subconjunctival space prior to conjunctival and tenons dissection is preferred so as to facilitate adequate separation of flap. Bipolar cautery is suitably applied to make a good scleral bed for glaucoma drainage device implantation. Wire vectis is used to create an adequate subconjunctival pocket so as to accommodate the valve plate in a proper position.

The Priming of Valve (Fig. 47.7)

The priming of valve is an essential procedure prior to the placement of the valve. A small quantity of balanced salt solution is pushed into silicon tube of AG valve with the help of a 27 gauze cannula mounted on a 2 ml syringe so as to open up the valve and ensure its initial and definitive unsealing and patency of the silicone valves. Inadequate opening of valve at this stage may lead to insufficient reduction in the IOP during immediate postoperative period as well as to a failure of valve functioning.

The tip of the cannula is introduced 3 to 4 mm into the tube since the pressure required to prime the tube is over 75 to 110 mmHg. One should ensure adequate holding of the valve at this stage to avoid implant pushing away. It is therefore suggested that the body of the valve be held with the other hand while the priming is performed. While pushing fluid into the valve, the initial spurt of fluid is observed.

The simultaneous decrease in the resistance of the implant to the outflow of the liquid is felt immediately. In certain cases, priming may need more pressure to attain

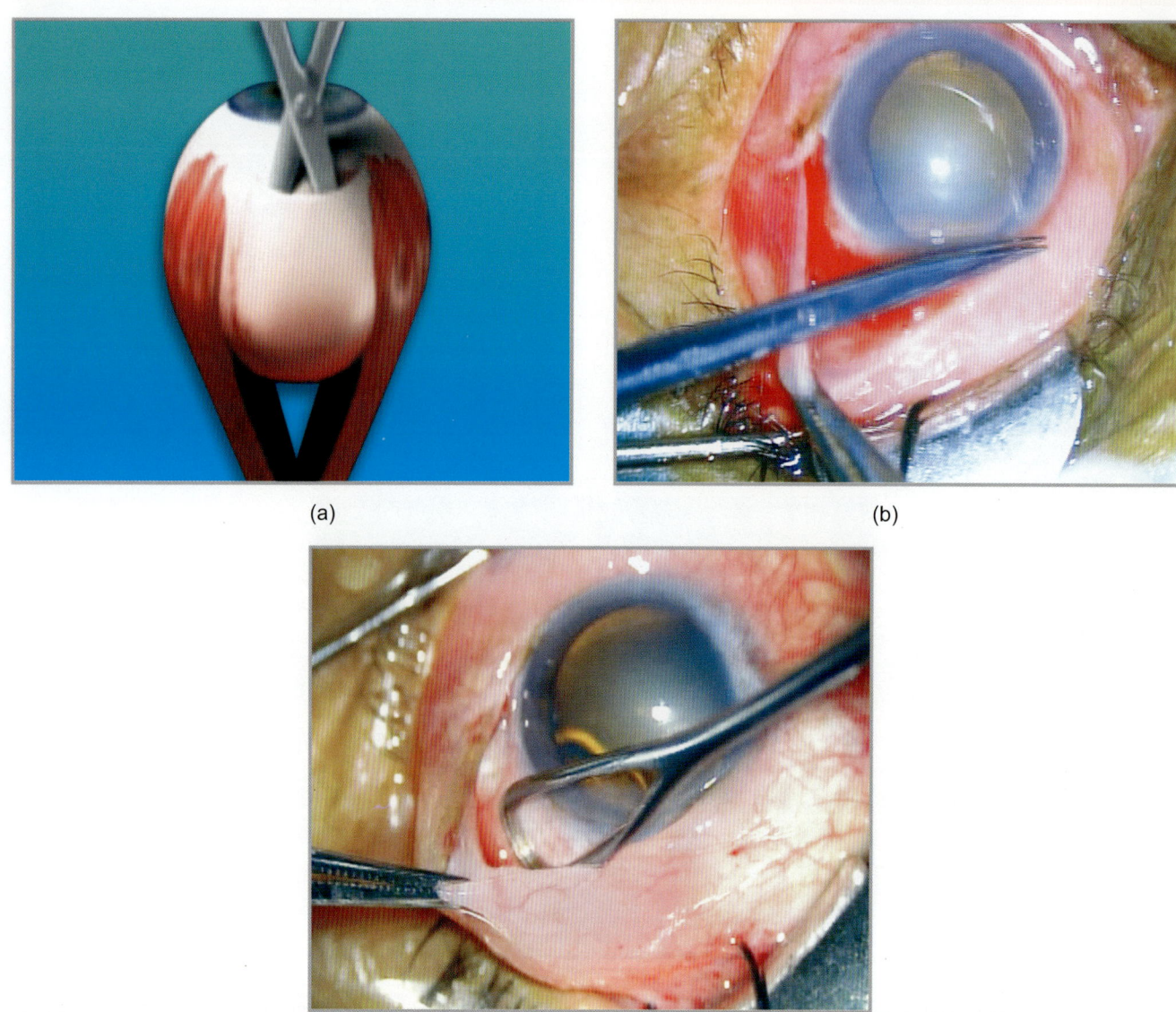

(a)

(b)

(c)

Fig. 47.6: (a) and (b) Conjunctival flap, (c) Creation of subconjunctival pocket for the insertion of AG valve plate

free and smooth flow probably owing to some variation in the assembly of the valve. However, the author did not encounter such a problem in his personal experience of several cases.

Anchoring of the AG Valve (Fig. 47.8)

Preplaced anchoring: The AG valve can be anchored with the help of 7–O Prolene/8–O monofilament polyamide suture. The author prefers to apply 7–O Prolene suture since it provides better grip to the valve over the sclera.

Parihar's Modified Technique of AG Valve Placement (Fig. 47.9)

In this technique, the author prefers to use a without lock straight needle holder with reverse movements both at the

time of preplaced anchoring of valve as well as while securing valve over sclera. Such reverse movements with straight needle holder facilitates smooth insertion of suture.

7 'O Monofilament Polypropylene suture on 3/8 circle tapered needle is passed through both the eyelets of the valve plate and tied over the plate by double knots.

Subsequently, AG valve is placed over sclera by reverse suturing into the subtenon space approximately 6 to 8 mm away from the limbus.

It is recommended to place scleral sutures by reverse pattern and parallel to the limbus, rather than perpendicular for obvious reasons of surgical comforts and ease. Such sutures can be tied over sclera without much discomfort. Over and above, parallel sutures ensure the desired position of the valve over the sclera since parallel sutures are unlikely to move alongwith the movements of the eyeball.

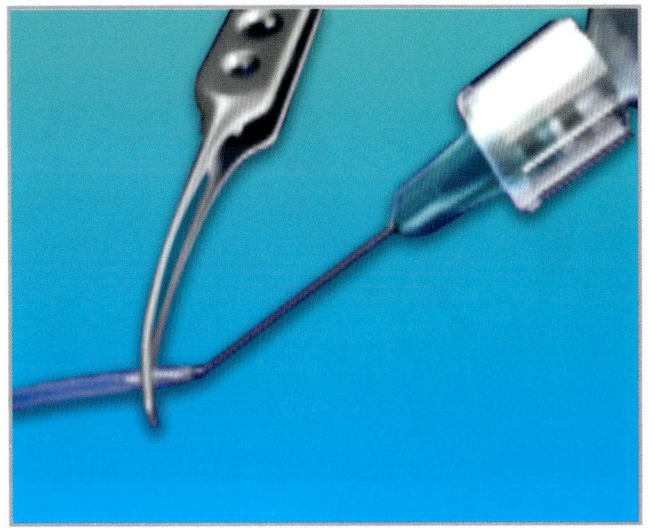
(a)

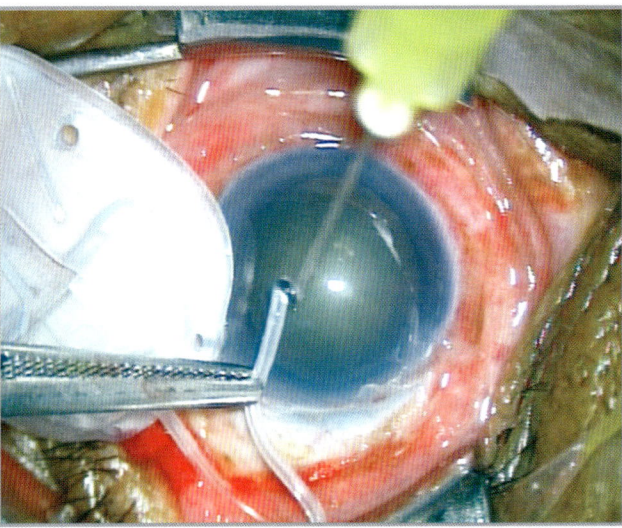
(b)

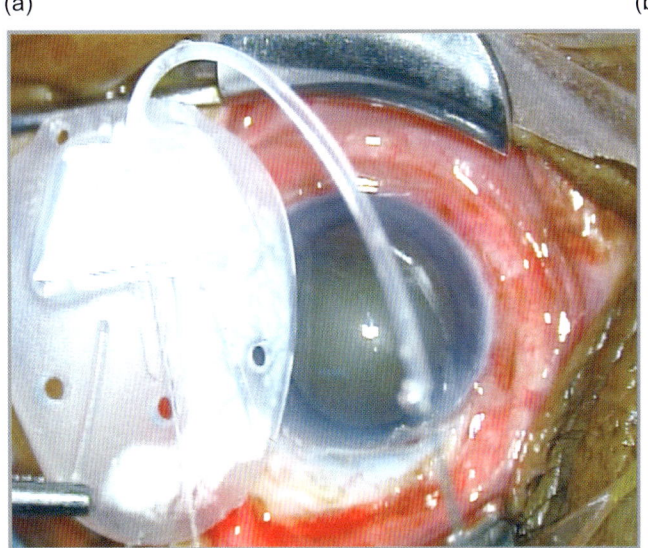
(c)

Fig. 47.7: Priming of the valve: (a) and (b) Insertion of fine cannula in the tube, (c) free flow of BSS through valve

Construction of Partial Thickness Scleral Flap

A small limbal based partial thickness scleral flap (Fig. 47.10) of about 4.5 mm² was fashioned to cover the silicone tube of AG valve prior to its insertion into the anterior chamber.

Advantages of Partial Thickness Scleral Flap and Sclerotomy over Patch Graft/Amniotic Membrane/Pericardium Graft

(i) Partial thickness scleral flap and subscleral sclerotomy technique is a safe procedure that offers some advantages over the conventional graft implantation technique.

(ii) Technically much simpler and easy.

(iii) No need of extra instrumentation, least expensive.

(iv) No need to procure preserved scleral or pericardium graft or amniotic membrane, hence less expensive.

(v) Partial thickness scleral flap does not produce any immunological reaction as it is possible with allografts or other materials.

(vi) Minimal inflammatory reaction, better control of IOP.

(vii) Easy to cover scleral flap by conjunctiva as compared to the allograft hence less foreign body sensation and better tolerance and less chances of tube extrusion or exposure.

Relative Indications of Patch Graft/Amniotic Membrane/Pericardium Graft over Partial Thickness Scleral Flap

Partial thickness scleral flap may not be suitable in cases of extensive conjunctival scarring such as in cases of chronic recurrent uveitis, rheumatoid arthritis, complicated glaucoma associated with scleral thinning like

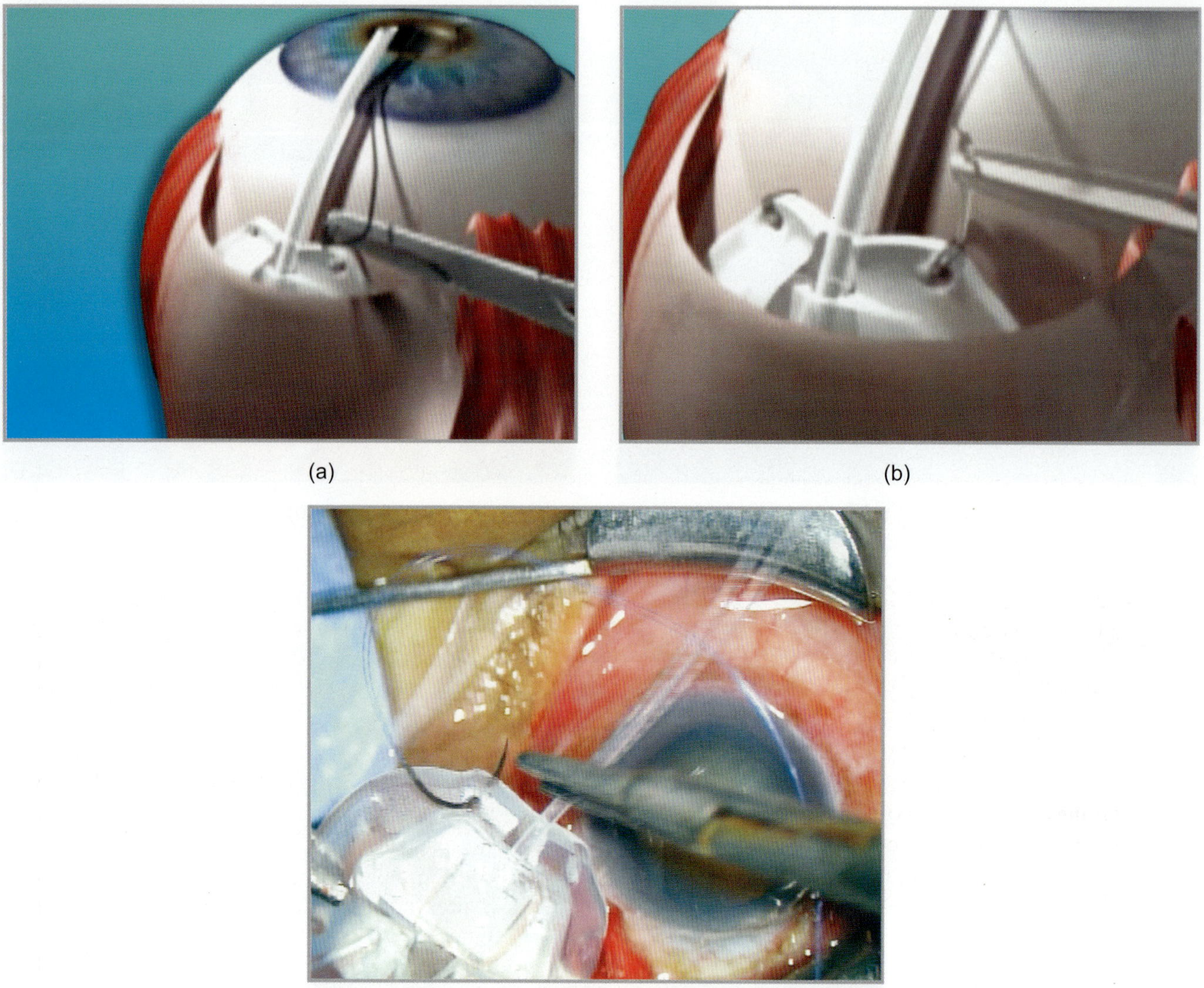

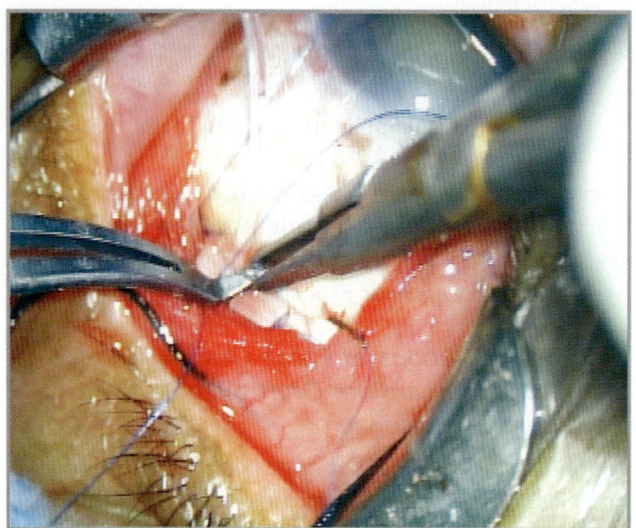

(a)

(b)

(c)

Fig. 47.8: (a) and (b) Anchoring of the AG valve with the help of 7–O Prolene monofilament polyamide suture, (c) Preplaced anchoring of the AG valve with the help of 7–O Prolene monofilament polyamide suture

Fig. 47.9: Securing AG valve over sclera

buphthalmos, chemical injuries and posttraumatic complicated glaucoma.

The remaining steps of valve implantation like shortening and entry of tube into the anterior chamber performed after completion of phacoemulsification surgery will be described subsequently, in detail.

PHACOEMULSIFICATION SURGERY

After the completion of placement of AG valve over the sclera and construction of a partial thickness scleral flap, the steps of phacoemulsification surgery are performed in a standard manner. The author prefers to apply direct phaco chop technique through clear corneal incision in adult cases, whereas phacoaspiration by coaxial/bimanual technique in soft or in paediatric cases. Single piece hydrophobic acrylic foldable IOL implant is an ideal choice. However, other types of foldable IOL implants can also be used.

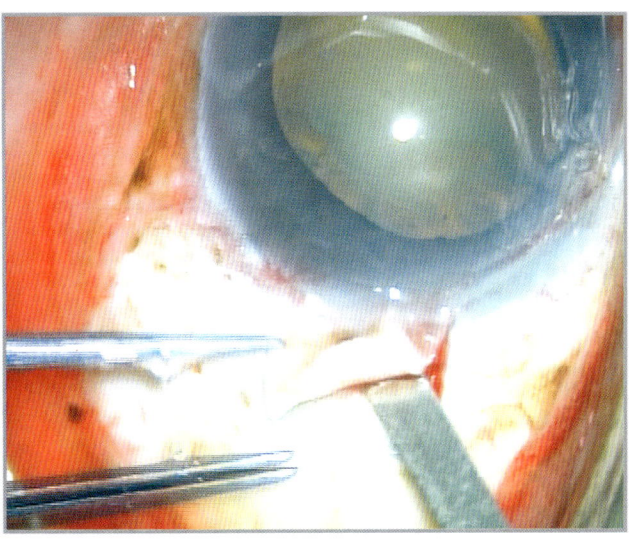
(a)

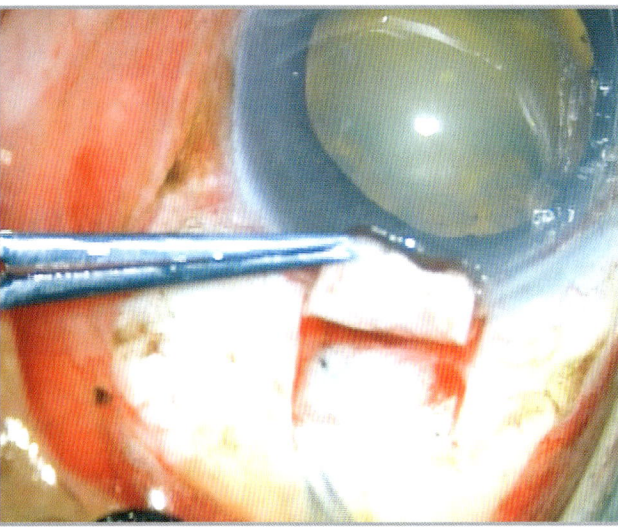
(b)

Fig. 47.10: (a) and (b) Construction of partial thickness scleral flap

(i) Site of clear corneal incision (Fig. 47.11b): The site of clear corneal incision is chosen according to the probable site of tube entry into the AC as well as on the surgical ease while performing phaco with sutured AG valve plate over sclera. The author prefers to construct two identical incisions each of 1 mm size with the help of 15 degree entry blades. Of these, one incision is converted into is 2.8 mm main incision after completion of rhexis and hydroprocedures. The chosen site remains distal temporal for the right eye and nasal for the left eye, respectively, provided the valve is being placed in the temporal quadrant. However, the site of incision will require modification according to the position of the valve in different quadrants.

(ii) Capsulorrhexis (Fig. 47.12): Most cases of coexisting cataract and glaucoma are invariably associated with a rigid and miotic pupil and hard cataract or both simultaneously. A miotic pupil may require mechanical stretching of the pupil with the help of iris hooks. In certain cases, dye enhanced rhexis may be necessary and beneficial. However, rhexis can be completed without much inconvenience.

(iii) Hydroprocedures and nucleus rotation: Hydroprocedures are very crucial requirements of a successful phaco and energy modulation. Gentle, meticulous and repeated efforts are essential to achieve complete and good hydrodissection and delineation.

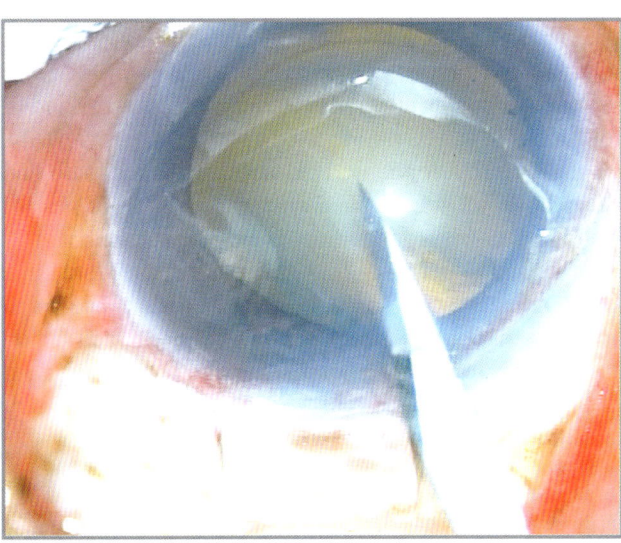
(a)

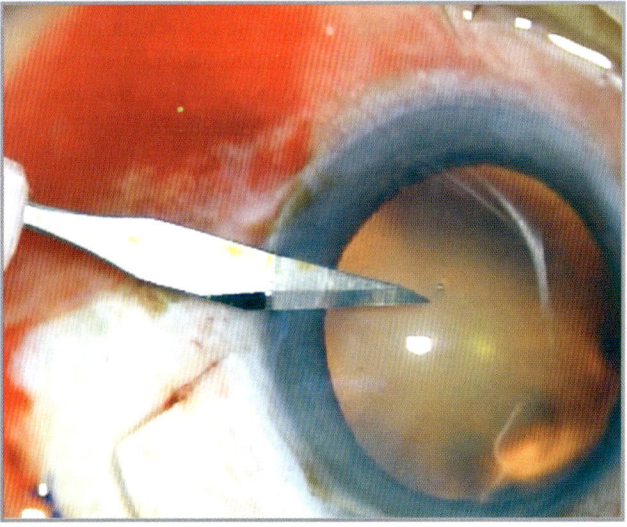
(b)

Fig. 47.11: (a) Clear corneal incision temporal to the scleral flap, (b) Side port clear corneal incision just adjacent to the scleral flap

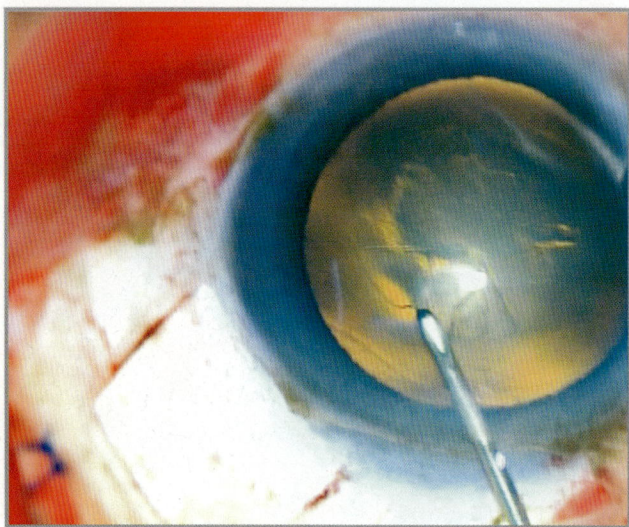

Fig. 47.12: Capsulorrhexis

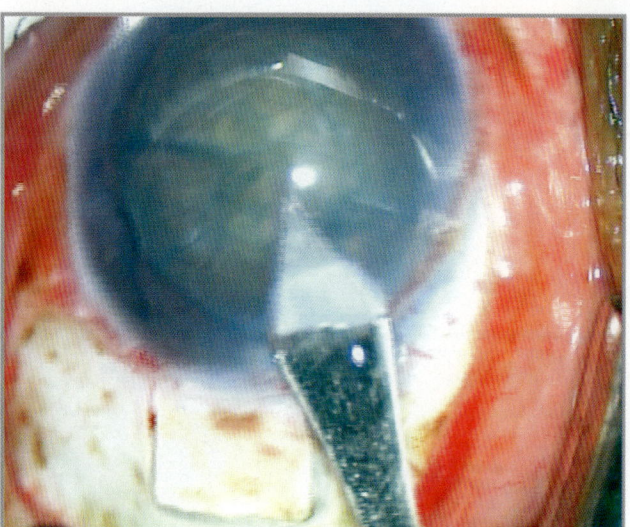

Fig. 47.13: Main incision for insertion of the phaco tip

The nucleus rotation demands utmost care since cataracts associated with glaucoma are invariably found to have intercapsular adhesions between the cortical plate and the fornices of the capsular bag. Forceful rotation in this situation may lead to intraoperative complications like zonulysis, posterior capsular rent or even nucleus dislocation into the vitreous cavity.

Main incision for insertion of the phaco tip (Fig. 47.13): After completion of hydroprocedures and nucleus rotation, the temporal incision is extended with the help of 2.8 mm keratome so as to facilitate entry of the phaco tip into the anterior chamber.

Nucleotomy (Fig. 47.14): Nucleotomy can be performed by any method. The author prefers to perform direct central chopping in most cases. Peripheral chopping may find difficulty in cases of a miotic pupil or a very hard and large nucleus. Sculpting also finds difficulty most of the time due to the complicated nature of the cataract which is invariably associated with other pathologies like thinning of the posterior capsule, zonular weakness and vitreous degeneration, hence is likely to have a higher incidence of intraoperative complications. Chopping is relatively safe as compared to other methods of nucleotomy since there is no pressure on zonules and vitreous while performing nucleotomy. As such, chopping requires less energy as compared to sculpting to complete the phacoprocedures. In our practice, we use moderate settings of aspiration, flow and phacopower (ranging from 10% to 30% on white staar technology).

Management of Residual Cortical Plate

Management of residual cortical plate (Fig. 47.15) can be done in three stages:

(i) Meticulous and adequate attention on hydro-procedure leads to sufficient softening of cortical matter. While performing nucleotomy, a repeated and gentle irrigation is very important to have smooth completion of I/A procedures.

The author continues to remove a significant chunk of cortex with the help of a zero degree phaco tip. However, it is better to use I/A mode if any other type of phaco tip is being used.

(ii) Use of capsule polisher: Use of capsule polisher to dislodge cortical plate from the periphery is very useful and highly recommended.

(iii) Final removal of residual cortical matter can be done either by coaxial or bimanual irrigation/aspiration cannula.

A high vacuum and adequate flow rate is recommended for this purpose.

IOL Implantation (Fig. 47.16)

IOL Implantation technique essentially remains same as in conventional phacoemulsification surgery. Any kind of foldable IOL can be implanted. However, in our view, the single piece hydrophobic IOL implant is most safe and acceptable to the eye, particularly in all types of complicated cases including coexisting glaucoma and cataract and undergoing highly complex procedures like GDD implantation. These IOL implants are known to have least inflammation, posterior capsular opacification as well as zero incidence of opacification of IOL implant even in cases of concurrent AG valve and phaco surgery and other complex situations.

Insertion of Valve Drainage Tube into the Anterior Chamber

After completion of phaco, the next step is to prepare the drainage tube for insertion into the anterior chamber.

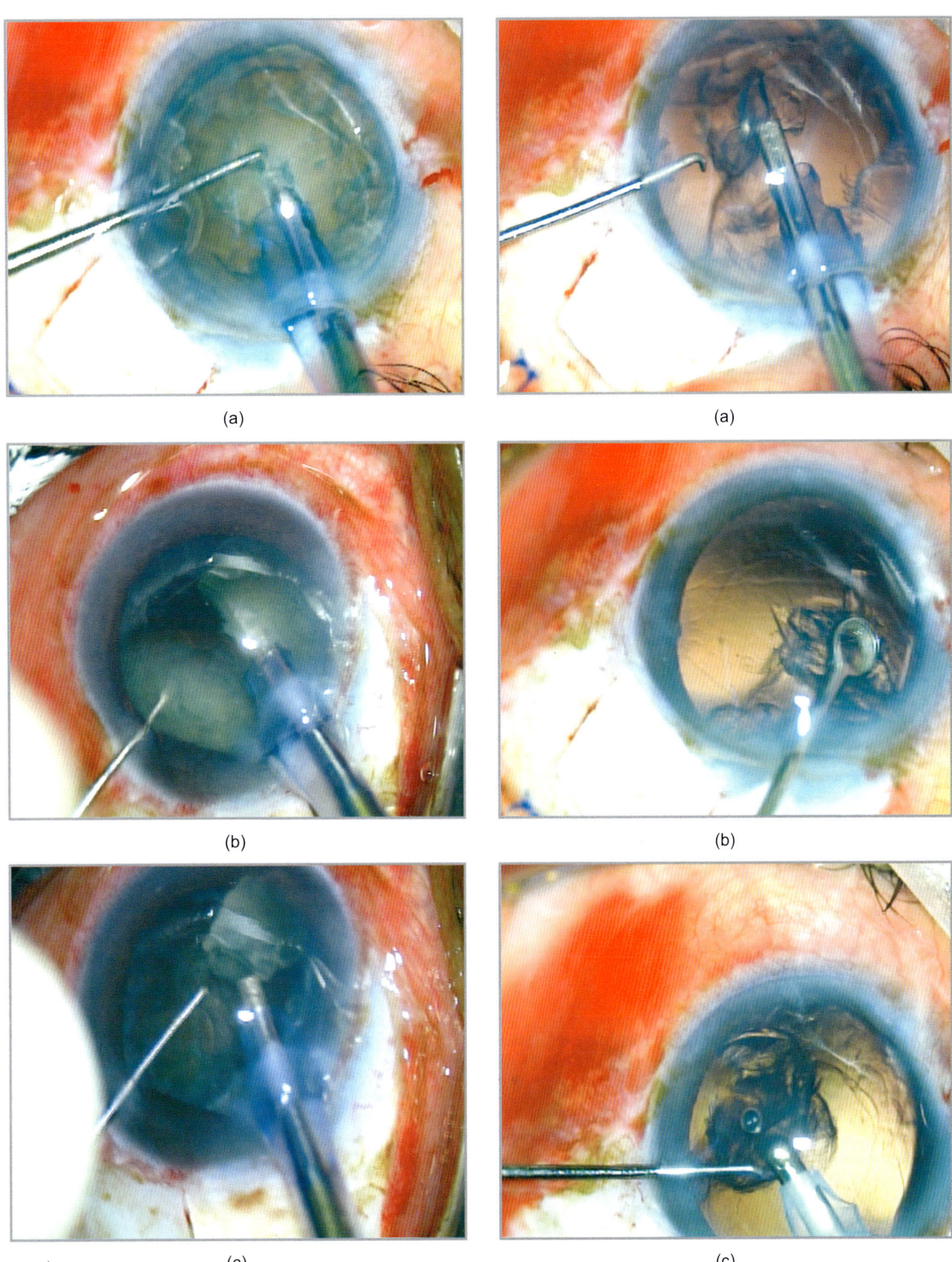

Fig. 47.14: (a) and (b) Nucleotomy by the direct chop technique, (c) Fragment aspiration

Fig. 47.15: (a) and (b) Management of the residual cortical plate, (c) Coaxial I/A removal of the residual cortical plate

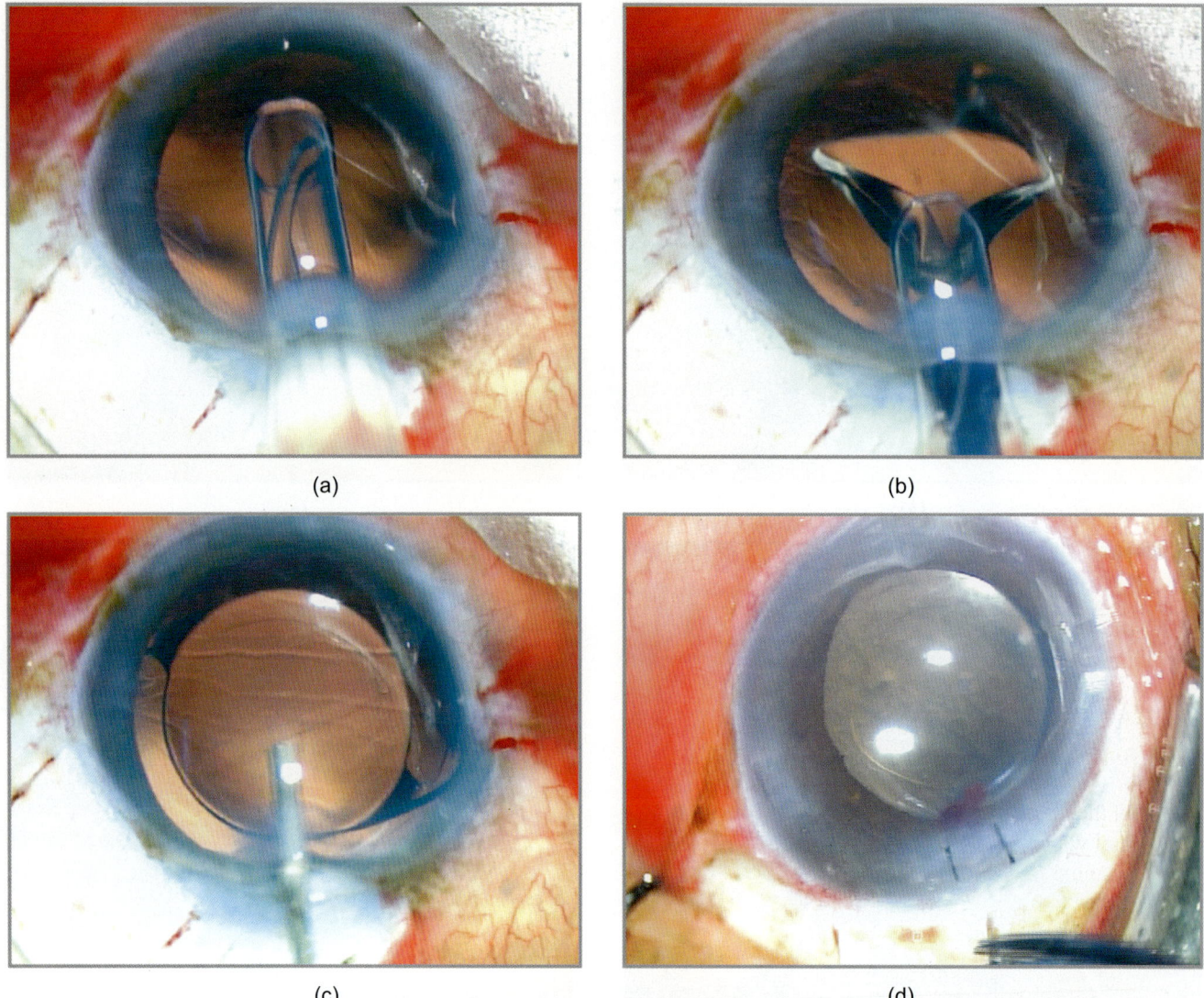

(a)

(b)

(c)

(d)

Fig. 47.16: (a) and (b) Single piece hydrophobic IOL implant is being implanted, (c) and (d) single piece hydrophobic IOL implant is in situ

Ideal Length of the Tube in the Anterior Chamber

The ideal length of the silicone drainage tube into AC is mainly based on the depth of the anterior chamber and other configurations which are likely to vary on the merits of each and every case. However, an ideal length is around two to three mm in the anterior chamber.

Essential criteria of adequate length: In general, the ideal position of the drainage tube should not have touched any structure in the anterior chamber including the posterior surface of cornea, iris or lens. It should not come in the zone of visual axis and should exactly traverse through trabecular meshwork. However, it is not possible to attain all the ideal situations in each and every case.

Preparation of Tube and Insertion Technique

The tube should be made short in such a manner that it achieves approximately 2–2.5 mm length in the anterior chamber. The distal tip of the tube should be cut in such a

manner that it attains on elongated bevel down position. Such a position has surgical ease while inserting into the AC as well as facilitates the least trauma to the corneal endothelium as well as adequate patency of the tube even in the event of an iris touch (Fig. 47.17).

HOW TO CONSTRUCT SCLEROTOMY/SCLERAL TUNNEL FOR VALVE TUBE INSERTION

The scleral tunnel or sclerotomy under partial thickness scleral flap can be performed prior to the commencement or after the completion of phaco procedure. However, in our view, it is most appropriate to design sclerotomy after completion of phaco and just before the insertion of the tube into the anterior chamber.

Needle or Blade

The Author has experimented and evaluated various methods of construction of scleral tunnel or sclerotomy

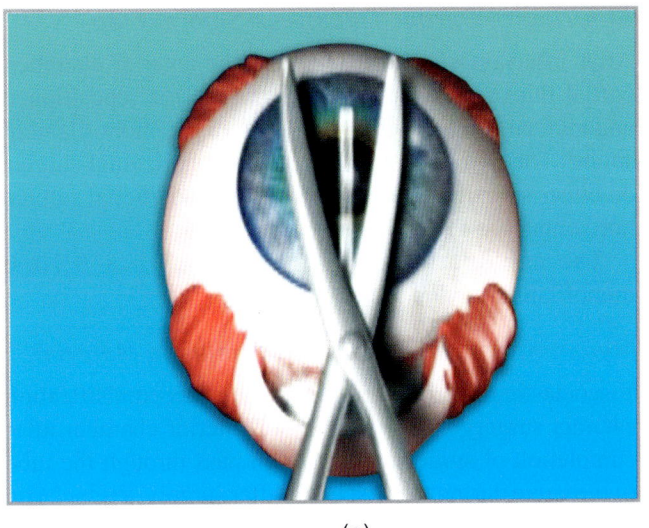
(a)

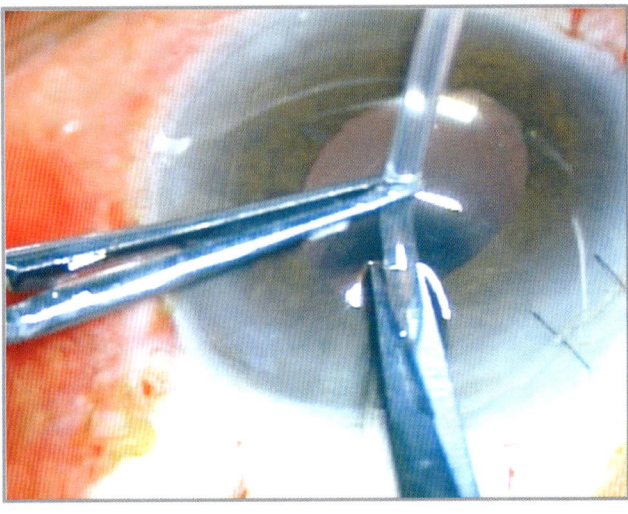
(b)

Fig. 47.17: (a) and (b) Preparation of tube: The tube is being shortened to achieve approximately 2–2.5 mm length in the anterior chamber

for the insertion of silicon tube into the AC. However, the most safe mode remains the use of a 22 gauze needle which is bent to a 45 to 60 degree angle and just short of the hub of the needle. It is very difficult to manipulate tube insertion through the sclerotomy created with the help of a 23 gauze needle. The side port entry blade can also be used for this purpose. However, one may not be sure about the exact width of the tunnel as well as of the subsequent stability of the tunnel which may be too loose, thereby resulting in a leaking tunnel in turn. The most suitable alternative to the needle is a 0.9 mm keratome which is used in micro phaco (phaconit/ MICS) procedures. The author found to have an excellent wound construction and a stable tunnel created with the help of MICS keratome.

Sclerotomy without Partial Thickness Scleral Flap (Fig. 47.18)

Sclerotomy can be fashioned without creating scleral flap. Direct insertion of a 22 gauze needle or the MICS blade under meticulous observation to ensure parallel movement of the tip of needle or blade at the subscleral plane may achieve desired results.

The Direction of the Needle

The direction that the needle should traverse while penetrating the anterior chamber should be parallel to the plane of the iris. The most ideal situation remains through angle of anterior chamber; however the final location of track will invariably vary from case to case, despite an identical approach in all cases. Construction of sclerotomy track in cases of angle closure glaucoma is very tricky and demands utmost accuracy and attention due to less space available in the anterior chamber. However, myopia and juvenile glaucoma do not pose much inconvenience while constricting track but scleral thinness must be kept in mind to

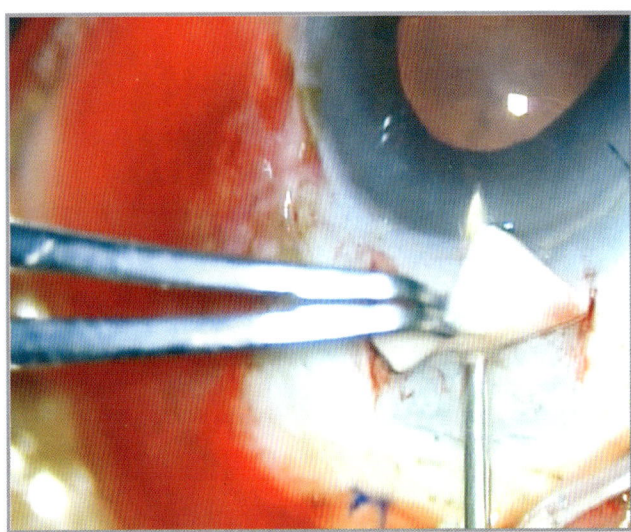

Fig. 47.18: 22 gauze needle track subscleral flap sclerostomy

avoid inadvertent perforation. However, it is better to keep the tube away from the cornea upto the maximum possibility.

Insertion of Silicon Tube into Anterior Chamber

Silicon tube (Fig. 47.19) can be inserted into the anterior chamber with the help of any forceps. Dr Mateen Ahmed has specially designed grooved and curved forceps which facilitate smooth insertion of the tube into the anterior chamber. However, McPherson forceps can also be used for this purpose.

The silicone tube of the AG valve drainage device is allowed to make entry into the AC through the sclerotomy created with the help of a 22 gauge syringe needle. The tube entry is ensured to remain parallel to the iris plane throughout its course and at its final position.

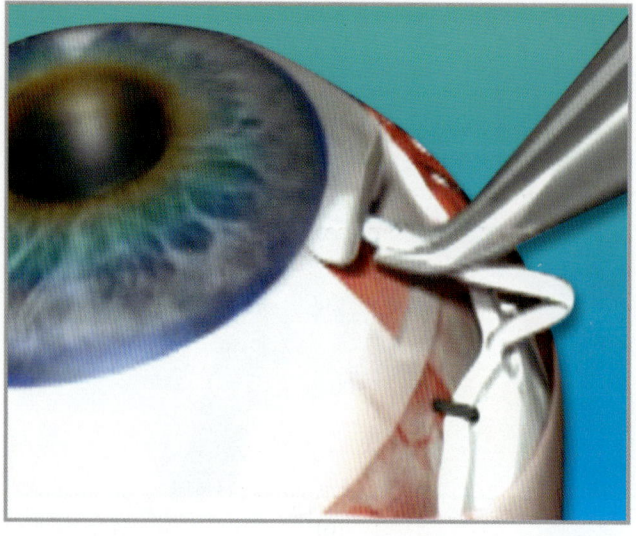

(a)

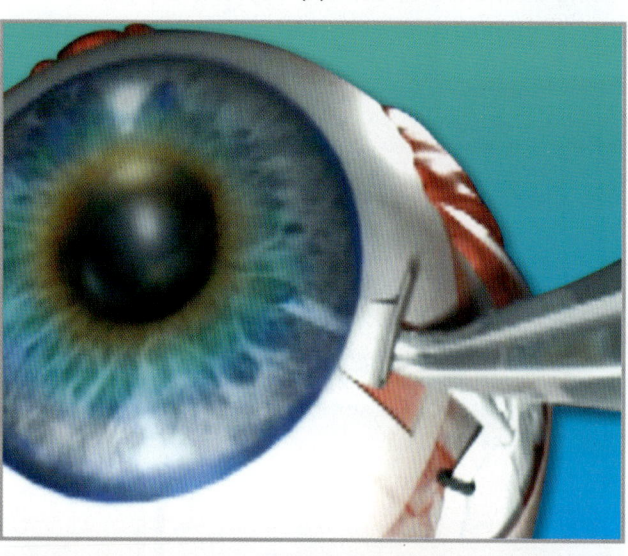

(b)

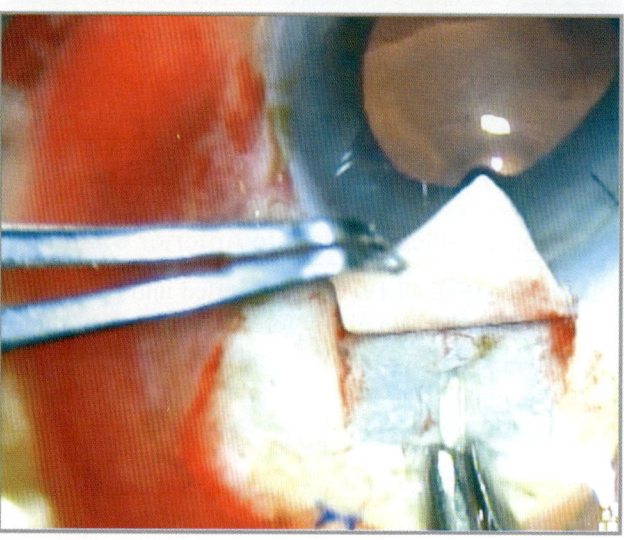

(c)

Fig. 47.19: (a), (b) and (c) Insertion of silicon tube into anterior chamber

Suturing of Partial Thickness Scleral Flap

After insertion of silicon tube into the anterior chamber, partial thickness scleral flap (Fig. 47.20) is repositioned and may be sutured with the help of 10 "0" monofilament suture. The author prefers to place two horizontal sutures on either side of the tube as well as two additional sutures horizontally at the end of the flap.

The conjunctiva can be secured with 8–0/10–0 monofilament nylon/vicryl suture.

Management of Residual Viscoelastic Material

Viscoelastic material used during the phacoemulsification cataract surgery can be left in the anterior chamber after completion of surgery, since it will pass through the tube of the valve during the first hours after surgery. Viscoelastic material in the anterior chamber minimises the risk of excessive hypotony and a shallow chamber during the immediate postoperative period as well as reduces the incidence of choroidal detachment.

POSTOPERATIVE TREATMENT AND FOLLOW-UP REGIMEN

At the end of surgery, the administration of a subconjunctival injection of 15 mg gentamycin and 4 mg of dexamethasone alongwith a small quantity of lignocaine is recommended.

Topical dexamethasone and neomycin 0.3% eye drops are given four times daily for 4 weeks and three times in a day for subsequent two weeks. Moderate cycloplegics like cyclopentolate is recommended twice a day for one week followed by once a day for the subsequent week.

No antiglaucoma medication is required during the initial phase of hypotony.

Detailed and meticulous postoperative examination is essential and very crucial and should be carried out in all cases at regular intervals during follow-up period. Emphasis should be given on assessment of visual acuity,

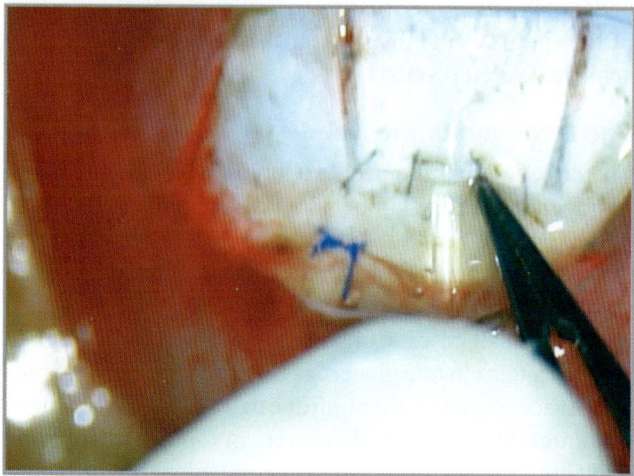

Fig. 47.20: Suturing of partial thickness scleral flap

extra-ocular movements, and IOP measurement the using non contact tonometer method. Detailed slit lamp, fundus, and other examinations should be carried out on day 1, 3 followed by one week interval for four weeks and monthly thereafter for six months and periodically thereafter as and when indicated. In cases of noncooperative or very young children, examination under GA should be carried out at a monthly interval for initial period of three months and thereafter, if indicated.

In terms of IOP, a complete success has been defined as an IOP of between 9 to 21 mmHg without medication, qualified success as IOP between 14 to 21 mmHg with one or more medications, and failure as a sustained secondary rise of (once stabilised to an optimal satisfactory level) postoperative IOP of >21 mmHg with one or more medications for more than one month. Complete failure can be defined as chronic hypotony (hypotony is defined as IOP less than 6 mmHg on any single visit), need of additional glaucoma surgery, development of phthisis bulbi or loss of light perception attributed to glaucoma.

It is very important to observe closely the immediate postoperative period, since the functional future of the valve could depend on such follow-up.

Frequent evaluation of the anterior chamber's depth should be done during the first 5 to 10 days period in which formation of the cyst that will wrap the body of the valve in the future is initiated. One should make sure that the depth of the anterior chamber is maintained more or less constant or increases as days go by.

Intraoperative Complications

Concurrent phacoemulsification and AG valve implantation surgery is a technically sound and viable procedure. The incidence and pattern of intraoperative complications do not magnify both in terms of quantum and pattern as compared to the singular phacoemulsification or AG valve implantation alone. We did not notice any significant intraoperative complications except difficulty in inserting AG valve tube into AC in the first attempt in less than 4% and traces of hyphaema in two per cent cases in the experience of more than 200 cases in the last five years. These problems were mainly observed in cases of cataract associated with angle closure or neovascular glaucoma, especially during the initial phase of learning curve. The incidence of such complications can be restricted further up to the bare minimum by introduction of viscoelastic materials into the anterior chamber through separate paracentesis just prior to the insertion of silicone tube into the anterior chamber.

Postoperative Complications

Combined AG valve implantation and phacoemulsification surgery do not face much intraoperative problems as well as the pattern and incidence of postoperative complications do not exceed that of singular phacoemulsification or glaucoma valve implant surgery. As such, in the last decade, both phacoemulsification and glaucoma valve surgery have witnessed a marked decline in the incidence and pattern of complications both in quantum and severity.

Postoperative complications can be grouped into immediate and early, intermediate and delayed postoperative complications.

Immediate and Early Postoperative Complications

The main constraint in glaucoma drainage device implant remains undue hypotony both in the immediate and during the intermediate postoperative period and complications following Ahmed glaucoma drainage device valve surgery in cases of nonresponsive refractory glaucomas. Other noted but infrequent postoperative complications are as follows:

(i) Hyphaema (Secondary): 1%
(ii) Choroidal detachment: 3–5%
(iii) Shallow chamber with hypotony: 5–7%
(iv) CME: 3–5%
(v) Corneal endothelial touch of drainage tube: 2–3%
(vi) Irido drainage tube adhesions: 1–2%
(vii) Iridocorneal anterior Synaechiae: 2–3%
(viii) Encapsulated bleb: 9–10%
(ix) Partial exposure of valve plate: 0.5 to 0.75%

Postoperative Status of IOP

Concurrent phacoemulsification with AG valve implantation has shown remarkable control of IOP even in long term follow-up in cases of refractive glaucoma, despite three or more drug regimen. In our experience, more than 90% cases continue to maintain complete success (IOP of between 9 to 21 mmHg without medication) following more than four years follow-up whereas qualified IOP control (IOP between 14 to 21 mmHg with one or more medications) was seen in remaining cases. We did not notice any failure so far.

CONCLUSION

The AGV implant has the advantage of achieving a lower rate of overdrainage without having to perform a two staged operation or to modify the surgical technique.

In our view, the Ahmed glaucoma drainage device valve has been found to be very effective in the management of refractory glaucomas in cases of coexisting glaucoma and cataract, irrespective of age and aetiology which provides good visual rehabilitation and control of IOP, with low incidence of complications.

BIBLIOGRAPHY

1. Rosenberg LF, Krupin T. Implants in glaucoma surgery: In: Ritch R, Shields MB, Krupin T, editors: The Glaucomas, 2nd ed. St. Louis: Mosby, 1996:1783–1807.

2. Alejandro N. Chung, Tin Aung, Jenn C. Wang, Paul TK Chew. Surgical outcomes of Combined Phacoemulsification and Glaucoma Drainage Implant Surgery for Asian Patients with Refractory Glaucoma with Cataract:Am J Ophthalmol 2004; 137:294–300.

3. Miller SJH. Genetic aspects of glaucoma. Trans Ophthalmol Soc UK 1966; 86:425–434.

4. Broadway D, Grierson I, Hitchings R. Racial differences in the results of glaucoma filtration surgery: are racial differences in the conjunctival cell profile important? Br J Ophthalmol 1994; 78:466–7

5. Aung T, Seah SKL. Glaucoma drainage implants in Asian eyes. Ophthalmology 1998;105:2117–22.

6. Da Mata A, Burk SE, Netland PA, Baltatzis S, Christen W, Foster CS.Management of uveitic glaucoma with Ahmed glaucoma valve implantation.Ophthalmology. 1999 Nov; 106(11):2168–72.

7. Ishida K, Netland PA.Ahmed Glaucoma Valve implantation in African American and white patients.Arch Ophthalmol. 2006 Jun; 124(6):800–6.

8. Watson JC, Kadri OA, Wilcox MJ.Effects of mitomycin C on glaucoma filtration capsules. Biomed Sci Instrum. 2005; 41:394–9.

9. Kurnaz E, Kubaloglu A, Yilmaz Y, Koytak A, Ozerturk Y. The effect of adjunctive Mitomycin C in Ahmed glaucoma valve implantation.Eur J Ophthalmol. 2005 Jan-Feb; 15(1): 27–31.

10. Sarodia U, Sharkawi E, Hau S, Barton K. Visualisation of aqueous shunt position and patency using anterior segment optical coherence tomography. Am J Ophthalmol. 2007 Jun; 143(6):1054–1056.

11. Carrillo MM, Trope GE, Pavlin C, Buys YM.Use of ultra-sound biomicroscopy to diagnose Ahmed valve obstruction by iris.Can J Ophthalmol. 2005 Aug; 40(4):499–501.

12. Budenz DL, Pyfer M, Singh K, Gordon J, Piltz-Seymour J, Keates EU. Comparison of phacotrabeculectomy with 5-fluorouracil, mitomycin-C, and without antifibrotic agents. Ophthalmic Surg Lasers 1999; 30:367–374.

13. Donoso R, Rodriguez A. Combined versus sequential phacotrabeculectomy with intraoperative 5-fluorouracil. J Cataract Refract Surg 2000; 26:71–74.

14. Hoffman KB, Feldman RM, Budenz DL, Gedde SJ, Chacra GA, Schiffman JC. Combined cataract extraction and Baerveldt glaucoma drainage implant: Indication and outcomes.Ophthalmology 2002; 109:1916–1920

15. Wedrich A, Menapace R, Radax U, Papanos P. Long-term results of trabeculectomy and small incision cataract surgery. J Cataract Refract Surg 1995;21:49–53.

16. Derick RJ, Evans J, Baker ND. Combined phacoemulsi-fication and trabeculectomy versus trabeculectomy alone: A comparison study using mitomycin-C. Ophthalmic Surg Lasers 1998; 29:707–713.

17. Donoso R, Rodriguez A. Combined versus sequential phacotrabeculectomy with intraoperative 5-fluorouracil. J Cataract Refract Surg 2000; 26:71–74.

18. Filous A, Brunova B. Results of the modified trabeculotomy in the treatment of primary congenital glaucoma. J Aapos 2002; 6:182–6

19. Hill R, Heur D, Baerveldt G, Minckler D, Martone J. Molteno implantation for glaucoma in young patients. Ophthalmol. 1991; 98:1042–1046.

20. Englert J, Freedman S, Cox T. The Ahmed valve in refractory pediatric glaucoma. Am. J. Ophthalmol.1999; 127:34–42.

21. Morod Y, Donaldson C, Kim Y, Abdolell M, Levin A. The Ahmed drainage implant in the treatment of pediatric glaucoma, Am. J. Ophthalmol. 2003; 135:821–829.

22. Hamush NG, Coleman AL, Wilson MR. Ahmed glaucoma valve implant for management of glaucoma in Sturge-Weber syndrome.Am J Ophthalmol. 1999 Dec; 128(6):758–60.

23. Al-Aswad LA, Netland PA, Bellows AR, Ajdelsztajn T, Wadhwani RA, Ataher G, Hill RA.Clinical experience with the double-plate Ahmed glaucoma valve. Am J Ophthalmol. 2006 Feb; 141(2):390–391.

24. Taglia DP, Perkins TW, Gangnon R, Heatley GA, Kaufman PL. Comparison of the Ahmed glaucoma valve, the Krupin eye valve with disk, and the double plate Molteno implant. J Glaucoma 2002; 11:347–353.

25. Tsai JC, Johnson CC, Kammer JA, Dietrich MS.The Ahmed shunt versus the Baerveldt shunt for refractory glaucoma II: longer-term outcomes from a single surgeon.Ophthalmology. 2006 Jun; 113(6):913–7.

26. Wilson MR, Mendis U, Paliwal A, Haynatzka V. Long-term follow-up of primary glaucoma surgery with Ahmed glaucoma valve implant versus trabeculectomy.Am J Ophthalmol. 2003 Sep; 136(3):464–70.

27. Wilson MR, Mendis U, Smith SD, Paliwal A. Ahmed glaucoma valve implant vs trabeculectomy in the surgical treatment of glaucoma: a randomised clinical trial. Am J Ophthalmol. 2000 Sep; 130(3):267–73.

28. Papadaki TG, Zacharopoulos IP, Pasquale LR, Christen WB, Netland PA, Foster CS. Long-term results of Ahmed glaucoma valve implantation for uveitic glaucoma. Am J Ophthalmol. 2007 Jul; 144(1):62–69. Epub 2007 May 9.

29. Melamed S, Fiore PM. Molteno implant surgery in refractory glaucoma. Surv Ophthalmol 1990; 34:441–8.

30. Jewelewicz DA, Rosenfeld SI, Litinsky SM. Epithelial downgrowth following insertion of an ahmed glaucoma implant. Arch Ophthalmol. 2003 Feb; 121(2):285–6.

31. Trigler L, Proia AD, Freedman SF.Fibrovascular ingrowth as a cause of Ahmed glaucoma valve failure in children. Am J Ophthalmol. 2006 Feb; 141(2):388–9.

32. Merrill KD, Suhr AW, Lim MC. Long-term success in the correction of exposed glaucoma drainage tubes with a tube extender. Am J Ophthalmol. 2007 Jul; 144(1):136–7.

33. Feldman RM, El-Harazi SM, Villanueva G. Valve membrane adhesion as a cause of Ahmed glaucoma valve failure. J Glaucoma 1997;6:10–12.

34. Lam DSC, Lai JSM, Chua JKH, et al. Needling revision of glaucoma drainage device filtering blebs. Ophthalmology 1998; 105:1127.

35. Eibschitz-Tsimhoni M, Schertzer RM, Musch DC, Moroi SE.Incidence and management of encapsulated cysts following Ahmed glaucoma valve insertion.J Glaucoma. 2005 Aug; 14(4):276–9.

36. Tannenbaum DP, Hoffman D, Greaney MJ, Caprioli J. Outcomes of bleb excision and conjunctival advancement for leaking or hypotonous eyes after glaucoma filtering surgery. Br J Ophthalmol 2004; 88:99–103.

37. Christmann LM, Wilson ME. Motility disturbances after Molteno implants. J Pediatr Ophthalmol Strabismus 1992; 29:44–8.

38. Wentzloff JN, Grosskreutz CL, Pasquale LR, Walton DS, Chen TC. Endophthalmitis after glaucoma drainage implant surgery. Int Ophthalmol Clin. 2007 Spring; 47(2):109–15.

39. Bayraktar Z, Kapran Z, Bayraktar S, Acar N, Unver YB, Gok K. Delayed-onset streptococcus pyogenes endophthalmitis following Ahmed glaucoma valve implantation. Jpn J Ophthalmol. 2005 Jul-Aug; 49(4):315–7.

40. Gutierrez-Diaz E, Montero-Rodriguez M, Mencia-Gutierrez E, Fernandez-Gonzalez MC, Perez-Blazquez E. Propionibacterium acnes endophthalmitis in Ahmed glaucoma valve. Eur J Ophthalmol. 2001 Oct-Dec; 11(4):383–5.

41. Gedde SJ, Scott IU, Tabandeh H, Luu KK, Budenz DL, Greenfield DS, Flynn HW Jr.Late endophthalmitis associated with glaucoma drainage implants.Ophthalmology. 2001 Jul; 108(7):1323–7.

42. Papadaki TG, Siganos CS, Zacharopoulos IP, Panteleontidis V, Charissis SK. Human amniotic membrane transplantation for tube exposure after glaucoma drainage device implantation. J Glaucoma. 2007 Jan; 16(1):171–2.

43. Ainsworth G, Rotchford A, Dua HS, King AJ.A novel use of amniotic membrane in the management of tube exposure following glaucoma tube shunt surgery. Br J Ophthalmol. 2006 Apr; 90(4):417–9.

44. Rai P, Lauande-Pimentel R, Barton K.Amniotic membrane as an adjunct to donor sclera in the repair of exposed glaucoma drainage devices. Am J Ophthalmol. 2005 Dec; 140(6):1148–52.

45. Chan CH, Lai JS, Shen SY. Delayed retrobulbar haemorrhage after Ahmed glaucoma implant: a case report. Eye. 2006 Apr; 20(4):494–5.

46. Tuli SS, WuDunn D, Ciulla TA, Cantor LB. Delayed suprachoroidal hemorrhage after glaucoma filtration procedures. Ophthalmology. 2001 Oct; 108(10):1808–11.

47. Kahook MY, Noecker RJ, Pantcheva MB, Schuman JS. Location of glaucoma drainage devices relative to the optic nerve. Br J Ophthalmol. 2006 Aug; 90(8):1010–3. Epub 2006 Apr 13.

48. Al-Aswad LA, Netland PA, Bellows AR, Ajdelsztajn T, Wadhwani RA, Ataher G, Hill RA. Clinical experience with the double-plate Ahmed glaucoma valve. Am J Ophthalmol. 2006 Feb; 141(2):390–391.

49. Brasil MV, Rockwood EJ, Smith SD. Comparison of silicone and polypropylene Ahmed Glaucoma Valve implants.J Glaucoma. 2007 Jan; 16(1):36–41.

50. Ishida K, Netland PA, Costa VP, Shiroma L, Khan B, Ahmed II. Comparison of polypropylene and silicone Ahmed Glaucoma Valves. Ophthalmology. 2006 Aug; 113(8):1320–6.

51. Nouri–Mahdavi K, Caprioli J. Evaluation of the hypertensive phase after insertion of the Ahmed Glaucoma Valve. Am J Ophthalmol. 2003 Dec; 136(6):1001–8.

52. Garcia-Feijoo J, Cuina-Sardina R, Mendez-Fernandez C, Castillo-Gomez A, Garcia-Sanchez J. Peritubular filtration as cause of severe hypotony after Ahmed valve implantation for glaucoma. Am J Ophthalmol. 2001 Oct;132(4):571–2.

53. Kee C. Prevention of early postoperative hypotony by partial ligation of silicone tube in Ahmed glaucoma valve implantation. J Glaucoma. 2001 Dec;10(6):466–9.

48

Phacotrabeculectomy: Different Techniques

Dr Mahipal S Sachdev, Dr Tanuj Dada, Dr Anand Aggarwal and Col JKS Parihar SM, VSM

INTRODUCTION

Both glaucoma and cataract are diseases with an increasing prevalence with age, and thus one often finds that they are coexistent in the elderly patient population. The association of glaucoma with cataract has become more frequent because of increase in life expectancy and the increased risk of cataract development in patients with glaucoma, especially with the use of antiglaucoma medications. The presence of cataract can affect the ability to assess glaucoma progression, and cataract extraction affects the intraocular pressure and effectiveness of glaucoma surgery. On the other hand, glaucoma surgery significantly increases the risk of the development of cataracts. For this reason, and to reduce the trauma induced by two surgical procedures, the prevailing trend is to perform a combined procedure, taking care of both pathologic conditions. Recent developments in bimanual small incision phaco-emulsification, the latest improvements in trabeculectomy and non-penetrating filtering surgery and implant drainage devices have favoured this trend for doing a combined surgery.

The goal of treatment in a glaucoma patient with cataract, is to achieve an adequate long term control of intraocular pressure (IOP), avoid postoperative IOP spikes which are deleterious to the health of the optic nerve head, obtain an optimal visual rehabilitation and improve the quality of life of the patient.

Cataract surgery alone has significant effects on the intraocular pressure. Following an early rise in the intra-ocular pressure, the IOP tends to fall in the long run. The effect is however small, averaging around 2–4 mmHg and one cannot depend on this as a means of lowering the IOP.

The combined surgical technique of phacotrabeculec-tomy has become the standard technique for management of eyes with co-existent cataract and glaucoma. Phacotrabe-culectomy is either done as a single site surgery with both phacoemulsification and trabeculectomy performed from the same site or more commonly as a two site surgery which entails performing a temporal phacoemulsification and a superior trabeculectomy. Separating the two incisions may decrease the inflammation and subsequent fibrosis induced by the surgery leading to a better survival of the filtering bleb. The combined single site surgery can be performed with the surgeon sitting superiorly, i.e without the need to change position intraoperatively.

The most important step before operating on a patient with cataract and glaucoma is the preoperative evaluation and decision making regarding the type of surgery to be performed.

PREOPERATIVE EVALUATION

In addition to the routine evaluation conducted for any cataract patient, patients with a coexistent glaucoma require evaluation of the ongoing medical therapy, diurnal IOP control on medication, corneal endothelial count, gonio-scopy, stereoscopic disc evaluation and visual fields (if possible). Conjunctival inflammation due to topical drug therapy, a low corneal endothelial count, miotic pupil, poor response to mydriatics, posterior synechiae, weakened zonules (esp. in eyes with pseudoexfoliation) and the raised IOP are some of the important factors which increase the degree of difficulty for the surgeon and may be responsible for a poor postoperative outcome.

Drugs such as pilocarpine and prostaglandin analogs must be stopped atleast 2 weeks prior to the surgery. The surgeon should arrange for iris hooks which are often required for intraoperative pupillary dilatation, especially in eyes with primary angle closure glaucoma and endocapsular rings should be kept handy if surgery is being planned in a case with pseudoexfoliation syndrome.

The decision to do a cataract surgery alone, or a combined procedure or to do a filtering surgery alone is decided by evaluation of the following factors:

- IOP control on current treatment
- Required target IOP for the patient
- Number of medications needed to achieve target IOP
- Extent of glaucomatous damage (disc and visual fields)
- Compliance to medical therapy
- Allergic reactions/significant side effects of topical therapy
- Socio-economic status of the patient
- Access to medical care facilities
- Effect of disease on quality of life of the patient.

OPTIONS FOR SURGICAL MANAGEMENT

Although there is still a controversy on the ideal protocol for surgery, combined surgery to tackle both cataract and glaucoma has become firmly established as a widely accepted modality of treatment. The advent of phacoemulsification has further allowed the reduction of incision size with a reduced complication rate. The advantages of such a combined approach include rapid visual rehabilitation, one time surgery, a reduced cost and more comfort for the patient. Cataract surgery has been successfully combined with both implant surgery and non-penetrating procedures. Further, the technique of cataract surgery that may be employed includes micro-incision bimanual phacoemulsification, standard phacoemulsification, extracapsular cataract extraction and manual small incision cataract surgery.

Since combined surgical procedures have reduced long term success rates as compared to that of trabeculectomy alone with increased incidence of postoperative inflammation, careful case selection is important. Combined surgery is best avoided in patients with secondary glaucoma, extensive conjunctival scarring, normal pressure glaucoma, advanced glaucomatous optic neuropathy and previous failed trabeculectomy. The other surgical option in such patients would be to perform a staged procedure with a trabeculectomy followed by cataract surgery in the second sitting. We use antimetabolites (mitomycin C 0.2 mg/ml) routinely in combined surgery.

The following options are available when dealing with a case with coexistent cataract and glaucoma:

- Cataract surgery alone
- Laser trabeculoplasty followed by cataract extraction
- Filtering procedure followed by cataract extraction at a later date
- Simultaneous cataract and glaucoma surgery – Combined extraction
- Extracapsular cataract extraction + Trabeculectomy
- Small incision cataract surgery (SICS) + Trabeculectomy

- Standard phacoemulsification + Trabeculectomy
- Single site
- Two site
- MICS (Phakonit) + Trabeculectomy
- Endoscopic cyclophotocoagulation + Cataract surgery
- Deep Sclerectomy + Cataract surgery
- Glaucoma drainage device + Cataract surgery

Cataract Extraction alone

It is probably the treatment of choice in patients on a low-dose, well tolerated medical regimen and with early or no glaucomatous optic nerve damage. There might be some danger in patients with moderate/advanced glaucomatous field damage because even a slight postoperative rise of the intraocular pressure (IOP) can threaten the remaining field of vision. These may be minimised using perioperative beta blockers and carbonic anhydrase inhibitors to blunt any IOP spike. On the other hand, cataract extraction in a patient of chronic angle closure glaucoma may result in lowering of the IOP and may allow the ophthalmologist to withdraw anti-glaucoma drugs. These patients should be followed up on a regular basis, as they can develop poor control of glaucoma any time in the future, requiring modification of therapy or filtering surgery.

Therefore, if the IOP is well controlled on a single topical drug with early glaucomatous optic nerve damage, cataract surgery alone can be performed.

Surgical Caveats

In patients with glaucoma, the corneal endothelium is already compromised. A dispersive viscoelastic device such as chondroitin sulfate or viscoadaptive like Healon 5 (23 mg/ml of sodium hyaluronate) should be used to maximise corneal endothelial protection. In addition, BSS plus with glutathione may be used to maintain integrity of the endothelial cells during surgery.

Poor pupil dilatation may be encountered especially in angle closure glaucomas and patients on long standing pilocarpine therapy. This requires additional surgical dilatation to achieve optimal visualisation. Stretching maneuvers or the use of iris hooks or rings for pupillary dilatation, multiple sphincterotomies are therefore recommended.

The weakness of the zonules and the increased contraction of the capsule in pseudoexfoliative glaucoma require additional intraoperative care and the need to use a capsular tension ring.

In glaucomatous eyes and especially in the pseudoexfoliation syndrome, there is a tendency for enhanced breakdown of the the blood-aqueous barrier, further aggravated by the use of pilocarpine and prostaglandins. Intense topical steroid therapy for a longer period of time may be required in the postoperative period, with occasional use of systemic steroids.

The surgeon has to be extra cautious in these cases as a posterior capsular rent with vitreous loss will aggravate the glaucomatous process, leading to inflammation and a rise in IOP.

During the course of cataract surgery, care should be taken to completely remove any viscoelastic used. Retained viscoelastic can cause significant intraocular pressure spikes in the immediate postoperative period which may further compromise a glaucomatous optic nerve.

In extracapsular cataract extraction (ECCE) or Manual SICS through a superior limbal approach, the limbal conjunctiva is incised during the surgery. The conjunctiva in this region is thus prone to scarring, which may preclude creation of a filtering bleb in this location. With the advent of phacoemulsification for cataract extraction and the clear corneal approach for access to the cataractous lens, the conjunctiva is not manipulated during cataract surgery. Phacoemulsification is performed with a significantly smaller incision than ECCE and therefore induces smaller amounts of astigmatism. Clear cornea, especially temporal, phacoemulsification cataract surgery is the preferred approach to maximise the options available for future glaucoma surgery.

Laser Trabeculoplasty Followed by Cataract Extraction

Laser trabeculoplasty followed by cataract extraction is another alternative to cataract surgery alone. Although argon laser (ALT) has been commonly used, diode laser, double frequency Nd:YAG laser, krypton laser, etc may also be used. This modality of treatment decreases the risk of immediate elevation of IOP in the postoperative period and may also reduce the requirement of antiglaucoma medications both prior to and following cataract surgery. Complications following ALT include hemorrhage from the trabecular meshwork during treatment, formation of peripheral anterior synechiae, uveitis and elevation of IOP. There is a decrease in the success rate of ALT with time and thus these patients require a long term follow up.

Another option is to do a selective laser trabeculoplasty (SLT) followed by cataract surgery. This is a new technique for laser trabeculoplasty which uses a Q switched double frequency (532 nm) YAG laser with a nanosecond pulse which does not cause any thermal damage and is selectively absorbed by the pigment granules in the trabecular meshwork. The advantage of SLT is that there is no thermal effect and therefore, it does not lead to scarring and can be repeated unlike ALT.

Filtering Surgery Followed by Cataract Extraction at a Later Date

When glaucoma is uncontrolled in spite of maximal tolerable medical therapy and/or laser trabeculoplasty, a trabeculectomy should be performed alone. This is also the case in eyes with advanced glaucoma that require a very low target pressure. Cataract extraction can be performed through a temporal clear cornea at a later date (preferably after 3 months). One can use a subconjunctival injection of 5FU (5 mg) away from the site of surgery and the bleb to prevent any subsequent compromise of the filtering bleb after the cataract surgery. There is a concern in such cases that cataract surgery may trigger inflammation and stimulate a fibroblastic response in the bleb leading to bleb failure.

Simultaneous Cataract and Glaucoma Surgery: Combined Extraction

Indications for a combined procedure include:
- When in spite of maximal tolerable topical medical therapy and/or laser trabeculoplasty, glaucoma control is poor in a patient with mild/moderate glaucoma.
- When the patient does not tolerate the medical therapy or is not compliant.
- When the patient cannot afford long term medical therapy.
- Advanced glaucomatous damage which cannot tolerate postoperative IOP spike.
- If there is uncontrolled glaucoma, but an urgent need to restore vision or when two separate surgeries are not feasible.

A combined procedure should not be performed in an eye with advanced glaucomatous damage with significant cataracts, even if IOP is well controlled because even a transient rise of IOP postoperatively, can threaten the residual field of vision.

When combining glaucoma surgery with cataract extraction, the surgery becomes technically more difficult than either surgery alone, there is more postoperative inflammation, the bleb formation is less reliable and the lowering of IOP may not be adequate to the amount of glaucomatous damage (i.e may not achieve target pressure).

Two site surgeries separating the phacoemulsification and the trabeculectomy sites have theoretical advantages of reducing inflammation at the site of the filter and thereby decrease the stimulus for the subsequent fibroblastic response. Standard two site phacotrabeculectomy requires two separate incisions, one for the cataract surgery and the other at the ostium under the scleral flap. In addition, the surgeon needs to adjust his position intraoperatively along with that of his assistants' and equipments (i.e. superior for trabeculectomy and temporal for phacoemulsification).

Surgical Technique

Although cataract extraction has also been successfully combined with nonpenetrating glaucoma surgery, endoscopic laser ablation and with implant surgeries our experience with these techniques is limited and we do a single or a two site phacotrabeculectomy.

The surgery should be performed under peribulbar anesthesia. Optimal pupillary dilatation is desirable to facilitate cataract extraction. Either a fornix or limbal based conjunctival flap may be used. Care should be taken to preserve the conjunctiva so that future filtering surgeries may be possible, if required.

For a limbal based flap, the conjunctiva is incised 8–9 mm behind the limbus. Wescott's scissors is used to separate the tenons and extend the conjunctival incision. For a fornix based flap, an incision is made in the conjunctiva at the limbus about 3–4 clock hours and extended posteriorly for a distance of around 7–8 mm. After dissecting the conjunctival flap superiorly, a triangular/rectangular scleral flap is marked with a sharp blade approximately 5 mm wide and 5 mm in height (Fig. 48.1a). Dissection is carried out with a steel crescent knife/diamond knife to the level of the cornea. We prefer using antimetabolites routinely in our cases. 0.2 mg/ml concentration of mitomycin C is used for 2–3 minutes under the scleral flap with a cellulose sponge after which the area is irrigated with balanced salt solution. The conjunctiva is then reposited back and cataract surgery started.

Phacoemulsification and Trabeculectomy

The cataract may be removed by the same incision (one site) or by a temporal incision (two-site). We prefer the two site approach as theoretically decreased astigmatism, minimal conjunctival manipulation, decreased inflammation and less fibrosis would be expected by separating the two sites. If the cataract is very hard and an ECCE is planned, then the surgery is carried out through the same wound as the trabeculectomy. The nucleus is delivered after extending the corneal wound on either side of the scleral flap.

Single site phacotrabeculectomy: In case the surgeon prefers the one site technique, then entry into the anterior chamber is made under the scleral flap with a 3.2 mm keratome and the phacoemulsification completed and the IOL implanted (Fig. 48.1b and c), before cutting the block of tissue under the scleral flap (Fig. 48.1d). A peripheral iridectomy is performed. The iris is reposited by gently stroking the cornea and the scleral flap secured with three 10–0 monofilament sutures (Fig. 48.1e). The conjunctival flap is sutured with running 8–0 vicryl sutures if a limbus based flap has been used. A fornix based flap is pulled down and sutured to the cornea with two 8–0 vicryl anchoring sutures and additional 10–0 nylon sutures to ensure that there is no leakage under the flap.

There is another way of performing the single site phacotrabeculectomy through the scleral tunnel. In this technique, scleral tunnel is constructed. The phacoemulsification is then performed through it. After implanting the IOL, the trabeculectomy window is cut near the inner posterior lip of the tunnel with the help of Kelly's punch. The tunnel is then sutured or left unsutured depending upon the case and the surgeon's preference. The scleral tunnel is then covered with the conjunctiva.

Two Site Phacotrabeculectomy: If a two site surgery is performed, the surgeon first makes a temporal entry with a 3.2 mm Keratome (Fig. 48.2a) or a diamond knife after making a side port entry with an MVR blade. The standard phacoemulsification is completed using the usual methods like stop and chop nucleotomy (Fig. 48.2b) or phaco chop nucleotomy. Its always helpful to make use of the power modulations available with the newer generation phaco machines like the burst or hyperpulse mode (40–50 pulses/sec) to minimise unwanted ultrasound energy being given into the eye and thereby protecting corneal endothelium. The cortex is removed by irrigation aspiration and IOL implanted under a viscoelastic. The viscoelastic should not be removed after IOL implantation. A square edged hydrophobic acrylic IOL is our choice for a phacotrabeculectomy (Fig. 48.2c).

The surgeon shifts back to the superior limbus to complete the trabeculectomy (Fig. 48.2d). A conjunctival flap is fashioned with Wescott's scissors. The bleeders

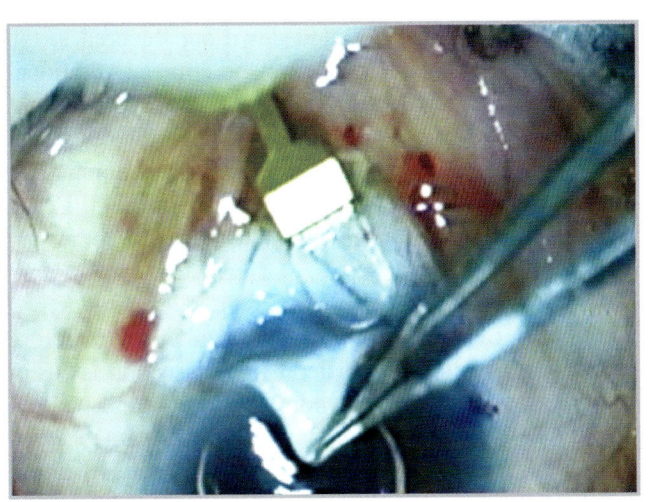

(a)

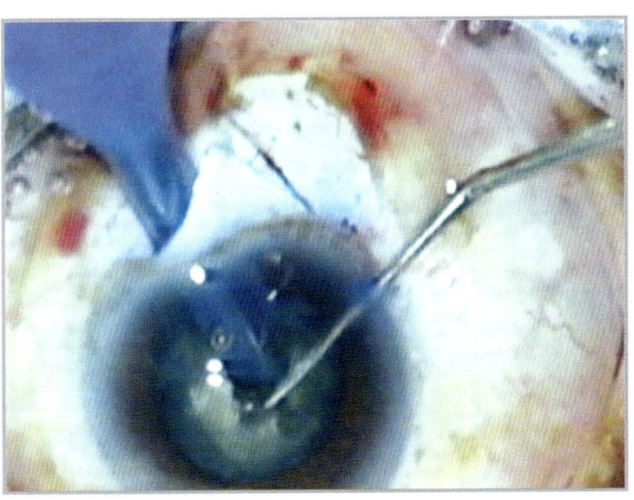

(b)

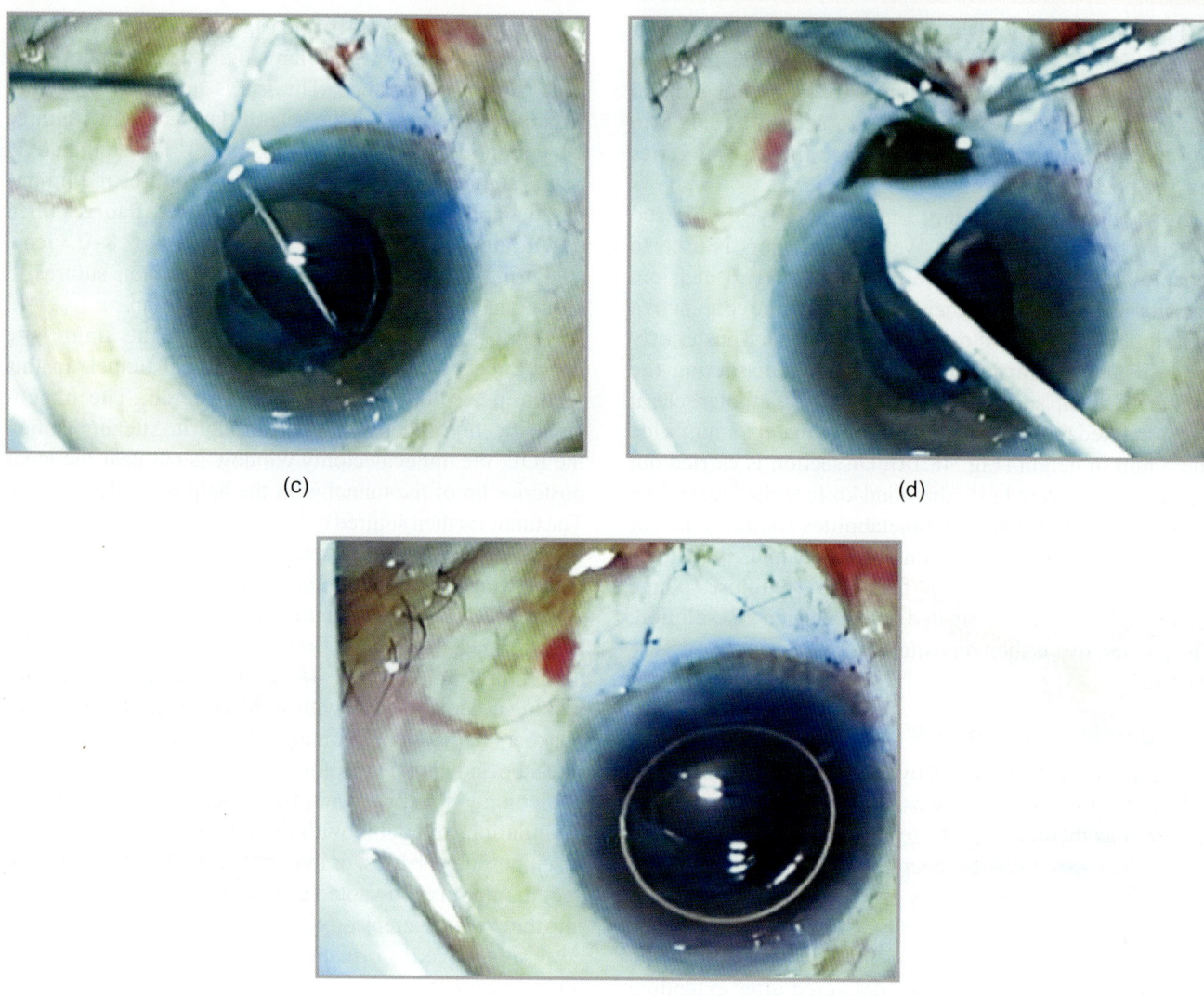

(c)

(d)

(e)

Fig. 48.1: (a) Single site phacotrabeculectomy: Scleral flap creation, (b) Phaco through scleral tunnel, (c) IOL implantation through scleral tunnel, (d) Creation of trabeculectomy ostium, (e) Final appearance after flap closure

are cauterised with bipolar cautery and a triangular flap 5 × 5 mm marked with a super sharp blade. The scleral flap is dissected to the level of the cornea with a crescent knife or a diamond blade.

The anterior chamber is entered with a sharp blade or an MVR knife, and a block of tissue 3.5 × 1 mm is cut with Vannas scissors. The scleral flap is lifted, the iris pulled out and a peripheral iridectomy performed. The scleral flap is closed with two/three 10–0 monofilament sutures. The viscoelastic can now be removed via the temporal corneal incision (Fig 48.2e) or can also be removed through the trabeculectomy fistula thereby avoiding the need to change position again using I and A. One 10–0 nylon suture should be applied to the corneal incision to prevent any possibility of leakage, if massage of the bleb is required in the postoperative period. A Kelly's descemet punch can also be used for cutting the block and releasable sutures may be used to allow titration of filtration after surgery.

If a limbus based flap has been used then the conjunctiva is closed by a running 8–0 Vicryl suture. For a fornix based flap, the conjunctiva is pulled down and secured at the edges with 8–0 Vicryl sutures to the cornea. Additional 10–0 nylon sutures may be placed to achieve watertight closure. Care should be taken to avoid covering releasable sutures with conjunctiva. In all cases, a subconjunctival injection of 0.25cc dexamethasone 4 mg/ml and 0.25cc gentamycin 40 mg/ml is given at the end of the surgery in the lower fornix.

Alternatively some surgeons prefer making conjunctival and scleral flap without anterior chamber entry before phacoemulsification. The scleral flap dissection is easier with the closed globe with normal tension and without the chance of anterior chamber leak. The surgeon then shifts to the temporal site to perform phacoemulsification and IOL implantation. After that the surgeon shifts back to the superior location to complete the trabeculectomy.

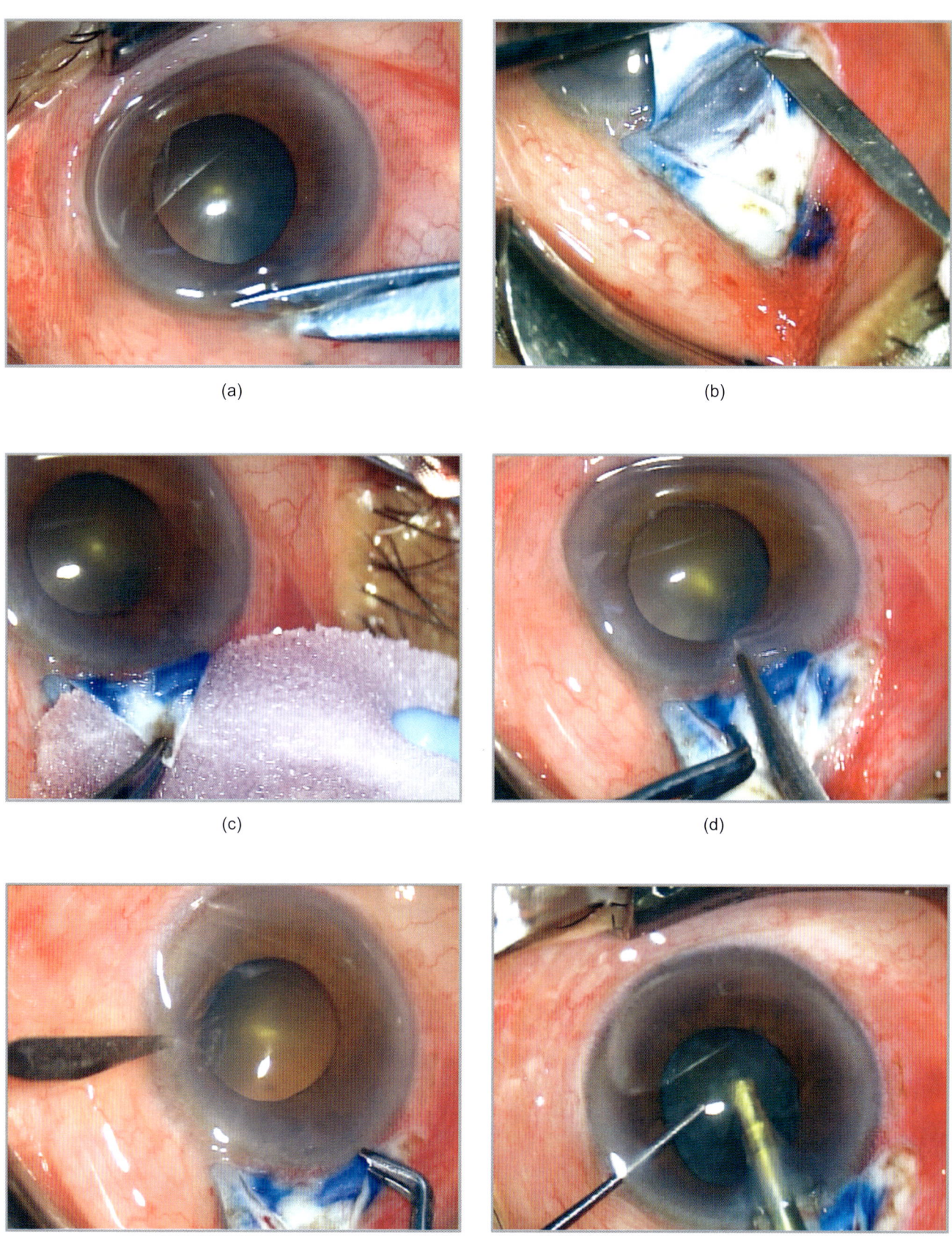

Fig. 48.2: (a) Two site phacotrabeculectomy: Fornix based conjunctival flap, (b) Partial thickness triangular scleral flap, (c) Mitomycin modulation of partial thickness scleral flap, (d) 1.0 mm entry for rhexis, (e) Side port entry for second instrumentation during phacoemulsification surgery, (f) Phacotrab: Nucleotomy by direct chopping

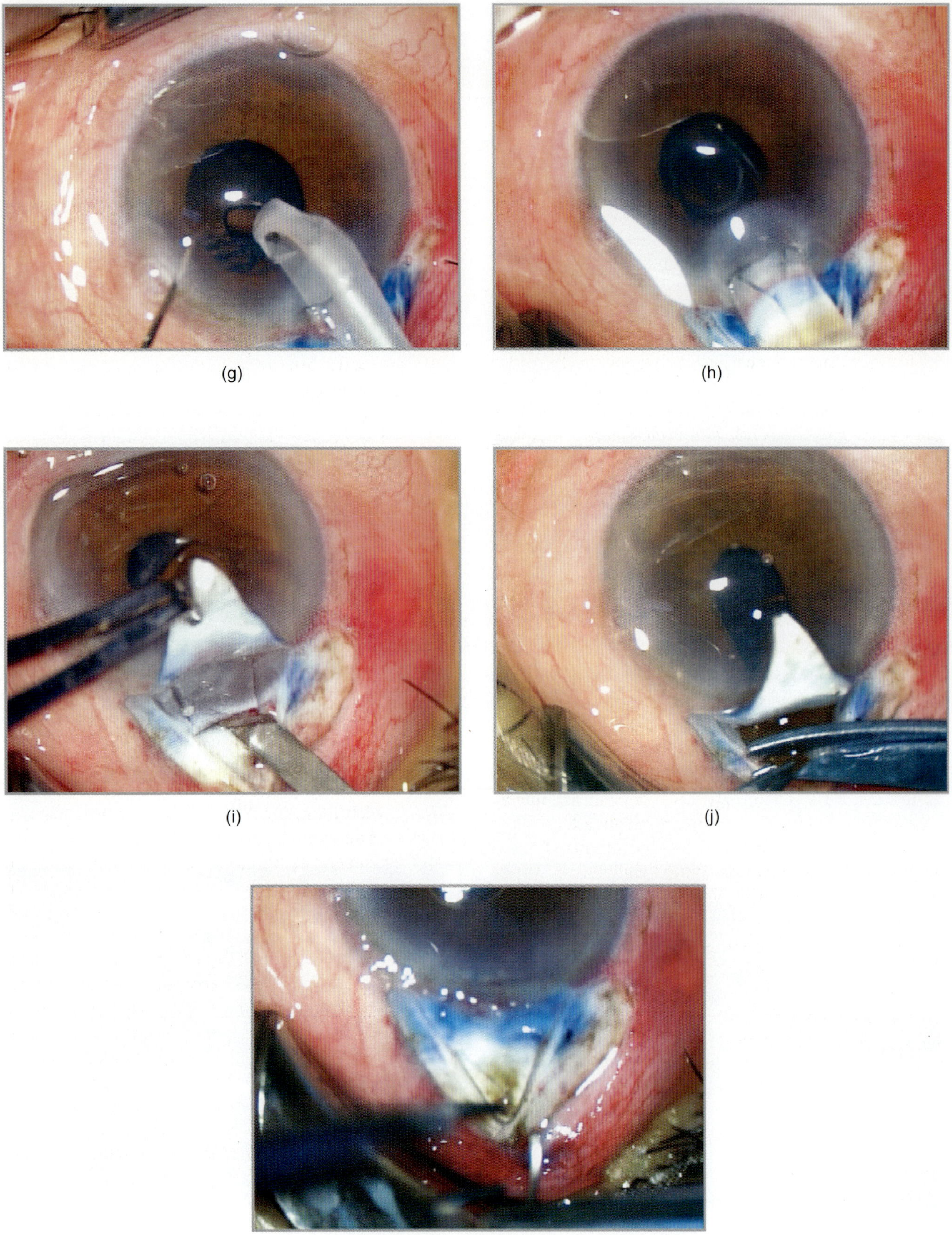

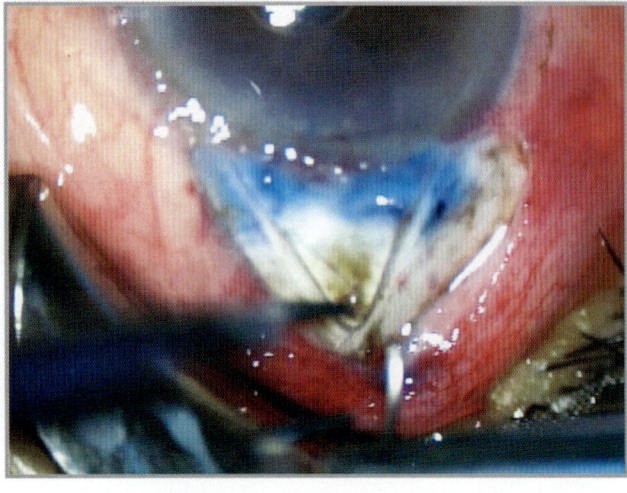

Fig. 48.2: (g) Phacotrab: I/A, (h) Phaco trab: IOL Implantation, (i) Excision of piece of trabecular meshwork, (j) Phacotrab: Iridectomy, (k) Suturing of partial thickness triangular scleral flap

Postoperative regimen includes 1% predinisolone acetate eye drops (6–8 times/day), 0.3% ciprofloxacin eye drops (3–6 times/day) and 1% tropicamide (HS).

Trabeculectomy alone followed by Second Stage Cataract Surgery

The success rate for combined procedures is lower than that reported for trabeculectomy alone. We generally advise to space the two surgeries by 3–6 months. One can also titrate the status of the filtering bleb intraoperatively during surgery by noting the staining of the filtering bleb with trypan blue when it is injected into the anterior chamber for capsulorrhexis. The trabeculectomy is done superiorly and the cataract removed by a temporal approach to avoid the bleb site. Since, there is leakage of fluid from the bleb site, the bottle height should be raised to an adequate amount. The use of a superpinky should be avoided as it can result in gross hypotony with shallowing of the anterior chamber. The corneal endothelium should be coated with a dispersive viscoelastic (Viscoat) or a viscoadaptive (Healon 5) to provide maximal protection. Subconjunctival injection of 5-FU or mitomycin drops may be considered if there is a tendency for bleb failure after the second stage cataract surgery.

Postoperative Management

A close watch for complications is needed in the immediate postoperative period. Due to the iris manipulation, there is an increased chance of severe postoperative fibrinous uveitis which requires intense topical and sometimes even systemic steroids and cycloplegics. Follow up examinations are recommended on the first postoperative day, 4th postoperative day and weekly thereafter in the first month. Topical corticosteroids in maximal strength are used two hourly in the first week and tapered gradually to be discontinued by 8–10 weeks. Topical antibiotic drops and short acting mydriatics are also used in the first postoperative month. Should releasable sutures be removed, antibiotic drops are continued till 2 weeks after the suture removal. Dilute pilocarpine therapy (0.25%) may be tried in patients who complain of glare due to a permanent mydriasis following the use of iris hooks during surgery. These patients require a long term follow-up as there is always a risk of failure of the filtering surgery with a subsequent rise in the IOP.

Management of Postoperative Complications

The complication rate of a combined procedure has been reported to be similar to that following trabeculectomy. Vision threatening complications include severe postoperative uveitis, suprachoroidal hemorrhage, hypotony, a flat anterior chamber, raised IOP and the need for a repeat surgery.

Postoperative Inflammation

Uveitis is generally more severe when the two procedures are combined together. It has been suggested that the incidence of fibrinous reactions is greater following a combined procedure. This complication usually encountered in the first three days following surgery is thought to be more frequent in eyes with myopia, hyphaema, iridectomy, and exfoliation syndrome. The reported incidence ranges from 5–27%. The incidence appears to be less with phacoemulsification and foldable lens implantation.

Hyphaema

The origin of this complication appears to be trauma to the iris or bleeding from the scleral flap. Usually it resolves within a week. More severe cases may mandate a surgical approach with bimanual irrigation- aspiration for hyphaema drainage.

Vitreous Loss

The incidence is similar to that following routine cataract surgery. However in this case, vitreous in the anterior chamber can block the internal ostium resulting in failure of the surgery. Hence, recognising this complication and a thorough anterior vitrectomy is advisable.

Elevated Intraocular Pressure

This is a common postoperative complication. Usually, the internal ostium is blocked by retained viscoelastic, blood or fibrin. Blockade of the internal ostium may be diagnosed by gonioscopy. Other rare causes include a suprachoroidal hemorrhage and malignant glaucoma. A conservative management is advised. An attempt may be made to encourage filtration by a gentle digital massage on the inferior sclera. This method should not be used, when a fornix based conjunctival flap has been used to avoid leakage. Bleb formation is noted as the digital massage forces aqueous out. If a dense fibrinous exudates is present, then intracameral tissue plasminogen activator may be used. Argon laser may be used to relieve the block in the ostium though occasionally, surgical revision is required. In addition, a tight closure of the scleral flap may result in inadequate filtration. If releasable sutures have been used, they should be removed. The time for removal is within 2 weeks in routine surgery and within 6 weeks if mitomycin C has been used intraoperatively. Additional digital massage may be needed to commence filtration. Removal is not advised in the first week as this is associated with hypotony and leak from the anterior chamber. Removal is safe in the second and third weeks provided the conjunctiva is not too avascular and thinned out. Removal of sutures should also be considered if the overlying conjunctiva is excessively vascular.

Hypotony

Causes include a leaking bleb, over filtration due to large internal ostium, cyclodialysis cleft, and aqueous under secretion due to iridocyclitis. The presence of a leaking bleb may be diagnosed by painting the suspected area with a fluorescein strip and examining the patient under the cobalt blue filter of the slit lamp. Such blebs are associated with an increased risk of infection. Management includes a pressure bandage, a large soft contact lens or scleral shell or cyanoacrylate glue. If all measures fails, resuturing of the conjunctiva may be required.

The use of antimetabolites is associated with hypotony. Usually the IOP tends to recover with time. Prolonged and untreated hypotony may lead to hypotony maculopathy and optic disc edema with a permanent drop in vision. This may require the use of a conjunctival autograft or a scleral graft to reinforce the area of the leak.

Failed/Failing Blebs

Failed blebs are flat and vascular. Such blebs are best managed by needling. The procedure may be performed under the slit lamp or the operating microscope. 0.2 ml of balanced salt solution is injected under the conjunctiva to elevate the conjunctiva to facilitate dissection. A 26G needle is inserted 1cm from the bleb and sideways movement is used to dissect the scar tissue. The sclerostomy wound may be entered if need be. Success is indicated by a reduction in IOP and egress of aqueous with formation of the bleb. Antimetabolites are usually used at the end of the procedure. We prefer the use of 5 fluorouracil 0.1 ml of 50 mg/ml solution injected 1cm from the bleb sites. Usually three injections are given on alternate days. 5 FU may be used alone without needling. Another option is to use topical mitomycin C soaked swabs for 3 minutes over the bleb.

Postoperative Glare and Diplopia

Use of iris hooks during surgery can lead to a permanent mydriasis and resultant postoperative glare and diplopia. Dilute pilocarpine therapy may be used initially although some patients may finally require a pupilloplasty with use of prolene sutures.

CONCLUSION

In conclusion, combined cataract and filtering surgery is a feasible and successful approach to treat coexisting glaucoma and cataract. The success rates being lower than that of filtering surgery alone, treatment needs to be individualised for each patient. Patients adequately controlled by medication/previous successful surgery may be rehabilitated by cataract surgery alone. Phacoemulsification is the preferred technique to remove cataract in a combined procedure. Patients undergoing a combined surgery benefit from the use of mitomycin C with a greater IOP reduction. All patients should be maintained on a long term follow-up with regular assessments of the intraocular pressure, optic disc and visual fields as the long term success and the IOP control achieved after a phacotrabeculectomy is less than that achieved with a standard trabeculectomy alone.

BIBLIOGRAPHY

1. Friedman DS, Jampel HD, Lubomski LH, Kempen JH, Quigley H, Congdon N, Verbin HL, Robinson KA, Bass EB. Surgical Strategies for Coexisting Glaucoma and Cataract. Ophthalmology 2002; 109(10):1902–1913.

2. Agarwal A, Agarwal A, Agarwal S. Phakonit. In: Agarwal S, Agarwal A, Agarwal A. editors. Phacoemulsification Vol1. New Delhi: Jaypee Brothers, 2004; 318–329.

3. Lee RK, Gedde SJ. Surgical Management of Coexisting Cataract and Glaucoma. International Ophthalmology Clinics 2004; 44(2):151–166.

4. Verges C, Jorge C, Cosme L. Surgical strategies in patients with cataract and glaucoma. (In) Current Opinion in Ophthalmology 2005; 16(1):44–52.

5. Casson RJ, Salmon JF. Combined surgery in the treatment of patients with cataract and primary open-angle glaucoma. J Cataract Refract Surg 2001; 27:1854–1863.

6. Jampel HD, Friedman DS, Lubomski LH, Kempen JH, Quigley H, Congdon N, Verbin HL, Robinson KA, Bass EB. Effect of Technique on Intraocular Pressure after Combined Cataract and Glaucoma Surgery. Ophthalmology 2002; 109(12):2215–2224.

7. Donoso R, Rodrfguez. Combined versus sequential phacotrabeculectomy with intraoperative 5-fluoracil. J Cataract Refract Surg 2000; 26:71–74.

8. Caporossi A, Casprini F, Tosi GM, Balestrazzi A. Long-term results of combined 1-way phacoemulsification, intraocular lens implantation, and trabeculectomy. J Cataract Refract Surg 1999;25:1641–5.

9. Hoffman KB, Feldman RM, Budenz DL, Gedde SJ, Chacra GA, Schiffman JC. Combined Cataract Extraction and Baerveldt Glaucoma Drainage Implant. Ophthalmology 2002; 109:1916–1920.

10. Dogru M, Omoto M, Fujishima H, Yagi Y, Tsubota K. Early visual results with rollable ThinOptx intraocular lens. J Cat Refract Surg 2004; 30:558–565.

11. Diaz-Valle D, del Castillo B, Jimenez A, et al. Endothelial changes with cataract surgery techniques. J Cataract Refract Surg 1998; 24:951–955.

12. Verges C, Cazal J, Cipres MC, et al. Endothelial cell density and corneal thickness in cataract surgery comparing continuous vs micropulsed ultrasound. Cornea [Epub ahead of print.].

13. Fine H, Packer M, Hoffman RS: Power modulation in new phacoemulsification technology: improved outcomes. J Cataract Refract Surg 2004; 30:1014–1019.

14. Cohen JS, Khatana AK, Osher RH. Combined Cataract Implant and Filtering Surgery. In:Steinert RF, editor. Cataract Surgery. Philadelphia: Saunders, 2004; 223–246.

15. Beckers HJ, De Kroon KE, Nuijts RM, Webers CA. Phacotrabeculectomy. Doc Ophthalmol. 2000; 100(1):43–7.

16. Vass C, Menapace R. Surgical strategies in patients with combined cataract and glaucoma. Curr Opin Ophthalmol 2004; 15:61–66.

17. Gayton JL, Karr MVD, Sanders V. Combined cataract and glaucoma surgery: Trabeculectomy versus endoscopic laser cycloablation. J Cataract Refract Surg 1999; 25:1214–1219.

18. Gosiengfiao DH, Latina MA. Avoiding complications in combined phacotrabeculectomy. Semin Ophthalmol. 2002 Sep-Dec; 17(3–4):138–43.

19. Lochhead J, Casson RJ, Salmon JF. Long term effect on intraocular pressure of phacotrabeculectomy compared to trabeculectomy. Br J Ophthalmol. 2003 Jul; 87(7):850–2.

20. Caprioli J, Park HJ, Weitzman M. Temporal corneal phacoemulsification combined with superior trabeculectomy: a controlled study. Trans Am Ophthalmol Soc. 1996; 94:451–463; discussion 463–468.

21. Chen PP, Weaver YK, Budenz DL, et al. Trabeculectomy function after cataract extraction. Ophthalmology 1998; 105:1928–1935.

22. Rebolleda G, Munoz-Negrete FJ. Phacoemulsification in eyes with functioning filtering blebs: a prospective study. Ophthalmology 2002; 109:2248–2255.

23. Greenfield DS, Miller MP, Suner IJ, et al. Needle elevation of the scleral flap for failing filtration blebs after trabeculectomy with mitomycin C. Am J Ophthalmol. 1996; 122:195–204.

24. Kleinmann G, Katz H, Pollack A, et al. Comparison of trabeculectomy with mitomycin C with or without phacoemulsification and lens implantation. Ophthalmic Surg Lasers. 2002; 33:102–108.

25. Siriwardena D, Kotecha A, Minassian D, et al. Anterior chamber flare after trabeculectomy and after phacoemulsification. Br J Ophthalmol 2000; 84:1056–1057.

26. Shingleton BJ, Chaudhry IM, O'Donoghue MW, et al. Phacotrabeculectomy: limbus-based versus fornix-based conjunctival flaps in fellow eyes. Ophthalmology. 1999; 106: 1152–1155.

27. Lemon LC, Shin DH, Kim C, et al. Limbus-based vs fornix-based conjunctival flap in combined glaucoma and cataract surgery with adjunctive mitomycin C. Am J Ophthalmol. 1998; 125:340–345.

28. Kozobolis VP, Siganos CS, Christodoulakis EV, et al. Two-site phacotrabeculectomy with intraoperative mitomycin-C: fornix-versus limbus-based conjunctival opening in fellow eyes. J Cataract Refract Surg. 2002; 28:1758–1762.

29. Berestka JS, Brown SV. Limbus-versus fornix-based conjunctival flaps in combined phacoemulsification and mitomycin C trabeculectomy surgery. Ophthalmology 1997 Feb; 104(2):187–96.

30. Borggrefe L, Lieb W, Grehn F: A prospective randomised comparison of two techniques of combined cataract-glaucoma surgery. Graefes Arch Clin Exp Ophthalmol 1999; 237: 887–892.

31. Sayyad F, Helal M, Maghraby A, et al. One-site versus two-sites phacotrabeculectomy: a randomised study. J Cataract Refract Surg 1999; 25:77–82.

32. Wyse T, Meyer M, Ruderman JM, et al. Combined trabeculectomy and phacoemulsification: a one-site vs two-site approach. Am J Ophthalmol 1998; 125:334–339.

33. Rossetti L, Bucci L, Miglior S, et al. Temporal corneal phacoemulsification combined with separate-incision superior trabeculectomy vs standard phacotrabeculectomy: a comparative study. Acta Ophthalmol Scand 1997; (Suppl):39.

34. Cohen JS: Combined cataract implant and filtering surgery with 5-fluorouracil. Ophthalmic Surg 1990; 21:181–186.

35. Budenz DL, Pyfer M, Singh K, et al. Comparison of phacotrabeculectomy with 5-fluorouracil, mitomycin C and without antifibrotic agents. Ophthalmic Surg Lasers. 1999; 30:367–374.

36. Shin DH, Ren J, Juzych MS, et al. Primary glaucoma triple procedure in patients with primary open-angle glaucoma: the effect of mitomycin C in patients with and without prognostic factors for filtration failure. Am J Ophthalmol 1998; 125:346–352.

49

Post Phaco Pseudophakic Bullous Keratopathy: IOL Exchange and Scleral Fixated IOL Implantation

Col JKS Parihar SM, VSM and Col Vijay Mathur

INTRODUCTION

Corneal Endothelium has an extremely important role in keeping the corneal stroma in a dehydrated state thus maintaining corneal clarity. Disruption of endothelial function or integrity leads to corneal oedema. Fluid within the stroma causes separation of corneal collagen fibrils, thus disrupting the lattice arrangement and resulting in loss of transparency. Many chemical changes too occur in the corneal stroma due to oedema like increase in levels of Beta Ig-h3, TN-C, fibronectin and fibrillin.

Corneal decompensation can occur following Phacoemulsification whenever endothelial cell count falls below the critical limit of $2,200/mm^2$. This can occur due to various reasons.

FACTORS INFLUENCING CORNEAL ENDOTHELIAL STATUS

Pre-existing Conditions

(i) **Fuchs' endothelial dystrophy:** Is a progressive bilateral condition in which there is gradually progressive diminution of endothelial cells. Detailed preoperative slit lamp examination to rule out 'endothelial excrescences' that are the hallmark of Fuchs' endothelial dystrophy should be done. Fellow eye examination should always be done. It should be suspected whenever a previously operated eye has developed bullous keratopathy.

(ii) **Pseudoexfoliation syndrome:** Is characterised by deposition of pseudoexfoliated material at the pupillary margin, poor pupillary dilatation due to iris atrophy, hard cataracts with large nucleus, glaucoma and pigment dispersion. Due to the combination of above factors, these cases require more manipulation and phaco energy leading to a greater loss of endothelial cells.

Intraoperative Factors

(i) **Descemet's stripping:** Massive Descemet's membrane detachment can be created during initial entry (by defective keratome), while inserting the phacoprobe or while IOL implantation. If left unrecognised and untreated, PBK can result.

(ii) **Endothelial damage due to surgical manipulation:** Poor surgical technique, excessive use of phaco power for hard cataracts and frequent collapse of the anterior chamber causes damage to endothelial cells.

(iii) **Posterior capsular rent:** Vitreous in the anterior chamber may touch the endothelium to cause endothelial cell loss. Excessive intraoperative surgical manipulation also contributes towards endothelial cell loss. Implanting an AC IOL has been shown to contribute towards endothelial cell loss by close proximity to the endothelium and a tendency to cause glaucoma and uveitis. Initial clinical features include excessive striate keratitis and corneal haze. This progressively increases till frank epithelial bullae appear and corneal thickness increases. Recurrent painful epithelial erosions occur due to frequent bursting of bullae. Corneal scarring due to long-standing oedema eventually results.

MANAGEMENT

Initial management may be medical. IOP lowering medication and hyperosmotic agents can be given to reduce corneal oedema. Bandage contact lens is useful whenever epithelial erosions occur. Ultimate treatment is surgical with removal of the offending IOL, clearing the anterior chamber of vitreous and doing penetrating keratoplasty. Implanting a PC IOL, if capsular remnants permit, or implanting a scleral fixed IOL (SF IOL) can best correct aphakia. In the author's view, the anterior chamber IOL implant is not preferred since in a complicated PBK, the end result with an AC IOL implant is not encouraging.

IOL POWER CALCULATION

Presents unique challenges as corneal decompensation results in irregular corneal surface and mires are not formed properly for keratometry. K readings from fellow eye can be helpful in such circumstances. However, biometry values from the other eye are known to cause a discrepancy, as only in 60% of eyes, biometry values of both eyes are equal. Moreover, previous surgery may have resulted in changes in K readings. If an AC IOL has been implanted it adds to the problem as all current formulae for IOL power calculation are only programmed for PC IOL.

SURGICAL TECHNIQUE

There are many techniques described. The choice depends upon the training of the surgeon performing the procedure and other adjunct procedures being performed. In cases of IOL exchange (AC/PC), after making the scleral flaps in horizontal meridian from where sutures will be passed, it would be better to explant the offending lens, do a complete vitrectomy before proceeding with SF IOL implantation. In cases where cornea is decompensated and PK is being planned, corneal button is removed and the whole procedure is done as an open sky technique.

Implanting an SF IOL invariably requires anterior/mid vitrectomy to be performed. This can be done by the three port pars plana technique or through the Limbal section. There are various techniques described for passage of sutures to anchor the IOL.

Ab Externo Technique

In this, the sutures are passed from out to in. This results in lesser chance of damage to ciliary body and is done under direct visualisation. A 10/0 prolene suture on a straight long needle is passed into the eyeball, 3.5 to 4.0 mm behind the limbus under a partial thickness scleral flap. From the opposite side, a 26G needle is introduced into the eye. Into the lumen of this needle, the straight needle with prolene suture is threaded and pulled out of the eye from the opposite side. The same is repeated with the other arm. The advantage being that sutures are passed before the eye is opened and there is minimal distortion of the globe. Now, the eye is entered at the 12 O'clock limbus and using a sinsky hook, the sutures are brought out of the eye. The suture is now cut and tied to haptics of the IOL. The limbal incision is extended and the IOL manipulated into the posterior chamber. This technique is difficult to perform if another lens is in place that needs to be explanted.

Ab Interno Technique

After making the scleral flaps as mentioned above, the anterior chamber is entered at the limbus. The eyeball is entered with the straight needle under one of the scleral flaps and this is taken out of the eye through the limbal incision. This suture is now passed through the eyelet on the haptic of scleral fixated IOL. A 26G needle is passed through the scleral flap on the same side and a straight needle is threaded into the lumen of this needle and taken out of the eye by a reverse movement. The same process is repeated on the other side with the other arm. The advantage of this technique is that there are no knots inside the eye. The disadvantage being that the globe is open for a longer time while manipulations are being carried out.

In both techniques, centration of the IOL is extremely important. It is preferable to decentre the IOL superiorly as the IOL tends to move downwards when the patient is in the upright position.

With both techniques, the limbal incision can be made with a self sealing scleral tunnel. It is however advisable to give a suture at the end, such that wound leak does not happen with postoperative hypotony.

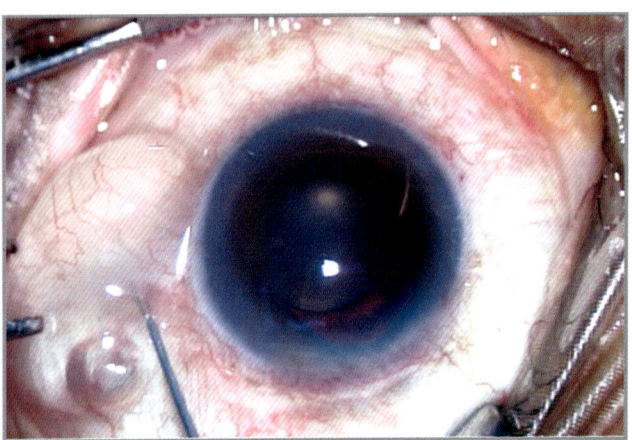

(a)   (b)

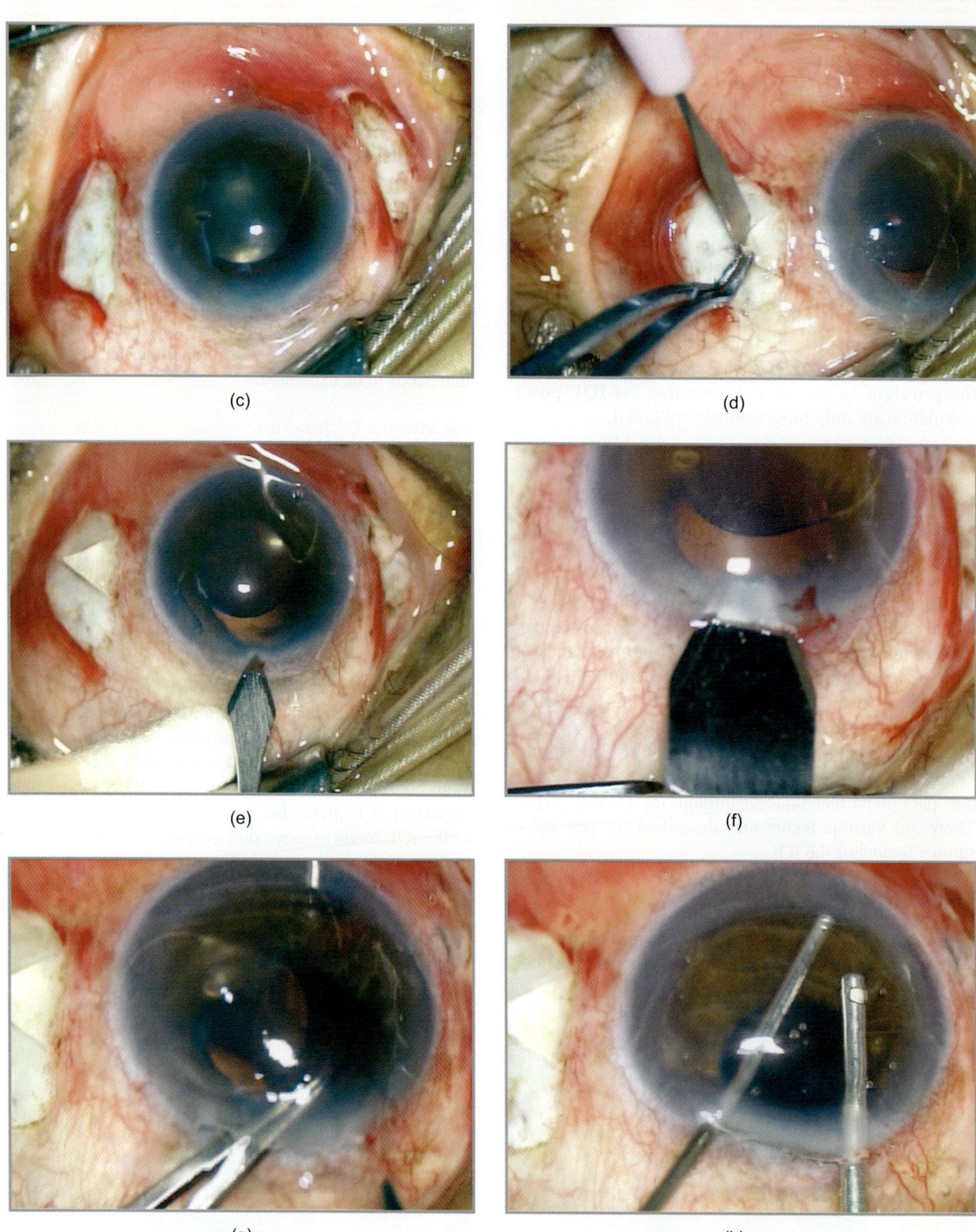

Fig. 49.1: (a) Postphaco PBK (PC IOL implant is placed in AC), (b) Subconjunctival infiltration of lignocaine 2% to raise the conjunctiva prior to the dissection, (c) Conjunctival pocket is created prior to the construction of partial thickness scleral flap, (d) Construction of a partial thickness scleral flap, (e) A 3.2 mm entry to construct incision for explantation of AC IOL, (f) A 6.0 mm Incision for explantation of AC IOL, (g) Explantation of AC IOL after fracturing iris entrapped haptics, (h) Vitrectomy prior to scleral fixated IOL implantation

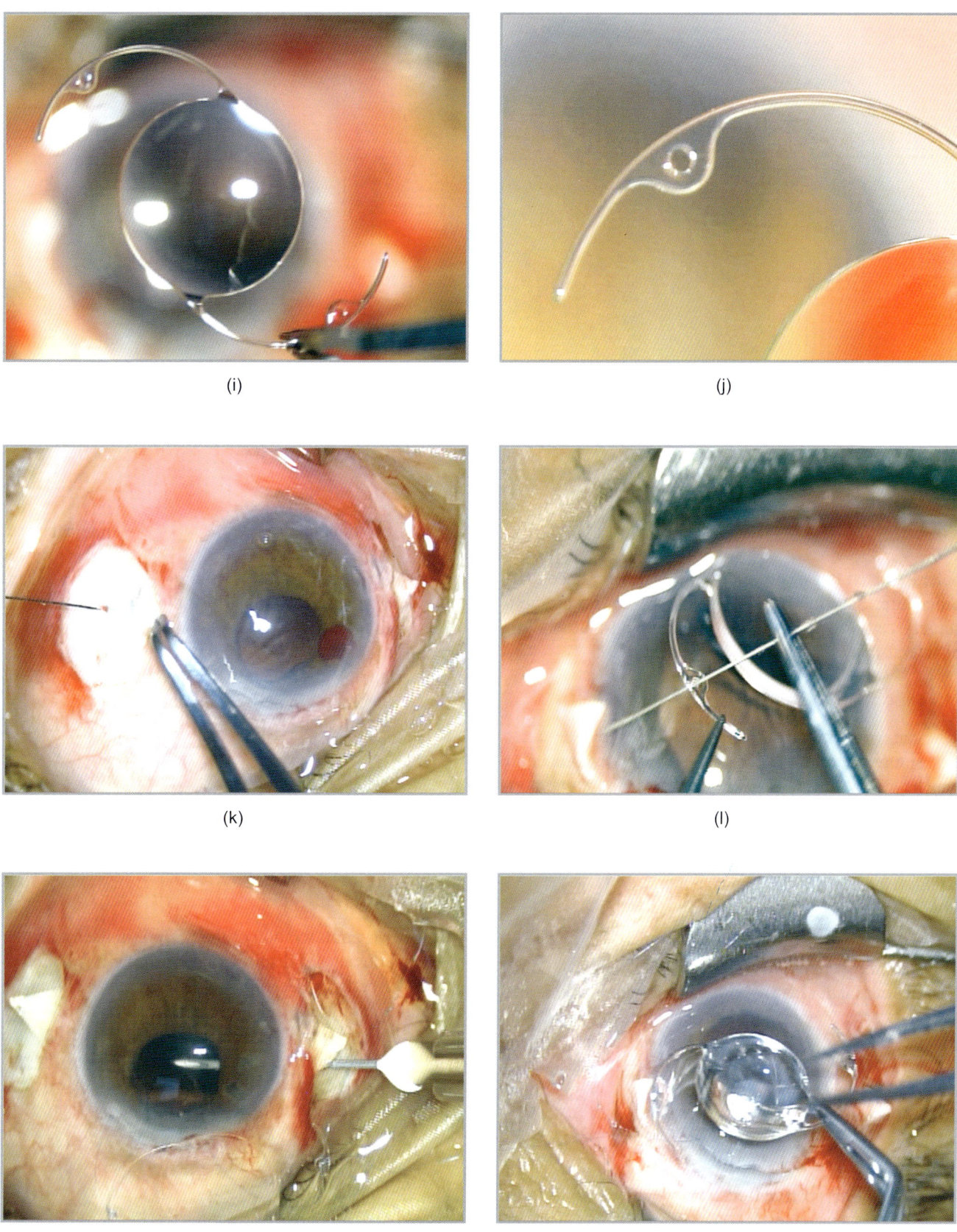

Fig. 49.1: (i) Scleral fixated IOL implant, (j) Magnified view of the eyelet of scleral fixated IOL implant, (k) 10 '0' prolene suture on straight needle through the scleral flap, (l): Anchor suture through the eyelet of scleral fixated IOL, (m) Reverse movement of 10 '0' Prolene suture with the help of a 26 guaze needle, (n) Insertion of a scleral fixated IOL

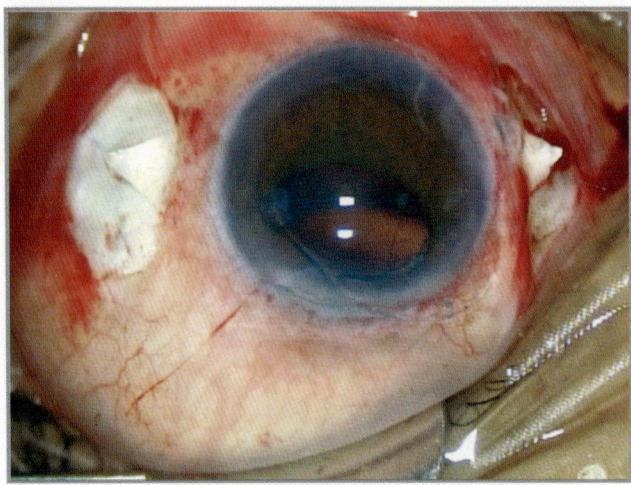
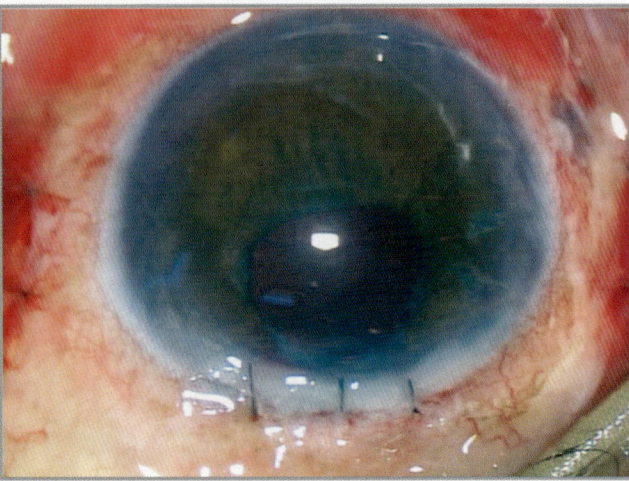

(o)   (p)

Fig. 49.1: (o) Insertion of scleral fixated IOL, (p) Scleral fixated IOL implant is in position

INTRAOPERATIVE CONSTRAINTS

Several problems can arise during the procedure:

Difficulty in Making Scleral Flaps

Scleral fixated IOL is generally carried out as a secondary procedure. Scarring and adhesions due to the previous surgery can lead to excessive bleeding and buttonholing of scleral flaps.

Intraoperative Haemorrhage

This can result from damage to the ciliary body while passing sutures. Bleeding can be torrential and the procedure may have to be abandoned. Postoperative vitreous hemorrhage can result from residual blood in the vitreous cavity. Small and self-limiting vitreous hemorrhages are often seen postoperatively due to mild intraoperative hemorrhages and do not require any active management.

Suture Related Problems

These are most commonly faced complications. The suture may get cut inadvertently or the wrong suture maybe tied to the incorrect haptic or suture may get entangled with the haptic of the IOL. These can be rectified readily and totally avoided by an attentive and diligent assistant. In the worst case scenario, the suture may have to be reapplied all over again.

Excessive Hypotony

Once the globe is open and anterior/mid vitrectomy has been done; there is a tendency for the globe to collapse. This can lead to a host of intraoperative difficulties like corneal haze, improper suturing, and difficult visualisation of the intraocular procedure. Chances of suprachoroidal hemorrhage increases significantly in an open hypotonic eye.

POSTOPERATIVE COMPLICATIONS

Endophthalmitis

Chances of endophthalmitis are higher in this technique due to:

(i) **Being a relatively prolonged procedure** where the globe is open and hypotonous for a long time and there are chances of contaminated fluids from the conjunctival sac finding their way into the eye. Keeping the eyeball firm and making a scleral tunnel will minimise this problem.

(ii) **Scleral sutures that are anchoring the lens, if exposed** act like a wick from which microbes can find their way into the eye causing delayed postoperative endophthalmitis. At times vitreous can get incarcerated into the suture track and act as a Nidus for the microbes.

SF IOL Malpositioning

Due the two-point fixation of the SF IOL in the horizontal meridian, downward displacement of the IOL is bound to occur. It is better to decentre the IOL superiorly during the procedure in order to counter this. Entry site of the suture also plays a major role in lens centration. A slight difference in entry sites of sutures into the eye can lead to tilting of the lens and gross astigmatism. Pseudophakodonesis can occur if sutures fixating the IOL are loose or improperly tied to SF IOL.

Lens Dislocation

This can occur if one of the sutures fixing the SFIOL slips out or erodes through the eyelet of the lens. Accidental suturolysis is possible (if the suture has not been buried) by an unsuspecting ophthalmologist, leading to the IOL dropping onto the retina.

Cystoid Macular Edema (CME)

Chances of CME are high due to the loss of posterior capsule with disturbance of the vitreous face and being an extensive procedure there is excessive release of pigment. This is a significant cause of poor visual recovery following a successful surgery.

Secondary Glaucoma

Can occur due to blockage of trabecular meshwork by vitreous in the anterior chamber, persistent hyphaema or dispersed pigment.

Retinal Detachment

Inadequate vitrectomy can result in traction at vitreous base and retinal tear with retinal detachment. Excessive manipulation of the globe can result in dialysis with detachment. All cases must be closely followed up postoperatively for early detection of retinal breaks.

Postoperative Uveitis

Severe inflammation of the eye can result. This can lead to choroidal effusion/detachment, cyclitic membrane formation, pigment deposit on IOL surface, opacification of IOL, secondary glaucoma and CME.

Corneal Decompensation

Excessive intraoperative manipulation, vitreous in the anterior chamber, persistent uveitis and persistently raised intraocular pressures can result in corneal decompensation and bullous keratopathy.

POSTOPERATIVE MANAGEMENT

Often aggressive postoperative management is required to control postoperative uveitis, glaucoma and CME. Systemic steroids and acetazolamide along with topical medication are needed to control uveitis and glaucoma. Laser trabeculoplasty is a useful procedure in cases not responding to maximal medication. Severe uveitis must raise suspicion of endophthalmitis. In case of doubt, immediate therapy in form of intravitreal injection of broad-spectrum antibiotics must be given as early as possible. Oral NSAID's are helpful in controlling CME. There is a need to closely monitor these patients for early detection of retinal breaks. Indirect ophthalmoscopy with indentation must be done as soon as wound healing has occurred. Prophylactic cryotherapy should be given to suspicious areas.

CONCLUSION

Scleral fixated IOL is a useful method of visual rehabilitation in cases that are developing complications like PBK and have no capsular support. It is a challenging and an extensive procedure that requires the anterior segment surgeon to go into the realm of the posterior segment surgeon.

BIBLIOGRAPHY

1. Vats DP, Parihar JKS, Singh VK, Trehan HS, Khan MA. "AC/PC intraocular lens exchange with penetrating keratoplasty in cases of pseudophakic Bullous Keratopathy". MJAFI 2006; 62: 11–13.
2. Lan-Hsing Chuang, Chi-Chun Lai. "Secondary intraocular lens implantation of traumatic cataract in open-globe injury". Can Jr of Ophthalmol 2005; 40: 454–459.
3. H. Mittelviefhaus, K. Mittelviefhaus. "Transscleral suture fixation of posterior chamber intraocular lenses in children under 3 years". Graefe's Archive for Clinical and Experimental Ophthalmology. Vol 238:2, 143–148; 2000.
4. R N Gaster, R C Troutman et al "Combined Penetrating Keratoplasty and Posterior chamber lens implantation in the absence of lens capsule". Tr Am Ophthalmic Society, vol LXXXVIII, 1990.
5. Saeed Akhtar, Anthony J Bron et al. "Ultrastructural morphology and expression of proteoglycans, tenacin-C, betaig-h3, fibrillin–1 and fibronectin in Bullous Keratopathy". Br Jr of Ophthalmology, 2001: 85; 720–731.
6. A L Young, GYS Leung, LL Cheng and DSC Lam. "A modified technique of scleral fixated intraocular lens for Aphakic correction". Eye,19; 2005, 19–22.
7. Renuka Srinivasan, Subashini Kaliaperumal, G Chandrashekar. "Comparison of scleral fixation IOL with Anterior chamber IOL". AIOC proceedings 2005; 89–90.
8. David K Berler, Mark A Freidberg. "Scleral fixation of Posterior Chamber lens implants combined with Vitrectomy". Tr Am Ophthalmic Society, vol LXXXIX, 1991.
9. Yeom IY, Chang JH, Jung YC. A Clinical Study on Implantation of Anterior Chamber Intraocular Lens and Posterior Chamber Intraocular Lens by Scleral Fixation in Eyes without Capsular or Zonular Support. J Korean Ophthalmol Soc. 1993 Oct; 34(10):950–955. Korean.
10. Lee V Y W, Yuen H K L, Kwok A K H. Comparison of outcomes of primary and secondary implantation of scleral fixated posterior chamber intraocular lens. British Journal of Ophthalmology 2003; 87:1459–1462.
11. Hu BV, Shin DH, Gibbs KA, Hong YJ. Implantation of posterior chamber lens in the absence of capsular and zonular support. Arch Ophthalmol. 1988 ; 106(3):416–420.
12. Kumar M. Arora, Sanga L. Sota L. D. Scleral-fixated intraocular lens implantation in unilateral aphakic children Ophthalmology (Ophthalmology) ISSN 0161–6420 1999, vol. 106, 2184–89.

13. .Apple DJ, Price FW, Gwin T, Imkamp E, Daun M, Casanova R, Hansen S, Carlson AN. Sutured retropupillary posterior chamber intraocular lenses for exchange or secondary implantation. The 12th annual Binkhorst lecture, 1988. Ophthalmology. 1989; 96(8):1241–1247.

14. Speaker MG, Lugo M, Laibson PR, Rubinfeld RS, Stein RM, Genvert GI, Cohen EJ, Arentsen JJ. Penetrating keratoplasty for pseudophakic bullous keratopathy. Management of the intraocular lens. Ophthalmology. 1988; 95(9):1260–1268.

15. Heilskov T, Joondeph BC, Olsen KR, Blankenship GW. Late endophthalmitis after transscleral fixation of a posterior chamber intraocular lens. Arch Ophthalmol. 1989; 107(10): 1427.

16. Stark WJ, Gottsch JD, Goodman DF, Goodman GL, Pratzer K. Posterior chamber intraocular lens implantation in the absence of capsular support. Arch Ophthalmol. 1989; 107(7): 1078–1083.

17. Pang MP, Peyman GA, Minatoya HK. Posterior chamber lens implantation following pars plana lensectomy and vitrectomy in severe proliferative diabetic retinopathy. Can J Ophthalmol. 1989; 24(4):175–178.

18. Kraff MC, Lieberman HL, Sanders DR. Secondary intraocular lens implantation: rigid/semi-rigid versus flexible lenses. J Cataract Refract Surg. 1987; 13(1):21–26.

19. Cowden JW, Hu BV. A new surgical technique for posterior chamber lens fixation during penetrating keratoplasty in the absence of capsular or zonular support. Cornea. 1988; 7(3): 231–235.

20. Lindstrom RL, Harris WS. Secondary anterior chamber lens implantation. CLAO J. 1984 10(2):133–136.

21. Lindquist TD, Agapitos PJ, Lindstrom RL, Lane SS, Spigelman AV. Transscleral fixation of posterior chamber intraocular lenses in the absence of capsular support. Ophthalmic Surg. 1989; 20(11):769–775.

22. Wong SK, Koch DD, Emery JM. Secondary intraocular lens implantation. J Cataract Refract Surg. 1987; 13(1):17–20.

23. Pannu JS. A new suturing technique for ciliary sulcus fixation in the absence of posterior capsule. Ophthalmic Surg. 1988; 19(10):751–754.

24. Lim ES, Apple DJ, Tsai JC, Morgan RC, Wasserman D, Assia EI. An analysis of flexible anterior chamber lenses with special reference to the normalised rate of lens explantation. Ophthalmology. 1991; 98(2):243–246.

25. Sen HA, Smith PW. Current trends in suture fixation of posterior chamber intraocular lenses. Ophthalmic Surg. 1990; 21(10):689–695.

25. Gaster RN, Troutman RC, Ong HV, Draga A, Belmont SC. Combined penetrating keratoplasty and posterior chamber intraocular lens implantation in the absence of a lens capsule. Trans Am Ophthalmol Soc. 1990; 88:326–342.

26. Koenig SB, Han DP, Mieler WF, Abrams GW, Jaffe GJ, Burton TC. Combined phacoemulsification and pars plana vitrectomy. Arch Ophthalmol. 1990; 108(3):362–364.

27. Girard LJ. PC-IOL implantation in the absence of posterior capsular support. Ophthalmic Surg. 1988; 19(9):680–682.

28. Duffey RJ, Holland EJ, Agapitos PJ, Lindstrom RL. Anatomic study of transsclerally sutured intraocular lens implantation. Am J Ophthalmol. 1989 Sep 15; 108(3):300–309.

29. Ruiz RS, Saatci OA. Posterior chamber intraocular lens implantation in eyes with inactive and active proliferative diabetic retinopathy. Am J Ophthalmol. 1991b 15; 111(2): 158–162.

30. Spigelman AV, Lindstrom RL, Nichols BD, Lindquist TD, Lane SS. Implantation of a posterior chamber lens without capsular support during penetrating keratoplasty or as a secondary lens implant. Ophthalmic Surg. 1988; 19(6):396–398.

31. Price FW Jr, Whitson WE. Visual results of suture-fixated posterior chamber lenses during penetrating keratoplasty. Ophthalmology. 1989; 96(8):1234–1240.

32. Johnson SM. Results of exchanging anterior chamber lenses with sulcus-fixated posterior chamber IOLs without capsular support in penetrating keratoplasty. Ophthalmic Surg. 1989; 20(7):465–468.

33. Girard LJ. Pars plana phacoprosthesis (aphakic intraocular implant): a preliminary report. Ophthalmic Surg. 1981; 12(1): 19–22.

34. Shin DH. Implantation of a posterior chamber lens without capsular support during penetrating keratoplasty or as a secondary lens. Ophthalmic Surg. 1988; 19(10):755–756.

Concurrent Phacoemulsification and Pars Plana Vitrectomy

Col VS Gurunadh, Brig Ajay Banarji, Col JKS Parihar SM, VSM and Wing Cdr HS Trehan

INTRODUCTION

Cataract is very closely related to both surgical as well as medical retinal pathologies. Cataract can predispose to surgical retinal conditions like retinal detachment with or without choroidal detachment and surgical retinal conditions can also cause a cataract. It is the presence of surgical retinal conditions that make the management of cataract an aspect of decision making which is different from the routine. The case scenario may be:

1. The presence of an ultrasonic retinal detachment and or vitreous hemorrhage in the presence of a total cataract.
2. The cataract permits retinal evaluation for a diagnosis but is not enough for a proper surgical maneuver.
3. There is also a case setting wherein the retinal condition has been diagnosed and the cataract has formed while awaiting surgery. The issue is clear. The debate is whether to opt for a two step procedure or for a single surgery combining cataract surgery with pars plana vitrectomy. This would have been a discussion in days when planned extracapsular cataract surgery was the rule. With the advent of advanced techniques of phacoemulsification and a revolution in pars plana vitrectomy this discussion is perhaps outdated.

In the first setting, the retinal details are not known and there is also the possibility of the ultrasound not picking up the correct diagnosis. In such a situation it might be prudent to go in for a two step approach.

Since the issue is that of a vitreous manoeuvre, cases where the decision is for taking up a conventional re-attachment procedure will not be discussed. In patients less than 20 years of age, pars plana lensectomy can be performed and hence these patients do not come under the purview of the discussion of combined phacoemulsification and pars plana vitrectomy.

INDICATIONS FOR COMBINED SURGERY

1. Vitreous haemorrhage (usually due to proliferative diabetic retinopathy or Eales' disease in India).
2. Vitreous haemorrhage with retinal detachment.
3. Rhegmatogenous retinal detachment not amenable to conventional re-attachment surgery due to:
   (a) Large breaks
   (b) Multiple breaks
   (c) Choroidal detachment
   (d) Proliferative vitreo-retinopathy > C 3 (Retina society classification).
4. Macular hole with or without detachment
5. Tractional retinal detachments.
6. Silicon oil filled eyes with cataract with or without re-detachment.

Silicon oil filled eyes are a special situation and the surgical decision is first directed to the removal of the oil with prevention of re-detachment and the vitreo-retinal technique takes precedence.

CONTRAINDICATIONS

1. The decision of the operating surgeon.
2. In cases of total cataract wherein there is doubt of the ultrasound diagnosis.

PREOPERATIVE EVALUATION

Routine investigations as for a cataract are done. The most important investigation is the measurement of the intraocular lens (IOL) power. There is no requirement to opt for a formula other than SRK II formula. The problem is the measurement of the axial length due to:

1. Hypotony

2. The retinal detachment

3. Co-existing choroidal detachment

The best option is to calculate the IOL power of the fellow eye.

Ultrasound A/B scan is anyhow performed and hence, the axial length should be re-assessed with the B-scan findings also.

At times, the degree of lens opacity can be exceedingly difficult to confirm preoperatively especially in the setting of a dense vitreous haemorrhage, poor papillary dilation, or a poor red reflex from retinal detachment. Sometimes the decision to remove the lens is made intraoperatively if the surgeon had under estimated the severity of the lens opacity preoperatively.

SURGICAL TECHNIQUE

Since the cataract is precluding the observation of the retina, the same has to be negotiated first.

This surgery should best be done by two surgeons if facilities exist. The phacoemulsification is usually faster when performed by a surgeon trained in the same. The vitreo-retinal surgeon gets more surgical time and is not tired with the procedure of the phacoemulsification before starting the posterior segment procedure.

The first procedure to be done is the placement of an infusion cannula. For this, limbal exposure would not be preferred unless one has access to a suture less vitrectomy set. In cases of retinal detachment, a 360° peritomy is required. After the insertion of an infusion cannula, attention has to be paid to phacoemulsification, except in cases where only the vitreous procedure has been planned and the surgeon faces difficulty in the form of lenticular opacification or lenticular clouding due to accidental lens damage.

Phacoemulsification

Incision

Since the limbus is exposed except in circumstances of sutureless vitrectomy, the incision for phacoemulsification is not a matter of debate and lies exclusively upon the discretion of the surgeons own preference. The author prefers to go ahead with clear corneal incisions. However a limbal or a scleral incision may retain better intraoperative corneal clarity during prolonged duration of VR surgery. The incision should be closed with a single 10–0 nylon or vicryl suture before the vitrectomy (Fig. 50.1).

Capsulorrhexis

In these cases because of the retinal pathology, the retro-illumination is usually poor. A dye assisted capsulorrhexis may be an ideal option. If the surgeon still faces a problem, the viewing of the anterior capsule can be improved by introducing the intravitreal endoilluminator through the side

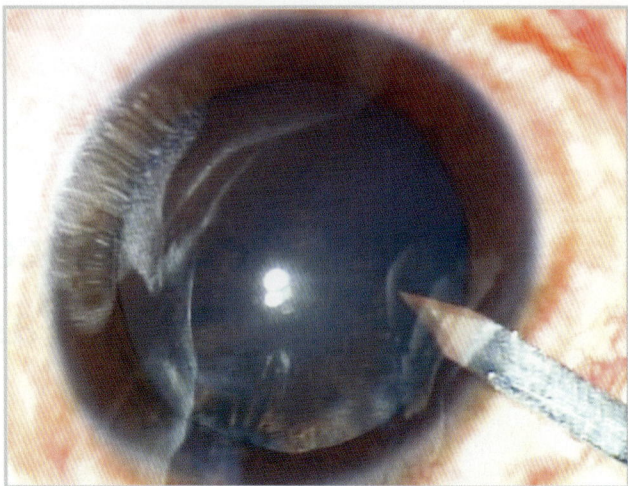

Fig. 50.1: Clear corneal incision after introduction of infusion cannula

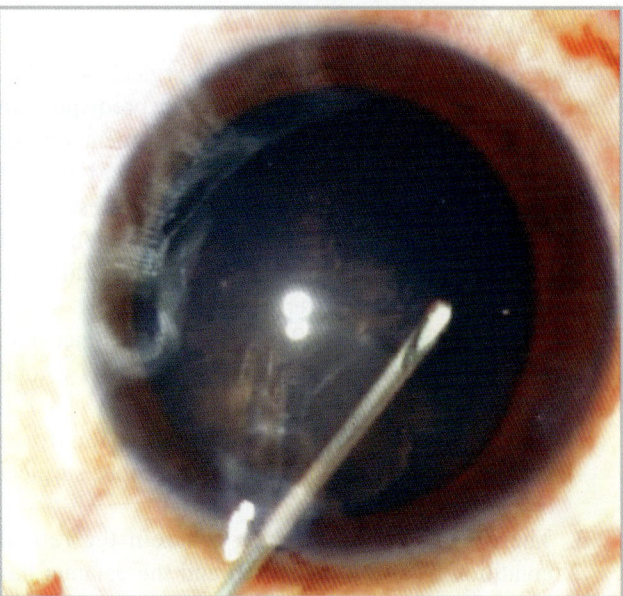

Fig. 50.2: Capsulorrhexis

port incision. A 5.0 to 5.5 mm continuous curvilinear capsulorrhexis should be made. However, the size of the capsulorrhexis is not important for the completion of the vitreous procedure. An intact smaller capsulorrhexis helps in the implantation of the IOL whenever the same is planned (Fig. 50.2).

It is only in the cases of lensectomy that the issue of sparing the anterior capsule comes up.

Hydroprocedures

There is no special procedure for performing the hydro-dissection and the hydro-delimitation in phacoemulsi-fication combined with vitrectomy. The procedure is left to the operating surgeon's preference. There is no need to fear a nucleus drop into the vitreous as the vitreous procedure would follow phacoemulsification.

Technique of Nucleotomy

Any type of nucleotomy technique can be performed. The technique with which the surgeon is comfortable should be employed. However, direct central chopping in cases of moderate to hard cataract and flip and chip, in cases of soft cataract are ideal choices. In certain cases of very soft cataract or in cases wherein a young individual is involved, phacoaspiration alone may be sufficient enough to remove the cataract (Fig. 50.3).

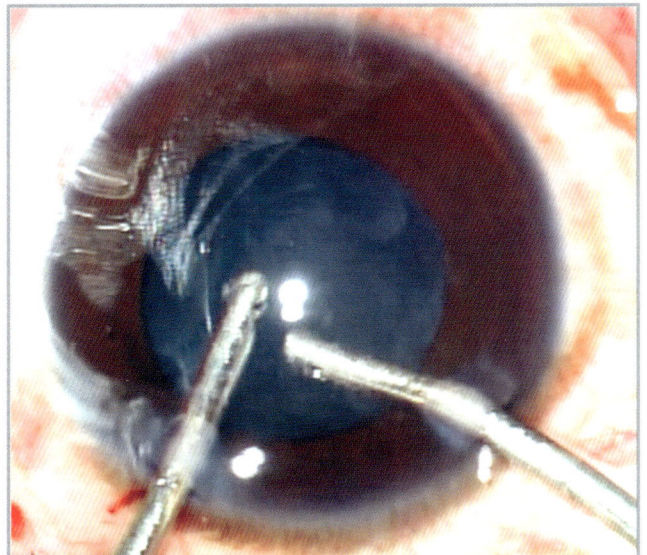

Fig. 50.3: Phacoaspiration of a soft traumatic cataract

I/A

Complete cortical clean up should be attempted. An intact posterior capsule is essential when planning implantation of a long acting intravitreal tamponade. Hence, posterior capsular polishing should be done with care (Fig. 50.4).

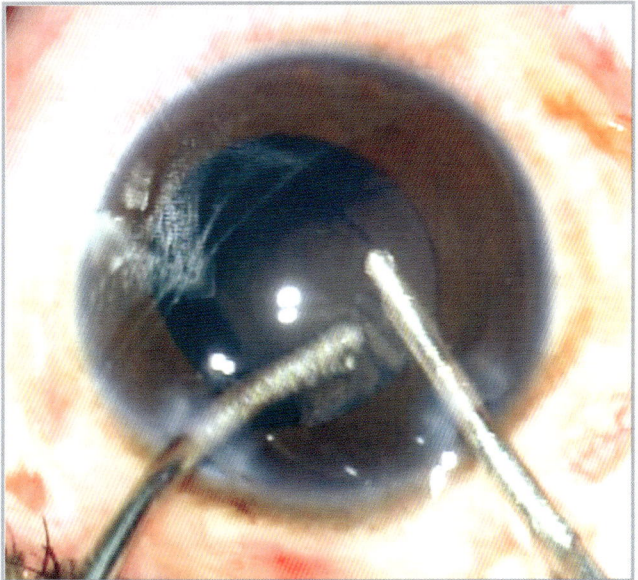

Fig. 50.4: Removal of sub-incisional sticky cortex

IOL Implantation

The decision to implant an IOL in combined procedures has to be made with reference to the integrity of the posterior capsule or as per the need of the subsequent procedure. Depending upon the situation, a foldable lens or a rigid lens can be implanted. However, implantation of silicon IOL implants should be considered an absolute contraindication, since it maybe adversely affected by Silicon oil injection. If the posterior capsule is intact, then a foldable lens can be implanted. When the posterior capsular integrity is doubtful, then it would be prudent to implant a rigid IOL with a 6 to 6.5 mm optic. In certain situations, like retained IOFB where removal of FB may be required through an anterior approach, the choice of IOL may be deferred to rigid lens despite an intact capsule. In our view, it is better to complete the VR procedure prior to the an IOL implantation, since it will provide enhanced surgical ease as well as the final status of the posterior capsule may be ascertained prior to insertion of an IOL implant. In certain situations where postoperative tamponade with gas or silicon oil is planned, it would be better to implant the lens before tamponade with gas or silicon oil.

In cases where the capsular support is doubtful as is the favourable outcome to the vitreous procedure, it may be prudent not to implant an IOL. This can be done at a later stage.

Role of AC maintainer

The AC maintainer can be used instead of an infusion cannula in eyes which are oil-filled and have undergone a previous pars plana vitrectomy (PPV), or along with an infusion cannula for the stabilisation of the eye. Pan-retinal photocoagulation of the retina in case with proliferative diabetic retinopathy has been performed by laser indirect delivery after cataract extraction on the table with the help of an AC maintainer. The AC maintainer is placed inferiorly through the corneal paracentesis.

Vitreous Procedure

After the cataract procedure is completed, the superior ports for vitreous procedure are made and the surgery is carried forthwith. Since the eye is pseudophakic or aphakic when the vitrectomy is started, the site of these ports from the limbus is not a matter of discussion. Any type of viewing can be utilised for the surgery.

Machine Considerations

The machine should be a complete high speed vitrectomy unit with diathermy, endo-diathermy, pneumatic and electric vitrectomy, air insufflation and silicon oil injector along with phacoemulsification. The later is usually a venturi type in these machines. This should not be a problem for an expert (Figs 50.5 to 50.12).

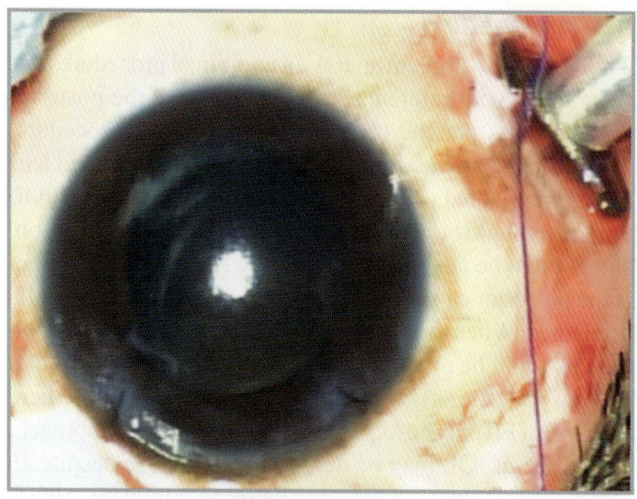

Fig. 50.5: Infusion Cannula is well placed. Corneal incisions are secured with 10 "O" monofilament suture prior to the commencement of vitrectomy

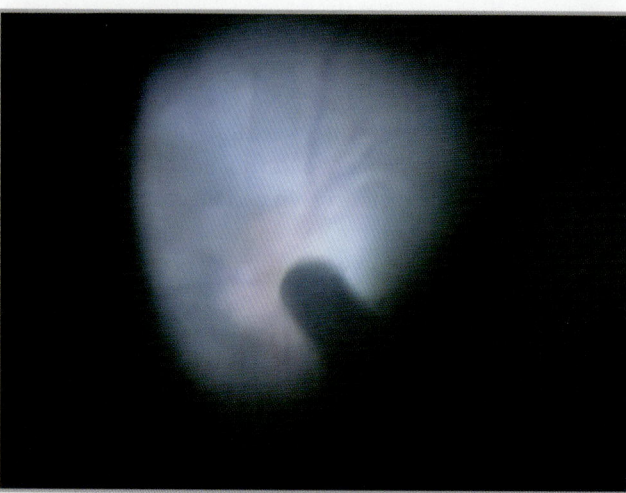

Fig. 50.6: Three ports pars plana vitrectomy is under progress

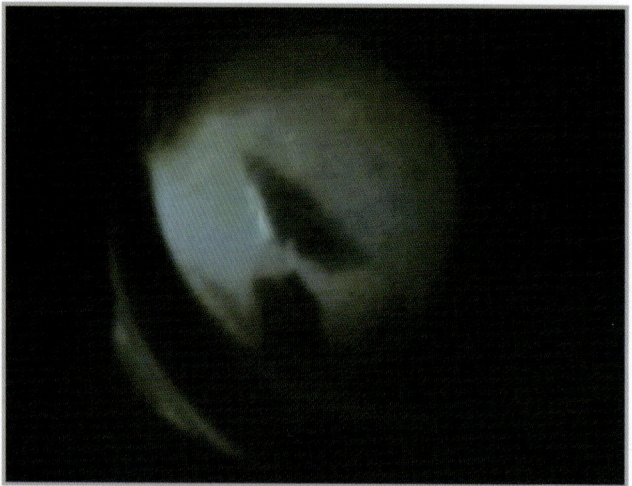

Fig. 50.7: Retained IOFB

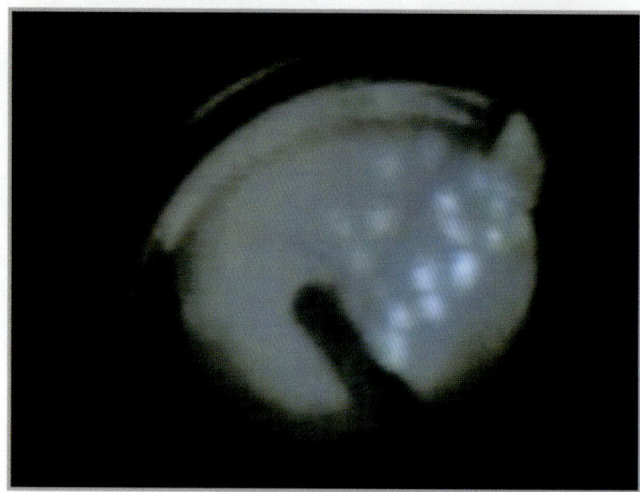

Fig. 50.8: Endolaser

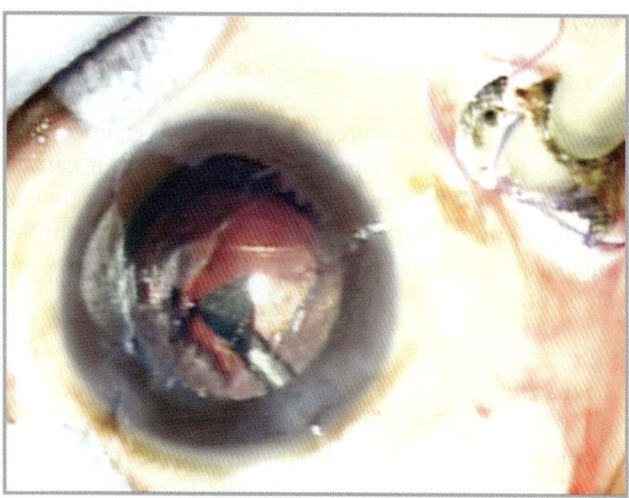

Fig. 50.9: Removal of retained IOFB with the help of an intravitreal magnet

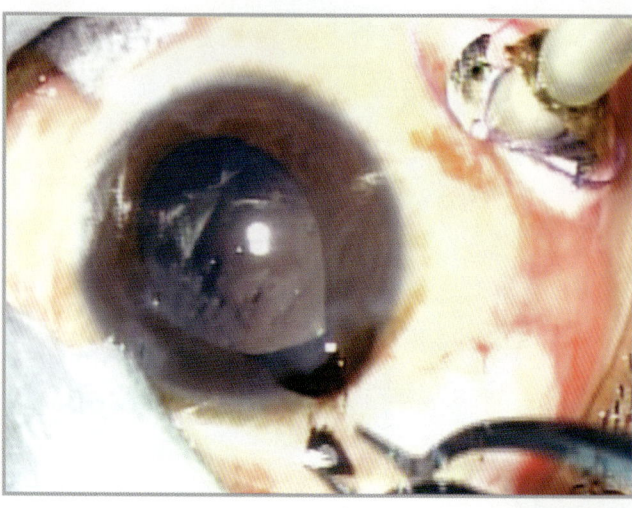

Fig. 50.10: Large metallic IOFB is removed through a limbal phaco incision

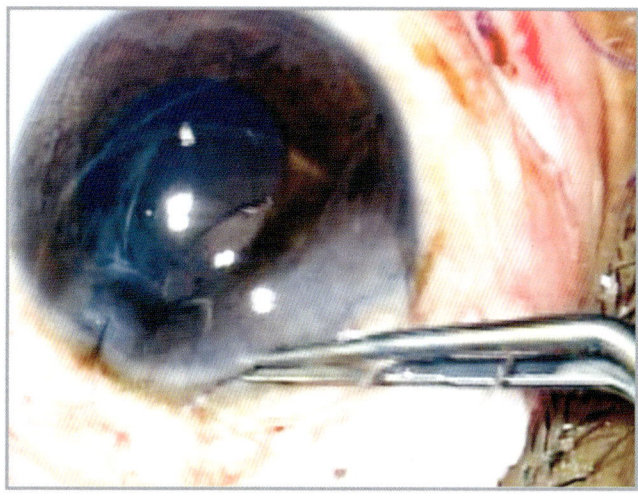

Fig. 50.11: Implantation of all PMMA rigid IOL implant

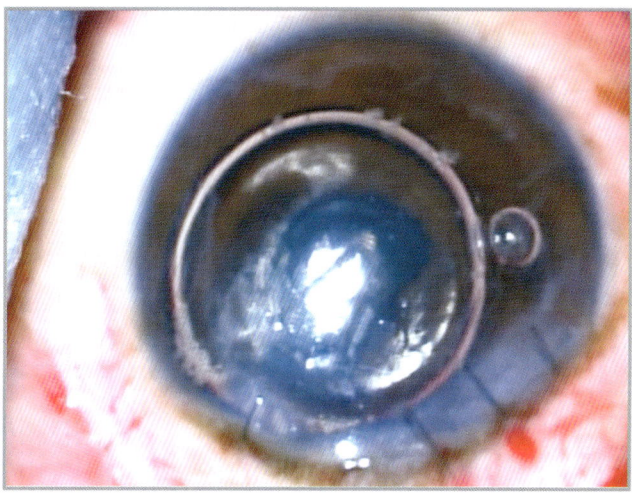

Fig. 50.12: PPV and phaco on completion of surgical procedure

PPV and Phacoemulsification with Foldable IOL Implantation in a Case of Post Eales' Complicated Cataract and Vitreous Haemorrhage

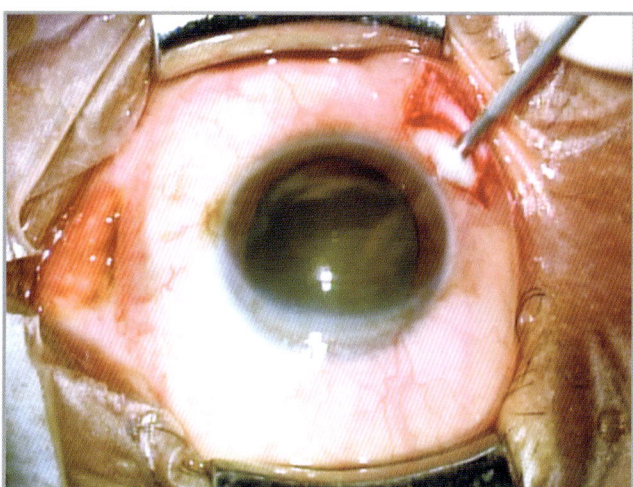

Fig. 50.13: Construction of pars plana irrigation port for PPV and phacoemulsification surgery

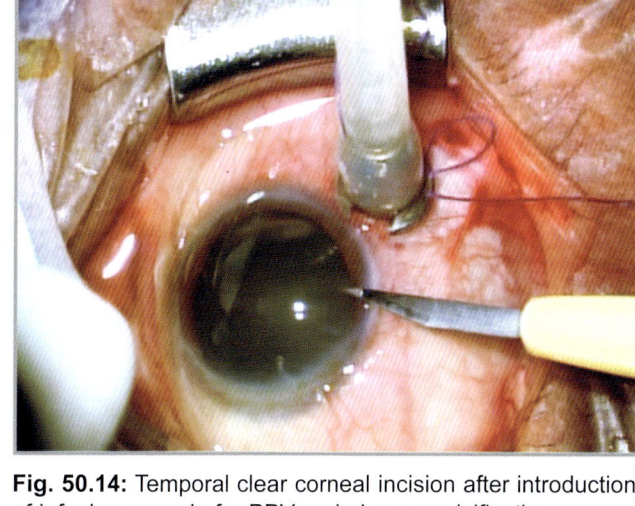

Fig. 50.14: Temporal clear corneal incision after introduction of infusion cannula for PPV and phacoemulsification surgery

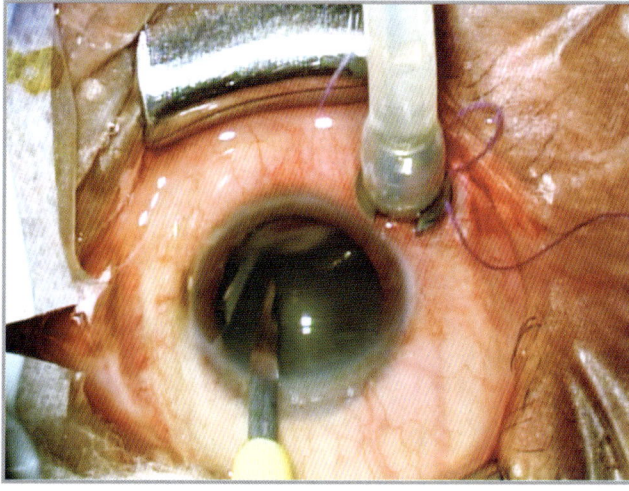

Fig. 50.15: Side port incision after introduction of infusion cannula for PPV and phacoemulsification surgery

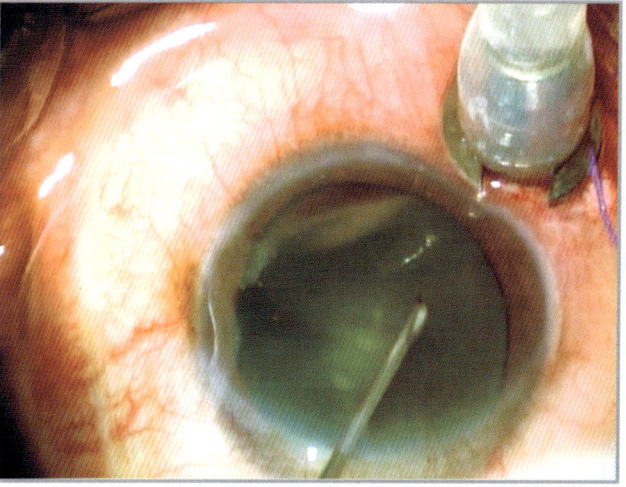

Fig. 50.16 : Capsulorrhexis after introduction of infusion cannula for PPV and phacoemulsification surgery

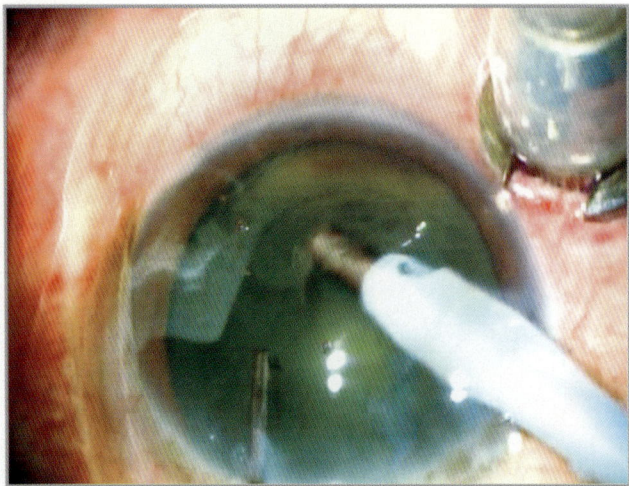

Fig. 50.17: Removal of superficial cortex prior to the commencement of nucleotomy

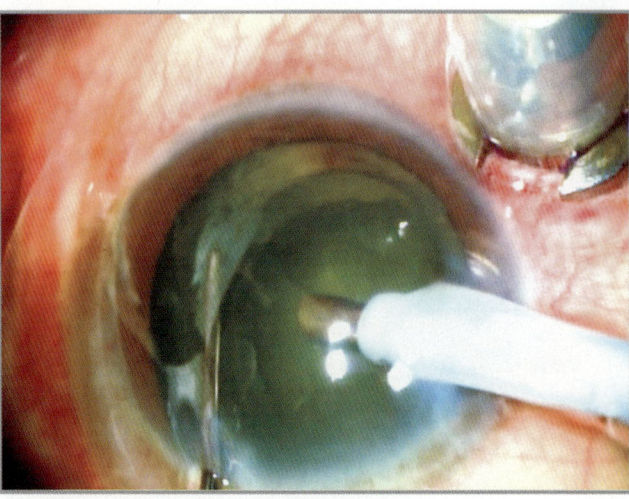

Fig. 50.18: Commencement of chopping for PPV and phaco

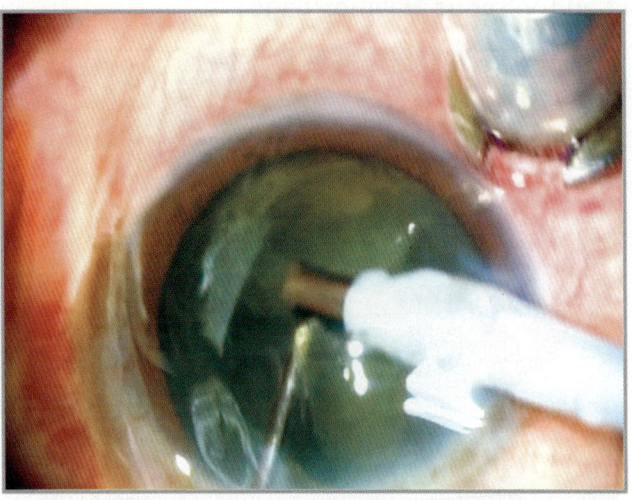

Fig. 50.19: Nucleotomy: PPV and phaco

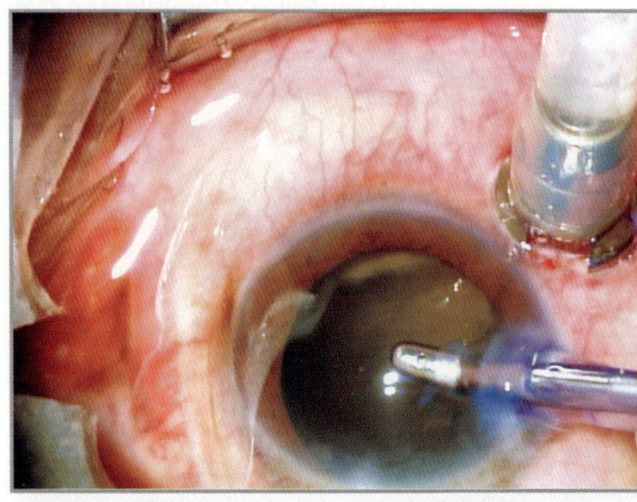

Fig. 50.20: Removal of cortex by irrigation and aspiration

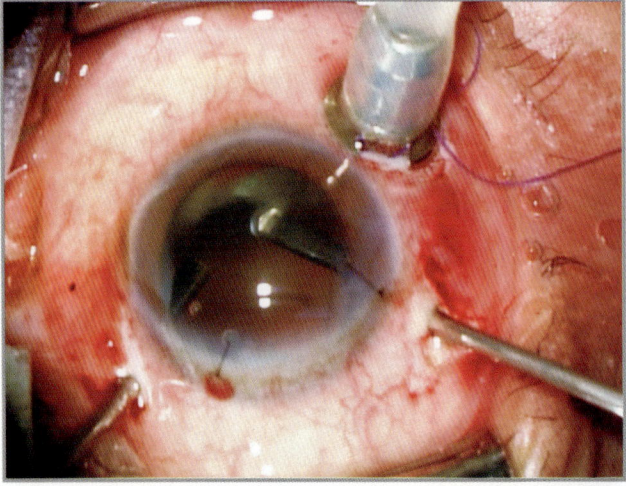

Fig. 50.21: Three ports pars plana vitrectomy is under progress. Corneal incisions are secured with 10 "O" monofilament suture prior to the commencement of vitrectomy

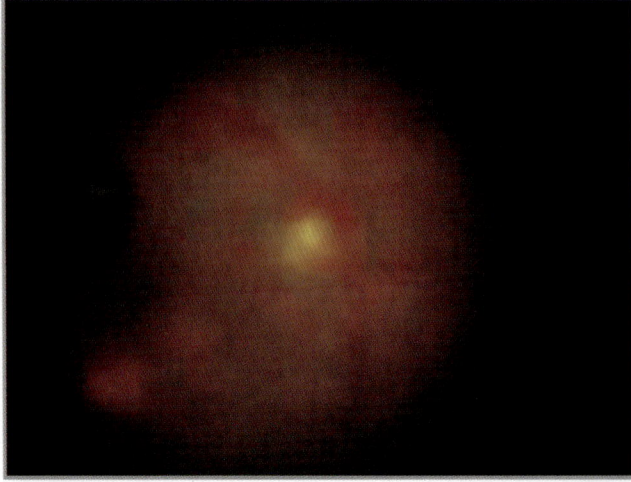

Fig. 50.22: Three ports pars plana vitrectomy is under progress: Posterior pole and disc are clearly visible following vitrectomy

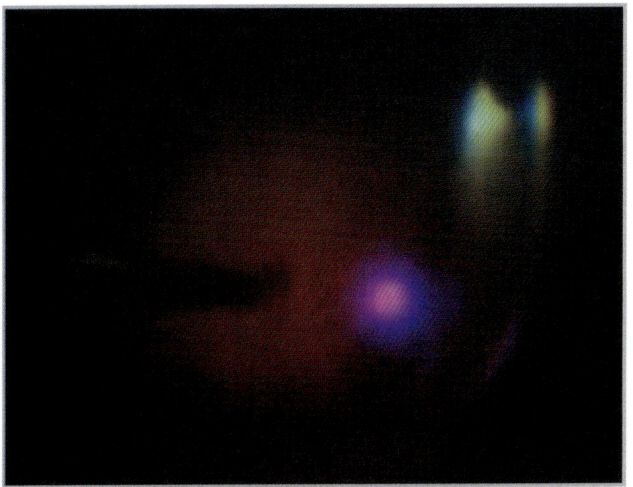

Fig. 50.23: Endolaser following vitrectomy

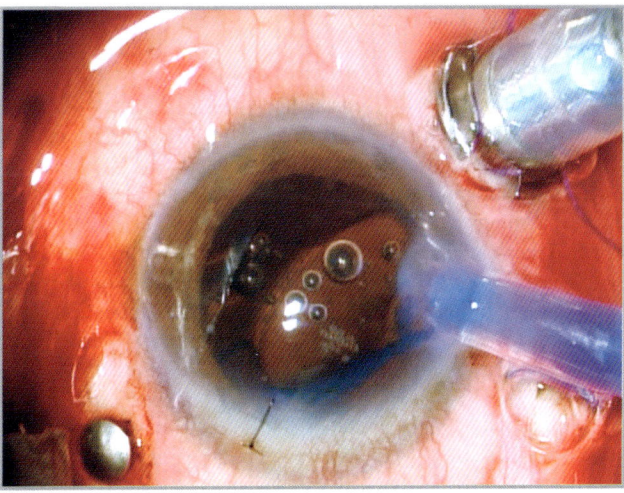

Fig. 50.24: Insertion of a single piece acrylic foldable IOL implant following PPV and phacoemulsification

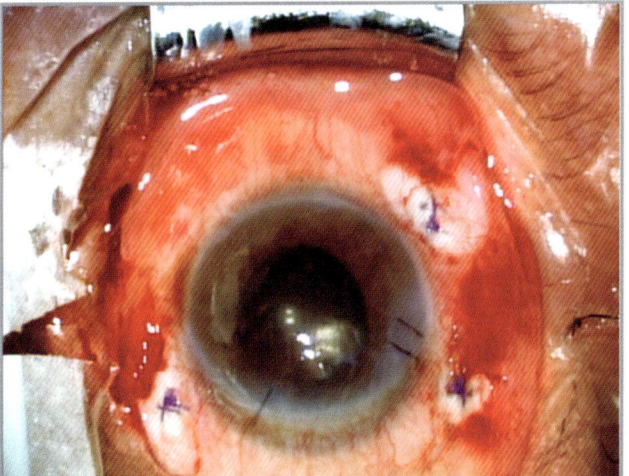

Fig. 50.25: All three PPV ports are well secured

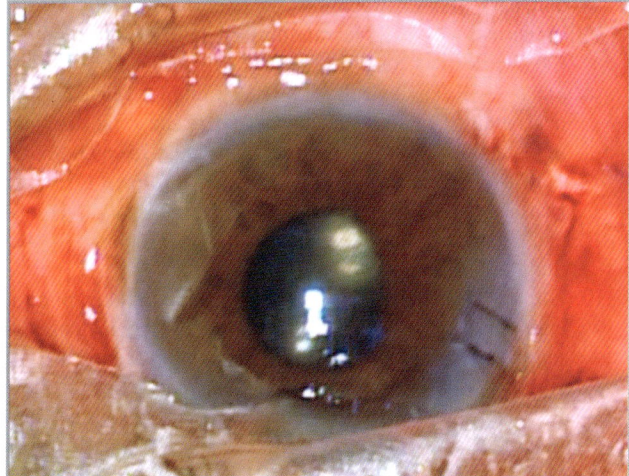

Fig. 50.26: PPV and phaco: Completion of surgical procedure

CONCURRENT MEDICAL MANAGEMENT

The incidence of postoperative reaction is more in these cases, as also is the severity. Most cases have preoperative inflammation. It would be prudent to administer preoperative steroids to these eyes. Preoperative hydrocortisone is also advisable as would be postoperative systemic steroids. Topical steroids should be given along with topical non-steroidal preparations and the duration is usually longer than in the routine cases of cataract. Topical cycloplegics are also required and these should be administered judiciously otherwise the IOL may be disturbed with the development of pupillary capture.

CONCLUSION

Combined phacoemulsification and vitrectomy is no longer a matter of controversy. The main indications being the merit of the case and the willingness of the treating surgeon. It is even possible to perform the combined surgery with a temporal approach. This does not mean that the two-step procedure is outdated. Given the varied nature of the vitreo-retinal pathologies there would always be an indication for a two-step procedure as there is for a single approach.

REFERENCES

1. Koenig SB, Han DP, Mieler WF, Abrams GW, Jaffe GJ, Burton TC. Combined phacoemulsification and pars plana vitrectomy. Arch Ophthalmol 1990; 108: 362–4.
2. Koenig SB, Mieler WF, Han DP, Abrams GW. Combined phacoemulsification, pars plana vitrectomy and posterior chamber intraocular lens insertion. Arch Ophthalmol 1992; 110: 1101–4.
3. Jain V, Kar D, Natarajan S, Shome D, Mehta H, Jayadev C,

Borse N. Phacoemulsification and pars plana vitrectomy: a combined procedure. Indian J Ophthalmol. 2007 May-Jun; 55(3): 203–6.

4. Demetriades AM, Gottsch JD, Thomsen R, Azab A, Stark WJ, Campochiaro PA, de Juan E Jr, Haller JA. Combined phacoemulsification, intraocular lens implantation, and vitrectomy for eyes with coexisting cataract and vitreoretinal pathology. Am J Ophthalmol. 2003 Mar;135(3):291–6.

5. Treumer F, Bunse A, Rudolf M, Roider J. Pars plana vitrectomy, Phacoemulsification and intraocular lens implantation. Comparison of clinical complications in a combined versus two-step surgical approach. Graefes Arch Clin Exp Ophthalmol. 2006 Jul; 244(7): 808–15.

6. Chung TY, Chung H, Lee JH. Combined surgery and sequential surgery comprising phacoemulsification, pars plana vitrectomy and intraocular lens implantation: Comparison of clinical outcomes. J Cataract Refract Surg 2002; 28: 2001–5.

7. Heiligenhaus A, Holtkamp A, Koch J, Schilling H, Bornfeld N, Lösche CC, Steuhl KP. Combined phacoemulsification and pars plana vitrectomy: clear corneal versus scleral incisions: prospective randomised multicentre study. J Cataract Refract Surg. 2003 Jun; 29(6): 1106–12.

8. Scharwey K, Pavlovic S, Jacobi KW. Combined clear corneal phacoemulsification, vitreoretinal surgery and intraocular lens implantation. J Cataract Refract Surg 1999; 25: 693–8.

9. Lam DS, Young AL, Rao SK, Cheung BT, Yuen CY, Tang HM. Combined phacoemulsification, pars plana vitrectomy, and foldable intraocular lens implantation. J Cataract Refract Surg. 2003 Jun; 29(6): 1064–9.

10. Hurley C, Barry P. Combined endocapsular phacoemulsification, pars plana vitrectomy and intraocular lens implantation. J Cataract Refract Surg 1996; 22: 462–6.

11. Benson WE, Brown GC, Tasman W, McNamara JA. Extracapsular cataract extraction, posterior chamber lens insertion and pars plana vitrectomy in one operation. Ophthalmology 1990; 97: 918–21.

12. Patel AK, Cacciatori M. Combined panretinal photocoagulation and cataract surgery in a patient with diabetes mellitus. Ophthalmic Surg Lasers Imaging. 2007 Nov-Dec; 38(6): 500–2.

13. Lahey JM, Francis RR, Kearney JJ. Combining phacoemulsification with pars plana vitrectomy in patients with proliferative diabetic retinopathy: A series of 223 cases. Ophthalmology 2003; 110: 1335–9.

14. Lahey JM, Francis RR, Kearney JJ, Cheung M. Combining phacoemulsification and vitrectomy in patients with proliferative diabetic retinopathy. Curr Opin Ophthalmol 2004; 15: 192–6.

15. Freeman WR, Azen SP, Kim JW, el-haig W, Mishell DR, Bailey I. Vitrectomy for the treatment of full-thickness stage 3 or 4 macular holes. Arch Ophthalmol 1997; 115: 11–21.

16. Lahey JM, Francis RR, Fong DS, Kearney JJ, Tanaka S. Combining phacoemulsification with vitrectomy for treatment of macular holes. Br J Ophthalmol 2002; 86: 876–8.

17. Androudi S, Ahmed M, Fiore T, Brazitikos P, Foster CS. Combined pars plana vitrectomy and phacoemulsification to restore visual acuity in patients with chronic uveitis. J Cataract Refract Surg 2005; 31: 472–8.

18. Brazitikos PD, Androudi S, Christen WG, Stangos NT. Primary pars plana vitrectomy versus scleral buckle surgery for the treatment of pseudophakic retinal detachment: A randomised clinical trial. Retina 2005; 25: 957–64.

19. Melberg NS, Thomas MA. Nuclear sclerotic cataract after vitrectomy in patients younger than 50 years of age. Ophthalmology 1995; 102: 1466–71.

20. Smiddy WE, Stark WJ, Michels RG, Maumenee AE, Terry AC, Glaser BM. Cataract extraction after vitrectomy. Ophthalmology 1987; 94: 483–7.

21. Hainsworth DP, Chen SN, Cox TA, Jaffe GJ. Condensation on polymethylmethacrylate, acrylic polymer and silicone intraocular lenses after fluid-air exchange in rabbits. Ophthalmology 1996; 103: 1410–8.

22. Meyers SM, Klein R, Chandra S, Myers FL. Unplanned extracapsular cataract extraction in post-vitrectomy eyes. Am J Ophthalmol 1978; 86: 624–6.

23. Sneed S, Parrish RK 2nd, Mandelbaum S, O'Grady G. Technical problems of extracapsular cataract extractions after vitrectomy. Arch Ophthalmol 1986; 104: 1126–7.

24. Cheung CM, Hero M. Stabilisation of anterior chamber depth during phacoemulsification cataract surgery in vitrectomised eyes. J Cataract Refract Surg 2005; 31: 2055–7.

Advancement in Phacoapplications

51

Bimanual Microincision Phacoemulsification Surgery
(Phaconit with Ultrathin IOL Implantation)

Col JKS Parihar SM, VSM

INTRODUCTION

Bimanual microincision cataract surgery is popularly known as MICS, phaconit, microphaco, bimanual microphaco, sleeveless phaco or ultra microphaco. Phaconit is being considered as the latest revolution in phacoemulsification cataract surgery. Phaconit or microincision phaco-emulsification cataract surgery is breaking all barriers to achieve smaller and smaller incisions for cataract surgery.

The problem in phacoemulsification is that we are not able to go below an incision of 1.9 mm, as the infusion sleeve takes up a lot of space, however, in this new technique of phaconit, phacoemulsification is being performed with the help of a phaco probe with a micro thin phaco tip of 0.9 mm or less and without the sleeve. The infusion line is also detached from the phaco handpiece and attached to the irrigating chopper through a 0.9 mm incision followed by implantation of an ultrathin acrylic foldable IOL or rollable intraocular lens which leads to negligible astigmatism and faster visual recovery than phacoemulsification with a foldable intraocular lens. Phaconit with rollable intraocular lens is a new break-through which will replace phacoemulsification with foldable lens in the coming years with the advent of better technology and instrumentation.

With more patient awareness, the time is not far away, when patients demand phaconit surgery with rollable IOL rather than phacoemulsification surgery with foldable IOL, thus making it absolutely necessary for ophthalmologists to convert to phaconit surgery.

Phaconit (Phakonit): What Does it Mean?

The word phaconit supports the basic concept of micro-incision which almost resembles the size of 20–21 gauze needle tip hence this technique can be called phaco with Needle Incision Technology (NIT) or PHACONIT. The popular term PHAKONIT also involves the fact that in this technique phaco is (PHAKO) being done with a needle (N) opening via an incision (I) and with the phako tip (T).

The Other Synonyms

  (i) Bimanual phaco
 (ii) Microincision cataract surgery
(iii) Microphaco
(iv) Microphacoemulsification
 (v) Bimanual microphaco
(vi) Sleeveless phaco

EVOLUTION OF MICROINCISION/BIMANUAL PHACOEMULSIFICATION CATARACT SURGERY

Since the inception of Phacoemulsification cataract surgery by Charles Kelman, the technique has undergone tremendous and unbelievable revolutionary changes in the recent past. Such changes have been intended to make cataract surgery more refined, rapid, and reliable with (rebound) faster recovery and rehabilitation as well as re-defining keratolenticular refractive status into emmetropia.

Recent changes in fluid dynamics, torsional phacoemul-sifier systems, newer softwares and inventions of newer generation IOL implants are phenomenal and road-breaking milestones. However, microincision bimanual, sub 1 mm incision and ultrathin IOL implants have been changing direction in context of rapidly advancing technique with the invention of monoaxial sub two mm phacoemulsification cataract surgery by torsional or aqualase system and newer generation of apodized or Diffractive IOL implants.

As such, the first reported ultrathin incision for cataract surgery goes back to 2000 years when a Roman surgeon had aspirated lens matter through a fine bore needle inserted through limbus. This was a modification in the technique of couching.

The modern concept of biannual phacoemulsification cataract surgery was derived from the technique of early eighties which comprised sleeveless small incision pars plana cataract surgery with the help of lensectomy by a fragmatome/ocutome.

The concept of micro phaco was further revolutionised in 1984. Then, the modified technique comprised cataract removal through sleeveless phaco using a 1.5 mm phaco tip and AC maintainer. However, the concept of irrigating chopper through the side port was yet to see the light of day at that particular time.

Dr Amar Agarwal from Chennai (India) has contributed significantly to make this technique more refined, precise up to the standard of sub one mm as well as to make it very much acceptable all over the world. The first sub one mm phacoemulsification was performed by him on August 15th, 1998. He also has the unique distinction of performing the first ever live phaconit surgery on August 22nd, 1998 at Pune, India, at the Phaco and Refractive Surgery Conference which was also witnessed by the author. However, the incision size had to be extended up to 3.2 mm for IOL implantation since ultrathin IOLs were not available at that time. Undoubtedly, it was the commencement of a journey towards the ultimate aim of postcataract surgery emmetropia or keratolenticular refractive surgery in the true sense.

Dr Amar Agarwal's technique did not involve any kind of anaesthesia. To make the incision sub one mm, he had separated the phaco tip from the infusion sleeve. The side port incision was used to introduce infusion fluid into the eye through a bent needle of 20 gauge which acted as the irrigating chopper. The balanced salt solution (BSS) was continuously poured over the eye by an assistant at the site of the incision so as to cool the phaco tip.

The next breakthrough was the invention of the ultrathin IOL implant. Wayne Callahan from the USA had designed the first ultrathin IOL which is based on the Fresnel principle. Thinoptx is the first such ultrathin IOL implant. Dr Jairo Hoyos from Spain has the distinction of performing the first such IOL implantation. Dr Amar Agarwal has modified this lens into a special 5 mm optic rollable IOL. Various surgeons continued to reform and modify the technique of phaconit. The initial problems were a significant surge mainly due to altered fluidics of phacomachine, application of smaller bore tip as well as of irrigation infusion devices, (irrigating choppers), etc. Dr A Agarwal popularised the use of pressure air pumps to infuse fluids through such smaller bore cannulae. Some other surgeons had advocated the use of AC maintainers or surge control devices. However, newer generation phacomachines equipped with modern software and phaco handpieces have made possible MICS to be more refined, comfortable, and widely-accepted.

In addition to the above mentioned changes, several other modifications have taken place in the recent past in this field. Various types of irrigating choppers, keratomes and blades were designed and innovated. The author (JKS Parihar) has modified various keratomes to make them amenable for appropriate maneuverability of surgical instruments and ultrathin IOL implantation through a sub 1.4 mm incision. He had designed keratomes of 0.9, 1.2, and 1.4 mm in Jan, 2002 for various applications. Authors had also designed 21, 22, 23 and 24 gauze irrigating choppers and bimanual I/A cannula during that period. Such instruments have been extensively used in several hundred cases on Ventury system phacomachines. Dr Amar Agarwal had used the 700 Micron tip to perform phaconit in 2005–06. Parihar (2002) is among the pioneers who had clubbed the phaconit technique with other ocular surgeries, namely concurrent phaconit and penetrating keratoplasty, Ahmed glaucoma valve and phaconit and phaconit with Ahmed glaucoma valve, keratoplasty, and stem cell transplantations as well as phaconit with PP vitrectomy in highly complicated situations.

Bimanual phaconit surgery is not merely the smaller incision surgical procedure but needs several modifications in machine settings, irrigating systems, phaco tip, phaco sleeves and instrumentations as well as the basic concept of phacoemulsification surgery. This very much resembles the phrase that "Paediatric cases are not miniature adults".

MODIFICATIONS IN PHACOEMULSIFIER SYSTEMS AND TECHNIQUES

Despite several merits, coaxial phaco is not free from certain inherent constraints like unpredictability in anterior chamber stability, postoperative induced astigmatism and endophthalmitis, though much less as compared to the conventional ECCE. Bimanual MICS is rapidly taking over the centre stage which may facilitate sub 1.5 mm cataract surgery.

Phacoemulsification cataract surgery involves ultrasonic vibration of the phaco needle. This vibration of the needle subsequently creates friction and heat, which is transferred to the surrounding tissue.

Efforts have been made to minimise adverse impact of heat and thermal injuries to ocular tissues by anterior chamber infusion provided through the silicone sleeve surrounding the phaco needle as well persistent and regular maintenance of the anterior chamber throughout the procedure. The various modifications in ultrasonic energy delivery system as well as inception of newer software and microprocessors have significantly contributed towards safe and cold phacoemulsification surgery. Typical phaco tips have diameters of approximately 1.2 mm. However, minimal incision for conventional coaxial phaco-mulsification surgery cannot be reduced to less than 2.5 to 3.00 mm so as to facilitate sufficient incision to allow adequate fluid inflow through infusion sleeves. As such, conventional foldable IOL implants cannot be implanted through less than 2.8 mm incision without any modification.

There has been significant improvement in the configuration as well as reduction in the size of these incisions in the recent past. Despite such evolution, conventional phacoincisions are still far away from the complete freedom of the threat of intraoperative anterior chamber instability, induced astigmatism as well as from postoperative endophthalmitis. Such constraints and the ultimate goal to achieve postsurgical emmetropia laid the foundation of phaconit or 'microincisional' cataract surgery (MICS) which can achieve cataract removal through a very small sub 1 mm microincision.

How to Perform Bimanual MICS using Basic Model Phacoemulsifier Machines

MICS can be performed by using any kind of phacoemulsifier. Undoubtedly, advanced machines are equipped with various programmes and modifications to handle peculiarities of MICS such as compromised fluidics, surge control and power modulation devices. Hence, the outcome is better and one can take up even very hard cataracts without much discomfort. Contrary to it, certain modifications in technique and machine settings allow a reasonably good outcome even with basic machines.

Suggested parameters on basic phacoemulsifier are as follows:

Peristaltic Systems

(i) Power: 40 to 50% of phaco power. It is preferred to perform chopping under the continuous mode followed by fragment aspiration under the pulse mode.

(ii) Flow rate: 22–28 ml/min

(iii) Suction: Removal of superficial cortex prior to chopping by using vacuum of 75 mmHG. Chopping is done at 150–175 mmHG followed by fragment removal at 100 to 125 mmHG. Use of an air pump may be required if a smaller gauze chopper like 21 gauze or less is used or managing grade three to four cataracts.

Ventury Systems

(i) Power: 25 to 35% of phaco power. It is preferred to perform chopping under the continuous mode followed by fragment aspiration under the pulse mode.

(ii) Flow rate: Machine based

(iii) Suction: Removal of superficial cortex prior to chopping by using vacuum of 50 mmHG. Chopping is done at 75–125 mmHG followed by fragment removal at 70 to 100 mmHG. Use of an air pump may not be required unless a smaller gauze chopper like the 22 gauze or less is used or managing grade three to four cataracts.

How to Prevent Thermal Burn in MICS

Thermal injuries at the site of incision and disproportionate corneal endothelial cell loss are major issues in case of the advanced bimanual MICS technique. Several factors have been considered responsible for such insults.

During phacoemulsification, ultrasonic vibration of the phaco needle creates friction and heat, which is transferred to the surrounding tissue. In the conventional, coaxial phacoemulsification surgery, anterior chamber infusion is supplied through a flexible silicone sleeve surrounding the phaco needle which maintains temperature equilibrium at the incision site. Adequate cooling during phacoemulsification at the site of incision and over the phaco tip demands sufficient fluid circulation through and around the lumen of the tip phaco. The adverse impact of thermal energy is maximum at the time of tip occluded with nuclear fragments which results in arrest of fluid circulation despite continuous release of ultrasonic energy resulting in an ultimate and sustained rise of temperature at the incision site.

Suggested measures to reduce or prevent thermal burn are as follows:

(i) Use of a cold BSS at 4° celsius minimises risk of thermal injuries at the site of incision.

(ii) Use of a half cut silicon sleeve allows protection of the incision site from maximum exposure to thermal energy at the site of contact. Over and above, fluid contact at this point also reduces thermal effect.

(iii) Use of microflow needles: Microflow needles possess external grooves which allow fluid to pass through spaces between the tip and the incision, thus providing cooling over the tip. In addition, less contact surface of tip and incision reduces heat liberation, thus preventing thermal injuries.

(iv) Adequate incision size: (neither too tight nor too loose): This allows the fluid to come out of the incision site and in cooling the phaco needle, however, incision size should not allow excessive leakage of fluid which may lead to surge and corneal endothelial injuries.

Modern higher end phacoemulsifiers are aiming towards least yet effective application of ultrasonic energy so as to minimise the risk involved with excessive US energy. WhiteStar (Sovereign), Millennium and Infinity (Alcon) are a few among such leading technologies.

'Ultra pulse' modulation of ultrasound is a unique feature of WhiteStar technology. Conventional phaco delivers pulse energy at fixed mode, hence system delivers pulse energy at sustained and fixed pattern of 50% duty cycle provided with the given system. In comparison, Whitestar technology allows for the adjustment of the duty cycle and pulse duration, hence modulation of quantum of energy and pattern of pulse delivery can be customised as per the need of the particular nucleus in a given situation. Thus amount of energy delivered becomes bare minimum which ultimately minimises risk of incisional thermal injuries.

Recent studies conducted by Soscia on cadaver eyes have demonstrated the thermal impact of various phacosystems on the incision while performing MICS. He had observed that wound temperature continues to remain below 45 degree (threshold for thermal injury) in any given clinical situation.

Author has been performing bimanual MICS regularly for more than a year using the WS technology with 1:1 micro pulses (50% duty cycle). We did not notice even a single incidence of thermal incisional burn out of 125 cases of MICS performed on WhiteStar during the last year.

The author has experienced MICS on the Millennium Microsurgical System (Bausch and Lomb, Rochester, NY) in 45 cases of various grades of nuclei.

Millennium Microsurgical System is equipped with several features to monitor ultrasonic energy delivery and to provide cold phaco. In addition to the conventional pulse mode, specially designed microprocessor system, fixed-burst mode, and multiple-burst mode are added features. These different options allow the surgeon to control the pulse width, frequency, energy, and duty cycle in a wide variety of combinations. The unique feature of Millennium is its Phaco handpiece of 28.5 kHz, much lower than 40 kHz as compared to the conventional phaco machines. This allows less thermal energy generation due to less friction and yet is more effective than a 40 kHz phaco handpiece due to its (peculiar) greater stroke length which may result in effective performance.

Wound temperatures produced during bimanual MICS with the Millennium were recently studied in cadaver eyes by Braga-Mele and Liu. It was observed that wound temperature remained below 45 degree even when the continuous ultrasound is applied for 3 minutes at 100% power. Hence, MICS on Millennium has good thermal control and a less risk of incisional burn. The torsional phaco system available on Infinity (Alcon) is a new revolutionary change in energy delivery system. The sonic oscillatory motion with longitudinal ultrasonic vibrations enhances emulsification potential of the Neosonix handpiece even at very less US energy application which is responsible for practically no thermal burn. Aqualase technology, based on fluid wave pulses delivery system is a newer concept to emulsify and delaminate the lens without using ultrasonic energy. Aqualase uses 4 micro liter pulses of heated balanced saline solution to delaminate and emulsify nuclear material, hence eliminates the risk of thermal injuries. Present aqualase system (Infinity) is capable of managing soft nucleus up to grade two. However, this promising technology may take over in the near future as the choicest technique.

Surge Control in Bimanual Phaco

The word Surge is derived from Latin word "Surgere" which means "to rise or" a sudden powerful forward or upward movement."

Optimal fluidic equilibrium is most essential while performing bimanual MICS. Unstable anterior chamber remains the main concern of every MICS surgeon, especially during the transitional period. The triad of infusion rate of the irrigating chopper or the I/A cannula, quantum of leakage through the incision and of fluid aspirated through the phaco tip are the most crucial factors that influence the fluid balance in bimanual MICS. An ideal fluid dynamics can be achieved by increasing the inflow or decreasing the outflow.

As such, most of the conventional longitudinal phacoemulsifiers are designed to act as coaxial phacoemulsifiers at specific parameters and fluidics. Average fluid inflow in a coaxial phacoemulsifier is about 50 to 55 ml/mt. This inflow maintains equilibrium with fluid outflow in normal circumstances. Any alteration or deviation from such set protocol leading to imbalance in inflow and outflow demands substitute measures to maintain fluid dynamics, particularly while handling bimanual MICS. The sizes of incisions and diameters of instruments are additional significant factors to induce surge in MICS.

Surge can be minimised or eliminated either by rescheduling fluid inflow directly proportionate to the fluid outflow or by reducing the outflow according to the inflow of fluids. Hence, surge can be controlled by following measures:

(i) Increased bottle heights (more than 110 cm) enhances fluid entry.
(ii) Infusion devices like anti-chamber collapser which injects air into the infusion bottle or air pumps like fish tank air pump to infuse more fluid to make proportionate balance with fluid outflow.
(iii) Cruise control devices.

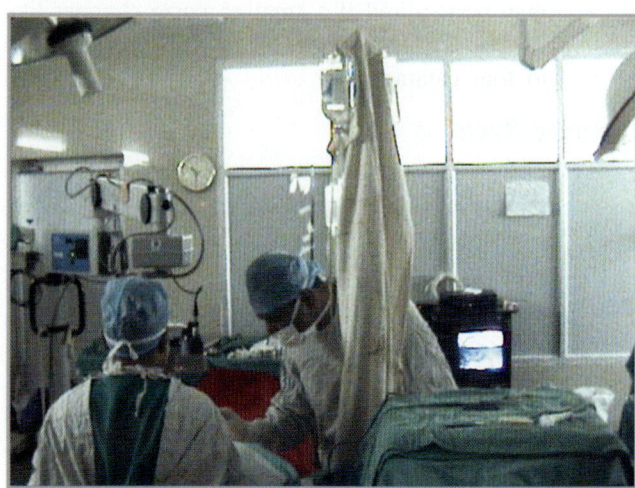

Fig. 51.1: Bottle height

Anti-chamber Collapser

A 18 gauze irrigating chopper is the most ideal anti-chamber collapser to maintain adequate infusion of irrigating fluid and to maintain sustained and a uniform depth of the anterior chamber during MICS. However, in cases of hard cataracts or small bore irrigating choppers or in cases of bimanual I/A devices, an anti-chamber collapser infuses air into the irrigating fluid bottles. This results in more fluid into the eye through the irrigating chopper during bimanual phaco. This ultimately maintains a good depth of the anterior chamber throughout the procedure. It makes phacoemulsification a relatively safe procedure by reducing surge even at high vacuum levels. Hence, smaller gauze cannula up to 21 gauze can safely be used along with this simple device.

Infusion Pumps (Fish Tank Air Pumps)

A very simple and readily available fish tank air pump is a very handy and useful device to prevent surge during MICS. This air pump can increase fluid inflow. The air pump is connected to the infusion bottle by the IV set. The air is purified with the help of a micropore filter and allowed to enter into the infusion bottle.

Infused air creates a positive pressure which enhances the quantity of fluid that circulates into the anterior chamber under positive pressure thereby eliminating surge.

TUR set: Transurethral resection tubings can be used instead of using IV tubing from the infusion bottle to facilitate enhanced quantity of fluid into the anterior chamber of the eye at any given point of time, to reduce surge.

Anterior Chamber Maintainer

Use of an anterior chamber maintainer can effectively reduce the surge. However, this converts MICS into a three-port phacoemulsification.

Specially Designed Phaco Tips/Needles

Specially designed needles like the flared tip needle, with the aspiration bypass system or microflow needles have a definite role to minimise fluid outflow from the anterior chamber.

Conversely, methods which reduce the fluid withdrawn from the eye include:

Cruise Control Devices (Outflow Restrictor)

Cruise control device manufactured by STAAR surgicals is a disposable outflow restrictor. This device is connected between the phaco handpiece and the aspiration tubing, hence can monitor and restrict flow. The device has its internal diameter of 0.3 mm which is placed behind the 2.0 cm long sleeve that allows the fluid to pass through a smaller lumen of 0.3 mm and restricts the fluid outflow through the lumen, thereby reducing surge without compromising the efficacy of the phacoemulsifier.

Vacuum Surge Suppressor

Vacuum surge suppressor manufactured by the VSS (Surgin Inc.) is a small disposable device that is fitted in the aspiration port of the phaco handpiece. This device is of immense merit in regulating the egress of fluid from the anterior chamber. The device deflates once vacuum increases which ultimately leads to minimal fluid quantity egressing out of the anterior chamber. This results in a decreased surge.

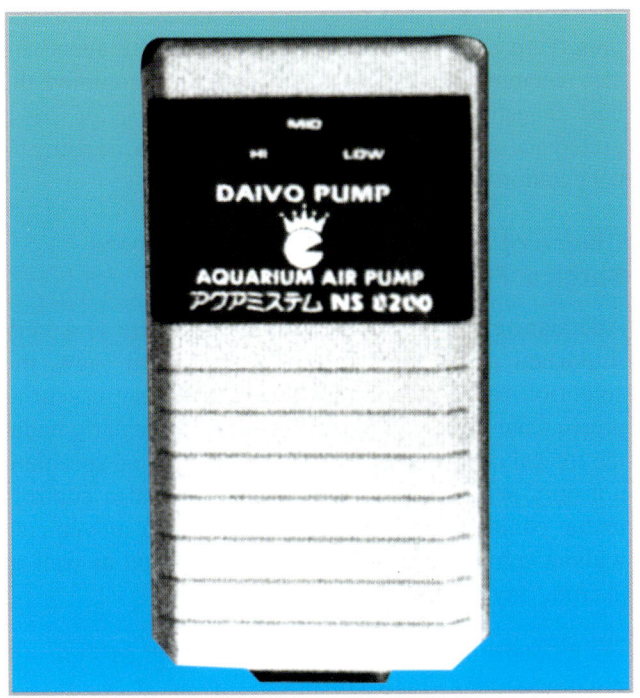

Fig. 51.2: Infusion pumps (fish tank air pumps)

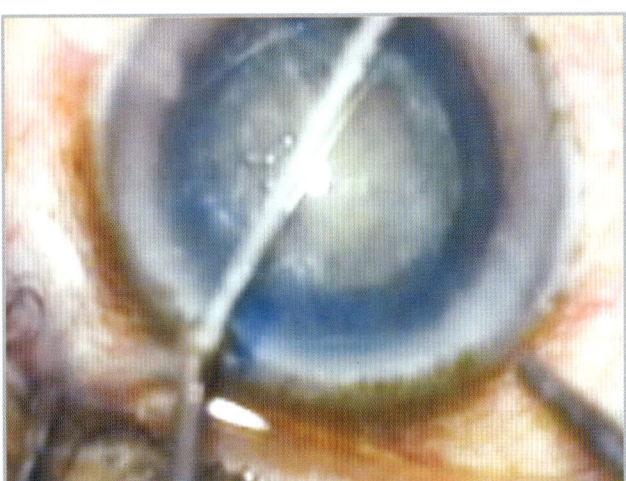

Fig. 51.3: Air pump enhanced irrigation flow through irrigating chopper

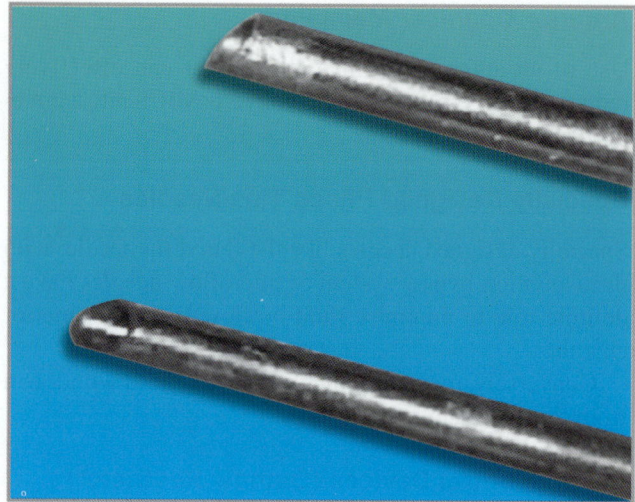

Fig. 51.4: Microincisonal phaco tip (0.9 mm tip seen with 1.2 mm tip)

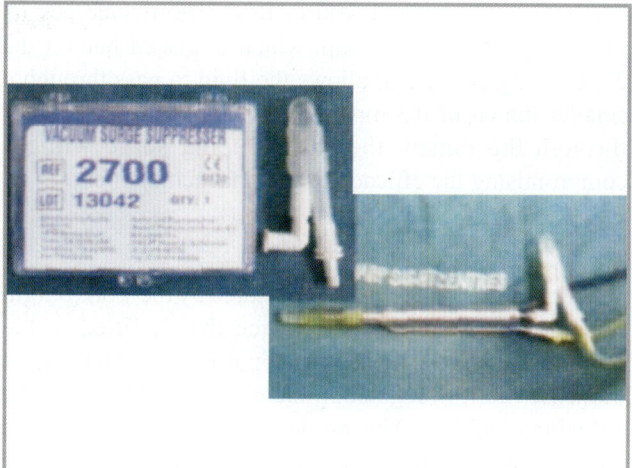

Fig. 51.5: Cruise control devices (outflow restrictor)

Foiled Super VAC Tubings

Foiled Super VAC tubings device regulates fluid flow resulting from occlusion in a dynamic fashion. The continuous change in direction of fluid flow through this foiled tube increases the resistance through the tubing only at high flow rates. Hence, it acts as an effective post-occlusion restricting device to control surge.

How to Transform into Bimanual MICS: Points to Ponder

MICS is not merely a procedure which involves a smaller incision but also separates the infusion line which is linked with the irrigating chopper. Though the procedure itself has several unique features in terms of modulation of system and technology, one can convert to MICS from coaxial phaco by adopting a meticulous approach. This approach can be directed towards following points:

(i) Understand, learn and know your phacoemulsifier system and surgical technique in detail.
(ii) Should be able to perform topical phaco as routine.
(iii) Surgeon should be a proficient coaxial phaco surgeon having good consistency in surgical performance. An excellent control over rhexis both with needle and forceps as well as a capability to perform straight phaco chop is a mandatory requirement.

PREOPERATIVE EVALUATION

Preoperative evaluation of cataract cases is essentially the same as desired for coaxial conventional phacoemulsification surgery. This has been discussed in length in the relevant previous chapters. However, it is advisable to avoid grade four or five cataracts at initial stage till the surgeon gains adequate experience and confidence to handle such cataracts.

SURGICAL TECHNIQUE

Anaesthesia

MICS can be performed under any kind of local anaesthesia or even without any anaesthesia (the no anaesthesia technique). As such, most of the good experienced and quick phaco surgeons rely upon topical anaesthesia. Dr Amar Agarwal has popularised and prefers the no anaesthesia technique. The author has also used the no anaesthesia technique which appears sound in a good number of cases. However, he prefers to use topical anaesthesia as his most favoured technique. In this technique, 4% or 2% topical lignocaine can be used. In addition to it, 3 to 5 ml of Xylocard in 500 ml of infusion fluid may be added. Intracameral preservative-free lignocaine or other anaesthetic agents are also recommended by various surgeons. In our opinion, the best anaesthetic technique remains the surgeon's own preference depending on his comfort as well as the patient's cooperation and acceptability to it.

Choice of a Speculum to obtain Adequate Surgical Field

Adequate exposure of the palpebral fissure is a very important and crucial requirement. In our view, the selection of a suitable speculum is a very essential prerequisite for any intraocular surgery particularly under the topical or no anaesthesia technique. A good speculum not only provides adequate exposure but also controls undue ocular as well as periocular muscle movements without compromising the position of eyeball as well as exerting any unwanted pressure over it.

Wire Speculum or Selfretaining Blade Speculum

A wire speculum can be used in cases of topical anaesthesia, however, in our experience, we find it suitable under limited

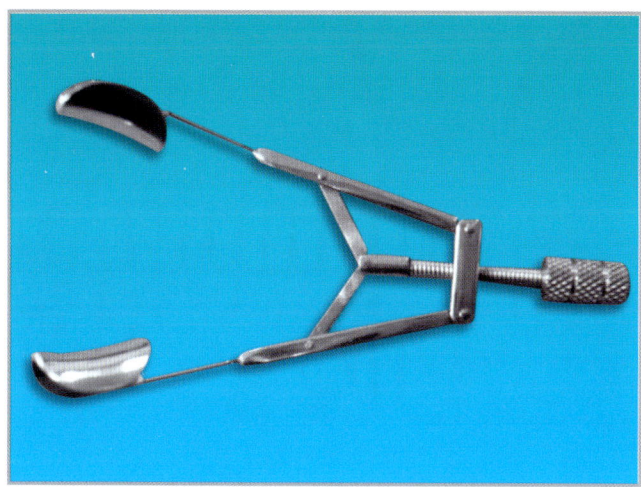

Fig. 51.6: Self-retaining blade speculum

choice, like in cases of elderly patients who do not have good or strong orbicularis muscle action, a small palpebral fissure and deep-seated eyeballs.

In contrast to the wire speculum, self-retaining blade haptics are much more convenient and suitable. Out of solid plate-like blades and strong rectangular metal-hook type speculums, solid plate-like blade speculum has strong preference in the author's choice and practice.

Such a speculum not only provides good exposure but also carries a great advantage while performing the procedure under topical anaesthesia. The author has stopped using any other instrument or metal rod to hold the eyeball during the procedure, particularly at the time of performing rhexis.

Incisions and Injection of Viscoelastic

Bimanual phacoemulsification surgery essentially requires two incisions for the phaco tip as well as for the irrigating chopper. For excellent surgical performance, both incisions should have a good configuration and valve effects. Hence, we do not label them as the main incision and side port. Some surgeons prefer to inject viscoelastics through a 26 gauge needle into the AC prior to the construction of the side port incision. The viscoelastic distends the eye which helps to construct a self-sealing clear corneal incision. However, the author has adopted the technique of constructing both incisions simultaneously as clear corneal valve incisions with the help of specially designed 0.9 mm trapezoid keratomes. This keratome and other instruments for phakonit are made by Joja surgicals and Ovation. However, good instruments for MICS are available from several Indian and international manufacturers like Appasamy, Huco (Switzerland), Microsurgical Technology (USA) and Gueder (Europe). The microdiamond knives of 09 to 1.0 mm can also be used. However, single use metal blades do this job very well.

In our practice, it works very well. There is no chamber collapse during the procedure at all, since both the incisions are self-sealing. Over and above, the second incision is continuously used to release excessive fluid pressure during hydroprocedures. Sites of incisions can be planned as per surgeon's own preference, since such small incisions practically do not induce significant astigmatism due to any specific site of incision. The author constructs both the incisions at around, 100 to 120 degree apart from each other.

The right hand incision which is generally used for the phaco handpiece is kept around 9.30–10.30 O'clock position in case of right eye and 1–2 O'clock for left eye. The second incision for irrigating chopper is being kept at 1 O'clock and 4 O'clock in the right and the left eye, respectively. The author does not shift himself temporally while constructing on incisions in the right eye, whereas he only makes 15 degrees left shift for making incision in the left eye. This is of great help to reduce shifting of operating microscope, phacomachine, and trolley which reduces the undue delay and discomfort in the operation room.

Rhexis, Hydroprocedures (Hydrodissection and Delineation) and Nucleus Rotation

A good circular rhexis and good hydroprocedures are essential and one of the most crucial factors for the success of a MICS surgery. There are several methods to construct rhexis in MICS. The 26–30 gauze bent needle cystitome is the most popular and convenient tool for this purpose. However, specially designed microrhexis forceps can also be used. Some surgeons use the stabilising rod, spatula, or Sinskey hooks to hold the eyeball during rhexis. The author has adopted the technique of performing rhexis without any support from the second incision. In our practice, we have observed that a good solid blade speculum and smooth and quick movement are highly productive. Another instrument through the second incision may be of support in stablising the eyeball during rhexis in cases of no anaesthesia MICS. However, the best option remains the surgeon's own preference.

After making both self-sealing corneal incisions of 0.9 mm and reforming the anterior chamber with viscoelastic substance, continuous curvilinear capsulorrhexis of 5.5 to 6 mm is made and hydrodissection and hydrodelineation is done in the usual manner. However, meticulous attention is required to avoid an undue rise in pressure in the anterior chamber during hydroprocedures due to excess fluid waves, since the microincision virtually acts as a sealed chamber; hence repeated gradual tapping to allow fluid egress from incisions is beneficial. Continuous monitoring of fluid wave passing under the nucleus is essential to avoid any undue pressure on the posterior capsule.

It is worth considering making both the incisions prior to the hydroprocedures. Nucleus rotation is mandatory prior to nucleotomy by chopping techniques.

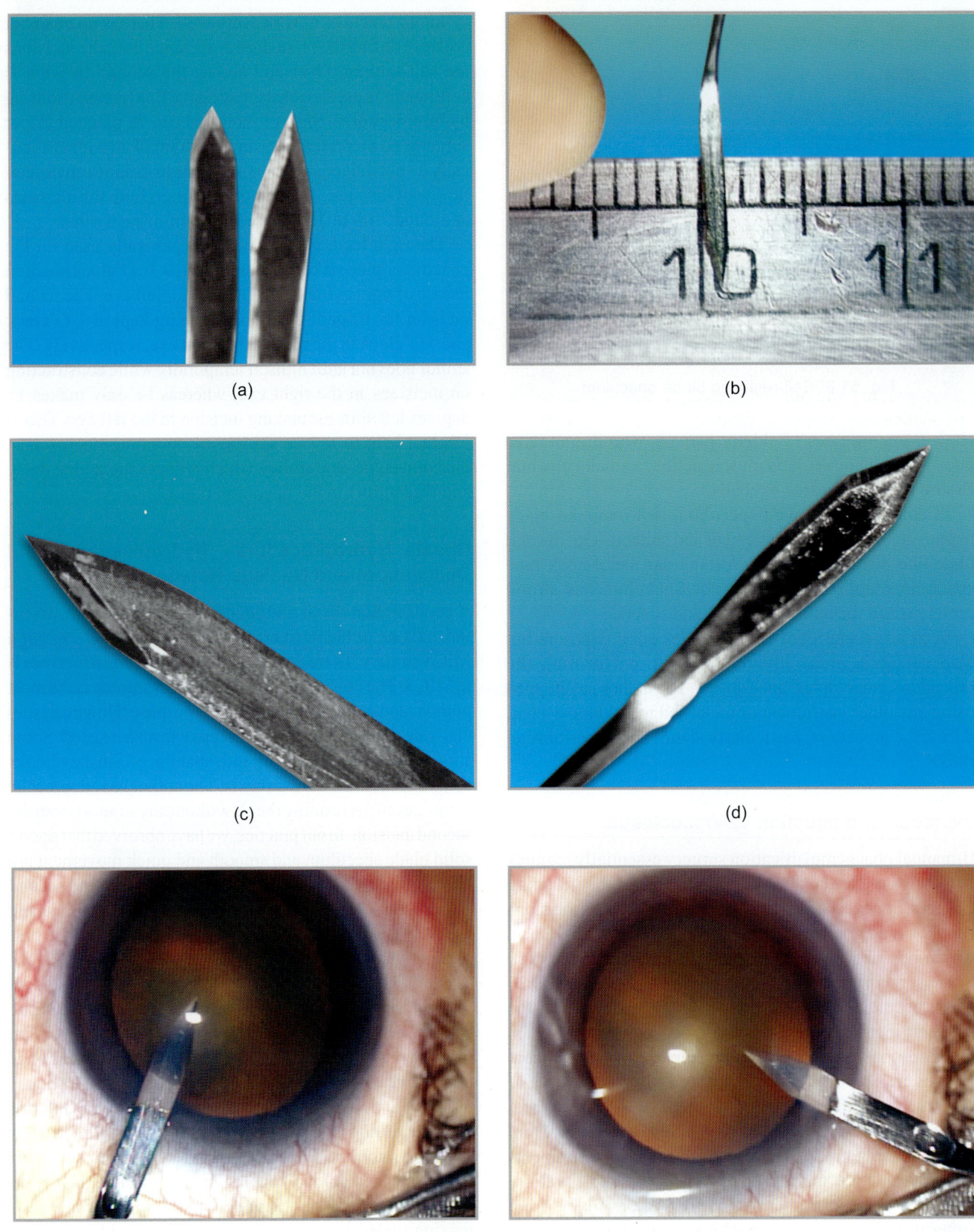

Fig. 51.7: (a) MICS blades, (b) 1.0 mm trapezoid keratome, (c) 0.9 mm trapezoid keratome, (d) Dual (0.9 mm proximal to tip and 1.2 mm at distal end) trapezoid keratome, (e) 0.9 mm trapezoid keratome incision for the irrigating chopper is being kept at 1 O'clock and 4 O'clock positions in the right and the left eye, respectively, (f) 0.9 mm, clear corneal incision at the 10 O'clock position in the right eye for the phaco handpiece is being constructed under topical anaesthesia

Nucleotomy (Phacoemulsification and Fragment Aspiration/Removal)

Bimanual phacoemulsification can be performed by applying any of the conventional nucleotomy techniques with certain modifications. However, most of the experienced phaconit surgeons prefer chopping /stop and chop over sculpting or divide and conquer techniques due to the obvious advantage of less dependency on fluidics at the time of chopping as well as quick and safe surgical performance. As such, bimanual MICS essentially requires an irrigating device through the second incision, hence chopping is a much more natural response in MICS.

Choice of Irrigating Chopper

One can choose an irrigating chopper of his own preference. Both terminal end and side opening choppers have their respective advantages and disadvantages. Conventional irrigating choppers are available in 20 gauze. These choppers are very much convenient and deliver good results in any grade of cataract and are most ideal and suitable for basic phacomachines. The author has designed very specific choppers of 21 to 24 gauze with both side and distal end opening flow. However, these choppers need significant modifications in techniques, particularly in the case of hard cataracts and using basic machines. The author has designed his own technique to use irrigating chopper up to 23 gauze in case of moderately dense nucleus of grade three without any assistance of air infusion devices.

The 24 gauze chopper is convenient with up to grade two nucleus with air infusion devices. Higher-end phaco machines and Ventury based phaco machines can safely be used along with 22 or 23 gauze choppers without using an air pump. The author recommends 20/21 gauze chopper for hard nucleus, whereas 22 to 23 gauze choppers designed by Joja surgicals, ovation or any other company can be used in the remaining types of cases.

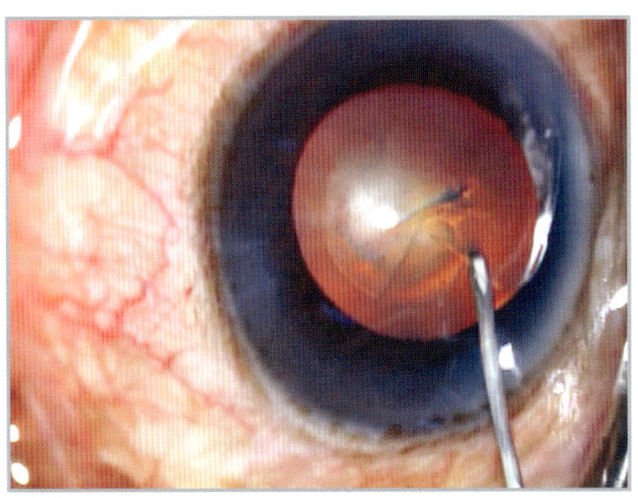
(a)

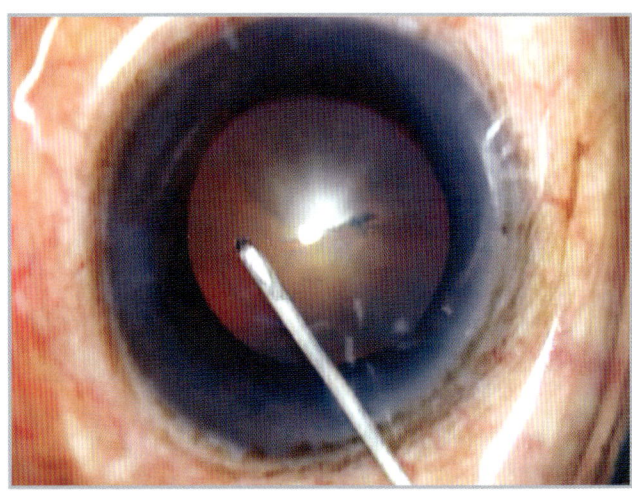
(b)

Fig. 51.8: (a) and (b) Continuous curvilinear capsulorrhexis (MICS)

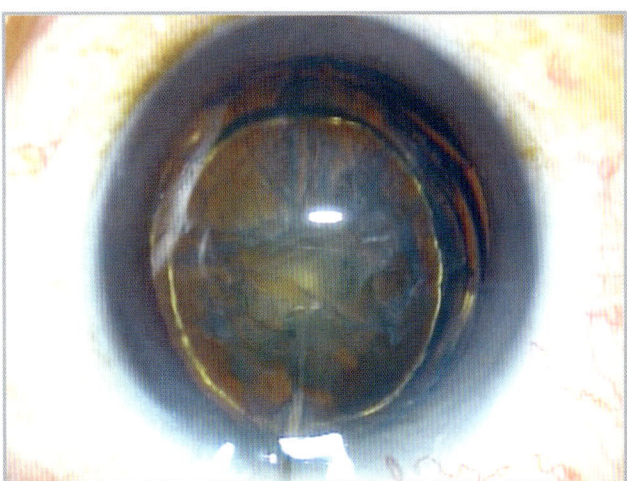

Fig. 51.9: Hydroprocedures (Golden ring appearance)

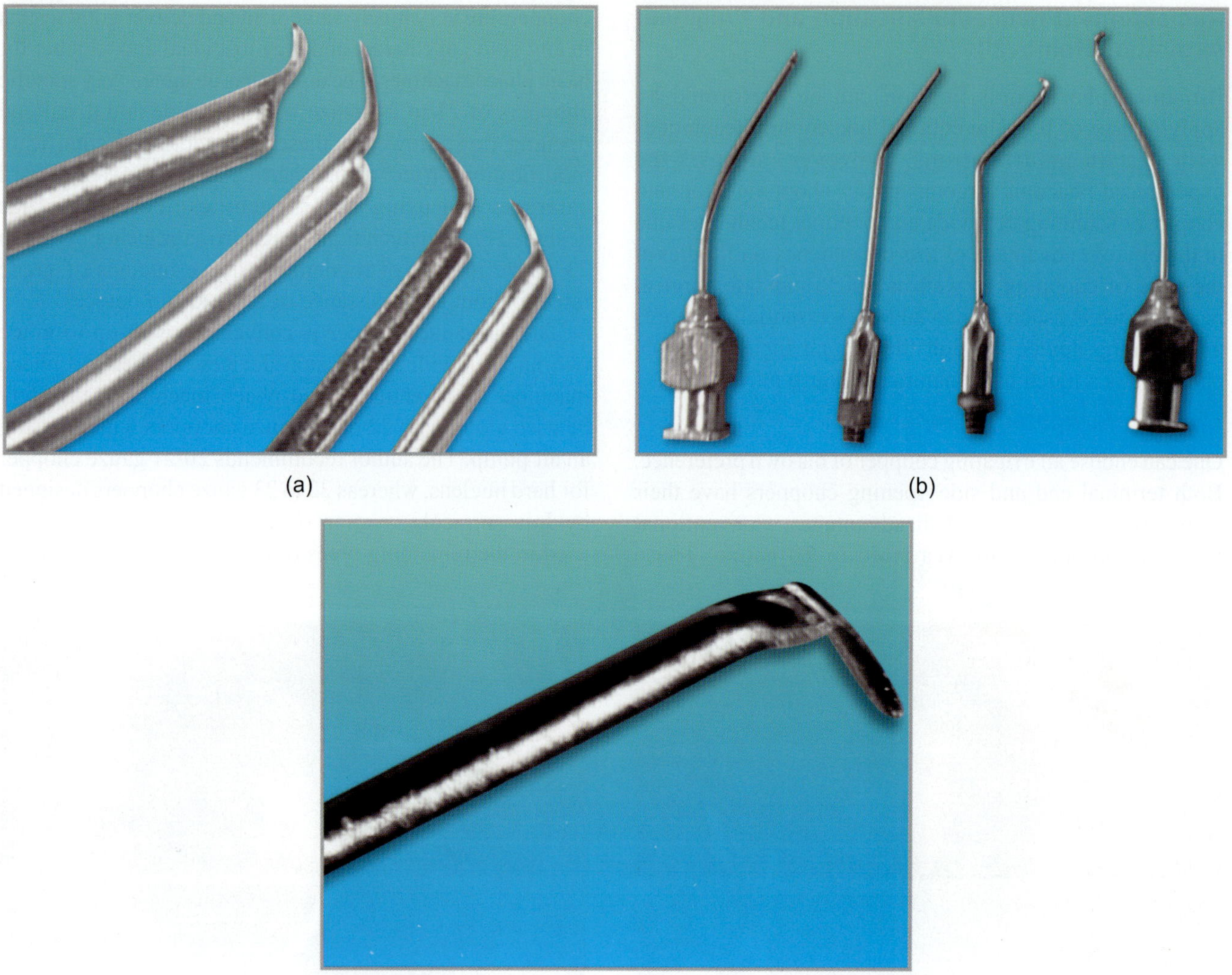

(a)

(b)

(c)

Fig. 51.10: (a) Irrigating choppers (end opening 20 to 23 gauge), (b) Irrigating choppers (20 to 23 gauge), (c) Irrigating chopper (front opening)

MICS: Nucleotomy

The essential deviation in the use of instruments in case of a bimanual MICS as compared to the coaxial phaco is the introduction of an irrigating chopper, before the phaco handpiece which is contrary to what is done in cases of coaxial phaco, since the infusion line is separated from the phaco handpiece and linked to an irrigating chopper. Hence, to maintain an intact and adequate AC depth, irrigating chopper has to be introduced before the entry of handpiece which is just the reverse sequence as compared to the coaxial phaco.

The phaco probe with only aspiration line and the micro phaco tip (0.9 mm or less) with a half cut infusion sleeve is introduced through the right hand clear corneal incision. US energy settings, based on the nucleus grading, being set prior to the introduction of the handpiece into the AC.

The phaco tip is directly embedded into the centre of nucleus while commencing movements from the superior edge, ensuring oblique and tangential movements aiming a slight and gradually progressive posterior inclination of the probe up to two-third to three-fourth thickness of the nucleus. The nucleus is slightly lifted in the bag itself to ensure adequate safety of the posterior capsule. The foot pedal is positioned at position two to hold the nucleus with vacuum. The irrigating chopper from the centre moves outward while ensuring the holding of nucleus which is followed by a final chop in a linear, inverted L-shaped motion. The author prefers to give a small burst of power at the time of linear movement of the irrigating chopper by pushing to position three so as to allow rapid and adequate crack or break in the nucleus, especially in cases of hard cataracts. However, chopping can be done even without giving US energy at the final rotational movement of the irrigating chopper.

Subsequent secondary and tertiary nucleotomies are performed to achieve multiple fragmentation of the nucleus

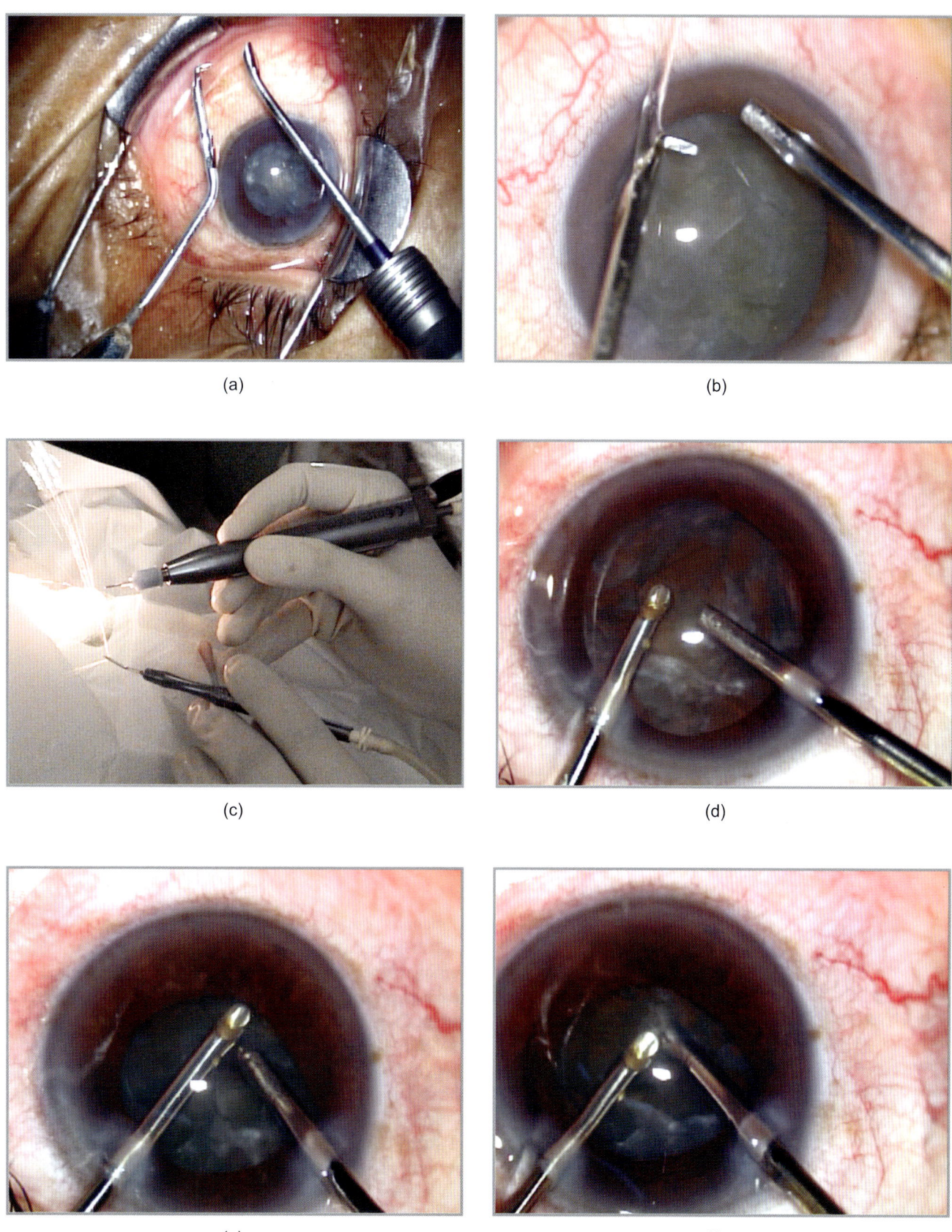

Fig. 51.11: (a) Irrigating chopper and Kelman MICS phaco tip, (b) and (c) Irrigating chopper and MICS phaco tip, (d) Bimanual MICS (phaconit) being performed. Nucleotomy by internal chopping: removal of superficial cortex, (e) Bimanual MICS, (phaco nit): nucleotomy by primary internal chopping, (f) Bimanual MICS, (Phaconit): Secondary internal chopping

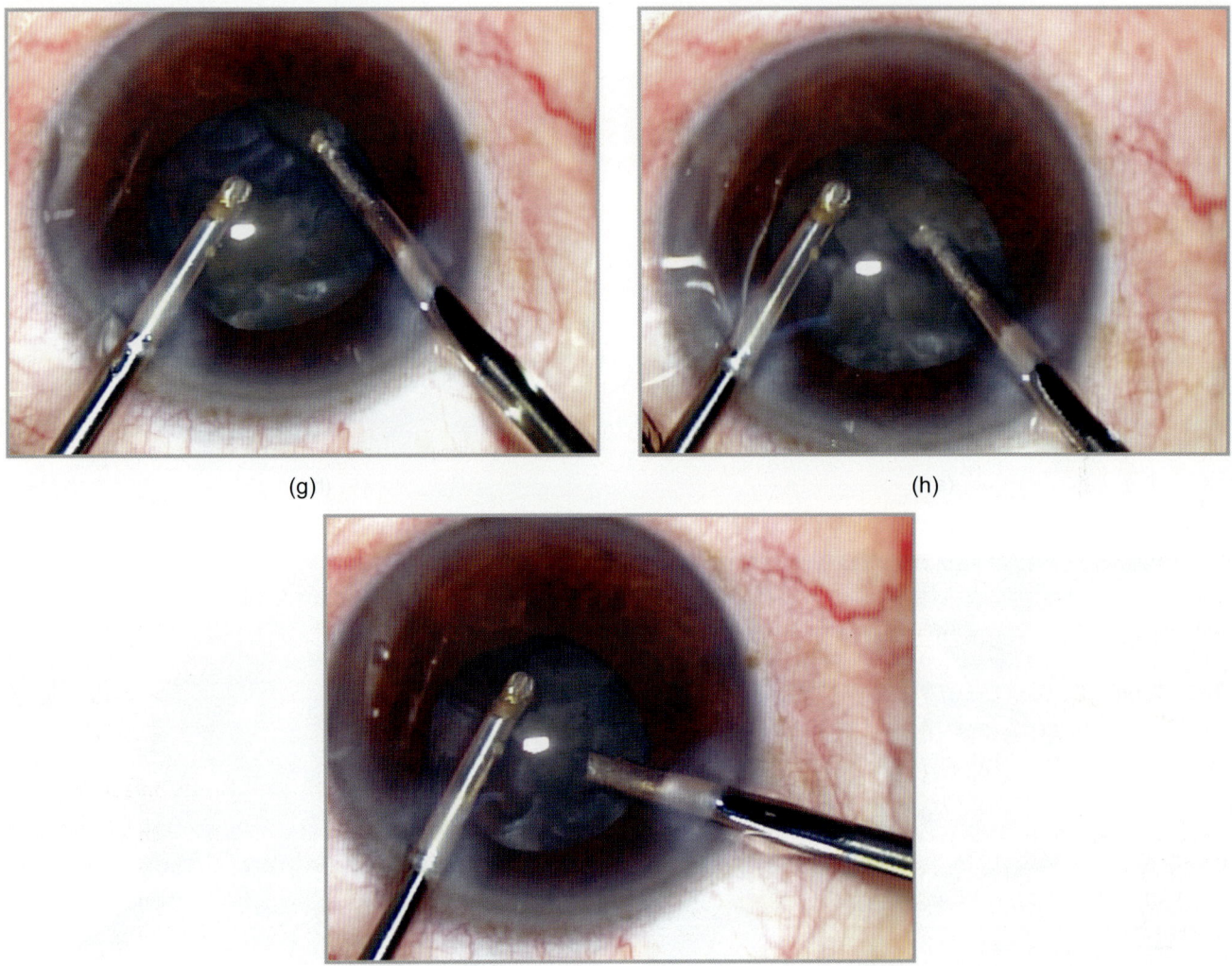

(g)

(h)

(i)

Fig. 51.11: (g) Bimanual MICS (phaconit): Tertiary internal chopping, (h) and (i) (Bimanual MICS (Phaconit): fragment removal

by several rotations. Each piece of the nucleus is slightly lifted in the bag and a short burst of US energy at pulse mode is given, subsequently enhancing nucleus fragment aspiration until the complete nucleus is emulsified and aspirated out. Cortical wash-up is done subsequently by applying the bimanual irrigation aspiration technique.

In case of peripheral chopping, the nucleus is lifted from the periphery and the margin is brought out of the bag using minimal power and high vacuum settings. It is followed by tangential chopping. The author recommends central chopping in case of a large nucleus as well as in cases of grade three or four nucleus, whereas peripheral chopping is much safer while handling a nucleus of up to grade two. Just lifting of nucleus from the periphery in case of soft nucleus followed by aspiration under very minimal power (less than 10%) is enough.

Recommended settings required to handle different grades of nuclei at various stages of nucleotomy and cortical washing are shown in the Tables 51.1 to 51.3.

Bimanual Irrigation and Aspiration (I/A) for Posterior Plate Removal and Cortical Cleaning

Bimanual irrigation and aspiration technique is very crucial and an essential mode of handling the posterior plate and removal of residual cortical matter. Bimanual irrigation and aspiration provides good opportunity to remove subincisional cortical matter at ease as compared to coaxial I/A due to obvious advantage of manoeuvrability and switching over irrigation and aspiration cannula to either of the incisions as per the desire and need arising in the given situation. This provides good hydration to facilitate removal of sticky cortex. However, one needs to be cautious while performing bimanual I/A, since it has different settings and techniques of movement of cannula in the AC.

It is recommended to practise bimanual I/A during routine coaxial phaco as well as to acquaint oneself with the procedure. The author has completely switched over to bimanual I/A in all procedures. Of course, this is essentially required in bimanual phaco to allow the I/A

Table 51.1: Phaconit: Effective phaco time and ultrasound energy requirement and its correlation with nucleus grading (Ventury/Peristaltic)

Nucleus Grading	Effective phaco time	US energy (%) (Chopping)	US energy (%) (Fragment emulsification/asp)
Grade I	10–20 sec	5	5
Grade II	25–30 sec	10	10–15
Grade III	30–40 sec	10–15	10–15
Grade IV	60–75 sec	20–25	20–30
Grade V	120–150 sec	30–35	25–30

Table 51.2: Phaconit: Effective Irrigation/Aspiration time and settings at fragment aspiration and cortical wash (Ventury system)

Nucleus Grading	Effective aspiration time	Vacuum (Fragment emulsification/asp)	Vacuum (Cortical irrigation/asp)
Grade I	20–30 sec	50–75 mmHG	200–250 mm
Grade II	45–60 sec	75–100	200–250 mm
Grade III	75–90 sec	75–100	200–250 mm
Grade IV	75–90 sec	100–125	200–250 mm
Grade V	120–150 sec	100–125	200–250 mm

Table 51.3: Phaconit: Effective Irrigation/Aspiration time and settings at fragment aspiration and cortical wash (Peristaltic system)

Nucleus Grading	Effective aspiration time	Vacuum (Fragment emulsification/asp)	Vacuum (Cortical irrigation/asp)
Grade I	45–60 sec	125–150 mmHG	200–250 mm
Grade II	60–75 sec	125–150 mm	200–250 mm
Grade III	90–120 sec	200–275 mm	200–250 mm
Grade IV	120–50 sec	200–275 mm	200–250 mm

through a sub 2 mm incision except in case of Infinity torsional (Alcon) system which allows coaxial sub two mm incision phacoemulsification.

Microincision Foldable IOL Implants

The MICS or phaconit is not merely a smaller incision cataract surgery technique but it also involves a technological evolution which demands several modifications at each and every step of surgery, equipments and IOL implants as well.

Rollable or ultrathin lens is an essential requirement of modern micro phaco surgery through the sub one mm incision. However, these IOLs need a little larger incision which may vary from 1.4 to 1.8 mm for IOL insertion. Characteristic features of the ideal IOL implant for MICS or phaconit surgery are as follows:

For an IOL to be considered as a MICS lens or MICS IOL, it should fulfil the following requirements:

(i) The IOL insertion should be possible through a sub 2 mm incision without compromising its mechanical, optical or structural qualities while being rolled or compressed into the injector system.

(ii) The IOL should have excellent biocompatibility despite its ultrathin structure.

(iii) In-the-bag stability.

(iv) Excellent visual outcome.

(v) No optical or chromatic aberration.

(vi) Least or no posterior capsular opacification (PCO).

(vii) IOL should have excellent optical performance without having induced halos, glare or night-vision phenomenon, no induced aberrations or scattering compared to conventional lenses.

Microincision Cataract Surgery Intraocular Lenses

Various models of ultrathin IOLs are available in the market. Commonly available micro IOL implants are as follows:

(i) ThinOptX Ultra Choice 1.0 IOL (ThinOptX Inc, Abrindon, Virginia, USA);

(ii) Acri. Smart lOLs (Acri-Tec GmbH, Berlin, Germany);

(iii) IOL tech microincision lens (lOL tech SA, Zeiss Meditec A, Jena, Germany);

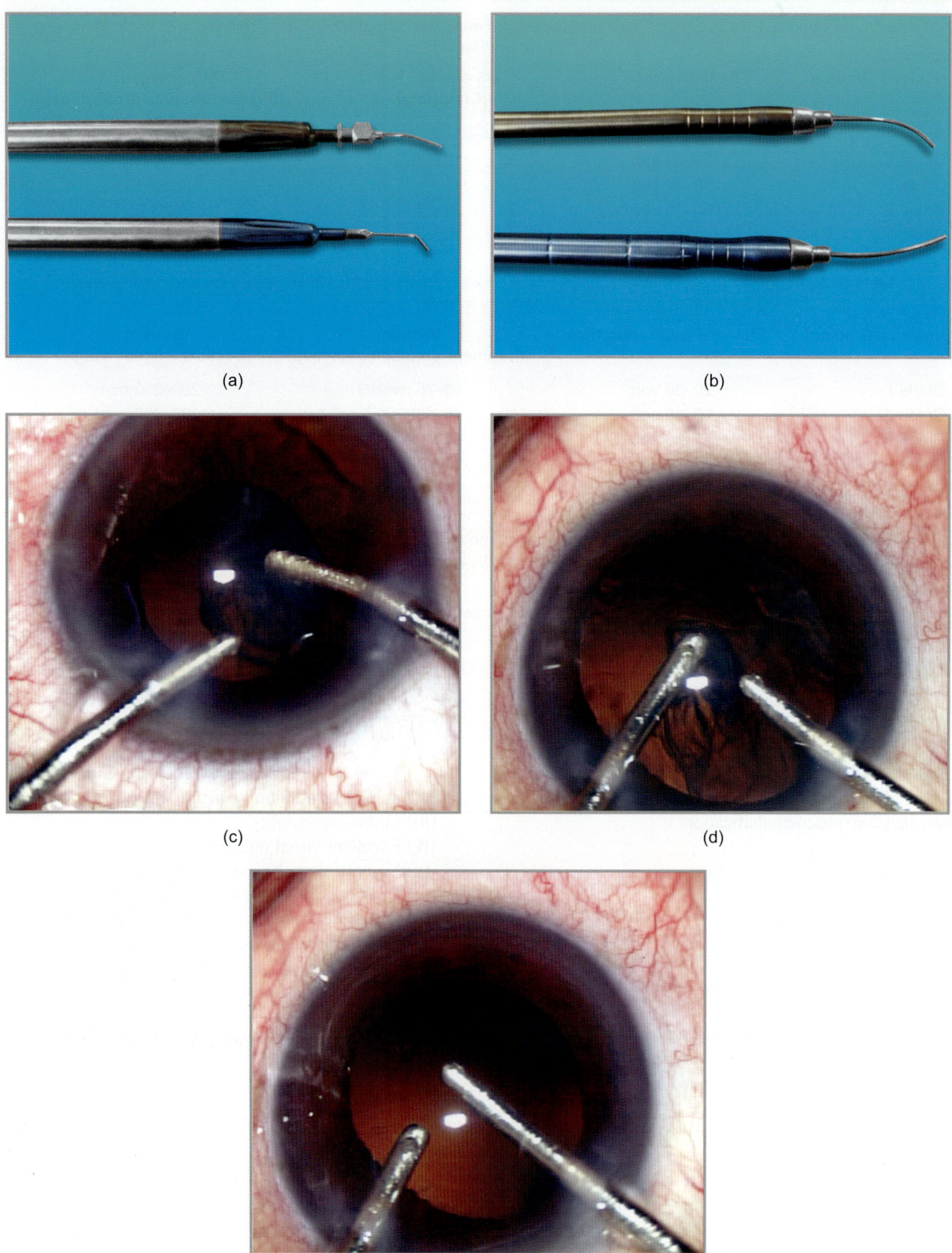

Fig. 51.12: (a) and (b) Bimanual irrigation aspiration system, (c), (d) and (e) Bimanual I/A: Removal of residual cortex

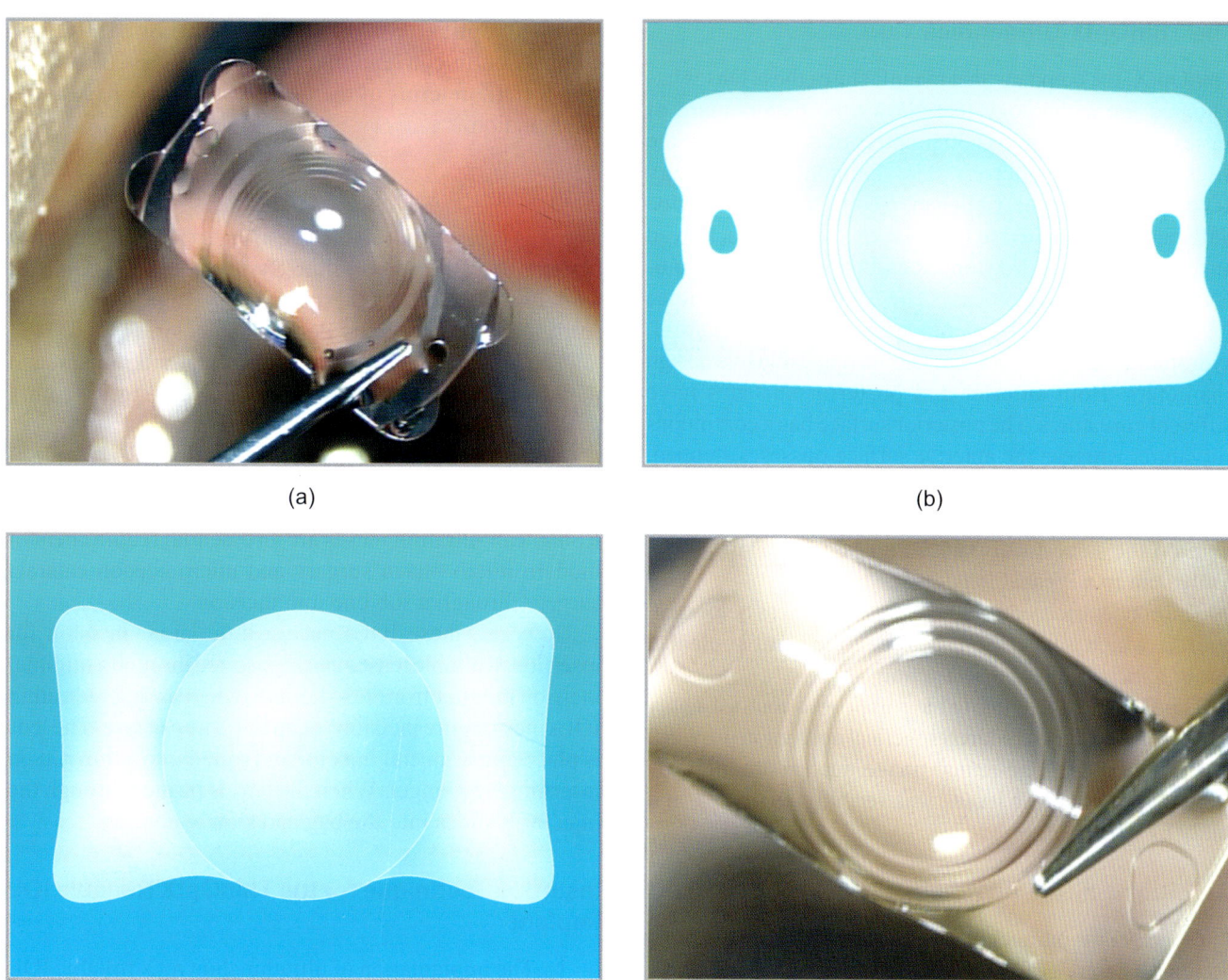

(a)	(b)
(c)	(d)

Fig. 51.13: (a) and (b) ThinOptX ultrathin rollable IOL, (c) Ultrathin IOL for MICS, (d) Micriol thin IOL for MICS

(iv) Care Flex IOL (W2O Medizintechnik AG, Bruchal, Germany);

(v) Tetra Flex KH-3500 microincision lens (Lenstec Inc, Florida, USA);

(vi) Acri Flex MICS 46CSE IOL (Acrimed GmbH, Berlin, Germany);

(vii) Super Flex and C-flex lOLs (Rayacryl Rayner Intraocular Lenses Ltd, UK);

(viii) Ultra smart lens (Appasamy, India);

(ix) Micriol (Care Group, India);

(x) Akreos AO (Bausch and Lomb) Microincision Lens

The specifications of commonly available thin IOLs given in Table 51.4

Table 51.4: Specifications of some thin IOLs

Specification	ThinOptX	Micriol care group, India	Acrismart	Ultrathin Appasamy
1. Incision size	1.4–1.5 mm	1.75–1.90 mm	1.75–1.90 mm	1.75–1.90 mm
2. Optic zone	5.5 mm	5.5 mm	5.5 mm	6.00 mm
3. Total length	11.2 mm	11.0 mm	11.0 mm	11.00 mm
4. Optic geometry	Biconvex/equiconvex	Biconvex/equiconvex	Biconvex/equiconvex	Equiconvex
5. Profile	Plate haptic	plate haptic	Sharp-edged	Plate haptic
6. Material	Hydrophilic acrylic 18% WC	Hydrophilic acrylic 24% WC	Acrylic 25% WC	HEMA material 26% WC
7. Insertion	Rollable	Foldable	Foldable	Foldable

The ThinOptX Ultrachoice 1.0

ThinOptX, the company that manufactures these lenses has patented the technology that allows the manufacture of lenses with plus or minus 30 dioptres of correction on the thickness of 100 microns. The ThinOptX technology developed by Wayne Callahan, Scott Callahan and Joe Callahan is not limited to material choice, but is achieved instead by revolutionary optics and unprecedented nanoscale manufacturing process. The ThinOptX Ultrachoice 1.0 is a single-piece, meniscus shaped plate haptic, hydrophilic acrylic intraocular lens having exclusive design characters. Both anterior and posterior surfaces have different curvatures. The posterior surface has a continuous curvature, whereas the anterior surface posseses stepped, concentric rings, each with a height of 50 micron. Each step is angled in such a fashion that it allows refraction of light on the same focal point in a design similar but not equivalent to a Fresnel lens.

The concentric steps keep the optic thickness below 450 micron, which allows the lens to be rolled and implanted through incisions less than 1.6 mm.

ThinOptX lens is found to have improved contrast acuity most probably due to reduced spherical aberration provided by the thin optic. The retinal image quality produced by the above intraocular lenses was recently evaluated in a study by Alio et al.

Acri.Smart Intraocular Lenses

The Acri.Smart intraocular lenses are available in various designs. It comprises of a single piece biconvex/equiconvex sharp-edged thickness and is made up of an acrylic material with a maximum water content of 25%. The refractive index of IOL varies from prehydrated 1.51 (at 25°C) to 1.46 following hydration.

The Acri.Smart intraocular lenses are found to have excellent optical and insertion performance. The IOL is resistant to any optical or structural changes following compression for insertion. Various studies have documented identical optical performance of Acri.Smart IOL in comparison to conventional AcrySof IOL and ThinOptX MICS IOL, in terms of the quality of retinal images after implantation.

Implantation Technique

The lens is injected into the eye using a specially designed system, the Acri.Smart Glide System (Acri-Tec GmbH). The system includes a special cartridge (Acri.Glide cartridge) and a specially designed injector.

The Acri.Smart Glide System facilitates the injection of the lens through a sub-2.0 mm incision (1.75 to 1.90 mm).

Implantation Techniques of Ultrathin and Rollable IOL Implants

Rollable or ultrathin lenses are an essential requirement of modern micro phaco surgery and microincision cataract surgery through a sub one mm incision.

However, these IOLs need a little larger incision for insertion. Rollable lenses can be inserted through a minimal incision ranging from 1.3–1.5 mm, whereas other ultrathin IOLs may require incisions of up to 1.8 mm of size. The lens is placed on a special injector and rolled into a thin rod on inserting the plunger. When the lens is pushed through the injector it slides into the bag and slowly unfolds.

Insertion Technique for the ThinOptX Rollable IOL Implant

1. The implantation of ultrathin thinOptX rollable IOL implant can be performed through a very small incision of 1.4/1.5 mm size by using the roller injector system, designed exclusively for this purpose.
2. The lens is taken out from the bottle. The lens is then held with a forceps (Fig. 51.15d).
3. The lens is then placed in a bowl of BSS solution that is approximately at body temperature. This makes the lens pliable.

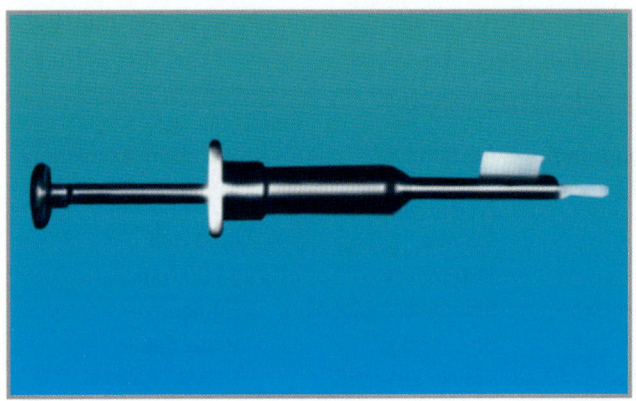

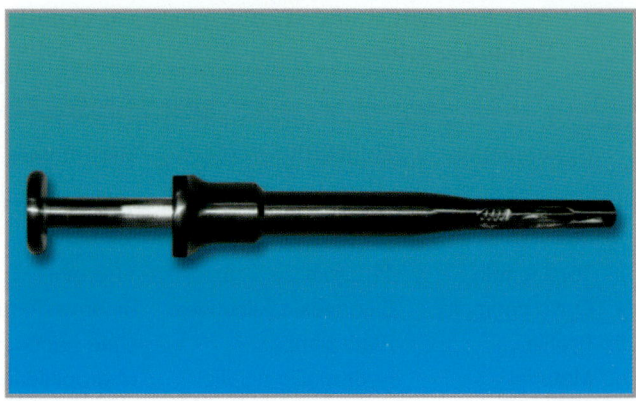

(a)   (b)

Fig. 51.14: (a) Acri.Smart glide system (cartridge, silicone plug and injector), (b) Acri. Smart glide system

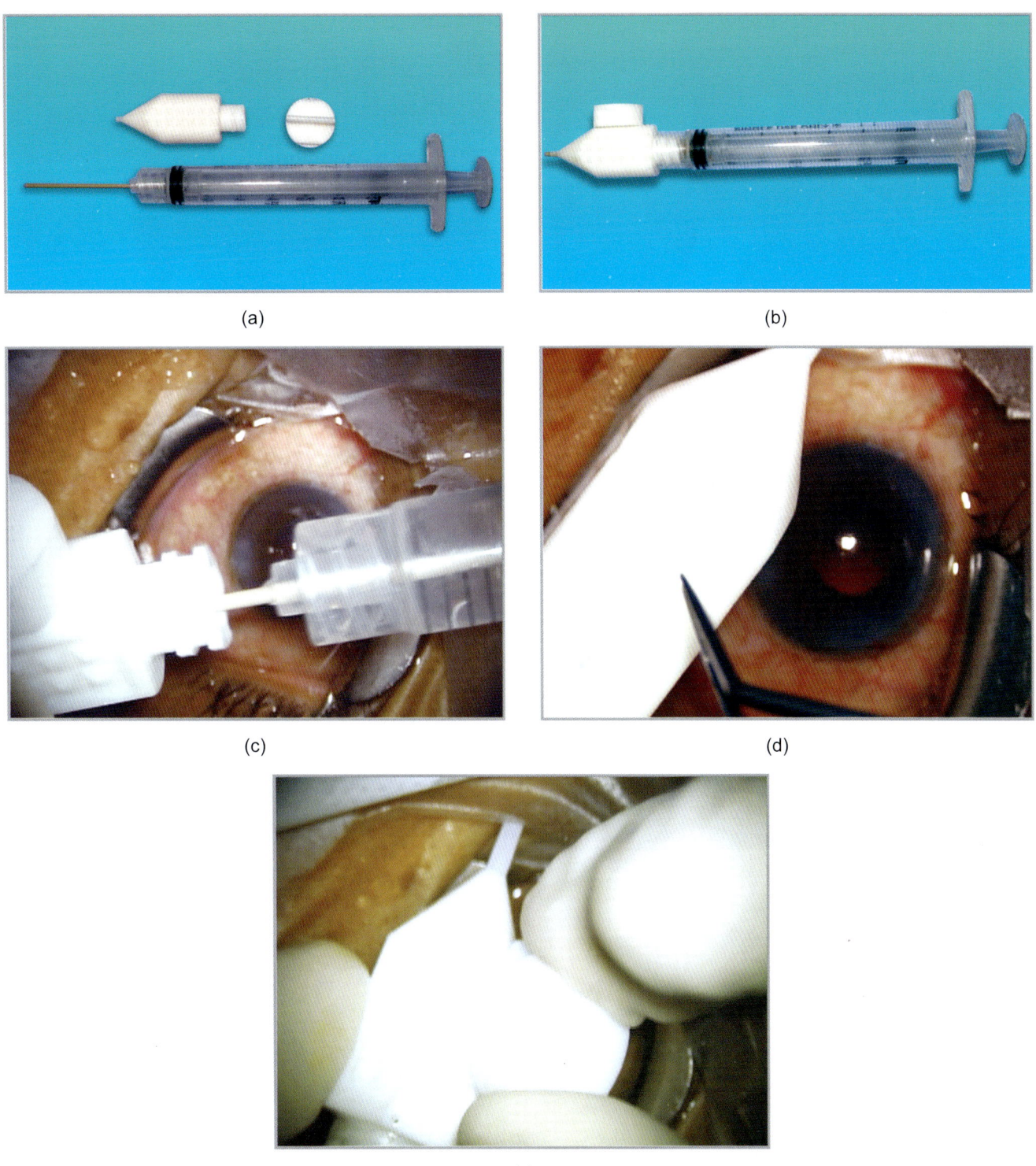

(a)

(b)

(c)

(d)

(e)

Fig. 51.15: (a) and (b) Thin roller injector, (c) Thin roller injector (head socket is made up of teflon), (d) Ultrathin IOL is being placed into the teflon socket of roller injector, (e) Ultrathin IOL is being compressed in the groove with the help of the cap of head of roller injector

4. The lens is then placed into a specially designed socket in an exclusively made roller injector for this purpose. The head of the roller injector is made up of teflon with a thin groove to accommodate IOL *in situ*. This groove can be covered with the help of a specially designed cap which exactly fits into the groove. Hence, the rollable IOL can safely be compressed in the groove with a gradual and downward pushing manoeuvre of the cap.

5. The compressed IOL is subsequently pushed gently into the anterior chamber through a forward motion of the plunger while maintaining the injector's

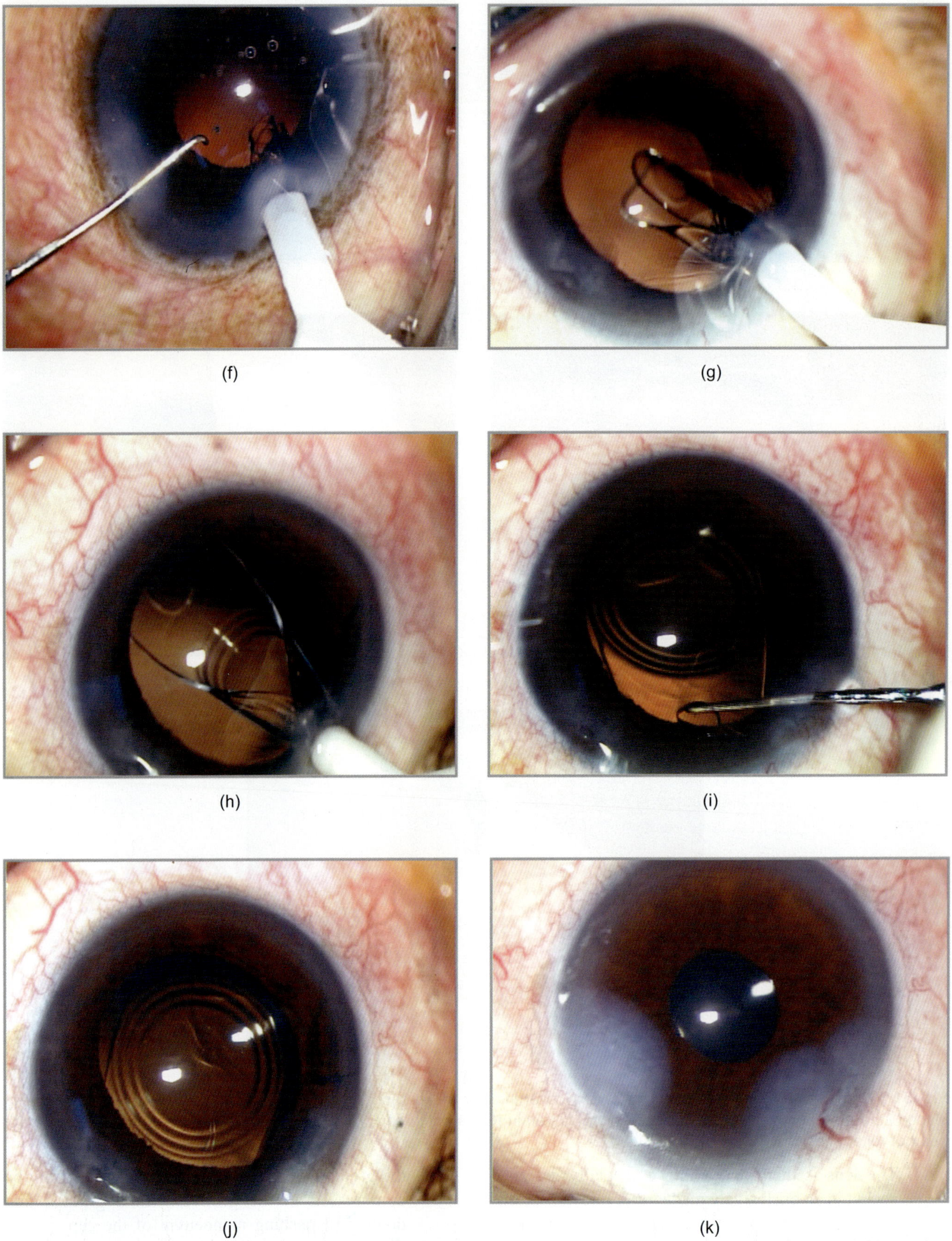

(f)

(g)

(h)

(i)

(j)

(k)

Fig. 51.15: (f) and (g) Ultrathin IOL is, being introduced into the anterior chamber, (h) The leading haptic of ultrathin IOL is being introduced into the capsular bag, (i) The trailing haptics of ultrathin IOL is being introduced into the capsular bag, (j) Ultrathin IOL is well placed in the capsular bag, (k) Stromal hydration

position only at the site of incision without placing the injector tip into the anterior chamber. When the lens is pushed through the injector it slides gradually into the bag and slowly unfolds.

The natural warmth of the eye causes the lens to open gradually. Hence, incision size can be restricted up to sub 1.5 mm. Viscoelastic is then removed with the bimanual irrigation aspiration probes. The tips of the footplates are extremely thin which allow the lens to be positioned with the footplates rolled to fit the eye.

Stromal Hydration

Stromal hydration is a good step to seal clear corneal incisions. A 24 to 26 gauze blunt cannula can be used for this purpose. The cannula is placed between the incision lips and a gentle stream of BSS is injected into the sides of the incision.

The author prefers to give a subconjunctival injection of steroid and antibiotics. The eye pad is kept on for two hours and removed subsequently. Frequent instillation of topical steroids and antiglaucoma medication is given on the same day. A good examination on a slit lamp the next day is advisable which is followed by a follow-up visit after four weeks.

IOL Tech Microincision Lens

lOL tech microincision lens (lOLtech SA, Zeiss Medi-tec A) is a single piece, square edged, 13 degrees angulated haptics, hydrophilic acrylic lens that has an overall length of 12.0 mm with an optic diameter of 5.5 mm. The IOL posseses an estimated A-constant of 119.3 in accordance with an anterior chamber depth of 5.77 mm. The large diameter and the angulations haptics minimise IOL decentration and optimise optical performance.

This lens can be implanted through a sub 2 mm incision using a disposable IOL injector.

SuperFlex and C-Flex Intraocular Lenses

SuperFlex and C-flex lOLs (Rayacryl Rayncr Intraocular Lenses Ltd) are made up of hydrophilic acrylic (a copolymer of 2-HEMA and methyl methacrylate, with ethylene glycoldimethacrylate as a cross linking agent). SuperFlex and C-Flex lOLs comprise of single piece biconvex/equiconvex sharp square edged thickness design. The IOLs are coated with benzophenone ultraviolet absorbing agent effective at between 220 and 360 nm. The IOLs have a 118.0 A-constant adjusted at the anterior chamber depth of 4.97 mm for both lenses.

The SuperFlex IOL has an overall length of 12.5 with an optical diameter of 6.25 mm, whereas the C-flex lens has an overall length of 12.0 mm with an optic size of 5.75 mm.

Implantation Technique

The SuperFlex lens can be implanted through a 2.0 mm incision using a single-use disposable injector and the C-flex lens can be implanted through a 1.8 mm incision using a single-use disposable injector.

CareFlex Microincision Cataract Surgery Intraocular Lens

CareFlex MICS Acrylic Lens (W2O Medizintechnik AG) is a single piece biconvex acrylic IOL with 26% water content. The IOL has an overall length of 10.5 mm with an optic diameter of 5.8 mm at zero degree angulation. The estimated A-constant is 118.0 at the recommended anterior chamber depth of 5.1 mm.

Ultrasmart Lens (Appasamy)

The Design of the Lens

The optics is equibiconvex and the special haptic design with slots prevents buckling or anteroposterior movement, postoperatively. The haptics structure is stiff enough to withstand the forces of capsule contraction.

The optical resolution is much better as compared to the Fresnel design. This design eliminates spherical aberration and improves the quality of the vision.

- The Nanotechnology Lathe produces the finest part of the optics, free from astigmatic aberration.
- The lens can be injected through a 1.8 mm incision. The smaller incision reduces the astigmatism. The delivery of the trailing haptics, the lens swallows by itself because of the water content and settles in its original position in the bag without using any effort or instrumentation.

Specifications:
- Optic diameter   : 6.00 mm
- Overall length   : 11.00 mm
- Positioning holes : No

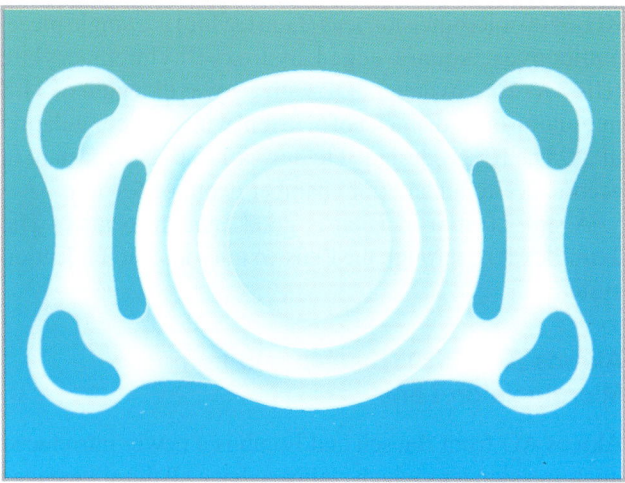

Fig. 51.16: Ultrasmart lens (Appasamy)

- Optic design : Equibiconvex
- A constant : 118.0
- Angulation : Zero degree

The lens can be injected through between a 1.8 mm incision. The smaller incision reduces astigmatism.

The lens is placed on a special injector and folded. The IOL is pushed gently through the plunger into the anterior chamber while maintaining the injector's position only at the site of incision without placing injector tip into the anterior chamber. When the lens is pushed through the injector, it slides into the bag and slowly unfolds. Hence, incision size can be restricted to up to sub two mm.

AcriFlex IOL for MICS

AcriFlex MICS Acrylic Lens 46 CSE (AcriMed GmbH) is a single piece sharp-edged, zero degree angulated acrylic-copolymer (25% water content) IOL with an overall length of 11 mm and a 5.5 mm optic size with a central thickness of 600 micron. The refractive index is 1.46 at 20°C. The estimated A-constant is 118.0/4.9 mm AC depth.

Implantation Technique

The insertion technique is similar to the Acri.Smart IOL insertion method.

Accommodative IOL for MICS: TetraFlex KH-3500

TetraFlex KH-3500 IOL is a haptic action based accommodative IOL which can be implanted through a sub 2 mm incision. This IOL generates good psuedophakic accommodation, which is based on forward movements of the IOL due to contraction of the ciliary muscles resulting in forward movements of specially designed flexible haptics.

The mechanism of accommodative action is slightly different in case of the TetraFlex IOL. Contrary to hinge optic principle, the peculiar design and configuration of haptics of TetraFlex IOL enhances forward movements of the IOL along with the entire capsular bag. The TetraFlex KH-3500 microincision lens (Lenstec Inc) is a single piece, equiconvex, square edged hydroxyethylmethacrylate (HEMA) 26% hydrated IOL with an overall length of 11.5 mm and an optic diameter of 5.75 mm with haptic angulation of 5°. The IOL is designed to have a 118.0 A – Constant in accordance to an anterior chamber depth of 5.1 mm.

A sub 2.0 mm incision is good enough to inject The TetraFlex IOL through the Lenstec microincision injection system.

Akreos AO MI-60 (Bausch and Lomb) Microincision Lens

Akreos AO from Bausch and Lomb is a newly introduced microincision lens which claims to have all the advantages of conventional Akreos AO as well as the merits of MICS.

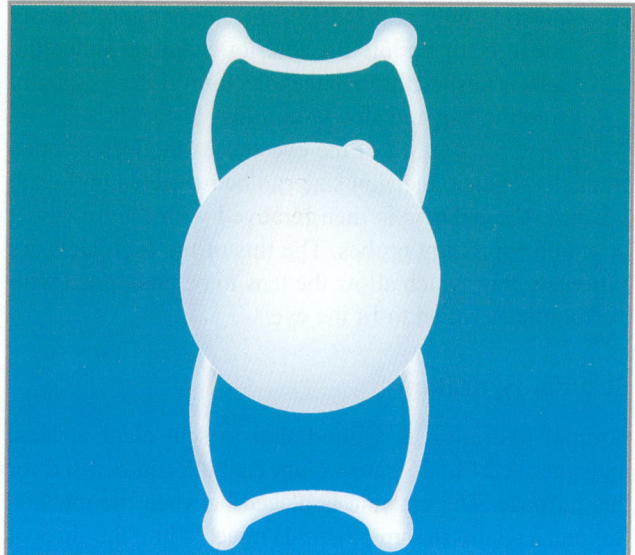

Fig. 51.17: Accommodative IOL for MICS: TetraFlex KH-3500

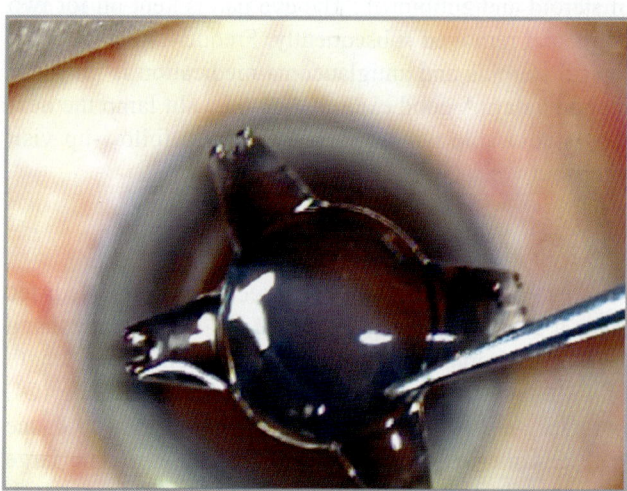

Fig. 51.18: (a) Akreos AO MI-60 (Bausch and Lomb) microincision lens

Properties/Specifications

(i) Made up of Akreos acrylic material which has an excellent track record of long-term experience of safety and biocompatibility since July 1998.
(ii) Specifications.

Overall diameter: 11.0 mm from 10.0 to 15.0 D, 10.7 mm from 15.5 to 22.0 D, 10.5 mm from 22.5 to 30.0 D

Dioptre range: 10.0 to 30.0 in 0.5 D

A-Constant

US Biometry: 118.4; Zeiss IOL Master: 118.9

ACD: 5.20

Surgeon factor: 1.45

Material: 26% hydrophilic acrylic UV blocker

Refractive index: 1.458 (hydrated)

Optic: Biconvex aspheric anterior and posterior

Optic body: 6.2 mm from 10.0 to 15.0 D, 6.0 mm from 15.5 to 22.0 D, 5.6 mm from 22.5 to 30.0 D

Haptics: One-piece with 10° average angulations

Merits

(i) Akreos AO MI-60 MICS can be implanted through a microincision of 1.80 mm size.

(ii) Made up of Akreos acrylic material with good biocompatibility.

Advanced Optics

Aspheric aberration-free optic designed for improved quality of vision.

3 Dimensional Stability

The innovative shape of the Akreos MI-60 has been designed to optimise its postoperative behaviour in the capsular bag and to allow proper positioning of IOL.

Akreos MI-60 includes a foundation zone formed by the optic and the base of the four haptics. This is the stable portion of the lens. It is surrounded by an absorption zone which bends under the contraction forces of the capsular bag. The conforming tip conforms to the curve of the periphery of the capsular bag and initiates the inflection of the absorption zone, which features an average 10° angulation.

Four Haptics: A Factor of Stability

The four-point fixation of the haptic is designed to provide stability, already clinically proven with the Akreos Adapt. This specific design allows for absorption of contraction forces of various intensities ensuring that the lens is well centred. The conforming tip conforms to the periphery of the capsular bag. Under capsular bag contraction, the two parts of the conforming tip approach each other, the absorption zone angle bends, protecting the optic from any movement.

Shaped to Fit the Capsular Anatomy

Similar to its predecessor, Akreos Adapt, the overall diameter of the Akreos MI-60 varies with the range of dioptres for consistent stability in the myopic (large), emmetropic (medium) and hyperopic (small) capsular bags.

Aspheric for Improved Quality of Vision

Spherical lenses create positive spherical aberrations. Aspheric and aberration-free lenses are found to have improved contrast sensitivity and overall optical superiority.

Anti-PCO Features

With its 360° barrier and square edge, Akreos MI-60 incorporates the same attributes as its Akreos predecessors to resisting PCO. Its 10 degree angulations are a further improvement, reinforcing the lens contact with the posterior capsule.

Early Capsular Adhesion and Durable Capsular Transparency

Adhesion of anterior and posterior capsules is achieved very quickly and visible on retroilluminated pictures two weeks after surgery. This early symphysis contributes to preserve the capsular bag transparency that is observed behind the lens optic. In addition, no fibrosis or capsular bag contraction has been noticed during the first year follow-up.

Surgical Technique

Akreos AO MI-60 MICS can be implanted through a microincision of 1.80 mm size by applying the wound-assisted injection technique. The remaining MICS technique is essentially basic and identical as required for implantation of any other MICS IOL implants.

The wound-assisted injection technique consists of using the corneal tunnel to inject the lens. It prevents the cartridge tip from being introduced into the anterior chamber. To minimise corneal stress, the internal cartridge diameter must fit the incision size. This allows the Akreos AO micro incision lens to be inserted through a 1.8 mm incision, as measured after lens injection, in a consistent manner; hence delivering maximum advantages of MICS without compromising the biocompatibility of lens material. The hydrophilic nature of the Akreos MI-60 lens and its softness help preserve the corneal integrity.

Choice of Injector

Akreos MI-60 MICS IOL is available with a specific injector designed for the wound-assisted injection technique.

We have however, found conventional injector which is being used for insertion of Akreos IOL as a better option after certain minor modifications in the delivery cartridge.

Modifications in the IOL Implant Delivery Cartridge

Delivery cartridge of Akreos can safely be converted into MICS System by converting tapered delivery end into a horizontal block pattern so as to allow the internal diameter of cartridge to remain in apposition to the internal diameter of corneal tunnel incision.

This allows MICS IOL to be delivered into anterior chamber without pushing cartridge inside the anterior chamber.

Loading Steps

The loading chamber is coated with an HPMC viscoelastic, a small amount in the opening of the cartridge tunnel, two lines in the lateral grooves.

The lens is removed from its holder by grasping the full optic with the forceps. The lens must be positioned at the

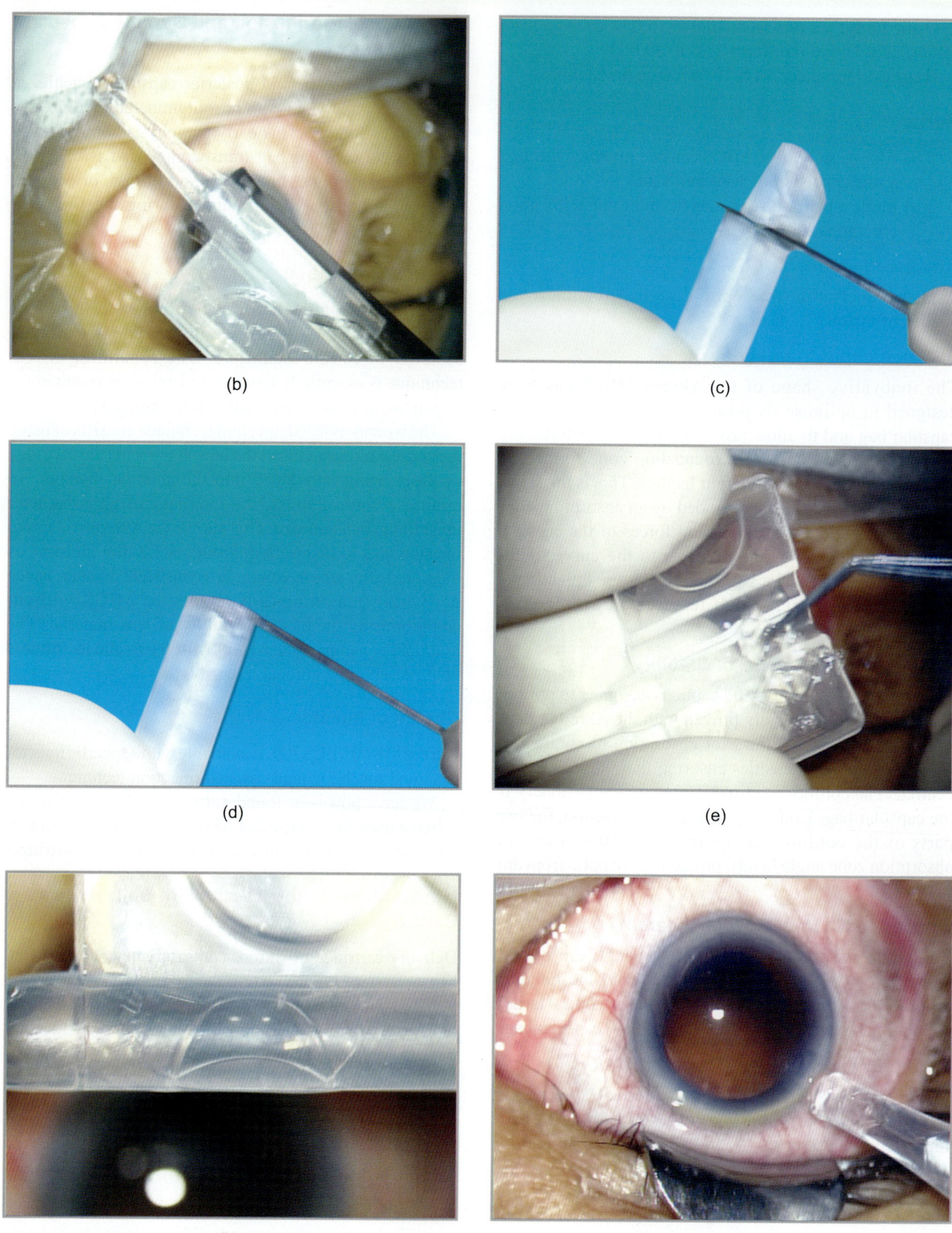

Fig. 51.18: (b) Akreos MI-60 MICS IOL loaded into standard injector, (c) Modifications in the IOL implant delivery cartridge, (d) Modified IOL implant delivery cartridge, (e) Loading of Akreos MI-60 MICS IOL into the modified cartridge, (f) Akreos MI-60 MICS IOL loaded into modified cartridge, (g) Modified injector cartridge is placed over the corneal tunnel incision

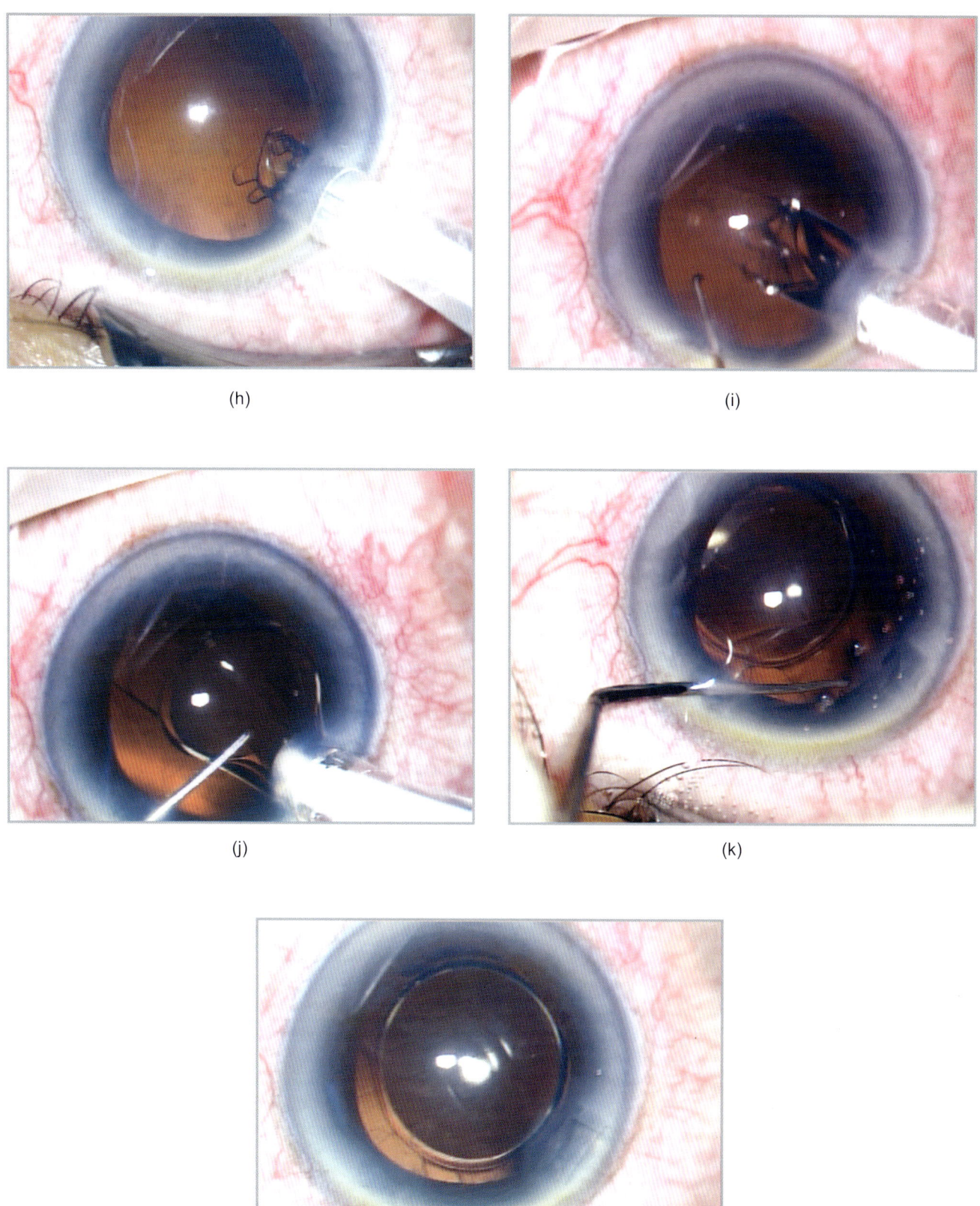

(h)

(i)

(j)

(k)

(l)

Fig. 51.18: (h) Commencement of delivery of MICS IOL into the AC, (i) Unfolding of MICS IOL into the AC, (j) MICS IOL is being positioned into the capsular bag, (k) Positioning of the trailing haptics into the bag, (l) Well placed MICS IOL

top of the holder, anterior face up. The position of the lens is checked before loading, the haptics must be oriented upwards.

The lens is placed in the centre of the loading chamber and the haptics are pushed down inside the lateral grooves.

The cartridge is closed and locked after having checked that no lens material is trapped between the wings.

The cartridge is placed in the injector and the plunger is advanced slowly until the silicone cushion has reached the tunnel opening. The lens is ready for injection.

IOL Implantation Technique

(i) Modified cartridge is placed over the incision site of corneal tunnel.
(ii) The compressed IOL is subsequently pushed gently into the anterior chamber through forward motion of the plunger while maintaining the injector's position only at the site of incision without placing the injector tip into the anterior chamber.

When the lens is pushed through the injector, it slides gradually into the bag and slowly unfolds.

The IOL may be positioned into the bag with the assistance of the second instrument (Synskey's hook or 'Y' pusher).

The remaining steps of postimplantation removal of residual viscous are essentially the same as applicable to other IOL implant surgery.

Conventional Foldable IOL Implants in MICS

The main concern with MICS remains the long-term behaviour, efficacy, adaptability and overall performance of ultrathin IOLs over other conventional acrylic hydrophobic IOL implants which are considered as the best option at present. Considering various factors, some surgeons have been using hydrophobic IOL implants following MICS after enlarging the incision up to 3 mm. Obviously such a technique will definitely loose merits of microincision cataract surgery. To enjoy the privilege and superiority of a sub 2 mm incision, successful attempts have been made by several surgeons to insert conventional hydrophobic IOLs like AcrySof through a two mm incision while using the same technique after certain modifications. In this technique, the tip of the injector cartridge is cut at the tip and made like zero degree phaco tip. This modified cartridge is just kept at the site of incision and the IOL is pushed through a 2.2 mm incision in the same manner as described for other thin IOLs.

Complications

The incidence of complications in phaconit surgery is as low as in the case of coaxial phacoemulsification technique. The procedure is very much convenient and acceptable to surgeons as well as to the eyes.

The author did not face any severe sight threatening complication in his personal experience. However, certain minor complications or problems are expected in any surgical procedure. Such events are as follows:

Intraoperative Complications

(i) Surge/chamber collapse: 5 to 8%
(ii) Iris chaffing: 01%
(iii) Corneal burn: 01%
(iv) Inadvertent posterior capsule rent (< 2 mm) 1 to 2%

Postoperative Complications (Early/Intermediate)

(i) Moderate corneal striate (disappear within 3 days) 5 to 8%
(ii) Uveitis (mild to moderate) 5%
(iii) Secondary glaucoma (after 2 weeks) 3.25%
(iv) Macular oedema (3.75%) which generally declines within three weeks postoperatively.

Delayed

(i) Secondary glaucoma (after 2 weeks) 2%
(ii) Macular oedema: 1 to 2%, usually associated with preexisting ocular or intraoperative complications.

Incidence of posterior capsular opacification is 2–2.5% within 9–12 months and up to 5% after 3 years. This incidence is based on other factors like grading of nucleus and intra or subsequent postoperative complications lile uveitis and glaucoma. The author had observed a relatively higher incidence of PCO up to 3.5 % in cases of Grade III nucleus and more than 5% in Grade IV nucleus densities. In contrast to this, very hard and soft cataracts have been found to have very less incidence of PCO which was up to 1.25% in his personal series.

Induced Astigmatism

In our experience, initial postoperative induced astigmatism ranges from +0.25 D to +0.75 D. However, it had regressed and stabilised within one to two weeks as compared to four to six weeks in cases of Acrylic IOL implantation through a 3 mm incision. Ultimate postoperative induced astigmatism was restricted up to +/– nil to 0.5 D as compared to ± 0.25 to 0.75 D in cases of Acrylic IOL implantation through a 3 mm incision. Best-corrected visual acuity of 6/5 was achieved by 3rd to 5th day.

Impact of Ultrathin IOL Implant over Near Visual Acuity

Ultrathin IOLs have been found to have better pseudophakic accommodation and near visual acuity as compared to conventional foldable IOL implants. In our experience, 70% patients had attained uncorrected visual acuity of N/10 after 6 months, whereas 85% were found to have N/12 during the same period. However, this had shown a marginal decline after one year, where up to 50% were found to have N/12 uncorrected near visual acuity. Despite such variations, all cases were found to have N/5 corrected visual acuity (Near vision correction ranged between 1.25 D Sph to 1.75 D Sph over distant vision correction).

Merits of MICS/PHACONIT (NIT JIT 23)

Bimanual MICS has several and definite merits over the conventional coaxial phacoemulsification:
- Closed procedure—less complications
- No to anaesthesia
- Ultra micro small incision: quick healing
- Least astigmatism/risk of endophthalmitis
- Ride and tide: no restrictions (earliest rehabilitation)

  (i) Least astigmatism: Minimal surgically induced astigmatism due to smaller size of incisions.
 (ii) Better retention of viscoelastics in the AC due to a practically sealed anterior chamber.
(iii) Smooth and stable intra cameral manipulations while performing capsulorrhexis, hydrodissection and hydrodelineation due to the fact that the smaller incision provides better AC stability and enhanced mydriasis over relatively larger incisions in case of coaxial phacoemulsification techniques.
 (iv) Increased intraoperative maneuvrability of phaco tip because separate fluid irrigation and aspiration lining facilitates fragment aspiration which is not adversely influenced by direction of fluid inflow.
  (v) Better control and efficacy during cortical removal, since bimanual I/A offers interchangeability of irrigation and the aspiration port. This is highly beneficial, particularly in handling subincisional cortex or densely adhered and sticky cortex and posterior plates. Another advantage is the ability to use the stream of irrigation fluid from the irrigating chopper as an instrument in the eye. If the lens material gets caught in the angle, one can automatically use fluid stream to wash it out rather than using another instrument.
 (vi) Less chances of inadvertent posterior capsular rent since fluid inflow through a separate irrigation port always directs the posterior capsule posteriorly. This protects the capsule against suddenly getting caught by the aspiration port.
(vii) Least pressure on zonules during I/A is hence very useful in cases of zonular dehiscence, subluxated cataracts, high myopia, miotic pupils, endothelial disease, pseudoexfoliation, postretinal detachment or vitrectomy surgery cataracts.
(viii) Theoretically surgeons believe that the smaller the incision, the less the likelihood that patients will develop endophthalmitis. A smaller incision leaks

less postoperatively and is less likely to draw in fluid from the eye, which can cause infection.
 (ix) Bimanual method of phacoaspiration and phacofragmentation achieves an effective utilisation of phacopower ranging from 5% to 40% (average 10–20%). This requirement of phaco-power was much less as compared to the standard phacoemulsification (30–50% phacopower).
  (x) Phaconit has definite superiority in terms of visual acuity and early rehabilitation over the standard phacoemulsification surgery.

Demerits/Constraints of MICS

The MICS technique had faced several constraints during the initial phase of conversion from coaxial phaco to bimanual phaco, since all phacoemulsifier systems have been designed to perform at specific fluid dynamics which is essentially required for smooth and efficient yet the most precise surgical technique. Certain modifications essentially required for MICS had definitely altered fluid dynamics of the machine, in terms of reduced inflow and outflow of fluids and vacuum parameters, as well. However, newer generation high end phacoemulsifier systems are well equipped with the latest software, microprocessor, and fluidic system which are specifically tailored for MICS technique, hence making the MICS a very safe and precise technique of cataract removal. Despite such modifications, certain under mentioned constraints of MICS still need attention:

  (i) The relatively tight incisions without sleeves may produce thermal injury at the site of incision.
 (ii) Fluid leakage through smaller incisions is difficult to regulate and may produce surge resulting in anterior chamber instability during phacoemulsification.
(iii) Compromised fluid in and outflow due to the use of smaller gauge instruments requires lower vacuum levels, as well as increased bottle heights and various surge control devices. Manufacturers are addressing these fluidic issues with new devices, such as larger-bore irrigating choppers (Micro-surgical Technologies, Redmond, WA), low compliance tubing (SuperVac, Staar Surgical, Monrovia, CA), pressurised inflow (Storz Premiere system, Bausch and Lomb, Rochester, NY), and postocclusion surge reduction (Cruise Control, Staar Surgical, Monrovia, CA).

Likely Disadvantages of Microincision/Rollable IOLs

  (i) Ring shadows/haloes: Observed by a number of patients, particularly when they are exposed to glare and motor vehicle lights. However, most of the patients remain comfortable.

(ii) YAG compatibility YAG capsulotomy is being considered difficult due to the ultrathinness of IOLs and a very close proximity to the posterior capsule. The incidence of PCO was found to be less than 10% after the follow-up period of more than three years. We did not notice any difficulty while performing YAG laser capsulotomy in these cases. Energy required for this procedure remained within 1.5 MJ. We have attempted to break the microincision IOL by direct exposure to YAG beam. However, IOL remained unaffected up to 2 MJ, except normal pitting. IOL sustained against tear up to direct exposure of 7 MJ. Hence, this may not be affected even during the YAG iridotomy procedure in case of direct exposure.

Position of the Implanted Intraocular Lenses

Changed IOL position in the bag is expected in certain number of cases following any IOL implant surgery due to changes in the bag particularly in the status of anterior capsule. However, we did not notice any altered position of ultrathin IOL in any case of MICS except in one case of concurrent phaconit and trabeculectomy where postoperative uveitis resulted in posterior synechiae which had tilted the IOL in the bag.

What is Next in MICS IOL Implants

Medennium Smart lOL (Medennium, Inc, Irvine, California, USA) is the latest breakthrough in the IOL technology which is yet to be made available for MICS in clinical practice. Medennium Smart lOL is based on the innovative idea to replace human crystalline lens material by compressible material so as to allow capsular bag to be filled by the material exactly in accordance with the optical and functional properties of human crystalline lens material. This innovative idea is another doorstep towards ultimate goal of cataract removal through the most the ultrathin micro prick opening into the anterior capsule. This concept is yet to address and establish the longterm physical, optical and biochemical stability of the material and capability of readjusting the dioptric power as well.

The Smart IOL is made up of a thermodynamic hydrophobic acrylic material with unique thermoplastic properties having chemically bonding wax to acrylic polymer which allows the IOL to remain in the solid state at normal temperatures. The thermoplastic properties facilitate temperature-induced changes in its shape.

Physical and Optical Properties

The refractive index of the material is 1.47. Effective glass transition function temperature is 20–30°C. Following implantation, the wax component melts at body temperature; hence adjusting the quantity of wax content so as to spread into the entire capsular bag of 10 mm and form a 3.5 mm thick intercapsular gelatinous polymer biconvex IOL in the bag. The complete process of transition takes less than 30 seconds.

The peculiarity of the insertion technique is to have pre-implantation warming of the IOL to allow it to mold into the 50 mm long rod. Once this rod-shaped IOL is inserted into the capsular bag and allowed to attend the body temperature inside the bag, it gets back to the predetermined shape and dioptre of an IOL with a diameter of 10 mm and 350 micron thickness. The Smart lOL is not yet available on a commercial basis until detailed clinical trials are conducted for appropriate evaluation.

CONCLUSION

Phaconit is an advancement in phacoemulsification surgery and is bound to overshadow the standard phaco procedure. It requires a better technology machine and instrumentation as well as better rollable lenses. On the surgeon's side, it requires a high degree of skill and dexterity to achieve an excellent surgical outcome.

BIBLIOGRAPHY

1. Alio JL, Rodriguez-Prats JL, Galal A. Microincision cataract surgery. Highlights of Ophthalomology International, Miami USA. 2004.
2. Alio J.L Rodriguez-Prats J.L Galal A.et al. Outcomes of Microincision cataract surgery versus coaxial phaco-emulsification. Ophthalmology 2005; 22 [Epubahead of print].
3. Alio JL, Schimchak P, Mico RM, Galal A. Retinal image quality after microincision intraocular lens implantation. J Cataract Refract Surg 2005; 31: 1557–1560.
4. Wehner W. Dehydrated prerolled acrylic lens for 1.5 mm incision. Proceedings of the ESCRS Meeting, Amsterdam, The Netherlands, 2001.
5. Wehner W. Clinical results with the Acri.Smart IOL implanted through a 1.4 mm incision. Proceedings of the ASCRS Meeting, San Francisco, California, USA, 2003.
6. Koch R. Cataract Surgery through a 2.0 mm incision; Results of bimanual phaco-chop technique and acrylic IOL implantation. Proceedings of the ASCRS Meeting, San Francisco, CA, USA, 2003.
7. Pandey SK, Werner L, Agarwal A, et al. Phakonit: cataract removal through a sub-1.0 mm incision and implantation of the ThinOptX reliable intraocular lens. J Cataract Refract Surg 2002; 28:1710–1712.
8. Alio J, Rodriguez-Prats JL, Vianello A, Galal A. Visual outcome of microincision cataract surgery with implantation

of Acri.Smart Lens. J Cataract Refract Surg 2005; 31:1549–1556.

9. Alio JL, Rodriguez-Prats JL, Galal A. Microincision cataract surgery and implantation of ThinOptX intraocular lens. Proceedings of the ESCRS Meeting, Paris, 2004.

10. Verges C. Bimanual microincision cataract surgery and implantation of IOL-tech MICS microincision lens. Proceedings of the ESCRS Meeting, Lisbon, 2005.

11. Sunita Agarwal, Athiya Agarwal, Mahipal S Sachdev, Keiki R Mehta, I Howard Fine, Amar Agarwal: Phacoemulsification, Laser Cataract Surgery and Foldable IOL's; Second edition Jaypee Brothers; 2000, Delhi, India.

12. Dogru M, Honda R, Omoto M, Fujishima H, Yagi Y, Tsubota K, Kojima T, Matsuyama M, Nishijima S, Yagi Y. Early visual results with the Rollable ThinOptX intraocular lens. J Cataract Refract Surg. 2004 Mar; 30(3):558–65.

13. Agarwal Amar, Agarwal Athiya, Agarwal Sunita. Rollable IOL enhances cataract surgery through 0.9 mm incision. Ocular Surgery News Europe /Asia Pacific Edition 2/1/2002.

14. P. Stodulka. 1.5 mm cataract surgery with rollable IOL – first 30 operations in the Czech Republic. Cataract Surgery Outcomes 2003.

15. Roibeard O'hÉineacháin. Anterior chamber maintainer adequate for micro surgery, ECRS; December 2002.

16. Dodick, Jck Is ophthalmology ready for lens implants through ultra-small incisions? Intraoperative control through a watertight incision and a truly astigmatic-neutral wound would be of value. Ophthalmology Times; December 15, 2001.

17. Shearing SP, Relyea RL, Louiza A, et al. Routine phacoemulsification through a one-millimeter nonsutured incision. Cataract 1985; 2:6–11.

18. Girard LJ. Ultrasonic fragmentation for cataract extraction and cataract complications. Adv Ophthalmol 1978; 37:127–135.

19. Fine IH, Packer M, Hoffman RS. New phacoemulsification technologies, J Cataract Refract Surg 2002; 28:1054–1060.

20. Hoffman RS, Fine IH, Packer M. New phacoemulsification technology, Current Opinion, Ophthalmol 2005; 16:38–43.

21. Soscia W, Howard JG, Olson RJ. Bimanual phacoemulsification through stab incisions: a wound-temperature study. J Cataract Refract Surg 2002; 28:1039–43.

22. Soscia W, Howard JG, Olson RJ. Microphacoemulsification with WhiteStar: a wound-temperature study. J Cataract Refract Surg 2002; 28:1044–1046.

23. Donnenfeld ED, Olson RJ, Solomon R, et al. Efficacy and wound-temperature gradient of WhiteStar phacoemulsification through a 1.2 mm incision. J Cataract Refract Surg 2003; 29:1097–1100.

24. Braga-Mele R, Liu E. Feasibility of sleeveless bimanual phacoemulsification with the Millennium microsurgical system. J Cataract Refract Surg 2003; 29:2199–2203.

25. Mackool RJ, Brint SF. AquaLase: a new technology for cataract extraction. Curr Opin Ophthalmol 2004; 15:40–43.

26. Olson RJ, Jin Y, Kefalopoulos G, et al. Legacy AdvanTec and Sovereign WhiteStar: A wound temperature study. J Cataract Refract Surg 2004; 30: 1109–1113.

27. Olson MD, Miller KM. In air thermal imaging comparison of Legacy Advan-Tec, Millennium, an Sovereign WhiteStar phacoemulsification systems. J Cataract Refract Surg 2005; 31:1640–1647.

28. Tsueoka H, Hayama A, Takahama M. Ultrasmall-incision bimanual phacoemulsification and AcrySof SA30AL implantation through a 2.2 mm incision. J Cataract Refract Surg 2003; 29:1070–1076.

29. Rose AD. Coaxial and bimanual phacoemulsification; considerations in patient and technique selection. Tech Ophthalmol 2005; 3:63–70. Detailed summary of one surgeon's technique and experience with bimanual phacoemulsification, including a wealth of practical information.

30. Fine IH, Hoffman RS, Packer M. Optimising refractive lens exchange with bimanual microincision phacoemulsification. J Cataract Refract Surg 2004; 30:550–54.

31. Chang DF. 400 mmHg High-vacuum bimanual phaco attainable with the Staar Cruise control device. J Cataract Refract Surg 2004; 30:932–933.

32. Stratas BA. Clear corneal paracentesis: A case of chronic wound leakage in a patient having bimanual phacoemulsification. J Cataract Refract Surg 2005; 31:1075.

33. Tsuneoka H, Shiba T, Takahama M. Ultrasonic phacoemulsification using a 1.4 mm incision: clinical results. J Cataract Refract Surg 2002; 28:81–86.

34. Agarwal A, Agarwal A, Agarwal S, et a/. Phakonit: phacoemulsification through a 0.9 mm corneal incision. J Cataract Refract Surg 2001; 27:1548–1552.

35. Olson RJ. Clinical experience with 21-gauze manual microphacoemulsification using Sovereign WhiteStar Technology in eyes with dense cataract. J Cataract Refract Surg 2004; 30:168–172.

52

Laser Phaco

Dr S Kelkar

INTRODUCTION

Cataract surgery has evolved considerably over a period of time and it continues to do so. From the time of ICCE to ECCE and phacoemulsification, the main aim of the surgeon has remained to find a better and less traumatic way to remove the cataractous lens and to achieve good postoperative visual recovery. Introduction and development of phaco was a big leap forward in this direction. Development in IOL technology has given an edge to phaco. Phacoemulsification with foldable intraocular lens is now a standard and well accepted procedure giving good postoperative visual results with minimum postoperative induced astigmatism. Refractive cataract surgery is not a new technique now. In the new millennium, what surgeons are looking forward to is to achieve total emmetropia with the full range of accommodation as in the virgin lens, thereby truly replacing the natural lens.

Though phacoemulsification has become a gold standard for cataract surgery, it is not without its own disadvantages. Use of ultrasound energy is associated with heat production and resultant endothelial damage and wound burns. This, along with a longer learning curve, makes the surgery not so easy to master. Advances in the phaco machine, fluidics and tip design have made things a lot simpler now-a-days. Still, search for new energy modes to remove cataract, which would be far safer than ultrasound, is high on the agenda of many scientist and companies. In this quest for newer technologies, laser is a natural choice for its ability to cause tissue breakdown with precision.

For more than two decades use of lasers in cataract removal is under investigation and the technology has been developed over the period to be made commercially available.

Laser cataract removal holds the promise of removing cataract with the help of a fiber optic probe through a tiny incision made in the capsule and removing the cataractous lens through it. This possibility has given big hope of achieving true accommodation with injectable IOLs. The extremely rapid development in laser technology has led to two types of solid-state laser systems for cataract extraction. The ER-YAG and Nd-YAG are currently being tested.

HISTORY OF LASER CATARACT SURGERY

The ability of lasers to remove tissues with a high degree of precision and the availability of a wide range of laser frequencies in the industry for a number of years now has prompted their use in cataract surgery. Both ultraviolet and infrared lasers were tried in the past.

Attempts to utilise lasers with different wavelengths (short ultraviolet as well as near infrared wavelengths) in cataract surgery were started in the mid-eighties.

Ultraviolet lasers were in use in ophthalmology for keratorefractive surgeries, and their ability to cut tissues with precision is well known. The 193 nm laser is a well established tool for precise cutting of the cornea. However, ultraviolet lasers were found not suitable for the laser cataract surgery. These wavelengths are not suitable for fiber optic delivery and in addition have a cataractogenic property making them hazardous to the surgical team.

Other ultraviolet frequencies used in the past were ultraviolet diode lasers, tuneable dye lasers and even the 5th harmonic Nd-YAG laser (213 nm). All these frequencies were found incompatible with fiber optic delivery and not useful for cataract removal. Based on a survey of recent literature, it can be stated that the use of both excimer and picosecond lasers was largely discontinued due to technical problems, high equipment costs, and considerable risks (e.g. primary and secondary radiation of the laser beam).

The Turning Point

In 1991 Dr. Jack Dodick in New York described the method of cataract removal using laser energy. A pulsed Q– switched Nd: YAG laser similar to capsulotomy lasers is used to ignite a plasma on a titanium target. This phenomenon is used to create shock-waves which are used to disrupt the nucleus of a cataractous lens.

Infrared lasers used in the past gave initial success in cataract removal. These were found to have the required cutting power as well as suitability for easy delivery through a hand held probe. In the past a two step technique using Nd-YLF laser was tried experimentally where laser delivered through the slit lamp causes softening of the lens which then could be aspirated subsequently in the operation room as the second step.

The extremely rapid development in laser technology has led to two types of solid-state laser systems for cataract extraction – the ER-YAG and Nd-YAG, that a currently being tested. Both these techniques hold the promise to the future. However, a considerable difference exists between these two laser systems which will be discussed in detail subsequently.

Basic differences in Erbium-YAG Laser and Nd-YAG Systems

The effect of the Erbium-YAG laser is based on tile high absorption of its wavelength (2936 nm) in water. The energy is kept to a minimum by using short pulses, in order to avoid an increase in temperature.

In contrast, tile Nd-YAG laser (1064 nm) works based on the principle which has been used for several years in YAG-capsulotomy – the generation of both plasma and shock waves.

Nd-YAG Laser Systems

Nd-YAG lasers are in use in the industry and in ophthalmology for many years. It was well established for many years and the properties and industrial usage of this laser were well known when it was attempted for the cataract surgery and it was found successful.

How the Technology Works?

A standard Nd: YAG laser is used to generate a six nano second laser pulse. This laser pulse is channeled and focused into a 300 micron quartz fiber. The fiber is inserted into an irrigating and aspirating handpiece through the aspiration channel. At the end of the aspiration channel, a titanium target is present. When the laser pulse strikes a titanium target, plasma is ignited. This is soon followed by a shock wave which is sufficient to fragment the nuclear fragments. At no time is the eye exposed to the infrared laser since the target acts as a backstop for light leakage.

Additionally this irrigating aspirating handpiece can be used to aspirate residual cortex and the epinucleus once the nucleus has been ablated.

Nd-YAG based laser systems are divided into two types
  (i) Direct acting system
  (ii) Indirect acting system.

Direct Acting System (PhotonLaser-Phacolysis)

These systems utilise lasers which come in direct contact with the cataractous tissue without any intervening interface.

The Photon Laser Phaco Lysis system (Paradigm Medical) which is a direct acting system is used as an Nd: YAG 1,064 nm laser to produce photo-acoustic ablation of cataract material under aspiration. The specially designed 1.8 mm diameter ski-shaped distal tip of the probe curves up to intersect the laser light emitted from the optical fiber. The laser energy travels from the phaco tip into an open area called photo fragmentation zone. This is a 2.5 mm zone around the tip of the laser probe. The breakdown of the nucleus takes place in this zone.

The aspiration inlet is placed in the face of the tip, creating a photon trap. Thus, all rays of laser photons that enter the aspiration port are internally reflected and kept within the probe tip. While some minimal heating of tissue occurs, the heat is very rapidly removed by aspiration and the temperature of the probe tip only rises by approximately 1° C.

The Nd:YAG system has the potential for deeper penetration and damage to the tissues internally. For this reason the peak intensity of the photon of laser phaco lysis system is kept more than 10,000 times below that required for the onset of plasma generation, the operative action during posterior capsulotomy. Therefore, the photon laser phaco lysis system represents an exceptionally safe modality in terms of capsular integrity.

Indirect Acting System (Dodick ARC Photolysis)

As the name suggests, this phacoemulsification laser system (ARC Laser Corporation) does not allow direct contact between the laser and the tissue to be broken down but the energy is transmitted indirectly to cause fragmentation of the tissue. It was Dr Jack M Dodick who pioneered this system and it goes by the name of 'Dodick laser Photolysis'.

Using this system, the pulsed Nd:YAG (1064 nm) laser is made to fall on the titanium mirror. Laser energy is transmitted from the source by a quartz fiber which then strikes a titanium target on the surface of which optical breakdown and plasma formation occurs. The optical breakdown causes shock waves to emanate toward the distal opening of the probe. It is at this opening that the shock waves make contact with the lens material, which is held in apposition with the tip of the probe by suction.

The shock waves disrupt the lens material at the mouth of the probe and the fragmented material is then aspirated out. Thus with this system, there is no direct exposure of the Nd: YAG laser to either the lens or surrounding tissues and heat produced is minimal.

Nd:YAG photolysis represents a low energy modality for cataract extraction. The heat generated is minimal requiring no cooling of the tip and the system works without the irrigation sleeve. This causes reduction in entry wound size required associated with minimum endothelial loss and wound burn.

"This system continues to work effectively even by keeping infusion separately from the laser emulsifying probe, thus making it possible to perform sub 1.2 mm incisions bimanual microphaco cataract surgery.

The author (Dr SB Kelkar) has evaluated the efficacy and adaptability of Laser phaco systems in 50 cases with grade 2+ cataracts of variable nature; peculiar to the scenario of Indian subcontinent specially the rural areas. All these patients had no other ophthalmic problem.These patients were posted for sutureless cataract surgery using the laser phaco. These patients were followed-up for 3 months.

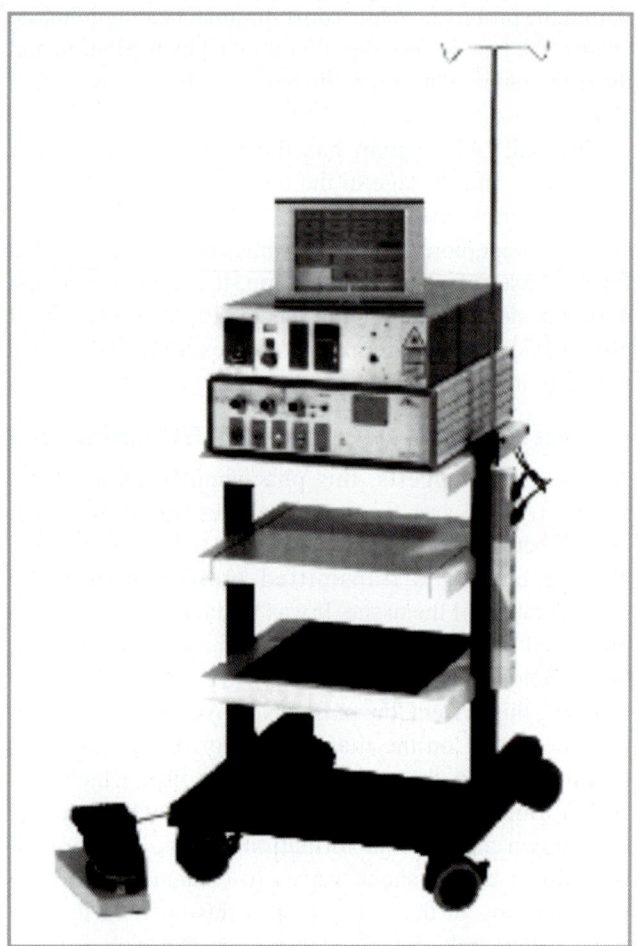

Fig. 52.1: Dodick ARC photolysis machine

He has designed a new probe using smaller fibers that will perform this procedure through a 1 mm incision.

Surgical Technique adopted by Dr SB Kelkar

Two 1.4 mm corneal paracentesis wounds were made, one for infusion and the other for a probe containing laser fiber and aspiration.

The nucleus was ablated with the help of repeated laser pulses. Approximately 300 shots were used at 10 mJ to ablate 2+ nuclear cataract.

Following the ablation of nucleus, the cortex was aspirated out with the same probe.

The incision was subsequently enlarged upto to 3 mm to implant foldable IOL implants.

It is hoped that this technology will spur the development of smaller incisions and perhaps foldable lenses to take advantage of this technology.

Out of 50 patients, 30 patients underwent uncomplicated laser cataract surgery and achieved BCVA of 6/12 or better.

The author could perform uneventful, uncomplicated laser cataract surgery in thirty eyes out of fifty cases. All these cases could achieve BCVA of 6/12 or better. However, the laser phaco was found unsuitable in the remaining cases, as the nucleus was found to be too hard for the laser phaco. Hence, the procedure was converted and conventional use phacoemulsifier system was used.

Two patients cases who underwent laser phaco had developed the PC rent. These patients had BCVA of 6/18 at the end of 2 months. No other complication were observed.

It could not be used for cataracts of more than 2+ hardness of the nucleus. Despite initial constraints of technology and cost efficacy, the system has some potential advantages:
- Smaller and a more ergonometric handpiece
- No moving parts inside the eye
- Same probe for I and A
- Disposable handpiece
- No clinically significant heat
- Eyes are not exposed to direct laser light – All light is enclosed in the handpiece
- Most cataracts of upto 2+ nucleus can be removed with 200 – 500 shots at 10 mJ
- Technology operates at only 1.5 Hz
- Corneal endothelium-friendly
- Glamour.

Laser phaco is still in its infancy, more research needs to be done to make the technique superior to US Phaco. In the author's view Nd: YAG Laser Phaco is a safe and effective mode of treatment available for cataract surgery but it does not have any remarkable advantages over US Phaco.

SYSTEMS USING ERBIUM LASER

Er:YAG laser phacoemulsification represents an emerging technology in cataract surgery. The potential advantages of the erbium laser over ultrasound include relative reduction in the energy requirement for cataract extraction and the absence of any potential for thermal injury to the cornea.

The Er:YAG laser was initially investigated for cataract surgery by Peyman and Katoh and Tsubota in the 1980s.

The Er-YAG laser is mid infrared laser of wavelength of 2.94 µm (2940 nm) in the infrared spectrum. It is highly absorbed by water. Since, the crystalline lens is composed of about 63% water, the Er: YAG laser is believed to be well-suited to achieve phacovaporisation of the lens.

Centauri Er:YAG developed by Premier Laser Systems (California) and MCL-29 developed by Asclepion-Meditec (Germany) are currently available.

Mechanism of Action of Er-YAG Laser

The mechanism of action of Er-YAG laser has been extensively studied. The explosive evaporation causes the cavitation bubble. This cavitation bubble implodes causing breakdown of the nuclear material. The ablation depth is 1 µm. However, as the laser energy from the successive pulses traverses this ablation zone to cause the micro cavitation beyond the first bubble the area of ablation is greater than 1 µm. In water, the cavitation bubble collapses but in the lens, the collapse of the bubble occurs more slowly. The laser beam can travel across the first bubble and form a second bubble in line with the first. If a third bubble forms it increases the effective range of the laser to 3 µm. A direct concussive effect of the laser energy emulsifies the lens material.

Advantages of Erbium Laser Phacoemulsification

Erbium laser phacoemulsification represents an emerging technology with several promising attributes.
- Suitable to up to grade two to three types of cataract.
- No heating of the anterior chamber and high protection of corneal endothelium.

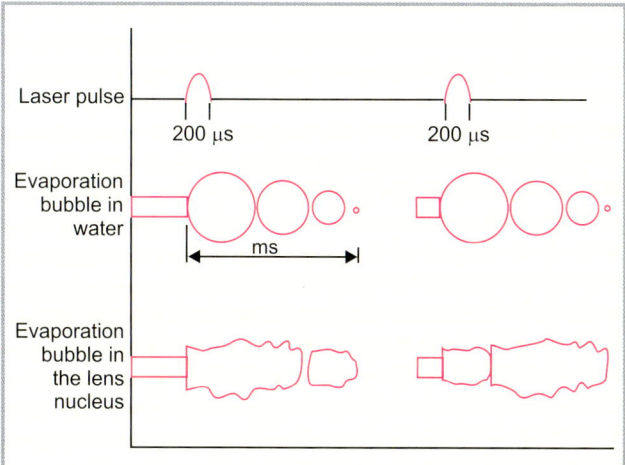

Fig. 52.2: Mechanism of action of Er-YAG laser

- One of the principal advantages of Er:YAG system is the absence of risk from thermal injury. Because the tip of the erbium laser system does not produce heat, the risk of corneal burn is eliminated and there is no need for a sleeve. Hence, endothelial cell loss is not very significant. The tip diameter can be smaller without the sleeve. The system provides the best absorption of laser under fluids.
- Less energy transmission to the eye.
- Potential reduction of incision size.
- smooth cutting capability – useful for capsulotomy.
- Smooth learning curve.

Limitations of Erbium Laser Phacosystem

- The current techniques are useful in soft cataract and they are less effective in dense nuclei making them incompatible in the Indian scenario where hard cataracts are a rule rather than the exception.
- Fibre material in erbium laser phacosystems is made up of zirconium fluoride and sapphire. Zirconium fluoride is sensitive to hydroscopic change. So cannot be autoclaved. Fibre is very expensive and has a variable life span. Sapphire is an alternative material. Fibers made of this can be autoclaved and last longer, but are more brittle and have relatively low transmission power.
- The existing system is not cost effective due to very high initial and running cost. Presently, laser cataract systems are priced well above the high end phaco-machines. This makes them not easily available for use.

Over and above, fibre material in erbium laser phaco systems are known to lose power during the course of surgery, requiring replacement. However, the future development in laser phaco system may help to make this small incision cataract surgery more accessible to more number of surgeons.
- Surgical time is much more and prolonged as compared to ultrasonic phacoemulsification or with other laser systems.
- Intraoperative complications—Potential risk of intra operative complications, particularly posterior capsule rent and other related risks.

MCL-29 Er: YAG Laser Developed by Asclepion-Meditec (Germany)

Positive results with the MCL-29 led to the development of the Phacolase (Asclepion-Meditec). This Er:YAG laser features a variable pulse energy from 5 mJ to 50 mJ, as well as a variable frequency from 10 Hz to 100 Hz. The Phacolase system is coupled to a megatron irrigation/aspiration (I&A) pump. The megatron has a peristaltic pump with venturi-like effect. The phacolase handpiece incorporates the laser fiber inside the aspiration port.

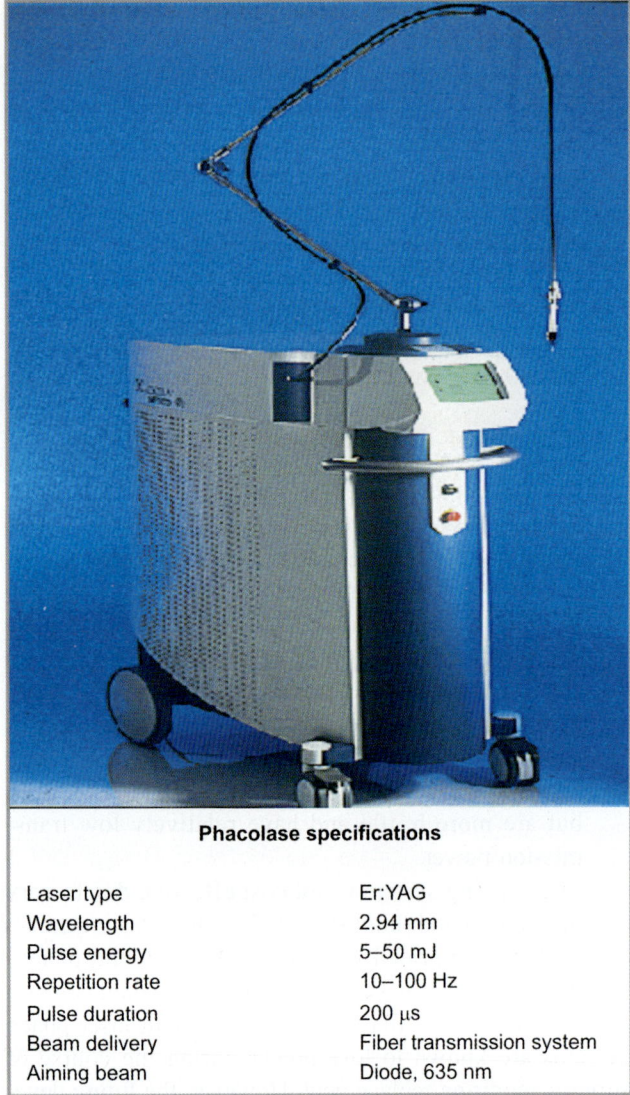

Phacolase specifications

Laser type	Er:YAG
Wavelength	2.94 mm
Pulse energy	5–50 mJ
Repetition rate	10–100 Hz
Pulse duration	200 µs
Beam delivery	Fiber transmission system
Aiming beam	Diode, 635 nm

Fig. 52.3: MCL-29 Er-YAG laser machine

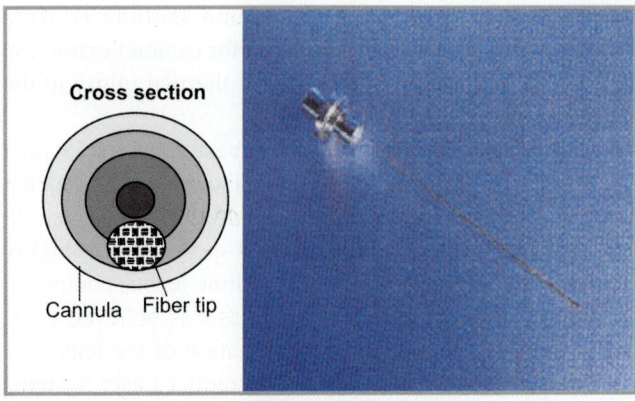

Fig. 52.4: Phacolase handpiece

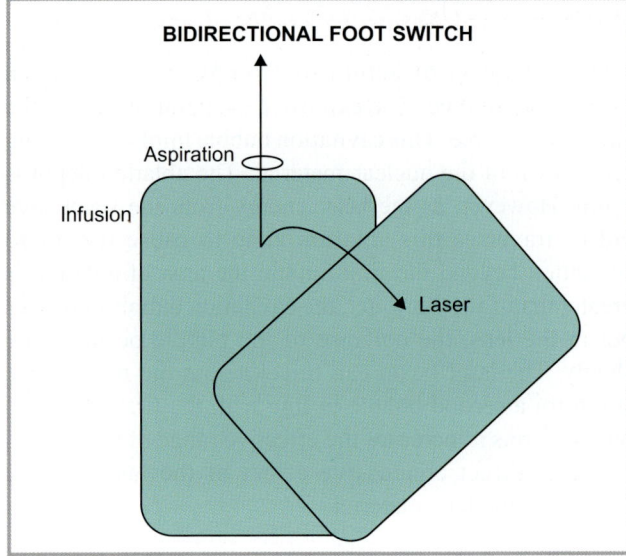

Fig. 52.5: Bidirectional footswitch of the phacolase machine

A bidirectional foot switch separates infusion and aspiration from laser energy. Moving the foot pedal laterally increases the repetition rate in a linear fashion. Pushing the pedal down provides linear control of vacuum.

CONCLUSION

Laser for cataract removal is still in its infancy stage. It is a new and novel approach, which holds promises and is expected to take centre stage in future.

BIBLIOGRAPHY

1. Kelman CD: Phacoemulsification and aspiration—a new technique of cataract removal, a preliminary report. Am J Ophthalmol 64:23–35, 1967.
2. "Use of Neodymium-YAG laser for removal of cataracts is reported". Ophthalmology Times 1: 1989.
3. "First Laser Phacolysis proves a success". Ophthalmology Times, 1991.
4. Dodick JM, Sperber LTD, Lally JM et al: Nd:YAC laser phacolysis of human cataractous lens—a case report. Arch Ophthalmol 111: 903–04,1993.
5. Aasuri MK, Basti S: Laser cataract surgery. Current Opinion in Ophthalmology 10:53–58, 1999.
6. Dodick JM: Laser phacolysis of the human cataractous lens. Dev Ophthalmol 22:58–64, 1991.
7. Dodick JM, Lally JM, Sperber LTD: Lasers in cataract surgery. Current Opinion in Ophthalmology 4(1):107–09,1993.
8. Dodick JM, Cristiansen J. Experimental studies on the development and propagation of shock waves created by the interaction of short Nd:YAG laser pulses with a titanum target—possible implications for Nd:YAG laser phacolysis of the cataractous human lens. Cataract Refract Surg 17:794–97, 1991.
9. Lewin PA, Bhatia R, Zhang Q et al: Characterisation of optoacoustic surgical devices. IEEE Transaction on Ultrasonics, and Frequency Control 43(4): 1996.

10. Alzncr H, Grabner G: Dodick laser phacolysis: termal effects. Cataract Refract Surg 25:800–03,1999.

11. "Laser Lens Lysis—a new approach to' very small incision cataract surgery" Cataract and Refractive Surgery Euro Times, Volume 6:1997.

12. Dorothy SP Fan, Dennis SC Lam, Kenneth KVV Li: Retinal complications after cataract extraction in patients with high myopia. Ophthalmology 106:688–92,1999.

13. Bath PE: Laserphaco—an introduction and review. Ophthalmic Laser Ther 3(2):75–82, 1988.

14. Bath PE, Kar H, Apple DJ et al: Endocapsular excimer laser phakoablation through a 1 mm incision. Ophthalmic Laser Thor 2(4):245–48, 1987.

15. Bath PE, Mueller G, Apple DJ ct si: Excimer laser lens ablation (letter). Arch Oththalmol 105:1164–65, 1987.

16. Bonnie SR, Puliafito CA: Erbium:YAG and Holmium:YAG laser ablation of the lens. Lasers Surg Method 15:74–82, 1994.

17. Cleary SF: Laser pulses and the generation of acoustic transients in biological material. In Wolbarsht ML (Ed): Laser Applications in Medicine and Biology New York: Plenum Press, 3: 175:219, 1977.

18. Maguen E, Martinez M, Grundfest W et ah Excimer laser ablation of the human lens a 308 nm with the fiber delivery system. Cataract Refract Surg 15: 409–14, 1989.

19. Muller-Stolzenburg N, Muller Gl: Transmission of 308 nm excimer laser radiation for ophthalmic microsurgery medical, technical and safety aspects. Biomed Tech (Berlin) 34(6): 131–38, 1989.

20. Muller-Stolzenburg N, Stange N, Kar Ht'al: Endocapsular cataract surgery using the excimer laser at 308 nm (in German with English abstract). Forlschr Ophlhalmol 86(6):561–65, 1989.

21. Nanevicz T, Prince MR, Gawande AA el al: Excimer laser ablation of the lens. Arch Ophthahnol 104: 1825–29, 1986.

22. Peyman GA, Katon N: Effects uf an Erbium:YAG laser on ocular structures. Ophthalmol 10:245–53, 1987.

23. Pita-Salorio D, Simon G el ah Erbium:YAG laser cataract surgery. Course presented at the American Society of Cataract and Refractive Surgery (ASCRS) Annual Meeting 1998.

24. Tsubota K: Application of Erbium:YAG laser in ocular ablation. Opthahmologica 200(3): 117–22, 1990.

53

Torsional Phacoemulsification: A Newer Technology of Application of Ultrasonic Phacoemulsification System

Col JKS Parihar SM,VSM

INTRODUCTION

The Ultrasonic phacoemulsification system remains the most acceptable and widely popular technology for the management of cataract by the phacoemulsification technique. The delivery of ultrasound energy is based on the vibratory mechanism in which the phaco tip needle moves forward and backward in a linear direction along the axis of the shaft. Surprisingly, this technology remains unchanged since its inception by Charles Kelman, M.D. in 1967.

Undoubtedly, this particular technology is time proven and very effective. However, the forward and backward movement in a linear direction along with the axis of the shaft restricts energy application in one dimension only in a traditional phaco tip. Over and above, there is a tendency to generate more heat at the tip and hub of the phaco needle; hence the system is vulnerable to the higher risk of thermal burn to the cornea as well as internal injuries. The repulsion of nuclear fragments during phacoemulsification is another disadvantage associated with conventional phacoemulsification systems. This undesirable effect of traditional ultrasound has required surgeons to use methods such as linear power (gradual increase in the tip stroke length) and the pulse mode in order to interrupt ultrasound and, thereby permit fluid removal to return the chattering particle to the tip of the ultrasonic needle.

A newer technology called torsional phacoemulsifier was introduced by Alcon laboratories USA in 2005, which claims to have several advantages over conventional ultrasonic phacoemulsification systems. Using a newly designed handpiece and computer software, this system provides a unique side to side shearing effect which almost eliminates repulsion, increases the cutting efficiency and flowability to very high levels as compared to the traditional phaco.

MECHANICS OF TORSIONAL PHACOEMULSIFICATION

The torsional phacoemulsification system provides different high end functions for different varieties of cataract. A special handpiece called OZil torsional handpiece and its software are available on infinity vision system of Alcon.

Understanding the Physics of Torsional Phaco

Successful phacoemulsification surgery is a delicate balance of complex forces. On the one hand, energy is required to separate and remove the hardened nuclear material while on the other hand, a significant imbalance of fluidics and/or energy delivery can cause unwanted trauma to the eye.

Torsional phaco utilises ultrasonic oscillations of an angulated or curved needle, which dramatically changes both the energy profile of the tip and the reaction of lens material contacted by the vibrating needle.

The unique design with the angled tip design makes the velocity at the tip three times that of its shaft. In the torsional mode, the handpiece oscillates from side to side at about 32,000 times per second. This side to side motion provides a much greater amount of energy at the tip than the amount of heat generated at the incision which ultimately transmits up to the lens material (than by the shaft to the surrounding infusion sleeve and incision, as compared to the traditional phaco). This peculiar movement of the tip provides more constant contact with the nucleus, shears off nucleus pieces, eliminates repulsion, and thereby increases cutting efficiency significantly.

With each oscillatory cycle, the distance travelled by the tip is approximately two times greater than the distance (arc) through which the shaft moves.

Hence, the effective outcome is at par with the impact of 64 kHz delivered by traditional longitudinal phaco system, despite the oscillations of 32 kHz in contrast to the traditional ultrasound which has the forward and backward motion of the tip at a speed of only 40 kHz. It is worth considering that in case of traditional longitudinal phaco, the energy is being utilised by nucleus only during forward movement and backward movement which produces only thermal energy without performing nucleotomy. Therefore, the traditional phaco generates much higher thermal energy as compared to the torsional phaco with less cutting abilities. Whereas in case of torsional phaco, the amount of energy being released at the tip is much greater than the amount of the heat generated at the incision. Over and above, the torsional phaco can be combined with the traditional linear ultrasound so that combination of power can be delivered for faster and safer removal of nucleus. This technique is far more useful in hard cataracts.

Fluidics of Torsional Phacoemulsification System

Torsional phacoemulsification system has a unique fluidics system as compared to the conventional phacoemulsification system.

The basic concept of phacosystem is to maintain the sustained position of lens material at the tip so as to ensure efficient and uniform application of energy into the nuclear tissue.

Appropriate equilibrium among vacuum pressure and aspiration flow rate is an essential need of a successful phacoemulsification procedure. Excessive use of fluids and very high aspiration and vacuum settings may lead to corneal oedema and chamber instability that could result in an inadvertent rupture of the posterior capsule. Such occurrences are not the unusual happenings with traditional longitudinal phacoemulsification systems.

As compared to the conventional phaco system, torsional phaco has decreased repulsion of lens material on the tip which decreases the amount of balanced salt solution required to draw lens material back to the tip. Torsional phaco need significantly less balanced salt solution during nucleus removal, approximately 44 to 48 ml as compared to the 58 to 62 ml used during longitudinal phaco, a reduction of more than 20% with torsional. The obvious advantage of this more than 20% reduction in fluid application is proportionately linked with less turbulence and chatter ultimately leading to improved efficiency, thereby minimising possibilities of corneal edema and thermal injuries.

How Torsional Phacoemulsification differs from the Conventional Phacoemulsification System

Difference in the US Energy System

Torsional handpiece works on 32 KHz as compared to the conventional phaco handpiece which works on 40 KHz.

However, despite the less power being delivered in the torsional handpiece, effective utilisation of energy in this

system is many folds. In the conventional system, movements of phaco tip are linear; hence energy delivered is used only on forward action, whereas in torsional rotatory movements US energy is more effective. Hence, despite 32 KHz energy at the tip, the ultimate effect on the nucleus is much higher. Rapidly oscillating torsional movement at 32,000 times per second liberates less energy at the phaco tip which makes it more effective in a hard nucleus and microphaco as well.

Less Thermal Energy Despite Two Fold Cutting Ability

Traditional, ultrasound has had a greater chance of causing thermal injury due to equal distribution of the velocity at the tip and at the shaft in the incision. The amount of motion in the incision is very small with torsional phaco compared with traditional phaco. When the torsional handpiece oscillates, only a small arc is created at the incision compared with the arc created at the angled tip which is almost three times higher. Hence, traditional phaco generates higher amount of thermal energy. It has been found that at 100% power and total occlusion (no flow) for 30 seconds, traditional ultrasound produces 65 to 75°C temperature at the incision, whereas the torsional ultrasound produces heat upto 45°C only at the site of incision.

1. It is also possible to use the OZil™ torsional handpiece, alternating between longitudinal and the torsional motion.
2. Torsional phaco can be combined with aqualase technology.
3. It is designed to minimise repulsion or chatter of nuclear material, thereby increasing flowability, and improving the effectiveness and safety of cataract removal.
4. Torsional phaco can be even more efficient at lower vacuum and flow rates settings. Hence, it is potentially the ideal technology to harness micro-coaxial cataract techniques.

COMPONENTS OF TORSIONAL PHACOEMULSIFICATION

Phacoemulsifier machine (Main console) and Handpiece

Torsional phaco technology system is a high-end triple function phacoemulsifier with following specific features:

(i) Traditional ultrasound
(ii) OZil handpiece for torsional phaco
(iii) Aqualase—pulsed water jet system for soft cataract.

The system has been provided with such different high-end functions for the different variety of cataract. Its specific available software utilises a unique side to side shearing effect. In addition to torsional phaco, this system can also provide Aqualase technology.

Aqualase uses pulses of balanced salt solution at 50 Hz to 100 Hz to dissolve the cataract. This modality may potentially demonstrate advantages in terms of safety and prevention of secondary posterior capsular opacification.

OZil Phaco handpiece for torsional phaco: The special handpiece called OZil torsional handpiece is a very light-weight and ergonomic handpiece which can deliver torsional ultrasonic oscillations, traditional longitudinal ultrasound, or a combination of both. Torsional handpiece utilises a unique side to side shearing effect which almost eliminates repulsion, increases the cutting efficiency and flowability to very high levels compared to the traditional phaco.

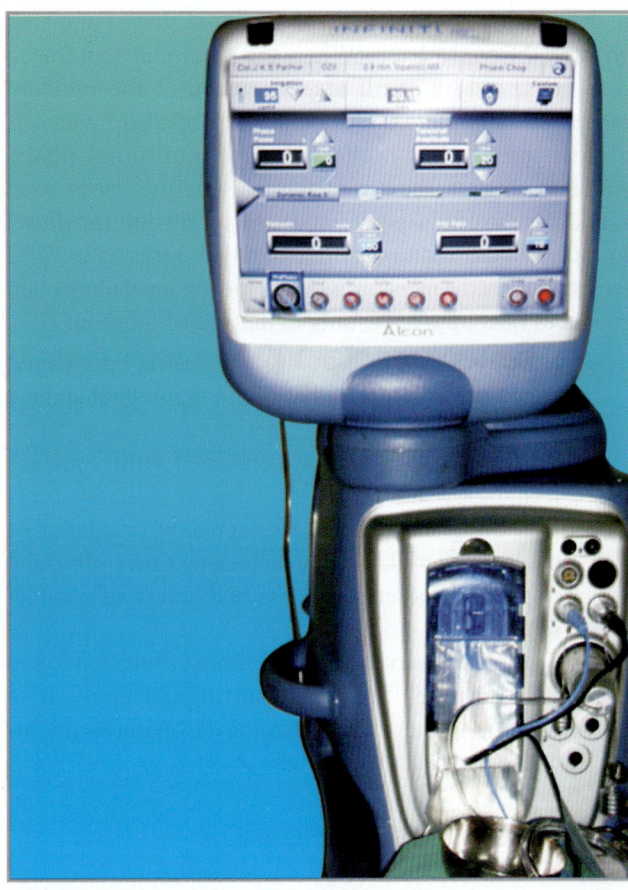

(a)

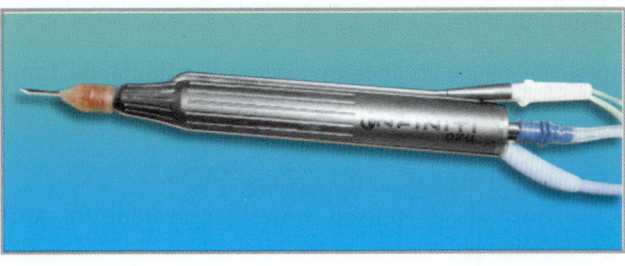

(b)

Fig. 53.1: (a) Infinity phacoemulsifier system, (b) OZil phaco handpiece for torsional phaco

The specifications of OZil torsional handpiece are as follows:
- (i) Made up of titanium
- (ii) Weight: 60 grams (Very light weight as compared to NeoSonix Handpiece—134 grams, LEGACY Ultrasound Handpiece—90 grams and other conventional handpieces those that are ranging from 150 to 175 grams)
- (iii) Length: 13 cm (5.25 inches).

Phaconeedle (Phaco Tip)

A kelman (bent) tip or Mackool tips can be used with torsional phacosystem. Torsional ultrasound energy can be delivered by using 0.9 mm angled Kelman tip instead of the 1.1 mm straight flare tip. Because of the downward curve, the design is more ergonomic providing lesser stress on the wound by keeping the handpiece more aligned to the incision. Kelman (bent) tip has 19 G needle similar to the standard tip but the distal end is bent to give it increased cutting ability.

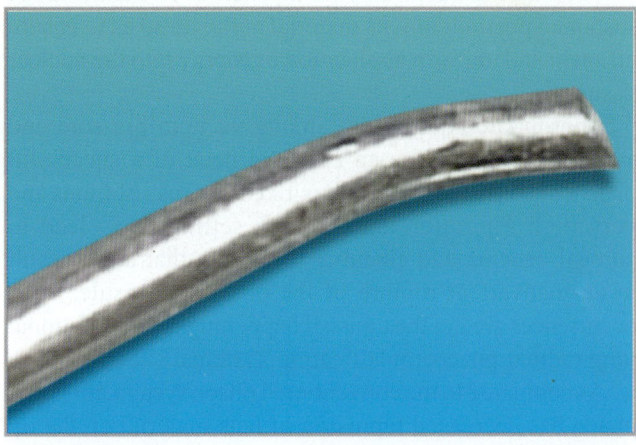

(a)

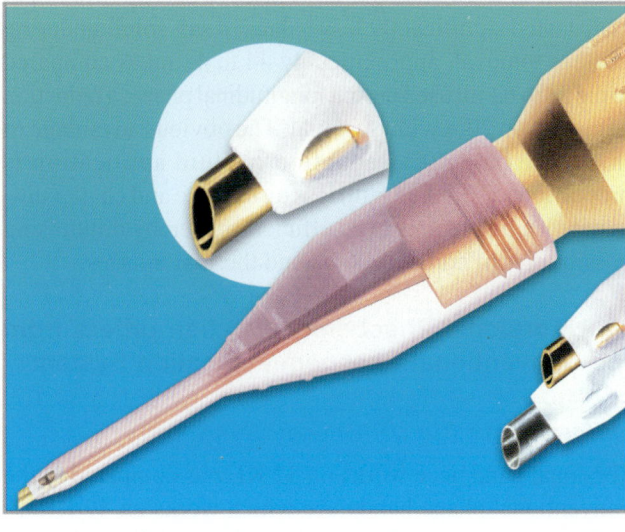

(b)

Fig. 53.2: (a) Kelman (bent) tip (b) Mackool tip

There is also transverse motion in addition to the normal longitudinal motion of the phaco tip. The bent edge is in more contact with the nucleus, thus able to transmit phaco power better, especially to the posterior part of the nucleus.

Mackool tip contain thin polymer tubing inside the infusion sleeve separating it from the vibrating needle.

This polymer, about 50–75 micron thick has a very less friction coefficient. The vibrating needle generates less heat when surrounded by this polymer thus heat transmission is reduced. This has a greater advantage in comparison with slightly increased infusion sleeve thickness.

Mackool tip are available in both standard as well as micro tip version.

Sleeves for Phaco Tip (Fig. 53.3)

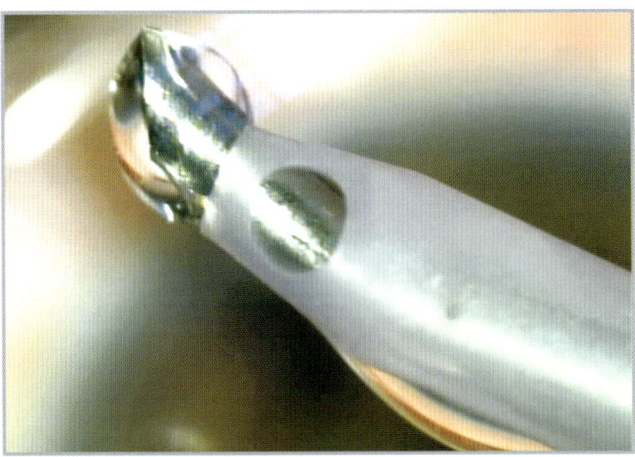

Fig. 53.3: 1.1 mm high infusion sleeve (shown with 1.1 mm flared ABS Tip)

TORSIONAL PHACOEMULSIFICATION SYSTEM

Merits

(i) The motion of tip generates significantly less energy simply because of the way it oscillates, rather than backward and forward.

(ii) Torsional phaco allows less risk of thermal injury. Thermal imaging studies using infrared thermography conducted by various workers have proved that temperature created at the incision due to torsional rotatory tip is well below the critical temperature to produce incisional burn.

(iii) Lack of repulsion is the main benefit of torsional phaco.

(iv) Torsional phaco prevents dispersion of nuclear fragments due to multidimensional delivery of ultrasonic energy and hence assures rapid, secured, and very effective emulsification.

(v) Quick and efficient phacoemulsification.

(vi) Excellent chamber stability. Anterior Chamber does not move at all throughout the procedure.

(vii) When nuclear fragments are not repelled and dispersed, there is a less chance of small fragments getting trapped in the angle, or under the fornices of capsular bag. Hence, possibilities of undesirable, unintentional residual lens material or fragment left over are practically nil.

(vi) Excellent performance even in very difficult situations like hard cataract, miotic pupil, subluxation or in case of floppy iris

(vii) Very effective for bimanual microincision phacoemulsification surgery.

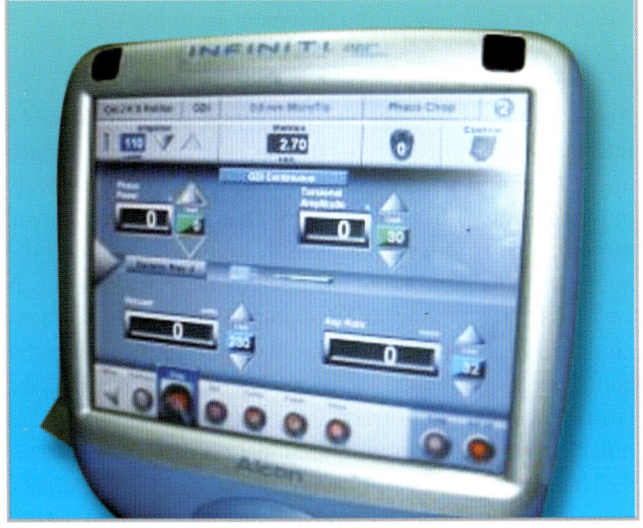

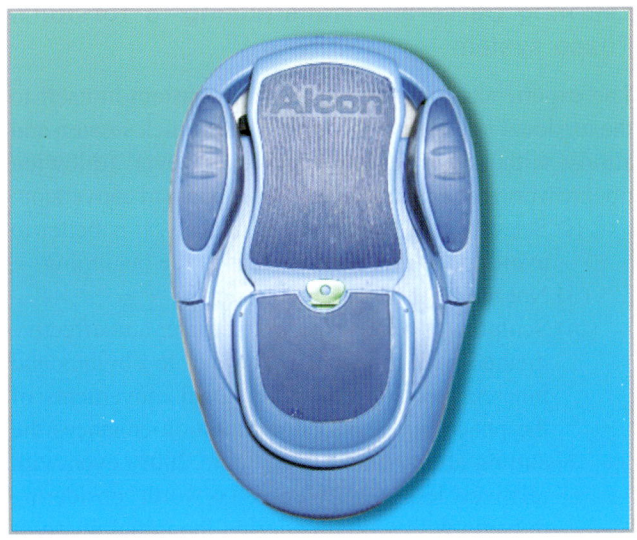

| (a) | (b) |

Fig. 53.4: (a) Infinity torsional phacoemulsifier, (b) Infinity foot pedal

Aim

(i) Attempt to introduce less irrigation fluid into the eye without compromising efficiency, maintaining as efficient a system as possible.

(ii) Maximum protection of corneal endothelium against fluid, thermal and dispersion of lens fragments. Achieve clear corneas.

(iii) Effective and good performance while performing bimanual microincision phacoemulsification surgery.

Aqualase

Aqualase uses pulses of balanced salt solution at 50 Hz to 100 Hz to dissolve the cataract with the help of a smooth polymer tip. This smooth polymer tip facilitates intra capsular bag aquaemulsification throughout the procedure, since the polymer tip carries least possibilities of likely tear in the posterior capsule.

Undoubtedly, Aqualase is the best technology for removing soft nuclei with some mild alterations in conventional phacoemulsification techniques. The aqualase technique can manage soft cataract of upto grade two more efficiently as well as maintain a greater degree of safety than ultrasound through the procedure without adversely influencing the final outcome. The aqualase technique provides an excellent spray and power washing of the capsule which is a unique feature of this method. This modality may potentially demonstrate advantages in terms of safety and prevention of secondary posterior capsular opacification.

APPLICATION OF TORSIONAL PHACOEMULSIFICATION SYSTEM IN DIFFERENT TYPES OF CATARACTS AND SITUATIONS

Learning Curve and Transitioning to Torsional Phaco system

The experienced phaco surgeon can accustom himself to the torsional phaco system within a very quick session and almost without any learning curve. However, following tips are worth considering during initial phase of conversion:

(i) Select a grade two or three nucleus. It is better to avoid too soft or hard nucleus at the beginning.

(ii) Not too tight or leaking incisions.

(iii) Sculpting is relatively a much easier and effective method with torsional phaco due to obvious and inherent peculiarities of torsional movements of the phaco tip. The torsional motion enhances the cutting ability and efficacy upto 200% even with relatively less power. Hence, it is worth considering to begin with sculpting during the initial phase of conversion to torsional phaco from conventional phaco.

(iv) Torsional and conventional phaco chop sandwich technique is an ideal technique during transition phase, since torsional tip may make chopping little difficult. In this technique initial holding of nucleus and chopping is being performed while using traditional ultrasound through same OZil handpiece to make quick chops and make the initial pieces which is followed by quadrant removal by changed torsional setting of 100% torsional phaco.

Customising Emulsification Techniques

(a) Sculpting

(b) Chopping

(c) Cartwheel Torsional (Col Parihar's technique)

Sculpting with Torsional Phaco

(i) Sculpting is relatively a much easier and effective method with torsional phaco due to obvious and inherent peculiarities of torsional movements of the phaco tip. The torsional motion enhances cutting ability and efficacy upto 200% even with relatively less frequency of 32 kHz with each side-to-side motion as compared to just the forward motion in conventional ultrasound frequency of 40 kHz. In true sense OZil torsional handpiece can provide enhanced efficiency of cutting strokes despite less US frequency.

(ii) Due to rotational movements of phaco tip, there is no repulsion of nuclear fragments away from the tip, which is a common problem with the conventional phaco system where dense nuclear fragments tend to be repulsed slightly away from the tip, particularly during sculpting. This results in an attempt to use more energy and tip push into the nucleus whereas torsional stroke is side to side so it shears the lens material and practically arrests the slipping away movement from the tip.

Phaco chop with Torsional Phaco

Application of torsional phaco in direct chopping needs a little modification at the initial stage of embedding of the phaco tip and holding, since torsional movements provide a relatively big crater even with the least energy. Over and above, torsional movement provides cyclic rotational movement to the nucleus; hence holding of the nucleus in such situations is very tricky, whereas traditional ultrasound enjoys easy lens holding due to back-and-forth movement resulting in better penetration and imbedding of the phaco tip into the nucleus. However, subsequent fragment aspiration and removal is much easier and faster with torsional phaco.

Hence, phaco chop can be performed by two techniques.

(i) **Torsional and conventional phaco chop Sandwich technique:** In this technique initial holding of the nucleus and chopping is being performed while using traditional ultrasound through same OZil hand-piece to make quick chops and make the initial pieces which is followed by quadrant removal by changed torsional setting of 100% torsional phaco.

(ii) Direct torsional phaco chop: Direct torsional phaco chop technique is an ideal and very good method in cases of dense hard nucleus. However certain sequential modifications in power settings make direct torsional chop possible even in cases of moderate grades of nucleus.

In this technique, initial holding of nucleus and chopping is being performed with the application of 30–40% torsional energy with zero US energy and 225 to 275 mmHg vacuum settings. Subsequent multiple secondary chopping continues with the same settings. However subsequent changed settings of 350 to 450 mmHg vacuum and 100% torsional phaco with 5 to 10% US energy can be used for smooth and quick quadrant removal.

Cartwheel Torsional Phaco (Col Parihar's Technique)

Torsional movements of the phaco tip provide great opportunity to emulsify lens nuclei even without having sculpting or chopping. Once nucleus is made free from superficial cortical matter, the nucleus has access and is free to rotate in a cyclic manner. This free and spontaneous cyclic rotation will allow nucleus emulsification and aspiration even without breaking by sculpting or chopping. The energy required is more or less the same as utilised in sculpting settings. This particular method is very effective for grade two to three cataracts.

Torsional Phacoemulsification

Torsional with different surgical techniques, postoperative results and improved outcomes.

Application of the Torsional System on Various Types of Nuclei

There has been significant change in the trends and patterns of cataract surgery throughout the world. We have experienced remarkable change in the type of cataract and density of nucleus encountered in phacosurgery in the recent past. This change has been witnessed primarily due to a change in the perception of cataract and phacoemulsification both at the ophthalmologist and the patient level due to obvious and enhanced expectations from the surgical outcome. Patients are demanding early removal of cataract rather as an alternative of refractive surgery as well ophthalmologists are also happy to see soft cataract. Despite this changed trend, newer challenges like post LASIK and PK cataract, complicated cataract, concurrent glaucoma and cataract are newer challenges.

Despite this wide spectrum, hard, complicated cataract and miotic pupil or floppy iris, the rubbery, Coca-Cola cataracts (Cataract with poor dilation and weak zonules) are still seen and are a nightmare for the ophthalmologist. The author enjoys the privilege, preference, and confidence on torsional phaco over conventional phaco in all these situations.

The torsional system has unquestioned superiority over any other system in any kind of cataract. Transition is very safe and smooth. However, each and every type of nucleus needs different type of settings as well as techniques. The author describes his own experience in different situations, but every surgeon will have his own settings and techniques.

Very Soft Nuclei

Aqualase is the best technology for the management of very soft cataract. Aqualase, with pre-chop, is a much more efficient, rapid and a very safe procedure particularly in cases of soft nuclei. Sculpting and torsional chopping are practically too difficult an option; hence the author does not recommend them as the preferred technique. However, torsional cartwheel method adopted by the author has definite superiority over other techniques. One need not use US energy at all. Superficial cortical matter can be safely removed with the help of the bimanual I/A system with settings of 400 to 500 mm of vacuum or with the help of torsional handpieces on zero US and 20% torsional power with 500–550 vacuum. Once the nucleus is free from superficial cortex it floats and moves freely in the bag. Torsional power can be readjusted to 100% with 600 vacuum settings to facilitate quick and safe emulsification and removal of floating, soft, and small nucleus. Residual cortical matter can be aspirated out with the help of bimanual I/A. One can use coaxial I/A system, however bimanual I/A provides better control and access to sticky cortex.

Absolutely watertight phaco incision enhances efficacy in this type of cataracts.

Grade II to III Nucleus

Grade II or III cataracts are ideal cataracts with any kind of emulsification system. However, the intraoperative ease and final outcome is much more superior and gratifying with the torsional phaco system. One can use conventional sculpting, stop and chop, direct chop or the cartwheel technique with moderate cataracts of grade II or III. Stop and chop can be done with exclusive torsional energy without any US or a standard combination of 20% longitudinal energy and 80% torsional power for the initial groove which is followed by exclusive torsional energy only. Recommended vacuum settings are 300 to 400 mmHg during initial groove followed by 450 to 500 for chopping. I/A can be performed having 500–550 mmHg settings. One can use coaxial or bimanual I/A system. However, the author prefers to use bimanual system for the simple reason of enhanced manoeuvrability and ease all the time, particularly while manipulating subincisional cortex.

Dense Nuclei

Management of dense nuclei remains a challenging task for any phaco surgeon. Stop and chop or direct chopping is the preferred technique over conventional sculpting techniques. Despite this, dense nuclei are always at the risk of intraoperative or postoperative events like PCR, fragment or nucleus drop as well as subsequent corneal endothelial cell loss due to excessive use of US energy, fluids, thermal burn,excessive time taken or intraoperative complications. In contrast to these hiccups, torsional phaco is a very smooth and pleasant experience even with very dense nuclei. The author prefers to apply the stop and chop technique while using a 1.1 mm flared tip. The gold standard of any phaco technique is to remain in the central safe zone, occlude the tip and attempt to rotate the nucleus fragments right upto the tip. As a contrast to the conventional phaco system where continuous foot adjustment between two and three is essential to maintain US energy equilibrium with traditional ultrasound, the torsional system just needs holding of nucleus in foot position two and slight turning movement of the tip of the needle to snugly hold the nuclear piece, resulting in a good occlusion.

This particular movement facilitates quick and safe fragment emulsification under activated torsional ultrasound. The most striking benefit is the total absence of repulsive effect which is a common occurrence in case of traditional ultrasound systems.

Using Torsional Phaco on Hard Brown Cataract

Management of hard brown nuclei remains a challenging task for any phaco surgeon. Stop and chop or direct chopping is the preferred technique to conventional sculpting techniques. Despite this, hard brown nucleus invariably faces a great risk of severe intraoperative or postoperative complications like PCR, fragment or nucleus drop as well as subsequent corneal endothelial cell loss due to excessive use of US energy, fluids,thermal burn, excessive time taken or intraoperative complications. In contrast to these hiccups, torsional phaco is a very smooth and pleasant experience even in the case of a very hard nucleus.

Phaco chop with Torsional Phaco in Hard Cataract

The author prefers to apply stop and chop technique while using 1.1 mm flared tip. As a contrast to the conventional phaco system where continuous foot adjustment between two and three is essential to maintain US energy equilibrium with traditional ultrasound torsional system just needs holding of the nucleus in the foot position two and slight

turning movement of the tip of the needle, flush the nuclear piece resulting in a good occlusion.

This particular movement facilitates quick and safe fragment emulsification under activated torsional ultrasound. The most striking benefit is the total absence of the repulsive effect which is a common occurrence in case of traditional ultrasound systems.

Torsional Phaco Settings

(i) **Choice of the Phaco tip:** 0.9 mm tapered, angled tip which facilitates smaller size of incision ranging from 2.8 to 2.6 mm without compromising fluid dynamics and safety.

(ii) **Machine settings for stop and chop on torsional phaco system:**
Superficial cortical cleaning
Energy and Vacuum settings: 300–350 mmHg for superficial cortex removal with no US energy and 40% torsional power so as to allow free floating movements of nucleus which is prerequisite to the nucleotomy.
Construction of the initial small groove: Combination of 20% conventional US energy + 80% torsional or 100 torsional with 10 % US energy on torsional mode with vacuum settings of 300–350 mmHg has been found very effective.
Chopping: Combination of 100% Torsional with 10% US energy on torsional mode with vacuum settings of 400–450 mmHg has been found very effective.
Fragment removal: 100% on torsional mode with no US energy and vacuum settings of 350–400 mmHg.

Since torsional ultrasound does not create any kind of repulsive forces at the tip, one may use continuous ultrasound without any apprehension of chatter of nuclear fragments at the tip.

Torsional Phaco in Difficult Conditions

Merits of Torsional Phaco in Difficult Conditions

(i) **Absence of chattering:** Even in the case of a very dense, hard brown nucleus, lens fragments remain on the tip and do not chatter.

(ii) Good, uncomplicated phacoemulsification surgery with good postoperative results are possible even in the case of a very dense hard brown nucleus, zonular dehiscence or in cases of poor endothelial cell count of less than 700 cells/mm^2.

MICROINCISION CATARACT SURGERY(MICS) USING TORSIONAL PHACO SYSTEM

The term MICS (micro incisional cataract surgery) refers to bimanual microincisional or sub 1 mm incision cataract

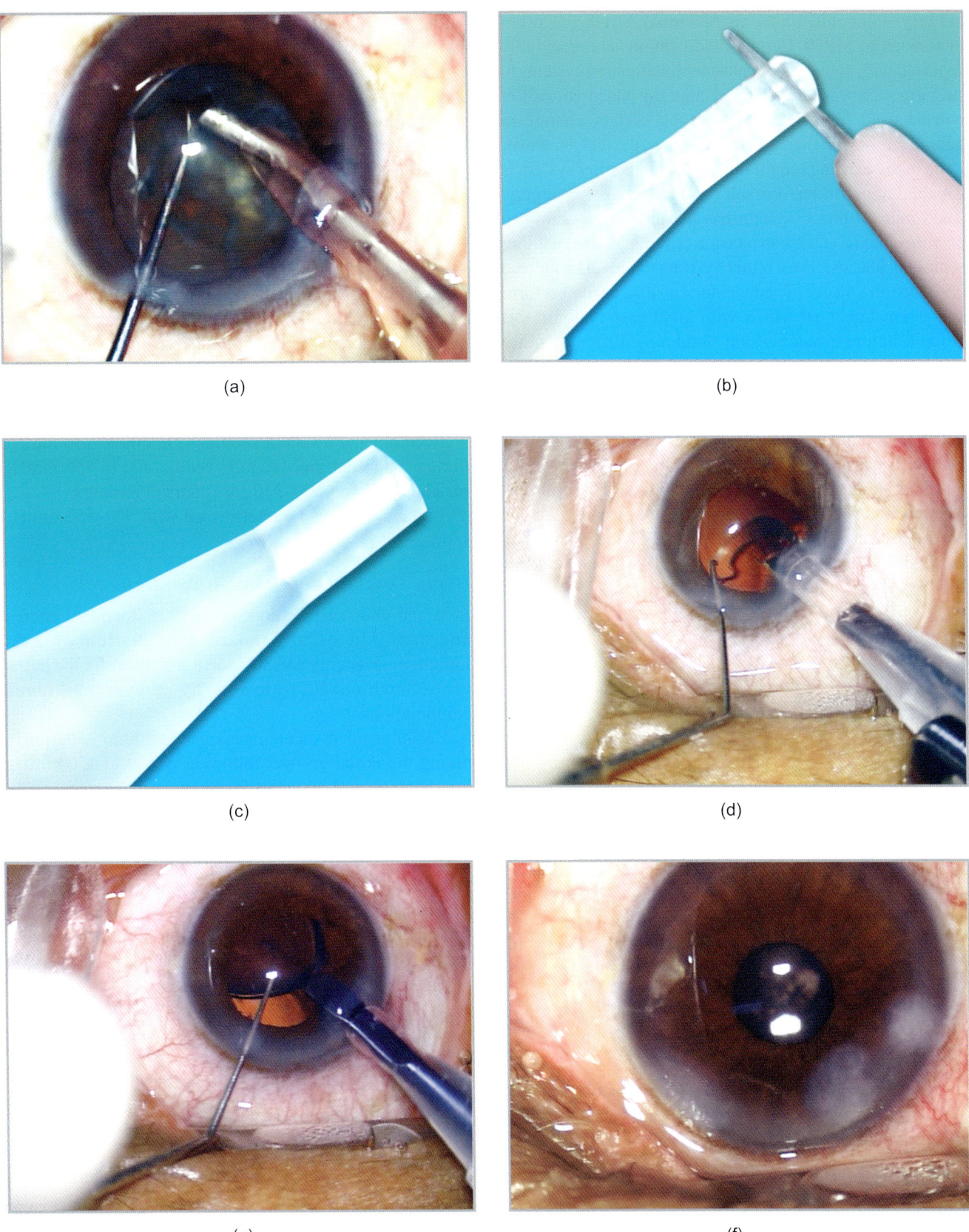

Fig. 53.5: (a) Co-axial sub 2 mm incision (1.8 mm) MICS, (b) Modifications in cartridge to insert a single piece hydrophobic AcrySof IOL through a 2.1 mm incision, (c) Modified cartridge to a insert single piece hydrophobic AcrySof IOL through a 2.1 mm incision, (d) IOL insertion through a 2.1 mm incision, (e) IOL insertion through a 2.1 mm incision, (f) Co axial sub 2 mm incision (1.8 mm) MICS : IOL implant is in situ

surgery. Phaconit, phakonit bimanual MICS are other synonyms of MICS. Certain modifications are essentially required with conventional phacoemulsification systems to perform such procedure. By and large any phaco-emulsifier can be used for MICS after having certain change in parameters or with fluid infusion/air pump devices. However none of the existing longitudinal phacoemulsifier system is capable enough to perform sub 1 mm coaxial MICS surgery. The torsional phaco system has the unique capability to perform coaxial sub 2 mm incision (1.8 mm) MICS without removing phacosleeves; rather by using torsional handpiece with the ultra sleeve. The machine can also easily perform sub 1 mm bimanual MICS with great ease and comfort without any assistance of any fluid/air infusion or other devices. Author has evaluated coaxial and bimanual MICS on torsional phaco system.

In our view coaxial MICS has produced excellent outcome without compromising the structural integrity of cornea. The procedure has been very smooth. After certain modifications in cartridge, single piece hydrophobic Acrysof IOL was placed through 2.1 mm incision. We did not notice any significant difference in the pattern of induced astigmatism between bimanual MICS and coaxial MICS performed on torsional system

Bimanual Microphaco with Torsional Phacoemulsification System

Torsional phacosystem has been found very effective to perform bimanual Microphaco. In the author's view, the torsional system is much more convenient and safer for MICS due to obvious added advantages of the torsional system over longitudinal phaco. One can easily proceed with ease in handling a nucleus of up to grade III–IV without compromising fluidics or need of any assistance of pressure infusion devices, air pumps or any surge control measures. Suggested techniques, type of instrumentation and machine settings, based on our experience are as follows:

(i) **Phaco tip:** 0.9 mm microphaco torsional phaco tip.
(ii) **Incisions:** 1.0 mm trapezoid keratome for both incisions.
(iii) Irrigating chopper 21 Gauze (side or distal end, both are acceptable)
(iv) **Bimanual I/A:** 21 Gauze.
(v) **Technique:** Direct/stop and chop for two to four grades of nucleus, where as cart wheel lift and aspiration for soft nucleus.

Settings for Soft Nucleus

Cartwheel lift and aspiration/aqualase technique.

US Energy settings

One need not use US energy at all. Superficial cortical matter can be safely removed with the help of bimanual I/A system with settings of 300 to 350 mm of vacuum or

with the help of a torsional handpiece on zero US and 20% torsional power with 500–550 vacuum. Once the nucleus is free from superficial cortex, it floats and moves freely in the bag. Torsional power can be readjusted to 100% with 350–375 mm vacuum settings to facilitate quick and safe emulsification and removal of a floating, soft, and small nucleus. Residual cortical matter can be aspirated out with the help of bimanual I/A. Absolutely watertight phacoincision enhances efficacy in these types of cataracts.

Grade II to III Nucleus

Grade II or III cataracts are ideal cataracts for MICS.

Stop and chop can be done with exclusive torsional energy without any US or a standard combination of 20% longitudinal energy and 80% torsional power for the initial groove which is followed by exclusive torsional energy only.

Recommended vacuum settings are 200 to 250 mmHg during the initial groove, followed by 400 to 450 mmHg for chopping and 300–350 for fragment removal.

Bimanual I/A can be performed with 500–550 mmHg settings.

Using Torsional on Hard Brown Cataract

Stop and chop can be done with 100% torsional energy and 15% US or a standard combination of 20% Longitudinal energy and 80% torsional power for the initial groove which is followed by above mentioned combinations.

Recommended vacuum settings are 200 to 250 mmHg during the initial groove, followed by 400 to 450 mmHg for chopping and 300–350 for fragment removal.

Bimanual I/A can be performed with 500–550 mmHg settings.

Management of hard brown nuclei by using MICS is a very challenging task for any phaco surgeon. In contrast to higher risk of complications in case of longitudinal phaco systems, torsional phaco is a very comfortable, safe, and rapid MICS procedure even in cases of hard brown cataract.

Coaxial/Mono axial Micro Phaco with Torsional Phacoemulsification System

The most common concept and understanding in relation to MICRO phaco remains bimanual MICS or phaconit which is true in case of traditional longitudinal phaco. Undoubtedly, bimanual MICS is a big leap towards ultramicro phaco which is the future of any technique and method of cataract removal. However, torsional phaco system is capable of performing sub two mm incision microphaco surgery with the help of a 0.9 mm tip and an ultra thin phaco sleeve. Hence certain modifications and compromises essentially required for bimanual MICS are not required in case of coaxial MICS. Over and above

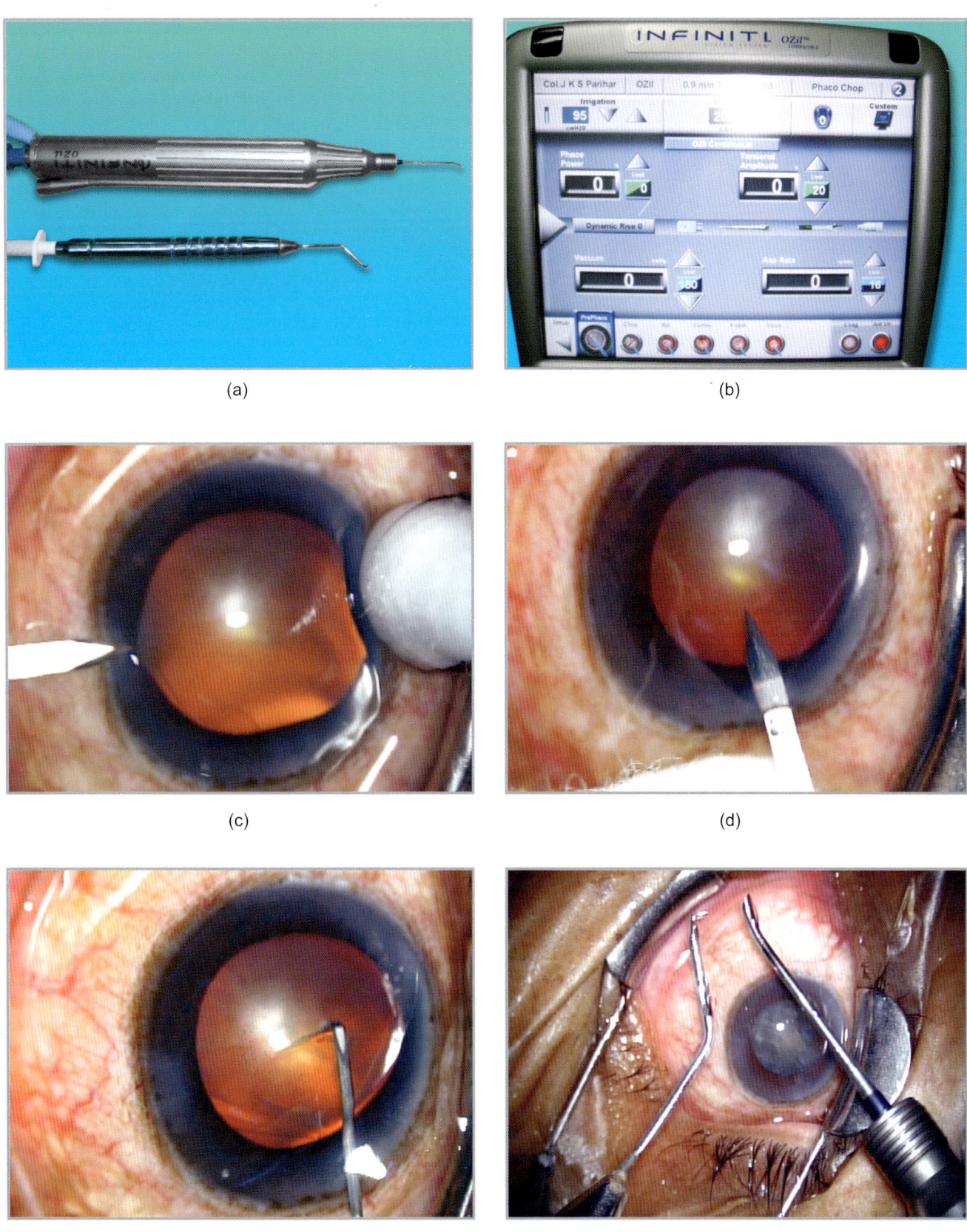

Fig. 53.6: (a) Bimanual sub 1 mm incision MICS with torsional phacoemulsification system (irrigating chopper and 0.9 mm micro phaco tip), (b) Machine settings for torsional bimanual MICS, (c) Bimanual torsional MICS: Incision, (d) Bimanual torsional MICS: Incision, (e) Bimanual torsional MICS: Rhexis, (f) Bimanual, torsional MICS: OZil handpiece with microtip and irrigating chopper

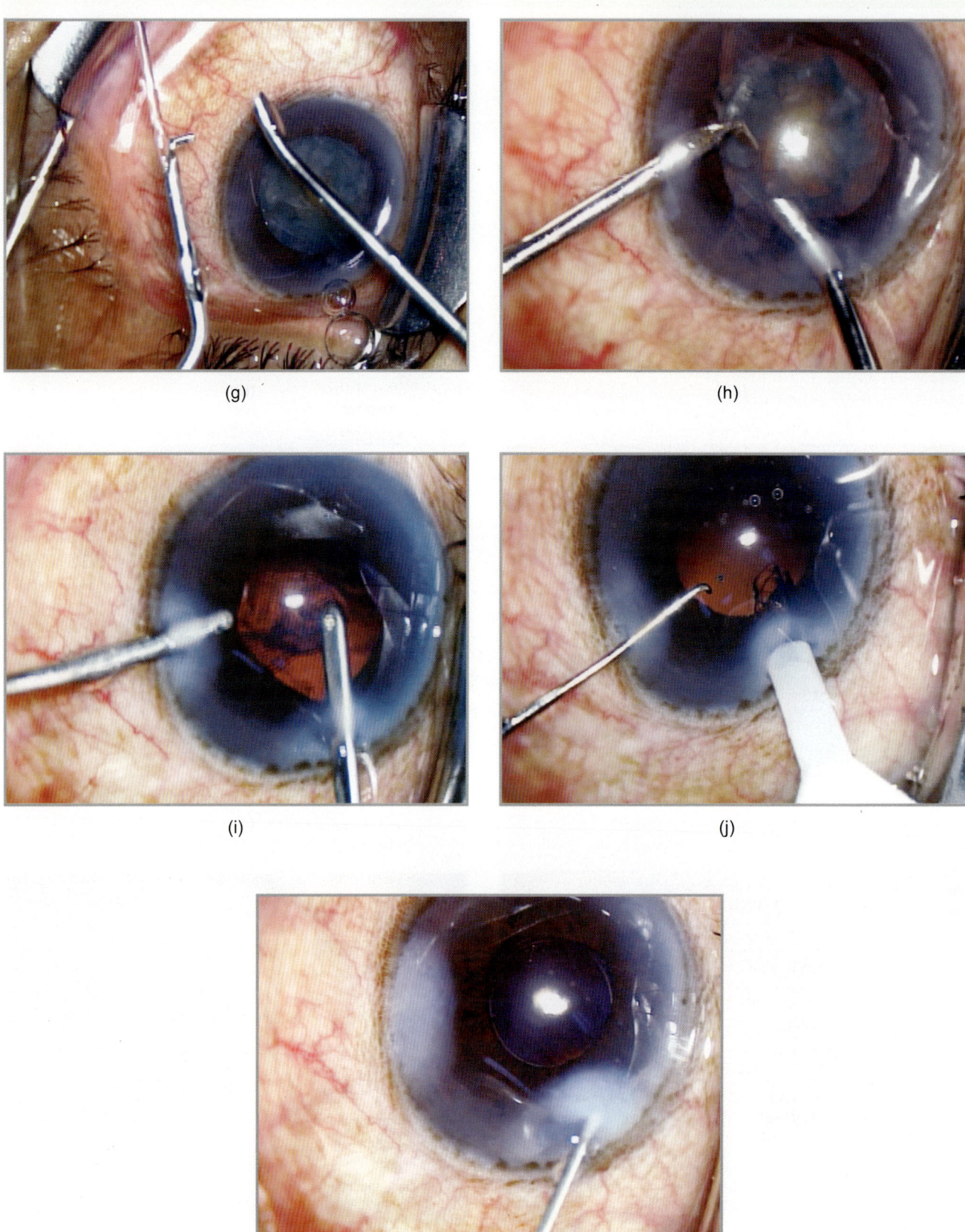

Fig. 53.6: (g) Bimanual torsional MICS: OZil handpiece with microtip and irrigating chopper, (h) Bimanual torsional MICS: chopping, (i) Bimanual torsional MICS: I/A, (j) Insertion of Ultra thin IOL implant, (k) Bimanual torsional MICS: Stromal hydration

certain undesirable effects of altered fluidics are automatically overruled in case of coaxial MICS.

BIMANUAL VERSUS MICRO-COAXIAL CATARACT SURGERY

Torsional phacosystem is capable of providing a good functional capability to high vacuum settings with a micro thin tip and a small incision; hence very effective for micro phaco surgery without creating thermal burn and any additional fluidic assistance or surge control devices like air pump or cruise control methods.

Standard phaco chop technique, applying 225 to 275 mmHg, to impale and hold the nucleus and subsequent settings of 350 to 425 mmHg remain effective in case of nuclear fragment removal.

Torsional phaco can be combined with a 0.9 mm tapered tip and a high infusion sleeve which can be readily accommodated through a 2 mm incision.

Monoaxial MICS Settings for Torsional Phaco with Ultra Sleeve

(i) Aspiration flow of 35 to 40 ml /min
(ii) Maximum vacuum of 275 to 400 mmHg
(iii) Infusion bottle height of 120 to 135 cm

Monoaxial MICS Settings for Torsional Phaco with High-in-fusion Sleeve

(i) Aspiration flow of 45 to 50 ml /min,

(ii) Maximum vacuum of 600 to 750 mmHg.
(iii) Infusion bottle height of 120 to 135 cm.

CONCLUSION

Torsional phacoemulsification technology dramatically improves the phacoemulsification procedure. The amount of energy used in this technology is much less as compared to the conventional phacosystems even in cases of very hard cataracts. Torsional phacosystem is capable of rapid, quick, and safe removal of any type of cataract irrespective of density or hardness of nuclei. The intraoperative fluid requirement is much less as compared to traditional phacoemulsification systems. The overall composite impact of minimal utilisation of ultrasound energy in Torsional delivery system, less fluidic circulation and least time taken in the surgical procedure results into a lessened risk of wound burn, enhanced safety to corneal endothelium as well as drastically reduces the risk of postoperative infections. The ability to utilise aqualase for soft lenses and torsional ultrasound for dense lenses makes the best combination of these two technologies to ensure the best surgical performance and the final outcome. Torsional phacoemulsification technology is a revolutionary change in the US delivery and fluid dynamics system in Phacoemulsification surgery. The ability to utilise aqualase for soft lenses and torsional ultrasound for dense lenses extends marked flexibility and enhanced performance in any given situation. This technology is going to replace the present concept and technology of phacoemulsification cataract surgery.

BIBLIOGRAPHY

1. Bond LJ, Cimino WW. Physics of ultrasonic surgery using tissue fragmentation: part II. Ultrasound Med Biol. 1996; 22:101–1 17.
2. Zacharias J. Role of jackhammer effect and cavitation in phaco. Presented at: Annual Meeting of the American Society of Cataract and Refractive Surgery; March 17–22, 2006; San Francisco.
3. Topaz M, Motiei M, Assia E, et al. Acoustic cavitation in phaco: chemical effects, modes of action and cavitation index. Ultrasound Med Biol. 2002; 28:775–784.
4. Cionni R. Torsional to longitudinal phacoemulsification comparison. Presented at: Annual Meeting of the American Society of Cataract and Refractive Surgery; March 17–22, 2006; San Francisco.
5. Mackool R. Lens removal/torsional phacoemulsification: advantages of nonlinear ultrasound. Presented at: Annual Meeting of the American Society of Cataract and Refractive Surgery; March 17–22, 2006; San Francisco.
6. Mackool R. Torsional phaco: the elimination of lens chatter and thermal energy. Presented as an Alcon booth presentation at: Annual Meeting of the American Society of Cataract and Refractive Surgery; March 17–22, 2006; San Francisco.
7. Yoo S. Conventional ultrasound versus torsional phacoemulsification. Presented at: Annual Meeting of the American Society of Cataract and Refractive Surgery; March 17–22, 2006; San Francisco.
8. Lehmann R. Outcomes and efficiency using torsional phacoemulsification versus traditional ultrasound. Presented at: Annual Meeting of the American Society of Cataract and Refractive Surgery; March 17–22, 2006; San Francisco.
9. Solomon K. Performance of the Infiniti System: torsional vs conventional phacoemulsification handpieces. Presented at: Annual Meeting of the American Society of Cataract and Refractive Surgery; March 17–22, 2006; San Francisco.
10. Solomon K. Longitudinal vs torsional phacoemulsification. Presented as a sponsored booth presentation at: Annual | Meeting of the American Society of Cataract and Refractive Surgery; March 17–22, 2006; San Francisco.
11. Alien D. Efficient surgery with a new torsional phaco mode. Presented at: Annual Meeting of the American Society of Cataract and Refractive Surgery; March 17–22, 2006; San Francisco.
12. Aguilera F. Comparing outcomes of linear phaco technology vs torsional phaco technology in the emulsification of

cataracts. Presented at: Annual Meeting of the American Society of Cataract and Refractive Surgery; March 17–22, 2006; San Francisco.

13. Boukhny M. Laboratory performance comparison of torsional and conventional longitudinal phacoemulsification. I Presented at: Annual Meeting of the American Society of I Cataract and Refractive Surgery; March 17–22, 2006; San Francisco.

14. Dunbar CM, Goble RR, Gregory DW, Church WC.

Intraocular deposition of metallic fragments during phaco: possible causes and effects. Eye. 1995; 9:434–436.

15. Cameron MD, Poyer JF, Aust SD. Identification of free radicals produced during phacoemulsification. J Cataract Refract Surg. 2001; 27:463–470.

16. Tjia K. Microcoaxial torsional phacoemulsification for 2.0 to 2.2 mm incision cataract surgery. Presented at: Annual Meeting of the American Society of Cataract and Refractive Surgery; March 17–22, 2006; San Francisco.

54

No Anaesthesia Technique in Phacoemulsification Cataract Surgery

Col JKS Parihar SM, VSM, Surg Cdr T Choudhary, Lt Col Shantanu Mukherjee
Maj Jaya Kaushik and Surg Lt Cdr AS Parihar

INTRODUCTION

Since its inception in India around circa 500 BC, the saga involving 'surgery for cataract' has travelled a long way. Susruta, the legendary Indian surgeon has been credited with the introduction of cataract surgery in the form of 'couching' technique, whereby the mature lens was simply spiked into the vitreous cavity by a sterile surgical spear. Techniques were refined over a period of time and within the last fifty years, there has been an explosive advancement pertaining to this sphere of ophthalmic surgery. It was not until 1884 that anaesthesia became a part of ocular surgery when cocaine eye drops were used to induce local anaesthesia.

Forty years ago, intracapsular extraction, general anaesthesia and sandbags were the rule. Following this, came the retrobulbar injection which combined with extracapsular cataract removal greatly reduced the risk to the patient, who because of his old age was usually not a good candidate for general anaesthesia. Retrobulbar anaesthesia was the first improvement; however, this was not without risks. Retrobulbar haemorrhage, muscle laceration, nerve laceration, and perforation of the globe were possible complications along with pressure on the globe, which had its own set of problems. The next advancement was the introduction of the scleral tunnel incision with phacoemulsification and the peribulbar injection. This greatly decreased the complications but allowed peribulbar haemorrhage and the occasional retrobulbar haemorrhage and positive pressure on the globe. Sub-Tenon's injections helped alleviate the haemorrhage aspect; however, the pressure exerted extraocularly continued to impose risks on the procedure.

Today, cataract surgery has become a day care procedure and the anaesthesia required has gradually moved on from general anaesthesia (used in the fifties) to periocular injectable anesthesia, topical anesthetic drops and to the latest but 'still evolving' concept of no anesthesia surgery. Infact, this is one aspect of ocular surgery that has come a full circle, from 'no anaesthesia' in ancient times to 'no anaesthesia' of our modern day.

CONCEPT OF NO ANAESTHESIA IN CATARACT SURGERY AND ITS APPLIED ASPECTS

Cataract surgery is one of the most commonly performed surgical procedures. With the now commonly used phacoemulsification and small incision surgical techniques- the duration of surgery has been grossly shortened. Additionally, cataract being a geriatric condition in most cases, there is a tendency to have co-existent associated morbidity. Therefore, if a surgical procedure can be theoretically performed under a no anaesthesia technique, it removes the chances of anaesthesia related complications. However, keeping the fact in view that a sudden approaching object or even a dust particle is enough to cause the eyelids to close immediately as a protective reflex, operating on an eye without any anaesthesia seems ridiculous. But it has been tried earlier. Dr Arthur Jacob (1790–1874), of Dublin, Ireland, was one of the leading ophthalmologists of his time. The initial descriptions of cataract surgery without anaesthesia go to his credit. His other significant contribution in cataract surgery was to introduce a curved needle for cataract surgery from a sewing needle (Jacob's needle).

The concept of 'no anaesthesia' in modern cataract surgery was reintroduced in the late nineties. Dr Amar Agarwal from Chennai has made significant contribution in popularising no anaesthesia in our recent past. He was the first to perform a live demonstration of no anaesthesia phacoemulsification surgery at Pune on 13 Jun 1998 as was witnessed by the principal author.

Dr Francisco Gutierrez-Carmona from Spain used cooled BSS during surgery which was popularised as "cryoanalgesia". Dr Tobias Neuhann from Germany preferred application of hydroxypropyl methylcellulose (HPMC) 2% to moist cornea during no anaesthesia surgery. Incidentally, his series were mainly confined to an elderly age group. This technique is also practiced by other surgeons from the USA, Brazil and Europe. The author has completely switched over to topical or no anaesthesia cataract surgery since last nine years of practice. Indeed, no anaesthesia works very well, and that too, without any discomfort in a group of a large number of patients.

APPLIED ANATOMY OF THE CORNEA

The ocular surface is one of the most sensitive structures with the highest density of sensory nerve endings. Cornea is most sensitive of all ocular structures, most sensitive to pain and the last to lose sensations under anaesthesia. It is perceived that the cornea has 300 times more innervations per sq mm in comparison to the skin. The nerves are numerous and are derived from the ciliary nerves, which are end branches of the ophthalmic division of 5th cranial nerve. Around the periphery of the cornea they form an annular plexus, from which fibers enter the substantia propria. They lose their medullary sheaths and ramify throughout its substance in a delicate network, and their terminal filaments form a firm and closer plexus on the surface of the cornea proper, beneath the epithelium. This is termed as the subepithelial plexus, and from it fibrils are given off which ramify between the epithelial cells, forming an intraepithelial plexus.

Peculiarities of Corneal Sensitivity

(i) Cornea is highly sensitive to touch, pain and temperature. The centre most part of cornea is highly sensitive. Also the horizontal meridian is more sensitive than the vertical meridian and the temporal area is more sensitive than the nasal area.

(ii) Sensitivity is lowest in the morning and increases as the day progresses. Altered pattern of oxygen concentration at the epithelium surface during closed eyes is one of the important reasons to have reduced corneal sensitivity in the morning.

(iii) Age, sex and race have shown significant influence on the pattern of corneal sensitivity. There is a gradual decrease in the nerve endings with age particularly after 55 to 60 years of age as well as in some pathological states. This decrease is more at the perilimbal area. Corneal sensitivity declines almost upto 50% at around 65–70 years of age. Arcus Senilis and decline in biochemical neurotransmitters like acetylcholine do play major role in this mechanism.

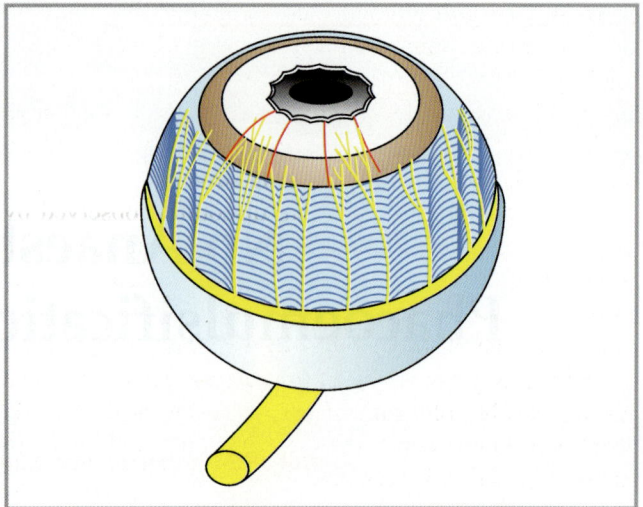

Fig. 54.1: Peculiarities of corneal sensitivity

Gender influence is seen on the corneal sensitivity as reduced sensitivity in females especially during the premenstrual and menstrual periods.

(iv) **Environmental factors:** Frequent and repeated exposure to ultraviolet rays (between 280 and 310 nm) is likely to reduce corneal sensitivity to a great extent—even more than 60 to 70%.

Cold injuries due to cryoanalgesia is a known factor; hence exposure to extreme cold climate may result in marked decrease in corneal sensitivity.

(v) **Racial factors:** Though cornea does not possess pigmentation, various studies related to contact lens application have established an inversely proportionate quantum of corneal sensitivity to the density of uveal pigmentation in the eye. It has been observed that corneal sensitivity in dark-brown eyes as in Indians, Asians and coloured population is 3 to 4 times less as against pigmented greenish-blue eyes of the Caucasians population. However, the exact genesis of reduced corneal sensation and its correlation with corneal thickness and density of pigmentation is not known.

WHY AND HOW "NO ANAESTHESIA" IS POSSIBLE IN PHACOEMULSIFICATION CATARACT SURGERY

Considering anatomical peculiarities of cornea, no anaesthesia phacoemulsification surgery is possible provided meticulous case selection and preoperative assessment is carried out. In addition, the role of absolutely flawless and quick surgery cannot be undermined. Since corneal sensitivity is least in the superior and the nasal quadrants, the incision designed at this meridian and manipulations just prior to the corneal site of peri limbal plexus are essential and the most crucial aspect of no anaesthesia procedure.

Dr Amar Agrawal conducted a collaborative study on no anaesthesia cataract surgery in comparison to topical and topical plus intracameral anaesthesia. In this study, major thrust was on evaluation of various factors related to the patient's response to the procedure, comfort and the stress levels for the surgeon during surgery.

He had analysed pain, touch, discomfort observed by patients during surgery under topical, no anaesthesia and topical plus intracameral groups, surgeon's response was also analysed by himself. The threshold of intraoperative pain in the no anaesthesia group was marginally higher, yet statistically not as significant as compared to topical and topical plus intracameral groups. Touch and discomfort level was almost comparable to pain threshold. Most of patients in this series remained comfortable.

MERITS OF NO ANAESTHESIA PHACOEMULSIFICATION SURGERY

(i) The choice of the anaesthetic method depends on several factors such as the personality of the patient, the type of cataract surgery, and the surgeons' skills and preferences.

(ii) Constraints and complications associated with various local anaesthetic procedures like infiltrative, topical, combination of topical and intracameral in phacoemulsification surgery can be minimised or completely avoided in cases of no anaesthesia cataract surgery technique.

Anaesthetic agents carry the inherent risks due to possible hypersensitivity reaction, over dosage, central nervous system toxicity and damage to the optic nerve or eyeball penetration during injection. Owing to simplicity and low cost, topical anaesthesia is being increasingly used for clear corneal phacoemulsification by experienced surgeons. There is no risk of globe perforation. Compared to regional anesthetic techniques such as peribulbar anaesthesia, the topical approach does not increase the vitreous pressure, and there is no effect on the optic nerve blood flow. Over and above, postoperative recovery pattern is rapid and much quicker. Although the topical anaesthetic agents without preservative are generally considered safe, they are not totally free from untoward adverse effects such as corneal epithelial and endothelial toxicity, retinal toxicity as well as idiosyncratic reactions like periocular swelling, erythema and the typical rash of contact dermatitis which may occasionally occur from ophthalmic use of some of these agents. In addition to the above mentioned complications, frequent and topical instillation of anaesthetic agents may also result in increased corneal thickness and opacification, persistent alteration of the stability of

Lacrimal and tear films as well as delay in healing of the epithelium in the presence of epithelial defects. Frequent instillation of topical anaesthetic agents may be the rare cause of endophthalmitis due to increased intracameral flow of microorganisms.

(iii) Quiet eye in the postoperative evening. It is not possible to recognise from far which eye has been operated.

(iv) No pad on the operated eye.

(v) No prick (injection) and its inherent risks.

(vi) Immediate visual rehabilitation.

(vii) Better patient satisfaction

DEMERITS/CONSTRAINTS OF NO ANAESTHESIA PHACOEMULSIFICATION SURGERY

(i) Surgeon has to learn practising surgery under dynamic and kinetic ocular status.

(ii) Every patient is not an ideal patient for no anaesthesia procedure.

(iii) Needs absolutely atraumatic, flawless and precise surgical performance on the part of the surgeon.

(iv) Operation theatre environment should be very calm and quiet. Even the slightest amount of noise or unpleasant communication may disturb the surgeon and the patient.

NO ANAESTHESIA AS PRACTICED BY THE AUTHOR

The author (JKSP) is practising no anaesthesia since 2002. Undoubtedly, the surgical technique has undergone a significant transformation since then, mainly owing to marked improvement in phaco fluid dynamics and instrumentation as well as cumulative surgical experience. In the recent past, almost 98% of my cataract cases have been subjected to either topical or no anaesthesia technique. Atleast 40 to 45% of these received the no anaesthesia technique. In my practice the no anaesthesia technique works very well.

Indications

(i) Quiet and very composed personality

(ii) Elderly patients

(iii) Moderate orbicularis action

(iv) Normal palpebral fissure

(v) Uncomplicated cataract

(vi) Very good pupillary dilatation

(viii) Grade two to three nucleus

Contraindications

(i) Very apprehensive patients/ extreme anxiety.

(ii) Poor intraoperative communication with patients due to language, hearing impairment or any other relevant factors.

(iii) Significant associated systemic diseases like uncontrolled hypertension, Bronchial Asthma, Parkinson's disease, mental retardation and dementia.

(iv) Extremes of age and relatively younger patients

(v) Monocular patients

(vi) Strong orbicularis action

(vii) Small palpebral fissure

(viii) Poorly dilating pupil

(ix) Shallow Anterior Chamber

(x) Hard brown cataract

(xi) Subluxated cataract

(xii) Co-existent glaucoma and Cataract to undergo concurrent combined glaucoma and cataract surgery.

(xiii) Complicated cataract.

(xiv) High myopia/Hypermetropia.

(xv) High risk of the Floppy Iris Syndrome.

(xvi) History of past retinal surgery.

(xvii) Intraoperative complications.

Preoperative Evaluation/ Assessment

(i) **Assessment of patients' personality, his perception of touch, pain and prick sensations:** It is essential to start the assessment of a patient as soon as he walks into the consultation chamber. His level of cooperation, apprehension related to the surgery, pain tolerance and ability to obey commands can be easily assessed in the first interaction without employing any special tests. Asking a patient how painful or uncomfortable an earlier surgery (if any) was, gives us a good clue to the mental disposition of the patient. We in our set-up lay the greatest stress on the opinion of our trained ophthalmic assistants regarding the patients

cooperation ability as it is they who carry out most of the "uncomfortable" tests on the patient like sac syringing, A- Scan biometry etc.

(ii) **Assessment of orbicularis action:** Orbicularis action is assessed to rule out any element of blepharospasm. A good idea is to applanate the cornea and record the IOP with and without a speculum inserted. A marked rise in the IOP with the speculum might indicate a patient's unsuitability for no anaesthesia.

(iii) **Adnexa:** Adnexa needs to be evaluated to rule out any cause of increased intra-orbital pressure in the form of an orbital lesion or a mass. We also need to evaluate the adnexa for the purpose of adequate ocular exposure at the time of surgery. All this ensures an ideal milieu for performing the surgery, which is absolutely essential for no anaesthesia.

(iv) **Evaluation of Cataract and Anterior segment:** This is only done for the purpose of satisfying the operating surgeon so that he is comfortable with the grade of cataract and the eye as a whole. A surgeon should adopt no anaesthesia only in those cases in which he is absolutely skilled and confident of handling.

Surgical Technique of No Anaesthesia Phacoemulsification Cataract Surgery

Preoperative Counselling

(i) Patients is informed about the presence of persistent appreciation of mild to moderate touch sensation.

(ii) All our patients selected for no anaesthesia are well conversed with our protocol, cooperative patients with a moderate cataract and no co-existing ocular morbidity. Since, we receive patients speaking different languages and sometimes not conversant

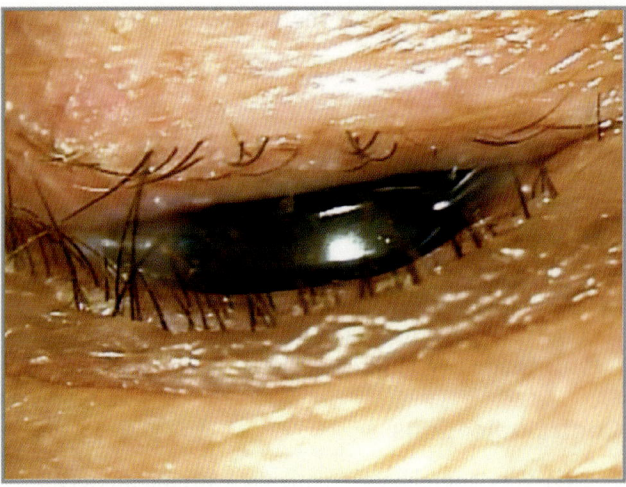

(a)

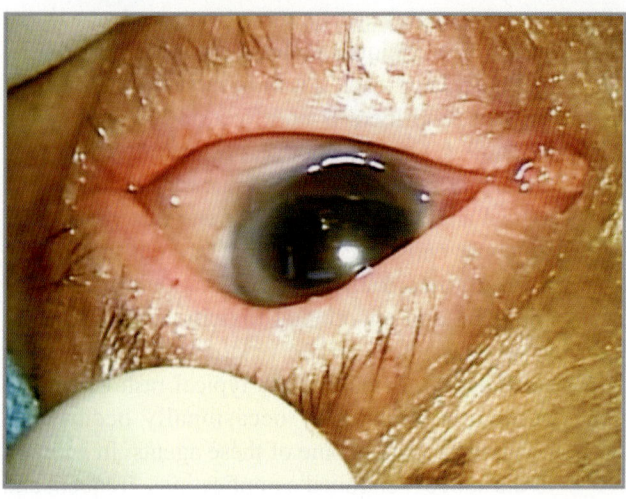

(b)

Fig. 54.2: (a) and (b) Strong orbicularis action with a very small palpebral fissure: Unsuitable for no anaesthesia/topical phacoemulsification surgery.

with either Hindi or English, we take up a patient for no anaesthesia cataract only if the patient and the surgeon have a common language of communication. We are extremely cautious of patients who "whistle in the dark" as described by Jaffe. These patients are the one who treat everything about their surgery casually and take a perfect outcome for granted. They enthral you with tales of their heroic pain tolerance and exhort you to try anything on them however, the moment they become horizontal on the operating table, their personality undergoes a U turn and they are the most demanding patients to handle. A patient who vehemently resists covering his nose/mouth with the drape is not a good candidate for no anaesthesia cataract.

(ii) Patients are asked to keep both eyes open under the drape, including the one not undergoing surgery and to keep them in a horizontal gaze. This can be achieved by fixing the patients eyes on the surgeons palm prior to surgery and subsequently looking towards the operating microscope light. However, there is no restriction on occasional movements of the eyes so as to avoid any undue stress on them during surgery.

The author's Preoperative Medication Protocol

No anaesthesia Phacoemulsification surgery invariably requires the same preoperative medications as for cataract surgery under topical or peribulbar anaesthesia. In our practice, we don't advocate any preoperative medications including systemic or topical antibiotics and sedatives. To achieve adequate mydriasis preoperatively, all patients are subjected to frequent instillation of phenylephrine (5%), Homatropine 2% or cyclopentolate (0.5%) along with Tropicamide (1%) eyedrops. Topical NSAID may also be used. However, some surgeons don't recommend NSAID drops since it may reduce corneal sensations hence surgery may not remain a no anaesthesia cataract surgery. In our practice we did not notice any significant difference in patient's appreciation of pain sensations with and without topical NSAID and thereby there is no harm in using topical NSAID.

Surgical Cleaning/Asepsis

While keeping both lids closed, periorbital skin surface excluding lids are cleaned with the help of application of 5% Povidone Iodine solution. However conjunctival sac was irrigated exclusively with the help of Ringer lactate or Balanced Salt Solution.

Choice of Speculum

A self retaining speculum consisting of metal plate blades and a screw is of immense value in cases of Phacoemulsification surgery during topical or no anaesthesia technique. Self retaining speculum can be adjusted in such a manner so as to restrict eye movements during surgery. While placing speculum great care is observed to avoid any touch on cornea or around limbus. While placing speculum blade over lower lid, patient is requested to look up and towards nasal side, whereas for placing the superior blade of speculum, patient is requested to look down and out. Simultaneously, great precautions are observed while removing the speculum at the end of surgery. Once the speculum is placed, patient is requested to look into the light or towards the surgeons palm while keeping both eyes open. The intensity of operating microscope light should be adjusted in a manner so as begin with a very low intensity initially and to gradually increase the intensity. The next step is to adjust the speculum screw so as to retain a horizontal plane position of eye as well as a moderate restriction of eye movements in vertical gaze.

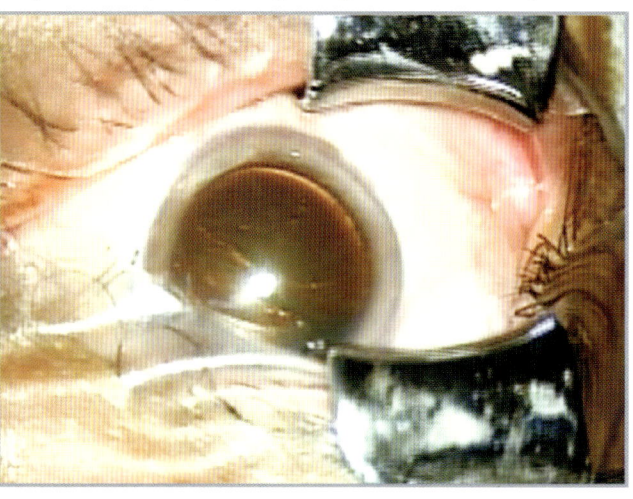

(a)

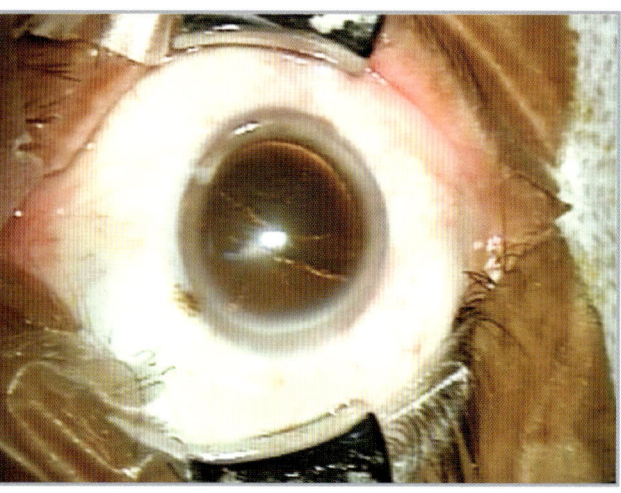

(b)

Fig. 54.3: (a) A speculum is being placed to retract lids (Touch on cornea is avoided by initiating insertion of speculum from lateral canthus when patient is looking towards the opposite direction), (b) Speculum is being well positioned

Incisions

The Principal author prefers to make two identical clear corneal incisions like side port incisions wide apart from each other. Great care is exercised to commence incision around one mm from the limbus and that they are confined away from the site of entry of perilimbal plexus and beginning of descemet's membrane. Of these two, the right sided incision is subsequently converted into a main incision. Before constructing incisions, adequate quantity of viscoelastics (Methylcellulose 2%) is placed over the cornea. To fix the eye, the patient is being requested to retain the eye position towards the light source. The next step is to apply gentle pressure over the speculum with the help of a Johnson's bud with the incision being constructed simultaneously. While doing so it is ensured that no direct touch of knife or cotton bud occurs over conjunctiva and cornea. The author does not use any instruments like-Sinskey hook or metal rod to fix the eye during the procedure. It is needless to stress the significance of avoiding epithelial injury due to iatrogenic insult at the site of incision. We recommend applying viscoelastics over the site of instrumentation to protect the surface against any inadvertent injury to it.

Capsulorrhexis

An ideal needle cystitome is very crucial to have a desired rhexis in any situation, especially in case of no anaesthesia cataract surgery. Good needle cystitome possesses a sharp bent tip, it should not have any knuckle or undue bend at

its tip. The tip should be at 90 degrees perpendicular to the shaft of the needle. Exact alignment of the hub, shaft, fulcrum and the bent tip position is of utmost significance to achieve atraumatic, smooth rhexis. Ultramicro rhexis forceps (23G) may also be used. The author prefers to design a rhexis with the help of a 26-gauge bent needle cystitome which is approximately 5.5 mm in size. The most important pre requisite is to maintain the horizontal position of the patient's head without extension or flexion of the chin throughout the procedure.

The next important issue is to retain the eye position in a straight horizontal gaze with least ocular movements. A tilted position of head or eye invariably leads to running/irregular or improper rhexis.

Hydroprocedures

Gradual sequential and slow Hydrodissection is recommended with BSS, since distended anterior chamber results in increased pressure, pain and forward push on iris lens diaphragm. This leads to shallowing of the AC and subsequent inadvertent iris prolapse from the site of incision.

Once adequate Hydrodelineation has been done, viscoseparation of the contents of the lens is carried out.

Nucleotomy

Pre-requisite of Ideal Nucleotomy

The maximal manipulation inside the eye occurs during the actual process of phacoemulsification. This is the step in which the widest instrument (the phaco tip), is going

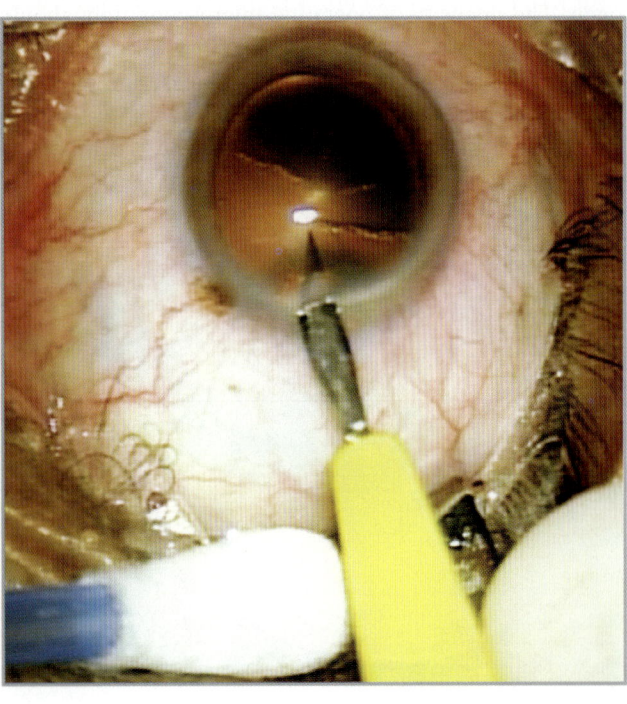

(a)

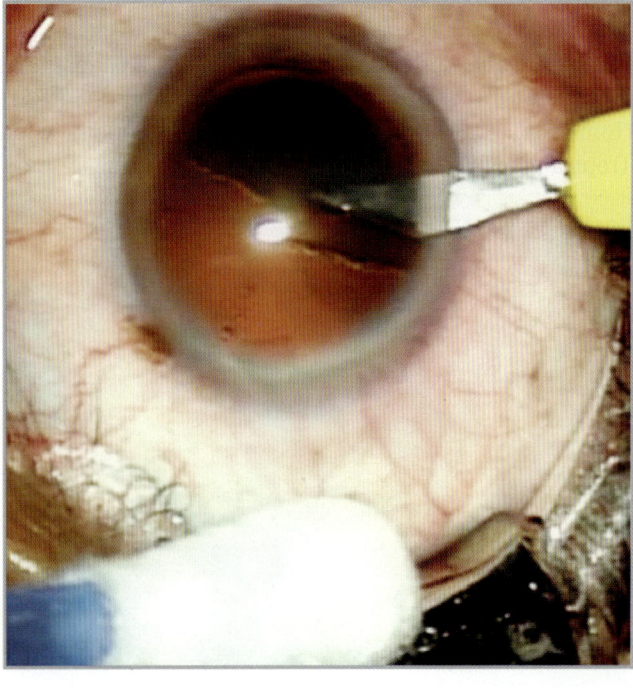

(b)

Fig. 54.4: (a) and (b) Incisions: Two identical clear corneal incisions like side port incisions wide apart from each other (Gentle pressure is being applied over the speculum with the help of Johnson's bud)

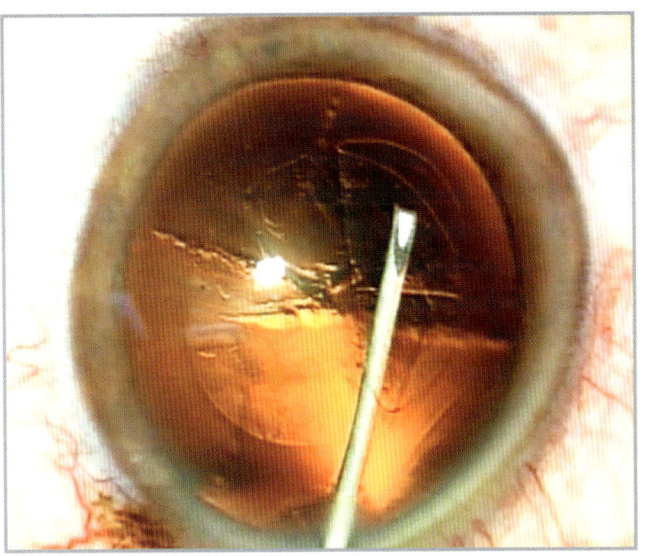

Fig. 54.5: Rhexis (Please note that no instrument is being used to fix eye ball

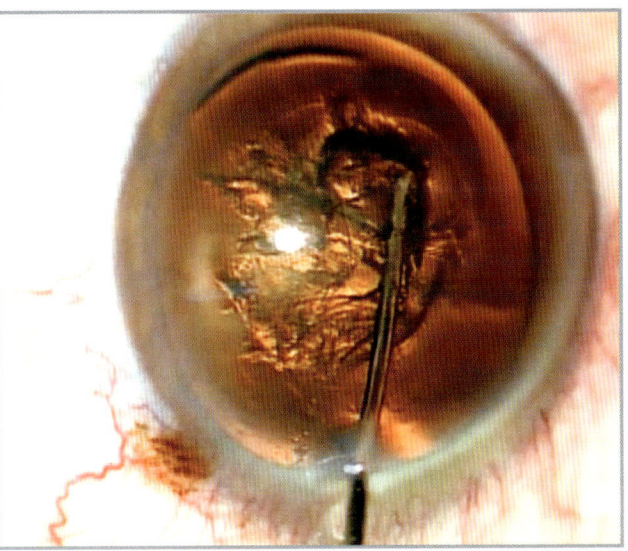

Fig. 54.6: Hydroprocedures

inside the eye through the main incision, causing it to stretch. Also, maximal amount of fluid turbulence in the anterior chamber occurs in this step and fluid currents strong enough to cause sensation on the iris innervations exist. The ideal nucleotomy for no anaesthesia cataract is therefore that which employs the mildest flow rates, minimal power and maximal vacuum. There should be no occasion or cause for repeated entry of instruments and the phaco tip into the eye.

Choice of Nucleotomy Technique

Chopping is most ideal: Central or paracentral. However, if the surgeon is comfortable and can achieve all essential benefits then any technique can be employed.

The author prefers to go ahead with paracentral chopping followed by central debulking while retaining the outer contour of nuclear fragment to facilitate smooth and atraumatic nuclear fragment rotation, thereby minimising the risk of inadvertent PCR and iris injuries.

Irrigation and Aspiration

Irrigation and Aspiration is being performed in a usual standard manner. Cortical clean up will either be co-axial or bi-manual.

Rigid IOL implants cannot be implanted through no or topical anaesthesia technique since insertion of these IOLs require a relatively large incision which is not possible to

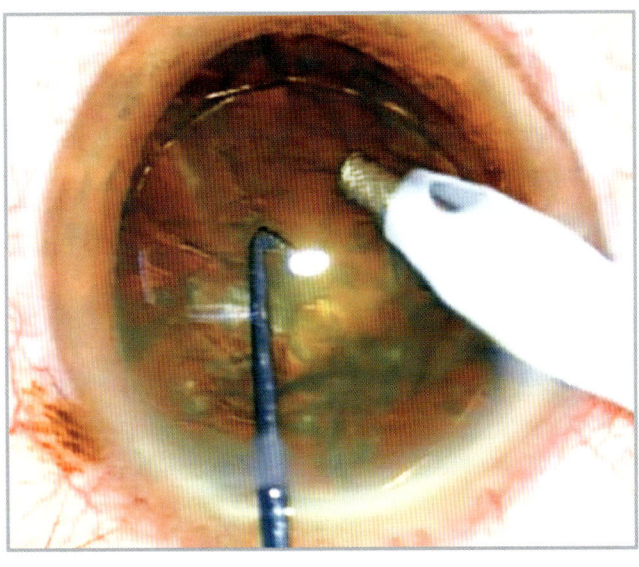

(a)

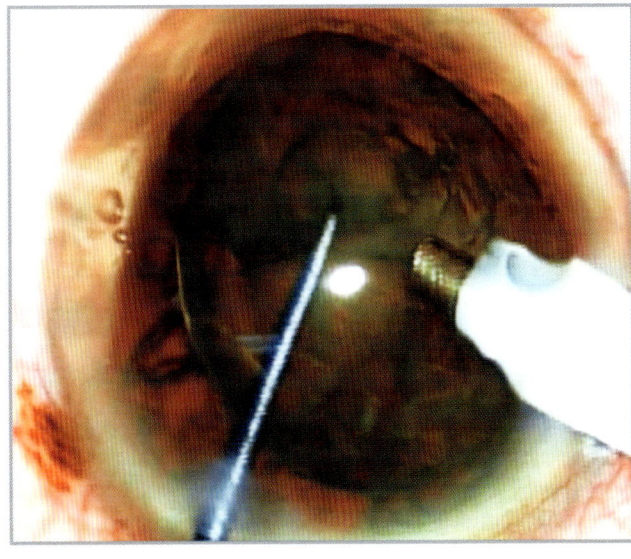

(b)

Fig. 54.7: (a) Primary nucleotomy by paracentral chopping, (b) Secondary/Tertiary nucleotomy by paracentral copping

fashion under no or topical anaesthesia. Hence, foldable Acrylic/Silicone single piece IOL implants remain the singular option for this technique.

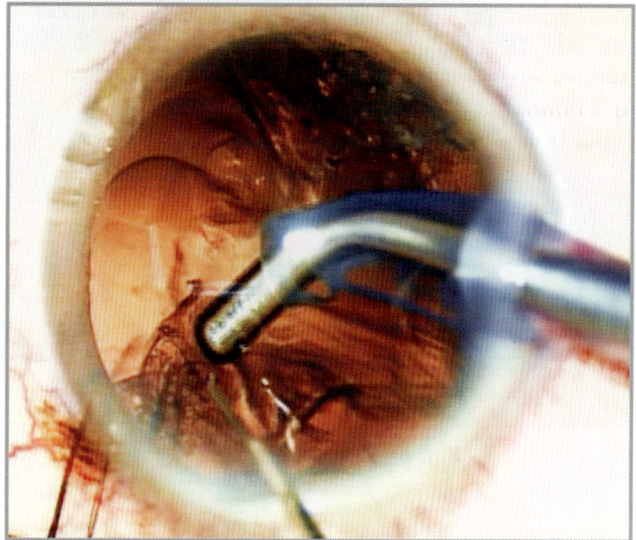

Fig. 54.8: Irrigation/Aspiration

The best choice of injector and IOL design is exclusively based on the fact that IOL insertion should be quick, flawless, should exert least pressure on incision as well as have a quick smooth and expected delivery of IOL into the capsular bag with very high order of consistency and precision. Undoubtedly, MICS lenses are a good choice but currently available injector systems are not very good for the no anaesthesia technique. The author has used all available IOLs and injector designs in no anaesthesia cataract surgery.

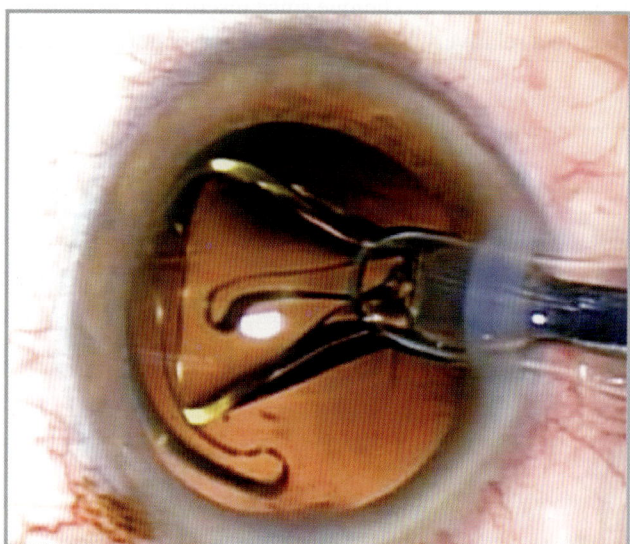

Fig. 54.9: IOL implantation

In our practice, FDA approved Single piece hydrophobic square edged IOLs and their injector systems have been found to be most suitable for no anaesthesia technique. However, the choice of IOL is exclusively the surgeon's

own preference and should be able to provide a desired surgical comfort to both the recipient and the surgeon.

Post IOL Implantation Wash

Care is taken during the post implantation wash to keep low aspiration settings, especially while using bimanual IA, as the chance of iris prolapse and chaffing are much more due to wound leak.

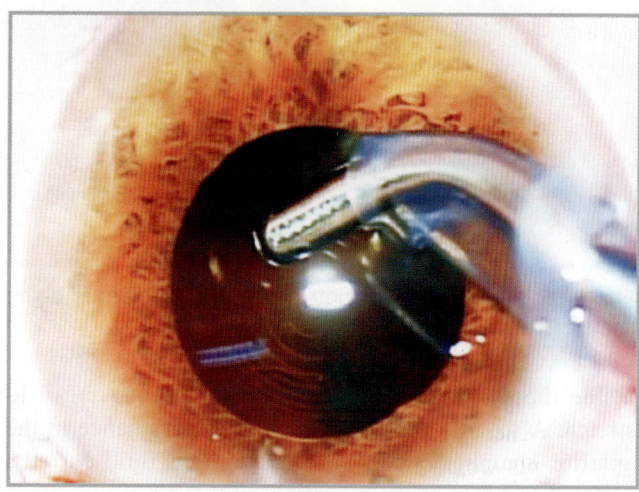

Fig. 54.10: Post IOL implantation wash

Stromal Hydration

Stromal hydration is a must as the incisions are more corneal than normal. After hydration, check the pressure of the eye by lightly tapping it on the sclera (not the cornea here as it is more sensitive and also an approaching instrument sets in the blink reflex). A high IOP can cause pain because of the iridial innervations.

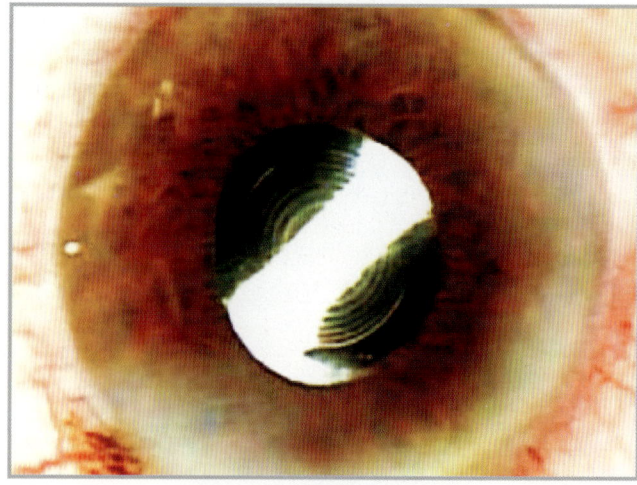

Fig. 54.11: Stromal hydration

Subconjunctival Injections/Eye Pad

Phacoemulsification surgery under Topical or No anaesthesia technique does not require subconjunctival injections or an eye pad. Since eye movements under the eyepad are too troublesome and annoying to the patients, as well as the absence of an eye pad provides good opportunity to start frequent instillation of topical medications at the earliest, thus minimises risks of postoperative inflammation.

Pre and Postoperative experience of Patients and Surgeons Comfort/Discomforts

In our practice, response to no anaesthesia phaco-emulsification surgery has been remarkable. Most of the cases remained asymptomatic or could not differentiate between effects of no anaesthesia or topical anaesthesia during phacoemulsification surgery.

Following criteria were analysed to assess the efficacy and acceptability of no anaesthesia technique.

Surgeon's Preoperative Response/Surgical Stress During Surgery

During his initial phase of commencement of no anaesthesia surgery, the author had experienced surgical fatigue due to frequent, uncontrolled movements of the patient's eye. Eye movements were quite significant probably because the surgical technique and phacoemulsifier systems were not that advanced or the surgeon himself was not mature enough in fine tuning the tricks of no anaesthesia phacoemulsification surgery. Over and above, we used wire speculum in place of a solid blade metal speculum at that time. Infact, solid blade metal speculum works very well to restrict undue eye movements during topical or no anaesthesia cataract surgery technique. At present the author has become well accustomed and does not feel any inhibition while performing no anaesthesia phacoemulsification surgery even in cases of moderately hard cataract of up to grade four nucleus. We conducted preoperative monitoring of the surgeons vital parameters in the form of pulse, respiratory rate and consistency of BP. These parameters definitely revealed fluctuations and variations during various steps of surgery and at the event of eye movements and during unpleasant or unwanted non surgical disturbances. However, such variations were marginal and insignificant to be compared with the topical anaesthesia technique. Infact, if the author has to operate under peribulbar anaesthesia a feeling of general anaesthesia is observed. We have become so accustomed to a little bit of ocular movements that their absence gives us an unusual feeling.

Recipient's Factors Related with Influence of No anaesthesia on Surgery

(i) Fear and apprehension against untoward effect on the eye during surgery due to inadvertent movement or poor cooperation from the recipient

Fear and apprehension against untoward effect on eye during surgery due to inadvertent movement or poor cooperation from the recipient remains a major factor in the patient's mind. This anxiety level has to be handled meticulously preoperatively. A well-informed patient on various aspects of no anaesthesia and phacoemulsification procedure, expected cooperation from the patient indeed relieve anxiety and subsequent feeling of touch, pain and discomfort substantially.

(ii) Touch

Response to feeling of touch sensation is the most common observation among patients undergoing no anaesthesia cataract surgery. This is mainly associated with an apprehension against inadvertent injury or untoward effect on eye due to inadvertent movement of the eye during various steps of surgery. The surgeon must be very cautious to avoid any touch onto the conjunctiva, cornea (especially at the central and optical zone of cornea) as well as repeated and coarse touch to the rest of ocular surface and adnexae. Precise and atraumatic entry of instruments through a viscous coated surface that too with minimal repetition of steps do play a major role in comfortable outcome of no anaesthesia cataract surgery. In our observation, touch sensation is well tolerated in more than 90% cases.

(iii) Sensations of pressure and distention

A Preoperative feeling of sensations of pressure on the eye and distention in the eye is one of the most common discomforts observed by the patient. Infact, these sensations are occasionally misinterpreted as pain and vary according to manipulations encountered during different steps and stages of the surgery. The surgeon has to exercise surgical movements and instrumentation with great care to avoid such feelings. Experience of mild pressure is noticed by most of the patients first due to pressure on the speculum with the help of cotton bud at the time of constructing the incision. Hence it is suggested to apply cotton bud on the body of solid blade of speculum slowly and in a linear fashion rather than compressing it in a sudden and downward direction. Administration of viscoelastics into the anterior chamber definitely produces sensation of distention and heaviness in the eye. A slow and gradual filling of viscoelastics into the anterior chamber and simultaneous egression of aqueous through the second incision by depressing the lower lip of incision minimises the gravity of pressure and distension sensations. Quality of IOL inserter system and size of incision thereof, are among the most crucial aspects related to the severity and extent of sensations of pressure and distention. In our experience, most patients had observed maximum discomfort at the time of IOL insertion. Size of incision, design of IOL delivery cartridges and delivery system amount significantly to minimise the feelings of discomfort and pressure exerted on the eye. It is better to have a slightly larger size of (0.20 mm larger than the size of cartridges) incision rather than it being too tight to allow an IOL inserter into the anterior chamber. The IOL should unfold into the bag in a flawless fashion without pressing the iris from behind and should not require manipulation by a second instrument to position the optics or any of the haptics. In our experience, the FDA approved single piece square edged hydrophobic intraocular lenses along with injector systems were found to be the most suitable deliverers of IOL with least discomfort to the patient and ease to the surgeon. However, it is the surgeon's own discretion to use any IOL and delivery system of his own choice.

(iv) Prick and foreign body sensations

Pricking and foreign body sensation is next to pressure and distention sensation among the order of frequency in no anaesthesia cataract surgery. However, most of the time pricking sensation is very minimal and not more than that of a small ant bite. A well informed patient as well as preoperative advisory and word of caution prior to surgical steps make the patient prepared to accept the fine prick and foreign body sensations. Commencement of construction of incisions, superficial epithelial abrasions due to instrumentation or a dry surface are common causes of the pricking sensation. However, iris touch or iris stroking remains the most common cause of intraoperative pricking sensation in a large number of patients. It is very interesting to note that about 30% patients do not appreciate any pricking sensation in spite of repeated iris stroking or touch. Indeed, it's a patient perception to react or tolerate any particular sensation. The author recommends to avoid any mechanical stroking of the iris as well as to exercise meticulous care while rotating the nucleus in the bag or during nuclear fragmentation and while removal of fragments out of the bag. We have noticed that the posterior surface of the iris reacts more to touch rather than stroking the iris on its anterior surface.

(v) Pain

Most patients are not able to distinguish pain sensations from the feeling of moderately significant touch of instrumentation, distention due to intracameral viscoelastics and fluids or from the prick and foreign body sensations. In common terms any unexpected intra operative happening is invariably described as pain. The author prefers to have continuous conversation with the patient during operation on various steps of the surgery and co-operation expected from patient during these particular occasions definitely are a big factor relieving the patient's anxiety. Lighter interaction during the course of surgery imbibes high confidence in the patient as well as diverts their attention from mental apprehension and fear of pain. A surgeon's confident voice makes a patient more confident and relaxed. We recommend such interactions in both topical and no anaesthesia phacoemulsification cataract surgery cases. Infact it is very difficult to quantify the spectrum of pain

during cataract surgery since it is a subjective assessment and response. Moderate pain may be considered as severe or very mild and vice versa, by two different individuals. A broad grading of pain can be graded as no pain (Grade 0), mild /minimal (1 to 3), Moderate (Mild to moderate/ Moderately moderate/ graded as 4 to 6, respectively), Severe (Moderately severe /bearable to excruciating and unbearable may be graded as 7 to 10). Dr Amar Agrawal has described pain on a 10-point visual analogue graphic pain scale with numeric and descriptive ratings awarded. In this scale, 0 is represented as no pain and 10 is represented as severe, "unbearable" pain. Undoubtedly, intraoperative pain is more in no anaesthesia cataract surgery as compared to surgery under topical anaesthesia in most of the cases, however the difference is not very significant. Infact, 20 to 30 % patients do not appreciate any pain, discomfort or foreign body sensations at all, whereas a large number of cases of topical anaesthesia or even peribulbar anesthesia experience pain and discomfort. In our view pain and discomfort in cataract surgery is more subjective than objective.

(vi) Postoperative irritable eye

In some cases, intraoperative epithelial abrasions or significant iris handling may lead to an irritable eye during the initial few hours postoperatively. It is wise to coat the cornea with the help of viscoelastics on the completion of surgery. Use of lubricants as a routine practice in all the cases of topical and no anaesthesia phacoemulsification surgery improves postoperative comforts as well as minimises the risk of pricking and foreign body sensation and irritable eye.

Complications

Though the encountered complications are no different from those in conventional phacoemulsification surgery, there are a set of complications more dreaded or common in a no anaesthesia cataract surgery.

Epithelial Injuries/Abrasions

As the eye of the patient is capable and liable to move because of lack of akinesia, there is an increased chance of an instrument causing epithelial injury or abrasion in case the patient moves the eye suddenly. To avoid this we minimise the instrumentation in the form of reducing their entry/exit from the eye to a minimum.

Inadvertent Extension of Rhexis

This complication is again the result of the dynamics of the patient's moving eye coming into play. At the time of capsulotomy, even a micro-movement of the eye of the patient can make the CCC run away into the periphery and into the zonules. Also if the orbicularis of the patient is in play, it causes an increased intraocular pressure, subsequent iris prolapse and the domino effect so dreaded.

Iris Prolapsed and Iris Chaffing

As described above, the ocular movement or raised intra-ocular pressure can cause iris chaffing or iris prolapse. Once it occurs, it is wise to leave heroics aside and give a 3 ml peribulbar block of 1% Ligniocaine. This is so, because the iris is one of the two maximally pain sensitive structures which we have to take into account in no anaesthesia surgery. Prolapse – squeesing – pain – squeesing - more prolapse - more pain-more squeesing- this vicious cycle is a sure recipe for trouble.

Endothelial/Descemets Injury

As the anterior chamber has an increased tendency to become shallow, the danger of endothelial injury and descemet's tear is real. Manoeuvring instrument's in or out of a moving eye can also strip off the descemets membrane.

Posterior Capsular Rent (PCR)

In our observation, carefully selected cases, good counselling, immaculate technique, optimal instrumentation and due caution can keep the rate of PCR no more than in a surgery performed under any other form of anaesthesia. The golden rule is to take the help of anaesthesia when anticipating such complications.

Pearls

(i) No touch on conjunctiva: Instrumentation or cotton bud sponges.
(ii) No Superior Rectus suture.
(iii) No application of cautery; Hence clear corneal incision is highly beneficial.
(iii) Eye is stabilised with the help of a blade speculum and the patient is asked to look into the light microscope. The author does not use any instrumentation like a metal rod to stabilise the eye as used in Dr Amar Agrawal's technique.
(iv) Actively go weeding out patients likely to have IFIS (Intraoperative Floppy Iris Syndrome). Ask for any history of prostate problems and intake of Urimax or similar drugs.

CONCLUSION

The speed and dexterity of the surgeon are paramount to the successful use of this technique, as is the proper patient selection. Incision and manipulations through the least sensitive (superior) part of the cornea are probably the most important factors. Further decrease in corneal sensation due to the dark iris of patients in India is another important factor.

No anaesthesia had revealed quite an uneventful performance in selected patients undergoing phaco-emulsification cataract surgery. It avoids any toxicity associated with topical and/or intracameral anaesthetic solutions. The surgical discomfort to the patient and the surgeon is minimal, pain; discomfort felt during the operation is invariably low and remains tolerable. Despite the fact that the cornea is one of the most sensitive structures, no anaesthesia phacoemulsification surgery works well in a selected group of cases under expert hands with certain modifications in the surgical technique. Absolutely flawless, atraumatic surgical intervention with precision in the form of construction of incision and subsequent surgical intervention through the least sensitive (superior) part of the cornea are probably the most crucial factors. Indeed no anaesthesia phacoemulsification surgery is very safe, effective in a selected band of patients and surgeons; and hence definitely worth considering.

REFERENCES

1. Greenhalgh D: Anesthesia for cataract surgery. In Yancff M, Ducker JS (Eds): Ophthalmology. St Louis: Mosby-Yearbook, 21.5–6, 1998.

2. Davis DB, Mandel MR: Anesthesia for cataract extraction. Int Ophthaimol Clin 34:13–30, 1994.

3. Haridas RP. Cataract surgery without anaesthesia: two descriptions by Arthur Jacob. Anaesth Intensive Care. 2009 Jul, 37 Suppl 1:36–41. Review.

4. Pandey SK, Werner L, Apple DJ, Agarwal A, Agarwal A, Agarwal S. No-anesthesia clear corneal phacoemulsification versus topical and topical plus intracameral anesthesia. Randomised clinical trial. J Cataract Refract Surg. 2001 Oct, 27(10):1643–50.

5. Agarwal A, Agarwal A, Agarwal S: No anesthesia cataract surgery with karate chop. Pliacoemulsification, Laser Cataract Surgery and Foldable lOLs (1st ed). New Delhi: Jaypee Brothers 145–53, 1998.

6. Millodot M: A review of research on the sensitivity of the cornea. Ophthal Physio) Opt 4:305–18, 1984.

7. Millodot M: Diurnal variation of corneal sensitivity. Br Ophthaimol 56:844, 1972.

8. Millodot M: Do blue-eyed people have more sensitive cornea than brown-eyed people? Nature 8:151–52, 1975.

9. P.S. Koch, Anterior chamber irrigation with unpreserved lidocaine 1% for anesthesia during cataract surgery. J Cataract Refract Surg 23 (1997), pp. 551–554.

10. Scott J, Huskisson EC: Graphic representation of pain. Pain 2:175–84, 1976.

11. Chalam KV, Murthy RK, Agarwal S, Gupta SK, Grover S. Comparative efficacy of topical tetraVisc versus lidocaine gel in cataract surgery. BMC Ophthalmol. 2009 Aug 17, 9:7.

12. Schutz JS, Mavrakanas NA. What degree of anesthesia is necessary for intraocular surgery? It depends on whether surgery is "open" or "closed". Br J Ophthalmol. 2009 Feb 11. Epub ahead of print.

13. Chuang LH, Lai CC, Ku WC, Yang KJ, Song HS. Efficacy and safety of phacoemulsification with intraocular lens implantation under topical anesthesia. Chang Gung Med J. 2004 Aug, 27(8):609–13.

14. Figueira EC, Sharma NS, Ooi JL, Masselos K, Lee KJ, Rosenberg ML, Francis IC, Alexander SL, Ferch NI, Stapleton F. The Lanindar test: a method of evaluating patient suitability for cataract surgery using assisted topical anaesthesia. Eye. 2009 Feb, 23(2):284–9.

15. Jonas JB, Pakdaman B, Sauder G. Frequency and predicting factors of surgical complications in cataract surgery performed under topical anaesthesia. Acta Ophthalmol Scand. 2006 Feb, 84(1):151–2.

16. Modi N, Shaw S, Allman K, Simcock P.Local anaesthetic cataract surgery: factors influencing perception of pain, anxiety and overall satisfaction. J Perioper Pract. 2008 Jan, 18(1):28–33.

17. Erdurmus M, Aydin B, Usta B, Yagci R, Gozdemir M, Totan Y. Patient comfort and surgeon satisfaction during cataract surgery using topical anesthesia with or without dexmedetomidine sedation.Eur J Ophthalmol. 2008 May-Jun, 18(3):361–7.

18. Crandall AS, Zabriskie NA, Patel BCK et al: A comparison of patient comfort during cataract surgery with topical anesthesia versus topical anesthesia and intracameral lidocaine. Ophthalmology 106:60–66, 1999.

19. Sharma NS, Ooi JL, Figueira EC, Rosenberg ML, Masselos K, Papalkar DP, Paramanathan N, Francis IC, Alexander SL, Ferch NI. Patient perceptions of second eye clear corneal cataract surgery using assisted topical anaesthesia. Eye. 2008 Apr, 22(4):547–50. Epub 2007 Feb 2.

20. Rengaraj V, Radhakrishnan M, Au Eong KG, Saw SM, Srinivasan A, Mathew J, Ramasamy K, Prajna N V. Visual experience during phacoemulsification under topical versus retrobulbar anesthesia: results of a prospective, randomised, controlled trial. Am J Ophthalmol. 2004 Nov, 138(5): 782–7.

21. Ang CL, Au Eong KG, Lee SS, Chan SP, Tan CS. Patients' expectation and experience of visual sensations during phacoemulsification under topical anaesthesia. Eye. 2007 Sep, 21(9):1162–7. Epub 2006 May 26.

22. Jain S, Ragoussi M, Rahman W, Grosvenor D. Incidence of visual sensations during cataract surgery under regional anaesthesia. Clin Experiment Ophthalmol. 2007 Nov, 35(8):784. No abstract available.

23. Venkatesh R, Muralikrishnan R, Au Eong KG.Visual sensation during phacoemulsification using topical versus regional anesthesia. J Cataract Refract Surg. 2005 Oct, 31(10): 1855–6.

24. Biró Z, Schvöller M. Subjective visual sensations during cataract surgery performed under topical anaesthesia. Acta Ophthalmol. 2008 Dec, 86(8):894–6.

25. Ismail SA, Mowafi HA. Melatonin provides anxiolysis, enhances analgesia, decreases intraocular pressure, and promotes better operating conditions during cataract surgery under topical anesthesia. Anesth Analg. 2009 Apr, 108(4): 1146–51.

26. Bertrand RH, Garcia JB, de Oliveira CM, Bertrand AL. Topical anesthesia associated with sedation for phaco-emulsification. Experience with 312 patients. Rev Bras Anestesiol. 2008 Jan-Feb, 58(1):23–34. English, Portuguese.

27. Balkan BK, Iyilikçi L, Günenç F, Uzümlü H, Kara HC, Celik L, Durak I, Gökel E.Comparison of sedation requirements for cataract surgery under topical anesthesia or retrobulbar block. Eur J Ophthalmol. 2004 Nov-Dec, 14(6):473–7.

28. Habib NE, Mandour NM, Balmer HG.Effect of midazolam on anxiety level and pain perception in cataract surgery with topical anesthesia. J Cataract Refract Surg. 2004 Feb, 30(2): 437–43.

29. Cok OY, Ertan A, Bahadir M. Comparison of midazolam sedation with or without fentanyl in cataract surgery. Acta Anaesthesiol Belg. 2008, 59(1):27–32.

30. Fernández SA, Dios E, Diz JC. Comparative study of topical anaesthesia with lidocaine 2% vs levobupivacaine 0.75% in cataract surgery. Br J Anaesth. 2009 Feb, 102(2):216–20.

31. Borazan M, Karalezli A, Akova YA, Algan C, Oto S. Comparative clinical trial of topical anaesthetic agents for cataract surgery with phacoemulsification: lidocaine 2% drops, levobupivacaine 0.75% drops, and ropivacaine 1% drops. Eye. 2008 Mar, 22(3):425–9. Epub 2007 Sep 7.

32. Borazan M, Karalezli A, Oto S, Algan C, Aydin Akova Y. Comparison of a bupivacaine 0.5% and lidocaine 2% mixture with levobupivacaine 0.75% and ropivacaine 1% in peribulbar anaesthesia for cataract surgery with phacoemulsification. Acta Ophthalmol Scand. 2007 Dec, 85(8):844–7. Epub 2007 Jul 28.

33. Ezra DG, Nambiar A, Allan BD. Supplementary intracameral lidocaine for phacoemulsification under topical anesthesia. A meta-analysis of randomised controlled trials. Ophthal-mology. 2008 Mar, 115(3):455–87. Epub 2007 Dec 3.

34. Ezra DG, Allan BD. Topical anaesthesia alone versus topical anaesthesia with intracameral lidocaine for phacoemulsi-fication.Cochrane Database Syst Rev. 2007 Jul 18, (3): CD005276. Review.

35. Välimäki JO.Is intracameral lidocaine really effective in cataract surgery? Eur J Ophthalmol. 2007 May-Jun, 17(3): 332–5.

36. P.S. Koch, Anterior chamber irrigation with unpreserved lidocaine 1% for anesthesia during cataract surgery. J Cataract Refract Surg 23 (1997), pp. 551–554.

37. Ugur B, Dundar SO, Ogurlu M, Gezer E, Ozcura F, Gursoy F. Ropivacaine versus lidocaine for deep-topical, nerve-block anaesthesia in cataract surgery: a double-blind randomised clinical trial. Clin Experiment Ophthalmol. 2007 Mar, 35(2): 148–51.

38. Di Donato A, Fontana C, Lancia F, Di Giorgio K, Reali S, Caricati A. Levobupivacaine 0.75% vs. lidocaine 4% for topi-cal anaesthesia: a clinical comparison in cataract surgery. Eur J Anaesthesiol. 2007 May, 24(5):438–40. Epub 2007 Jan 4.

39. Amiel H, Koch PS. Tetracaine hydrochloride 0.5% versus lidocaine 2% jelly as a topical anesthetic agent in cataract surgery: comparative clinical trial.J Cataract Refract Surg. 2007 Jan, 33(1): 98–100.

40. Gombos K, Jakubovits E, Kolos A, Salacz G, Németh J. Cataract surgery anaesthesia: is topical anaesthesia really better than retrobulbar ? Acta Ophthalmol Scand. 2007 May, 85(3):309–16.

41. Perone JM, Popovici A, Ouled-Moussa R, Herasymyuk O, Reynders S. Safety and efficacy of two ocular anesthetic methods for phacoemulsification: topical anesthesia and viscoanesthesia (VisThesia). Eur J Ophthalmol. 2007 Mar-Apr, 17(2):171–7.

42. Ryu JH, Kim M, Bahk JH, Do SH, Cheong IY, Kim YC. A comparison of retrobulbar block, sub-Tenon block, and topical anesthesia during cataract surgery. Eur J Ophthalmol. 2009 Mar-Apr, 19(2):240–6.

43. Fazel MR, Forghani Z, Aghadoost D, Fakharian E. Retrobulbar versus topical anesthesia for phacoemulsification. Pak J Biol Sci. 2008 Oct 1, 11(19):2314–9.

44. Budd JM, Brown JP, Thomas J, Hardwick M, McDonald P, Barber K. A comparison of sub-Tenon's with peribulbar anaesthesia in patients undergoing sequential bilateral cataract surgery. Anaesthesia. 2009 Jan, 64(1):19–22. Erratum in: Anaesthesia. 2009 Feb, 64(2):231. Budd, M [corrected to Budd, J M].

45. Rodrigues PA, Vale PJ, Cruz LM, Carvalho RP, Ribeiro IM, Martins JL. Topical anesthesia versus sub-Tenon block for cataract surgery: surgical conditions and patient satisfaction. Eur J Ophthalmol. 2008 May-Jun, 18(3):356–60.

46. Gutiérrez-Carmona FJ, Alvarez-Marín J.Randomised comparative clinical study of cryoanalgesia versus topical anesthesia in clear corneal phacoemulsification. J Cataract Refract Surg. 2005 Jun, 31(6):1187–93.

47. Chung SA, Kim CY, Chang JH, Hong S, Kang SY, Seong GJ, Lee JB Change in ocular alignment after topical anesthetic cataract surgery. Graefes Arch Clin Exp Ophthalmol. 2009 Sep, 247(9):1269–72. Epub 2009 Apr 30.

48. Sharwood PL, Thomas D, Roberts TV. Adverse medical events associated with cataract surgery performed under topical anaesthesia. Clin Experiment Ophthalmol. 2008 Dec, 36(9): 842–6.

49. Judge AJ, Najafi K, Lee DA, Miller KM, Corneal endothelial toxicity of topical anesthesia. Ophthalmology 104 (1997), pp. 1373–1379.

50. G.O.D. Rosenwasser, Complications of topical ocular anesthetics. Int Ophthalmol Clin 29 (1989), pp. 153–158.

51. Garcia-Arumi J, Fonollosa A, Sararols L, Fina F, Martínez-Castillo V, Boixadera A, Zapata MA, Campins M. Topical anesthesia: possible risk factor for endophthalmitis after cataract extraction. J Cataract Refract Surg. 2007 Jun, 33(6): 989–92.

52. Unal M, Yücel I, Altin M.Pain induced by phacoemulsification performed by residents using topical anesthesia. Ophthalmic Surg Lasers Imaging. 2007 Sep-Oct, 38(5): 386–91.

53. Kongsap P, Wiriyaluppa C.A comparison of patient pain during cataract surgery with topical anesthesia in Prechop Manual Phacofragmentation versus phacoemulsification. J Med Assoc Thai. 2006 Jul, 89(7):959–66.

54. Eke T, Thompson JR. Serious complications of local anaesthesia for cataract surgery: a 1 year national survey in the United Kingdom. Br J Ophthalmol. 2007 Apr, 91(4): 470–5. Epub 2006 Nov 23.

55. Hadden PW, Scott RC. Cardiac arrest during phacoemulsification using topical anesthesia in an unsedated patient. J Cataract Refract Surg. 2006 Feb, 32(2):369. No abstract available.

56. Liu DT, Lee VY, Chan WM, Lam DS. Pain induced by phacoemulsification without sedation using topical or peribulbar anesthesia. J Cataract Refract Surg. 2006 Jan, 32(1):2.

57. Rosenwasser GOD: Complications of topical ocular anesthetics. Int Ophthaimol Clin 29:153–58, 1989.

58. T. Kim, G.P. Holley, J.H. Lee et al., The effects of intraocular lidocaine on the corneal endothelium. Ophthalmology 105 (1998), pp. 125–130.

Contemporary Issue in Phacoemulsification Surgery

55

SICS and Phaco:
Compare and Contrast

Dr Pushpa Varma

INTRODUCTION

Cataract is a major cause of preventable blindness since ancient times. Despite giant leaps in medical technology, no therapeutic agent has been discovered which can cure or prevent cataract. Therefore, surgery remains the only modality of treatment and a constant evolution in the surgical techniques to extract cataract and restore fruitful vision is always underway.

Manual SICS is definitely a breakthrough in a country like India. In our country, we are overburdened with mature and hard cataract and according to the size and hardness of the nucleus, we design the incision length which may vary from 5.5 mm to 7.0 mm or even 7.5 mm in manual SICS.

In manual SICS, S stands for small, but for all practical purposes, in normal SICS, S is not always small to us. The S's for us are – Safe, Sutureless, Stressless, Stable, Secure and Self sealing cataract surgery with a short learning curve.

It is a very useful alternative technique to phacoemulsification which complements the surgeons.

HISTORY OF MANUAL SICS

Kelman predicted that incisions 3 mm wide will be astigmatism neutral because of their visual size. But with the introduction of IOL implants, enlargement of incision became necessary upto 6.5–7.0 mm for lens implantation.

Kratz was the surgeon who made the incision posteriorly in the sclera, increasing appositional surfaces to enhance wound healing. Girard and Hoffman were the first to call the posterior incision a "scleral tunnel incision".

Dr Gerald T. Kuner was the first to successfully achieve nuclear division in the anterior chamber in 1983 using a constricting wire loop. Subsequently came the

Luther Fry's phaco sandwich technique and **Peter Kansas** Phaco Fracture.

Dr Richard Kraty developed the scleral pocket incision. The incision consisted of a posteriorly placed incision with a scleral tunnel and corneal wedge. However, these incisions had to be closed with sutures. Initially, radial interrupted sutures were used and later single stitch closure technique involved X-stitch, horizontal anchor suture of Masket and the infinity suture of Howard Fine.

Michael McFarland in 1990 demonstrated the first sutureless closure of the scleral tunnel wound. **Paul Ernest** recognised that the long scleral tunnel incision terminated in a corneal entrance and that the posterior lip of the incision (corneal lip) acted as a one-way valve imparting the self-sealing characteristics.

Koch (1991) in Warwick, Rhode Island described incisional funnel, indicating that there were certain characteristics of self-sealing incisions with respect to length and configuration that imparted not only self-sealability but also astigmatism neutrality to these incisions.

Gimbel in 1984, developed a technique for anterior capsulotomy called capsulorrhexis, hydrodissection was first described by **Michael Blumenthal** and hydrodelineation was introduced by **Aziz Y. Anis**.

ADVANTAGES OVER CONVENTIONAL ECCE

(a) Better wound stability.
(b) Reduction of induced astigmatism (stability of refraction).
(c) Greater patient compliance with early visual rehabilitation.
(d) Less chances of anterior chamber collapse during surgery.
(e) Dreaded complications, like expulsive hemorrhage can be avoided.

(f) Suture and suture-related complications like iris prolapse, endophthalmitis, bleeding and epithelial defects can be avoided.

(g) Minimal postoperative visits.

ADVANTAGES OF SICS OVER PHACOEMULSIFICATION

(a) Universal applicability.

(b) Easier learning Curve.

(c) Less instruments required.

(d) Useful alternative to phacoemulsification in case of machine failure.

(e) Minimal surgical complications.

(f) Faster procedure as compared to phaco.

CRITERIA FOR IDEAL CASE SELECTION FOR MANUAL SICS

(a) Cornea: Good clarity, normal thickness, healthy endothelium.

(b) Normal anterior chamber depth.

(c) Well dilated pupil.

(d) Intact zonules.

(e) Type of cataract:

    (i) Immature cortical cataract.

    (ii) Nuclear sclerosis grade II and III.

As the surgeon learns this technique, gradually he can master this procedure virtually in all types of cataract.

CONTRAINDICATIONS FOR MANUAL SICS

(a) Dislocated lens and subluxated lens with inadequate zonular support.

(b) Corneal conditions:

    (i) Congenital abnormalities of cornea like micro cornea.

    (ii) Endothelial dystrophies and conditions with low endothelial cell count.

    (iii) Peripheral thinning of cornea.

(c) Ocular inflammations

    (i) Scleritis, scleral ectasia or ciliary staphyloma.

    (ii) Inflammatory Conjunctival scarring disorders.

    (iii) Systemic disorders—Any bleeding diathesis, predisposing the patient to hyphaema from the scleral tunnel.

From the above considerations, it is clear that contraindications to SICS are minimal, but in practical terms, the major limiting factors are the skill and experience of the surgeon.

PREOPERATIVE PREPARATION AND ANAESTHESIA

(a) A medical clearance is obtained. Wide spectrum antibiotic drops are instilled topically every four hours a day before surgery. Mydriasis is achieved using cyclopentolate 1% or tropicamide 1% along with phenylephrine 5–10% drops. Topical 0.03% flurbiprofen or diclofenac sodium 0.1% every 20 minutes thrice will maintain intraoperative mydriasis.

(b) Peribulbar or retrobulbar anesthesia, anything can be given. The surgery can be performed even under topical anesthesia. But the important point is not to give bulbar massage or pressure with super pinky. The need is for normotensive or hypertensive eyeball. Hypertonic state of the eyeball also facilitates the following:

    (i) Introduction of MVR for side port entry or AC maintainer.

    (ii) Dissection of sclerocorneal tunnel.

    (iii) For CCC, hydroexpression of epinucleus, cortex or blood.

BASIC STEPS OF MANUAL SICS

(a) The steps of manual SICS are:

    (i) Superior rectus bridle suture

    (ii) Conjunctival flap (fornix based)

    (iii) Sclerocorneal tunnel construction

       • External incision

       • Sclerocorneal tunnelling

       • Internal incision

    (iv) Anterior capsulotomy

    (v) Hydrodissection and hydrodelineation

    (vi) Nucleus prolapse from the capsular bag

    (vii) Nucleus extraction from the anterior chamber

    (viii) Cortical clean up

    (ix) Implantation of the IOL into the bag

    (x) Wound closure.

Superior Rectus Bridle Suture

Superior rectus bridle suture is given to manoeuvre the globe forward and downwards. It not only fixes the globe during the initial steps of surgery like tunnelling and paracentesis, it also provides a counteraction force during procedures like nucleus extraction and epinucleus delivery, thereby enhancing the efficiency of these techniques.

Conjunctival Flap

A small fornix based conjunctival flap is preferred. A small flap of approximately 8 mm length and 4 mm width is often sufficient. First, give a small radial cut with the scissors. Do a good undermining dissection of it along with Tenon's capsule, and then cut along the limbus for 6–8 mm. The important point is to clear all the Tenon's attachments from the sclera. Otherwise, the first external scleral groove incision may not be in perfect depth in all lengths.

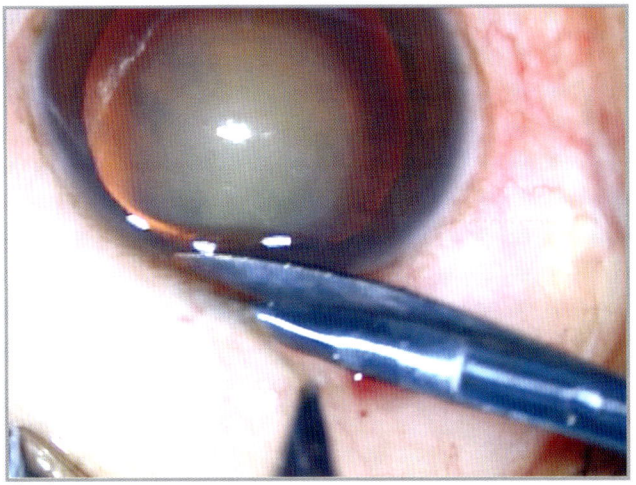

Fig. 55.1: Fornix based conjunctival flap

A gentle and just adequate cautery (wet field cautery is always better) is applied.

Sclerocorneal Tunnel Construction

External Incision

In manual SICS, incision is the main concern. The very goal of this surgery lies on the self sealing property of the incision. Paul Ernest introduced the concept of an internal corneal lip (three plane incision) acting as a one-way valve. This corneal lip not only imparted a self-sealing nature to this incision but also prevented the development of hyphaema and delayed filtering blebs.

The classical incision is a three-step incision, shaped like Z. One limb of the Z is the vertical gutter at the external site of incision. The second limb is the horizontal dissection and the third limb is the angled entry into the anterior chamber.

Instruments that are commonly used to making the external groove are razor blade fragments or a No. 15 surgical knife or crescent knife or a guarded diamond knife.

The vital statistics that go into the making of a manual phaco incision include:

  (i) **Site of the external incision:** The external incision should be based 2–3 mm posterior to the limbus.

 (ii) **Placement of the external incision:** The scleral tunnel incision is usually placed at the 12 O'clock position.

Advantages and Disadvantages of Temporal Incision

• Greater access to the incision.
• The eye does not need to be turned down.
• Iris plane is parallel to the microscope light, so red glow is excellent and visualisation is enhanced.
• Being farthest from the visual axis, it is more refractively stable.

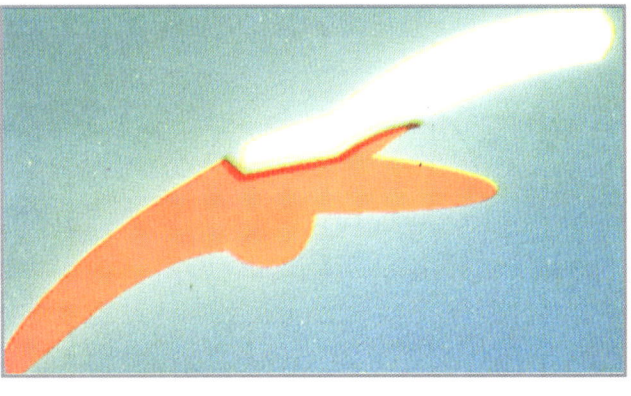

(a)

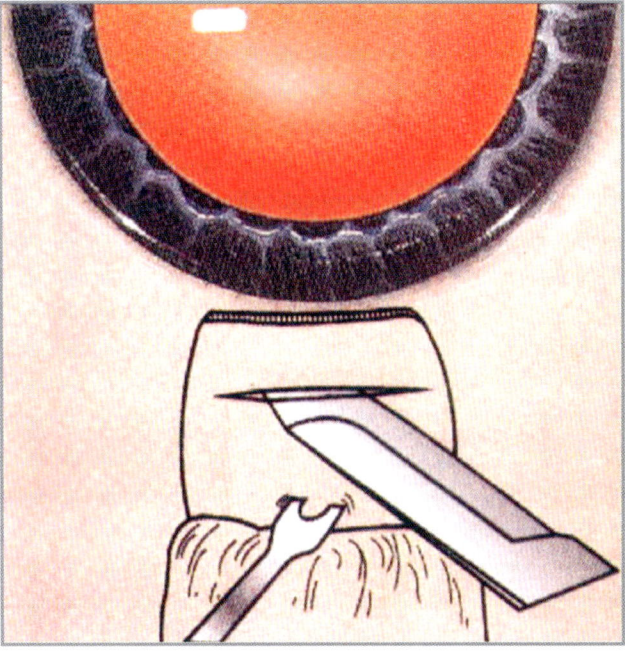

(b)

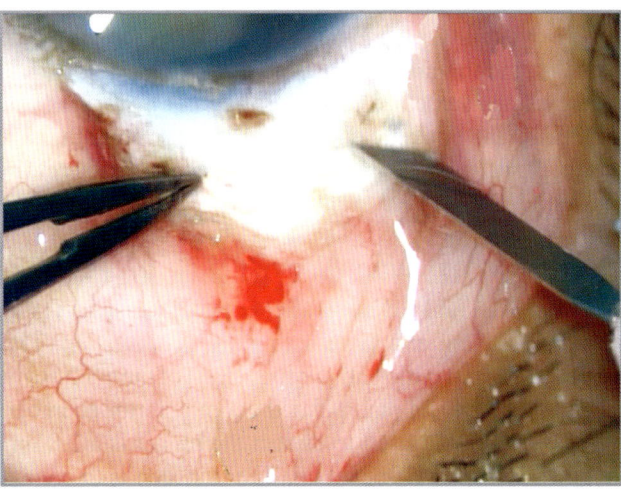

(c)

Fig. 55.2: (a) Three plane Incision, (b) External incision (SICS), (c) Frown shaped external incision

Types of incisions

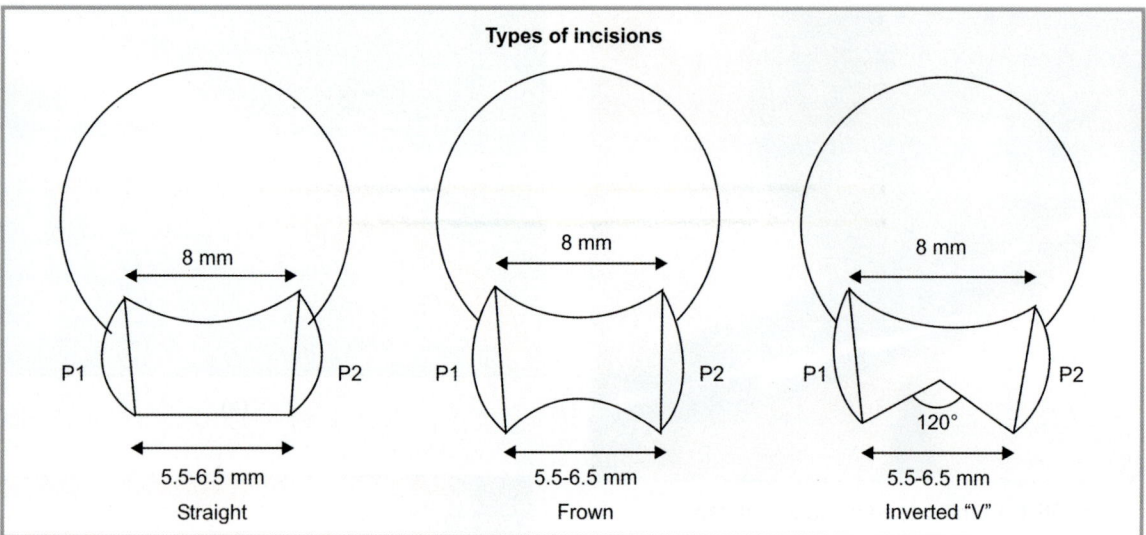

Fig. 55.2: (d) Types of incisions

The disadvantage of the temporal incision is the higher risk of complications and the uncomfortable position to work.

(iii) **Style of incision:** Can be in the form of:
- Straight
- Frown
- Inverted 'V' or Chevron.

Frown incision is the most stable and is supposed to prevent the sliding between the roof and floor of tunnel, thereby minimising astigmatic shift.

(iv) **Length of incision:** The length of the external incision should equal the size of the IOL that has to be introduced through it.

(v) **Depth of tunnel dissection:** The thickness of the roof of tunnel should be about 300 μ or 1/3rd to 1/2 of scleral thicknesses.

(vi) **Length of the tunnel:** The tunnel length is usually 4 mm. Too long tunnel lengths compromise visibility preoperatively. Too short tunnel length tend to make the incision leaky.

Remember, external incision is the gateway for adequate and efficient pocket tunnel dissection. A smooth, well defined, sharply cut, uniform scleral groove is therefore, desirable.

Sclero-corneal Tunnelling

The tunnel should have a smaller external incision, a large internal incision and large side pockets dissection. This configuration of outlet, allows the largest of the nuclei to be accommodated and manipulated out of anterior chamber.

The instrument used to dissect the tunnel is a 2.8 mm angled crescent with bevel up. The first step is to engage the tissue on the anterior edge at the depth of the groove.

Now dissect little at the external scleral lip. Split the sclera from the centre, as it is easier. The tip of the blade

should be tilted anteriorly to follow the anterior curve of the limbus and then the cornea; 1.5 to 2.0 mm of the clear cornea is dissected. Once the straight tract is created, the crescent is moved sideways to right and left, keeping in dissected plane side pockets in sclera and cornea are dissected by turning the blade 60–70° away from the 12 O'clock meridian.

During tunnelling within the sclera, the forward surface of the blade should just be visible. If it is very clearly visible, the tunnel is too superficial, and if it is barely visible, the tunnel is too deep. During tunnelling forward, one should raise the tip and depress the heel of the blade to prevent premature entry into the anterior chamber. Never hold the scleral tip during any point of dissection of tunnel.

Side Port Entry

One side port entry is usually made using a 15° super blade at the 10 O'clock position or perpendicular to the tunnel, in the clear cornea.

The stab entry should be 2 mm wide. It provides an alternative entry for the capsulotome and aspiration of subincisional cortex with reformation of the anterior chamber at the end of surgery.

Internal Corneal Incision

This is done using a sharp 2.8 mm or 3.2 mm angled keratome. Anterior chamber being maintained deep either by ACM flow or by viscoelastic; the angled keratome is introduced into the pre-dissected sclero-corneal pocket tunnel.

Once the Keratome tip reaches the extreme anterior limit of the tunnel, the bowel of the keratome is lifted to dip the tip into the anterior chamber, with forward movements, the keratome held parallel to the iris. The keratome is next turned 80° to 90° sideways to accomplish the lateral ends of the internal incision.

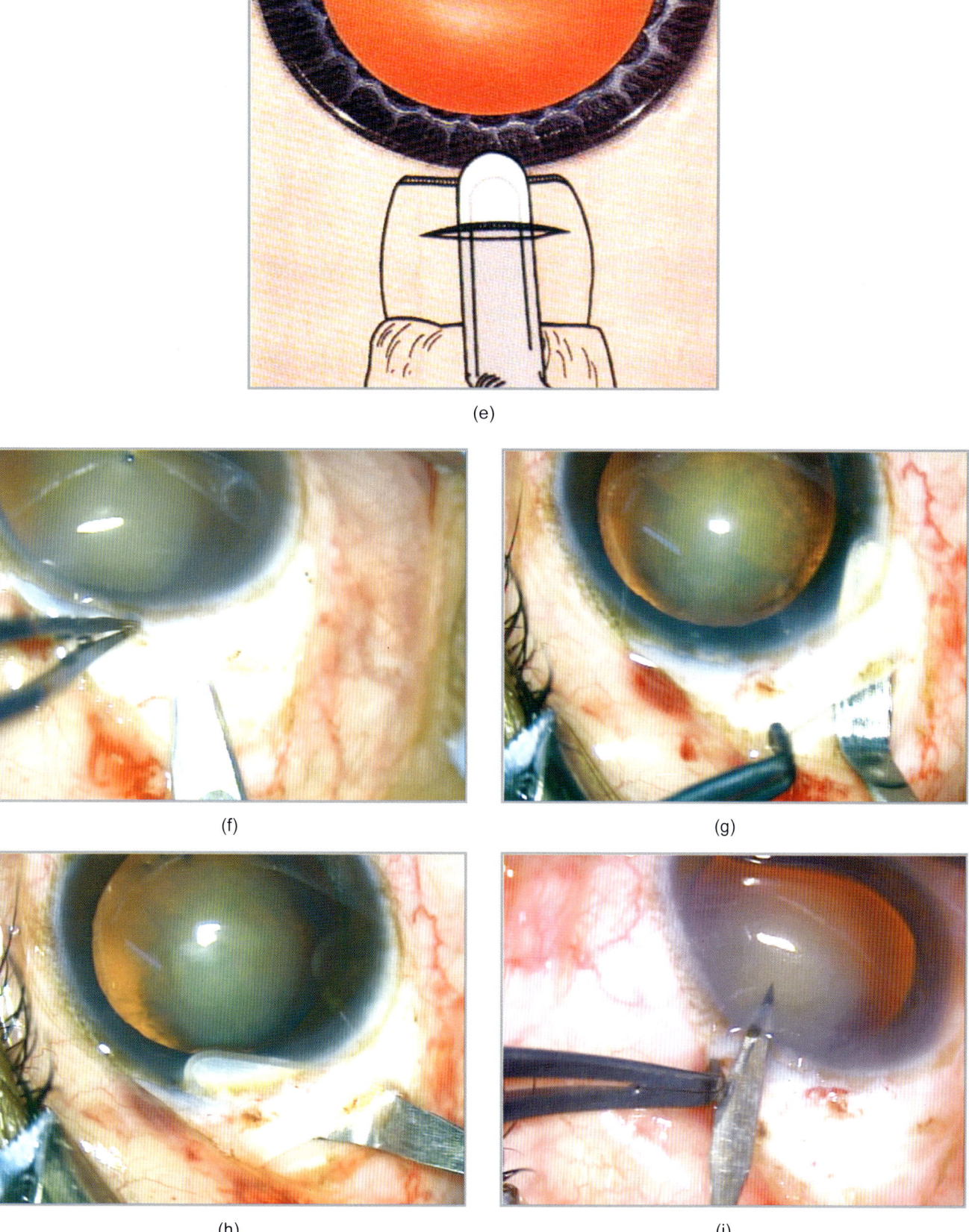

Fig. 55.2: (e) Sclero-corneal tunnelling (SICS), (f) Sclero-corneal tunnel, (g) SICS : Internal pocket, (h) SICS: Internal pocket, (i) SICS: Side Port Entry

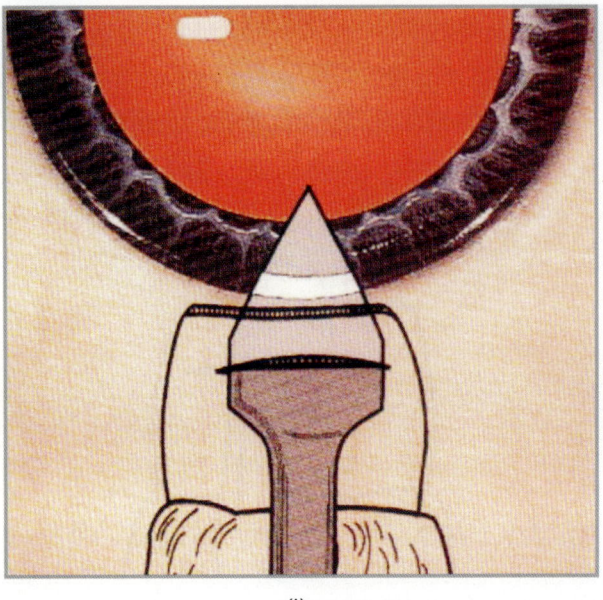

(j)

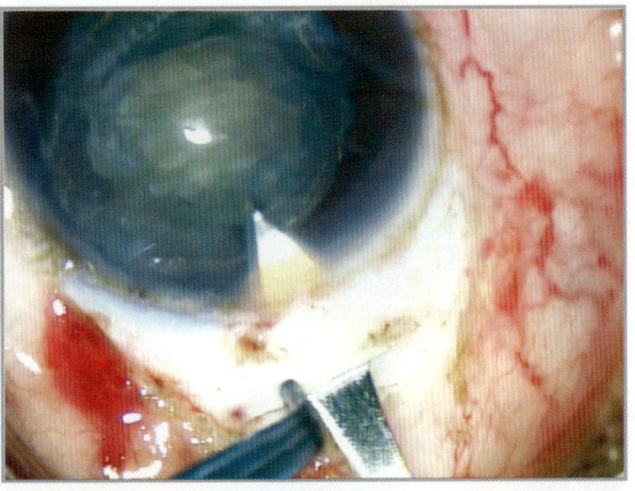

(k)

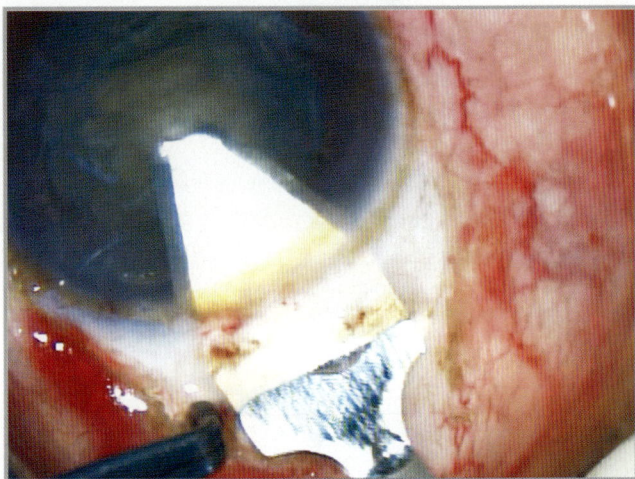

(l)

Fig. 55.2: (j) Internal Incision (SICS), (k) Internal corneal incision (3.2 mm entry), (l) Extension of the internal corneal incision (5.25 mm entry)

CAPSULOTOMY

Four types of capsular openings can be made:
1. CCC
2. Envelope
3. Can-op-rhexis
4. Can opener.

Continuous Curvilinear Capsulorrhexis

It is the ideal and preferred type of capsulotomy except for a few contraindications. There are several advantages of capsulorrhexis.

Intraoperative

1. The capsule can be stretched considerably.

2. Limits the risk of tear or radial cracks during the operation.
3. Hydrodissection is safe.
4. The intraoperative stress on the zonules is minimal
5. Easier cortical aspiration.
6. IOL can be positioned safely and symmetrically in the bag.
7. IOL can be placed on the rhexis in cases of posterior chamber rupture (sulcus fixation).

Postoperative

1. Prevents IOL from displacements and effects of mechanical pressure.
2. Produces an extensive contact area between the haptics of the IOL and the anterior capsule which reduces the possibility of decentring.

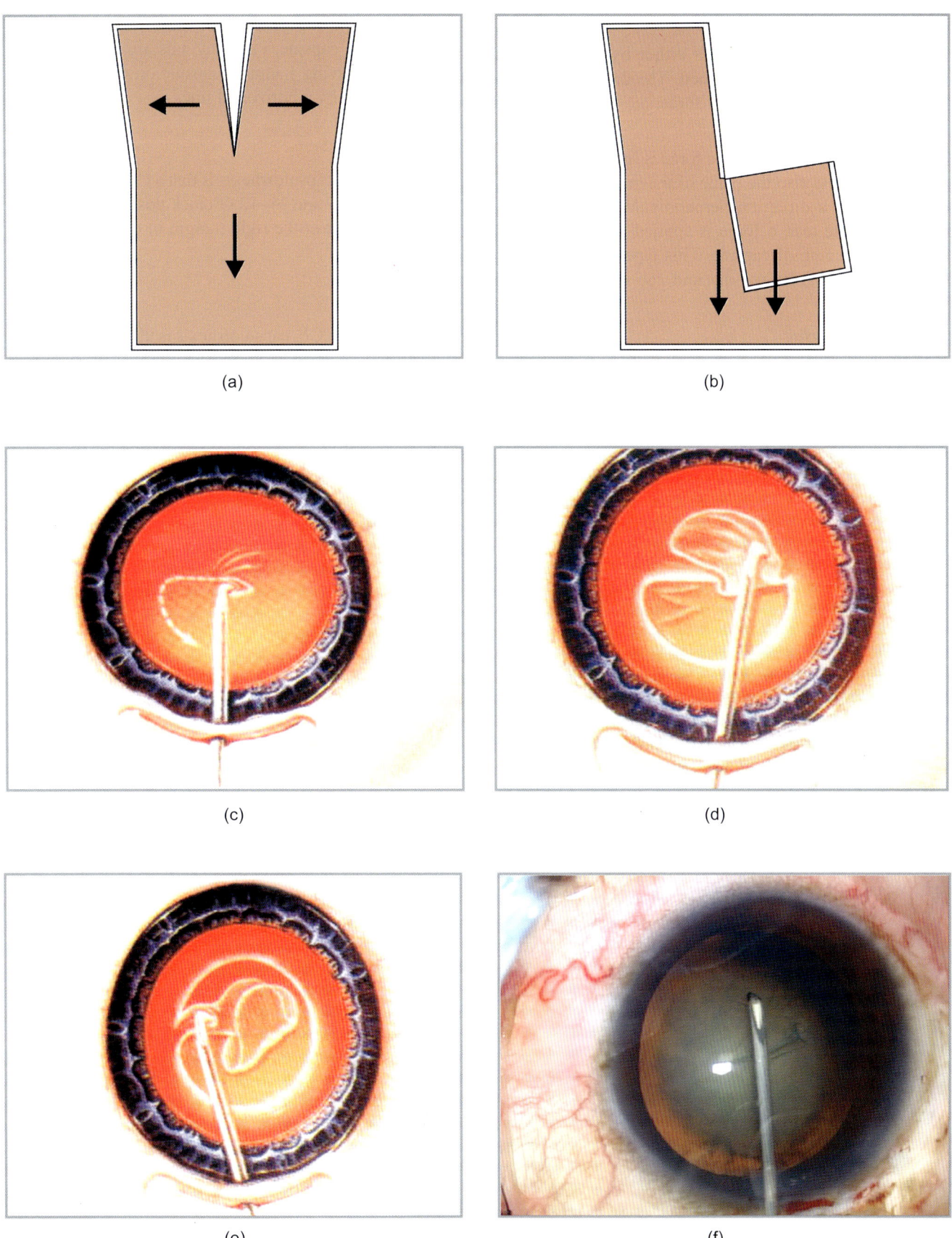

Fig. 55.3: (a) Capsulorrhexis: Tearing by Ripping, (b) Capsulorrhexis: Tearing by shearing, (c) Continuous curvilinear capsulorrhexis, (d) Continuous curvilinear capsulorrhexis, (e) Continuous curvilinear capsulorrhexis, (f) Continuous curvilinear capsulorrhexis

Mechanics of Capsulorrhexis

A planar material can be torn either by stretching or shearing once the tear is initiated. The difference lies in the magnitude and direction of force.

Tearing by Ripping

The plane of application of the force is in the plane of the material which is also the plane of the maximum strength of capsule. In a direction perpendicular to the desired direction of the tear, a force is applied to overcome the maximum strength of capsule. This type of tearing once started, will progress rapidly and can easily go out of control.

Tearing by Shearing

Here, the effective angle of the applied force at the tearing vertex is perpendicular to the plane of the material. The applied force is in the direction of the least resistance of the planar material, so only minimal force is needed to tear it. There is lesser chance of extending to the equator than if stretching is used.

Technique

A bent 26 G needle/cystitome is used to make a capsulorrhexis through either the main tunnel or side port entry. With the tip of bent needle, an initial puncture is made in the centre of the capsule and the cut extended horizontally to the nasal or temporal side of the lens.

A cystitome is inserted just below the capsule, raising it. to form a small capsular flap. The cystitome is then placed above the flap and the flap is directed clockwise or anti-clockwise to make the capsulorrhexis. The size of the rhexis should at least be 6 mm with the part of the tear joining the first part from the outside. Care should be taken to keep the anterior chamber deep all the time while making the rhexis. For better visualisation of the anterior capsule, staining can be done using tryphan blue, fluorescein and indocyanine green.

Envelop Technique

Is preferred over can opener in cases of morgagnian, intumescent black/brown or hypermature cataract. A scratch

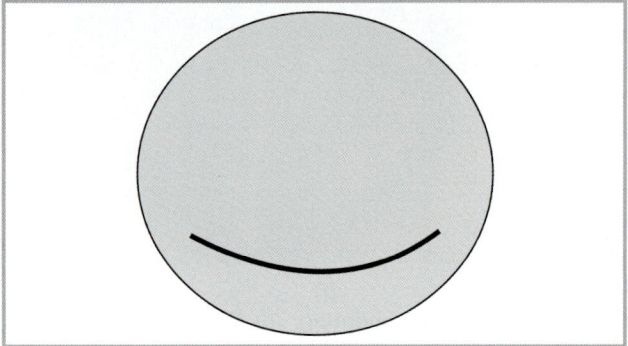

Fig. 55.4: Envelope capsulotomy

mark is made at this juncture of the lower 2/3rd and the upper 1/3rd of capsule. Fine tiny cuts are given medially and laterally saving 1 mm of capsule on either side, cuts are then joined by a horizontal line.

Can-Op-Rhexis

Another type of capsulorrhexis is that a CCC may be given relaxing cuts at 7 and 11–12 O'clock positions for nuclear manipulation out of the rigid margin in cases of hard and large nuclei.

Can Opener

In any form of ECCE, capsulorrhexis is ideal as it facilitates implantation of the IOL in the bag. However, in certain situations, can opener Capsulotomy may be employed in manual SICS.

(a) Those who have not mastered capsulorrhexis.
(b) Even while learning capsulorrhexis, conversion to a can opener capsulotomy can be made at any stage following the peripheral extension of capsulorrhexis.
(c) In certain situations where rhexis is difficult like
  (i) Mature cataracts
  (ii) Small pupils
  (iii) Calcified or fibrosed anterior capsule
  (iv) Cases of grade III or grade IV nuclear sclerosis.

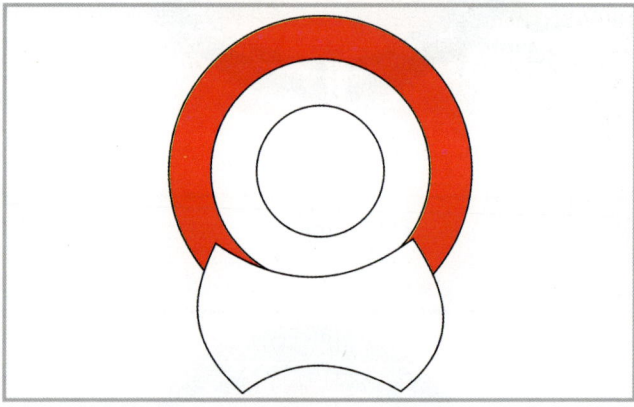

Fig. 55.5: Can-op rhexis

HYDROPROCEDURES

Comprise of hydrodissection and hydrodelineation. The aim is to separate the lens nucleus, epinucleus and the cortex from the capsule and the lens lamella from the cortex and its different layers.

Hydrodissection

For dissection, 1 cc of ringer lactate / BSS is taken in a 2 cc syringe and is injected behind the rhexis margin. The bolus of fluid injected between the anterior capsule and cortex dissects all around the capsular bag and separates it from the nucleus. Indication that the dissection has occurred

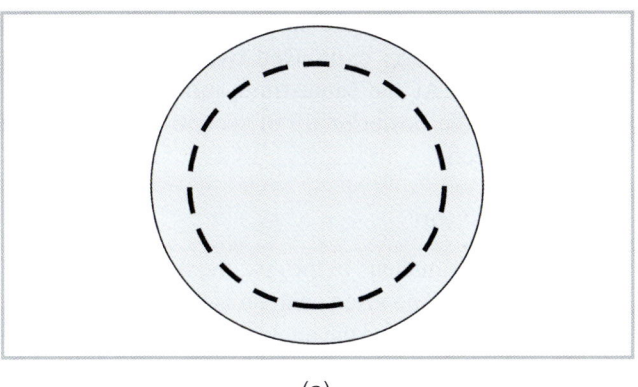
(a)

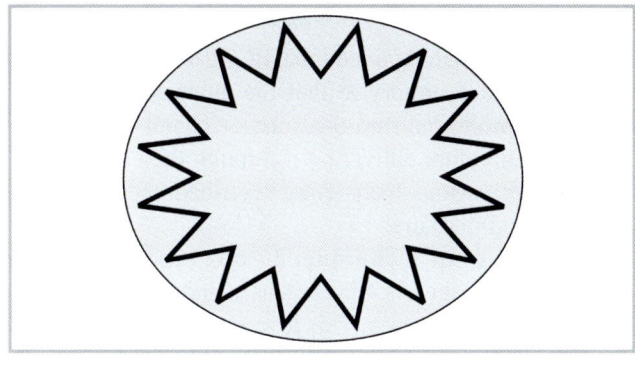
(b)

Fig. 55.6: (a) and (b) Can opener capsulotomy

is shallowing of the anterior chamber, signifying entrapment of fluid in the subcapsular layer of the lens.

Hydrodelineation

In hydrodelineation, fluid is injected between the epinucleus and nucleus. The fluid wave appears as a golden ring under the surgical microscope. A straight cannula or the one with 2 side ports is passed into the nucleus until it meets resistance where the soft outer nucleus ends and a firm inner nucleus begins. At the point of resistance, the cannula is pulled back a fraction of an mm and fluid is injected. Thorough hydrodelineation reduces the size of the nucleus which in turn enables the surgeon to deliver it out of a small incision.

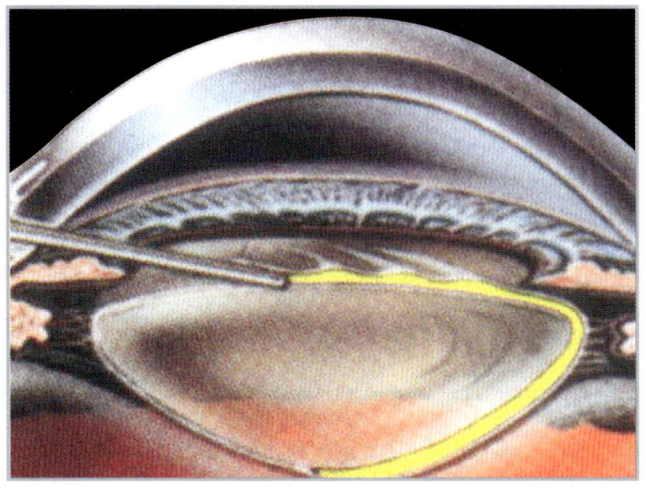
(a)

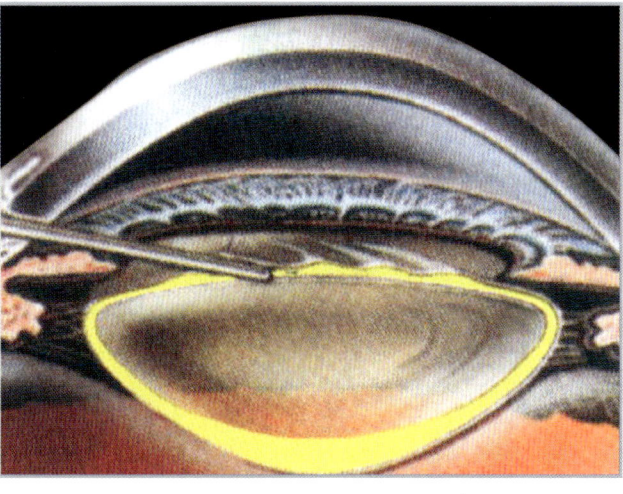
(b)

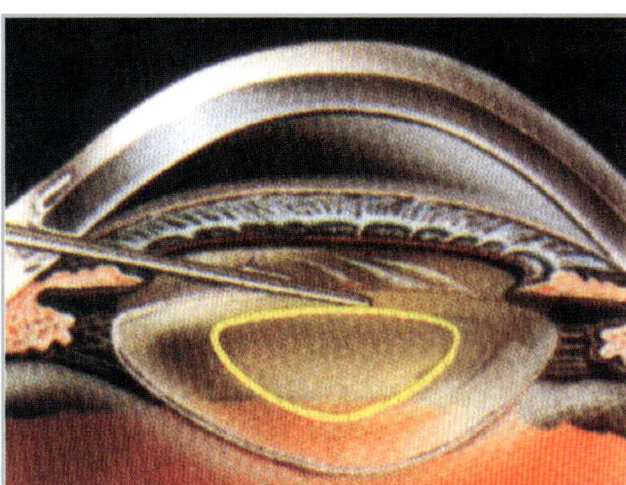
(c)

Fig. 55.7: (a) and (b) Hydrodissection, (c) Hydrodelineation

Nucleus Prolapse from Capsular Bag

SICS differs from the conventional ECCE and Phacoemulsification cataract surgery in that the nucleus needs to be essentially prolapsed into the anterior chamber from the capsular bag before delivering it through the incision.

There are various techniques described and practised. The preferred ones are:

1. **Tipping up technique:** In this procedure, after retracting the iris, the nucleus is nudged towards the 6 O'clock position. This lowers the superior pole of the nucleus, and the superior pole is tipped up with the iris spatula. The viscoelastic is injected between the nucleus and the posterior capsule. The nucleus is then rotated with the iris spatula and is eventually prolapsed into the anterior chamber.

2. **Tyre levering technique:** It is useful if the nucleus is larger than the capsulorrhexis or capsulotomy. The nucleus is nudged posteriorly towards the posterior capsule at the 9 O'clock equator so that the 3 O'clock equator comes out of the capsular rim slightly. The nucleus is then lifted up at 3 O'clock with iris spatula and rotated out of the capsular bag.

3. **Tumbling of the lens:** In this technique, the viscoelastic or BSS is injected under the anterior capsule rim at 9 O'clock. The pooling of viscoelastic or BSS behind the nucleus pushes the nucleus out of the rim at 3 o'clock. The nucleus is further pressed at 9 O'clock which pops the nucleus at 3 O'clock.

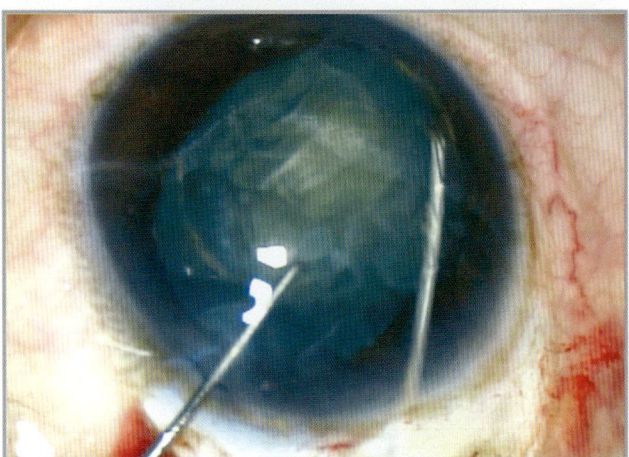

Fig. 55.8: Prolapse of nucleus in to AC

NUCLEUS EXTRACTION

Once the nucleus is prolapsed into the anterior chamber, it can be extracted through the tunnel by the following methods:

Micro-vectis Method

When the nucleus is in the anterior chamber, viscoelastic is injected both above and below the nucleus. A microvectis

that is 3–4 mm is introduced under the nucleus, following which the nucleus is expressed by applying forward pressure gently. At the same time, minimal amount of depression of the posterior lip of wound is done by the shaft of the vectis.

Viscoexpression

After delivery of nucleus in the AC, the AC is again filled with viscoelastic. The visco cannula is introduced through the main incision, behind the nucleus and positioned below the inferior pole of the nucleus. The viscoelastic is then reinjected and simultaneously the scleral tip is depressed with the cannula. This positive pressure pushes the nucleus out of the eye.

Phacosandwich Technique

This is used when the nucleus is soft. Using a vectis which goes behind the nucleus and a broad iris spatula that goes in front of the nucleus, the nucleus is sandwiched between the two instruments and is brought out.

Phaco-fracture Technique

The nucleus is fragmented by placing the spatula beneath and the nucleotome on top of the nucleus. Pressure is then created by slowly pressing the nucleotome against the spatula, until this section of the nucleus is fragmented into four pieces which remain within the nucleotome, and which, with the help of the spatula, are extracted from the anterior chamber with a "sandwich" technique.

Modified Fish-hook Technique

After extending the inner incision like a smile fashion, a 26 G needle bent like a hook is mounted on a 2 cc viscoelastic filled syringe. We enter in the anterior chamber injecting visco to make it deep. A downward pressure by the hook and visco is applied at the 12 O'clock position on the nucleus. By this maneuver, the nucleus at 12 O'clock is pushed downward and inferiorly. Later on, it will tumble inside the bag and the hook goes posterior to the nucleus. Now, inject the viscoelastic to push the posterior capsule back. This creates a space to make the tip of hook anteriorly to get embedded in the mid-substance through the posterior surface of nucleus. After hooking the nucleus, an active (by hook) pressure and passive (by visco) pressure would help to extract the nucleus from the tunnel.

Modified Blumenthal's Technique

An anterior chamber maintainer system is used. The advantage of ACM is that it constantly maintains a positive intraocular pressure during surgery. The eye is thus maintained in a physiological state. The length of the incision is equal to the size of the endonucleus.

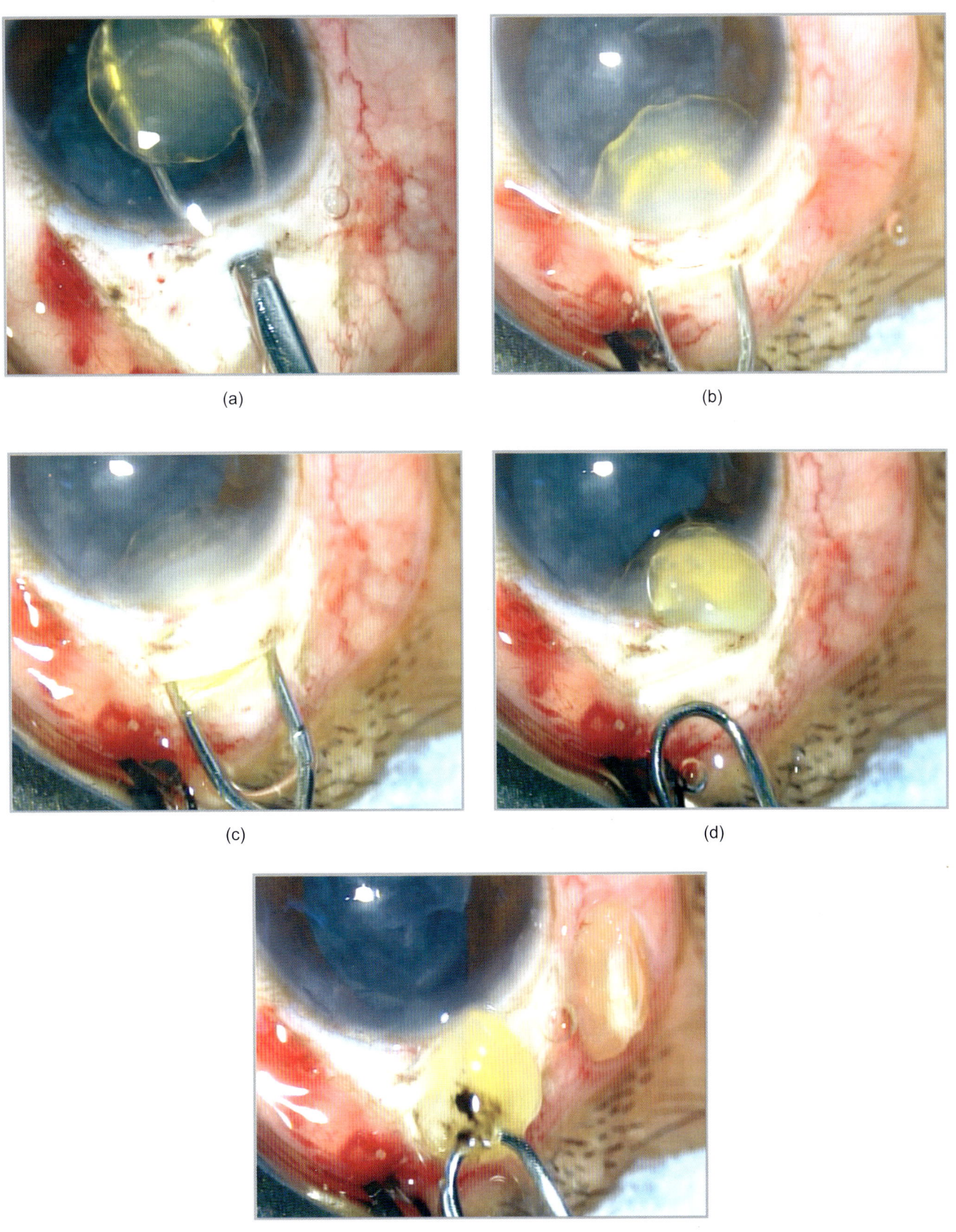

Fig. 55.9: (a) Nucleus extraction (Micro-Vectis technique), (b) Nucleus expression: Nucleus is being engaged in the tunnel, (c) Nucleus extraction SICS, (d) Nucleus extraction SICS, (e) Nucleus extraction SICS

The MVR entry is made at 6 O'clock position parallel to limbus, away from the vascular arcade of cornea. The ACM, a hollow steel tube with 0.9 mm outer and 0.65 mm inner diameters is entered with bevel-up and then turned 180° so that the bevel faces the iris. The ACM is always inserted from the temporal side. The tube of ACM is attached to BSS bottle suspended 60–70 cm above the patient's eye. Once the reduced sized nucleus has been brought out in deep AC, a lens glide is passed from 12 O'clock behind the nucleus. Once the glide is in position, the ACM flow is switched on fully. The tip of forceps is used to apply a firm pressure on the lens glide on the scleral side of section. The nucleus will be taken up by the section and the adjacent pockets. A few intermittent taps on the lens glide will see the nucleus delivered out, deepening the AC. A few more taps will allow the cortex and epinucleus to be washed out of eye. We pull out the ACM at this stage. Simcoe cannula is further used for cleaning up the remaining cortex.

CORTICAL CLEANUP

Cortical removal can be accomplished using either the automated systems or manual irrigation aspiration (I/A) devices depending upon the preference of the surgeon or the demands of the situation.

A large variety of manual irrigation aspiration cannulae are available in the market, but the most commonly used one is the Simcoe cannula. Cortical aspiration should ideally start from the 6 O'clock position and gradually proceed towards the 5, 4, 3, 2 O'clock positions and 7, 8, 9 10 O'clock positions or vice versa depending upon the preference of the surgeon or the demands of the situation.

Implantation of IOL into the Bag

It is preferable to place the IOL after inflating the bag with viscoelastics. The only important point is to clean the tunnel thoroughly before introducing the IOL through the tunnel.

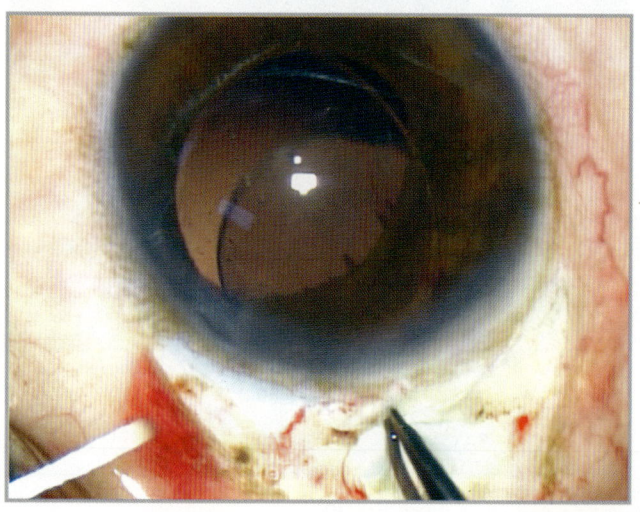

(a)

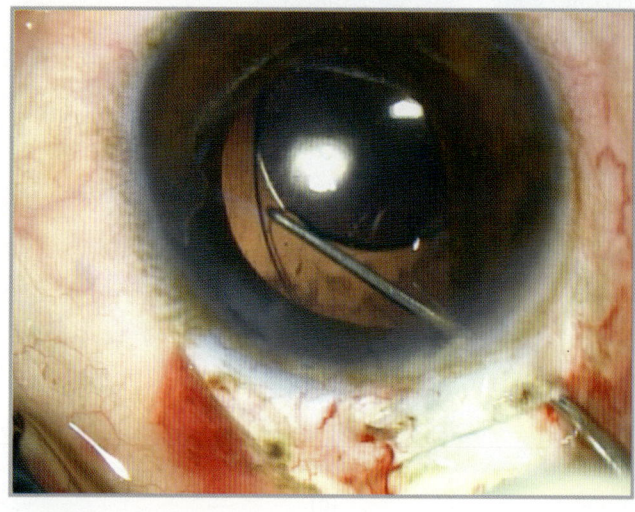

(b)

(c)

Fig. 55.10: (a) Implantation of all PMMA IOL (5.25 mm), (b) Implantation of all PMMA IOL (5.25 mm) into the bag, (c) All PMMA IOL (5.25 mm) is positioned in the bag

Otherwise, sometimes blood clot or lens cortical particles may go inside along with the lens and cleaning them is difficult.

Removal of viscoelastic from the bag and the anterior chamber should be followed by tunnel washing.

Suturing

Suturing is required if
(a) There is a leaking tunnel
(b) Tunnel is more than 6.5 mm in length
(c) Premature entry
(d) Triple procedure has been done
(e) Pediatric cataract (due to a thin sclera).

Suturing Technique

1. Appositional/Radial/Vertical sutures
2. Horizontal.

1. Vertical Sutures

They appose the external lip of the wound, which results in internal separation of the corneal lip because of pulling of the sclera and cornea in a new unphysiological position.

2. Horizontal Sutures

They are less likely to disturb the alignment of internal entry incision so as to cause less astigmatism than vertical sutures.

Types of Horizontal Sutures
• Shepherd's single horizontal suture
• Horizontal anchor suture
• Fines infinity suture.

Complications of Manual SICS

Wound construction

The complications that may be encountered are related to the wound placement, the length and the depth of incision.

(a) Placement
(i) Anterior incision → Poor self-sealing effect
↓
Wound leak
ATR Astigmatism

(ii) Posterior incision
• Wide tunnel
• Risk of bleeding
• Risk of premature entry
↓
Difficulty in nucleus delivery and instrument manipulation

(b) Incision Length
(i) Short incision → Difficulty in nucleus delivery
↓
Endothelial damage
Iris damage

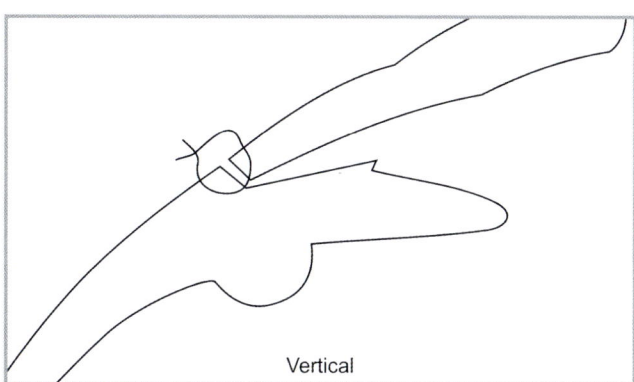
Vertical

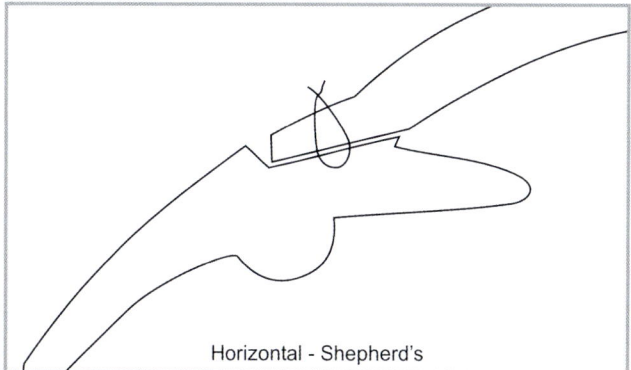
Horizontal - Shepherd's

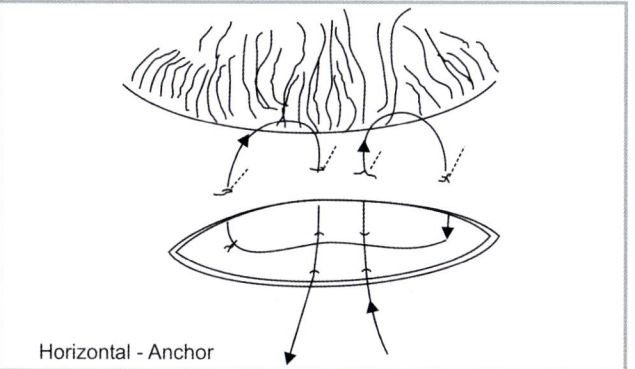
Horizontal - Anchor

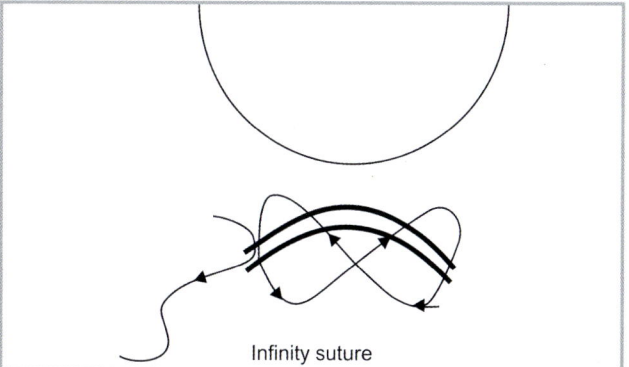
Infinity suture

Fig. 55.11: Suturing techniques in SICS

(ii) Long incision → Poor approximation
$$\downarrow$$
Wound leak
Induced ATR astigmatism

(c) Incision depth

   (i) Button holing: Occurs due to superficial dissection of the scleral flap.

   (ii) Premature entry: Occurs because of deep dissection of the scleral flap.

   (iii) Scleral disinsertion: A very deep roof incision can cause scleral disinsertion by complete separation of the inferior sclera from the sclera superior to the incision.

Descemet's Membrane (DM) Stripping on Entry

DM strips may occur when fluid or viscoelastic is injected through the paracentesis if the cannula tip is placed in the corneal canal of the paracentesis. The injected fluid causes inter-lamellar hydrodissection of the cornea creating a space between the deep stroma and DM.

Paracentesis

(a) Too far central into the cornea   → DM Stripping
(b) Too far peripheral into the sclera   → Bleeding
(c) Too small for instruments DM   → Stripping
(d) Too large   → Leakage

Capsulotomy

The size of the capsulorrhexis should be adequate depending on the size of nucleus.

   (a) Small Capsulorrhexis
     • Difficulty in prolapsing the nucleus and cortical aspiration
     • Zonular dialysis
     • Residual cortex

   (b) Large Capsulorrhexis: Problem for in-the-bag placement of IOLs

Hydrodissection

Ideally, hydrodissection should be attempted in all the four quadrants. If the hydrodissection procedure is performed forcibly at any one site, there is a grave risk of undue pressure in the posterior capsule leading to PCR and chances of nucleus drop.

Nucleus Prolapse

Difficulty in prolapsing the nucleus from the bag into the anterior chamber can cause:

   (a) Endothelial damage
   (b) Iridodialysis
   (c) Damage to iris
   (d) Zonular dialysis
   (e) Posterior capsule tear.

Nucleus Delivery

Following problems can occur during delivering the lens, if the size of tunnel is inadequate:

   (a) Endothelial damage.
   (b) Iris sandwich can occur when the 6 O'clock iris gets trapped between the vectis inferiorly and the nucleus superiorly.

Hyphaema

Can be caused either in the initial steps of the surgery by a more posteriorly placed scleral incision or a deeper placed incision or later due to iris injury, especially due to iridodialysis during the nucleus delivery.

CONCLUSION

Manual SICS carries several advantages over conventional ECCE technique in terms of quick procedure, smaller incision, minimal suture and astigmatism, thus offering a very safe alternative option, particularly in case of mass community work. Over and above, SICS carries several advantages of phacoemulsification and can be considered particularly during learning the curve, in case of impending conversion or mechanical constraints.

Manual SICS is definitely a breakthrough in a country like India where ophthalmic surgeons are overburdened with mature and hard cataract. SICS is going to replace conventional ECCE as the preferred option.

BIBLIOGRAPHY

1. Kansas P. Phacofracture. In: Rozakis G W, editor. Cataract Surgery- Alternative Small Incision Techniques. New Jersey, USA: SLACK Incorporated.1990;45–70.

2. Dada T, Sharma N, Vajpayee R B, Dada V K. Conversion from phacoemulsification to extracapsular cataract extraction: Incidence, risk factors,and visual outcome. J Cataract Refract Surg 1998; 24:1521–24.

3. Blumenthal M, Askenazi I, Fogel R, Assia E I. The gliding nucleus. J Cataract Refract Surg 1993; 19: 435–37.

4. Oshika T, Nagahara K, Yaguchi S, Emi K, Takenaka H, Tsuboi S, et al. Three year prospective, randomised evaluation of intraocular lens implantation through 3.2 and 5.5 mm incisions. J Cataract Refract Surg 1998; 24:509–14.

5. Thomas R, Braganza A, Raju R, Lawrence, Spitzer K H. Phacoemulsification – A senior surgeon's learning curve. Ophthalmic Surg 1994; 25(8):504–9.

6. Thomas R, Naveen S, Jacob A, Braganza A. Visual outcome and complications of residents learning phacoemulsification. Indian J Ophthalmol 1997; 45:215–19.

7. Sackett D L, Haynes R B, Guyatt G H, Tugwell P. Clinical Epidemiology, Little, Br Prajna NV, Chandrakanth KS, Kim R, Narendran V, Selvakumar S, Rohini G, et al . The Madurai intraocular lens study II: clinical outcomes. Am J Ophthalmol 1998; 125:14–25.

8. Yorston D, Foster A, Wood M, Foster A. Does prospective monitoring improve cataract surgery outcomes in Africa? Br J Ophthalmol 2002; 86:543–7.

9. Holladay JT, Dudeja DR, Koch DD. Evaluating and reporting astigmatism for individual and aggregate Data. J Cataract Refract Surg 1998; 24:57–65.

10. Burgansky Z, Isakov I, Avizemer H, Bartov E. Minimal astigmatism after sutureless planned extracapsular cataract extraction. J Cataract Refract Surg 2002; 28:499–503.

11. Kimura H, Kuroda S, Mizoguchi N, Terauchi H, Matsumura M, Nagata M. Extracapsular cataract extraction with a sutureless incision for dense cataracts. J Cataract Refract Surg 1999; 25:1275–9.

12. Naeser K. Popperian falsification of methods of assessing surgically induced astigmatism. J Cataract Refract Surg 2001; 27:25–30.

13. Sawhney S. Theoretical validity of vector analysis for aggregate astigmatic data. J Cataract Refract Surg 2002; 28:385–6.

14. own1 Keener GT. The nucleus division technique for small incision cataract extraction. In: Rozakis GW, Anis AY, et al, editors. Cataract Surgery: Alternative Small Incision Techniques. Thorofare (N.J): Slack Inc; 1990. 163–195.

15. Fry LL. The Phacosandwich Technique. In: Rozakis GW, Anis AY, et al, editors. Cataract Surgery: Alternative Small Incision Techniques. Thorofare (N.J): Slack Inc; 1990. 71–110.

16. Kansas P. Phacofracture. In: Rozakis GW, Anis AY, et al, editors. Cataract Surgery: Alternative Small Incision Techniques. Thorofare (N.J): Slack Inc; 1990. p. 45–70.

17. Blumenthal M. Manual ECCE, the present state of the art. Klin Monat Augenheilkd 1994; 205: 266–270.

18. Thomas R, Kuriakose T, George R. Towards achieving small-incision cataract surgery 99.8% of the time. Indian J Ophthalmol 2000; 48: 145–151.

19. Ruit S, Poudyal G, Gurung R, Tabin G, Moran D, Brian G. An innovation in developing world cataract surgery: sutureless extracapsular cataract extraction with intraocular lens implantation. Clin Experiment Ophthalmol 2000; 28:274–279.

20. Natchiar G. Manual Small Incision Cataract Surgery. Madurai, India: Aravind Publications, 2000.

21. Hennig A, Kumar J, Yorston D, Foster A. Sutureless cataract surgery with nucleus extraction: Outcome of a prospective study in Nepal. Br J Ophthalmol 2003; 87(3):266–270.

22. Gogate P M, Deshpande M, Wormald R P. Is manual small incision cataract surgery affordable in the developing countries? A cost comparison with extracapsular cataract extraction. Br J Ophthalmol 2003; 87:843–846.

23. Gogate P M, Deshpande M, Wormald R P, Deshpande R D, Kulkarni S R. Extracapsular cataract surgery compared with manual small incision cataract surgery in community eye care setting in Western India: a randomised controlled trial. Br J Ophthalmol 2003; 87:667–672.

24. Prajna NV, Chandrakanth KS, Kim R, Narendran V, Selvakumar S, Rohini G, et al. The Madurai intraocular lens study II: clinical outcomes. Am J Ophthalmol 1998; 125:14–25.

25. Hennig A, Kumar J, Singh AK, Singh S, Gurung R, Foster A. World Sight Day and cataract .University of Illinois Eye Centre. "Cataracts." Retrieved August 18, 2006. SICS

56

Phakic IOL

Lt Col Nitin Vichare and Col JKS Parihar SM, VSM

INTRODUCTION

Search is always on to find a reliable and predictable method to correct refractive errors in patients. Prescribing glasses or just contact lenses may not be suitable to all patients due to cosmetic reasons or the restrictions they pose in day to day life. With increasing awareness, many patients want complete cure for their refractive errors. More and more patients are choosing surgical correction of refractive error and expect trouble free clear vision postoperatively.

Keratorefractive surgery has evolved considerably over a period of time. Manipulation of cornea to change refractive status of eye is a logical choice considering that major refractive power of eye is contributed by cornea which is easily accessible for surgical remodelling. Various surgical techniques evolved over a period of time include RK, PRK, LASIK, LASEK, newer Epi-LASIK as well as intra corneal implants and refractive lens exchange.

LASIK involving laser ablation of the cornea is arguably the most commonly practised laser refractive surgery which is also preferred by patients. It has a high level of comfort, stable predictable results and an ability to perform bilateral treatments in a single sitting. However, when it comes to higher grades of refractive errors it tends to have unpredictable results and higher chances of postoperative keratectasia. Phakic IOL where intra ocular lens is implanted in a phakic eye can be a viable alternative in such case.

HISTORY OF THE PROCEDURE

The Phakic myopia lens was introduced by Strampelli and later popularised by Barraquer in the late 1950s. The design was of a biconcave angle-supported lens. These lenses were abandoned following serious angle- and endothelium-related complications. In the mid 1980s, Baikoff introduced newer design angle supported lens Kelman-type haptics.

These angle supported lenses had less postoperative complications.

Fechner and Worst introduced a phakic myopia lens of iris claw design in 1986 (now called Artisan/Verisyse).

The concept of placing the IOL in the posterior chamber near the true anatomical location and near the nodal point of eye is not new. Fyodorov introduced and popularised the soft phakic lens in the space between the iris and the anterior surface of the crystalline lens.

INDICATIONS

Any refractive error which is unsuitable for laser refractive surgery could be considered for phakic IOL.
  (i) Myopia beyond –12 D.
 (ii) Hyperopia beyond + 4 D.
(iii) Initial corneal thickness of less than 480 micron/ estimated residual corneal thickness of less than 270 microns after laser ablation.
(iv) Suspected cases of early keratoconus.

CONTRAINDICATIONS

  (i) Myopia other than axial.
 (ii) History of uveitis/presence of anterior or posterior synechiae.
(iii) Corneal dystrophy.
(iv) Glaucoma or an IOP higher than 20 mmHg.
 (v) Personal or family history of retinal detachment.
(vi) Evidence of nuclear sclerosis or developing cataract.
(vii) Anterior chamber depth less than 3 mm.
(viii) Endothelial count less than 2000 cells/sq cm.

ADVANTAGES

  (i) No risk of iatrogenic keratectasia/tear film abnormality as following laser ablation.
 (ii) Minimum handling of cornea.

(iii) Rapid healing with stable postoperative refraction

(iv) A reversible and adjustable procedure

Surgery for phakic IOLs does not require costly equipment and a good anterior segment surgeon can easily adjust to this refractive surgery.

Phakic IOLs when implanted inside the eye, are closer to the nodal point of eye. This has an advantage that the effective optic zone is 1.25 times on the corneal surface. Larger effective optic zone gives better image clarity. Also, as spectacles are dispensed with magnification or minification of image due to glasses done away with. This gives added quality of vision in such patients.

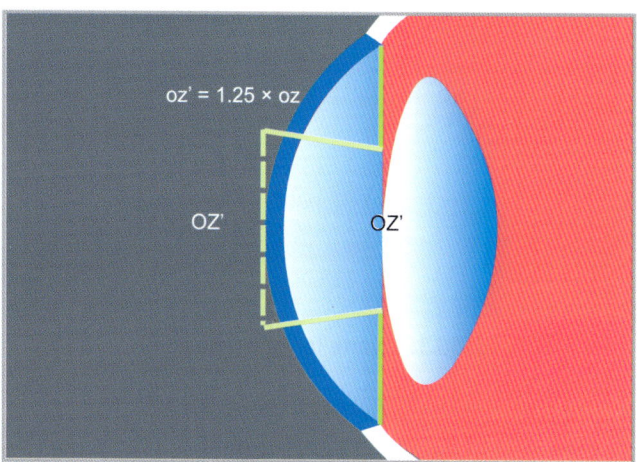

Fig. 56.1: Optical principle of Phakic IOL

PREOPERATIVE EVALUATION

Surgical procedure for phakic IOLs places great demand on the surgeon and utmost care has to be taken so as to avoid or minimise damage to angle structures, iris or crystalline lens. This requires knowledge of anatomy as well as precise preoperative measurements.

Subjective Refraction

Subjective correction and glasses prescription for BCVA at a standard vertex distance of 12 mm.

K Value

Keratometric value in the principal meridian with average K reading and astigmatism.

Corneal Diameter

Horizontal and vertical corneal diameters measured from white to white distance. Helps in sizing the optic diameter of lens.

Anterior Chamber Depth (ACD)

The anterior chamber depth should not be less than 3 mm. This helps in maintaining a safe distance from endothelium.

Endothelial Cell Count

Endothelial count should not be less than 2000 cells/sq cm.

Newer anterior segment imaging methods find relevance in evaluation. These non invasive techniques like AC OCT or Pentacam give multiple readings and are patient friendly

PHAKIC IOL POWER CALCULATION

Implantation of a phakic IOL is a refractive surgery with high patient expectation. Accurate power calculation is essential to avoid postoperative refractive surprises.

Essential parameters are:

(i) Spectacle power calculation at a vertex distance of 12 mm

(ii) AC depth

(iii) K value

Since implanting phakic IOL causes placement of new IOL over crystalline lens, the axial length remains unchanged.

Various formulae have been proposed. Simplified formulae in use are as follows.

Holladay Formula

Also called as vergence formula takes into account both pre treatment refraction and the desired post treatment refraction.

$$IOL = \frac{1336}{\dfrac{1336}{1000 + Kref} - ELP} - \frac{1336}{\dfrac{1336}{1000 + Kref} - ELP}$$

$$\frac{1000}{PreRx} - V \qquad \frac{1000}{DPostRx} - V$$

Definition of variables:

ELP = Expected lens position in mm (distance from corneal vertex to principal plane of intraocular lens)

IOL = Intraocular lens power in D

Kref = Net corneal power in diopters (0.996885 × keratometric)

PreRx = Preoperative refraction in D

DPostRx = Desired postoperative refraction in D

V = Vertex distance in mm of refraction.

Azar / Wong Simplified Phakic IOL Formula

P iol = 1.06 L + KLM

K = keratometry reading

L = preoperative spherical equivalent corrected at corneal plane

M = IOL position or effective lens position (ELP) in meters

Calculating IOL power and its sizing is very complex and various nomograms are available so that the surgeon can pick the ideal IOL. Manufacturers also provide data and softwares on Internet through company web site where data can be feed to get the IOL power.

TYPES OF PHAKIC IOLs

Angle Supported Phakic PMMA IOL

Baikoff Angle Supported Phakic IOLs (ZB, ZB5M, NuVita)

It was Baikoff (1987) who modified the Kelman four point multiflex implant to introduce angle supported phakic IOLs. The first generation lens, ZB lens, were rigid PMMA lens with 4.5 mm optic with overall diameter 13 mm. initial designs were associated with higher endothelial cell loss, pupil ovulation, night vision problems associated glare. Subsequent modifications in design leads to newer second generation lenses called ZB5M.

Third generation lenses subsequently introduced are called NuVita MA20 lens. It is a PMMA lens with 4.5 mm optic zone with larger curved footplate and no optic shoulder. It has an antiglare coating. These modifications are supposed to give better centration and night vision.

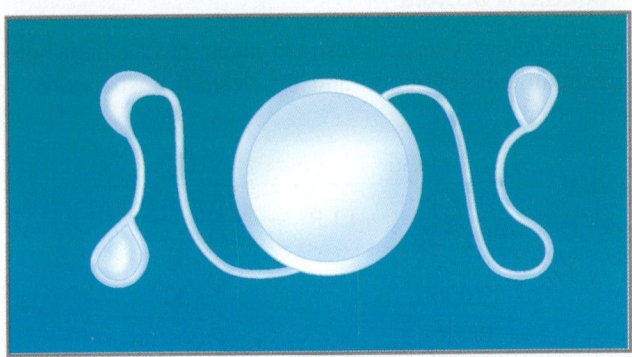

Fig. 56.2: NuVita M20

ZSAL – 4 and ZSAL–4/PLUS lenses (Morcher GMBH, Germany)

PMMA rigid plano concave lenses with z shaped haptics. Overall diameter 12.5 mm with optic diameter 5.5 mm with effective optic zone 5 mm to reduce night vision problems.

Phakic 6, 6H and 6H2 lens (Ophthalmic Innovations International, CA)

Phakic 6 and 6H IOLs are rigid PMMA lens with optic of 5.5 mm to 6 mm. Haptic size ranges from 11.5 to 14 mm in increments of 0.5 mm. In addition the IOL is heparin coated for better biocompatibility.

Angle Supported Phakic Acrylic Foldable IOL

Vivarte Foldable IOL (Ciba vision, USA)

One piece three point angle supported lens (tripod support) was the first foldable angle supported phakic lens to be

introduced in the market. The lens has an optical zone of 5.5 mm with overall diameter of 12–13 mm. Lens power ranges from –7 D to –25 D. the lens has a soft, hydrophilic, acrylic optic attached to rigid acrylic haptics which provides stability to lens when placed in the anterior chamber.

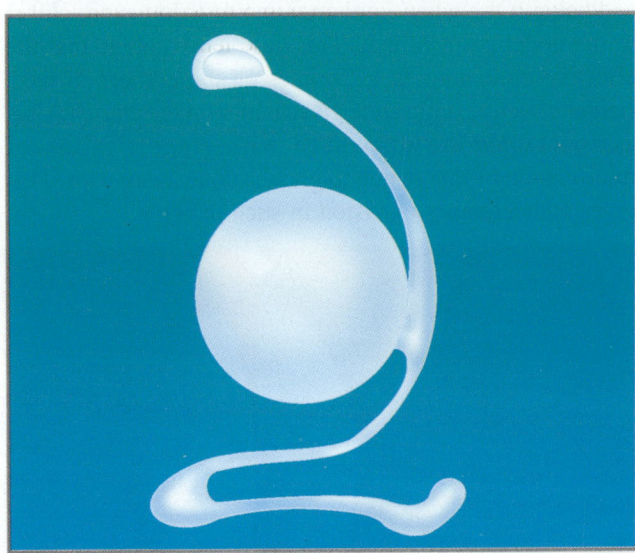

Fig. 56.3: Vivarte foldable phakic IOL

Kelman Duet IOL (Tekia, Irvine, CA)

It is a foldable angle supported phakic IOL with two independent parts. Tripod haptic is made of PMMA and silicon optic of 5.5 mm with OD 12–13 mm. This IOL is implanted in two steps. First, the haptic is inserted and placed in the anterior chamber and the position is adjusted. Optic is injected subsequently using an injector. Haptic has small haptic tabs which fit in the tabs of optic. Once both the pieces are inside, the eye optic is fixed to haptic tabs.

Iris Fixated Phakic IOL

Artisan/Verisyse Iris Claw Lens

Based on the design of Worst iris claw lens, these lenses have a claw like structure by which they are fixated to the iris tissue. There design is supposed to keep them away

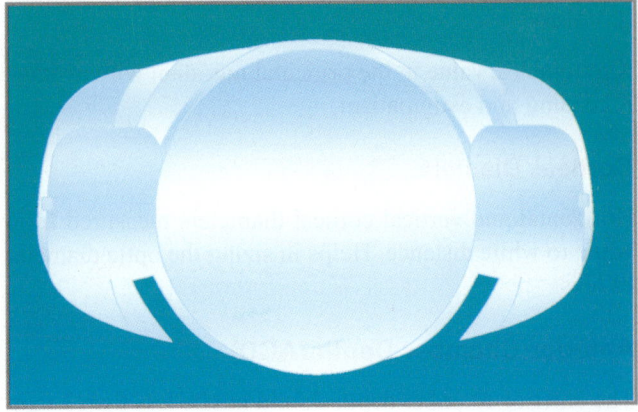

Fig. 56.4: Verisyse IOL

from corneal the endothelium and avoid contact with crystalline lens.

They are made of PMMA. The optical part of Verisyse lens comes in two different sizes: 5.0 mm and 6.0 mm optic depending on the pupillary diameter. With a power range available from –3.0D to –23.5D in 5 mm optic and –3.0 D to –15.5 D in 6 mm optic. Verisyse lenses for hyperopia correction are available in power range of +1.0 D to +12.0 D.

To reduce surgically induced astigmatism, foldable version of Verisyse with silicon optic and PMMA haptic which can be introduced through a 3 mm incision have been made available. Toric Verisyse IOL for correction of preexisting astigmatism have been available since 2001.

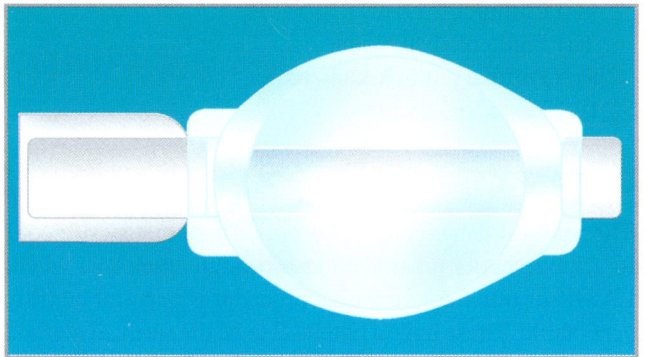

Fig. 56.5: Foldable Verisyse IOL

Posterior Chamber Phakic IOL

ICL or Implantable Contact Lens (STAAR Surgical)

Posterior chamber plate haptic design lens are made of highly biocompatible collagen copolymer, a compound combining acrylic and porcine collagen (less than 0.1% collagen). It has a refractive index of 1.45, the polymer material is soft, elastic and hydrophilic. These lenses are very thin with the optical zone 60 micron thick and haptic 500–600 micron. The optical zone diameter 5.5 mm with overall diameter varies 11.5 to 13 mm. Available powers are –3.0D to –23.0 D for myopic lenses and +3.0 D to +21.5 D for hyperopic lenses. The design is such that the posterior surface is concave so as to vault over the anterior capsule.

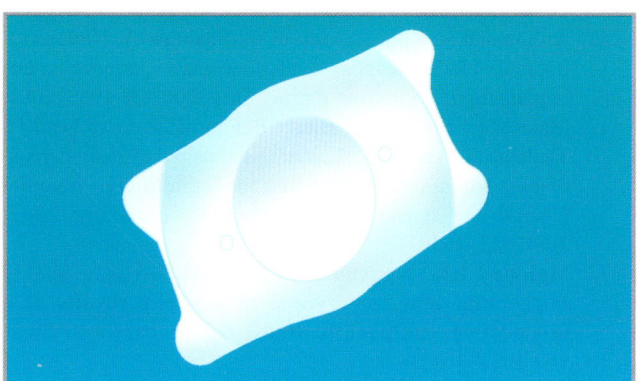

Fig. 56.6: Posterior chamber phakic IOL

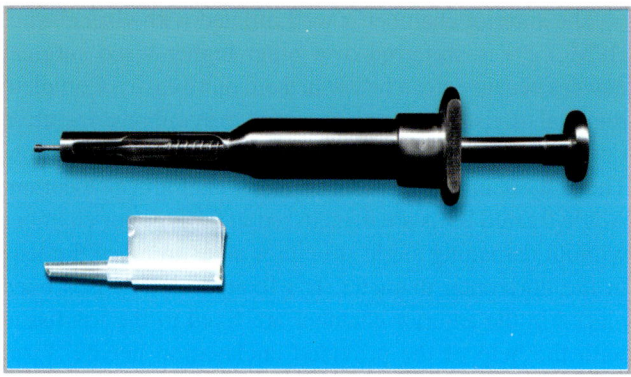

Fig. 56.7: Injector system

Insertion technique of these lenses requires great care while loading them into the cartridge. There are markers on the haptic to help in the proper placement of lenses. Toric version of ICL have also been made available.

PRL or Phakic Refractive Lens (Ciba vision)

PRL made from ultra thin silicon copolymer with refractive index of 1.46. The material is soft, elastic and hydrophobic. It is available in power range –3.0D to –20.0D for myopia and +3.0 D to +15.0 D for hyperopia. It has no anatomical fixation site and is supposed to 'float' in posterior chamber.

OPERATIVE PROCEDURE

The decision to implant phakic IOLs has to be taken with utmost care after considering all the factors and patients willingness. Good preoperative evaluation and IOL power calculation is a must so that the surgeon is prepared for the procedure with ideal IOL.

Patent iridotomies are essential prerequisites before implanting phakic IOL. This is to prevent papillary block which might occur postoperatively. Laser iridotomies are done 2 weeks preoperatively ideally at 10 o' clock and 1 o' clock and their patency is confirmed before surgery. Alternatively, surgical iridotomy can be done intra-operatively either with scissors or vitrectomy cutter.

Patient started on topical antibiotics and NSAIDs topically two days prior to surgery. Surgery can be undertaken under topical or peribulbar anesthesia as per surgeons/patient choice. Preoperatively pupil is constricted with Pilocarpine 2% when an angle supported or iris fixated IOL is planned. For the posterior chamber IOL adequate pupillary dilatation is achieved with topical mydriatic agents.

The incision site and size is planned preoperatively. The size of incision depends on the optic size in cases of non-foldable IOLs while the standard 3.2 mm incision is planned in cases of foldable phakic IOLs so as to pass the tip of the cartridge easily. The incision is generally planned on the axis of the steepest meridian so as to reduce postoperative induced astigmatism.

The anterior chamber is well inflated with viscoelastic. HPMC 2% is preferred over other higher visco surgical devices because it can be washed out more easily. Complete removal of viscoelastics is essential to avoid postoperative rise in IOP and to prevent anterior chamber inflammation. The IOL is inserted carefully in its anatomical location. Angle fixated IOLs are maneuvred in the anterior chamber without damaging angle structures so as to place the lens in the horizontal diameter. Iris fixated claw lenses once placed in the anterior chamber are fixed to the iris tissue with the help of the provided enclavation needle. Firm anchoring with out pupillary distortion is achieved.

The posterior chamber phakic IOL is first loaded in the cartridge before making the incision as its proper loading is essential for its smooth injection and placement. Various markers are made over the lens so as to assist in its proper placement. Markers are provided over optic in cases of toric IOLs for assisting in proper alignment.

After implanting the IOL, viscoelastic is washed off completely. The section is closed with 10–0 nylon sutures if a rigid IOL is implanted.

Postoperatively, the patient is placed on topical steroids and NSAIDs. Cycloplegics are avoided to prevent displacement of IOL.

COMPLICATIONS

Main complications of phakic IOLs

Angle Supported Lenses

(i) Glare and halos
(ii) IOL rotation

(iii) Pupil ovulation
(iv) Endothelial cell loss
(v) Iris atrophy

Iris Supported

(i) Chronic sub clinical inflammation
(ii) Endothelial cell loss
(iii) Traumatic or spontaneous dislocation
(iv) Iris atrophy
(v) Secondary glaucoma

Posterior Chamber

(i) Cataract
(ii) Pigment dispersion
(iii) Pupillary block glaucoma
(iv) Posterior luxation

SUMMARY

The phakic IOL has given a new option to refractive surgeons to achieve better results in cases of high ametropia where LASIK or other conventional procedures may not be fully acceptable. These have a potential to be the surgical method of choice with very few complications. The fact that it can be reversed in cases of unacceptable results gives it an edge over other surgical methods. However, a steep learning curve may prevent its use by everyday anterior segment surgeons. With newer models of phakic IOLs, availability of foldable and toric lenses and more experience gained over a period, phakic IOL will be valuable in the treatment of higher grades of refractive errors.

REFERENCES

1. Chang DH, Davis EA. Phakic intraocular lenses. Curr Opin Ophthalmol. 2006 Feb;17(1):99–104.
2. Lovisolo CF, Reinstein DZ. Phakic intraocular lenses. Surv Ophthalmol. 2005 Nov-Dec;50(6):549–87.
3. Dick HB, Tehrani M . Phakic intraocular lenses. Current status and limitations Ophthalmologe. 2004 Mar;101(3):232–45.
4. Comaish IF, Lawless MA. Phakic intraocular lenses. Curr Opin Ophthalmol. 2002 Feb;13(1):7–13.
5. Marinho A, Pinto MC, Vaz F. Phakic intraocular lenses: which to choose. 7: Curr Opin Ophthalmol. 2000 Aug;11(4):280–8.
6. Holladay JT. Refractive power calculation for intra ocular lenses in phakic eye. Am J Ophthalmol 1993; 116: 63–66.
7. Baikoff G, Arne JL, Bokobza Y, et al. Angle fixated anterior chamber phakic intraocular lens for myopia of –7 to –19 diopters. J Refract Surg 1998; 14: 282–293.
8. Allemann N, Chamon W, Tanaka HM, Mori ES, Campos M, Schor P, Baikoff G. Myopic angle-supported intraocular lenses: Two-year follow-up. *Ophthalmology*. 2000;107: 1549–554.
9. Aguilar-Valenzuela L, Lleo-Perez A, Alonso-Munoz L, Casanova-Izquierdo J, Perez-Molto FJ, Rahhal MS. Intraocular pressure in myopic patients after Worst-Fechner anterior chamber phakic intraocular lens implantation. J Refract Surg. Mar-Apr 2003;19(2):131–6.
10. Pérez-Santonja JJ, Alió JL, Jiménez-Alfaro I, Zato MA. Surgical correction of severe myopia with an angle-supported phakic intraocular lens. J Cataract Refract Surg. Sep 2000; 26(9):1288–302.
11. Ardjomand N, Kolli H, Vidic B, El-Shabrawi Y, Faulborn J. Pupillary block after phakic anterior chamber intraocular lens implantation. *J Cataract Refract Surg*. 2002;28:1080–1081.
12. Malecaze FJ, Hulin H, Bierer P, Fournie P, Grandjean H, Thalamas C, Guell JL. A randomised paired eye comparison of two techniques for treating moderately high myopia: LASIK and artisan phakic lens. *Ophthalmology*. 2002; 109:1622–1630.
13. Maloney RK, Nguyen LH, John ME. Artisan phakic intraocular lens for myopia: Short-term results of a prospective, multicentre study. *Ophthalmology*. 2002; 109:1631–1641.
14. Asano-Kato N, Toda I, Hori-Komai Y, Sakai C, Fukumoto T, Arai H, et al. Experience with the Artisan phakic intraocular

lens in Asian eyes. J Cataract Refract Surg. May 2005; 31(5):910–5.

15. Menezo JL, Peris-Martinez C, Cisneros AL, Martinez-Costa R. Phakic intraocular lenses to correct high myopia: Adatomed, Staar, and Artisan. 1: J Cataract Refract Surg. 2004 Jan; 30(1):33–44

16. Alio' JL, de la Hoz F, Perez-Santonja JJ, et al. Phakic anterior chamber lenses for correction of myopia: a 7-year cumulative analysis of complications in 263 cases. Ophthalmology 1999; 106: 458–466.

17 Landesz M, Worst JGF, Siertsema JV, Van Rij G. Correction of high myopia with Worst myopia claw intraocular lens. J Refract Surg 1995; 11: 16–25.

18 Fechner PU, Singh D, Wulff K. Iris-claw lens in phakic eyes to correct hyperopia: preliminary study. J Cataract Refract Surg. Jan 1998; 24(1):48–56.

19 Senthil S, Reddy KP. A retrospective analysis of the first Indian experience on Artisan phakic intraocular lens. Indian J Ophthalmol. Dec 2006; 54(4):251–5.

20. Menezo JL, Cisneros AL, Rodriguez-Salvador V. Endothelial study of iris-claw phakic lens: Four-year follow-up. *J Cataract Refract Surg*. 1998; 24:1039–1049

21. Pineda-Fernandez A, Jaramillo J,Vergas Jetal. Phakic posterior chamber intra ocular lens for high myopia. J Cataract Refract Surg 2004; 30(11): 2277–2283.

22. Kohnen T. Searching for the perfect phakic intraocular lens. J Cataract Refract Surg. Sep 2000; 26(9):1261–2.

23. Arne JL, Lesueur LC. Phakic posterior chamber lenses for high myopia: functional and anatomical outcomes. J Cataract Refract Surg. Mar 2000; 26(3):369–74.

24. Assetto V, Benedetti S, Pesando P. Collamer intraocular contact lens to correct high myopia. J Cataract Refract Surg. Jun 1996; 22(5):551–6.

25. Rosen E, Gore C. STAAR collamer posterior chamber phakic intra ocular lens for myopia and hyperopia. J Refract Surg 1998; 24: 596–606.

26. Baikoff G, Colin J. Intraocular lenses in phakic eyes. Ophthalmol Clin North Am. 1992; 5:789–795.

27. Zaldivar R, Ricur G, Oscherow S.The phakic intraocular lens implant: in-depth focus on posterior chamber phakic IOLs. Curr Opin Ophthalmol. 2000 Feb; 11(1):22–34.

28. Jimenez-Alfaro I, Benitez del Castillo JM, Garcia-Feijoo J, Gil de Bernabe JG, Serrano de La Iglesia JM. Safety of posterior chamber phakic intraocular lenses for the correction of high myopia: Anterior segment changes after posterior chamber phakic intraocular lens implantation. *Ophthalmology.* 2001; 108: 90–99.

29. Dejaco-Ruhswurm I, Scholz U, Pieh S, Hanselmayer G, Lackner B, Italon C, Ploner M, Skorpik C. Long-term endothelial changes in phakic eyes with posterior chamber intraocular lenses. *J Cataract Refract Surg*. 2002; 28:1589.

30. Kaya V, Kevser MA, Yilmaz OF .Phakic posterior chamber plate intraocular lenses for high myopia. J Refract Surg. 1999 Sep-Oct; 15(5):580–5.

31. Pesando PM, Ghiringhello MP, Di Meglio G, Fanton G. Posterior chamber phakic intraocular lens (ICL) for hyperopia: ten-year follow-up. J Cataract Refract Surg. Sep 2007; 33(9):1579–84.

32. Gonvers M, Othenin-Girard P, Bornet C, Sickenberg M. Implantable contact lens for moderate to high myopia: Short-term follow-up of 2 models. *J Cataract Refract Surg*. 2001; 27:380–388.

57

Medicolegal Aspects of Intraocular Surgery: General Information and Formal Informed Consent

Col JKS Parihar SM,VSM and Col FEA Rodrigues

INTRODUCTION

Ophthalmology is a science which has seen such drastic changes that we are almost flooded with volumes of information. This evolution of modern day ophthalmic surgery has changed many long held beliefs and assumptions following the cataract surgery. It is imperative on our part that we disseminate this information to our patients so that we clear most of their queries and also remove any misconceptions about the same not only for the benefit of the patient but also for the medicolegal aspect in the current scenario. It is a mandatory requirement under the Consumer Protection Act that the patient is well informed about the pros and cons of cataract surgery and in this regard furnishing detailed yet concise information to the patient will do away with most of the medicolegal claims in the court of law if the situation does arise.

The information on cataract surgery can be disseminated to patients by bringing out an information brochure which will provide information about 'cataract surgery and its various aspects' to the patients and their relatives. This information brochure will also guide the patients about the how, what and when of the cataract surgery.

A prototype of the information brochure along with the consent form has been given here which is being used in all the cataract cases operated at this tertiary eye care centre. The consent form tries to highlight all major complications and this can be explained to the patient in brief.

In short, providing all the basic information about the cataract surgery to the patient will go a long way in building a healthy relationship between the doctor and the patient.

An information booklet has been designed by us which is in circulation in the armed forces medical setup. An attempt has been made in this booklet to provide useful and comprehensive information to the patients and their relatives about cataract, its management including preoperative preparations, informed consent, operative procedures and postoperative management as well rehabilitation protocol depending upon visual and professional requirements. The booklet is available in English as well as Hindi. This booklet is reproduced here for reference. The information given here will act as a guideline for the phaco surgeons who can further modify it as per their requirements.

CATARACT SURGERY: GENERAL INFORMATION

What is Cataract?

A cataract refers to the clouding (opacity) of the normally clear lens that is situated behind the pupil (dark centre) of the eye. A cataract usually occurs as a natural consequence of ageing. Direct or indirect injury (trauma) to the eye or many systemic or ocular (eye) diseases may also lead to cataract formation. It causes gradual deterioration of vision and "glare", particularly in bright sunlight or when driving at night.

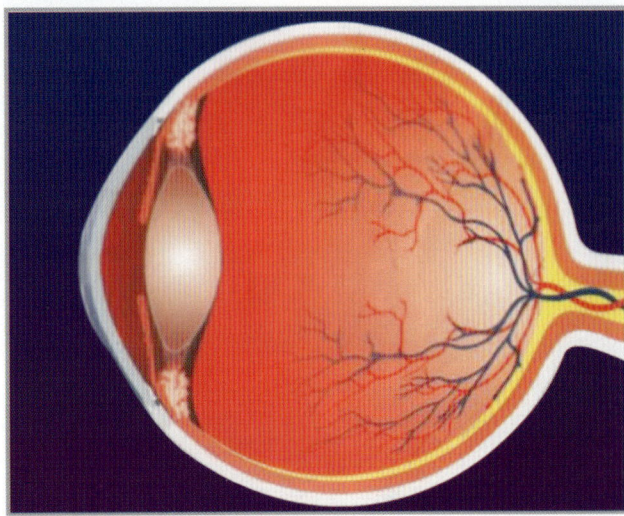

Fig. 57.1: Normal human eye

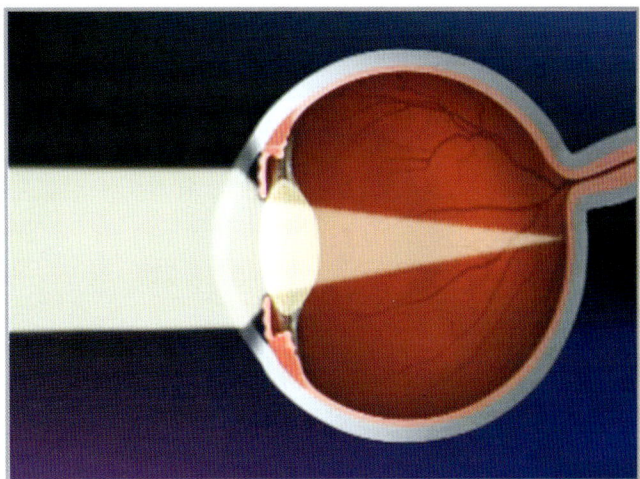

Fig. 57.2: Image formation in a normal human eye

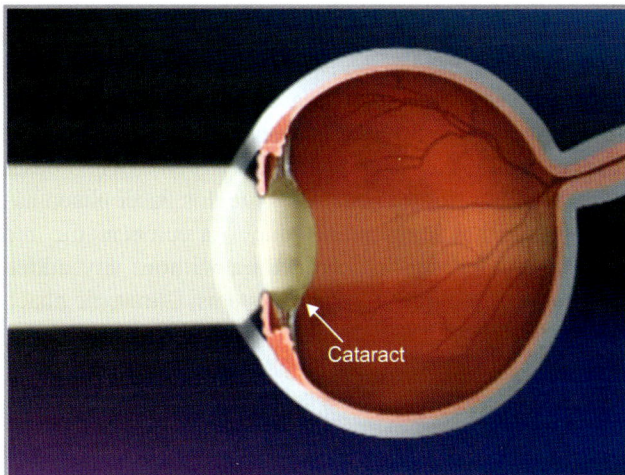

Fig. 57.3: Blurred image formation in a cataractous human eye

Management of Cataract

There is no other treatment except surgical removal of cataract.

Purpose

The purpose of cataract surgery is to restore clear vision. It is indicated when cloudy vision due to cataract has progressed to such an extent that it interferes with normal daily activities.

Alternative Procedures that are available

Surgery is the only way to remove a cataract.

Do Cataracts have to be "Ripe" before an Operation is Advised?

No. Earlier forms of cataract surgery carried substantial risks and the surgery was only recommended when the cataract was quite advanced. Nowadays, with the use of small incision techniques (Phacoemulsification), surgery is recommended when the patient has unacceptable visual acuity. As such, amount of energy required for emulsification of lens in the phacoemulsification technique is directly proportionate to the density and hardness of the nucleus. Hence, early intervention leads to least intra and postoperative complications and quick visual rehabilitation.

What is Phacoemulsification Surgery for Cataract?

Phacoemulsification surgery is a procedure where the lens is emulsified with the help of ultrasonic energy and then aspirated through a narrow port. This can all be achieved through a 2–3 mm incision. Following this procedure a suitable foldable lens is implanted. The incision site may be left without sutures or may be closed with one suture depending upon the status of the eye at the end of surgical procedure.

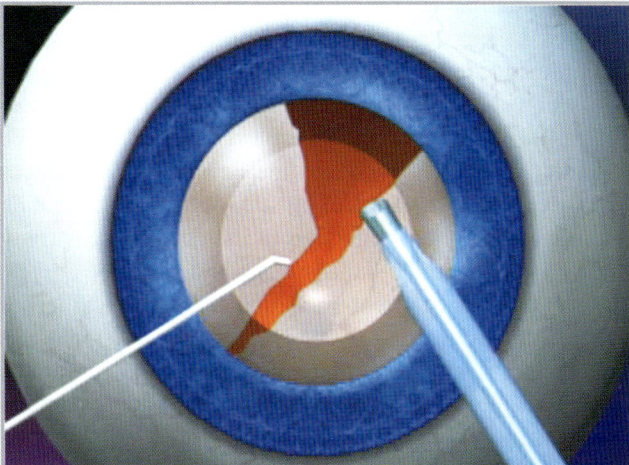

Fig. 57.4: Phacoemulsification surgery by chopping (breaking of lens nucleus by ultrasonic energy)

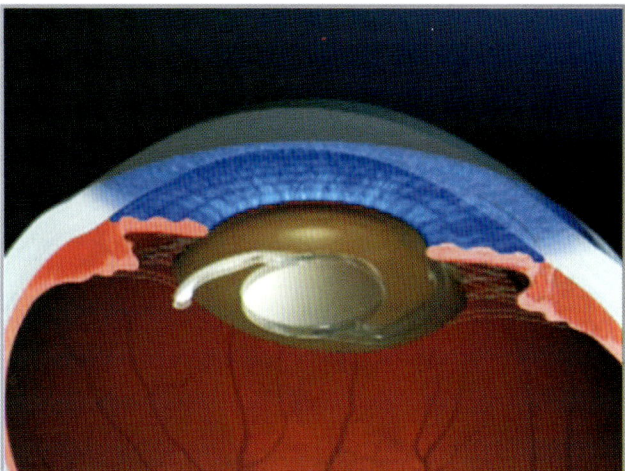

Fig. 57.5: Foldable intraocular lens is implanted following phacoemulsification surgery

Are Cataracts Removed by Laser?

Laser has been used in the experimental stage for removal of cataract, however, even in case of laser phaco, the same kind of incision and surgical technique is involved except the fact that the nucleus is emulsified with the help of laser in place of ultrasonic energy. Despite this, laser phaco has not attained much acceptance due to a cumbersome and very prolonged surgical procedure without any added advantage over ultrasonic phaco systems. Ultrasonic phaco system has been in use all over the world till now.

What are Intraocular Lens Implants?

These are artificial lenses (synthetic acrylic, silicone, or PMMA lenses) placed within the eye to correct the vision for distance and/or near. Synthetic acrylic or silicone lenses are foldable lenses so the incision remains tiny, thus causing minimal, if any, distortion or astigmatism. Conventionally, we use foldable intraocular lenses except in certain

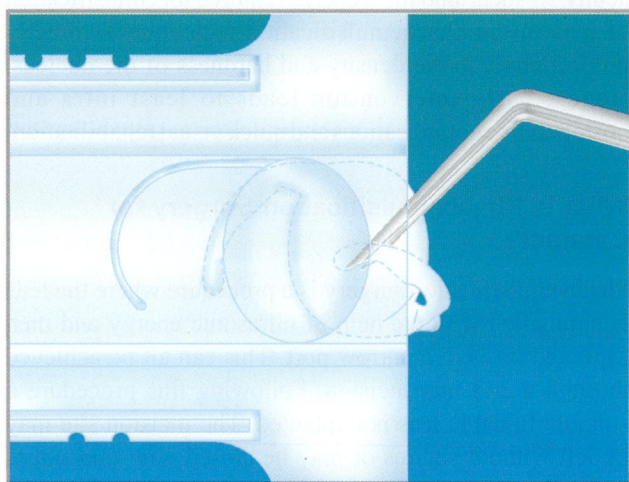

Fig. 57.6: Foldable posterior chamber Intraocular lens Implants

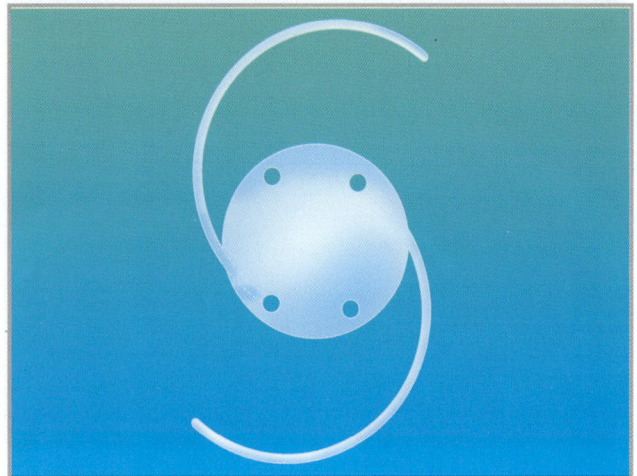

Fig. 57.7: Rigid (nonfoldable) posterior chamber IOL

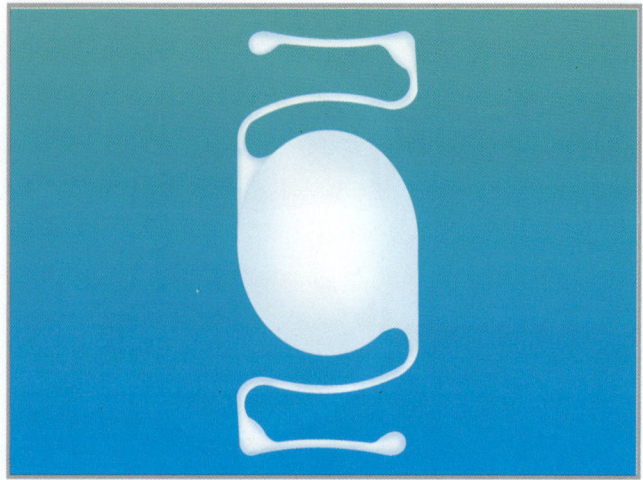

Fig. 57.8: Anterior chamber IOL

unprecedented situations where nonfoldable PMMA lenses may remain the solitary option.

What do you mean by Monofocal, Multifocal or Accommodative Intraocular Lens Implants?

Conventional acrylic or silicone foldable IOL implants provides good visual acuity only for one particular visual purpose. Such IOL implants are designed to have good visual acuity for common purposes like viewing distant or intermediate objects. Hence, they are popularly known as monofocal lenses. However, monofocal IOL implants do not possess accommodation quality; hence despite good distant vision following surgery, one needs to have glasses for near work like reading as required by most of us after the age of 40 years or so. In contrast to this, accommodative IOL carries certain amount of accommodation by the virtue of flexible support; hence moderate type of near work can be performed without any correction for near. However, one definitely requires spectacle correction for prolonged or very fine near work. Accommodative lenses tend to loose accommodative capability in due course of time due to changes in the posterior capsule. Multifocal lenses comprise multiple concentric rings of variable power for a different focus of vision. This allows great freedom from glasses for casual distant and near vision. However, glasses are essentially required for very fine near work. The major drawback and constraints of most multifocal IOLs remain significant glare and reduction in the contrast sensitivity and poor vision under dark or less illumination.

Over and above, accommodative and multifocal lenses are not suitable for high visual demand professionals, as well as in cases of abnormal and high corneal curvatures (astigmatism of more than 1 dioptre). Such IOLs demand precision and accuracy of a very high order, both in terms of pre and intraoperative consistency and proficiency.

To summarise, monofocal IOL implants remain the sheet anchor and the first choice in most of the cases.

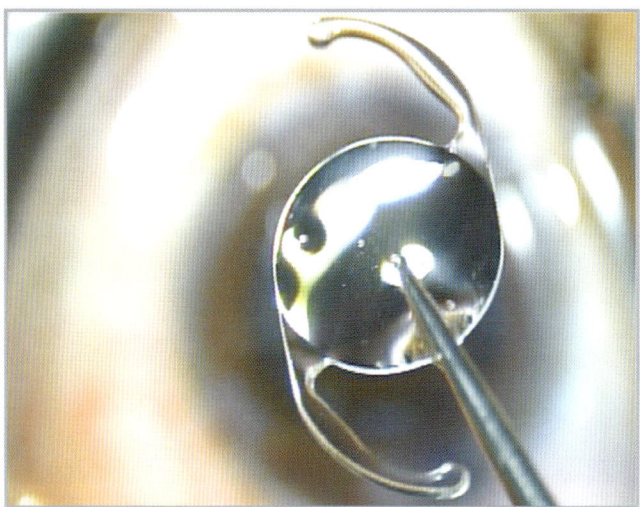

Fig. 57.9: Single piece hydrophobic acrylic foldable intraocular lens implant

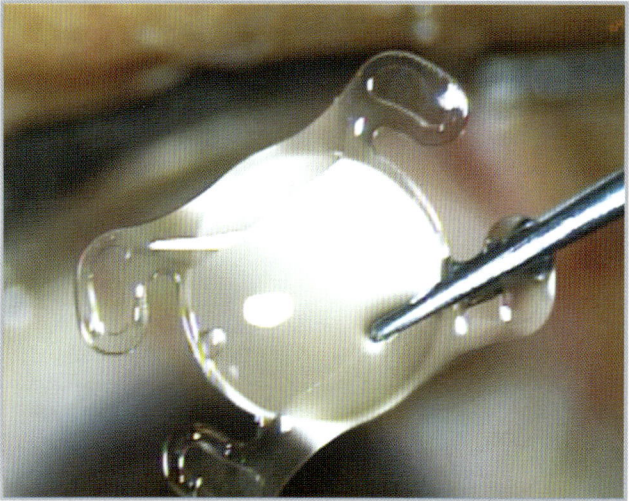

Fig. 57.10: Square edged hydrophilic acrylic foldable intraocular lens implant

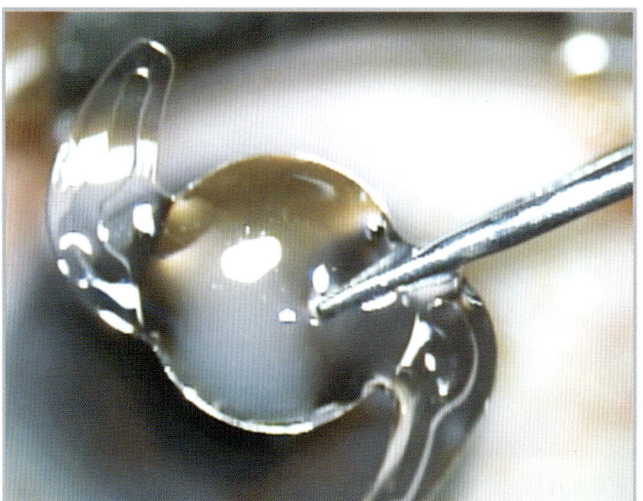

Fig. 57.11: Hydrophilic acrylic foldable intraocular lens implant with modified square edged haptics

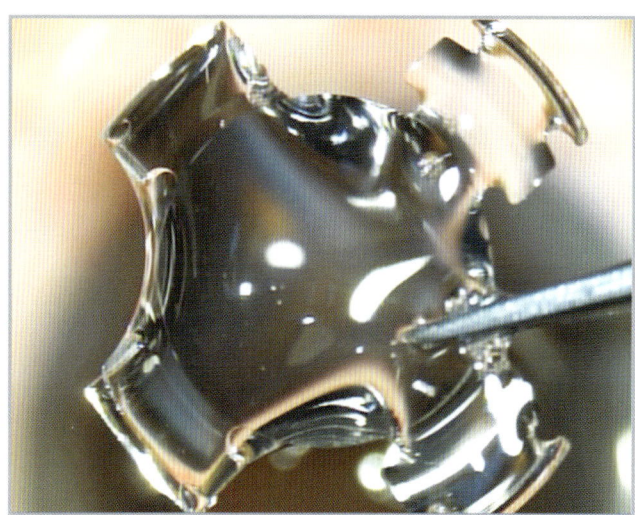

Fig. 57.12: Accommodative acrylic foldable intraocular lens implant

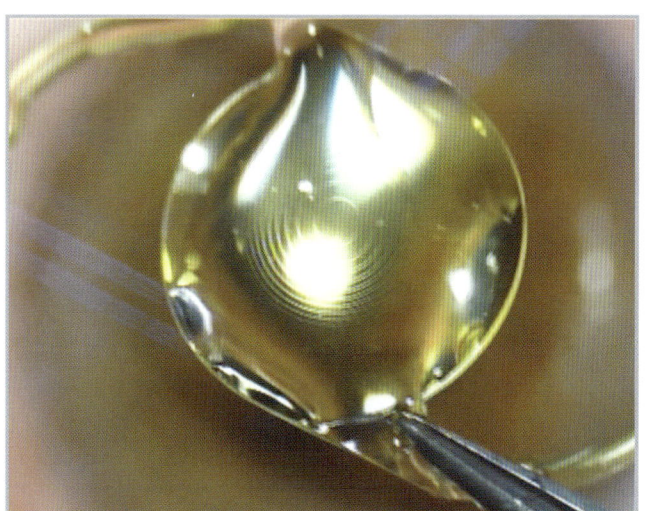

Fig. 57.13: Full range vision apodized diffractive multifocal intraocular lens implant

What does the Operation Involve?

It is usually performed in less than twenty minutes using local anaesthesia in the eyelid. The procedure can also be performed without injection under topical instillation of anaesthetic drops in selected and motivated cases. Topical anaesthesia is being preferred in this institution as the first choice of anaesthesia technique. By and large, the procedure is very safe and painless. Patient gets into operation theatre walking and comes out of the theatre in the same manner soon after the surgery. A small patch is being kept over the eye for three hours so as to protect the anaesthetised eye from inadvertent exposure to dust which may lead to injury and infection. The patient himself can remove the patch afterward and should commence instillation of desired eyedrops as advised by the operating surgeon.

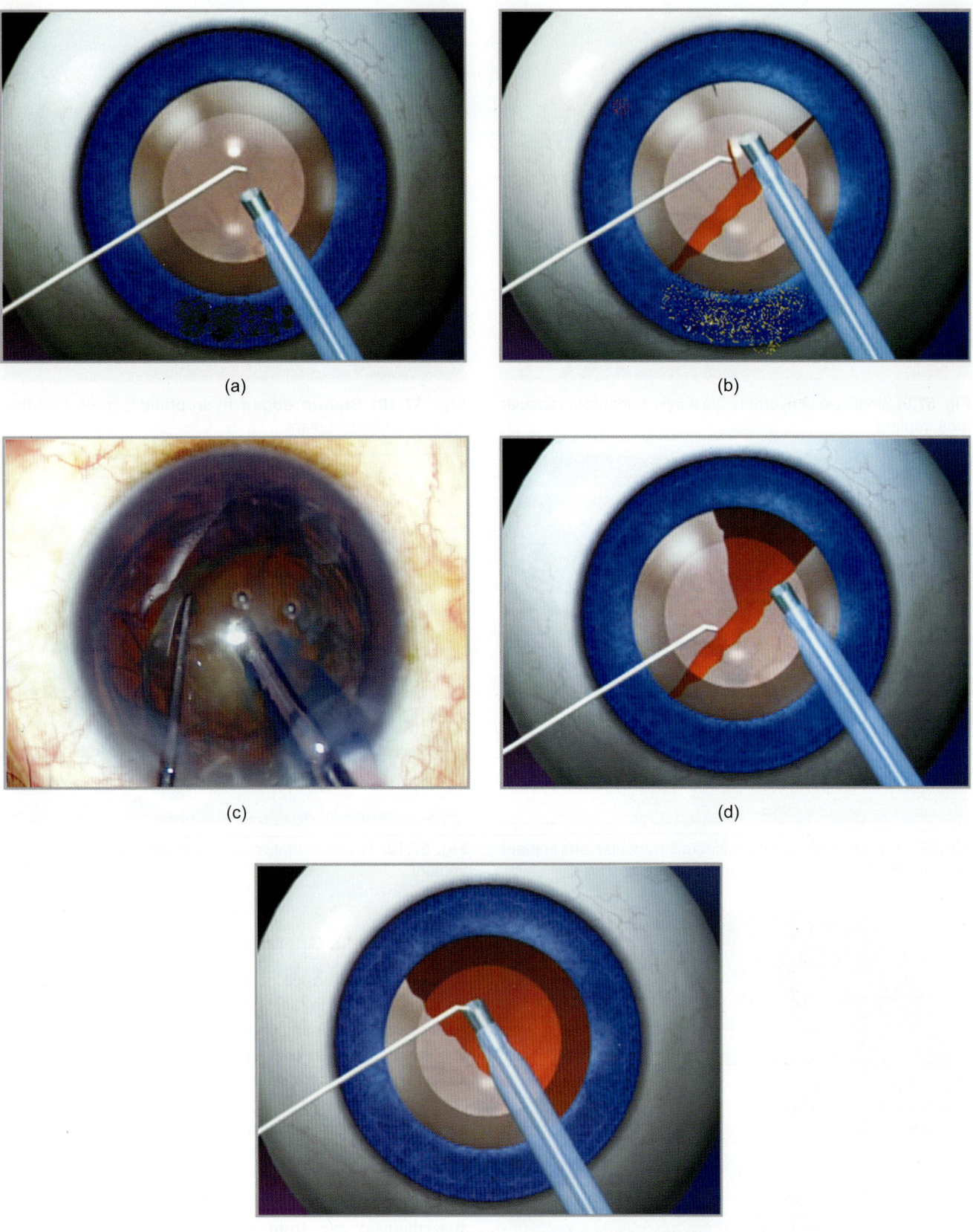

Fig. 57.14: (a) Phacoemulsification surgery by chopping (breaking of lens nucleus by ultrasonic energy), (b) Phacoemulsification surgery by chopping (breaking of lens nucleus by ultrasonic energy), (c) Phacoemulsification surgery is in progress (breaking of lens nucleus by ultrasonic energy), (d) Phacoemulsification surgery by chopping (breaking of lens nucleus by ultrasonic energy), (e) Phacoemulsification surgery by chopping (breaking of lens nucleus by ultrasonic energy)

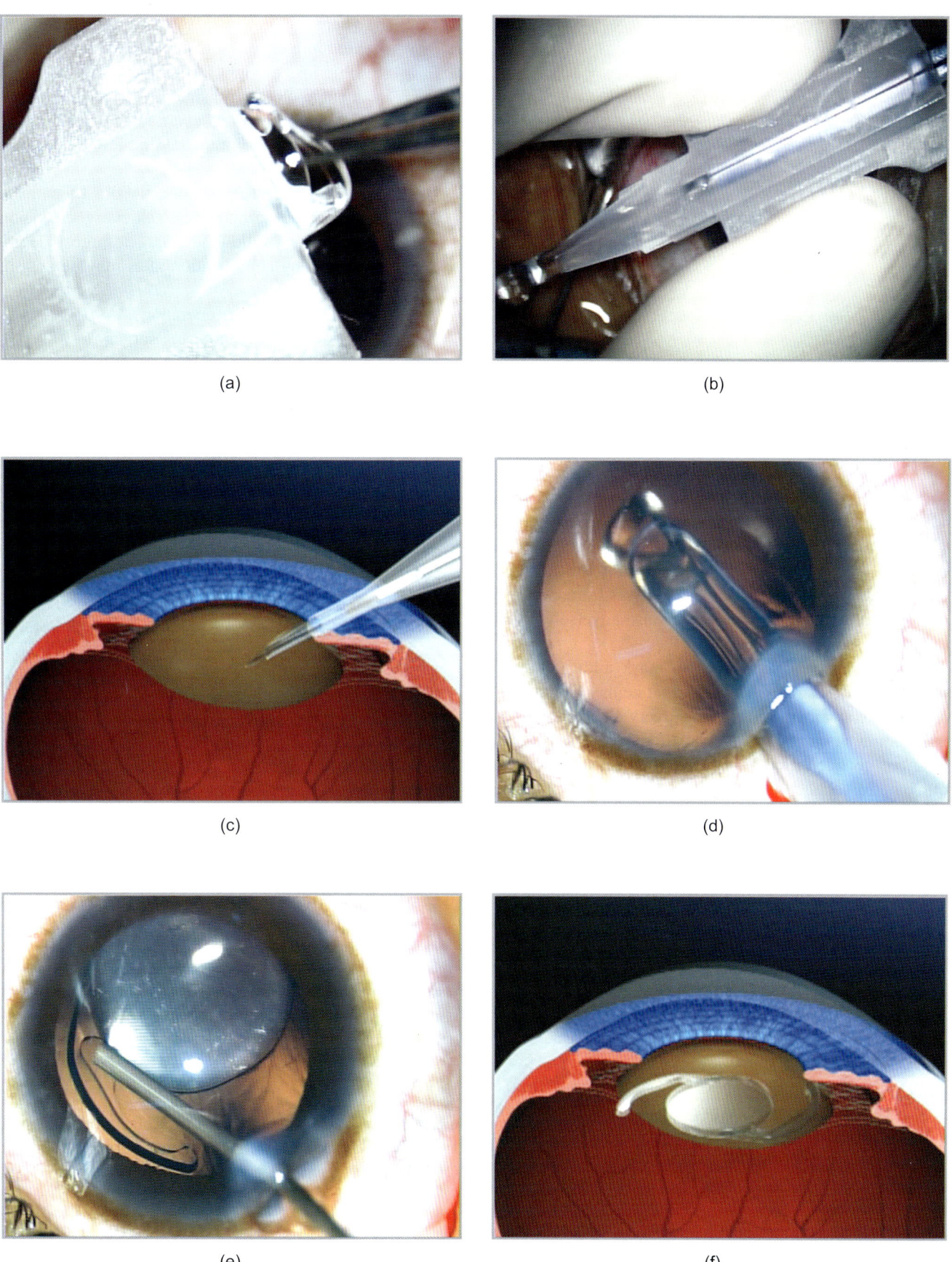

Fig. 57.15: (a) and (b) Loading of a foldable IOL implant in the injector system prior to the implantation into the eye, (c), (d) and (e) Insertion of a foldable IOL implant is in progress, (f) The foldable IOL implant is in the bag

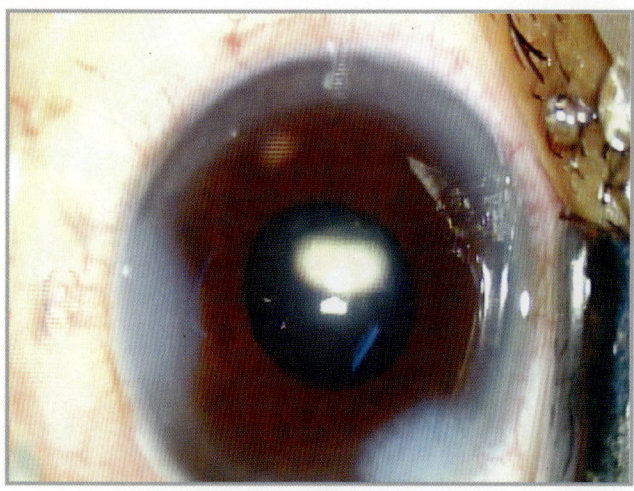

(g)

Fig. 57.15: (g) The foldable IOL implant is in the bag

How Successful is the Operation?

Current techniques can ensure that over 95% of patients would achieve an excellent corrected normal or near normal vision of up to 6/6 or even better, provided there is no other associated eye disease involving the cornea, intraocular pressure, retina or optic nerve. Intraoperative or postoperative complications may also adversely affect the visual outcome.

The presence of cataracts can mask additional eye problems, such as retinal damage, that neither doctors nor patients are aware of prior to the surgery. Such conditions will continue to impair sight even after cataract removal if they are not identified and treated. Hence, the eventual outcome of cataract surgery will depend on the outcome of other problems.

Serious or Frequently Occurring Risks

(a) All operations being invasive procedures carry some obvious risks. Considering such unprece-dented and unpredictable risks involved, cataract surgery is not performed simultaneously on both the eyes at the same sitting. To avoid risking blindness in both eyes in the event of infection or other catastrophe, the first eye is allowed to heal before the cataract is removed from the fellow eye.

(b) There are many complications that can arise from a cataract operation; however, the vast majority of people have successful surgery. We wish to give you the opportunity to think about the risks of cataract surgery before consenting to your operation.

    (i) The minor complications include an increase in pressure or inflammation inside the eye; these problems are usually temporary and easily treatable.

    (ii) There are, however, some complications that are more serious and could lead to an irreversible loss of sight in the operated eye. These include bleeding inside the eye at the time of the operation, or a severe infection inside the eye that arises within the first few weeks after surgery.

(c) It has been observed that about 90% of patients with otherwise normal eyes, achieve good vision (6/12 or better) following cataract surgery. However, following complication rates may be kept in mind:

    (i) Events during the operation

      Any complication during surgery 5–7%

      Capsule rupture and vitreous loss 4–5%

      Tiny lens fragments in the back (vitreous) cavity of the eye, all of which can lead to loss of sight (less than 01%).

    (ii) Immediate postoperative period (within 48 hrs)

      Any complication at this time: 10–15%

      Corneal swelling: 3–5%

      Leaking wound less than: 1%

      External infection: 0.05%

      Internal infection (endophthalmitis): 0.02%

    (iii) Sight-threatening complications (within three months of surgery):

      Internal infection (endophthalmitis): 0.05–0.1%

      Retinal detachment 0.2%

Risks with Local Anaesthetics

Local anaesthetics are a very safe type of anaesthetics. Very rarely people have an allergic reaction to the local anaes-thetic itself, but the patient will be asked about allergies beforehand.

Will I Never use Glasses again?

In this procedure, routine work is possible without glasses. Using a monofocal intraocular lens implant, (fixed power lens) the patient will require glasses for distance and/or near. Usually, the dependence of glasses is greatly reduced.

What are the Restrictions of Activity?

Generally, we recommend patients to refrain from driving for a week and/or heavy lifting from a bending position. Otherwise, the patient can immediately resume fairly normal activity.

Can an Operation be done without Stitches?

Yes, it can be done. However, recent studies indicate that the "sutureless" techniques may carry an increased risk of infections, which may be seriously visually threatening. Therefore, one suture can be placed in the cornea until the incision is healed. However, the decision to place sutures depends upon the wound status and the surgeon's discretion at the time of surgery.

Can a Cataract Grow Back?

No, however in about 10 to 15% of cases some scarring can occur behind the lens (opacification of the posterior capsule of natural lens, over which an artificial IOL implant is placed), causing a slow deterioration of vision. This scarring is easily removed by laser treatment as an outdoor procedure under topical anaesthesia (instillation of anaesthetic agent in the form of eyedrops). This procedure is painless and is over within a few seconds.

PREOPERATIVE WORK UP FOR CATARACT SURGERY

1. On arrival to the eye OPD, the patient is first examined in the eye OPD and a detailed history of the eye, systemic and family history of illness is recorded. Subsequently, examination of the eye is carried out under following steps:
   (a) Recording of visual acuity with and without glasses.
   (b) Intraocular pressure is recorded either by placing an instrument over the eye under topical anaesthesia or by noncontact method. The patency of lacrimal sac (tear drainage system) is simultaneously checked.
   (c) Subsequently, the pupil is dilated with the help of topical eyedrops to evaluate the status of lens and retina (the light sensitive part of the eye having connection with brain). The dilatation takes from 30–45 min.
2. If the lens is found to be cataractous on examination under magnification on a slit lamp, the surgeon decides the type of artificial lens suitable for the type of cataract. Then specific work-up for cataract surgery is done.
3. The power of the lens to be implanted is calculated with a machine in the eye department (IOL Power calculation/A-scan biometry).
4. The patient is then required to get certain basic investiga-tions before the surgery. These investigations are carried out in the MI room/pathology lab and the patient is required to come in with an empty stomach. The investigations required are:
   (a) Blood—Hb, TLC, DLC, BT, CT, ESR, blood sugar fasting and postprandial (two hours after breakfast)
   (b) Urine—RE (routine)
   (c) ECG

5. Following the investigations, the patient is referred to the anaesthesiologist for a PA checkup (pre-anaesthetic checkup) at the PA checkup room situated on the ground floor near the MI room. PA checkup is carried out every day and is required to assess the general condition of the patient and rule out any medical or surgical illness. Although the eye surgery is done under local anaesthesia, yet general assessment prior to the surgery is a mandatory requirement. In a way, the patient benefits since he undergoes a basic health checkup.
6. Once the patient is cleared for surgery from the anaesthesia standpoint, he is given a date for the surgery.
7. The patient is required to come one day prior to the surgery when he is once again seen over the slit lamp. The patient may be admitted or can be called directly to the OT for surgery and operated as a day-care surgery depending on the convenience of the patient. Daycare surgery is the most preferred and a convenient option in general, for cataract surgery under local anaesthesia.

Common Medical Terminology used with Medicine Prescriptions

(a)	OD	:	Once in a day
(b)	BD	:	Twice in a day
(c)	TDS	:	Thrice daily
(d)	QID	:	4 Times a day
(e)	AC	:	Before meals
(f)	PC	:	After meals
(g)	HS	:	At bedtime
(h)	P and B	:	Pad and bandage

PREOPERATIVE ADVICE (BEFORE SURGERY)

Consent

Formal and informed written consent is obtained.

Trimming of Eye Lashes

Generally, not done in our institution. However, there is no problem if eye lashes are trimmed as they grow back to normal length within 3–4 weeks.

Three Days Prior to the Day of Surgery (Medication)

Ciprofloxacin or any suitable antibiotic eyedrops applied locally 6 hourly in both eyes with effect from three days prior to the surgery.

One day Prior to the Day of Surgery

(a) Ciprofloxacin or any other prescribed antibiotic eyedrops locally to be instilled at a 6 hourly interval in both the eyes. However, the patient should not be disturbed if sleeping.

(b) Ibuprofen (ocuflur) eyedrops 8 hourly in the eye to be operated upon with effect from 7 PM.

(c) Tab Diazepam 1 Tab at 2200 Hr (10 PM, optional in very few selected cases depending upon the level of anxiety).

(d) Tab Ciprofloxacillin 500 mg or any other suitable antibiotic orally at 2200 Hrs.

Medications/Advice for the Day of Surgery

(a) You may take a cup of tea with two biscuits or light breakfast two hours before the surgery.

(b) Take the medicines as per the instructions. It is requested to continue all antihypertensive and other medications as prescribed by the cardiologist/physician/anaesthesiologist. However, antidiabetic medication should not be taken on the day of surgery.

(c) Tab Ciprofloxacillin 500 mg orally, twice a day (with effect from morning on the day of surgery).

(d) Requested to have hair wash with shampoo since the next head bath will be after a week (no kajal, hair oil, cosmetics should be applied).

(e) Please instill dilator eyedrops like Cyclopentolate/Tropicamide and FLUR three times at every 15 minutes interval in the eye to be operated upon for one hour prior to the arrival at OT.

(f) Kindly remove all jewellery, especially ear rings, nose rings, watch and finger rings before going to the OT (operation theatre).

(g) The patient is requested to urinate before being taken to the OT.

INTRAOPERATIVE CARE (DURING SURGERY)

1. The anaesthesiologist constantly monitors during all major eye procedures. All patients are operated under continuous cardiac monitoring. Intravenous (IV drip) is regularly maintained so as to meet any unforeseen eventuality or to administer any medication immediately without disturbing patient and surgeon both.

2. The operation is made painless by proper local anaesthesia. The patient usually falls asleep.

3. In case the patient feels pain or discomfort, it is requested that the patient feels free to talk to the surgeon immediately. It is instructed that the patient does not move his/her head. However, the patients can move their legs after prior intimation to the operating surgeon.

POSTOPERATIVE CARE AFTER PHACO EMULSIFICATION CATARACT SURGERY

Immediate Postoperative Instructions

(a) The patient may feel drowsy after the surgery due to the effects of the medicine given before or during the operation. However, most of the patients remain comfortable and alert during the operative period and the immediate postoperative period. The patient may walk comfortably soon after surgery. However, patients may choose to rest for one to two hours. The patient must not turn to the operated side while lying down for two days. One may turn to the unoperated side.

(b) You can take oral fluids followed by meals of your preference.

(c) You may sit up slowly. Please inform if you have a sensation of nausea or vomiting. In case you need to go to the toilet, you may do so with some assistance. Avoid straining and jerks.

(d) Do not stop the treatment you are taking for diabetes, high blood pressure, heart disease, etc., unless specifically instructed. Please ask if you have any doubts.

(e) The dressing is generally changed on the next day. This allows the surgeon to get a close look. However, it may be removed on the same day based on the advice given by the surgeon. In this event, all topical drops will commence from the same day. The eye may appear red and give minimal discomfort for a few days.

(f) Postoperative vision is variable during the 1st week. It takes 2 to 3 weeks before the best vision is achieved. There may be a need for stitch removal prior to the prescription of glasses for final correction.

(g) Frequent instillations of eyedrops are carried out for the first few days. The attendant may see the procedure for cleaning the eyes and medication.

(h) Treatment instructions prescribed are valid till the next follow-up visit or for the period specified, whichever is earlier.

Precautions to be Taken after Surgery
Caution against

(i) Injury
(ii) Infection
(iii) Inflammation and
(iv) Increased intraocular pressure

(The first two are in the hands of the patient and the remaining two will be taken care of by operating surgeon.)

Use

(i) All eyedrops and medicines as prescribed. This will continue at least for a period of 6 to 8 weeks. It is preferable to take the help of someone to instill the eyedrops.

(ii) You may continue to wear your old glasses till the new pair is prescribed 4–6 weeks after surgery.

Watch for Symptoms

(i) **Normal symptoms:** The following symptoms are normal and are not a cause for alarm. These are slight redness, mild watering, mild irritation, glare and a slight drooping of the upper eyelid. These will remain to some extent for 6–8 weeks.

(ii) **Alarming symptoms:** In case of increasing pain and redness; increasing stickiness or discharge from the eye; injury, decrease in vision or flashes of light in the operated eye, contact your surgeon immediately.

Stop the Medicine

If it hurts too much or if you develop allergy (itching, redness, swelling or rash), consult the doctor.

Avoid

(i) **Avoid sleeping on the operated side :** To avoid any pressure on the operated eye.

(ii) **Injury:** Rubbing, squeesing your eye. Do not rub or apply pressure to eye. Idea is to save it from infection and injury.

(iii) **Infection:** Cleaning of eye with sterile cotton and saline/water once a day at least for one week or as advised.

Cleaning the Eyes

Any discharge/collection in the morning may be gently wiped using sterile moist cotton Johnson's buds. (Boil the cotton/Johnson's buds in a clean bowl for 20 minutes and use it when cooled). Watering from the operated eye is usual for a few days which can be wiped using a clean handkerchief or cottoned away from the eye without touching it. The patient's hands should be washed scrupulously with soap and should not be wiped with a towel or a cloth.

Protection

The patient may wear the protective eye shield at night for the first week. Protective glasses may be worn during the daytime, especially outdoors, to avoid any discomfort that you may have from bright light and also to prevent any injury to eye.

Face Wash

For the first few days, avoid splashing water directly into the eye. The patient may use a clean, soft, wet towel to wipe your face. However, incidental inadvertent entry of water while, cleaning the face should not be taken very seriously. In such situation, prescribed antibiotic + steroid eyedrops may be used immediately.

Trimming

Trimming of hair is permitted after two weeks of the operation.

Bathing

Body bath (below the neck) may be resumed on very next day. However, one should avoid taking a shower or a bath in the bathtub for the first week after surgery.

Head Bath

One may wash the hair with the head tilted backwards to avoid any water splashing into the eye. A proper head bath may be taken after a week.

Makeup

Avoid eye makeup for 6 weeks.

Diet

There are no dietary restrictions and the patient may take routine diet. However, the restrictions prescribed as per preexisting systemic problems, like diabetes and high blood pressure must continue. Avoid constipation by taking more fluid, green vegetables, cereals and fruits. A mild laxative may be used, if necessary.

Watching TV/Movie in Theatre

No restriction. May resume on the same day, however adequate distance to be observed from the TV.

Reading/Writing/Working on Computers

No restriction. May be resumed soon after the operation.

Return to Normal Activities

May resume normal routine at home including diet on very same day.

Driving

Avoid driving, especially for one week unless the surgeon permits you.

Games

(i) **Indoor games like playing cards/chess etc:** No restriction, may be resumed soon after the operation.

(ii) **Outdoor games:** After one month.

(iii) **Contact sports:** Contact sports, etc. after 1–2 months.

(iv) **Golf:** After two to three weeks depending upon pace of recovery.

Physical Exercise

Normal daily activities including walking may be resumed soon after the operation. However, strenuous activities like jogging, lifting weights, bending exercises and aerobics should be avoided at least for 6 to 8 weeks.

Swimming

After six weeks.

Gardening

Avoid for six to eight weeks.

Job

(a) **Indoor office work/public meetings:** The patients may get back to their routine jobs within four to seven days after surgery.

(b) **Outdoor public meetings:** After one week.

Travelling

(a) **Air/Train:** No restriction

(b) **Road travelling:** Long distance travelling on improper roads to be avoided for 2 weeks. Road traveling of a short distance on private transport is permitted.

Sex

Sex life may be resumed a week or two after the operation and after consulting the patients eye surgeon.

CONSENT FORM FOR CATARACT SURGERY
ARMY HOSPITAL (RESEARCH AND REFERRAL) DELHI CANTT

1. I, hereby give consent for cataract surgery by extracapsular extraction of cataractous lens by conventional ECCE/ phacoemulsification or by SICS (Small incision cataract) technique on myself the father/mother/wife/son/daughter in right/ left eye under any kind of anaesthesia/no anaesthesia.

2. I fully understand that the surgery is performed for restoration of vision and that the surgical technique will be considered by my surgeon on case to case basis depending on the grading of cataract and corneal clarity. I will not hold any responsibility on the operating team for any decision taken intraoperatively in good faith and in the best of interest to restore vision including of conversion, additional procedures or total abandon of operation in a very rare and unforeseen situation.

3. A posterior chamber intraocular lens will be implanted subject to the intraoperative viability of posterior capsule. In case of inadequate posterior capsule for intraocular lens implantation, an anterior chamber intraocular lens will be implanted and in exceptional circumstances where the surgeon feels so, the eye can be left aphakic for a secondary lens implantation at a later date.

4. I also understand that the postoperative vision is subject to various preoperative, intraoperative and postoperative factors for which the operating surgeon cannot be held responsible.

   The various intra or postoperative complications that can affect the outcome of the surgery are:

   (a) Intraoperative complications:
   - (i) Intraoperative bleeding both at the time of local anaesthesia infiltration or during surgery which may be very minimal from the superficial tissue or severe intraocular like expulsive haemorrhage.
   - (ii) Rupture of the posterior capsule of lens
   - (iii) Vitreous prolapse
   - (iv) Dislocation of lens nucleus in toto or its fragments
   - (v) IOL displacement/dislocation

   (b) Postoperative complications:
   - (i) Anterior or posterior uveitis (inflammation inside the eye).
   - (ii) Corneal oedema and bullous keratopathy.
   - (iii) Postoperative glaucoma.
   - (iv) Iris prolapse, wound dehiscence.
   - (v) IOL displacement/dislocation.
   - (vi) Postoperative infection or endophthalmitis
   - (vii) Cystoid macular oedema (swelling of the central part of retina)
   - (viii) Retinal detachment
   - (ix) High postoperative astigmatism (irregular curvature of the cornea, i.e the outer transparent layer of eye responsible for clear light pathways)
   - (x) Aberrations in IOL power calculation leading to unexpected residual number of spectacles.
   - (xi) Posterior capsular opacification: May require YAG laser capsulotomy.

   The risks involved in the surgery had been duly explained to me in the language I understand and I accept the same.

(Signature of the patient if adult)   (Signature of the individual)

    Date   : ....   No........................ Rank....................

    Place   : ....   Name..

    Witness : ....   Unit: ....

    Date   : ....

    Place   : ....

CONCLUSION

Despite several noted complications and events encountered during the process of cataract surgery, modern techniques of cataract surgery have emerged as outstanding procedures of choice. This has resulted in tremendous change in the postcataract surgery scenario to near normal lifestyle as compared to the good old days of cataract surgery which would have left patients with highly uncomfortable thick glasses in the spectacles and lots of restrictions in routine activities as well as in professional requirements in various fields. The incidences of complications are very less and we do expect an excellent outcome in more than 97% cases. However, gentle care during postoperative period ensures swift and smooth recovery towards normal lifestyle. This information brochure has been designed to provide overall view as well as broad guidelines. However, specific queries and problems should be discussed with an ophthalmic surgeon as and when required.

BIBLIOGRAPHY

1. Elder MJ, Suter A."What patients want to know before they have cataract surgery", British Journal of Ophthalmology 2004, 88 (3), 331–2.
2. Hingorami M, Wong T, Vafidis G. (1999), "Patients and doctors" attitudes to amount of information given after unintended injury during treatment: cross-sectional questionnaire survey", British Medical Journal 1999, (318). 640–1.
3. Kavanagh S, Cowan, J. "Reducing risk in healthcare teams: an overview", Clinical Governance: An International Journal 2004, (9:3)200–4.
4. Minassian DC, Reidy A., Desai P, Farrow S, Vafidis G, Minassian A. "The deficit in cataract surgery in England and Wales and the escalating problem of visual impairment: epidemiological modelling of the population dynamics of cataract", British Journal of Ophthalmology 2000, (84:1) 4–8.
5. NHS Executive, "Action on cataracts, good practice guidance"2000, available at: www.dh.gov.uk/assetRoot/04/01/45/14/04014514.pdf, [Manual Request] [Infotrieve]
6. Reidy A, Minassian DC, Vafidis G, Joseph J, Farrow S, Wu J., Desai P., Connolly A. "Prevalence of serious eye disease and visual impairment in a north London population: population-based, cross-sectional study", British Medical Journal1998, (316)1643–6.
7. Royal College of Ophthalmologists, "Cataract surgery guidelines" 2004, available at www.rcophth.ac.uk/scientific/docs/cataract04.pdf,.

58

Phacosurgery:
As Experienced by Recipients

Surg Cdr TR Bera and Col JKS Parihar SM, VSM

INTRODUCTION

We deal with patients mostly of the geriatric age group. In the recent times of course, we are getting patients of relatively younger age groups for various reasons. The definition of surgery requiring cataract is changing fast and so is the spectrum of patients.

We operate our patients under local anaesthesia and sometimes even under no anaesthesia. Patients remain fully conscious and can listen to all conversations. Even this may cause some additional apprehensions in the mind of the patient and some discomfort for the surgeon at a later date, when the patient tries to clarify what he had heard during surgery. We must keep this in mind and thus be careful during the whole procedure.

EXPECTATIONS OF THE PATIENT

In this age of communication, patients can easily acquire fairly good knowledge about their ailments and can even find out various management options available to them. The whole gamut of information is easily available to them at the click of the mouse. In fact, a good percentage of the patients these days actually read about the procedure they undergo from either magazines, or local newspapers.

Gone are the days when the patients would listen from the treating surgeons about the advantages of a particular procedure and options and accept them as gospels. These days, the patient often comes to the surgeon with a particular procedure in mind and insists for it. A time has come when the patient's form an idea about the surgical skill of the treating surgeon from the procedures he performs/does not perform and the result he achieves. Hence, the surgeons of the modern era have no choice but to keep pace with the latest procedures and the art of balancing on a tight rope.

Surgeons are often left with the option of humbly discussing with the patient his specific condition and explain that under the circumstances a particular procedure will have better chances of improved vision and early recovery. Some patients even come equipped with adequate knowledge of advantages and disadvantages of each procedure and can take an active part in the decision-making discussion. This is particularly true in case of those patients who do not hesitate to visit a number of specialist surgeons and gather a variety of opinions on the subject. They remain on the verge of total confusion and sometimes even manage to create a certain degree of confusion even in the mind of an experienced surgeon. Whether the surgeon likes it or not he has to learn to deal with these patients and to design his ways smoothly under a given situation and eventually satisfy the patient with an acceptable visual outcome.

Those days are past when the patients used to visit the ophthalmologist with finger counting close to the face vision or keeping his finger crossed about the ultimate outcome and final visual and professional rehabilitation. Though in the developing countries like in the Indian subcontinent these patients have not disappeared altogether but a new breed of patients has emerged which desires to undergo the surgery for better vision even when their vision is quite acceptable for normal day-to-day activities. Minimal impairment in the quality of vision in these cases interferes with their professional output. These days patients are ready to undergo surgery early when they have only glare effect while driving at night.

Patients belonging to a variety of professions approach for early surgery so that they can perform better in their profession. One internationally famous film director in Calcutta reported with complaints of inability to distinguish different hues of the same colour, which interfered with the quality of his professional output. He gladly underwent cataract surgery for better clarity of vision even when his visual acuity was reasonably well in the Snellen's chart.

Similarly, professional people belonging to other visual art may require early surgery. While people having professions like pilot, police and defence forces require early surgery to maintain the visual standard required to continue in their respective services.

Till few years back, cataract surgery used to be considered a very delicate surgery and a number of restrictions were imposed on the patient for a long period. Even patients were often instructed not to perform certain acts during their lifetime following intraocular lens implantation surgery. Jumping and diving into a pool was a definite no-no for those patients. Things have changed since then. Better methods of cataract surgery with IOL implantation are available today. In their enthusiasm to impress the patient the surgeons are claiming that following in-the-bag phacoemulsification cataract surgery there is no need for any restriction for the patient. Through the efficient media, the message has reached the masses. Now it is our turn to keep the promise.

A number of patients now report with mild to moderate impairment of vision for surgery with a demand to perform the procedure in a manner so that they can continue in their profession after the surgery. Obviously their professions demand a variable degree of physical activity. I remember a middle-aged football coach who reported for surgery and demanded for the quality of surgery that can enable him to continue to coach the boys, as it was his bread and butter. He also explained that football coaching often involves jumping and heading the ball among many people often resulting in mild to moderate collisions. A practical demonstration of the bicycle-kick is often required to explain the trainee the body maneuver. He enthusiastically explained the head-down posture required for the shot and the final fall on the back with the resultant jerk, which he may (and the IOL) have to sustain.

Similarly, a young paratrooper with a traumatic cataract reminded us of his activity and intention to continue with it. They have all heard that the modern technique of cataract surgery is absolutely safe and can be done in a manner where usually no restrictions are imposed on the patient even after surgery with pseudophake in position (because it is securely in-the-bag). The modern surgeon has to learn to take up such pressures and accept the demands as challenges in this era of information highways. However one should not hesitate to restrict some activities for the benefit of the patient in some cases.

APPREHENSIONS OF THE PATIENT BEFORE AND DURING SURGERY

The ophthalmic surgeon primarily deals with elderly patients, some of whom are extremely apprehensive. However, most of them surprisingly behave in a gentle manner when prepared for surgery properly. It is better to prepare the patient preoperatively for some pain at the time of injection, rather than telling them that it is an absolutely painless surgery and will not cause any pain whatsoever. Some patients with poor tolerance become instantaneously unhappy after injection when not prepared adequately.

No prick topical anaesthesia cataract surgery has become a trend in the modern day ophthalmology practice. But it is better to select cases for such procedure during preoperative assessment period very meticulously. Some patients cooperate better while some behave in an erratic manner causing discomfort for the patient as well for the surgeon. Ophthalmic surgeons must keep in mind that the cataract surgeries are performed under local anaesthesia and patients can hear the conversation throughout the procedure. Some patients remain quite alert and observant throughout until they are draped and thereafter listen to everything till the end of the surgery.

It is thus advisable for the surgeon not to discuss about the complications with any assistant or colleague during the surgical procedure. Patients remain extremely apprehensive and note every word they hear during surgery. It is always better to discuss the management of a complication later with a colleague after the patient has left the operating room. Otherwise, patients put up embarrassing questions to the surgeon at a later date and even drag the surgeon to the courtroom. Patient becomes particularly unhappy if the postoperative vision is not very good and unhesitatingly attributes it to the operative complication and surgical competence of the surgeon.

Similarly, once a lens is selected for implantation, it is better not to discuss about its poor design or difficulty in implantation with a colleague in the presence of the patient. As it is the surgeon who always decides about implanting a particular brand of lens, it is his responsibility to choose the most suitable one. In case the outcome of the surgery is not to the satisfaction of the patient, he/she has the right to inquire why that particular brand was used when the surgeon was not conversant with it. We have to always remember that the patient is under local anaesthesia and can follow all discussions that take place in the OT room.

It is always better to exchange a few words with the patient prior to the surgery and during the procedure. It relaxes the patient; at the same time it gives an idea about the general physical state of the patient. Patients with cardiac ailments may develop any systemic complication at any stage of the procedure. Allergic reaction also remains a possibility. It also distracts the patient's mind from the minor discomfort of surgery.

At times of course, once the surgeon starts the conversation, a talkative patient takes off and then it becomes extremely difficult to stop the patient from talking. In this respect I remember a very interesting conversation we had in our OT.

Mr. Ganguly an elderly but energetic patient was placed on the OT table, like any other case for cataract surgery. As usual, only a peribulbar local anaesthesia injection was given to the patient and he was fully conscious and alert. To make the respectable patient feel more comfortable the gentle surgeon made the mistake of initiating a conversation with him, little realising that the octogenarian is actually a chatterbox. An otherwise quiet operation theatre and a whole lot of cooperative listeners probably enthused the patient further.

At the outset, the octogenarian expressed his displeasure and vehemently complained about the indecent OT etiquettes. Apparently, the preoperative room assistants were rather merciless and had the guts to request him to strip completely and change over to the OT gown before he was sent inside the OT for surgery. He was upset as nobody dared to do that to him at home in the last many decades.

By then, the surgeon realised that he had made a mistake by encouraging the patient in the conversation and replying to all his queries patiently. He decided to reverse his decision and politely requested the patient to keep quiet for sometime so that he can concentrate in his work and perform finer steps of the surgery in a more meticulous manner. The patient kept quiet for a brief period.

Then suddenly, surprising the surgeon, the octogenarian asked for the lady doctor whose voice he was hearing for sometime. The extra decent surgeon produced the lady doctor to avoid annoying the respectable patient. The request for the lady was also taken sportingly as the testosterone level was expected to remain on the lower side at that age under normal circumstances. The lady doctor announced her arrival with a greeting followed by a laugh. The elderly patient apologised to the lady that he was not in a position to shake hands with her as he was completely draped with sterile sheets.

After a pause he asked "from which state are you?" The lady doctor replied ' Andhra'. The surgeon added' Uncle, she is from the state of 'Chandra Babu Naidu'. The patient replied, 'Oh! That fellow, who talks more than me'.

In the meantime another elderly patient placed on the other table in the same OT started talking to his surgeon. He was explaining the surgeon that he was a footballer and was presently a football coach for two clubs. He reminded the surgeon to perform the surgery in a manner so that he can continue jumping and heading the ball to train his boys (this is the same patient about whom I have mentioned before in this chapter). At this juncture our octogenarian from the other table decided to join the conversation. "For which club in Calcutta have you played ?" he asked with an authoritative voice. "Have you heard about Dinanath Ganguly, who had scored a hat-trick for Mohun Bagan (the oldest and a popular football team of Calcutta) playing against the British team in 1936?" he continued. The surgeon, a quiet introvert had very little interest in football. But by then the two co-patients were engrossed in the football memories of the first half of the last century. The whole OT staff enjoyed the unusual conversation and the attitude of the octogenarians. The surgeon's request to keep quiet for better surgical results went unheeded. However, the outcome of the procedure was quite acceptable.

RAINBOW UNDER THE DRAPE: PHACOSURGERY AS EXPERIENCED BY THE PATIENT UNDER THE DRAPE

Each and every person has a different perception and analysis to the given situation. It is something like modern art or a children's visualisation and imagination of some image inside the clouds or on the tree. For the same shadow one can imagine a wide spectrum of images extending from a dancing doll to a lioness or even a flowing river.

We have provided a questionnaire to a group of patients belonging to different sections of the society and pertaining to specific aspects of phacoemulsification surgical procedures. All patients were requested to respond to the questionnaire as per their experiences on the operation table.

In addition to the structured questionnaire, patients were free to comment on any other observations deemed worth noting. We have tried to cover a large section of society including administrators, technocrats, legal experts, medical professionals (interestingly, intraoperative perception of phaco was varying to a great extent not only among the pilots, educationists and others but also amongst the surgeons, anaesthesiologists, pathologists, medical administrators and ophthalmologists). Here are a few glimpses from such experiences.

Phaco as Experienced by a General Surgeon

We requested one of our patients who himself was a general surgeon, to describe his experience while undergoing surgery and he obliged. We constantly interacted with him and allowed him to describe his experience in his own words. The conversation vis-a-vis the steps were as follows:

(i) I can see a variety of colourful particles in front of my eye (eye washed with betadine and ringer-lactate).

(ii) You are scratching inside my eye but there is no pain (capsulorrhexis is being performed).

(iii) Red and blue glow is moving in front of my eye. (hydrodissection and hydrodelineation being performed).

(iv) You are moving the lens in circles (nucleus rotation).

(v) You are cracking a nut inside the lens matter, red and blue glow is seen occasionally (fragmentation of the nucleus by chopping method is carried out).

(vi) Opaque matter is gradually getting clear. Nuclear fragments being removed.

I can see an undulating surface with humps and bumps in front. (This medical officer was familiar with the hill terrain of Northeast Indian states. Hence as and when he saw the undulating surfaces in front, he compared it with the Chola of Sikkim and sometimes with the Bhomragiri hills of Tezpur). (North East part of India).

(vii) You are cleaning materials from inside the eye, I can see rainbow glow in front of my eye. (Epinucleus and cortical matter being removed).

(viii) Two needle shadows are seen performing in front. (patient insisted that the instruments appear to come from below? Instruments were possibly casting a shadow in the upper retina resulting in lower visual field images).

(ix) I can see a bright light in front with central blue and peripheral yellow and red coloured zones. (Cortical matter is being removed with I/A probe.)

(x) You are injecting some fluid inside my eye. I can see an undulating surface in front. (Visco is being injected to inflate the bag).

(xi) I can see a bright light. A very bright dazzling object is unfolding inside the eye. (Foldable intraocular lens being implanted in the bag).

(xii) Now something is twisted and tilted inside the eye. Possibly, you are trying to take the lens in the proper place. (IOL is being rotated and positioned).

(xiii) I can see bright colours moving in front. AC cleaned with I/A probe.

(xiv) I can see a coloured circle with blue, yellow, green and red zones. (Procedure completed).

(xv) You have closed my eye, everything has become dark.

Phaco as Experienced by a Pilot

The author has experienced the appreciations of pilots on phacoemulsification surgery while under the drape.

In our view, a pilot being exposed to the open sky and horizon as well as viewing the world as a panorama, appears to be cool and well composed except for the one and only worry of a remote possibility of getting deprived of flying in case of poor visual recovery. However, a thorough and well explained preoperative counselling invariably makes them comfortable.

The undermentioned script is the compilation of intraoperative visual experience of seven pilots who have undergone phacosurgery in our setup.

The initial steps of surgery upto the incision remained unnoticed without any specific observation. The rhexis manoeuvre was experienced as the commencement of slow and gradual movements of a plane from the parking area. The hydroprocedures were observed as a sudden dipping of the plane into clouds. The nucleotomy by ultrasound was observed as a supersonic plane is flying on a rainy day with a rainbow and showers of bluish and orange colours. Insertion of the intraocular lens implant was experienced as landing of a flight after having slow gliding movements and unfolding of the IOL was experienced as opening of brakes and tyres. Iris stroking was experienced as shivering or blow of cold and biting wind. No other specific observations were conveyed to the operating surgeon.

Phaco as Experienced by an Erstwhile Cricket Legend on the Table

The author has had an opportunity to experience the visual appreciations of an erstwhile cricketer while undergoing phacoemulsification surgery. Indeed, eyes see what the brain knows. A kaleidoscope of visual impressions of a single given situation varies to a great extent. This reminds the author of his own early childhood experience of viewing clouds and searching for different images of a bird, a tree, a tiger, and even hills and goddess in the same cloud.

The phacoemulsification surgery performed under topical anaesthesia and that to without the influence of sedatives keeps the patient alert and responsive to the surroundings. The surgeon too remains over responsive to any call from the patient as well as from the surroundings.

Most sportsmen (except boxers) are well composed, and carry sportsman spirit in real sense even under conditions of severe stress and strains. Team spirit carried by them is also phenomenal. Hence, it becomes a relatively easy task to handle such patients on the operation table.

His very first reaction to the surgeons request on being requested to lie down on the operation table was, "once again on the cricket pitch but this time for a beneficiary match as the batsman who faces the ball which is bowled, stroked and scored by the operating surgeon himself but goes into my account. Pitch appears to be unknown yet friendly with an equal bounce. The operating surgeon had requested him to keep a close track on various observations and convey accordingly at the appropriate moment once being requested upon to do so."

The conventional draping which was followed by povidone irrigation was observed as a peculiar situation of the commencement of match under rainy shower pitch with covers on. The surgeons request to continuously observe the light source of operating microscope during the procedure was remarked as taking guard and setting the position of the side screen. However the next steps of two clear corneal incisions under the support of cotton buds remained unnoticed. Visco injection was appreciated as a sudden pressure inside the eyeball. Capsulorrhexis movement was followed as some circular movement over the side screen. Hydroprocedures were noticed as sudden diminution of light and the patient promptly conveyed, 'appears you are going to play under bad light conditions'.

However, the surgeon explained to him about this change in the intensity and colour of light due to clouding of lens matter as well as its impact on softening of the lens. Nucleus rotation was commented upon as reshuffling in field settings. The initial cortical clearing produced the impression of a bowler who is running towards the bowling crease. The phaco tip being embedded into the nucleus was observed as the completion of bowling action just short of its delivery. The first chopping was commented as batting strokes on back foot. Nucleus rotation and subsequent chopping and fragment removal was just like forward stroking and subsequent running between the wickets followed by scoring in the different directions. Final cortical irrigation/aspiration were concluded as lofted strokes. IOL insertion was appreciated as a gentle sweep on the third man. The author enjoyed each and every moment of conversation.

Phaco as Experienced by a Writer/Poet on the Table

Recently, the author (JKSP) had got an opportunity to operate upon on an elderly Urdu poetess. The poetess was very much comfortable and remained cheerful throughout the entire period of the procedure which was performed under topical anaesthesia. In fact, she kept on narrating visual perceptions of surgical steps experienced by her in the tune of their comparison with expressions narrated in classical gazals romantic poems in Urdu). The initial steps of placing the surgical drape was interpreted as "Doctor why are you taking me through clouds before taking into pleasant and beautiful valley of good visual experience" (Haseen lamhe dikhane ke pahle badalon se kyon gujaar rahe hon).

The next step of irrigation of conjunctival sac with betadine and subsequently with the help of BSS was interpreted as colours of holi (festival of exchange of greetings by applying colours to each other).

The steps of capsulorrhexis remain unnoticed but hydrodissection was experienced as dark bluish shadow. The most interesting conversation was experienced during nucleotomy and subsequent irrigation and aspiration which was narrated as a journey through a colourful path in heaven (Jannat ki rangeen and haseen vadiyaen ke nazare). The steps of insertion of the intraocular lens implant was experienced as the appearance of rising blue moon in the sky (Neela chand aasman main utar raha hai).

UNFORGETTABLE PHACO NIGHTMARE AS EXPERIENCED ON EITHER END OF THE TABLE

Each and every case possess some peculiarities either related with the eye, systemic conditions or related with the patient's personality, pre, per and postoperative behaviour. Each and every surgeon faces such challenges particularly while handling cataract surgery under topical anaesthesia. The spectrum of such problems carry a wide spectrum of initial apprehension, fear of the unknown environment and procedure as well as myths and facts aired through the experiences earned by relatives, friends and others in the surroundings. Informed, well explained and detailed preoperative deliberations are most rewarding. Eye to eye contact during preoperative evaluation clears several apprehensions. The most important factor which is generally not discussed preoperatively remains the issue of draping and covering the face and nose. A large number of patients find it too difficult to adjust under this new environment. It is very wise and prudent to enquire about the patient's sleeping habits well in advance. A patient who covers his face while sleeping under bed sheets, blanket or quilt remains comfortable during surgery under local anaesthesia. However, the other group with just reverse habits are very difficult patients, thus need preoperative counselling and are requested to practise the exercise of covering nose and face under bed sheets atleast for 30 minutes.

The author experienced three major instances related with claustrophobia of covered face. Incidentally, all three were female patients and that to from the VVIP group. The first experience was with the wife of a very senior general officer who himself was a surgeon. The lady had just refused to have any cover over the face under any circumstances. The patient was quite annoyed and was willing to leave the operation theatre without undergoing surgery. This was the authors maiden and most horrifying experience. The surgeon was really cursing himself to have this patient on table as well as realised the gravity of not enquiring about this specific problem of covering the face. The ultimate answer to this situation was just keeping half side of the face out of drape as well as support of intranasal oxygen. However the second eye operation was uneventful as the surgeon and the patient were both nicely educated and acquainted. The postoperative remark and right so from the patient was that "I have taught you how to handle a difficult patient". The second patient, again a wife of a retired admiral from the navy and a professor in English, was very cooperative, motivated and yet affirmative during preoperative counselling. She had conveyed her concern about claustrophobia against dark if eyes and nose were covered. However, surgeon did not realise the gravity of this problem and thought of managing with the support of intranasal oxygenation. Nothing worked. She was just not able to tolerate in any circumstances. The answer was to make an additional window in the drape before the other eye. She kept watching microscope light and surgical movements through out the entire course of procedure. Indeed it was a great lesson. The same trick was applied during the surgery performed on the fellow eye after the gap of one year. This time it was a great and pleasant affair for both of us.

The third experience was also with a lady, wife of a very senior officer, who was claustrophobic about each and every thing related with surgery. She had refused to undergo even recording of intraocular pressure by any method, had a great problem while being exposed to IOL master for calculation of IOL power. She had categorically conveyed her unwillingness against any kind of infiltrative anaesthesia yet desired to have an absolutely painless procedure. Over and above she was very keen for multifocal and very much against wearing any kind of spectacles later on. The worst for surgeon was her determination to get her surgery done by the author only.

The author planned surgery under topical anaesthesia supported by mild sedative and analgesics. However the lady luck stroke against surgeon as soon as patient entered the operation theatre. She was not at all willing to lie-down on operation table. With great difficulty this task could have been completed. The next bouncer was her unwillingness to get the face cleaned and draped. Surgeon had realised his biggest mistake of not planning this surgery under general anaesthesia. Patient had her morning breakfast; hence there were no possibility of administering the general anaesthesia. Options were either postponed surgery and plan for GA later on or to go with it after sedation. The author requested anaesthesiologist to provide sedatives which was followed by oxygenation and subsequent draping and surgery as well. It was the author's good fortune that everything had undergone very well including postoperative unaided visual acuity of 6/6 and N/5 respectively. This is not the end of the story. The fellow eye was still awaiting surgery. However the rich lesson learnt from previous experience made the task easy. God was not that unkind to surgeon. Both eyes have got excellent recovery.

DESTINY AND FATE OF THE SURGEON IS DECIDED BY AN UNKNOWN POWER

Ophthalmic surgeons of the modern era may have reservations to accept this topic in any chapter of a phacoemulsification cataract surgery book. However such humble acceptance in the strength of the Almighty is not very uncommon in the eastern part of the world and amongst the people of the Indian subcontinent in particular.

Often we operate on a difficult case and manage to do it well and eventually achieve a good result. While sometimes we land up with a complication in a simple case. Often complication occurs when we attempt to perform a new procedure or due to overconfidence we do a particular step a little casually. But in some case we land up in unexpected complication in spite of our best efforts to perform the case with all concentration and in a meticulous manner. All these various situations force me to keep another factor in mind. We can only try to achieve the perfect result but without the blessing of somebody we fail to achieve the desired outcome.

It happened many times when surgeons messed up a case on the OT table and expected a horrible result. But to their surprise, a reasonable outcome may be seen next morning and eventually an unexpectedly better result. The reverse is also not very uncommon. All of us must have faced many unexpected surprises on the postop morning after performing a meticulous surgery. Patients gradually developing a variety of unexpected complications in some apparently clean and uncomplicated cases are also not very uncommon, whereas some patient recovers uneventfully. When such operative complications occur or during postoperative period, a case turns bad in a so-called VIP patient it adds embarrassment and undue stress on our mind for a different reason. But as such having any complication in any of our cases certainly upsets each and every one of us.

We have seen many a turn in our practice during a long span of professional career. Today to some extent, one may get convinced that along with our effort to treat a case somebody else's blessing is also equally important in the overall benefit of the patient and to achieve a good visual outcome. No wonder, when I first entered my professor's room after joining the ophthalmology speciality I noticed a caption in front "We treat, God Cures".

WHERE WE ARE HEADING FOR VISION 2010–2020

Now let us see where we are heading for. Only a couple of years back some of us were happy performing extra capsular cataract surgery. Then came the wave of phacoemulsification cataract surgery. By the time we struggled and picked up the procedure and started to do it with some degree of confidence our more adventurous colleagues started to switch over to micro incision phaconit cataract surgery. With the availability of the rollable IOL commercially in the market, it is certain to become popular in the due course. Even the manufacturers of the phaco machine could not ignore the demand for long and have already come up with cool microincision pulse mode (CMP) in their latest version of the machines. The process of performing cataract surgery through a smaller and smaller incision is not likely to stop even here.

No wonder, one can foresee that in near future, the ophthalmic surgeon will be able to perform cataract surgery by a fine needle incision by laser ablating the lens matter or emulsifying and aspirating it through ultra thin needle probe. May be some day, there will be no need for the surgeon to be present in the OT table next to the patient. The procedure will be performed in a mechanical manner and thereafter there will be no need for the surgeon to be present in the OT as the remote mechanism takes over.

There is no end to such imagination. Certainly, we are likely to see further improvement in cataract surgery advancing at a galloping speed in this century.

59

Journey beyond the Rainbow: An Ophthalmologist's view from under the Sheets—Eye Drape

(An Ophthalmologist's personal experience of undergoing Phacosurgery on himself)

Col Rangin Banerji

INTRODUCTION

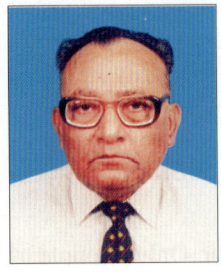

Colonel Rangin Banerji is one of the very senior ophthalmologists of the Armed Forces Medical Services and hails from the Eastern part of India. He was born in 1925 at Patna (Bihar/India). He is a graduate and postgraduate from the Patna Medical College (1955 and 57 respectively) and subsequently acquired the qualifications of DO (London) and FRCS (UK). He served in the Army Medical Corps as a Senior Adviser in Ophthalmology till his retirement in 1982. Col Rangin Banerji is amongst one of the pioneers in the fields of IOL implantation in Armed Forces Medical Service.

He has recently undergone phacoemulsification cataract surgery in both eyes which was performed by the author. This particular event has triggered off his thought process to pen down his experience of the last fifty years as well as the experiences he faced under the drape as an ophthalmologist. The golden moments of his memory are true glimpses and a rich treasure worth preserving for the author.

JKS Parihar SM, VSM

19 APRIL, 2005

Both of us, my wife and I needed cataract operation, and as usual with our Indian tradition I was supposed to be the first in line. Somehow, in keeping with our domestic demand-availability of daughter and the convenience of the surgeon, I got my wife operated first. So I saw the finished product –no scar – no mark of incision, etc.

When it was my turn, after having been associated with ophthalmology for half a century, and grown up in a doctor's family, I had my own premonitions galore-getting

rid of 'septic foci' which I have witnessed in several cases who were rendered completely edentulous prior to operation. All varieties of teeth irrespective of the state of their anchorage were taken away. That was when in the pre-war days there were no antibiotics, and the only agents then in use were prontosil rubrum and prontosil album, the chemotherapeutic drugs discovered by the Domagk brothers and exploited totally by a famous German firm – Schering's probably. Those were the days when cataracts were done solely under freshly prepared cocaine eye drops (4%). I had my own secrets like a broken-retained root which one of my dentists had refused to extract- due to my age 78. The denture and gum interface was raw so that I was having recurrent apical abscesses, which made me prepone the start of antibiotics-ciprofloxacin in my case-to a week before my operation. Further I managed my own damage-control exercise to minimise the rawness of the gum at that area, by insulating a part of the denture. The next worry was a slightly 'above normal' random blood sugar level, which on further scrutiny at another laboratory pronounced me to be euglycaemic.

Blood pressure was under medication and controlled. Kidneys functioned normally and prostrates gave no trouble. The next worry was my 'Spastic colon' which necessitated therapy with mepevrine derivatives. I had abjured the medications totally and adjusted my bowels with increased roughage, some more abdominal exercise and avoidance of some food items. But the nagging doubt was what if something happened when I was on the table. It seemed ciprofloxacin cleared my periapical problem. Drops mydriatics locomotion was a bit unsteady, but with helpers like my family members entry to the OT was uneventful barring the mental turmoil I was in, one tablet of calmpose notwithstanding. Once wheeled in near the table, I was helped up and thanks to my partial hearing loss-high frequency only and without either my glasses or hearing aid, I was spared the pains of scrutinising the area around, which I too had monopolised in my days in different hospitals in India and abroad, albeit without this array of present gadgetry. I was then immured in soft words of encouragement while my head was strapped and hands pinioned too, so that I was on a supine position for the electric chair!! But I was made very comfortable and with the ambient sound level being at a minimum, I was at peace. A prick-in the dorsum of palm, and another, a double puncture maybe or a corrective manoeuvre and I felt more at ease. What it was I could not judge, could have been pethidine plus calmpose or phenergan or a special cocktail for a senior on the table!! Anyway (A small quantity of injection pentazocine was used : author):

Some drapes were put, some drops squirted, some pressure around the orbital margins. I was wondering what was being done multiple puncture or one injection alone Van Lint's type. I tried to focus my brain to my thoughts, but they would not. I gave up. (A single prick peribulbar block was used by the author in this particular situation). There was a dark scum over my eye. Surely, I wondered they would be operating with lights, but I can't see it. Then there was a swirl of fluid inside, some more, some silence—some moments later, pressure again?? I do not know nor could I connect. I tried to relax, and relax I did. The drapes were taken off, the arms freed, and I was put up with a patch on my right eye. All was over. Why I could not see the light of the operating microscope I do not know, nor do I need to know at this stage. Some mysteries are best left unravelled. I am due for my second eye after a month. Till then I do not wish to know.

DAY ONE: AFTERNOON

I asked my wife to remove the strapped pad, though the Surgeon had told me to remove it a few hours after operation. I got it removed as the air conditioned dry air of the room had dried the pad-eye interface, and I felt I would feel better without it.

We have postage stamp sized balcony where I took my usual perch facing south. Suddenly it seemed it was Dussera time with street light lit prematurely festooned with a halo—all light, as a matter of fact, and the crowd on the road and traffic had suddenly multiplied and there was a surfeit of twins of all colours and in all size men and women and even cars, in Identical shapes with complementary colours. However much as I tried to get them to a reasonable order the images stayed apart. Closing one eye-the operated eye was the only answer. Then I realised that the retrobulbar had been far too accurate in its destination—the muscle cone and that the extra ocular muscles were

still under the haze of the drug boosted as it must have been with hylase. With dilated pupil—a little too much perhaps—effect of neo-synephrine (?), I did not force matters but managed. Later, when I moved indoors I had to alternate between the two eyes to pick up a point of interest on the TV screen. Later on, as and when the tempo of the scenario on the screen got interesting, the diplopia did not trouble me that much.

There was a bit of rawness within the muscle-cone which a painkiller took care of. I could not resist looking in on the operated eye with a focused torch. There was no striate keratitis no tension marks, AC was normal and the lens seemed in situ. There was however a thin suggestion of suffusion upto the anterior boundary of Tenon's—perhaps seepage of some secretions-blood—or tissue fluids! With betnesol drops and flur drops the suffusion cleared away slowly. By day two—diplopia was tolerable too, and by day three I could not feel it at all.

DAY FIVE: 24TH APRIL, 2005

I am still comfortable with my glasses-baseline myopia of minus three/three point five; inasmuch as I feel that my VA is the same as in the unoperated eye. Theoretically though, my unoperated eye is 6/6 or 6/9, I can feel the difference when I compare it with the operated eye. There is a thin scum of dirt – more precisely as if one is looking through a filter of grey – to borrow from an artist's palette- Payne's grey a shade, or a shade of van dyke brown or raw umber or burnt sienna depending on the degree of sunlight and presence of clouds. The operated eye, however seems endowed with a colour enhancer- like blue or pale magenta or violet, and the difference between the two eyes is marked. I have nearly 90% vision in my operated eye without any fresh correction, but the quality of this surpasses that of the contralateral eye so far as the coloured veil is concerned and its sullied nature, as compared to the pristine sheen of the colours perceived by the operated eye.

Though I am writing this less than a week after operation, I feel, I am fully rehabilitated so far as my vision is concerned, so that the 10% deficit in VA of the right eye is overshadowed by the unoperated eye. But the sheen of colours perceived by the operated eye makes it stand out in contrast and hence is by far more preferred by me. Once the haze of cloudiness disappears, after operation on that eye, I shall not be so prejudicial vis a vis one—eye or the other.

Till then, I hope my system behaves and the surgeon is not posted out.

Dated 24th April 05.

Rangin Banerji

Flat E2, 33/31 James Long Sarani, Calcutta 700034.

60

Ophthalmology— Then and Now: An Overview of the Past Fifty Years

Col Rangin Banerji

INTRODUCTION

Colonel Rangin Banerji's personal experience of more than 50 years of ophthalmic practice reflects the entire spectrum of transformation of ophthalmology from initial days of non microscopic surgery to the most advanced era of sub 1 mm incision. His brief biodata is given in Chapter 55.

OPHTHALMOLOGY—THEN AND NOW: AN OVERVIEW OF THE PAST FIFTY YEARS

This is an overview of the strides that ophthalmology has gone through in the last half a century and more. Why the cut-off period of 50 years, is a cogent question, that I need to answer now—as I have been an active member of this fraternity for the last fifty years, which I steered myself into, several years after graduation, after freelancing in army as a GDMO.

Secondly, I have been at the receiving end of the knife twice before, but last week I had my cataract operation, from a young eye specialist who was born the year I became a fledgeling eye specialist. This episode makes these short memories more seminal and poignant.

Having been brought up in a small town in a dust-bowl district in north Bihar, where we had no electricity, no water connection and not enough qualified doctors around, and beset as we were with annual visitations of plague, cholera, endemic filarial and malaria and no antibiotics, and tablets were hand rolled and mixtures were dispensed- some say with pure Ganges water for greater efficacy—the scenario was totally different. I used to watch my father-an allopathic doctor treating medical cases, lancing abscesses, extracting some teeth too and tapping hydroceles a very common malady along with filarial elephantiasis in that area of sub Himalayan Terai area and endemic goiter. He had also done cataract operations, for a few years when he was in

government service. A retinoscopy set that I use still, is his–Zeiss's lenses!!

Occasionally when there were fairs in the open ground across our house – Ramna area, I have seen itinerant surgeons doing the couching operation. During my service tenure in India and Nepal eye camps – I have seen such lenses at the bottom of the vitreous cavity cocooned in their casing of exudates and retino-lental adhesions, and an uncomplaining patient.

So my learning process started a long way back, may be several years after my birth, when I could relate to the outside world. This is therefore, an acknowledgement of the different Gurus that I have had over so many decades including the latest one – my surgeon, the present one. I am still learning Agyanatimirandhashya gunanjanashalakaya/ chakshur-unmilitam jena tasmaih sree guravey namah (one who leads a blind and ignorant person into the light of learning and opens his eyes – I bow my head to that sage, the guru). I shall confine my impressions basically to the area of cataract surgery and its added fringe areas.

There were no antibiotics, and the only mild eye drops were mercurochrome drops in aqueous solution, silver proteinate and nitrate (Argentii fortis), guttae acid acetic, acid boric et zinc, dionin, zinc et alum, picric acid, etc. Copper sulphate sticks for 'grattage' of trachoma follicles. For Phlyctenular conjunctivitis, the only medicine was smothering the nodule with calomel powder – hydrarg perchloride of mercury. There were no anti-histamines even. Benadryl the first entrant came during the war years. For allergy – calcium was used intravenously-calcibronat, calcium gluconate, etc.

Freshly prepared cocaine drops (4%) were used locally till the patient was brought to the table. Van lint's and O'Brien's methods of facial akinesia came later with a lot of fanfare. The patients had to have their head washed and sometimes shaved, and pupils had to be dilated with homatropine. Those old people who were addicted to opium were problem cases as their pupils were pinpoint and resistant to the usual mydriatics. Case selection was cautious septic foci-removal of all offending teeth – a clinical side room test of urine for sugar and albumin.

Some patients who reacted adversely to cocaine slumped silently to the ground. They all walked to the table, the reluctant ones reminded with vicious pinches on their fundamentals.

Instruments that went in the AC were segregated and subjected to immersion in pure Lysol for several minutes, then absolute alcohol – same time then transferred to a boiling point of distilled water same time – hand held by the chief sweeper in charge of the OT and finally cold distilled water. I am not sure of the exact drill – the minutiae – but that was the overall impression I carry.

Surgeons rarely changed their street cloths, except their hat and coat and worked with their waist coats and ties on, plus the shoes. Masks were optional and gloves not in use at all.

As I have always used surgical gloves, I would not know why they were not in universal use. I have seen Barraquer (senior) using linen gloves in thye late fifties. Surgeons in the UK did not use them, unless doing a DCR or exenteration of orbit, etc.

An all purpose speculum was used. Graefe knife section, very rarely a De Beer's knife section with a small conjunctival flap depending on the surgeon's expertise was done. The trouble with a new Graefe knife was that if one was not very alert, the blade cut through the cornea like a Saemisch' section much to the awe of the surgeon. Iridectomy was not mandatory one or two. A lens expressor was placed over the limbus externally at 6 O'clock and a gentle nudge given to the lower pole of the hypermature lens, so that its lower edge came up a little. In went the forceps – intracapsular and the lens grasped and tumbled out coaxed and cajoled all the way.

There were three types of surgeons—the one who went in for planned intracapsular extractions, the one opting for planned extracapsular, and the hit and miss types. A bit of age related or induced 'intention tremor' of the hands was an added advantage in case of manipulating the lens. Erysiphake came along and there were some converts. Then came Pau Krawitcz's cryophake which I had the privilege of witnessing in person, the Polish surgeon and his creative talent in the fifties in Glasgow where I was working then. We were all sceptical then. Years later when I was in Poona, in the sixties, Brigadier C S Krishnamurthy then the adviser, would rush in with a carbon dioxide snow pencil to hand over to me for use in a prototype that he had devised for cryoextraction which was a pioneering venture in army, till Appasamy of Chennai brought out their versions.

Around this time came the concept of zonulolysis-Barraquer's epoch making innovation which made intra-capsular extraction seem like a child's play. It was widely accepted and used, like viscoelastic substances now. It seemed intracapsular extraction had come to stay.

But the pioneering work of Ridley and Choyce of Britain changed the scenario totally, so that intraocular lens implants came to stay. I started off with Fyodorov Zacharvo type II –iris plane lenses popularly known as "Sputnik" lenses with their three loops for below the iris and three pods for above the iris, way back in the eighties in the Command Hospital, Calcutta. Later I graduated to the two loop posterior chamber ones. I must admit changing over from intracapsular to extracapsular was quite a painful learning process. But I learnt and progressed further. As a natural corollary came the concept of phacoemulsification now an established reality. With foldable lenses and no stitches , it seems we have come into a new era. The days of one hand, two hand manipulation and chop/cut /slash / and such appellates will make way for other more innovative expressions.

There are no picture postcard type surgeries. It is upto you to make them so simple as if they were textbook copies!! Those who studied Fasanella's complications of ocular surgery were a divided lot – those that abjured surgery for what the complications can do to their reputation or the patient, and those that kept the complications in mind, but never let them influence them in a negative manner. In our days when there were no antibiotics and no corticosteroids, we did manage postoperative complications, by first blaming the patient, who in turn blamed god's mercy, and we resorted to measures like: auto-haemotherapy, injection of boiled milk I.M. (tinted with methylene blue to prevent oral misuse), and finally leeches for reducing inflammation in orbital cellulites and periorbital oedema. I have mentioned leeches as I have seen them being used by my father in acute moribund cases, in the early forties by asking 'jonkwalis' to come over. Auto-haemotherapy has been used by me in several cases of obscure and resistant posterior uveitis where everything including massive retrobulbar injections of cortisone had failed and the old patient pleaded with me to carry on regardless, which I did, and he made a remarkable recovery full of twists and turns and heartache. It was providence perhaps-the greatest doer.

Now of course with cortisone antibiotics and intravitreal route and vitrectomy being so commonplace, the scenario has changed. But so has medicine changed to without its thrills of discovery and fighting the unknown. We chart our course through scans, MRIs print out analysis, 3D assessments and even studies of the degree of optic disc cupping et al. Surgeons do not have enough time to answer the nagging worries and doubts of a case that needs surgery. They do not have time, and time is money. At my age, I am at my wit's end at times how to convince a patient to go back to the surgeon for the questions she or he puts to me knowing that I have abjured surgery. No wonder I shall at any time, opt for the army surgeons.

MEMORIES ARE STILL FRESH: MY EXPERIENCE AT COMMAND HOSPITAL (EC), CALCUTTA (1981–82)

I joined the Command Hospital on 3rd January 1981, after a stint in the Military Hospital Namkum, which was supposed to be my last posting, as I had not desired any extension. I feel, like my AFMC tenure which was an afterthought by the 'powers to be in AHQ', and as it was aborted just before my planned departure for No. 5 Air Force Hospital, Jorhat, and I had to go to Poona midway, this posting too was a late afterthought, as I am not a son of the soil' having been born in UP and brought up in Bihar.

I retired from the hospital on 31 March 1982, and started private practice from the very next day from Russel street, courtesy Mr. H. N. Shah I have not looked back since, not even in anguish. I stopped active surgery and shunned it for the last six years, and am fully devoted to part time charitable or non paying consultation only, and the balance of my time is taken up with my writing (One autobiography is with editors and one book-fiction English published in 1988), and latterly serious painting-oils and watercolours.

The highlight of my tenure in the hospital here was my induction into intraocular lens implants, on a self taught basis in 1981. I started inserting iris plane implants– Fyodorov Zacharov Mk II, after intracapsular operation, which was silently acknowledged by few of my genre, I being the pioneer in that field in eastern India and according to one of the top ophthalmologist when approached by one of my patients lined up for surgery, and approached for his second opinion, advice, was told that ' if you wish to be a guinea pig you can go to Banerji…'

I implanted quite a number of these implants, and carried on merrily.

The then DDMS – Maj. General S M Ghose AVSM (now deceased) arranged for the then chief minister Sree Jyoti Basu to visit the command hospital, which he did on 18 March 1982, when he was brought to the Eye Dept. By then, and this time, I was fully into implants, and had commissioned the mothballed operating microscope (Zeiss) which was kept in the OT so that the then neurosurgeon Gen. Suraj Prakash could also use it.

Jyoti Babu was shown some of the cases operated by me and implanted by me, and The statesman of 18th March 1982, carried a front page photograph which came out in print with his hands on the focusing knobs) with the caption "The CM focusing a machine to "examine" a patient's eye in command hospital, Calcutta (report on page 3). Being a front page photograph in the leading newspaper, it made quite a few heads turn with ire and envy.

I retired on 31 March 1982, and went into practice mainly surgery that too implants in a big way in the city of Calcutta, as the first Indian doctor to have ventured in this field. A batch of Japanese doctor had implanted two/three cases in 1981, in Woodlands under the sponsorship of Mr.H.M.Shah. My first case of two looped posterior chamber implant after ECCE, was the late Dr. Binoy Ranjan Sen, ICS retd, and the longest serving director general of Food and Agriculture Organisation of Rome, and an international celebrity in 1983.

I wish to remember another event, my visit to the President of India. This was due to the efforts of Lt General J.M.Grover AVSM, who was then the Physician to the President His Excellency Giani Zail Singh. General Grover requested me to examine the president, and opine on his eye. This I did after General Grover put up a mini diagnostic setup for eyes with a Haag Streit Slit lamp et al right next to the study in Rashtrapati Bhawan. Thus, I did examine Giani Zail Singhji on 12 March 1983, with mydriatics also, and spent nearly an hour with him, and explained to him the need for cataract surgery, in his case and the pros and cons of implant surgery in his case. He took my advice and did get the operation done by Dr. Daljit Singh of Amritsar later, who was using the controversial Jan worst's lobster claw lenses exclusively.

Having, said this much, I feel I have had a long and very satisfying innings, and though out of surgery and the mainstream, I am enjoying my leisure and painting avidly, the latter hobby in spurts of mood allowing.

Twenty-two years is a long time and going back memory lane was a nostalgic journey for me. Most of the colleagues I worked with are gone, and a fair number of my AFMC students have retired!! I am carrying on regardless!! Perhaps I shall shortly launch a website for my paintings and Inshaallah I hope the book should be in print next year.!!

Colonel Rangin Banerji, Retd.
Flat E2, 33/31 James Long Sarani, Calcutta 700034.
Ph:2468 3318

25 April, 2005

61

An Untold Story: Transformation of an Ophthalmic Surgeon into Military Phaconit Surgeon Beyond Drape

Col JKS Parihar SM, VSM

INTRODUCTION

Self-introspection and going down memory lane and re-living the past is not beating one's own drum, but is in accord with human desire to share wonderful experiences. His journey has its own story in the form of varied experiences that have been enriching. The tracing of pages of yesteryear on professional experiences and training not only enlightens us, but also infuses us with renewed energy to act, react to situations and grow with the everyday evolving subject in respect to our own observations and the change in technology. This helps one in maturing one's thought process. It is wiser to learn the lesson from another's leaf rather than commit the folly on your own as our predecessors have refined techniques that have stood the test of time.

YAGNOPAVEET (BAPTISM) AS AN OPHTHALMIC SURGEON

It is fascinating to just pause and readjust the clock back to April 1977. It started as a dark day that came as an earthquake and saw my dream shattered for I had always thought of becoming a cardiothoracic surgeon and here I was grappling with the idea of peering into peoples eyes. When I was in my second prof, my elder brother who was then 24 years old sustained a blunt injury to his eye while riding his scooter in a remote town in MP. The closest help was in Indore around 250 km away, where I was studying. I ran from pillar to post to have my brother's eye evaluated and everyone from my closest friend to the senior residents to Dr PK Sethi, the lecturer on call examined it. Finally in the morning, Dr MC Nahata, Prof and HOD of Ophthalmology, who was held in high esteem professionally and had an almost legendary standing amongst his peers, examined my brother. He was admitted to MYH Hospital (affiliated to MGM Medical College,

Indore) as a case of traumatic cataract. The immediate concern was that of acute uveitis/iridocyclitis. To come to this diagnosis a slit lamp, which was a rarity in those days, was set up in the basement. The finding of acute cells and flare and KPs would have confirmed my worst nightmare. I immediately consulted people around me as well as interacted with Parsons for the first time. My prayers were answered when Dr Nahata reiterated that my brother's eye was devoid of any signs of inflammation. Subsequently my brother was subjected to major surgery as per that era and looking at it retrospectively he probably underwent lens aspiration. The surgery was heroic for the surgeon was devoid of an operating microscope, viscoelastics, and intraocular lens. Later, he also underwent some form of glaucoma surgery. It being my third year, I was naïve to the subject of ophthalmology and could not comprehend the consequences of monocular aphakia.

This particular incident spurred me to consider myself as a future ophthalmologist who would take the challenge of traumatic cataract head on. My Ophthalmic training at MGM Indore was a great experience.

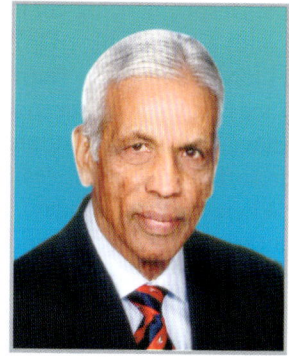

Dr MC Nahata

Those days the training used to be holistic and encompass professionalism, personality and conduct.

Prof MC Nahata happened to be a strong, exceptionally meticulous and thorough professional and an administrator par excellence with a graceful personality. His linguistic abilities and the command of his subject are a source of inspiration to us all till today. His charismatic personality, conduct, administrative capabilities and perfect command on language and subject was phenomenal and remains the source of inspiration for all of us till date.

Most of us tried to emulate his personality whenever we could. His presence was and will always be a source of inspiration to all those who knew him. His surgical skill and clinical acumen was admirable. His charismatic figure and his ability to transpire confidence have definitely transformed his students like me to take up big challenges in the field of ophthalmology with resolve and courage. Prof Nahata remains the evergreen source of inspiration and strength for me. I am proud to add that most of his students excel in the ophthalmologic sphere and have become reckonable figures in the same. Dr PC Mittal and Dr PK Sethi were known for their quick and ready accessibility for our regular problems during our formative years. Dr Pushpa Varma (she was and still is a very charismatic personality in the Dept of Ophthalmology at MGM Indore) was more a senior friend than a teacher and acted as a definitive source of encouragement and learning. Incidentally, she shares her birthday with Sir Harold Ridley (10th July). In contrast, during the 80s when I was doing my residency, residents nowadays perform their first intraocular surgery as ECCE with PC IOL implantation under VISU 200 Carl zeiss microscope with an observer tube to watch and learn. They are exposed to the techniques of Phacoemulsification from the day one and perform Phaco in the latter half of their second year. What a contrast! However, I still feel we were more clinicians rather than technocrats as compared to the present lot. A generation gap exists despite our flexibility to adapt to newer technology in toto.

My third span of learning was at the Medical college Jabalpur (MP). Dr AK Mukerji happens to be very close and affectionate to me. Despite is being controversial and the several personal odds faced by him, Dr AK Mukerji was extremely cordial towards me. One learns from each and every personality and I did too, with a deep sense of gratitude. Dr Meeta Shrivastava, at the same institute continued to be very accessible to sort out minor hassles faced during my training period. Wherever I stand today, Medical College Jabalpur carries a very big role, by far. Endurance, zeal and perseverance definitely emanated from there.

CONVERSION INTO A MILITARY OPHTHALMIC SURGEON

I had the opportunity to commence my solo ophthalmic practice at a high altitude in 1984, where courtesy the army,

I took my ophthalmoscope right upto 19000 feet to evaluate fundus changes. Regular ophthalmic OPD and few ophthalmic surgeries included intra ocular surgeries performed at 14300 feet height. A unique study on Ophthalmic Manifestations in Army equines at High altitude was conducted in unison with a veterinary surgeon serving with me at that time. Incidentally, that happens to be my first scientific publication. Looking back, someone had commented, "Seems you are only fit for ophthalmic practice on silent mules". I took that as a compliment. My father happens to be a Veterinary surgeon and it was with humble gratitude to all those silent animals, the care rendered by my father to them that provided us our bread and butter and saw me through my medical education that has brought me to this stage.

In the beginning, I saw a limbal based conjunctival flap with AB externo incision having three pre placed 7 "0" silk suture and Intracapsular Cataract extraction either by Aruga or by Cryo. I used to be totally confused as far as those three pre- placed sutures were concerned. Imagine seven to nine sutures to secure the incision! Assisting the Senior Adviser in this situation for several hours and then operating yourself with an identical technique was indeed a Herculean task. Brig (Colonel at that time) DC Roy, (Senior Adviser) a teacher and a senior, who was a disciplinarian to the core and yet was soft and tender by heart happened to be an ideal boss to reshape my carrier at the onset. This association provided me the art of tremendous patience and great stamina to keep my cool under duress. Good nursing care was an essential requirement those days. Hospitalisation for 7 to 10 days used to be a routine, alongwith bilateral bandage for 24 hours with no head movement. The next two days would involve confinement to the bed with a unilateral bandage. The mere thought of having to use a bedpan in the sixth or seventh decade of life is a mortifying thought at that age. Despite such prolonged and meticulous care, postoperative period used to have symptomatic eyes in the form of congestion, lid swelling and irritability.

A great revolution took place when I switched over to Fornix based incision and no preplaced suture under a new and modern boss like Colonel KA Ahmed. He also taught me ophthalmic photography and Anterior Chamber IOL in 1987 under three X magnification loupe. I learned how to use an operating microscope and performing ECCE at that time.

My journey towards regular ECCE with PC IOL implantation began in 1989 under Brigadier SP Saksena who happens to be the former Professor of Ophthalmology, at AFMC Pune and was then Commandant of the Military Hospital, Jabalpur where I was working. It used to be a great attraction using a three X magnifying loupe for the initial incision, capsulotomy and nucleus delivery followed by using an operating microscope for cortical wash.

I did my first PC IOL in 1989. However, the person who influenced my career to a great extent remains Lt General SC Verma PVSM (Rtd).

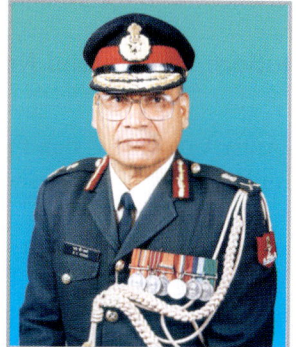

Lt General SC Verma PVSM

Lt Gen Verma, at that time Col Verma was most energetic and thorough professional. His capability to blend clinical acumen with sound theoretical knowledge was remarkable. I still remember his elliptical scleral - limbal incision, quick nucleus delivery and 3 to 4 sutures of 8 "0" silk or monofilament. Surgery for him used to be over within 10 minutes whereas my procedure had three plane corneoscleral incisions, ECCE and finally 9 to 11 sutures of 10 "0" Polyamide taking almost an hour's duration. He continued to be a guiding and decisive force for shaping my ophthalmic skills over several years.

ENTERING INTO THE ORBIT OF PHACO SURGEONS

I started practising small incision cataract surgery in 1993–94 with mixed memories of increased risk of intraoperative complications as well postoperative corneal problems, faced by us while performing the older conventional procedures. Simultaneously, Phaco-fever was on the rise.

My Journey towards Phacoemulsification began in 1995 at RP Centre for Ophthalmic Sciences, All India Institute of Medical Sciences New Delhi under Professor SK Angra.

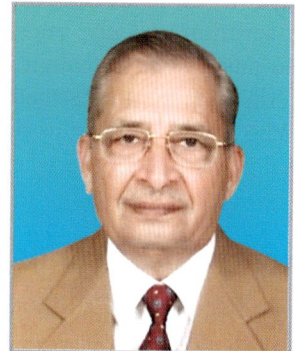

Prof SK Angra

Prof SK Angra is a thorough gentleman and is equipped with a vast knowledge in the realm of ophthalmology. He

happens to be a stalwart in his field and is equipped with a great persona. He not only taught me lens and cornea but was also instrumental in the transformation of my conduct and personality which I still cherish. Those days even RP Centre had only three regular phaco-surgeons. It was a Sangam of three rivers.

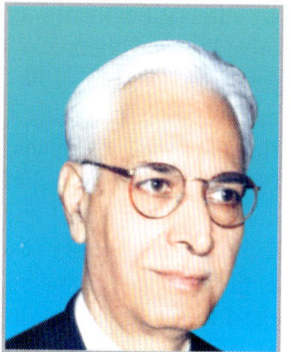

Prof VK Dada

We remember Dr VK Dada for his strict OT protocol, and even a mosquito would not have entered the OT without taking prior permission and a scrub. Even the back of observer and assistant was strictly restricted towards the panel of Phacoemulsifier. Touching the panel of a Phaco machine was a great achievement. Retrospectively, I had realised the significance and essentiality of such meticulous protocol to make procedures absolutely contamination free. He used to narrate and compare Phaco with Lord Krishna's Flute. He also infused theoretical knowledge of all the aspects of Phaco into our thought process. We had started dreaming, breathing and eating phaco all the time only because of him.

Dr RB Vajpayee was another giant of a wave who was very explosive but was on a different phaco plane as compared to the other two Phaco giants.

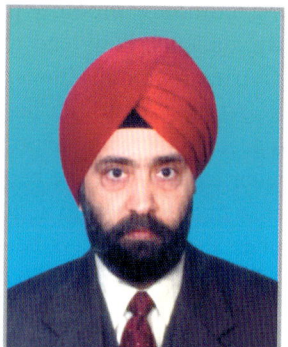

Dr Mahipal Sachdev

Dr Mahipal Sachdev was another great revolutionary in the field in Indian phaco in the mid nineties. He has been a role model Phaco surgeon for most of us. His dynamic, aggressive approach towards Phaco has remained a source of inspiration for several surgeons.

TIDE AND RIDE: MY FIRST INDEPENDENT PHACO SURGERY

My first independent phaco surgery was scheduled for 07 Jun 1996 at Army Hospital; Delhi cantt. The preparation involved reading each step of the procedure, dwelling into the nuances of the machine settings and the effect of the bottle height on my surgery. For me it was like a mission to the moon and involved several hours of my daily existence. I commenced my surgery on 07 Jun 1996 at 1000hrs, with a basic microscope and phaco machine. There was no one to guide me on that day, since I happened to be the only trained phaco surgeon. Imagine my relief once the rhexis and hydro procedure were complete. I was thrilled as I was going to handle the phaco handpiece. Pressure was enormous when I started sculpting, and the cracking of the nucleus was a big moment. I then started the ultrasonic fragment removal and with aspiration of every fragment, the pressure on me dwindled as the possibility of a nucleus drop dimmed. The moment came when all the fragments of the nucleus were out and only the cortical plate was left. It was a very mixed feeling. I could not believe that I had single handedly sailed the Phaco tide. It marked my entry into the Phaco club. Subsequent steps were managed with ease. However, Foldable IOL was not on the cards that day. I achieved the distinction of implanting Foldable IOL implant only after three months.

My journey was very smooth for the first fifty cases, but subsequently I had my share of series of complications. It reminded me of Dr Dada's words that every phaco surgeon has to perform Pind Dan (tribute to heavenly abode for parents /grand parents, a Hindu Myth in which a few Rolled Balls made up of Wheat and Barley are thrown into a river) by rolling nucleus fragment into the vitreous. I don't think any one of us would have traveled the phaco journey without this very unpleasant consequence. However when I compare modern phaco surgeons including my own students, they tend to pick up phaco very fast without too many complications. When I narrated this fact to one of my students he had asked me my reasoning on this account and I had retorted that either the present lot are better learners or have better teachers than we had. However in my heart I know it not to be true. My teachers are legends and will always be a mile ahead by their experience. For a new surgeon who begins his career directly using an operating microscope and sees phacoemulsification as a first line procedure for cataract management there is no infighting in his thought process to convert from a non operating microscope to an operating microscope. He doesn't know about ICCE at all. Retrospective self analysis has brought out the fact that phaco was a very little known procedure and linked with lots of myths, hallows and aura for the time. The present scenario is different. I feel proud to note that we Indians are rich in experience and technology in phaco our viz counter parts else where. More importantly, the present lots of trainers are more open, bold and willing to share all good or bad experiences with their trainee.

A Great Revolution: Topical and No Anaesthesia Technique

Undoubtedly, Dr Amar Agarwal has significant contribution in popularising Topical and no anaesthesia technique in the last 8 years.

After my initial success it was time for me to experience phaco surgery under no anaesthesia. I attempted this technique in a few cases but alas my initial experience was not very encouraging. It seems that I and my patients were both not tuned to this heroic exercise at that particular span of time. Hence, I switched over to topical anaesthesia as an alternative option. Interestingly, my conversion to topical from peribulbar technique was through my journey to no anaesthesia. 2% Lignocaine jelly was the preferred approach those days and I was not at all comfortable with the jelly since it was more prone to create corneal epithelial toxicity and getting it doubly autoclaved was not possible. Since Dec 2002, my preferential technique remains topical 2% Lignocaine/Proparacaine supplemented with 4 ml of Xylocard in 500 ml BSS being used as irrigating fluid. I found this anesthesia to be very safe and widely acceptable by all patients including those having complicated cataracts, miotic pupils or very hard cataract of grade VI, small palpebral fissure or even in the presence of a strong action of the orbicularis oculi muscle action. The surgeon may remain comfortable while handling even intraoperative complications like vitreous prolapse under this anaesthesia. After enjoying full confidence in topical anaesthesia I again used the No Anaesthesia technique in more than 150 cases. However, both I and my patients remain more comfortable and experienced less intra operative secretions of adrenaline under topical anaesthesia. Undoubtedly no anaesthesia cataract surgery is possible. I still feel that the choice of anaesthesia or no anaesthesia should be left to the patient's discretion. In my view either topical anaesthesia or no anaesthesia technique carries more or less the same merits with the former being slightly more advantageous. Who knows when the tide of time will change the mental block that I have when I compare the two.

BIMANUAL MICRO PHACO SURGERY

Other than the no anesthesia technique, Dr Amar Agarwal has significant contribution in popularising bimanual micro phaco in this part of the world. A procedure conceived in 1984 with a convention coaxial system remained in hibernation until 1998. He has also given thrust to topical and no anaesthesia cataract surgery. I also started dreaming of bimanual phaco in late 2000. I commenced bimanual phaco with a normal phaco tip with no sleeve. An irrigating chopper was used having a 20 gauze diameter with fluid via a separate line. I continued to use the phaco infusion line with handpiece to provide continuous cooling. These cases were performed under peribulbar anesthesia. Since I was using the Protégée Ventury system I could manage initial cases without much discomfort except for moderate chamber instability. However I realised very soon that I was not using the fluidics of the machine and exchanged the irrigating chopper for machine fluidics. It provided me more flexibility and ease which was evident as better postoperative out come.

I was unhappy with the existing side port blades and microphaco blades which used to be in practice to fashion sub one mm incision. These blades were not able to provide good stability of the chamber. Fluid dynamics as well as insertion of Thin or Rollable IOL implant was also very difficult since the corneal valve incision did not carry a good enough width to inject the IOL through a small incision. My own experience and constraints faced had given me thoughts to design a special trapezoid micro phaco blade of dimensions; 0. 9, 1.0. 1.2 and 1.4 mm. I was also encouraged to design special bimanual I/A System and irrigating choppers of variable gaze of 21, 22, 23 and 24. I have been using these ultra fine choppers and I/A since Jan 2003. However, lots of readjustment in machine parameters and fluidics was essentially required for small bore choppers and irrigating cannula which I could learn only after combination and trial. The air pump had become an essential need for 23 and 24 gauge systems or for use in grade four Cataracts. Later on we started using bimanual micro phaco in all sorts of complicated cataracts and combined surgeries such as traumatic subluxated lens, Phaconit trab and Glaucoma valve and nit combinations. We are very confident and sure that bimanual micro phaco is going to replace Co axial technique and IOLs.

LARGER CANVAS THAN THE SURGEON HIMSELF

Phacosurgery is like walking on a tight rope. The surgeon's margin of error involves a mere 6-8 microns which is the difference between his triumph and tragedy. This razor sharp edge can prove to be the surgeon's waterloo. Still I would prefer to analyse and narrate those unpleasant moments faced by me as an experienced surgeon after a creditable account of successful performances for self retrospection and leave them for wisdom of my readers. Most such events are described in detail in a chapter on complications of phacosurgery. I do not think any of us would have traveled the phaco journey without this very unpleasant consequence.

Why does a Surgeon Get Complications/ Unpleasant Outcome?

Complications emerge out of surgical performances mainly due to the following reasons/factors

Surgeon's Factors

  (i) Less experienced surgeon
 (ii) Over confident surgeon
(iii) Innovative surgeon

Mechanical/Instrumental

Patient's Factors

 (i) Preexisting ocular /Systemic conditions
(ii) Uncooperative patient

Postoperative

 (i) Attributable to intraoperative hurdles
(ii) Attributable to pre existing ocular /systemic conditions

Inadvertent Hiccups

1. Surgeon's factors

In our view, "Surgeon's factors" are the most significant and are responsible for any unpleasant eventuality both during, intra as well as postoperative phase.

  (i) **Less experienced surgeon:** Less experience or learning curve is invariably associated with a higher incidence of complications. Incidentally, most of the learners are over cautious during the initial period of learning both in terms of selection of cases as well as of the surgical technique. Hence a surgeon encounters relatively less problems during this particular phase.

The most common problem during the beginner phase is inadequate exposure to the machine, fluidics, and significance of microscope settings as well as inappropriate machine settings. Over and above shaky confidence, failure to recognise early signs of impending problems and timely intervention remains the key issues.

The relatively newer surgeon will face maximum problem during rhexis and nucleotomy particularly while making the trench. The inability to titrate energy requirement and machine settings, based on nucleus grading and excessive mechanical force remains the main constraint. The magnum of such incidences is compounded further particularly in cases of deranged ocular status as seen in myopia, high hypermetropia and glaucoma or uveitic patients.

In our view, the best surgeon knows when to stop rather to drive and dive into the problems. The surgeon should be able to identify the earliest signs of the impending problem and must take immediate decision in the patient's interest.

(ii) **Over confident / Innovative surgeon:** In our view, surgeon should have a balanced and realistic approach. Over or under confident surgeon with unrealistic attitude remains the main contention of an unpleasant outcome following any surgical procedure.

After having an uneventful learning curve the surgeon may be over confident or less attentive towards the selection of cases and surgical techniques. This simulates hill driving where maximum accidents take place while driving down slope rather than climbing up. Learning curve is like conquering the steep heights while the subsequent phase is like fast driving on the down slope. The amount of energy, concentration spent on the learning phase is now out and surgeons tend to pay lesser heed leading to complications. We have observed a higher incidence of complications during initial 75 to 125 cases followed by a second phase of 5000–5100 cases. Probably the second phase is when the surgeon tends to be more innovative and takes up challenges in the form of accepting more complicated cases as well as intends to revolutionise the surgery. It is essential to be progressive and innovative for the progress of medical science and to reach the pinnacle of precision. However, the surgeon has to weigh and balance between the pace and extent of innovation over safety, the patient's interest and the final outcome in toto. Retrospectively, the author has realised to go slow, steady with a safe and comfortable smooth take off, traveling safety as well as have an uneventful landing. After having experienced more than 15000 phacosurgeries, the author prefers to perform uncomplicated planned ECCE in a highly complicated, very hard black (Grade 5–7)cataract, poor corneal reserve, corneal opacities and miotic pupil of less than 2.5 mm of size. After all these patients are not demanding an unaided 6/5 and N/5 vision on the very next day owing to the complicated status of the eye. In our view a patient who has allowed cataract to advance up to a dense brown stage falls into the category of an easy going personality rather preferring to avoid surgery due to the unknown fear of risk and complications. Viewing this reality, it is very fair to provide a smooth recovery phase following conventional ECCE rather than a stormy and prolonged phase following an eventful phacoemulsification surgery in extremely adverse situations which may be associated with severe intraoperative complications like a nucleus drop or corneal decompensation or secondary glaucoma. Earlier the author was accepting challenges and risk of performing phaco in each and every case with reasonable success. However, this modified approach has practically attained more than 99% precision as well as patient satisfaction. After all the patients comfort and a good outcome is more important than a surgeon's ego and a rigid belief to perform phaco in each and every case.

2. Mechanical /Instrumentation related factors

Mechanical /Instrumentation related factors are among the most significant and crucial factors in terms of leading a trail of unfavourable outcome.

These factors can be grouped as follows:

(i) **Lesser known machine and technology both at initial and advanced stage of surgeons career:** Lesser known machine and technology remains the key issue at any stage of surgeons profile including both at initial and advanced stage. The beginner faces the constraints of less practical experience of identifying machines in terms of good performance and user friendly attitude as well as the financial angle if he is entering into private practice. One has to weigh and club all the advantages with a sincere attempt to minimise demerits. The most basic and less expensive machine may not be very user friendly and simultaneously a very expensive or most advanced technology may not be acceptable to the demands of a beginner both in terms of finances as well as the surgical technique adopted by a beginner. If you have learned to drive a Mercedes, you may not be able to switch over to an old Indian car of a basic model. It is worth considering to begin with a good quality basic or intermediate Phacomachine and to combine it with use of a basic technique of phacoemulsification. It is very-very important to learn about and know your machine and also live with it and that too with harmony. Experienced surgeons also face problems with their machine while upgrading the machine status and are yet unable to acquire the desired and customised parameters according to the need of their techniques and modifications. The author too had faced a shot span of inconsistency while shifting from intermediate model ventury system to a higher end peristaltic and finally to the most advanced and latest torsional technology. It is good to observe the guide line provided by the manufacturer and their experts but it definitely demands significant modifications and adjustments based on surgeons own technique and type of cataract handled by him. A blue chip surgeon in a most posh locality of a metro gets much different and highly sophisticated case as compared to a beginner in the same town in a different locality. A so-called hard cataract encountered by a western surgeon or by a reputed surgeon in a metro may be quite soft to a suburban or smaller town surgeon and vice versa. In the authors view, the hardness of nucleus and complexity of the cataract is inversely proportional to the socio- economic status of the patient. Hence parameters customised by the top most ophthalmic surgeons of our country may not be suitable for a beginner or an average surgeon. You have to learn and adopt a driving technique which is appropriate for you on your machine as well as suitable for you on the path traveled.

(ii) **Substandard quality and inconsistency of machine and instrumentation:** Substandard quality of machine and instrumentation remains a major source of concern with any procedure and phacoemulsification is not an exception to this rule. Needless to stress on the significance of application of a good Phacomachine. A sustained and consistent delivery of customised desired performance of machine is absolutely essential to achieve a good outcome. Inconsistency in display, delivered ultrasonic energy, aspiration and other parameters are a major issue of concern with relatively cheaper and basic machines; hence surgical outcome remains debatable in these situations.

Substandard quality of instrumentation like rough edges of a cannula, irrigation handpiece, chipped phaco tip, too sharp and eroded edges of a chopper, sinskey hook, blunt tip of rhexis cystitome, partly blocked cannula are all an essential attribute towards the added risk of intraoperative complications. Hence a close and meticulous evaluation of surgical instruments is of immense value.

(iii) **Mechanical failure:** Mechanical failure is one of the most unfortunate and unprecedented occurrence which may turn into a disaster irrespective of the quality of ones machine. Sudden surge due to occlusion of tubings, tip may lead to an about turn from a great performance to a nightmare in the form of corneal touch, Iridodialysis, posterior capsular rent, dropped nucleus or even an IOL, choroidal haemorrhage and so on. It is absolutely essential to keep a constant watch on your machine settings and commensurate ones performance so as to anticipate any problem at the earliest.

3. Patient related factors

Patient related factors are equally responsible and they adversely influence the ultimate surgical outcome in any procedure, however such factors are more significant in case of phacoemulsification surgery which demands a very high order of precision and accuracy and more so as it is being performed under local or topical anaesthesia, patient remains alert, vigilant and over cautious to the surroundings and to any happenings throughout the surgery. A meticulous evaluation of the patient's own apprehensions, anxieties and other factors are of immense value.

Surgeon should not be dogmatic on the choice of topical anaesthesia over peribulbar since, certain patients may not be comfortable under topical. The choice of anaesthesia is a matter of mutual interest and consent. A young individual, particularly a young lady patient, apprehensive, over anxious and being a labile hypertensive carries a higher risk of intraoperative complications under topical anaesthesia and hence are not a good choice for surgery under topical anaesthesia.

Certain ocular status like strong orbicularis muscle actions, small palpebral aperture High hypermetropic (smaller eye), shallow anterior chamber, miotic pupil, very hard cataract, associated congenital anomalies, any previous history of intraocular surgery are not a good choice for topical, since such eyes do carry the higher risk of intraoperative complications which may not be possible to handle without adequate regional anaesthesia.

Inadvertent and sudden abnormal postural movement of head and body is likely to enhance the risk of complications. Certain patients are claustrophobic on covering fellow eye or even placing a drape over the face. Intraoperative changes in the breathing pattern, holding one's breath and to avoid conveying the conditions of the urinary bladder are added precipitating factors.

The surgeon should keep a vigilant watch on all these above mentioned factors. Any deviation in the intraoperative position of iris diaphragm, status of posterior capsule and vitreous phase should immediately be attended in the context of any precipitating factors.

4. Postoperative

Postoperative complications are, by and large, linked with a preexisting ocular and systemic problem or an eventful surgical performance. Such problems have been discussed in length in previous para and chapters related with complications of phacosurgery. It is very rare and unusual to observe any postoperative failure without any previous background as described earlier.

5. Inadvertent hiccups

Inadvertent hiccups despite all precautions and meticulous efforts are most unfortunate and unprecedented eventualities one may face during the course of ones surgical practice. The author wishes to summarise such unpleasant moments encountered during the last 12 years of his phaco wedding period with the intention of sensitising the readers.

(i) Indecisiveness on merits of the case: Phaco or no Phaco.

(ii) Chamber collapses due to leaking irrigating line, kinked tube or slightly loose tip.

(iii) Working on wrong settings while presuming working on your own customised settings.

(iv) Greedy surgeon: Despite odds and complications still dragging on.

(v) Failure to anticipate the gravity of complications and subsequent management strategy.

(vi) IOL dislocation or Subluxation which could have been avoided.

(vii) Extensive hyphaema due to stroking of iris.

MY EXPERIENCE IN HANDLING PATIENTS WHO HAD COMPLICATIONS, DURING AND AFTER SURGERY

Each and every surgeon who operates is bound to face complications and unpleasant situations sometime in his professional career. The operating surgeon should not hide any unpleasant operative moment from the patient or from his attendant. As such, the patient has all right to know about the procedure and its ultimate outcome. Over and above, the results of intraocular surgery are invariably visible to the patient both structurally as well as functionally. A good central circular pupil may not be noticed by a patient but an eccentric and irregular peaked pupil or chaffed iris will definitely draw their attention. In the same manner, an irritable and inflamed eye cannot be overlooked by the patient. Over and above, if the visual acuity is short of normal, it will invariably be brought to notice by the patient. Hence, it is wiser to approach and convey to the patient about an eventful happening yourself rather than it being conveyed by someone else. I feel patients may loose trust in the surgeon's actions if the problems are swept under the carpet. Gradual and guarded information is more beneficial to the patient to prepare himself to adjust during the prolonged and unpleasant phase of recovery. The author invariably discusses intraoperative constraints of significant nature on the table itself in a very tactful manner like seeking permission to proceed with a larger size IOL in place of a foldable IOL on the basis of pleading merits and better stability of IOL in a situation where posterior capsule support is inadequate or a small window which may disturb the position of foldable IOL in due course of time. The author propounds the placement of 10 '0'suture in the case of a 3 mm incision if the incisional integrity is debatable. We have found that even patients who had a nucleus or IOL drop or endophthalmitis respond well if they are communicated with in the form of a positive discussion. As such most of the complications can be handled effectively with reasonable visual outcome. I feel that an honest, sincere and a truthful approach while keeping the patients interest above all remains the only key to success.

HOW TO PREPARE FOR THE GIANT LEAP OR PERFORMING PHACO SURGERY ON THE HIGHLY ELITE OR ENTERING INTO BLUE CHIP VVIP GROUP OF CLIENTELE

An ophthalmic Surgeon Performing Phaco on his better Half's Eye

I consider my decision to perform phacosurgery upon one's better half as the most challenging and controversial task. Undoubtedly, the dictum says to refrain yourself from riding on emotional waves while treating a patient. Conventionally, surgeons refrain themselves from operating upon their near and dear one with obvious reasons to avoid any hasty intraoperative decision which may be influenced by interpersonal relationships. I fully endorse and subscribe to such views in principle. However, every convention and rule has some exception. I feel my decision to operate on my wife itself was an exception. This decision was not intended for heroism but was exclusively based in her interest. My wife had developed bilateral posterior sub capsular opacities, which were detected in 2002 just a week after tonsillectomy under general anaesthesia as a sudden blurring of the vision in both eyes of recent onset. She preferred to take her consultation from Col PK Sahoo, Professor and Head at AFMC Pune at that time. This showed the level of confidence I enjoyed on the account of her assessment of my professional capability. Col Sahoo diagnosed a thin posterior sub capsular lenticular opacities with unaided vision of 6/9 in both eyes.

Since this was at an early stage, the only advice was just to wait and watch. I am still not sure about the etiology of this cataract and as to whether it was a pre existing opacity or a sequel of a complex drug reaction to any of the anaesthetic agent. She was reexamined after six months. This examination had revealed progressive lenticular changes that deserved impending surgical intervention. My wife was not at all keen to undergo cataract surgery despite my pursuance. I kept on insisting to get the earliest intervention anywhere and of course from any surgeon of her preference including Dr Mahipal Sachdeva, Dr Keki Mehta or Col DP Vats even though I was very sure that she would remain the most comfortable and cooperative in my hands. Time passed away and we had shifted to Kolkata and in the interim my abilities also soared in her eyes. By now, the cataract in her Left eye had become hyper mature. Imagine a phaco surgeon who could not persuade his wife to undergo cataract surgery in time! It was time to veto and surgery was ordered immediately but of course the choice of surgeon and the place of surgery were still wide open. Lady luck finally shone on my behalf and my wife decided to get operated by yours truly. She had decided in my favour. It was the second occasion to win a franchise (first was at the time of marriage). Preoperative workup was itself difficult, especially the difficulty faced in IOL power calculation. I knew the surgery would be difficult under topical due to apprehension, a strong orbicularis action as well as the presence of a hyper mature cataract which makes rhexis almost impossible under topical.

Once the surgery was finalised, the decision was conveyed to the Commandant who happened to have tremendous confidence in my so-called professional capabilities. He readily agreed to my decision but suggested I perform surgery on a holiday so as to involve the least number of people thereby keeping my wife comfortable. The next step was to consult the head of anaesthesiology, which happens to be my very close friend and well wisher. The procedure was scheduled on Sunday at 3 o' clock. The date and time was not disclosed to anyone in the department except the two Operation Room assistant and that too on the very same day at 11 'O' clock with strict instructions of confidentiality.

We had a quick lunch at 1400 hrs. I could see that she was a little bit nervous and the same was palpable on my face too. I decided not to think about the endeavor ahead anymore. It was 1430 hrs when we began from our home to the hospital. She just met my son who preferred to remain at home. Once we arrived at the OT, the OT matron over-took charge.

I have a set protocol of not accompanying any patient while getting into the main OT. The same protocol was maintained. I entered into the OT well in advance to ensure that all arrangement was made. Once everything was organised, I asked my ORA to get her inside. After five minutes I saw her entering the OT. She was looking frightened and very nervous in an OT dress. I was a bit stressed for the moment but then recovered my nerves. The next step was painting-draping.

Once draping was over, the initial anxiety at both ends was over.

Peribulbar anaesthesia was given. The anaesthesiologist was very keen to administer sedation but I declined the offer. It was time to commence surgery now. I switched off emotionally and left everything to God and destiny. The most difficult moment was rhexis and despite using planned trypan blue turned out to be smaller in configuration. As expected it had a tendency to extend and thus had to be completed with the help of Utrata. Phaco per se did not give much discomfort to either of us except that she kept shifting her head once in a while. The readjustment of head was definitely an annoying task but somehow I could manage. I was happy to see an intact posterior capsule just prior to the implantation of the IOL. The Acry Sof natural was on the cards even though we had been using a single piece AcrySof more often. This was my first exposure to natural Acry Sof. The IOL implantation and the remaining steps were uneventful. I guess it was to be the first AcrySof natural IOL implantation by an

ophthalmologist on his own wife. I was relieved from a major responsibility of finishing yet another uneventful surgery. She attained a Visual acuity of 6/12 two hours following surgery. Topical medication was started immediately. However, the path to success was not so smooth. She had observed marked blurring of vision the very next morning. It was the time to see moderate uveitis with significant vitreous haze, an unexplained event. A nervous moment. I have yet to find an answer. Was it a reaction to trypan blue or something with the IOL? As such, all the fluids and drugs used during surgery are double autoclaved in our setup for every patient irrespective of their status. However, I was sure that I was not handling endophthalmitis. I switched over to aggressive therapy in the form of hourly topical steroids along with adjuvant systemic steroids. She responded within one day though the steroids continued till the stipulatory period.

PCO was evident after three years which was essentially managed with YAG capsulotomy. The story doesn't end here. Three years following surgery; the other eye was due for surgery. The place had changed from Kolkata to Delhi and that too the Phacomachine from ventury (Strotz) to a White Starr. I was in a quandary over the selection of an IOL. Should it be an AcrySof natural again or an Apodized Restor? This decision was a little difficult and controversial in the form of matching the apodized with a monofocal IOL. I decided to choose the apodized IOL this time over the natural. It may have been the memories of a postoperative stormy period of previous surgery that were influencing my thought process.

The day and time chosen was afternoon again on a holiday but this time it was clubbed with one more VIP.

The procedure was uneventful and performed under topical anaesthesia. Rhexis was performed without trypan blue assistance. Dame luck was definitely shining on me on this occasion. She had an absolutely uneventful recovery throughout the postoperative period. She enjoys an excellent full range of vision in her right eye as well as an improved unaided 6/6 vision in her left eye with N/6 near vision. This interesting phenomenon in young individuals may be linked with a good neural adaptation in the fellow eye due to the presence of an apodized IOL.

I am still not sure about the correctness of my decision on operating twice on my nearest and dearest. However, it is better to leave certain queries unsolved for critical evaluation. So long everything went along fine it was the most appropriate step.

My Experience to Handle VVIP: Before, during and after Surgery

Every surgeon has a dream to handle highly sophisticated or complicated cases with success. Once a surgeon has attained a certain standard of surgical as well as communication skills he tends to accept these challenges. No doubt, dealing with a VVIP is always linked with glamour and accolades. However, the scene is not so rosy. The risk involved is the ability to fulfill the demands against all odds and is not at all a comfortable choice. The surgeon is always under deep surveillance from all the corners. However, all these constraints and risks don't deprive you of taking up such challenges. Life is full of risk, competition and challenges. One has to face such occasions with a brave face. The surgeon has to accept this as *Neel Kantha* (Dark blue neck as Lord Shiva is popularly known for holding poison, which came out of *Samundra manthan* (Churning of Sea) prior to Amrit (The essence of immortality) a famous episode from ancient mythology where Good and Evil forces (Deva and Asur) had a tug of war of getting Amrit out of sea. Hence, for the betterment of man kind and nature as a whole, Lord Shiva did not allow the poison to spill over the earth. In the same manner, the surgeon has to hold this responsibility to serve mankind without prejudice, without expecting any gain in return.

How Should a Surgeon Handle VVIP Preoperatively

A famous phrase states that, "let a thirsty person come to the well and drink rather than let the water flow to him." This should be the right approach. Surgeons should not try to hunt and attempt to grab at the occasion. A greedy feeling should not come in the way of a final decision. The author has never attempted to force any patient to get their surgery done by him irrespective of the status of the individual, may it be an ordinary citizen or a VVIP. I believe that all patients have a right to choose the surgeon, the place and if allowed the procedure of his or her own preference. The surgeon should not attempt to glorify himself at the cost of others. Every surgeon puts in his best efforts in a given particular situation. It is the preexisting, intraoperative and postoperative response as well as other unprecedented factors that decide the fate. I feel this approach pays rich dividends in the long run.

Self Assessment Prior to the Final Yes

Self assessment prior to the final yes to accept the challenge is a very important and crucial factor. Surgeon should have an unbiased and true introspection of his own surgical capability, confidence and infrastructure which should fulfill the demands of the specific situation. An overall assessment of the infrastructure and availability of support to handle even the worst possible complication is very crucial and mandatory. The first and foremost important thing is to look within your own self and try to get answers to the above mentioned queries. If your conscience allows then one can consider taking up the patient.

Remember You are under Scrutiny

The most important fact which a surgeon may not notice is that while interacting with a patient it's not only the surgeon assessing the patient but it is also the patient evaluating the surgeon. For a surgeon, the patient may be one of several, but for the patient it is this singular occasion when he or she develops trust and decides to place his or her trust in the surgeon. It is always an unsavory moment should the patients eye be operated on for a second time. There must be a feeling of ease between the surgeon and the patient. I feel the first meeting with the patient during the preoperative evaluation carries the key. The professional honesty and self confidence can readily be observed by the patient and his attendants too.

Preoperative Counselling

Preoperative counselling should have a detailed and honest assessment of the disease and situation. All the pros and cons of the procedure should be highlighted. A realistic assessment of the final outcome should be provided rather than a fabricated assurance which may not be able to hold ground.

No Publicity/Propaganda

Preoperative publicity/propaganda invariably makes the situation tense and uncomfortable to both the patient as well as to the surgeon. It is wise and in the best interest of the patient to maintain a quiet environment prior to the procedure. Our actions speak louder than our words.

Prepare Oneself for the Big Leap

The surgeon should prepare him self for the big leap. Mental coolness and calmness is very essential as over anxiety is likely to affect the final outcome of surgery.

Self confidence is absolutely essential to ensure the best of the outcomes.

Check, Cross Check Your Setup and OT Protocol

A meticulous scrutiny of instruments, equipment and OT protocol is very crucial. The strict vigilance on sterility and asepsis should be doubly ensured. I feel that all items, drugs and fluids should be used after double autoclaving as a routine in all the cases.

It is better to keep a full setup in running condition to handle any kind of operative or systemic complications. As such, most of the VVIPs belong to an elderly age group and hence, they are quite vulnerable to unpleasant occurrences. Surgeons should keep a complete setup which includes vitrectomy, endolaser, posterior segment microscope and VR instrumentation in running condition so as to handle any eventuality if need be. If a surgeon himself is not conversant or confident to handle such complications like a nucleus or a lens drop, a vitreo retinal surgeon must be available in the OT to handle them immediately. In addition to the above, another Phaco-machine, instrument set, different types of IOLs including AC, All PMMA IOL and foldable IOL of different designs to suit the intraoperative need should readily be available. This kind of preparation definitely gives a lot of confidence to the surgeon.

How to Face the Big Day of Surgery

The author prefers to keep VVIP surgery exclusively singular. The time schedule should be framed and adjusted as per the mutual ease rather than following a strict pattern of early morning surgery.

A good beginning wins half the battle. It is better not to receive the patient or his relatives outside the OT. Let this job be done by administrators. Sometimes over anxious or enthusiastic attendants may disturb the surgeon and the patient.

The operating surgeon should concentrate on his OT protocol and surgical plan rather than making heroic appearances outside.

Before getting the patient inside to the main theatre, the surgeon should ensure that machines, instruments, position of the OT table, microscope, assistants, emergency support systems as well as backup lights are readily available. There should be no undue traffic inside the OT. After reassuring that all is in place, the surgeon should scrub up and make himself available at the table prior to the arrival of the patient.

Arrival of VVIP Patient Inside the Theatre

Arrival of a VVIP patient inside the theatre is a very jittery moment for both the surgeon and the patient. Despite all preparations both are anxious to some extent. A warm greeting and a word of assurance helps ease things out.

The anaesthesiologist should provide I/V infusion line and cardiac monitoring, in addition to standby emergency measures. The use of mild analgesics and sedatives may be required depending upon the situation.

The surgeon should allow his assistant to perform the initial draping and relevant preparations. He should not be dogmatic about topical or peribulbar anaesthesia. It should be left to the merit of the case and the surgeon's comfort. However, it is worth considering the use of peribulbar in cases of a miotic and rigid pupil, hard cataract, strong orbicularis action or an over anxious patient.

The selection of surgical technique and type of IOL should strictly be as per the given situation and intra-operative demands. The patient's interest is supreme. Treat any VVIP as a patient and not as a VVIP. Don't get panicky while thinking of the end result of surgery and concentrate

on the step which you are performing. Never compromise on the basic principle and need of the procedure. If you are making an incision, just concentrate on the site and configuration of the incision. It is better to have flexibility on surgical planning as the situation warrants.

Postoperative Care

Postoperative care and protocol should also be maintained as per the standard schedule or the need of the situation.

Last but not the least

After having faced all possible challenges and accorded the highest professional achievements in the field of Phacoemulsification surgery I was destined to operate my fathers' eyes in Dec 2008. My mother had commented prior to his first surgery "there are several good surgeons around, rather than a boy who used to eat clay during his early childhood" Thankfully, my father carries tremendous faith on my capability as a professional.

I planned and managed to go with Phacosurgery and a Multifocal IOL in both the eyes. It was a wonderful and the most memorable moment of my life. I consider this trust as the richest gift from my parents.

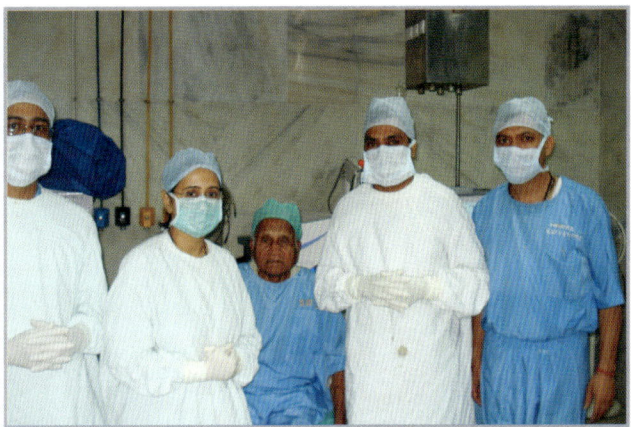

Author and his team in OT with his father soon after surgery under topical anaesthesia

CONCLUSION

Journey towards learning, practising, adaptability and heights are never ending. I still consider myself standing at the take-off point of this path which terminates ahead on the horizon. It is better not to think of oneself to be at the pinnacle of his or her career, but to be humble and thank God for all the skills he has presented us with for the service of mankind.

Index

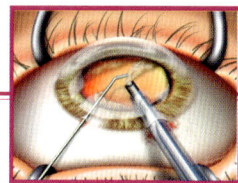